DIAGNOSIS *and*
TREATMENT PLANNING *in*
DENTISTRY

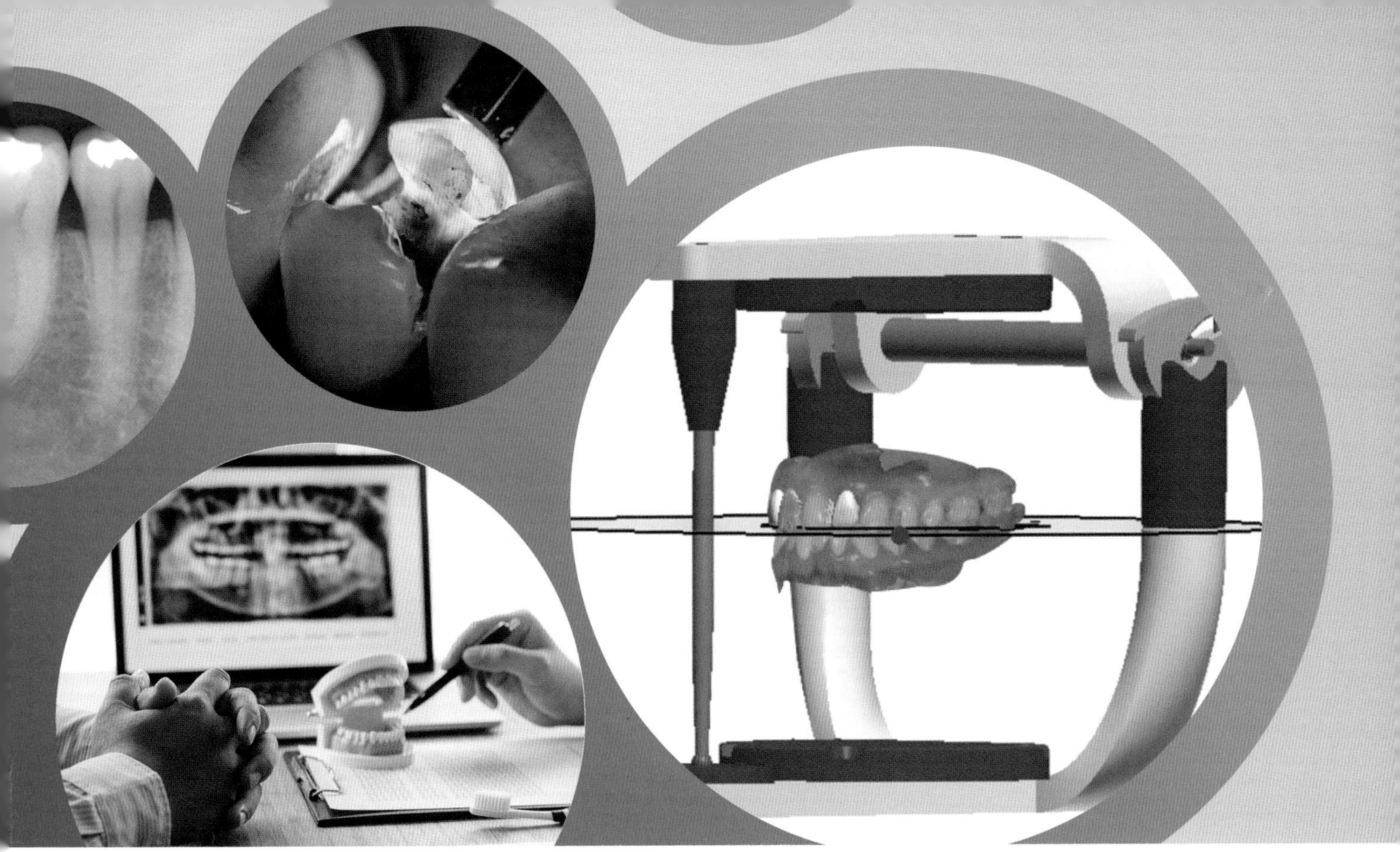

DIAGNOSIS *and* TREATMENT PLANNING *in* DENTISTRY

FOURTH EDITION

STEPHEN J. STEFANAC, DDS, MS

Professor emeritus, Department of Periodontics and Oral Medicine
The University of Michigan School of Dentistry
Ann Arbor, Michigan

SAMUEL P. NESBIT, DDS, MS

Clinical Professor, Department of Operative Dentistry
University of North Carolina School of Dentistry
Chapel Hill, North Carolina

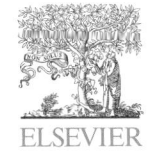

ELSEVIER

Elsevier
3251 Riverport Lane
St. Louis, Missouri 63043

DIAGNOSIS AND TREATMENT PLANNING IN DENTISTRY,
FOURTH EDITION

ISBN: 978-0-323-80975-7

Notice

Practitioners and researchers must always rely on their own experience and knowledge in evaluating and using any information, methods, compounds or experiments described herein. Because of rapid advances in the medical sciences, in particular, independent verification of diagnoses and drug dosages should be made. To the fullest extent of the law, no responsibility is assumed by Elsevier, authors, editors or contributors for any injury and/or damage to persons or property as a matter of products liability, negligence or otherwise, or from any use or operation of any methods, products, instructions, or ideas contained in the material herein.

Previous editions copyrighted 2017, 2007 and 2001.

Senior Content Strategist: Lauren Boyle
Content Development Manager: Ranjana Sharma
Publishing Services Manager: Deepthi Unni
Project Manager: Sindhuraj Thulasingam
Design Direction: Brian Salisbury

Printed in India

Last digit is the print number: 9 8 7 6 5 4 3 2 1

Carlos Barrero, BDS, MS
Acting Chief of Dental Service
W.G. (Bill) Hefner Salisbury
Department of Veterans Affairs
    Medical Center
Salisbury, North Carolina

Erika Benavides, DDS, PhD
Diplomate, American Board of Oral and
    Maxillofacial Radiology
Clinical Professor and Radiology Discipline
    Coordinator Associate Chair
Department of Periodontics and Oral
    Medicine
University of Michigan School of Dentistry
Ann Arbor, Michigan

Lee W. Boushell, DMD, MS
Division Director Predoctoral Clinical
    Education
Associate Professor
Department of General Dentistry
East Carolina University School of Dental
    Medicine
Greenville, North Carolina

Jennifer L. Brame, EdD, BSDH
Director, Graduate Dental Hygiene
    Education Program
Clinical Professor
Division of Comprehensive Oral Health
University of North Carolina Adams School
    of Dentistry
Chapel Hill, North Carolina

Zachary Brian, DMD, MHA
Adjunct Assistant Professor
Pediatric and Public Health
University of North Carolina Adams School
    of Dentistry;
Adjunct Assistant Professor
Health Policy and Management
University of North Carolina Gillings School
    of Global Public Health
Chapel Hill, North Carolina

Angela Broome, DDS,MS
Associate Professor
Diagnostic Sciences
University of North Carolina
Chapel Hill, North Carolina

Cassandra Callaghan, BBA, MS
Chief Information Officer Dental
    Informatics
University of Michigan School of Dentistry
Ann Arbor, Michigan

Wendy Clark, DDS, MS
Assistant Professor
Prosthodontics
University of North Carolina Adams School
    of Dentistry
Chapel Hill, North Carolina

John William Claytor Jr., DDS, MAGD
Executive Director
North Carolina Caring Dental
    Professionals
Shelby, North Carolina

Christine Downey, MS, DDS
Clinical Associate Professor
Craniofacial and Surgical Care
University of North Carolina Adams School
    of Dentistry
Chapel Hill, North Carolina

Ibrahim Duqum, DDS, MS, FICD
Associate Professor of Prosthodontics
Director for Clinical Curriculum
Division of Comprehensive Oral Health
University of North Carolina Adams School
    of Dentistry
Chapel Hill, North Carolina

**Gregory K. Essick, DDS, PhD,
D.ABDSM**
Adjunct Professor
Comprehensive Oral Health
    – Prosthodontics
University of North Carolina Adams School
    of Dentistry
Chapel Hill, North Carolina

Margherita Fontana, DDS, PhD
Clifford Nelson Endowed Professor of
    Dentistry
Cariology Discipline Co-coordinator
Director of Global Initiatives in Oral and
    Craniofacial Health
Department of Cariology, Restorative
    Sciences, and Endodontics
University of Michigan School of
    Dentistry
Ann Arbor, Michigan

Nisha Frances Ganesh, DDS, MAEd
Associate Clinical Professor
Department of General Dentistry
University of Maryland School of
    Dentistry
Baltimore, Maryland

**Shin-Mey (Rose) Y. Geist, DDS, MS, FDS
RCSEd**
Associate Professor
Divisions of Clinical Dentistry and
    Integrated Biomedical Sciences
University of Detroit Mercy School of
    Dentistry
Detroit, Michigan

Furat George, BDS, MS
Adjunct Clinical Professor
Department of Biologic and Materials
    Sciences, and Prosthodontics
University of Michigan School of
    Dentistry
Ann Arbor, Michigan

Sarah E. Getch, PhD
Program Director
Health Service Psychology
Assistant Provost of Accreditation
Kansas City University
Kansas City, Missouri

Gretchen Gibson, DDS, MPH
Director, Oral Health Quality Group
Office of Dentistry
Veterans Health Administration
Fayetteville, Arkansas

**Carlos Gonzalez-Cabezas, DDS,
MSD, PhD**
Richard Christiansen Collegiate Professor
    of Oral and Craniofacial
Associate Dean for Academic Affairs
Professor
Department of Cariology, Restorative
    Sciences and Endodontics
University of Michigan School of
    Dentistry
Ann Arbor, Michigan

Jennifer B. Harmon, RDH, MS
Associate Professor
Division of Comprehensive Oral
    Health
University of North Carolina Adams
    School of Dentistry
Chapel Hill, North Carolina

Jennifer Hartshorn, DDS, FSCD
Clinical Associate Professor
Preventive and Community Dentistry
University of Iowa College of Dentistry
Iowa City, Iowa

Tate H. Jackson, DDS, MS
Former Vice Chair, Craniofacial and Surgical
    Care
Former Program Director, Orthodontics
Adjunct Assistant Professor
Orthodontics
University of North Carolina Adams School
    of Dentistry
Chapel Hill, North Carolina

Lynn Johnson, PhD
Professor
Department of Periodontics and Oral
    Medicine
University of Michigan
Ann Arbor, Michigan

Erinne Kennedy, DMD, MPH, MMSc
Assistant Professor, Director of Pre-Doctoral
    Education
College of Dental Medicine
Kansas City University
Joplin, Missouri

**Lorne D. Koroluk, DMD, MSD, MS,
FRCD(C)**
Associate Professor and Director
Orthodontics
University of North Carolina Adams School
    of Dentistry
Chapel Hill, North Carolina

Lewis Lampiris, DDS, MPH
Former Associate Dean for Community
    Engagement and Outreach
Adjunct Associate Professor
Pediatric and Public Health
University of North Carolina Adams School
    of Dentistry
Chapel Hill, North Carolina

Pei-Feng Lim, BDS, MS
Clinical Associate Professor
Diagnostic Science (Orofacial Pain)
University of North Carolina Adams School
    of Dentistry
Chapel Hill, North Carolina

Leonardo Marchini, DDS, MSD, PhD
Professor and Chair
Department of Comprehensive Care
Case Western Reserve University School of
    Dental Medicine
Cleveland, Ohio

Cindy L. Marek, Pharm D, FACA
Professor Emeritus
The University of Iowa College of Dentistry;
The University of Iowa College of Pharmacy
Iowa City, Iowa

Antonio Moretti, DDS, MS
Professor, Periodontology
Division of Comprehensive Oral Health
University of North Carolina Adams School
    of Dentistry
Chapel Hill, North Carolina

Stephanie M. Munz, DDS, FSCD
Clinical Associate Professor and Associate
    Chair
Hospital Dentistry
Program Director General Practice
    Residency
Department of Oral and Maxillofacial
    Surgery/Hospital Dentistry
University of Michigan School of Dentistry
Ann Arbor, Michigan

**Carol Anne Murdoch-Kinch, DDS, PhD,
FDS, FRCS(Ed)**
Professor and Dean
Indiana University School of Dentistry
Indianapolis, Indiana

Romesh P. Nalliah, DDS, MHCM, FACD
Associate Dean for Patient Services
Clinical Professor
University of Michigan School of Dentistry
Ann Arbor, Michigan

Samuel P. Nesbit, DDS, MS
Clinical Professor
Department of Operative Dentistry
University of North Carolina School
    of Dentistry
Chapel Hill, North Carolina

Linda C. Niessen, DMD, MPH, MMP
Founding Dean and Professor
Kansas City University College of Dental
    Medicine
Vice Provost for Oral Health Affairs
Kansas City University
Joplin, Missouri

Gustavo Oliveira, DDS, MS
Clinical Associate Professor
Operative Dentistry and Biomaterials
Division of Comprehensive Oral Health
University of North Carolina Adams School
    of Dentistry
Chapel Hill, North Carolina

Jonathan Reside, DDS, MS
Assistant Dean of Admissions
Office of Admissions and Student Life;
Assistant Professor (Periodontology)
Comprehensive Oral Health
University of North Carolina Adams School
    of Dentistry
Chapel Hill, North Carolina

Allen Samuelson, BA, DDS, Certificate
Associate Professor
Craniofacial and Surgical Services
University of North Carolina Adams School
    of Dentistry
Chapel Hill, North Carolina

Kimberly A. Sanders, PharmD, BCPS
Clinical Assistant Professor
University of North Carolina Eshelman
    School of Pharmacy;
Assistant Professor
University of North Carolina Adams School
    of Dentistry
Chapel Hill, North Carolina

**Larry W. Segars, PharmD, DrPH, FCCP,
FACE, BCPS**
Chair and Associate Professor of
    Pharmacology
Department of Basic Sciences
College of Osteopathic Medicine
Kansas City University of Medicine and
    Biosciences
Kansas City, Missouri

Helen Sharp, PhD, CCC-SLP
Director and Professor
School of Communication Sciences and
    Disorders
Pacific University
Forest Grove, Oregon

Stephen J. Stefanac, DDS, MS
Professor emeritus, Department of
    Periodontics and Oral Medicine
The University of Michigan School of
    Dentistry
Ann Arbor, Michigan

Domenica Sweier, DDS, PhD
Clinical Professor
Director of Predoctoral Clinical Education
University of Michigan School of Dentistry
Ann Arbor, Michigan

Peter Tawil, DMD, MS, FRCD(C)
Graduate Program Director, Endodontics
University of North Carolina
Chapel Hill, North Carolina

Jeff Wang, DDS, DMSc
Adjunct Clinical Associate Professor
Periodontics and Oral Medicine
University of Michigan School of Dentistry
Ann Arbor, Michigan
United States;
Associate Professor
School of Dentistry
Taipei Medical University;
Associate Professor
Graduate Institute of Clinical Dentistry
National Taiwan University
Taipei, Taiwan

Pamela Zarkowski, JD, MPH
Provost and Vice President for Academic
    Affairs
Professor
Practice Essentials and Interprofessional
    Education
University of Detroit Mercy School of
    Dentistry
Detroit, Michigan

To our wives and families for their love and support.

And to our students and their patients—past, present, and future—who have been the real inspiration for this work.

We are excited to present the fourth edition of *Diagnosis and Treatment Planning in Dentistry*. All chapters from the third edition have been updated with new material. In addition, there is a new chapter, *Digital Tools for Diagnosis and Treatment Planning*. This chapter will help readers understand the large number of digital tools that dentists are using when examining and planning care for their patients. We have also added three new instructional videos on the ebooks+ for interpreting panoramic and cone beam computed tomographic images.

The overall purpose of this book has not changed: it is to provide the reader with the fundamental knowledge needed to create treatment plans for adolescent and adult patients. To this end, the authors advocate an organized, sequential methodology beginning with a detailed and thorough patient history and examination, followed by the compilation of a comprehensive diagnosis including risk assessment, then focusing on educating and engaging the patient in a thorough informed consent discussion that culminates in the formulation of a plan of care. The concept of person-centered care and attendant ethical principle of autonomy is threaded throughout the book. The governing principle derived from this concept is *to educate the patient and empower them to make the best oral health care decision for that time and life circumstance.*

The book is organized into four sections. Section 1 presents an overview of patient examination and diagnosis. This includes the collection of patient information, its evaluation, and the development of diagnosis and problem lists for patients. The comprehensive patient diagnosis serves as the foundation for the construction of the treatment plan.

Section 2 covers the treatment planning process. The important concepts of risk assessment, prognosis, and treatment outcomes are also presented with continued emphasis on evidence-based dentistry. To assist clinicians, we have added the new chapter about using digital tools to diagnose and to formulate a treatment plan for patients. A key chapter follows, outlining the development of the treatment plan in the context of patient and dentist considerations and treatment objectives. The rationale for phasing and sequencing the plan of care is described in detail and guidelines are offered for organizing the plan into phases and properly sequencing the steps in the plan. The chapter on interprofessional treatment planning introduces shared decision making and communication with other health professionals and presents examples of conditions that are best managed by an interprofessional team. The section concludes with a chapter that addresses the ethical and legal issues surrounding the planning and execution of dental treatment. Particular attention is focused on the doctor–patient relationship, obtaining informed consent from patients, maintaining the dental record, and professional ethics and jurisprudence.

Section 3 covers, in detail, the five phases of the treatment plan. We believe the concept of phasing treatment is critical to managing patient care, especially for patients with complex needs. Managing the patient's general physical health before and during treatment represents the *systemic phase* of treatment. The chapter on the *acute phase* presents a discussion of the diagnosis and management of frequently encountered urgent treatment needs. The *disease control phase* focuses on the management of dental caries, initial therapy for periodontal disease, and the resolution of other oral infections and pathologies. The chapter discussing the *definitive phase*, often the core of the treatment plan, includes discussions of orthodontic care, advanced periodontal treatment, single tooth restorations, and replacement of missing teeth. Implant-based treatment has become a mainstay in contemporary dental practice and is an important focus in this chapter. Finally, in the chapter on the *maintenance phase*, developing a long-term relationship with the patient to promote and preserve oral health after completion of active therapy is discussed.

Section 4, *Planning Treatment for Unique Patient Populations*, offers chapters written by experts on the oral health care of each group. These seven chapters provide the clinician with specialized guidance in assessing and planning for the oral health of individuals in these groups. The chapter on *Patients With Special Needs* is placed strategically at the beginning of the section. It provides detailed insight into the management of patients with complex general and oral health problems and is an introduction to the chapters that follow. We have updated the remaining chapters that address the unique requirements of patients who are substance dependent, are anxious or fearful, have psychological disorders, are an adolescent or older adult, and are motivationally compromised or financially limited. To treat patients in these groups successfully, the clinician must often make modifications in the planning and delivery of dental care.

We have continued many features that we introduced in previous editions of the book. These include:

- The use of full color images to illustrate and support important concepts. Although still available in both hard copy and electronic versions, the electronic version seamlessly links with additional figures, tables, and other resources.
- Additional electronic content, accessible through the ebooks+, and includes instructional videos.
- *In Clinical Practice* boxes distill information in terms of specific clinical situations faced by the practicing dentist, providing concrete illustrations in a format that can be easily and quickly reviewed when planning treatment.
- The *What's the Evidence?* boxes link clinical decision making and treatment planning strategies to current research. This feature provides a lively and broadly informative approach to the topics discussed and includes citations to relevant articles in the literature.
- The *Ethics in Dentistry* boxes in some chapters focus the reader on clinical situations where ethical decision making is required.
- *Suggested Readings* that can be found at the end of many chapters provide a bibliography of authoritative texts and links to relevant manuscripts, monographs, and other resources.

- *Review Questions* can be used by students and instructors to summarize and reinforce important concepts presented in the book. *Suggested Projects* provide thought-provoking and clinically useful exercises for the practicing dentist.
- Key terms are set in boldface at their first appearance in the text and are listed and defined in the *Glossary* located at the back of the book.

Students appreciate applying what they have learned. To this end, the fourth edition contains clinically relevant multiple-choice questions similar to those used for the US Integrated National Board Dental Examination.

Throughout the book, we have focused on the treatment planning process and, aside from the mechanics of how to compose a treatment plan, have not dealt with how to perform procedures and techniques. As was true in the earlier editions, there is an intentional emphasis on a generalist rather than a specialist-driven mode of treatment planning. Treatment modalities are generally discussed in the context of related clinical conditions and problems—rather than the context of a particular dental specialty. We believe that this taxonomy is clinically relevant and realistic in the contemporary practice of general dentistry and should be appropriate for dental students who are training or who have been trained in comprehensive care-based academic curriculums. We continue our focus in the fourth edition of a universal and world-centered view of treatment planning.

We recommend that the student or entry-level practitioner begin their perusal of the text with Sections 1 and 2 to help grasp key treatment planning concepts and to appreciate the information that is essential to have in place before treatment planning can begin. Section 2 should be useful to both the novice and the experienced practitioner, providing guidance on how to design, phase, and sequence a plan, and the necessary components to do so. Section 3 provides essential tools for the student and the novice regarding the five phases of treatment planning. It may act as a framework for the experienced practitioner to "recalibrate" their treatment planning process and it can provide useful information on how to manage patients with acute or active oral health problems, such as the patient with active caries and high caries risk. The individual chapters in Section 4 should be especially helpful to the experienced practitioner because they try to make sense of selected patient problems or specific treatment planning challenges. In time, all of the chapters in Section 4 may be relevant to each reader.

However you choose to approach this text, the authors invite you to share in their enthusiasm and the deep sense of professional accomplishment that comes with successful treatment planning. Putting together the puzzle—finding the best way to treat a patient with complex medical, dental, psychosocial, and financial needs—can be an immensely complicated and immensely rewarding undertaking at the same time. Putting all these pieces together and merging the art and science of dentistry with planning care that is patient-centered can sometimes seem to be a mystical process. The mission of this text is to demystify that process. Enjoy the journey!

Stephen J. Stefanac
Samuel P. Nesbit

ACKNOWLEDGMENTS

The authors wish to thank all the contributors to *Diagnosis and Treatment Planning in Dentistry*. A project of this size could not have been done without their help and expertise. We also wish to thank the authors who did not return for the fourth edition: Jason Armfield, Robert Barsley, Sean Buchanan, Deborah DesRosiers, Mark Fitzgerald, Sharon Nicholson Harrell, Lynn Carol Hunt, Edwin Parks, Chet Smith, and John Valentine. We valued your work and retained much of it in this edition. We also want to thank everyone at Elsevier for their professional support and for giving us the opportunity to create a fourth edition.

Dr. Nesbit wishes to thank the following colleagues at the University of North Carolina Adams School of Dentistry who generously shared their time and expertise: Jamie Burgess-Flowers, Brandon Johnson and Drs. Terry Donovan, Scott Eidson, Kent Moberly, Mauro Nunes, Ricardo Padilla, Glenn Reside, and Apoena Ribeiro. He also wishes to recognize Drs. Ali Altak, Zaid Badr, Glen Karunanayake, and Lisiane Susin who provided figures for this edition.

Dr. Stefanac wishes to thank several individuals at the University of Michigan School of Dentistry who provided illustrations, reviewed manuscripts, and provided support. These included Drs. Albert Chan, Patricia Doerr, Neville McDonald, Gustavo Mendonça, Won Oh, Phil Richards, and Mr. Ken Rieger. Finally, several faculty staff, and patients were actors in photos and videos. Thank you for contributing your time and expertise.

CONTENTS

VIDEO TOC

DIAGNOSIS *and* TREATMENT PLANNING *in* DENTISTRY

Patient Evaluation and Diagnosis

Patient Evaluation and Assessment

Stephen J. Stefanac and Margherita Fontana

📶 Visit eBooks.Health.Elsevier.com

Accurate diagnostic information forms the foundation of any treatment plan. This information comes from several sources: patient history and physical examination, clinical and radiographic examination, and other diagnostic sources. The dentist must critically analyze the information before recommending treatment options to the patient. The goal of this chapter is to discuss both the types of data that the dentist in general practice typically collects and the ways in which the dentist evaluates and documents this information in preparation for creating a treatment plan. There are several types of patient examinations (Box 1.1) and the focus of this chapter is on the comprehensive assessment of a patient.

OVERVIEW OF THE DIAGNOSTIC PROCESS

The diagnostic process is begun by gathering information about the patient and creating a patient database that will serve as the basis for all future patient care decisions. Although the components of each **patient's database** vary, each includes pieces of relatively standard information, or **findings**, that come from asking questions, reviewing information on forms, observing and examining structures, performing diagnostic tests, and consulting with other dentists and healthcare providers.

Findings fall into two general categories. **Signs** are findings discovered by the dentist during an examination. For instance, the practitioner may observe that a patient has swollen ankles and difficulty in breathing when reclined, signs suggestive of congestive heart failure. Findings that are revealed by the patients themselves, usually because they are causing problems, are referred to as **symptoms**. Patients may report common symptoms such as pain, swelling, broken teeth, loose teeth, bleeding gums, or esthetic concerns. When a symptom becomes the motivating factor for a patient to seek dental treatment, it is referred to as the **chief complaint** or **chief concern**. Patients who are new to a practice or presenting for emergency dental care often have one or more chief concerns (Figure. 1.1).

The clinician must evaluate findings individually and in conjunction with other findings to determine whether the finding is significant. For example, the finding that a patient is being treated for hypertension may not be significant alone, but when accompanied by another finding of blood pressure measuring 180/110 mm Hg, the level of importance of the first finding increases. Questions arise as to whether the patient's hypertension is being managed appropriately or whether the patient is taking the prescribed medication regularly. Obviously, further questioning of the patient is in order, generating even more findings to evaluate for significance. The process of differentiating *significant* from *insignificant* findings can be challenging for dental students and recent graduates. For example, a student may believe a dark spot on the occlusal surface of a tooth to be significant, whereas a faculty member might discard the finding as simply a stained fissure, not requiring treatment. Thankfully, this differentiation and selection process becomes easier as the clinician gains experience from examining and treating more and more patients.

The process of discovering significant findings leads to a list of **diagnoses** and **patient problems** and a comprehensive patient diagnosis that ultimately forms the basis for creating a treatment plan (Figure. 1.2). Diagnoses are precise terms that identify a particular disease or problem from signs or symptoms. Examples include diabetes, caries, periodontitis, and malocclusion. Problems can initially defy a precise diagnosis but are important issues to be addressed when planning treatment. Examples include pain, swelling, difficulty chewing, or dissatisfaction with appearance. Additional examples of common diagnoses and problems are discussed in Chapter 2.

The dentist should be able to provide several types of examinations for adolescent and adult patients. Most new patients to a dental office without urgent concerns will require a **comprehensive examination** before beginning treatment. A comprehensive examination includes a review and analysis of the patient's health history and chief concerns, radiographic examination of the teeth and surrounding tissues, and clinical evaluation of the intraoral and extraoral hard and soft tissues. A **periodic examination** is performed at regular intervals, commonly during recall visits, for patients who have had a comprehensive or prior periodic examination. Activities include updating general and oral health histories and examination of extraoral hard and soft tissues. A **problem-focused examination** is limited to evaluating a specific problem or concern presented by the patient—for example, the evaluation of pain, swelling, broken teeth, or damaged restorations. Finally, a **posttreatment assessment examination** is may be performed when a treatment plan is completed or when significant caries or periodontal disease is controlled.

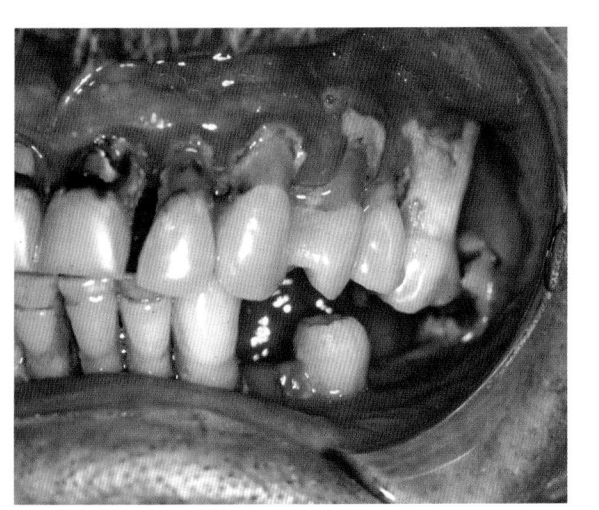

Fig. 1.1 This patient reported symptoms of tooth pain and bleeding gums. Many signs—dark teeth, receding gingival tissue, and poor oral hygiene—suggest serious dental problems.

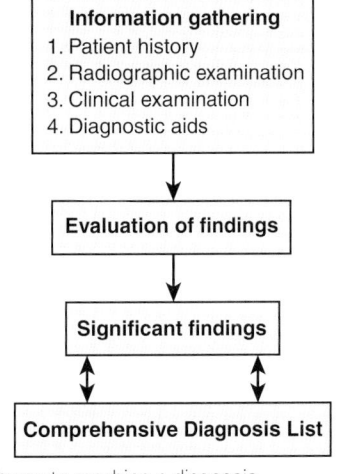

Fig. 1.2 The pathway to reaching a diagnosis.

Experienced practitioners may not always evaluate patients in a linear, sequential fashion. Instead, they move back and forth between discovering findings, evaluating for significance,

and making a diagnosis and they may begin to think about treatment options before gathering all the data. Despite this normal process, the novice practitioner (and even the experienced one) is *highly* advised against proposing treatment recommendations to patients before creating and analyzing the entire patient database. Typically, the patient initiates the discussion during the examination process. For example, examination of a sensitive tooth may elicit a query from the patient as to whether it can be saved and at what cost. Saying "yes" and "in two appointments" may prove embarrassing when subsequent radiographs reveal extensive decay and the need to extract the tooth. To prevent such errors, the inquisitive patient should be gently reminded that the examination is not yet complete and that, as more information is gathered, it will be possible to answer questions more completely.

Gathering and recording information about the patient often requires more time and attention than any other aspect of treatment planning. To prevent missing important findings, the dentist should gather data in an organized, systematic manner. Each practitioner must develop a consistent and standardized method for gathering historical information about the patient, obtaining radiographs, and performing the clinical examination. It is essential that any data gathered be both *complete* and *accurate*. If deficiencies occur in either completeness or accuracy, the validity of the final treatment plan may be suspect.

The sheer number of findings that arise when evaluating a patient with many dental problems or a complicated health history and many medications can overwhelm the newly qualified practitioner. Staying focused on each stage of information gathering and being careful to record information in an organized and systematic fashion for later analysis help to prevent confusion. This section discusses the four major categories of information required to begin developing a treatment plan: the patient history, clinical examination, radiographic examination, and other diagnostic aids.

INFORMATION GATHERING

Patient History

The distinguished Canadian physician Sir William Osler wrote, "Never treat a stranger."[1] His words underscore the need for a thorough patient history; experienced dentists learn everything they can about their patients *before* beginning treatment. Obtaining a complete and accurate patient history is part of the art of being a doctor. It takes considerable practice and self-study to become a talented investigator. No set amount of historical information is required for each patient. The volume of information collected and the complexity of the data collection process naturally depend on the severity of the patient's problems. As more information comes to light, additional diagnostic techniques may need to be used.

In dental offices, persons other than the dentist have access to patient information. The entire office staff should be aware of the confidential nature of patient information and cautioned about discussing any patient's general or oral health history other than for treatment purposes. The author is reminded of an example of a lapse in confidentiality. When updating the health history, a staff member learned that a patient had recently become pregnant. Later in the day, the patient's mother was in the office and another staff member congratulated her on her daughter's pregnancy. At first the mother was elated, but later was hurt that her daughter had not told her herself. The incident provided an uncomfortable reminder of the importance of keeping patient information confidential both inside and outside the office.

In the United States, the Health Insurance Portability and Accountability Act of 1996 (**HIPAA**) requires practitioners and healthcare organizations to prevent unnecessary use and release of **protected health information (PHI)**.[2,3] Patient PHI includes medical findings, diagnoses and treatment notes, and any demographic data that could identify the patient, such as an address, phone number, or personal identification number. HIPAA permits the use of a patient's PHI for treatment purposes, obtaining payment for services, and other organizational requirements, such as quality assurance activities or assisting legal authorities. Patients must be given, and sign, an acknowledgment that they have received information about how the practitioner or organization will use the PHI and whom they can contact if they believe their health information has been inappropriately used or released. Under HIPAA, patients also have the right to inspect, and even amend, their health records.

Techniques for Obtaining a Patient History

The two primary methods for obtaining the patient history are (1) questionnaires and forms and (2) patient interviews. A secondary method involves requesting information from another healthcare practitioner.

Questionnaires and forms. The use of questionnaires and forms during the examination process offers several advantages. Questionnaires save time, do not require any special skills to administer, and provide a standardized method for obtaining information from a variety of patients. Many types of forms are available commercially or practitioners can create their own.

Unfortunately, using a form to gather information has several disadvantages. The dentist only gets answers to the questions asked on the form and important findings may be missed. The severity of a condition may not be reflected in a simple positive response. Patients may misinterpret questions, resulting in incorrect answers. It may be necessary to have the forms printed in other languages to facilitate information gathering. The more comprehensive the questionnaire is, the longer it must be, which can be frustrating to patients. With the implementation of **electronic health records (EHR)**, patients may now enter their health information directly into electronic forms (see Chapter 4). One advantage of using this method is that the initial questionnaire can be brief, with the patient being prompted for more information if there is a positive response to a higher-level question. This individualized approach to delving into the positive responses would be difficult to duplicate efficiently with

a paper form. Finally, with a questionnaire or form, patients can more easily falsify or fail to completely reveal important information than when confronted directly in an interview.

Patient interviews. A major advantage to interviewing patients is that the practitioner can tailor questions to the individual patient. The patient interview serves a problem-solving function and develops quite differently from a personal conversation. There is a level of formality to the discussion, which centers on the patient's health and oral care needs, problems, and desires. To obtain accurate information and avoid influencing the responses, the dentist must be a systematic and unbiased information gatherer and have excellent communication skills. Most dentists are consciously aware of not showing **explicit bias**, which is expressing overt bias toward a patient based on their age, race, gender, socio-economic status, gender affiliation, appearance, or occupation for example. What is more common, and often unrecognized, is **implicit bias**, an unconscious bias toward these patient characteristics.[4] As a result, clinicians must actively keep such bias in check to be able to interact effectively with a diverse patient population.

Being a good listener is key to facilitating information flow from the patient. The desired outcome of the interviewing process is the development of a good rapport with the patient by establishing a cooperative and harmonious interaction. If the interviewer does not speak the patient's language, it may be necessary to have translation services available. A sign language translator may be also required if the patient is hearing impaired. Older patients may require more time for interviewing, particularly if their health histories are complex.[5]

The dentist can ask two general types of questions when interviewing: open and closed. **Open questions** cannot be answered with a simple response, such as "yes" or "no." Instead, open questions get the patient involved and generate reflection by asking for opinions, past experiences, feelings, or desires. Open questions usually begin with "what" or "how" and should avoid leading the patient to a specific answer.

Examples:
- How may I help you?
- What do you think is your biggest dental problem?
- Tell me about your past dental care.
- Tell me more about your heart problems.

Closed questions, on the other hand, are usually simple to answer with one or two words. They permit specific facts to be obtained or clarified but do not give insight into patient beliefs, attitudes, or feelings.

Examples:
- Do any of your teeth hurt?
- Which tooth is sensitive to cold?
- When were your teeth last examined?
- Do you have a heart problem?

In general, the examiner should use open questions when beginning to inquire about a problem. Later, closed questions can be asked to obtain answers to specific questions. The skilled clinician knows when to use each type of question during the interview. Examples are presented in the following sections. The *In Clinical Practice* box features tips on how to be an effective interviewer.

IN CLINICAL PRACTICE

Principles for Effective Interviewing

- Eye contact is important, therefore you should position the dental chair upright and sit facing the patient. Raise or lower the operator's stool so that your eyes are at the same level as the patient's.
- Use open-ended questions when seeking further information about positive responses to items on the health questionnaire.
- If the patient is hesitant or does not answer, explain why you are asking the question.
- Be an objective, unbiased interviewer. Avoid adding personal feelings. The primary goals during the interview are to accumulate and assess the facts, not to influence them.
- Be an attentive, active listener. The "golden rule" of interviewing is to listen more than speak.
- Use verbal facilitators like "yes" and "uh huh" to encourage patients to share information.
- Be aware of the patient's nonverbal communication, such as crossing arms or legs or avoiding making eye contact.
- At the conclusion of the interview, summarize what you have learned from the patient to confirm accuracy.
- See Video 1.1 Effective and Ineffective Interviewing on eBooks.Health. Elsevier.com.

Components of a Patient History

Demographic data. Demographic data include basic information, such as the patient's name, address, phone number, physician's name and phone, third party (guardian or insurance) information, national identification information, and so on. Demographic data, like any other historical information, must be accurate, complete, and current. Errors in recording insurance information, such as an incorrect policy number or failure to clarify who is responsible for payment, can be costly to a dental practice.

Useful additional information includes work, mobile, and evening telephone numbers, and seasonal and electronic mail addresses. The patient reports most of this information on demographic questionnaires and forms at the first visit. The office staff may also interview the patient if additional information is required or if information requires updating. Although commercial forms can be used to record and organize demographic information, many practices have designed their own. Dental practices that use an electronic health record instead of a paper record may scan paper forms or have the patient enter information into a computer or handheld device that is linked directly to the patient information system.

Chief concern or complaint and history. The **chief complaint** or **chief concern** is the primary reason, or reasons, that the patient has presented for treatment. For most patients, the chief complaint is usually a symptom or a request. Any complaints are best obtained by asking the patient an open-ended question, such as, "What brought you to see me today?" or "Is there anything in particular you are hoping I can do for you?" This is more effective than limiting the patient's response by asking a closed question, such as: "Is anything bothering you right now?" or "Has it been a long time since you've seen a dentist?" Record chief complaints in quotes to signify that the patient's own words are used. Careful attention to the chief complaint should alert the practitioner to important diagnoses and provide an appreciation for the patient's perception of their problems, including level of knowledge about dentistry.

The **history of present illness (HPI)** is the history of the chief complaint, which the patient usually supplies with a little prompting. When possible, the dentist should keep the questioning open, although specific (closed) questions help clarify details.

Example 1:

Chief complaint

"My tooth hurts." (*a symptom*)

HPI: The patient has had a dull ache in the lower right quadrant that has been increasing in intensity for the past 4 days. The pain is worse with hot stimuli and chewing and is not relieved by aspirin.

Example 2:

Chief complaint

"I lost a filling and need my teeth checked." (a symptom and a request)

HPI: The patient lost a restoration from an upper right molar 2 days ago. The tooth is asymptomatic. Her last dental examination and prophylaxis were 2 years ago.

Resolving the patient's chief complaint as soon as possible represents a "golden rule" of treatment planning. When a new patient presents in pain, the dentist may need to suspend the comprehensive examination process and instead focus on the specific problem, make a diagnosis and, quite possibly, begin treatment.

At times, the chief complaint may be very general, such as, "I need to chew better," or "I don't like the appearance of my teeth." In such instances, the practitioner must carefully dissect the issues of concern to the patient. Often, what initially appears to be the problem may be a more complex issue that will be difficult to manage until later in the treatment plan. During the course of treatment, the dentist should inform the patient regarding what progress is being made toward resolving the initial chief complaint.

General health history. The dentist must obtain a health history from each patient and regularly update this information in the record. A comprehensive health history contains a review of all of the patient's past and present physical illnesses and psychiatric disorders. Information about a patient's health history can prevent or help manage an emergency. Some systemic diseases may affect the oral cavity and the patient's response to dental treatment, including delaying healing or increasing the chance of infection. Conversely, some oral diseases can affect the patient's general health.[6] Because many patients see their dentist more frequently than they see their physician, the dentist should use the patient's general health history and physical examination to screen for significant systemic diseases, such as hypertension and diabetes.

Most dental practices screen for potential health problems by asking all new patients to complete a health questionnaire (Figure 1.3). When reviewing the health questionnaire, the dentist must look for conditions that may affect head and neck

Health History Form

ADA American Dental Association®
America's leading advocate for oral health

Email: Today's Date:

As required by law, our office adheres to written policies and procedures to protect the privacy of information about you that we create, receive or maintain. Your answers are for our records only and will be kept confidential subject to applicable laws. Please note that you will be asked some questions about your responses to this questionnaire and there may be additional questions concerning your health. This information is vital to allow us to provide appropriate care for you. This office does not use this information to discriminate.

Name: Home Phone: *Include area code*   Business/Cell Phone: *Include area code*
Last   *First*   *Middle*   (   )   (   )
Address: City: State: Zip:
Mailing address
Occupation: Height: Weight: Date of Birth: Sex: M   F

SS# or Patient ID: Emergency Contact: Relationship: Home Phone: *Include area code*   Cell Phone: *Include area code*
                                                                                  (   )   (   )

If you are completing this form for another person, what is your relationship to that person?

Your Name   *Relationship*

Do you have any of the following diseases or problems: (*Check DK if you Don't Know the answer to the the question*)   **Yes No DK**

Active Tuberculosis..   ☐ ☐ ☐
Persistent cough greater than a 3 week duration ....   ☐ ☐ ☐
Cough that produces blood..   ☐ ☐ ☐
Been exposed to anyone with tuberculosis ....   ☐ ☐ ☐
If you answer yes to any of the 4 items above, please stop and return this form to the receptionist.

Dental Information *For the following questions, please mark (X) your responses to the following questions.*

	Yes	No	DK		Yes	No	DK
Do your gums bleed when you brush or floss?	☐	☐	☐	Do you have earaches or neck pains?	☐	☐	☐
Are your teeth sensitive to cold, hot, sweets or pressure?	☐	☐	☐	Do you have any clicking, popping or discomfort in the jaw?	☐	☐	☐
Is your mouth dry?	☐	☐	☐	Do you brux or grind your teeth?	☐	☐	☐
Have you had any periodontal (gum) treatments?	☐	☐	☐	Do you have sores or ulcers in your mouth?	☐	☐	☐
Have you ever had orthodontic (braces) treatment?	☐	☐	☐	Do you wear dentures or partials?	☐	☐	☐
Have you had any problems associated with previous dental treatment?	☐	☐	☐	Do you participate in active recreational activities?	☐	☐	☐
Is your home water supply fluoridated?	☐	☐	☐	Have you ever had a serious injury to your head or mouth?	☐	☐	☐
Do you drink bottled or filtered water?	☐	☐	☐	Date of your last dental exam:			
If yes, how often? *Circle one:* DAILY / WEEKLY / OCCASIONALLY				What was done at that time?			
Are you currently experiencing dental pain or discomfort?	☐	☐	☐	Date of last dental x-rays:			

What is the reason for your dental visit today?

How do you feel about your smile?

Medical Information *Please mark (X) your response to indicate if you have or have not had any of the following diseases or problems.*

	Yes	No	DK		Yes	No	DK
Are you now under the care of a physician?	☐	☐	☐	Have you had a serious illness, operation or been hospitalized in the past 5 years?	☐	☐	☐
Physician Name: Phone: *Include area code* ( )				If yes, what was the illness or problem?			
Address/City/State/Zip:							
				Are you taking or have you recently taken any prescription or over the counter medicine(s)?	☐	☐	☐
Are you in good health?	☐	☐	☐	If so, please list all, including vitamins, natural or herbal preparations and/or dietary supplements:			
Has there been any change in your general health within the past year?	☐	☐	☐	_____			
If yes, what condition is being treated?				_____			
				_____			
Date of last physical exam:				_____			

A

Fig. 1.3 (A) Health history form, front.

Medical Information *Please mark (X) your response to indicate if you have or have not had any of the following diseases or problems.*

(Check DK if you Don't Know the answer to the question) **Yes No DK**

Do you wear contact lenses?.. ☐ ☐ ☐

Joint Replacement. Have you had an orthopedic total joint
(hip, knee, elbow, finger) replacement?... ☐ ☐ ☐
Date: _____ If yes, have you had any complications? _____

Are you taking or scheduled to begin taking an antiresorptive agent
(like Fosamax®, Actonel®, Atelvia, Boniva®, Reclast, Prolia) for
osteoporosis or Paget's disease?.. ☐ ☐ ☐

Since 2001, were you treated or are you presently scheduled to begin
treatment with an antiresorptive agent (like Aredia®, Zometa®, XGEVA)
for bone pain, hypercalcemia or skeletal complications resulting from
Paget's disease, multiple myeloma or metastatic cancer?.................. ☐ ☐ ☐
Date Treatment began: _____

Allergies. Are you allergic to or have you had a reaction to:
To all **yes** responses, specify type of reaction. **Yes No DK**

Local anesthetics _____ ☐ ☐ ☐
Aspirin _____ ☐ ☐ ☐
Penicillin or other antibiotics _____ ☐ ☐ ☐
Barbiturates, sedatives, or sleeping pills _____ ☐ ☐ ☐
Sulfa drugs _____ ☐ ☐ ☐
Codeine or other narcotics _____ ☐ ☐ ☐

Yes No DK

Do you use controlled substances (drugs)?.. ☐ ☐ ☐

Do you use tobacco (smoking, snuff, chew, bidis)?.......................... ☐ ☐ ☐
If so, how interested are you in stopping?
Circle one: VERY / SOMEWHAT / NOT INTERESTED

Do you drink alcoholic beverages?.. ☐ ☐ ☐
If yes, how much alcohol did you drink in the last 24 hours? _____
If yes, how much do you typically drink i n a week? _____

WOMEN ONLY Are you:
Pregnant?.. ☐ ☐ ☐
Number of weeks: _____
Taking birth control pills or hormonal replacement?........................ ☐ ☐ ☐
Nursing?.. ☐ ☐ ☐

Yes No DK

Metals _____ ☐ ☐ ☐
Latex (rubber) _____ ☐ ☐ ☐
Iodine _____ ☐ ☐ ☐
Hay fever/seasonal _____ ☐ ☐ ☐
Animals _____ ☐ ☐ ☐
Food _____ ☐ ☐ ☐
Other _____ ☐ ☐ ☐

Please mark (X) your response to indicate if you have or have not had any of the following diseases or problems.

	Yes	No	DK
Artificial (prosthetic) heart valve	☐	☐	☐
Previous infective endocarditis	☐	☐	☐
Damaged valves in transplanted heart	☐	☐	☐
Congenital heart disease (CHD)			
Unrepaired, cyanotic CHD	☐	☐	☐
Repaired (completely) in last 6 months	☐	☐	☐
Repaired CHD with residual defects	☐	☐	☐

Except for the conditions listed above, antibiotic prophylaxis is no longer recommended for any other form of CHD.

	Yes	No	DK		Yes	No	DK
Cardiovascular disease	☐	☐	☐	Mitral valve prolapse	☐	☐	☐
Angina	☐	☐	☐	Pacemaker	☐	☐	☐
Arteriosclerosis	☐	☐	☐	Rheumatic fever	☐	☐	☐
Congestive heart failure	☐	☐	☐	Rheumatic heart disease	☐	☐	☐
Damaged heart valves	☐	☐	☐	Abnormal bleeding	☐	☐	☐
Heart attack	☐	☐	☐	Anemia	☐	☐	☐
Heart murmur	☐	☐	☐	Blood transfusion	☐	☐	☐
Low blood pressure	☐	☐	☐	If yes, date:_____			
High blood pressure	☐	☐	☐	Hemophilia	☐	☐	☐
Other congenital heart defects	☐	☐	☐	AIDS or HIV infection	☐	☐	☐
				Arthritis	☐	☐	☐

	Yes	No	DK
Autoimmune disease	☐	☐	☐
Rheumatoid arthritis	☐	☐	☐
Systemic lupus erythematosus	☐	☐	☐
Asthma	☐	☐	☐
Bronchitis	☐	☐	☐
Emphysema	☐	☐	☐
Sinus trouble	☐	☐	☐
Tuberculosis	☐	☐	☐
Cancer/Chemotherapy/Radiation Treatment	☐	☐	☐
Chest pain upon exertion	☐	☐	☐
Chronic pain	☐	☐	☐
Diabetes Type I or II	☐	☐	☐
Eating disorder	☐	☐	☐
Malnutrition	☐	☐	☐
Gastrointestinal disease	☐	☐	☐
G.E. Reflux/persistent heartburn	☐	☐	☐
Ulcers	☐	☐	☐
Thyroid problems	☐	☐	☐
Stroke	☐	☐	☐

	Yes	No	DK
Glaucoma	☐	☐	☐
Hepatitis, jaundice or liver disease	☐	☐	☐
Epilepsy	☐	☐	☐
Fainting spells or seizures	☐	☐	☐
Neurological disorders	☐	☐	☐
If yes, specify:_____			
Sleep disorder	☐	☐	☐
Do you snore?	☐	☐	☐
Mental health disorders	☐	☐	☐
Specify: _____			
Recurrent Infections	☐	☐	☐
Type of infection: _____			
Kidney problems	☐	☐	☐
Night sweats	☐	☐	☐
Osteoporosis	☐	☐	☐
Persistent swollen glands in neck	☐	☐	☐
Severe headaches/migraines	☐	☐	☐
Severe or rapid weight loss	☐	☐	☐
Sexually transmitted disease	☐	☐	☐
Excessive urination	☐	☐	☐

Has a physician or previous dentist recommended that you take antibiotics prior to your dental treatment?... ☐ ☐ ☐

Name of physician or dentist making recommendation: _____ Phone: *Include area code*
( )

Do you have any disease, condition, or problem not listed above that you think I should know about?.. ☐ ☐ ☐
Please explain:

NOTE: Both doctor and patient are encouraged to discuss any and all relevant patient health issues prior to treatment.
I certify that I have read and understand the above and that the information given on this form is accurate. I understand the importance of a truthful health history and that my dentist and his/her staff will rely on this information for treating me. I acknowledge that my questions, if any, about inquiries set forth above have been answered to my satisfaction. I will not hold my dentist, or any other member of his/her staff, responsible for any action they take or do not take because of errors or omissions that I may have made in the completion of this form.

Signature of Patient/Legal Guardian: _____ Date: _____

Signature of Dentist: _____ Date: _____

FOR COMPLETION BY DENTIST
Comments: _____

B

Fig. 1.3, cont'd (B) Health history form, back. (Copyright 2015 American Dental Association. All rights reserved. Reprinted with permission.)

findings, treatment, patient management, or treatment outcomes. Interviewing the patient, first with open-ended questions about the problem and later with closed questions, usually clarifies positive responses to the questionnaire. Although it is beyond the scope of this book to present all the systemic conditions that can affect dental treatment, several are discussed in Chapter 8, including guidelines for consulting with the patient's physician if the dentist has detected significant findings.

Whether using a preprinted questionnaire or an interview technique, the general health history should include a **review of systems**.[7] The information gained through the review of systems enables the dentist (1) to recognize significant health problems that may affect dental treatment and (2) to elicit information suggestive of new health problems that have been previously unrecognized, undiagnosed, or untreated. Commonly reviewed systems and examples of some significant findings are shown in Table 1.1.

Medication history. Including both prescription and nonprescription medications in the medication history also provides valuable insight into the patient's overall health. Any over-the-counter medications, herbal remedies, vitamins, or nutritional supplements used should also be included. The medication history can corroborate findings from the health history or may suggest new diseases or conditions that need further investigation. Some medications are, in themselves, cause for limiting, delaying, or modifying dental treatment. The dentist may consult one of several reference sources to help determine the indications and potential problems that may arise from the use of various drugs. Several references, available on electronic media or on the Internet, provide rapid access to information (Figure. 1.4).

Personal history. The patient's social, emotional, and behavioral history represents one of the most important and challenging areas to investigate. The patient's occupation, habits, financial resources, and general lifestyle can significantly influence attitudes about dentistry. It is important to investigate the patient's attitudes about the profession, including priorities, expectations, and motivations for seeking treatment. The personal history is also a prime source of information about the patient's financial status, time availability for treatment, and mode of transportation to dental visits—any or all of which may have a bearing on how dental treatment is planned or executed. Much of the personal history will overlap with the oral health history, especially concerns relating to fear of dental treatment (covered in depth in Chapter 15) and concerns about the cost of treatment (discussed in Chapter 19).

The personal history also includes information about the patient's nutrition and dietary habits, with the primary goal of

TABLE 1.1 **Review of Systems With Examples of Significant Findings for Dentists**	
System	**Examples of Significant Findings for Dentists**
Constitutional symptoms (e.g., fever, weight loss)	Unexplained weight loss, fatigue and malaise, fever, recent trauma
Eyes	Vision loss
Ears, nose, mouth, and throat	Hearing loss, sinus problems
Cardiovascular	Hypertension, chest pain, shortness of breath
Respiratory	Cough, shortness of breath, wheezing
Gastrointestinal	Gastroesophageal reflux disease, unhealthy diet, food avoidance, and allergies
Genitourinary	Pregnancy
Musculoskeletal	Arthritis and joint pain, inability to sit/recline
Integumentary (skin and/or breast)	Skin lesions
Neurological	Headache, seizures, fainting
Psychiatric	Depression, anxiety, bipolar disorders, side effects of medications
Endocrine	Diabetes, thyroid problems
Hematologic/lymphatic	Anemia, coagulation problems, liver diseases
Allergic/immunologic	Medication allergies, seasonal allergies

▼ **Local Anesthetic/Vasoconstrictor Precautions**

No information available to require special precautions

▼ **Effects on Dental Treatment**

Key adverse event(s) related to dental treatment: Mouth sores, swallowing difficulty, gingivitis, gum hyperplasia, xerostomia (normal salivary flow resumes upon discontinuation), abnormal taste, tongue disorder, tooth disorder, and gingival bleeding (see Dental Health Professional Considerations)

▼ **Effects on Bleeding**

No information available to require special precautions

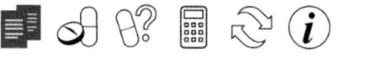

Fig. 1.4 Example of drug information from an application viewed on a mobile device. (Courtesy Wolters Kluwer Clinical Drug Information, Inc. Dental Lexi-Drugs. Wolters Kluwer; 2014.)

determining the level of fermentable carbohydrates consumed.[3] Frequently used screening questions include:

"What do you drink during the day?"

"What do you eat for meals and for snacks?"

"Where is there sugar in your diet?"

The health questionnaire can be used to evaluate the personal history for information about habits such as smoking, alcohol, and drug use, and the clinician should quantify the extent of use. Often, however, these questions are best pursued verbally, during the patient interview. For cigarette smokers, the number of packs of cigarettes is multiplied by the number of years the patient has smoked (½pack a day for 10 years is a 5 pack-year smoking habit). A patient's behavior or medication profile may suggest the presence of some type of psychological disorder, a topic discussed further in Chapter 16.

Oral health history. The oral health history incorporates such areas as the date of last dental examination, frequency of dental visits, types of treatment received, and history of any problems that have emerged when receiving dental care. Common problems include syncope (fainting), general anxiety, and reactions to drugs used in dentistry. Patients should also be questioned about their oral hygiene practices. Experienced dentists spend whatever time is necessary to investigate the oral health history of the patient because of the strong influence it can have on future treatment.

While obtaining the oral health history, the dentist should first determine the general nature of the patient's past care. Has the patient seen a dentist regularly or been treated only on an episodic basis? What kind of oral healthcare did the patient receive as a child? The frequency of oral healthcare can be an important predictor of how effectively the patient will comply with new treatment recommendations. If the patient has visited the dentist regularly, which types of treatment were provided? Was the patient satisfied with the treatment received? Did the dentist do anything in particular to make treatment more comfortable? It is also important to establish whether the patient has had any specialty treatment, such as orthodontic, endodontic, or periodontal care, in the event additional such treatment is required in the future.

Investigation into the patient's dental history supplements the clinical examination, during which new findings may be identified. The dentist should establish the explanation for any missing teeth, including when they were removed. Knowing the age of suspect restorations may yield important perspectives on the quality of previous work, how well previous treatment has held up, the patient's oral hygiene, and the prognosis for new work. The age of tooth replacements may also have a bearing on whether the patient's dental insurance will help pay for any necessary replacement.

Clinical Examination

Developing an accurate and comprehensive treatment plan depends on a thorough analysis of all general and oral health conditions that exist when the patient presents for evaluation. A comprehensive clinical examination involves assembling significant findings from the following five areas.

- Physical examination
- Intraoral and extraoral soft tissue examination

- Periodontal examination
- Examination of the teeth
- Radiographic examination

Physical Examination

The dentist has several tools that can be used to evaluate the patient's overall physical condition. Obtaining the patient's blood pressure and pulse rate represents one objective method. A more subjective, but equally valuable, approach involves simply evaluating the patient's appearance, looking both at general physical attributes and, more specifically, at the head and neck area. During this process, the clinician is searching for variations from normal that are not being managed by a physician and may have significance in a dental setting.

Unlike the physician, who examines many areas of the body for signs of disease, the dentist in general practice usually performs only a limited overall physical examination that only includes evaluation of:

- Patient posture and gait
- Exposed skin surfaces
- Vital signs
- Cognition and mental acuity
- Speech and ability to communicate

With careful observation and findings from the health history, the dentist can detect many signs of systemic diseases that could have treatment implications and may suggest referral to a physician. For example, a patient who has difficulty walking may be afflicted with osteoarthritis or have a neurologic problem, such as Parkinson's disease or the after-effects of a stroke. The appearance of the skin, hair, and eyes may suggest diseases such as anemia, hypothyroidism, or hepatitis.

Vital signs. Measuring vital signs provides an easy and objective measurement for physical evaluation. Blood pressure and pulse rate measurements should be obtained at every patient visit.[8] With the advent of accurate automated blood pressure measuring devices, measuring blood pressure and pulse rate has become a relatively simple process. Since the automated blood pressure device is being used for diagnostic purposes, it should be able to be regularly calibrated for accuracy and accept multiple cuff sizes. This contrasts with more inexpensive, personal blood pressure monitoring devices.

Blood pressure measurements can vary considerably between individuals. Ideally, the measurement is taken in a quiet room and the patient has an empty bladder, has not smoked, drunk coffee, or exercised for 30 minutes.[9] In addition, several other factors can affect the results (see Table 1.2).[10,11] Target blood pressure values for adults are listed in Table 1.3.[9] The dentist is primarily concerned when the patient has high blood pressure. Low blood pressure measurements (<60 mm Hg, diastolic) may be seen in some individuals, but such measurements are not usually significant unless the patient has other health problems or reports symptoms of light-headedness and fainting. Repeated high blood pressure readings may signify hy**pertension**, a disease that can lead to serious health problems such as heart failure, stroke, and kidney failure. Major risk factors for hypertension include smoking, diabetes, increasing age, gender (higher risk in men and in postmenopausal women), ethnicity,

TABLE 1.2 Correct and Incorrect Techniques and Their Effect on Blood Pressure Measurement

Correct Technique	Incorrect Technique	Possible Increase in BP (mm Hg)
Patient's bladder is empty	Full bladder	10–15
Proper size BP cuff	Cuff too small	2–10
Bare arm	Cuff over clothing	10–40
No talking	Conversation	10–15
Arm supported and at heart level	Unsupported arm not at heart level	10
Patient's back Is supported	Unsupported back	5–10
Feet flat on the floor	Unsupported feet	5–10
Legs uncrossed	Crossed legs	2–8

BP, Blood pressure.
Williams, J. S., et al. Videos in clinical medicine. Blood-pressure measurement. *N Engl J Med*. 2009;360(5):e6.
Ogedegbe, G., Pickering, T. Principles and techniques of blood pressure measurement. *Cardiol Clin*. 2010;28(4):571–586.
Pickering, T. G., et al. Recommendations for blood pressure measurement in humans and experimental animals: part 1: blood pressure measurement in humans: a statement for professionals from the Subcommittee of Professional and Public Education of the American Heart Association Council on High Blood Pressure Research. *Circulation*. 2005;111(5): 697–716.
O'Brien, E., et al. European Society of Hypertension recommendations for conventional, ambulatory and home blood pressure measurement. *J Hypertens*. 2003;21(5):821–848.

TABLE 1.3 Classification of Hypertension Based on Blood Pressure Measurement

Category	Systolic (mm Hg)		Diastolic (mm Hg)
Normal BP	<130	and	<85
High normal BP	130–139	and/or	85–89
Grade 1 Hypertension	140–159	and/or	90–99
Grade 1 Hypertension	≥160	and/or	≥100

BP, Blood pressure.
From Unger, T., et al. 2020 International Society of Hypertension global hypertension practice guidelines. *J Hypertens*. 2020;38(6):982–1004.

family history of hypertension, and high levels of certain lipids in the blood.

The pulse rate can be measured either manually or automatically with an electronic blood pressure cuff. An advantage of manual measurement, typically obtained by palpating the radial artery, is that the *character* of the pulse, in terms of regularity and strength, can also be detected. The normal heart rate is 60 to 100 beats per minute and is strong in character. High pulse rates, greater than 100 beats per minute range, may reflect an anxious patient or one who is under stress, has been smoking, or has just engaged in moderate exercise, such as rushing to the dentist's office. Individuals who are very physically fit or those who have severe heart problems may demonstrate a pulse rate lower than 60.[12]

Abnormal pulse measurements that cannot be explained by findings from the health history or from such circumstances as those previously listed may be significant and a sign of a cardiac arrythmia. The primary concern for the dentist is the possibility of uncontrolled cardiac, pulmonary, or thyroid disease. For example, a rapid but weak pulse can be a sign of a failing circulatory system. A weak, thready, and irregular pulse may signal a health crisis or emergency. Other conditions that may cause an irregular pulse rate include atrial fibrillation, dehydration, and medication side-effects.[13]

Although not regularly measured at the examination visit, the dentist will occasionally check a patient's oral temperature and respiration rate. Normal oral temperature is 98.6 °F (37°C) and may vary as much as ±1 °F during the day. Patients who have severe oral infections may feel feverish and have an elevated temperature. The respiration rate in adults is normally in the range of 12 to 20 breaths per minute. Shallow, irregular, or rapid breathing may be a sign of severe heart or lung disease, whereas breathing at a very rapid rate may indicate that the patient is apprehensive. Some practitioners record height and weight measurements for children, with the latter being especially useful for calculating medication dosages and body mass index (BMI).

Intraoral and Extraoral Soft Tissue Examination

Evaluation of head and neck structures for evidence of tissue abnormalities or **lesions** constitutes an important part of a comprehensive examination. This is typically accomplished by looking for variations from normal and by palpating the tissues to detect abnormalities. Figure. 1.5 illustrates normal head and neck anatomy. The following instruments and materials should be available before the examination is begun:

- Dental mirror
- Cotton gauze squares
- Tongue depressor
- Millimeter ruler

The extraoral examination begins with the patient positioned sitting upright with head unsupported to facilitate observation. The following extraoral structures of the head and neck should be evaluated in a systematic fashion: facial form and symmetry, the exposed skin, temporomandibular joint, eyes, ears, nose, major salivary glands, regional lymph nodes (Figure. 1.6), and the thyroid gland. The location and characteristics of any lesions should be noted in the patient record (Box 1.2). (See Video 1.2 Head and Neck Examination on eBooks.Health.Elsevier.com.)

After the extraoral examination, the dentist evaluates the intraoral structures, which include the lips, buccal mucosa and vestibule, tongue, floor of the mouth, salivary glands, hard and soft palate, and oropharynx (Figure. 1.7).

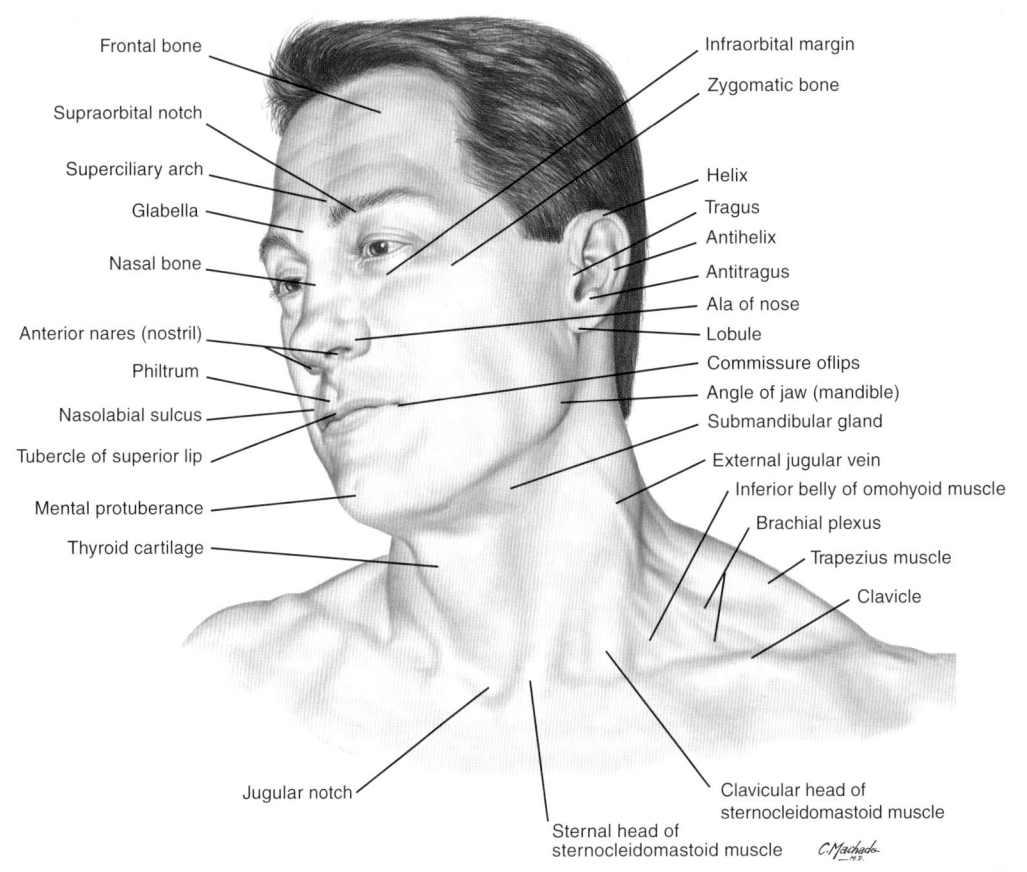

Fig. 1.5 Normal head and neck anatomy. (Netter illustration from www.netterimages.com. Elsevier Inc. All rights reserved.)

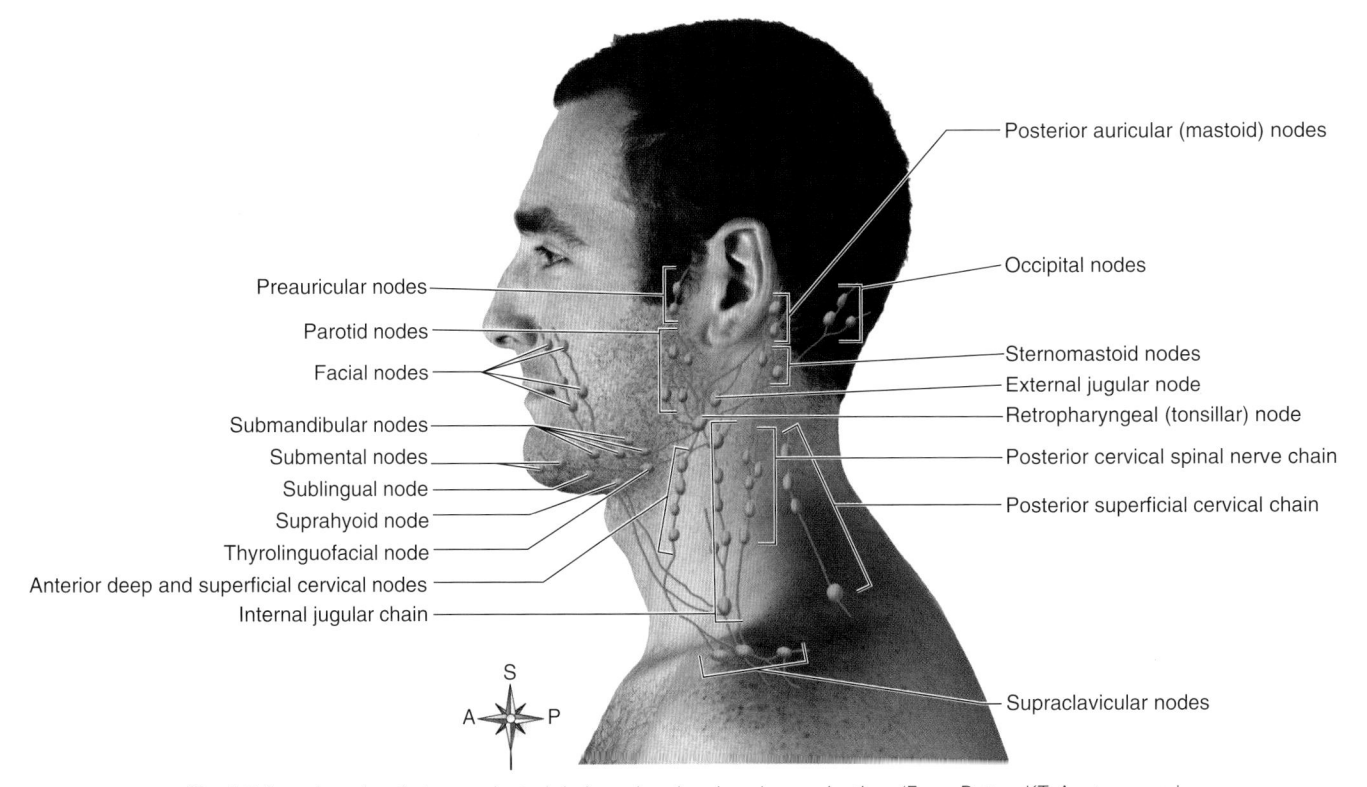

Fig. 1.6 Lymph nodes that are palpated during a head and neck examination. (From Patton KT: Anatomy and physiology, ed 10, St. Louis, 2019, Elsevier. Original figure: Fig. 20.29.)

BOX 1.2   **Characteristics of Surface Lesions**

Location
Size
Color
Shape
Borders
Surface contour
Surface texture
Consistency
Drainage/bleeding
Blanching with pressure
Fixed/moveable

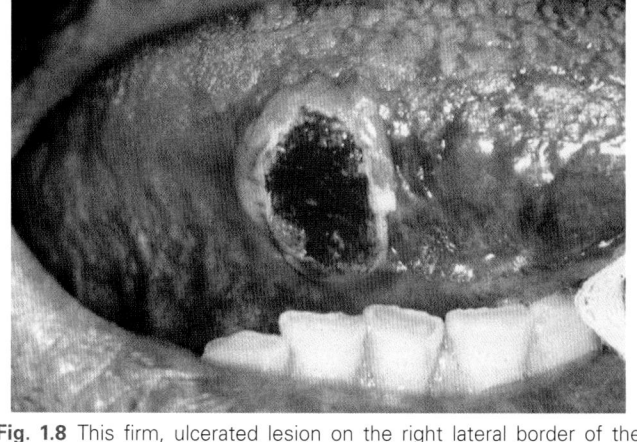

Fig. 1.8 This firm, ulcerated lesion on the right lateral border of the tongue was found in a patient who had used tobacco for more than 30 years. After biopsy and histologic evaluation, the lesion was diagnosed as a squamous cell carcinoma.

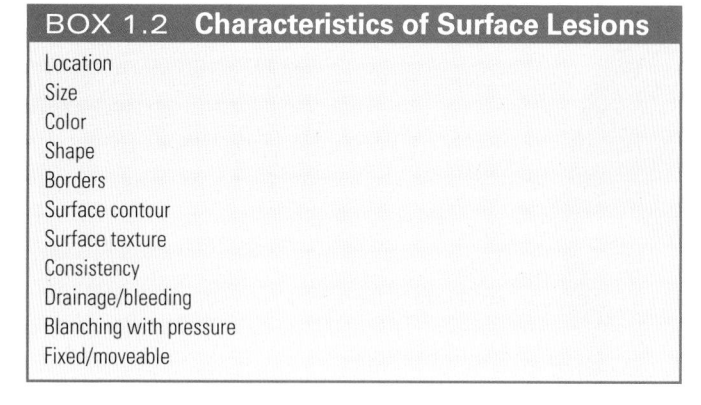
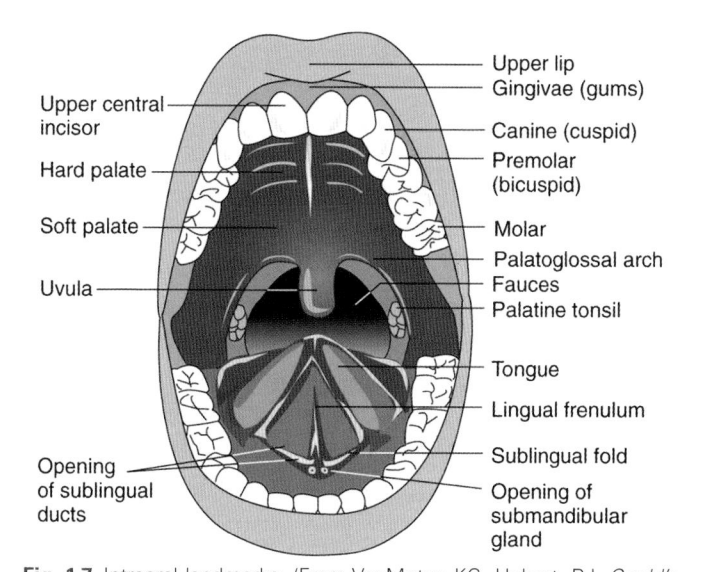

Fig. 1.7 Intraoral landmarks. (From VanMeter, KG, Hubert, RJ. *Gould's Pathophysiology for the Health Professions.* 5th ed. St. Louis: Saunders; 2015)

The significance of positive findings from the head and neck examination may be difficult to determine without further evaluation or biopsy. Common findings, such as small ulcerations, can be observed for 5 to 10 days to see whether they resolve. The patient can usually provide important historical information, such as how long the lesion has existed and whether it is associated with symptoms of pain or other discomfort. Along with this information, a history of repeated sun exposure or tobacco or alcohol use may elevate the significance of skin and oral lesions, suggesting the possibility of cancer (Figure. 1.8).

Periodontal Examination

Evaluating the periodontium is an important part of a comprehensive examination. Problems with the supporting structures of the teeth can affect the entire treatment planning process. The dentist records findings from the examination on a periodontal chart as part of the record. (See Video 1.3 Periodontal Examination on eBooks.Health.Elsevier.com.)

The examination begins with an overall assessment of the patient's oral hygiene and the appearance of periodontal soft tissue. Significant findings include areas of plaque and food accumulation on the teeth. Using disclosing solution can further reveal the presence and distribution of plaque and calculus, but this is best accomplished at the conclusion of the examination so that tissue color can be examined in its natural state. The clinician should look for deviations from healthy soft tissue, such as inflammation or rolled gingival margins.

The dentist next checks each tooth for excessive mobility, which may be related to loss of periodontal attachment or trauma from occlusion. Radiographs and periodontal probing depths provide information about the level of periodontal hard and soft tissue support. A full mouth periodontal charting (Figure. 1.9) includes identification of probing depths; the gingival margin; presence of bleeding on probing and areas of gingival recession; mucogingival problems, such as deficiencies of keratinized tissue; abnormal frenulum insertions; and the presence, location, and extent of furcation involvement. The relationship between periodontal pocket depth and attachment loss are demonstrated in Figures. 1.10 and 1.11.

Examination of the Teeth

See Video 1.4 Examination of the Teeth on eBooks.Health. Elsevier.com.

General assessment. Patients usually perceive the examination of their teeth as the most important reason to be evaluated by the dentist. The procedure is also important from the dentist's point of view because dental problems are common patient complaints. For an effective examination, it is important that the teeth are relatively clean and free from stain, plaque, and calculus, otherwise significant findings may be missed. For patients with extensive plaque and calculus, it may be best to perform a cursory examination of the dentition, begin periodontal treatment to clean the teeth, and have the patient return to finish the examination at a later appointment.

The following instruments should be readily available for use when examining the teeth (Figure. 1.12):
- Ruler
- Dental mirror
- Dental explorer
- Periodontal probe

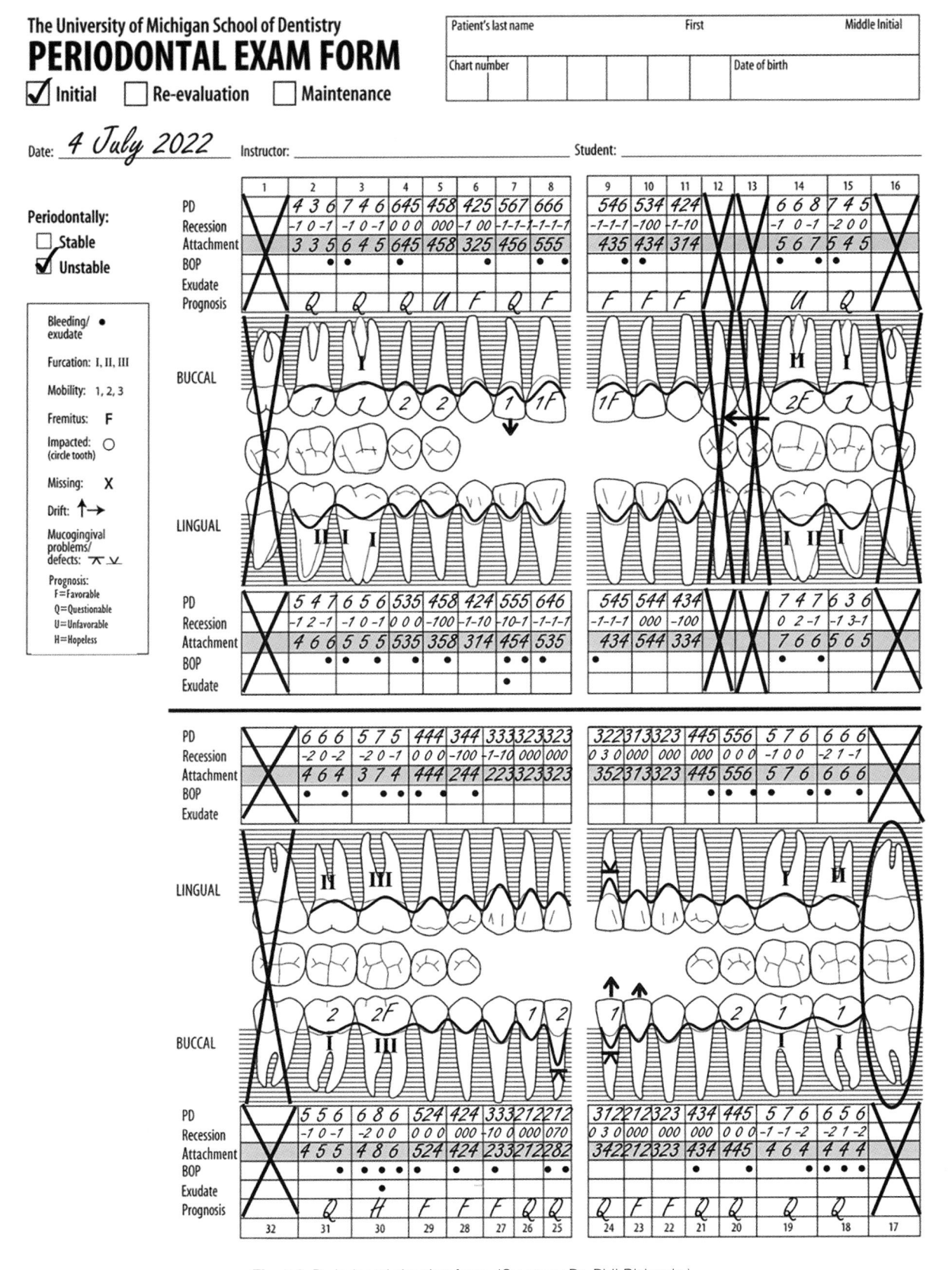

Fig. 1.9 Periodontal charting form. (Courtesy Dr. Phil Richards.)

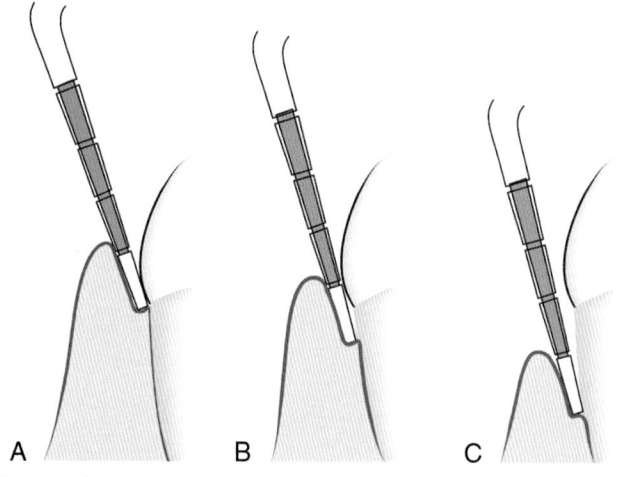

Fig. 1.10 Same pocket depth with different amounts of recession and attachment loss. **(A)** Gingival pocket with no recession and attachment loss. **(B)** Periodontal picket of similar depth as in **(A)** but with some degree of recession and attachment loss. **(C)** Pocket depth same as in **(A)** and **(B)** but with still more recession and attachment loss. (From Newman MG, Takei H, Klokkevold PR, et al. *Carranza's Clinical Periodontology.* 12th ed. St. Louis: Saunders; 2015.)

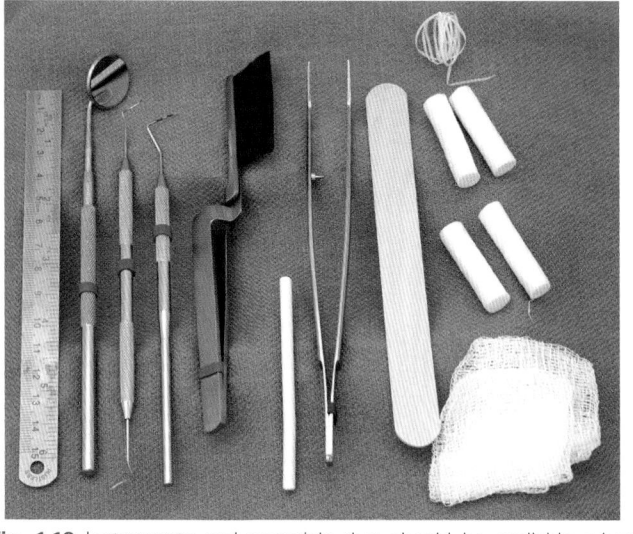

Fig. 1.12 Instruments and materials that should be available when examining a patient include a ruler, mouth mirror, dental explorer, periodontal probe, articulating paper with forceps, air/water syringe tip, cotton forceps, wooden tongue blade, dental floss, cotton rolls, and gauze squares.

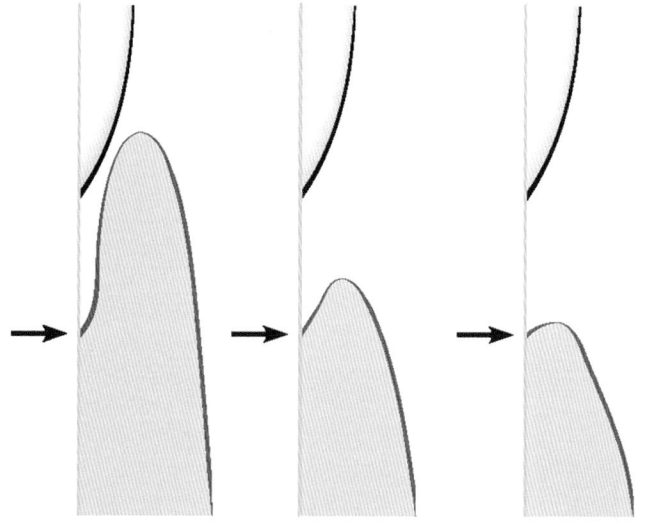

Fig. 1.11 Different pocket depths with the same amount of attachment loss. Arrows point to bottom of the pocket . The distance between the arrow and the cemento-enamel junctions remains the same, despite varying pocket depths. (From Newman MG, Takei H, Klokkevold PR, et al. *Carranza's Clinical Periodontology.* 12th ed. St. Louis: Saunders; 2015.)

- Miller forceps and articulating paper
- Cotton forceps
- Cotton rolls and gauze
- Air/water syringe
- Dental floss
- Wooden tongue blade

In addition, an electric pulp tester and refrigerant spray (for cold testing) will help to evaluate the pulp vitality of individual teeth. Although optional, the dentist's use of magnifying loupes or glasses can help identify signs of dental disease. However, early learners should consider the potential impact that magnification can have on the ability to differentiate between

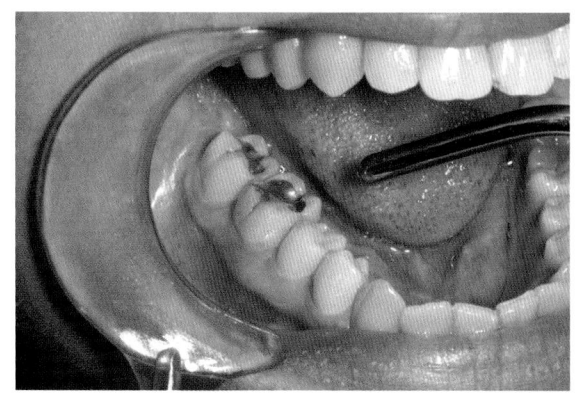

Fig. 1.13 It is important to dry the teeth before examination to avoid missing any significant findings.

anatomical characteristics of deep pits and fissures and dental disease, or the impact on the perceived severity of dental disease.[14,15]

Before beginning the examination, the dentist should review any significant findings from the dental history, especially chief concerns involving the teeth. The patient should be asked again about any dental problems, including teeth that might be sensitive to being dried with air. The dentist should review any available radiographs during the examination so that radiographic findings can be correlated with those found clinically. For efficiency and to maintain asepsis, it will be advantageous to record findings on a worksheet that can later be disposed of or to have an assistant available to record findings during the examination.

Each tooth is then evaluated sequentially, usually from the maxillary right to the mandibular left. First, air-dry a sextant of teeth and, if necessary, use cotton rolls to maintain dryness and isolation (Figure. 1.13). Next, the type and extent of all existing restorations is recorded. Any missing teeth are noted and any replacements for them, such as implants, fixed or removable partial dentures, or complete dentures, are evaluated. The patient should be questioned about the history of any missing teeth. If the patient has removable prostheses, they can be evaluated in the mouth at this time and then removed. Use dental floss to check the integrity of each interproximal contact. Non-endodontically treated (vital) teeth with large restorations or those that are symptomatic should be percussed with the end of the mirror handle and/or evaluated with cold or an electric pulp tester. Finally, assess teeth for general condition, noting overall numbers and types of restorations and any irregularities of tooth color, morphology, or ability to function.

The patient can be questioned about any concerns they have about the appearance of their teeth. Common esthetic concerns include tooth discoloration, crowding of teeth (especially the lower anterior teeth), spaces between teeth (referred to as **diastemas**) and variations in tooth size and shape. There may also be a loss of tooth structure, usually enamel, from exposure to acid, referred to as **erosion** (Figure. 1.14). This is most frequently caused by dietary sources and, less commonly, regurgitation of stomach acid as a result of gastroesophageal reflux disease.

Occlusal examination. Before examining individual teeth, the dentist should evaluate the dentition as a whole by examining the patient's occlusion. Looking at each arch separately, the clinician first checks for shifts of the dentition from the midline. Are the marginal ridges even or are teeth extruded or intruded from the occlusal plane? Have teeth moved mesially or distally into any edentulous spaces? Is there evidence of excessive wear

to the teeth? Instruct the patient to occlude in the maximum intercuspal position, so that the amount of overbite and overjet in the incisor area can be evaluated. Note the angle classification (Figure. 1.15) by examining the relationships between the maxillary and mandibular canines and molar teeth.[16] At this time, also note in the record any open bite or cross-bite. Instruct the patient to move the mandible from side to side and forward to study which teeth guide the occlusion in lateral and protrusive excursions. The dentist can then manipulate the lower jaw to evaluate the centric relation and look for interferences in lateral

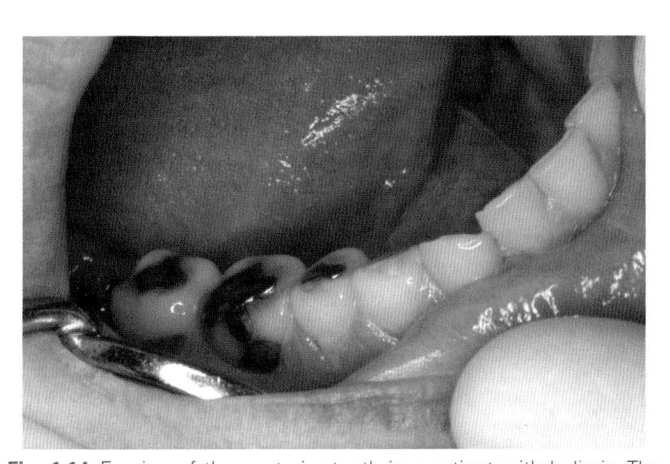

Fig. 1.14 Erosion of the posterior teeth in a patient with bulimia. The restoration appears to protrude from the occlusal surface because of the loss of tooth structure.

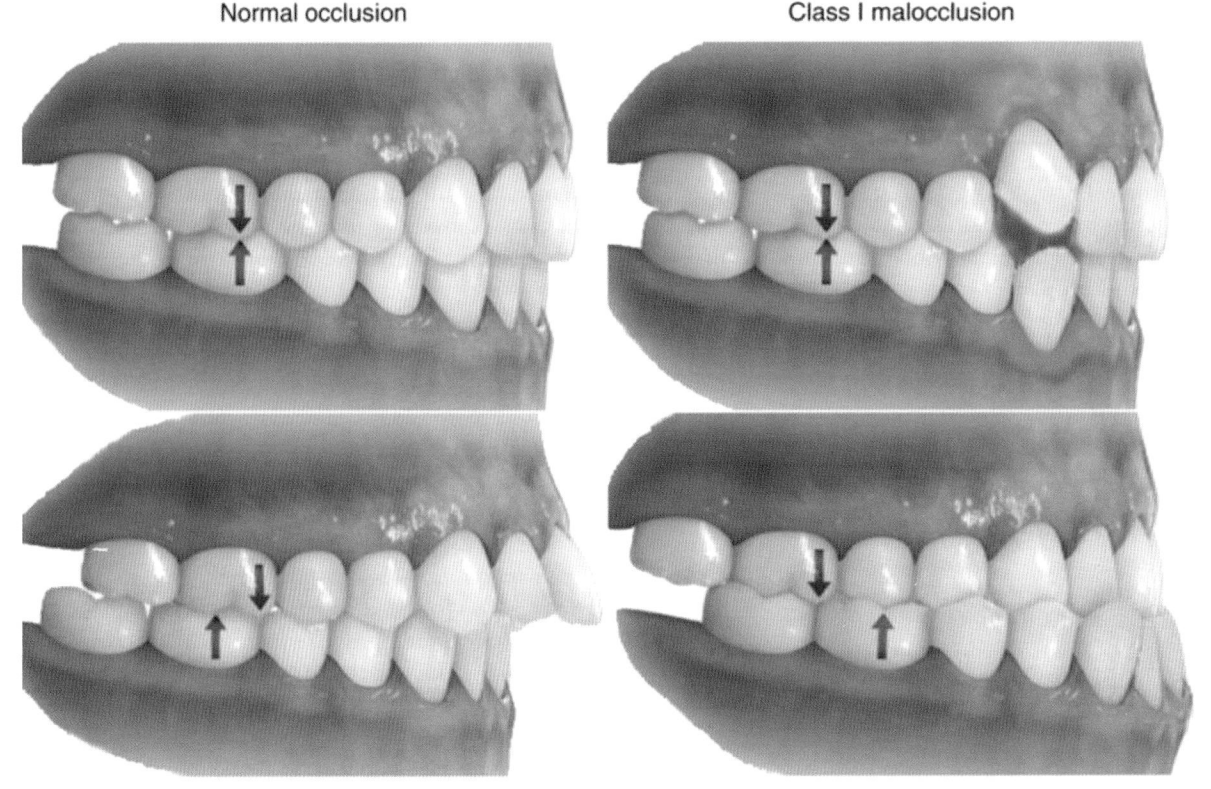

Fig. 1.15 Angle's classification. From Orthodontics, Principles and Techniques, 6th ed. 2017. https://evolve.elsevier.com/cs/product/9780323378321?role=student. Figure 8-2

and protrusive movements. At this point in the examination, question the patient about any pain or tenderness in the temporomandibular joint and associated muscles. The patient should be evaluated for visual, palpatory, or auditory evidence, such as "pops," "clicks," or crepitation. Any deviation on opening should be noted. Finally, ask the patient to demonstrate how wide they can open their mouth. A more detailed investigation is warranted if the patient has pain, an inability to chew, or a limited opening (<30 mm). The examiner should note any signs of abnormal tooth wear caused by excessive function (referred to as **attrition**). This is frequently a result of **bruxism**, or grinding the teeth, often at night (Figure. 1.16).

Caries assessment. The examination of teeth for caries lesion detection (i.e., identifying existing caries lesions) and assessment (i.e., characterizing the severity and activity of lesions once they have been detected) is the basis for evidence-based caries management (Chapter 3).[17] The ability to detect and differentiate between the various stages of caries lesion severity depends on the caries detection method and/or the clinical criteria being used. Many criteria have been developed for the examination and assessment of teeth for caries lesions, including visual and/or tactile-based criteria.[18] In the past, tactile criteria, based on use of the explorer under force to confirm cavitation ("catch"), were commonly used for the identification of dental caries and for many decades were considered the gold standard for caries detection.[19] In today's practice of dentistry, however, forceful use of a sharp explorer for the sole purpose of detecting caries lesions is highly discouraged.[20] As a result, examination of the teeth using predominantly visually based criteria is currently the most commonly recommended method for caries detection.[18,21]

The following steps should be followed when visually examining teeth for caries lesion detection and assessment:

1. Ask patient to remove any intraoral appliances (e.g., removable prostheses).
2. Clean surfaces with a toothbrush and water (in some patients, flossing between tight contacts may be needed and/or a more extensive prophylaxis may be necessary).
3. Isolate with cotton rolls if saliva will interfere with drying.

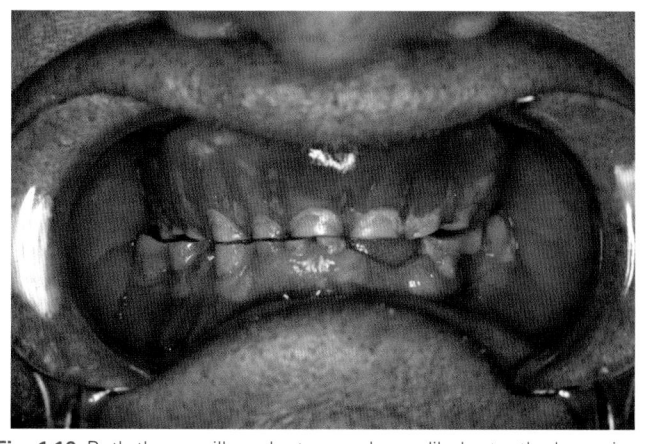

Fig. 1.16 Both the maxillary denture and mandibular teeth show signs of excessive attrition from bruxism in this patient who ground his teeth at night.

4. Examine all teeth and surfaces in order, first when the tooth is wet and then after gently air drying for 5 seconds.
5. The explorer is only an aid to visual caries examination and should never be used with force for caries detection. The appropriate use of the explorer includes only the following:
   - to clean debris or remove plaque gently,
   - to help confirm caries lesion cavitation very gently (break of the surface, Chapter 2) *only when in doubt,*
   - to aid in determination of lesion activity (e.g., soft dentin or rough-opaque enamel, Chapter 2), and
6. after the tooth has been sealed or restored, to help assess the dental material's integrity and retention.
7. After defects on tooth surfaces have been detected and assessed for severity, based on appearance and location, determine their origin—in other words, whether they are caries lesions or other defects, such as wear, fluorosis, and erosion. If they are caries lesions, then a determination of degree of activity (i.e., progressing or arrested) is necessary to complete the diagnosis of caries (see Chapter 2 for specifics).
8. Record findings.

Radiographic Examination

Conventional and digital radiographs provide valuable information about teeth and jaws and are used to document the patient's dental condition prior to treatment. Before ordering any radiographs, the dentist should review the patient's oral health history and perform the clinical examination. When possible, any radiographs made by a previous dentist should be obtained, particularly those less than 3 years old.

The dentist determines which type of radiograph to obtain based on patient age, clinical findings, and oral health history. Certain factors place a patient at higher risk of oral health problems (see Chapter 2 for caries risk assessment), necessitating a more extensive radiographic survey; see Box 1.3. Radiographs should be made only when the diagnostic benefits outweigh the risks of exposure to ionizing radiation. The American Dental Association and the US Food and Drug Administration (FDA) have issued a series of recommendations to assist practitioners with this decision (eTable 1.1).

Dentists in general practice commonly use several types of radiographs to examine patients for signs of pathologic conditions, caries, periodontal or periapical problems, and remnants of missing teeth, and to examine the quality of existing dental restorations. The primary intraoral exposures are periapical, interproximal (or bite-wing), and occlusal projections. The dentist can select from several types of extraoral radiographs, with the panoramic being most frequently used for examining areas not readily visualized with intraoral radiographs.

Periapical radiographs should show the crown and root of a particular tooth and the surrounding bone. Useful for imaging the teeth, detecting caries, and documenting signs of periodontal and periapical disease, these radiographs are limited by their size and the need to be placed in the mouth. A complete mouth survey of a completely dentate patient usually consists of 14 to 18 periapical radiographs along with four interproximal radiographs (Figure. 1.17).

BOX 1.3 Clinical Situations for Which Radiographs May Be Indicated

Positive Historical Findings
- Previous periodontal or endodontic treatment
- History of pain or trauma
- Family history of dental anomalies
- Postoperative evaluation of healing
- Remineralization monitoring
- Presence of implants, previous implant-related pathosis, or evaluation for implant placement

Positive Clinical Signs/Symptoms
- Clinical evidence of periodontal disease
- Large or deep restorations
- Deep carious lesions
- Malposed or clinically impacted teeth
- Swelling
- Evidence of dentofacial trauma
- Mobility of teeth

- Sinus tract (fistula)
- Clinically suspected sinus pathosis
- Growth abnormalities
- Oral involvement in known or suspected systemic disease
- Positive neurologic findings in the head and neck
- Evidence of foreign objects
- Pain and/or dysfunction of temporomandibular joint
- Facial asymmetry
- Abutment teeth for fixed or removable partial prosthesis
- Unexplained bleeding
- Unexplained sensitivity of teeth
- Unusual eruption, spacing, or migration of teeth
- Unusual tooth morphology, calcification, or color
- Unexplained absence of teeth
- Clinical erosion
- Peri-implantitis

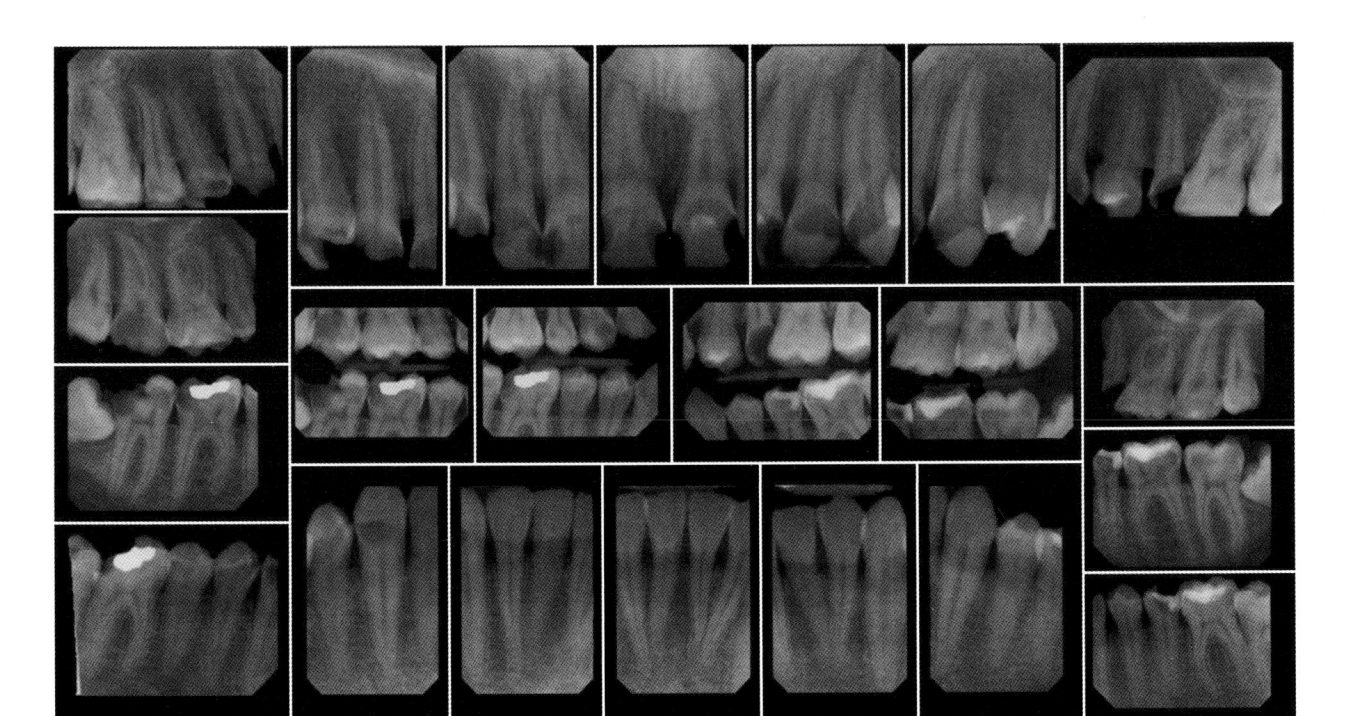

Fig. 1.17 A 22-image complete mouth survey consisting of 18 periapical and 4 bite-wing radiographs. The patient exhibits radiographic signs of rampant dental caries, impacted mandibular third molars, and erosion of the maxillary anterior teeth. (Courtesy Dr. Erika Benavides.)

Horizontal and vertical **interproximal** or **bite-wing radiographs** show the coronal portion of the teeth in both arches and the alveolar crestal bone. Most frequently used for the detection of interproximal caries and for evaluating crestal bone height, bite-wing radiographs are also valuable as a screening tool for patient evaluation before deciding to take posterior periapical radiographs.

Occlusal radiographs are placed over the teeth in the occlusal plane. In adults, their use is limited to visualizing palatal lesions and searching for impacted or supernumerary teeth.

The radiograph can also be helpful in documenting expansion of bone in the mandible or salivary stones in the ducts of the submandibular gland (Figure. 1.18).

The **panoramic radiograph** (also referred to as a **pantomograph**) displays a wide area of the jaws and hence enables evaluation of structures not visible in intraoral projections (Figure. 1.19). Relatively easy to take, panoramic radiographs may help detect developmental anomalies, pathologic lesions of the teeth and jaws, bone fractures, sinus disease, and temporomandibular joint disorders. In adults, dentists most commonly

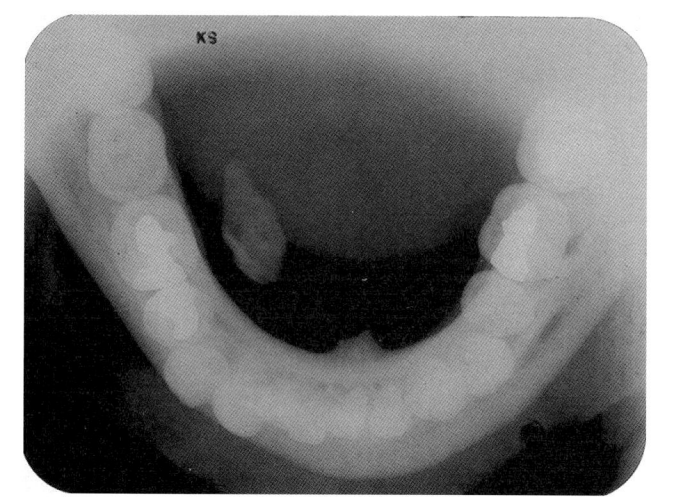

Fig. 1.18 A mandibular occlusal radiograph showing a sialolith in the patient's right submandibular gland duct.

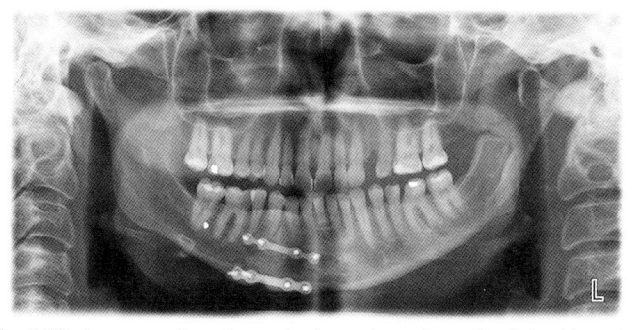

Fig. 1.19 A panoramic radiograph of a patient after a fist fight. Note the fracture on the right anterior mandible repaired with surgical plates. On the left ramus, there is a displaced condylar neck fracture, a fracture of the anterior ascending ramus, and signs of a displaced fragment superimposed over the angle of the mandible.

use this radiograph to evaluate third molar position or the condition of edentulous areas of the jaws before fabricating removable prosthodontics or placing implants. Because of the lower resolution and superimposition of structures, a film-based panoramic radiograph does not provide the fine detail necessary to diagnose early caries or accurately document periodontal bone loss. Digital panoramic radiographs are approaching the diagnostic yield of intraoral radiographs and may be used in combination with bite-wing images. Some panoramic equipment can make extraoral posterior bite-wing images, which can be useful for patients with restricted mouth opening or those who cannot tolerate having intraoral radiographs taken.[22] See Video 1.5 Systematic Interpretation of Panoramic Radiographs on eBooks.Health.Elsevier.com.

There are several situations in which three-dimensional imaging information is beneficial in diagnosis and treatment planning. Some examples include the placement of dental implants, precise localization of impacted teeth, evaluation of the relationship of third molar roots to the mandibular canal before surgery, assessment of buccolingual expansion caused by pathologic jaw lesions, or the analysis of jaw relationships in orthodontics. In the past, this information could be gained

only from medical **computed tomographic (CT)** examination, but today, **cone-beam CT (CBCT)** scanners dedicated to maxillofacial imaging are available (Figure. 1.20). This equipment permits acquisition of three-dimensional images with a lower radiation dose than with a medical scanner. See Video 1.6, What is CBCT? and Video 1.7, CBCT Anatomy on eBooks.Health. Elsevier.com. Additional information about digital imaging and CBCT can be found in Chapter 4.

Other Diagnostic Aids

Study Casts

Study casts are used during the examination stage to document and analyze the patient's dentition before providing treatment. Individual casts show the position and inclination of teeth and can be used to create matrices for fabricating temporary restorations. Study models should be obtained and mounted on an articulator to evaluate occlusal relationships whenever prosthodontic treatment is planned. The dentist can also use mounted casts to evaluate the necessity for preprosthetic surgery, especially in the edentulous patient with large maxillary tuberosities. Casts can also act as visual aids for presenting information to patients.

Diagnostic Wax-Ups and Altered Casts

Diagnostic wax-ups on study casts help the practitioner and patient visualize the tooth form, contour, and occlusion that will result from the proposed treatment. Wax-ups are especially useful when missing teeth are to be replaced or existing teeth significantly altered. The casts are usually mounted on an articulator to evaluate the waxing in the proposed functional relationship.

Altered casts should be made on duplicate models of the original study casts. Study casts are useful for establishing ideal relationships for jaw segments in planning orthognathic surgery or extensive fixed prosthodontic treatment. When the new relationships have been finalized, templates (thermoplastic shims) can be made from the altered casts to act as guides for tooth preparation or the location of tooth and jaw position during surgery.

Many dentists obtain digital scans of the teeth and arches, which are used for orthodontic and esthetic analysis and patient case presentation (see Chapter 4).

Occlusal Splints

When patients exhibit signs of temporomandibular dysfunction (TMD), such as jaw muscle pain or chronic headaches, it may be advisable to construct an occlusal splint to relieve symptoms. In such a situation, the occlusal splint becomes both a treatment modality and a diagnostic aid. If the pain persists after splint therapy, the clinician may need to reevaluate the initial working diagnosis of TMD and search for alternative causes for the pain.

Caries Excavation

Caries excavation, in addition to being an operative procedure, can also be used as a diagnostic technique. For example, it may be necessary to remove caries from a severely decayed tooth, often before endodontic therapy, to determine whether

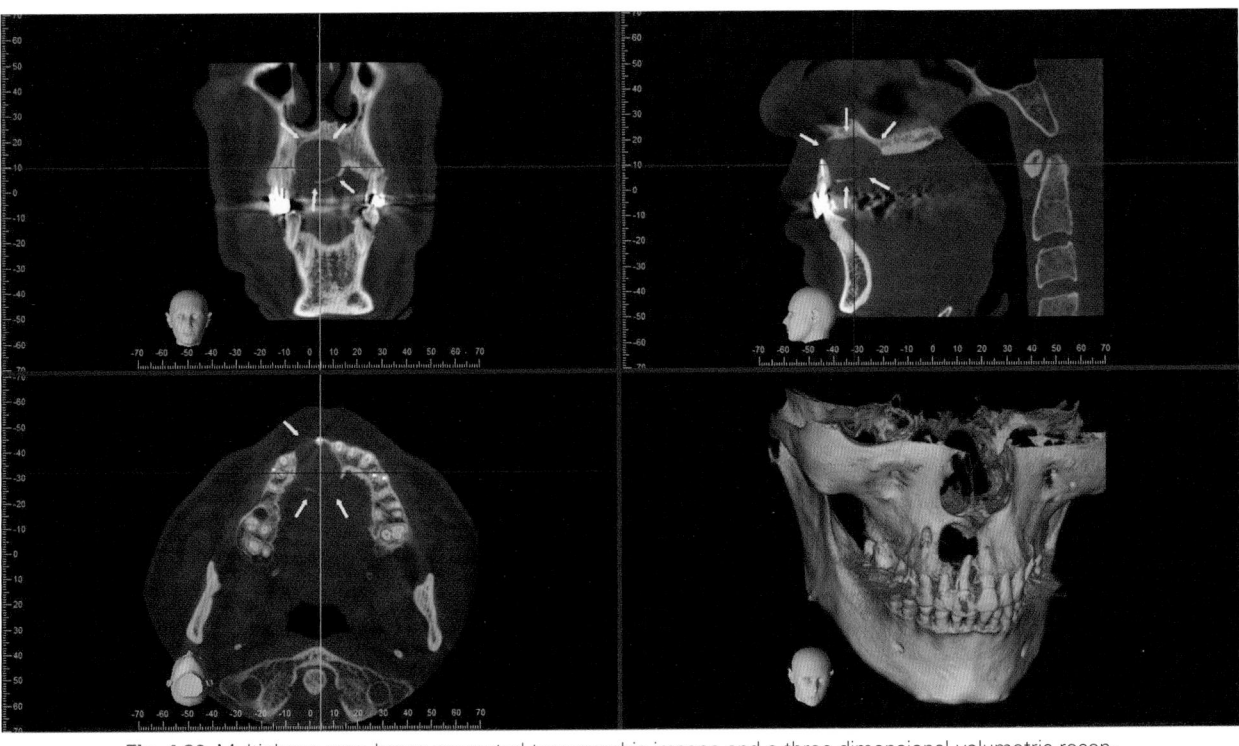

Fig. 1.20 Multiplanar cone beam computed tomographic images and a three-dimensional volumetric reconstruction of a large, well-defined, low-density periapical lesion associated with an endodontically treated maxillary right central incisor. The lesion is causing expansion and perforation of the buccal and palatal cortical plates. (Courtesy Dr. Erika Benavides.)

the tooth can be restored. Extensive treatment for a tooth may be contraindicated if it is not restorable and the tooth should be extracted. The issue of restorability is discussed in greater depth in Chapters 9 and 10.

Consultation

When is consultation with another dentist or a physician about the patient necessary or advisable? In general, if the primary care provider has questions concerning the patient's general health or the diagnosis or treatment of the patient's oral problems, it is in everyone's best interest to seek further guidance. For example, it may be appropriate to contact the patient's physician to establish any medical diagnoses and to consult about the capacity of the patient to withstand dental treatment. When a consultation is sought, it must be implemented with the patient's understanding and consent. More information about communicating with other dentists and healthcare providers can be found in Chapter 8.

Biopsy

Biopsy procedures are indicated to diagnose persistent oral lesions or to ensure that a previously diagnosed condition is still benign. The procedure consists of removing all or part of a lesion and submitting the tissue for histologic evaluation by a pathologist. Dentists should not hesitate to biopsy lesions themselves or to refer the patient for further evaluation and treatment, especially when the lesions are suggestive of oral cancer or some other serious condition.

Medical Laboratory Tests

A significant number of patients with serious systemic disease present for oral healthcare. Many may be taking medications that alter their blood coagulation time or immune system. In other situations, the dentist may suspect that a patient has an untreated systemic problem, such as leukemia or diabetes, that can only be confirmed with laboratory tests. Certain surgical procedures may require laboratory testing before treatment is provided. In these situations, the dentist usually refers the patient to their healthcare provider for testing and requests a copy of the test results.

Screening for diabetes, high blood pressure, high cholesterol, and other chronic conditions may be performed by members of the dental profession in the future.[23] Practitioners should be cautious, however, about performing tests for conditions about which they would be unable to counsel the patient adequately. The patient should instead be referred to a general medical health provider for evaluation.

Microbiologic and Other Testing Systems

The use of microbiologic tests in dental offices currently is limited, but in the future they will become more widely used, especially as a tool for diagnosing caries susceptibility and periodontal disease activity.[24]

Caries susceptibility can be evaluated by measuring the quantity of cariogenic bacteria, such as *Streptococcus mutans* and lactobacilli. A sample of the patient's saliva is placed on a special agar medium, which is then incubated. The patient's caries risk is related to the number of bacterial colonies that grow on the plate. A low salivary flow rate (<1 mL/min of stimulated saliva) and low salivary buffering capacity represent risk factors for increased caries activity. The evaluation of substances in a patient's saliva has the potential to act as a noninvasive test for several oral and systemic diseases.

Determining levels of enzymes and inflammatory mediators in blood serum or gingival crevicular fluid can provide evidence of active periodontal disease. Deoxyribonucleic acid (DNA) probes can also be used to screen for signs of disease-causing periodontal pathogens.[25]

Documentation

All examination results and diagnoses must be clearly documented in the patient's record. Record entries need to be accurate, complete, and consistent between patients. This can be challenging if there are multiple clinicians in a dental office or in an environment with a large turnover in clinicians and patients, such as a dental school. Consistent paper or electronic forms are helpful, as are standardized abbreviations. See eTable 1.2 for a full list of abbreviations in dentistry in the expanded chapter on ebooks+.

Progress or treatment notes document each appointment. These notes can include appointment-specific diagnoses, evidence of health history review, details of treatment provided, patient behavior, and plans for the next visit (Box 1.4). Entries must be stated clearly and objectively. Treatment detail should include the teeth or soft tissue area treated, medications administered, and details surrounding the treatment procedures. Any potentially life-threatening condition or medical problem that could have a significant impact on the dental treatment should be displayed in a prominent place in the record. Examples include allergies and the need for premedication.

The retention of study models for all patients presents storage problems. No specific guidelines for retention exist, but many dentists retain casts for patients who have had orthodontic treatment or extensive prosthodontic work. It is possible to digitize models and store the data electronically. The models can then be recreated later if necessary.

Color photographs and digital images of patients are excellent methods for recording patient findings, both before and after treatment. Some practitioners, especially orthodontists, routinely take photographs of all their patients. Intraoral video cameras are used to educate patients about specific problems in their mouths. Many systems can instantaneously print still images that can be given to the patient or placed in the record. See Chapter 4 for more information.

Several varieties of worksheets and dental charts are available for recording findings, diagnoses, and treatment recommendations. The choice of forms is a personal decision. Ideally, entries should be made in pen for permanence, with black ink to facilitate photocopying. The union of digital photographs and digital radiography with electronic charting and procedural notes has led to the creation of an **electronic patient record**.

Physical and electronic patient records must be maintained in good order and be retrievable even after the patient has left the dental practice. Good record keeping, complete examination documentation, and the ability to retrieve the record represent essential elements in dental practice. In the event of litigation, good documentation can protect the dentist by demonstrating a high level of professional competence. Good records help prevent litigation, win a malpractice suit, or decrease damages. In the United States patients who change practitioners have a legal right to obtain copies of recent radiographs. Finally, an additional important reason for maintaining a complete diagnostic and treatment-related information/file for each patient is that the dentist may have the unpleasant duty of providing dental records, postmortem, for the purpose of patient identification.

> ### BOX 1.4   Example of a Treatment Note entry
>
> **Treatment Note**
> **Problem:**
> Caries distal upper right first molar
> **Health status:**
> Reviewed: Treated hypertension BP 125/85 mm Hg
> **Treatment:**
> 1.7 cc 2% lidocaine 1:100,000 epinephrine infiltration, rubber dam isolation.
>   DO composite, shade A-2, placed over glass ionomer liner
> **Patient evaluation:**
> Patient was apprehensive but cooperative
> **Next visit:**
> Composite restorations for maxillary incisors. Check bite splint.

▌REVIEW QUESTIONS

- What are the major categories of information required to begin to create a treatment plan?
- Describe techniques that can be used and techniques to be avoided when interviewing a dental patient.
- What are the components of a patient history? What information is included in each of those components?
- List indications for obtaining study casts as part of the initial examination of the patient.
- When the dentist requests a consultation with a physician or other healthcare provider, what information is the dentist seeking and how will it be recorded in the patient record?

REFERENCES

1. Terezhalmy GT, Schiff T. The historical profile. *Dent Clin North Am.* 1986;30(3):357–368.
2. Moore W, Frye S. Review of HIPAA, Part 1: History, Protected Health Information, and Privacy and Security Rules. *J Nucl Med Technol.* 2019;47(4):269–272.
3. Moore W, Frye S. Review of HIPAA, Part 2: Limitations, Rights, Violations, and Role for the Imaging Technologist. *J Nucl Med Technol.* 2020;48(1):17–23.
4. National Center for Cultural Competace Georgetown University. Concious and unconcious bias in heathcare - Two types of bias. https://nccc.georgetown.edu/bias/module-3/1.php. Accessed August 30, 2021.
5. Stein PS, Aalboe JA, Savage MW, Scott AM. Strategies for communicating with older dental patients. *J Am Dent Assoc.* 2014;145(2):159–164.
6. Kane SF. The effects of oral health on systemic health. *Gen Dent.* 2017;65(6):30–34.
7. Centers for Medicare and Medicaid Services (CMS), Evaluation and Management Services Guide. Publication MLN906764, Feb 2021.
8. American Dental Association. Hypertension. *Oral Health Topics* 2020; https://www.ada.org/en/member-center/oral-health-topics/hypertension.
9. Unger T, Borghi C, Charchar F, et al. 2020 International Society of Hypertension global hypertension practice guidelines. *J Hypertens.* 2020;38(6):982–1004.
10. O'Brien E, Asmar R, Beilin L, et al. European Society of Hypertension recommendations for conventional, ambulatory and home blood pressure measurement. *J Hypertens.* 2003;21(5):821–848.
11. Pickering TG, Hall JE, Appel LJ, et al. Recommendations for blood pressure measurement in humans and experimental animals: part 1: blood pressure measurement in humans: a statement for professionals from the Subcommittee of Professional and Public Education of the American Heart Association Council on High Blood Pressure Research. *Circulation.* 2005;111(5):697–716.
12. Little J, Miller C. Rhodus N. *Little and Falace's Dental Management of the Medically Compromised Patient.* 9th ed. Elsevier; 2018.
13. Heart Arrythmia. 2021; https://www.mayoclinic.org/diseases-conditions/heart-arrhythmia/symptoms-causes/syc-20350668.
14. Wilde S, Campos PH, Marcondes AP, et al. Optical magnification has no benefits on the detection of occlusal caries lesions in permanent molars using different visual scoring systems: An in vitro study. *J Clin Exp Dent.* 2020;12(5):e479–e487.
15. Motschall KDS, Ballantine J, Eckert G, Fontana M. Magnification effect on caries detection and treatment by early learners. *AADR//CADR Annual meeting.* 2016;(Abstract 0829).
16. Graber N.V.R., Vig K., Huang G. Orthodontics, Current Principles and Techniques. 6th ed 2017.
17. Fontana M, Cabezas CG, Fitzgerald M. Cariology for the 21st Century: current caries management concepts for dental practice. *J Mich Dent Assoc.* 2013;95(4):32–40.
18. Pitts NB, Stamm JW. International Consensus Workshop on Caries Clinical Trials (ICW-CCT). Final consensus statements: agreeing where the evidence leads. *J Dent Res.* 2004;83. Spec No C:C125–128.
19. Radike AW. Criteria for the diagnosis of dental caries. American Dental Association. *Proceedings of the Conference on the Clinical Testing of Cariogenic Agents.* Chicago, The American Dental Association; 1968:87–88. 3rd ed.
20. American Dental Association. Treating caries as an infectious disease. *J Am Dent Assoc.* 1995;126:2-S–4-S.
21. Gimenez T, Piovesan C, Braga MM, et al. Visual Inspection for Caries Detection: A Systematic Review and Meta-analysis. *J Dent Res.* 2015;94(7):895–904.
22. Chan M, Dadul T, Langlais R, Russell D, Ahmad M. Accuracy of extraoral bite-wing radiography in detecting proximal caries and crestal bone loss. *J Am Dent Assoc.* 2018;149(1):51–58.
23. Genco RJ, Schifferle RE, Dunford RG, Falkner KL, Hsu WC, Balukjian J. Screening for diabetes mellitus in dental practices: a field trial. *J Am Dent Assoc.* 2014;145(1):57–64.
24. Dahlén G. Microbiological diagnostics in oral diseases. *Acta Odontol Scand.* 2006;64(3):164–168.
25. Al Yahfoufi Z, Hadchiti W, Berberi A. Deoxyribonucleic acid probes analyses for the detection of periodontal pathogens. *J Contemp Dent Pract.* 2015;16(9):727–732.

2

Common Diagnoses in Dentistry

Samuel Nesbit, Angela Broome, Shin-Mey (Rose) Geist, Ricardo Padilla, Pei-Feng Lim,
Gregory K. Essick, Antonio Moretti, Jonathan Reside, Margherita Fontana,
Lee Boushell, Stephen Stefanac, and Nisha Frances Ganesh

Visit eBooks.Health.Elsevier.com

OUTLINE

PATIENT DIAGNOSIS

DIAGNOSES AND PROBLEMS

Armed with the significant findings from the examination process, the dentist now begins to assemble a list of diagnoses for the patient. **Diagnoses** are precise, scientific terms used to describe variations from normal. They can be applied to a systemic disease, such as Type 2 diabetes, or a specific oral health condition, such as localized periodontitis stage 3 grade C. Other examples of diagnoses include occlusal caries, irreversible pulpitis, squamous cell carcinoma (SCCA), and Class II malocclusion. Often, more than one finding may be necessary to formulate a diagnosis. For example, a tooth that appears darker than the others may or may not be a significant finding. This finding, concurrent with a tooth that tests negative to electric pulp testing and the radiographic appearance of a periapical radiolucency, would strongly suggest pulpal necrosis.

Several *types* of diagnoses are possible. When several findings point clearly to a specific disease entity, the clinician may make a **definitive diagnosis**, indicating a high level of certainty. On the other hand, when the findings suggest several possible conditions, the process of distinguishing between the list of possibilities is referred to as a **differential diagnosis**. For example, the differential diagnosis of a lump on the patient's palate might require differentiation between possibilities such as a maxillary exostosis, a salivary gland tumor, or an odontogenic infection. Without more information, such as findings from a radiograph or a biopsy result, it may be impossible to reach a definitive diagnosis. A "golden rule" of treatment planning is that a diagnosis should be made before treatment begins. When the diagnosis is uncertain, but it is prudent to begin some type of treatment, a **working** or **tentative diagnosis** may be made. Diagnostic tests, consultation with other providers, or reevaluation of the patient will usually be required either to confirm the diagnosis or to change to a new, more definitive, diagnosis.

On many occasions, a precise diagnosis that matches a significant finding may not be achievable. For example, a patient may reveal that they have limited funds available for dental treatment. This is a significant finding that may affect the treatment plan but it does not fit the classic definition of a diagnosis. Such issues are typically referred to as **problems**. Patient problems can be general or specific issues that suggest the need for attention. Common examples of patient problems include dental pain of undetermined origin, fear of dental treatment, or the patient who requires the assistance of a caregiver to brush the teeth.

BENEFITS OF A DIAGNOSIS AND PROBLEM LIST

Foundation for the Treatment Plan

When generating a patient's treatment plan or plan of care each treatment on the plan must be justified by one or more diagnoses or **reasons for treatment**. The patient's diagnosis is the essential basis for any treatment plan. A treatment plan that lacks this foundation is often missing key components. Important patient concerns and/or oral health problems may be overlooked and remain untreated.

Organization

Diagnoses and problems can be sorted and organized more readily than findings. The dentist typically lists the important issues first, such as the chief concern, with other diagnoses following in order of significance. This process of prioritization sets the stage for developing a sequenced treatment plan.

Professional Competence

Documenting diagnoses in the record provides an important safeguard against avoiding the appearance of providing unnecessary treatment. In the event of malpractice litigation, dentists who list this information fare better than those who do not. A discussion of standardized codes is featured in the In Clinical Practice box.

Diagnostic Codes

Shin-Mey (Rose) Geist

As discussed throughout this chapter, the dentist should arrive at a diagnosis, whether definitive or tentative, before beginning a patient's treatment. Each treatment procedure should be rationalized with a specific diagnosis or set of diagnoses. The benefits of utilizing a standardized system of diagnostic nomenclature and coding are significant and include: accurate data recording; effective and efficient communication; treatment outcome tracking; evaluation of treatment outcomes; quality improvement; and third-party accounting, billing, and payment. As dental patients become more medically complex, frequently with multiple health care providers and insurers (also known as patient benefit plans or the third-party payers), standardized terminology and coding for diagnoses and treatment procedures have become essential. The increasing use of electronic health records (EHR) and electronic dental records requires encoded standard health terminology. Universally accepted diagnostic codes provide a foundation for integrating interprofessional (IP) patient care (see Chapter 6), and coordinating services between dental care providers and other health care providers.

Three dental coding systems have been utilized in US dentistry: the Code on Dental Procedures and Nomenclature, also referred to as Current Dental Terminology (CDT); the International Statistical Classification of Diseases and Related Health Problems, also called the International Classification of Diseases (ICD); and the dental subset of the Systematized Nomenclature of Medicine Clinical Terms (SNOMED CT) known as Systematized Nomenclature of Dentistry (SNODENT).

CDT was developed by the American Dental Association (ADA) to achieve uniformity, consistency, and specificity in accurately reporting dental treatment procedures and to enable efficient processing of dental claims. The first CDT code set was published in 1969 as the Uniform Code on Dental Procedures and Nomenclature in *The Journal of the American Dental Association*. Since then, updates have been released periodically by the ADA. In 2000 the CDT Code was designated as a Health Insurance Portability and Accountability Act (HIPAA) standard code set. Any claim submitted on an HIPAA standard electronic dental claim form must use dental procedure codes from the version of the CDT code in effect on the date of service.

The ICD evolved from the International Lists of Diseases and Causes of Death created and revised decennially beginning in 1891. After World War II, the World Health Organization (WHO) assumed the responsibility for maintaining and updating these lists. ICD-10-CM is the American version of ICD-10, that became the HIPAA standard on October 1, 2015. Federal regulations specify only ICD-10-CM codes as valid on claim submissions. ICD-10-CM is updated annually to include new diagnostic codes including dental diagnostic codes. In 2012, in response to the growing expectation of government and non-government dental benefit plans for providers to report diagnoses for services to patients, the American Dental Association updated the dental claim form. The form now allows reporting of up to four ICD diagnosis codes per each CDT procedure code. Since 2019 government-sponsored dental benefit plans such as Medicare or Medicaid have required ICD-10-CM diagnoses for fee reimbursement. Currently, not every dental benefit plan has to meet these requirements. It is expected that in the near future, diagnoses will be required for all dental procedure reimbursement by third party payers.

The SNOMED CT document was released in 2002 as a convergence of the College of American Pathologists' (CAP) SNOMED reference terminology (SNOMED RT) and the United Kingdom's Clinical Terms Version 3 (formerly known as the Read Codes). The CAP began the development of the Systematized Nomenclature of Pathology (SNOP) in 1965. In 1974 SNOP was expanded from a pathology-centric nomenclature to a broader version called the Systematized Nomenclature of Medicine (SNOMED). SNOMED RT was the version updated in 2000 that contained a broad range of basic sciences, laboratory, and specialty medicine terminology for the EHR environment and was cross-mapped to ICD-9-CM. In 2007 an international nonprofit organization, the International Health Terminology Standards Development Organization (IHTSDO), was created in Denmark to continue the updating, maintenance, and distribution of the SNOMED CT.

The ADA began development of the Systematized Nomenclature of Dentistry (SNODENT) in the 1990s. In 2007 the ADA began the process of updating SNODENT for electronic dental record use and for inclusion as a subset of SNOMED CT by cross-mapping SNOMED CT, ICD-9, and ICD-10. In 2012 the ADA and IHTSDO reached a licensing agreement for use of SNODENT as the dental subset of SNOMED CT. As a component of IHTSDO, the ADA is collaborating with the WHO to ensure that the oral health codes within ICD-11 are complete and are comparable and compatible with SNODENT.

As the EHR environment and the process of requiring diagnoses for dental benefit plan claims have evolved, these three coding systems have quickly become interoperable. For example, starting in 2021, CDT coding manual has been labeled as CDT Current Dental Terminology instead of the previous CDT Dental Procedure codes. The 2021 CDT update also incorporated a new section ICD-10-CM *Diagnoses for Dental Disease and Conditions*. Although the formal use of SNODENT is currently limited to test environments*, it continues to be influential in shaping the annual updates of the ICD-10-CM.

* SNODENT submitted to the Office of the National Coordinator for health Information Technology by Jean Narcisi/American Dental Association https://www.healthit.gov/isa/uscdi-data/snodent

Patient Education

At the conclusion of the examination, the dentist should inform the patient about their oral condition. A list of diagnoses and problems provides a convenient and straightforward way to share this information. Discussing diagnoses and problems with the patient becomes part of the process of obtaining **informed consent** to provide treatment.

Standard of Care

Dental professional organizations typically include in their codes of ethical principles the expectation that the dentist will arrive at a diagnosis and inform the patient of that diagnosis before beginning treatment. Most dental boards now explicitly require a documented diagnosis of the patient's condition before the dentist begins treatment.

THE COMPREHENSIVE PATIENT DIAGNOSIS

The patient's comprehensive diagnosis list or patient diagnosis is a compilation of any of the patient's problems or concerns that require (1) *recognition*, (2) *management*, or (3) *treatment*.

Not all diagnoses will require therapeutic or surgical intervention at the time of initial treatment planning. Some diagnoses need only to be identified and *recognized* at this juncture. A frequently encountered example is the patient with an amalgam tattoo. Any pigmented lesion in the oral cavity warrants our attention. However, when the history, clinical appearance, and lack of symptoms are consistent with a diagnosis of an amalgam tattoo, the usual course of action will be to record the presence, location, and appearance of the tattoo and to compare that description with the appearance of the tattoo at future periodic (recare) visits. Initial photographic images can facilitate this process. The diagnosis is explained to the patient and

the patient is reassured about the benign nature of the discoloration. No biopsy is necessary at this time.

A patient who, according to the American Heart Association guidelines, is at the highest risk of endocarditis will require antibiotic premedication for dental procedures for which tissue manipulation is expected. By taking into account issues relating to the patient's general health (i.e., the potential for endocarditis) we are not treating the patient's medical condition, but rather we are *managing* the patient's general health needs by providing dental treatment in a manner consistent with professional practice standards and in the patient's best general health interests.

The majority of a patient's oral health diagnoses will be *treated* through some form of direct chemotherapeutic, surgical, or restorative intervention.

Most patient diagnoses can be expected to fall into the following categories. Although it would be extremely unusual for any one patient to have issues in all of these categories, the general dentist can expect to encounter all of the following diagnoses regularly (Box 2.1):

The patient's chief concern
General health issues that impact on dental treatment
Diagnoses that evolve from the patient's oral health history
Diagnoses that evolve from the patient's personal history
Findings from the intraoral and extraoral exam
Findings from the radiographic exam

BOX 2.1 Example of a Patient Diagnosis List

The following is an example of a diagnosis list for a dental patient. For clarity, acronyms and abbreviations are either avoided or explained. Tooth numbers are not included to avoid confusion with varying numbering systems. In this example, the diagnoses are generally broad (not tooth or surface specific) with the presumption that specific clinical findings relating to tooth and surface lesions are identified in the patient's record.

1. Chief concern: fractured maxillary right incisor with exposed dentin and reversible pulpitis
2. Type 2 diabetes well controlled with oral hypoglycemic
3. Hypertension well controlled with medications
4. Allergic to penicillin and latex
5. Current smoker (30 pack/year smoking history)
6. Sporadic dental treatment history; last cleaning 3 years ago
7. Actinic keratosis on the lower lip
8. Hyposalivation
9. Multiple primary and secondary carious lesions (see charting for teeth and surfaces)
10. High caries risk
11. Localized moderate marginal periodontitis
12. Gingival recession on the facial surfaces of most posterior teeth
13. Root sensitivity on maxillary right canine
14. Maxillary left second molar with cervical caries penetrating into the pulp—necrotic pulp and chronic apical periodontitis[a]
15. Partial edentulism
16. Hypererupted maxillary left first molar
17. Upper and lower removable partial dentures (RPDs)—fractured clasp and poor retention with upper RPD

[a]Current American Academy of Endodontics designation: asymptomatic apical periodontitis

Disorders of the temporomandibular joint (TMJ) complex

Skeletal and occlusal abnormalities

Periodontal pathology

Pathology of the pulp or apical periodontium

Caries and noncarious abnormalities of the teeth

Esthetic concerns and problems

Defects or problems with restorations, an oral prosthesis and/or implants

COMMON DIAGNOSES

A. DIAGNOSES DERIVED FROM THE PATIENT'S CHIEF CONCERN AND OTHER CONCERNS

As described in Chapter 1, a patient interview should begin with an investigation of the patient's **chief concern**. A chief concern expressed as a request such as "I need a check-up and cleaning" would not normally be carried over to the patient's diagnosis because it would be a routine part of the patient's plan of care. Any chief concern that will require patient-specific action by the dental team, however, should be included in the diagnosis (Figure. 2.1).

A patient who presents to the initial examination visit with a chief concern described as "a toothache" definitely needs to have that problem recorded in the diagnosis. The way the problem is recorded, however, will vary with the findings that are available to the dentist at the initial visit. If, during the course of the initial examination, definitive tooth, pulp, and apical diagnoses can be determined, it will be appropriate to include all of those in the patient's diagnosis. If the diagnosis for the "toothache" is suspected but unconfirmed, it may be listed in the diagnosis as a tentative or working diagnosis. If the diagnosis for the "toothache" is undetermined at the initial exam and it is difficult to speculate on a diagnosis, it is appropriate to include the problem as *tooth pain of undetermined origin* in the diagnosis list.

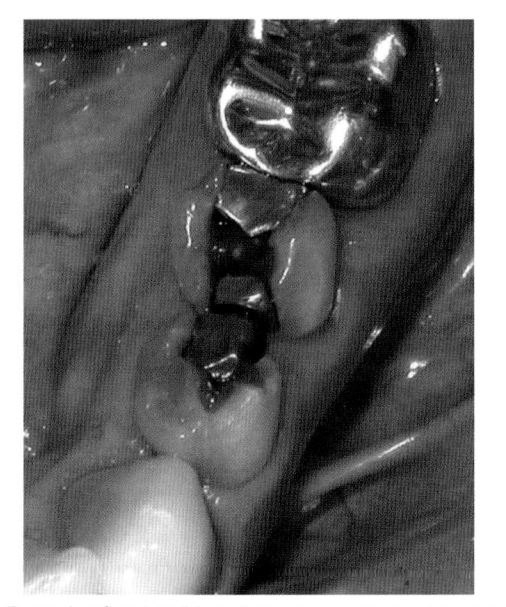

Fig. 2.1 Example of oral problem that would warrant urgent treatment if symptomatic. (Courtesy Dr. Lee Boushell)

If the chief concern is not an acute problem, that does not necessarily diminish its importance. Certainly, if the patient presents with a chief concern of "I don't like my smile; my teeth don't look good" that concern needs to be included in the diagnosis.

A patient may present with more than one concern and may have multiple treatment desires or objectives. Therefore, *any* patient concern, not just the chief concern, that may need to be addressed by the dental team is appropriate to include in the diagnosis list.

B. GENERAL HEALTH DIAGNOSES

A wide variety of diagnoses can be made concerning a patient's general health condition. Many of these diagnoses will be self-reported by the patient on the general health history questionnaire. The dentist may have additional concerns after reviewing the medication list, interviewing and examining the patient, and evaluating the vital signs. If any findings contradict the patient's own appraisal/report of their general health, it may be necessary to contact the patient's primary health care provider. Similarly, a patient who presents with signs or symptoms of an undiagnosed or untreated medical problem will need to be medically managed before, during, and following dental treatment (Figure. 2.2).

Any general health issues that may have an impact on the treatment plan or the delivery of dental treatment should be included in the diagnosis. When possible, an objective qualifier should be added to indicate both the type of problem and the level of disease control.

For example:

Asthma with last attack 25 years ago versus asthma with weekly attacks

Stable or unstable angina

Controlled or uncontrolled hypertension

Type 2 diabetes mellitus with the Hb A1C 7.0 measured 1 month ago

History of head and neck radiation with total radiation to the jaw bones

History of intravenous bisphosphonate use for the last 5 years in conjunction with breast cancer

History of deep vein thrombosis, currently taking warfarin

An overview of medical problems and their management in the context of dental treatment is set forth in Chapter 8 (Systemic Phase of Treatment). Selected general health diagnoses are also detailed in Chapters 13 (Patients With Special Needs), and 18 (Geriatric Patients). Additionally, Chapter 14 discusses substance abuse problems; Chapter 15 addresses patients with dental anxiety; and Chapter 16 focuses on psychological disorders.

C. PSYCHOSOCIAL CONSIDERATIONS THAT INFLUENCE THE TREATMENT PLAN

Patient considerations are modifiers to treatment planning that are behavioral in origin and can often be included in the realm of **social determinants of health**. The personal history

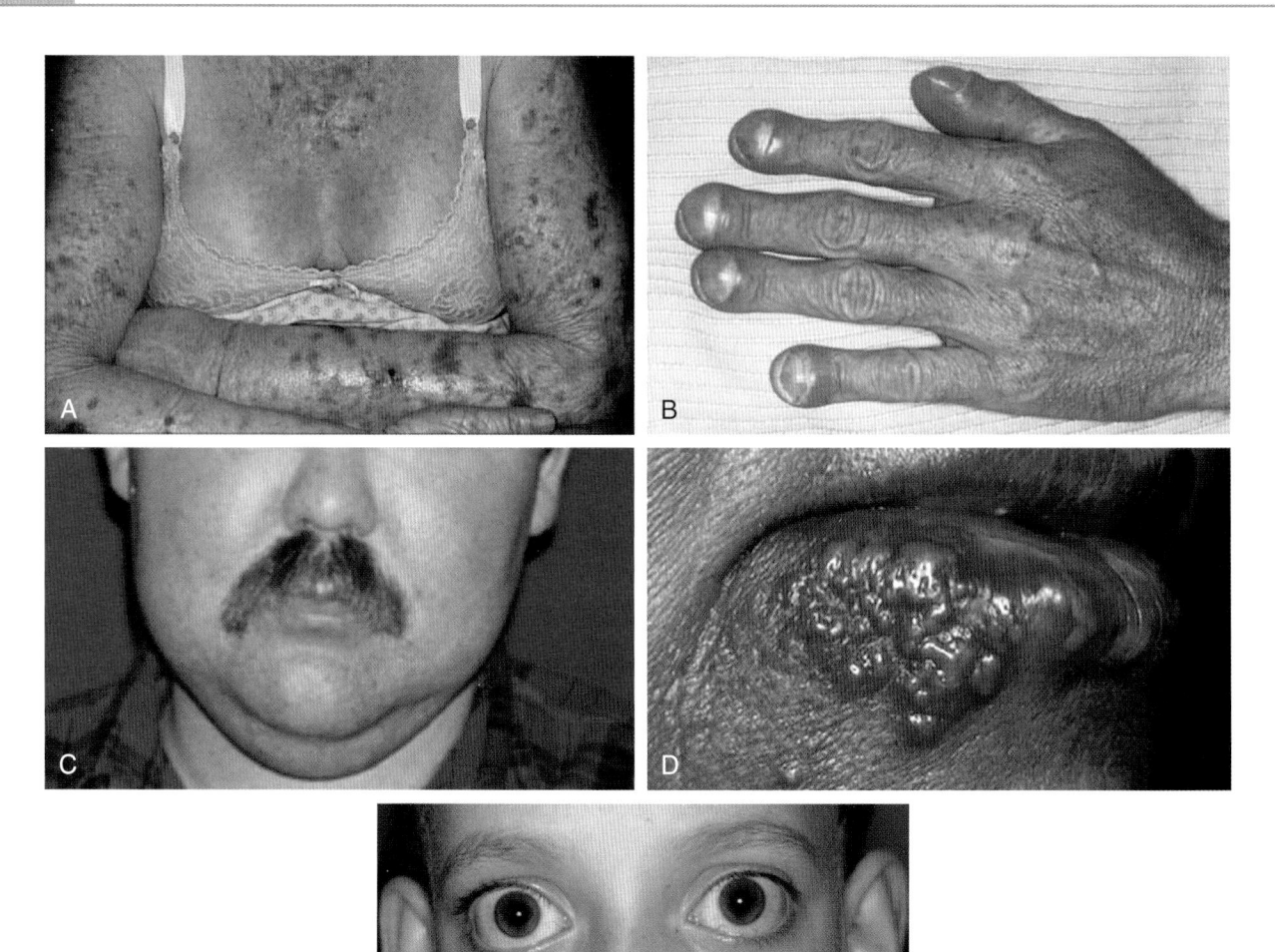

Fig. 2.2 **A-E**, Physical signs of medical conditions that may have a significant impact on the dental treatment plan. (**A**, From Darrell S. Rigel: CANCER of the SKIN, Second Edition, 2011 **B**, **D**, From Little JW, Falace DA, Miller CS, Rhodus NL: *Dental Management of the Medically Compromised Patient*, ed 8, St Louis, 2013, Mosby. C, From Bricker SL, Langlais RP, Miller CS: *Oral Diagnosis, Oral Medicine, and Treatment Planning*, ed 2, Hamilton, 2002, BC Decker. **E**, from Sapp JP, et al.: *Contemporary Oral and Maxillofacial Pathology*, ed 2, St Louis, 2004, Mosby.)

and the oral health history can be a rich source for this information. Additionally, patient considerations will be revealed in the course of conversation over multiple dental visits as the dental team and the patient become better acquainted. Some patient considerations, especially those that reflect the patient's motivation and abilities to accept recommendations and execute behavioral changes, will be fully revealed only after extensive interaction with the patient.

Throughout this book, the importance of including and weighing patient considerations while discussing treatment options and formulating treatment proposals is emphasized. An understanding of patient choices and preferences is essential to the development of a treatment plan that will be acceptable to the patient and addresses their expectations. This understanding is also critical if the patient is to be fully involved in the treatment planning and not only compliant, but energetically engaged in the treatment process as well. With the patient invested and engaged, the probability of success is also much improved and the patient is more likely to recognize and appreciate the benefits of the treatment.

The following is a list of some of the patient considerations that can have significant impact in planning treatment for a patient. Such factors, when they are believed by either the patient or the dentist to limit the scope of treatment or to require modification in the way treatment can be delivered, should be identified and recorded in the patient's diagnosis:

- Patient's level of knowledge relating to oral health issues and problems
- Patient's ability to establish and maintain effective oral self-care practices
- Patient's motivation to embark on dental treatment and the ability to sustain that effort
- Sufficient patient physical and mental stamina to engage in treatment in the face of competing personal priorities and family and society demands
- The resources – including time and money – necessary for participation in the treatment
- Reliable means of conveyance to and from the dental office
  Note: Chapter 19 specifically addresses the needs of patients who are motivationally or financially challenged.

D. EXTRAORAL DIAGNOSES

If a patient walks (or is assisted) into the dental operatory for an initial oral examination, any tremors, imbalance, or abnormalities of posture, gait, sight, hearing, or cognition should be addressed with the patient or care giver. As discussed in Chapter 1, the initial oral examination of the dental patient includes taking vital signs and a visual and palpatory assessment of exposed skin surfaces of the head, face, and neck. On occasion, the patient may request an opinion concerning an abnormality that is identified during this stage of the initial examination; for example, the discovery of a pigmented lesion on the skin that the patient had been previously unaware of. If there is any question about the diagnosis in the dentist's or the patient's mind, it will be appropriate for the dentist, to refer the patient to other related specialty clinicians for evaluation and treatment. The dentist also should be cognizant of any underlying health problems that may affect treatment planning or the manner that dental treatment will be delivered. This section highlights some of the more common conditions that may become apparent during an extraoral examination that are *likely to have a significant impact on treatment planning for the patient.* The topics in this section are organized and sequenced in the order in which the extraoral examination is usually carried out. For a more comprehensive and detailed analysis, the reader is referred to the current literature on the specific topic.

Abnormalities Apparent Through General Observation

Parkinson Disease *(PD)*

This degenerative disorder of the central nervous system causes involuntary, uncontrolled movements. The disorder progresses to widespread motor function impairments and sensory, emotional, and cognitive dysfunction.

Classic signs include body rigidity, short dragging footsteps, and trembling hands, arms, and legs. Sometimes the jaw, tongue, and lips are also affected with tremors. These patients often have challenges arranging transportation to the dental office, walking to the dental operatory, holding the mouth open during dental procedures, and performing daily oral self-care procedures (see Chapter 18 for more information).

Arthritis

Both osteoarthritis and rheumatoid arthritis may affect multiple joints of the body, causing difficulty in walking and in head and neck movement. Impairment of the joints in the dominant hand may contribute to ineffective oral hygiene. When the temporomandibular joints are affected, the range of jaw movement may be limited, especially in the presence of pain. Patients with rheumatoid arthritis are at increased risk of developing periodontitis (see Chapter 3).

Cerebrovascular Accident

A cerebrovascular accident (CVA), also known as a stroke, occurs when there is a disruption in the blood supply and oxygen deprivation to a portion of the brain, causing the death of some brain cells (infarction). The immediate cause of the disruption is often either a blood clot (thrombus or embolus) or bleeding (rupture of a blood vessel). The patient may exhibit a temporary (and sometimes permanent) speech or motor deficit on the side of the body controlled by the affected portion of the brain. In the dental setting, the patient may manifest aphonia, dysphonia, dystonia, dysphagia, and hemiplegia, and may have difficulty carrying out the activities of daily living independently. The patient may need assistance with oral hygiene activities due to impaired manual dexterity. When treating a patient with dysphagia it is prudent to place the patent in an upright or semi-supine position to avoid silent aspiration and its complications.

Neuromuscular Disorders

Neuromuscular disorders are a group of diseases related to nerves, muscles, or both that result in impaired movement and, with some conditions, sensory or other neurologic dysfunctions. Examples include multiple sclerosis, Huntington disease, myasthenia gravis, muscular dystrophy, and idiopathic inflammatory myosis. These disorders may pose challenges to oral health care depending on the nature of the deficit, the severity of the disease, and the side effects of treatment medications. Dental treatment concerns often mirror those of PD or post-stroke patients.

Irregularities in Vital Signs

Hypertension (high blood pressure reading). Patients may present at the initial visit with a history of hypertension, or hypertension may be suspected when the dental team assesses the blood pressure (see Chapter 1). When hypertension has no known cause, it may be identified as essential hypertension, primary hypertension, or idiopathic hypertension. Secondary hypertension is attributable to an underlying cardiac abnormality. Hypertension is a risk factor for heart attack, stroke, and chronic kidney disease. Its high prevalence and low rate of diagnosis and treatment have been major public health concerns. Oral health care providers have the responsibility to refer patients with persistent elevated blood pressure, including those resistant to treatment, to a medical provider for evaluation, diagnosis, and treatment. If a patient presents to the dental office with an extremely elevated blood pressure, referral to a local Emergency Department may be in order. Many antihypertensive medications have adverse oral effects, most notably hyposalivation, that can have a significant impact on a patient's oral health. Nifedipine and amlodipine, both calcium channel blockers, are well known to be associated with plaque-sensitive gingival enlargement.

Irregular pulse (arrhythmia; includes rhythm, intensity, and rate abnormalities). Arrhythmia is a general term for a group of conditions characterized by an irregular heartbeat. Some arrhythmias are genetic and others are acquired. Some are trivial; others can be life threatening. Severe arrhythmia can be precipitated by intense pain or by a variety of drugs or drug interactions. A patient's underlying cardiac condition may also play a role in the precipitation of a life-threatening arrhythmia. For example, in susceptible patients certain antibiotics, such as amoxicillin, can cause QT elongation and may precipitate a *torsade de pointe* (Tdp), a severe ventricular fibrillation, and sudden cardiac arrest.

To avoid precipitating severe arrhythmia it is important that the dentist identify patients who are at risk through their health and medication histories. Atrial fibrillation (AFib or AF) is a common medical condition among older patients. Patients with this condition take anticoagulants (warfarin or direct oral anticoagulants [DOAC]) to prevent thrombosis, thus raising the concern of postoperative prolonged bleeding.

Abnormalities Apparent on the Hands or Exposed Skin Surfaces

Arthritic Hands

The hands (Figure. 2.3) can provide insights into the patient's general health. Swollen and inflamed joints can be signs of many autoimmune diseases, such as rheumatoid arthritis, Sjögren syndrome, and systemic lupus erythematosus. The disease or its treatment may influence oral health or oral health care; for example, additional help may be needed for effective oral hygiene. Treatment modifications may be necessary.

Bruises (Ecchymosis)

Bruises on the skin (Figure. 2.4) can be a sign of an acquired or hereditary bleeding disorder or taking antithrombotic agents and may warrant further investigation or treatment plan modification. They can also be the result of trauma or physical abuse.

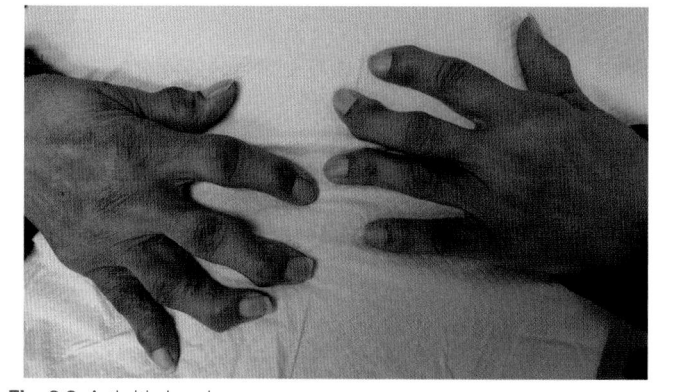

Fig. 2.3 Arthritic hands.

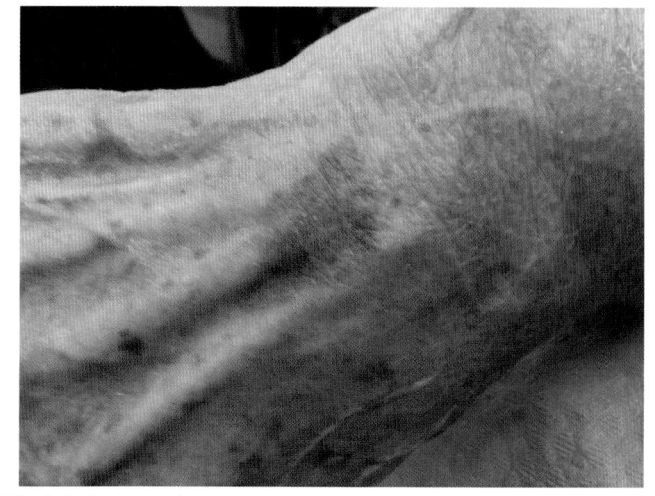

Fig. 2.4 Ecchymosis.

Splinter Hemorrhages

Splinter hemorrhages are dots or vertical streaks of hemorrhages under the nails (eFigure 2.1). Nail trauma is the most common cause but skin disorders, systemic or infectious diseases and medication use can also be responsible. Examples of systemic diseases that cause this condition include endocarditis, nail psoriasis, antiphospholipid syndrome and systemic lupus erythematosus. Aspirin, warfarin, DOACs (Direct Acting Oral Anticoagulants) and kinase inhibitors (such as sunitinib and sorafenib) are medications that can cause splinter hemorrhages.[1]

Pitting (or Dependent) Edema

Pitting edema is an abnormal accumulation of fluid in the extracellular space of lower limb tissue resulting in swelling that can be dimpled with finger pressure (eFigure 2.2). This may occur during pregnancy or may be associated with serious health problems such as congestive heart failure, kidney failure, and liver cirrhosis.

Nevi

It is not uncommon to find dark brown or black macules or papules on the skin of the face and neck (eFigure 2.3). The most common diagnosis of these lesions is *nevi* (plural for nevus). These most common benign tumors of the skin consist of clusters of nevus cells in the epidermis or dermis. By examining their clinical presentation, nevi can be differentiated from other common benign lesions of skin, such as dermatosis papulosa nigra and seborrheic keratosis, or from more serious conditions, such as malignant melanoma, pigmented basal cell carcinoma (BCCA), or SCCA. Oral health care providers play an important role in recognizing and identifying these pigmented lesions. When clinical findings are not discriminatory, referral to a dermatologist for evaluation and biopsy is indicated.

Seborrheic Keratosis

Seborrheic keratoses (eFigure 2.4) are light or dark brown lesions that are flat or slightly elevated on the skin of older individuals. The lesions vary in size but are usually less than 1 cm in diameter and have a velvety to finely verrucous surface. The dentist should be able to differentiate this condition from premalignant or malignant skin lesions; if in doubt, the patient should be referred to a dermatologist.

Solar (or Actinic) Keratosis and Solar Cheilosis

Solar keratosis is a premalignant skin condition caused by prolonged sunlight exposure. It usually occurs in older individuals with a light skin complexion. With this condition ultraviolet light causes the skin to become scaly, rough, and slightly elevated and red (eFigure 2.5). **Solar cheilosis** (aka solar cheilitis) is solar keratosis that occurs on the lower lip producing an indistinct vermillion and skin border and a patchy appearance on the vermillion. The dental team should recommend strategies to prevent the development of lip or skin cancer including reducing sun exposure, wearing wide-brim hats, using sunscreen agents. Actinic keratosis or solar cheilosis should be referred for biopsy to rule out malignancy.

Basal Cell Carcinoma

BCCA is a common neoplasm often found on the skin of adults who have a history of long exposure to sunlight (eFigure 2.6). In spite of being malignant, this condition rarely metastasizes. The patient should be referred to a dermatologist for definitive diagnosis and treatment.

Squamous Cell Carcinoma

SCCA, a malignant neoplasm of epidermal or epithelial origin, has potential for distant metastasis (eFigure 2.7). Although less common than BCCA on the skin of the head and neck, it has significantly higher morbidity and mortality. Early detection and treatment are the key to survival. Oral health professionals should be prepared to recognize a variety of clinical presentations of early SSCA. If detected, timely referral for further evaluation is warranted.

Melanoma

Melanoma, a malignant neoplasm of melanocytes in the basal layer of the epidermis and epithelium, occurs primarily in the skin of the head and neck region (eFigure 2.8). Excessive exposure to sunlight is a major risk factor. Although melanoma rarely occurs in the oral mucosa, given its serious nature, it must be included in the differential diagnosis of any intraoral pigmented lesion. Biopsy is warranted for a pigmented oral lesion that changes in size or pattern in a short period of time. Pigmented lesions that exhibit asymmetrical outlines, irregular or poorly-demarcated borders, a variety of colors, diameter greater than 6 mm, or evolution in size, outline, or color (the "ABCDEs of melanoma") should be considered suspicious for this disease.

Urticaria

Urticaria, also known as hives, is a transient skin condition characterized by red or white bumps on the skin with intense itching (eFigure 2.9). The most common cause is an Ig-E mediated allergic reaction to drugs or food. A less common cause can be an autoimmune disease in which the hives appear and resolve repeatedly over months or years. Emotional stress, temperature, and sun exposure have also been linked to episodes of hives. In many cases the cause remains unknown.

Angioedema

Although a result of the same mechanisms of urticaria, in which the edema is localized and limited to the superficial portion of the dermis, angioedema involves a wider and deeper portion of the dermis and subdermis, resulting in swelling over a larger area (eFigure 2.10). The causes of angioedema are similar to those of urticaria. Both are short-lived phenomena, lasting only a few hours. A local anesthetic may be the cause of angioedema and of anaphylaxis—a potentially life-threatening medical emergency (see Malamed's *Medical Emergencies in the Dental Office* for in-depth discussion).

Contact Dermatitis (Dermatitis Medicamentosa)

Contact dermatitis is a T cell-mediated delayed hypersensitivity reaction in which an antigen comes into contact with the skin and is linked to skin protein, forming an antigen complex that leads to sensitization (eFigure 2.11). Upon re-exposure of the epidermis to the offending antigen, the sensitized T cells initiate an inflammatory cascade. Within 24 to 48 hours after contact, pruritic erythema, vesicles, and bullae form. As the inflammation dwindles, a crust forms on the affected area, which heals in about 3 weeks.

Common antigens causing this reaction include poison ivy, nickel, and some fragrances. Patients who are sensitive to acrylic or metals in dental prostheses may develop this reaction.

A variety of topical medicaments, including antibiotics, steroids, anesthetics, and antifungals are frequently encountered as the cause of allergic contact dermatitis. Neomycin and lidocaine are most often reported.

Herpes Zoster (Shingles)

Herpes zoster is a skin eruption spreading in a belt-like pattern. It is a recurrent episode of varicella zoster virus infection in individuals who contracted chickenpox in childhood and harbor the virus in the sensory nerve ganglia (eFigure 2.12). Reactivation occurs spontaneously later in adult life when the immune system may be suppressed. The distribution of the lesions is confined to one or a few dermatomes (tissue innervated by sensory nerves from the affected ganglia) with sharp demarcation from other dermatomes. When occurring in the head region, the lesions follow the distribution of the trigeminal nerve branches. Intraoral cases may be extremely painful and debilitating and, in severe forms, may result in destruction of periodontal tissues on the affected side (see Suggested Readings at the end of the chapter for information on the diagnosis and management of herpes zoster).

Abnormalities in the Head, Face, and Neck Region
Thyroid Gland Enlargement/Goiter

Enlargement of the thyroid gland may be diffuse or nodular and may be unilateral or bilateral (Figure 2.5). An enlarged thyroid

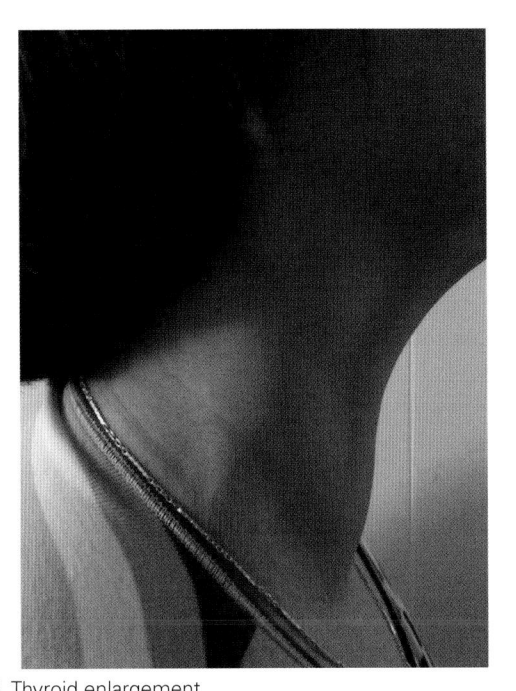

Fig. 2.5 Thyroid enlargement.

gland may function normally or may be associated with hyper- or hypothyroidism. When thyroid enlargement is newly discovered in the course of the initial oral examination, referral to an endocrinologist or primary medical care provider is in order. Laboratory testing can reveal the status of the gland. Visibly prominent thyroid enlargement, or goiter, may also be classified in terms of the cause, which can be iodine deficiency, autoimmune disease (Hashimoto thyroiditis, Graves disease), or benign or malignant neoplasia. The dental team must be attentive to the possibility that a patient with a goiter and clinical signs of hyperthyroidism may develop an acute life-threatening medical emergency while in the dental chair (see Malamed's *Medical Emergencies in the Dental Office* for extended discussion).

Lymphadenopathy (Lymphadenitis/Lymphoid Hyperplasia/Calcified Lymph Nodes)

Enlargement of cervical lymph nodes, also known as lymphadenopathy, can be the result of various antigenic stimuli including infectious agents or unidentified agents. The term **lymphadenitis** refers to inflammation in the nodes, in which the nodes become enlarged or tender. Lymphoid hyperplasia consists of enlargement of normal lymphoid aggregates, often caused by an antigenic stimulus. It is not uncommon for these reactive lymph nodes to become calcified, producing a radiopaque image on panoramic radiographs. Neoplasms can originate in or metastasize to the lymph nodes, causing enlargement. Detection and diagnosis of cervical lymphadenopathy can help identify the underlying disease and may greatly influence the outcome, especially in the case of head and neck cancer. The dentist must have the clinical skills necessary for detecting and diagnosing cervical lymphadenopathy and must be able to recognize instances in which the patient should be referred to other health care providers.

Carotid Atherosclerosis

Atherosclerosis is a degenerative disease of the arteries characterized by formation of atheromas or plaques in the luminal wall consisting of necrotic cells, lipids, and cholesterol crystals (eFigure 2.12). The coronary and carotid arteries are among the most commonly affected. The plaques formed in the carotid artery wall may rupture, causing thrombosis and possible embolism, which can cause a stroke. Plaques with high risk of rupture are characterized as "high risk" or "vulnerable" plaques. Carotid plaques may become calcified and visible on dental extraoral images. Computed tomography (CT) and magnetic resonance imaging (MRI) images provide more reliable capability for prediction of the risk of rupture. The significance of calcified carotid atheromas is controversial. An oral health professional has the responsibility to inform the patient's health care provider about the presence of calcified carotid atheromas so that a decision on further investigation or intervention can be made.

Cleft Lip and Cleft Palate

Cleft lip and palate are defects that arise during gestation as a result of improper merging of soft tissues and/or bones (eFigure 2.13). Both hereditary and environmental factors may be involved in cleft formation. Cleft lip results from the failure of the medial nasal and maxillary processes to fuse. Clefts of the lip may range from a small defect in the vermilion border to a large lesion that extends into the nose. Clefts can be unilateral or bilateral. Palatal clefts result from the incomplete union of the palatine processes of the right and left maxillary bones and, in some cases, may also involve the nasal septum. Cleft palate may manifest simply as a bifid uvula (involving only soft tissue) or may traverse the entire length of the hard and soft palates, involving both bone and soft tissue. Individuals may exhibit cleft lip alone, cleft palate alone, or clefts of both lip and palate.

E. INTRAORAL SOFT TISSUE DIAGNOSES

In this section, some of the most common conditions found during an intraoral soft tissue examination of the patient will be delineated. Because most of these conditions occur in more than one location in the oral cavity, they are organized here by origin rather than by location.

Developmental Lesions
Ankyloglossia

Ankyloglossia (also known as tongue-tie) is a condition in which the lingual frenum is attached too far anteriorly toward the tip of the tongue, preventing the tip of the tongue from reaching the hard palate when the mouth is open (Figure 2.6). Depending on the severity of the condition, individuals may experience aberration in speech. When ankyloglossia causes speech, swallowing, or other functional problems, surgical correction may be needed.

Hairy Tongue

Hairy tongue is a condition in which the filiform papillae become markedly long, resulting in an appearance similar to a long-tufted carpet (eFigure 2.14). The long filiform papillae may trap chromogenic bacteria, fungi, and food pigmentations,

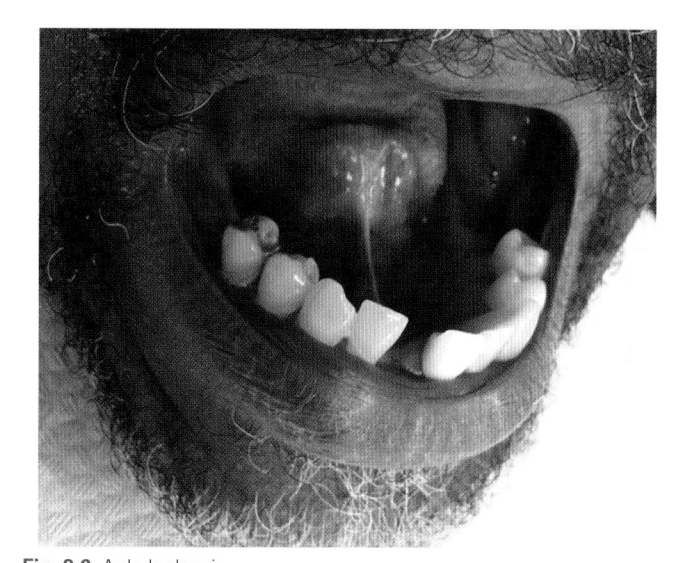

Fig. 2.6 Ankyloglossia.

giving the tongue various colors: white, brown, or black. Gently brushing the tongue with the toothbrush or using a tongue scraper will usually eliminate the discoloration commonly associated with the condition.

Varix/Varicosity

Varix or **varicosity** refers to dilation of a vein (eFigure 2.15). Common locations for varix in the head and neck region are the ventral surface of the tongue and the lower lip in older adults. Varices appear as purple or blue papules, nodules, or tortuous dilated veins that blanch with pressure. No treatment is required but the dentist must be able to differentiate varicosities from other vascular or pigmented lesions found in the oral cavity.

Torus and Other Exostoses

Exostoses are benign protuberances of bone that may arise on the cortical surface of the jaws (eFigure 2.16). A torus (plural: tori) is an exostosis that occurs in one of two locations intraorally. **Torus palatinus** is an exostosis in the midline of the hard palate and may appear as a solitary mass or may be multilobular. **Torus mandibularis** appears on the lingual surface of the mandible near the canines and premolars and may be unilateral or bilateral. Exostoses also appear as nodular masses on the buccal surface of the alveolar process. They can be solitary or multiple and sometimes become confluent, forming a shelf-like protuberance. If removable prostheses are planned, surgical removal may be required.

Cleft Palate

Cleft palate (see earlier Section D, *Extraoral Diagnoses* and eFigure 2.13) can occur as an intraoral lesion in the absence of a cleft lip.

Traumatic and Reactive Lesions

Chewing/Biting of Oral Mucosa

The formal name for this condition is **morsicatio**, the Latin word for "bite." These lesions, caused by chronic chewing of the mucosa, are usually habit- or stress-induced and may occur in children or adults (eFigure 2.17). Patients with this condition exhibit areas of thickened white and shredded mucosal surface interspersed with thin pink or red serrated areas, most commonly in the buccal or labial mucosa or on the lateral border of the tongue.

Linea Alba

The **linea alba** is a linear white thickening of the buccal mucosa (frictional hyperkeratosis) that occurs along the occlusal plane (eFigure 2.18). Less commonly, linea alba may be present on the lateral border of the tongue. It does not wipe off when rubbed with gauze. Linea alba may present with a scalloped shape, representing occlusal indentations. It may be more prominent early in the morning suggesting a nocturnal habit of drawing or pulling the cheek between the maxillary and mandibular teeth.

Traumatic Ulcers

An ulcer is a lesion characterized by focal loss of epithelium. **Traumatic ulcers** result from a cut, abrasion, or a bite of the mucosa (eFigure 2.19). They often appear as yellowish areas reflecting the fibrinous exudate that forms a pseudomembrane over the denuded connective tissue in the days following the causative action. The ulcers have red borders caused by inflammation and vary in size and shape. They usually heal in 1 or 2 weeks.

Hyperkeratosis

Hyperkeratosis is a term referring to a microscopic layer of thickened parakeratin and/or orthokeratin of the oral mucosal epithelium (eFigure 2.20). Because the thickened keratin layer exhibits a whitish clinical appearance in the moist environment of the oral cavity, the term hyperkeratosis is often used clinically to refer to white areas on oral mucosa without annotation as to the cause of the condition. The most common cause of hyperkeratosis is chronic irritation, or *frictional keratosis*. These lesions must be monitored. If the patient, dentist, or hygienist observes changes in lesion color, shape, borders, or surface texture, a biopsy may be appropriate.

Amalgam Tattoo

Amalgam in the gingiva, alveolar mucosa, palate, or buccal mucosa may produce a tattoo—a dark blue or black discoloration—ranging in size from a few millimeters to approximately 1 cm (eFigure 2.21). The amalgam tattoo is usually an incidental finding. Radiography of the lesion sometimes reveals radiopaque granules consistent with metal fragments. The dental team must be able to differentiate conclusively an amalgam tattoo from other types of intraoral pigmented lesions.

Nicotine Stomatitis

This lesion occurs on the posterior hard palate and anterior soft palate of smokers, especially pipe smokers (eFigure 2.22). It is caused by heat on the mucosa and not actually by the nicotine itself. Nicotine stomatitis consists of papules with an opaque, white surface and red dot in the center. The whiteness represents hyperkeratosis and the red dot is the dilated opening of an inflamed salivary gland duct. Papules often become confluent, forming a white plaque with interspersed red spots. The patient should be strongly encouraged to discontinue smoking (see Chapter 10).

Pyogenic Granuloma

Pyogenic granuloma is an overgrowth of young, highly vascular granulation tissue that; it is a reaction to chronic irritation or dental plaque (eFigure 2.23). (Note: The name is a misnomer; the condition does not produce pus and it is not a granuloma per se.) During pregnancy or puberty, hormonal changes may cause exaggerated tissue reactions to oral irritants or dental plaque. When pyogenic granuloma occurs during pregnancy, it is sometimes called a "pregnancy tumor." Pyogenic granuloma can occur at any age, however, and in males and females. Clinically it appears as a bright red enlargement caused by the vascularity of granulation tissue and the frequent thinning or loss of the overlying epithelium. The lesion, which bleeds easily, can occur anywhere in the oral mucosa or on the skin. The dentist must discern the cause for the granuloma (e.g., fractured tooth, faulty restoration, foreign body, dental infection) and resolve the problem.

Fibroma

The term "fibroma" usually refers to a reactive overgrowth of fibrous tissue and is not a true neoplasm. Clinically, it is a well-circumscribed firm swelling on the lip or buccal mucosa, usually less than 1 cm in dimension (eFigure 2.24). Patients usually report a history of trauma in the area; in such cases the term "traumatic fibroma" is widely used. Excisional biopsy should be considered if the patient considers the lesion to be unsightly, or if it is repeatedly traumatized, or if the patient habitually rubs or manipulates the lesion.

Hematoma

A hematoma consists of extravasated blood pooling under the epithelium or deep in the connective tissue or muscle, usually the result of blunt trauma (eFigure 2.25). The superficial hematoma of the oral mucosa appears as a dark red papule or nodule that ruptures easily. It occurs more often in individuals with bleeding disorders. It can be expected to resolve spontaneously. Administration of an inferior alveolar nerve block will, on occasion, cause a hematoma.

Mucocele (Mucous Extravasation Phenomenon/Mucous Retention Cyst/Ranula)

See Section F, *Salivary Gland Abnormalities.*

Infection/Inflammation
Parulis /Gingival Abscess

Parulis is a small abscess on the gingiva, originating from an apical or periodontal abscess, and is sometimes called a "gumboil." Clinically, it is a localized and often acute swelling on the gingiva with fluctuation (eFigure 2.26). A yellow point appears at the center of the swelling before spontaneous drainage. The parulis will resolve when the source of the infection is eliminated.

Patent Sinus Tract (Draining Fistula)

A **sinus tract** or **fistula** is an abnormal pathway between two spaces or a pathway that leads from an internal cavity to the surface of the body. In dentistry this is a common occurrence in the presence of an unresolved dental infection (chronic dental or periodontal abscess). The sinus tract may be intraoral (from the apex or periodontal ligament space of a tooth to the oral cavity) (eFigure 2.27), orofacial (draining to the external skin surface) or oroantral (draining from the maxillary sinus into the oral cavity). If the infection source (commonly a necrotic pulp) is not removed, the drainage of pus is likely to continue. In the presence of a chronic but inactive infection, an asymptomatic papule of granulation tissue may form on the gingiva at the site

of the sinus tract opening. In time, the papule may be replaced by scar tissue and persist in the form of a fibroma.

Herpes Infection (Primary Herpetic Gingivostomatitis/ Recurrent Herpes/Herpetic Ulcers)

At least eight types of herpes virus are known to infect humans, including herpes simplex virus type 1 (HSV-1), herpes simplex virus type 2 (HSV-2), and varicella zoster virus (VZV) (eFigure 2.28). HSV-1 and HSV-2 target epithelial cells, causing skin and mucosal lesions. When epithelial cells are infected, the viruses replicate, enter the neurons, and travel to the nerve ganglia where they remain latent until reactivated under certain triggers. They then travel back to the skin or mucosa, causing lesions. Both HSV-1 and HSV-2 can infect perioral skin and oral mucosa. The first (primary) infection is often subclinical. Some cases are preceded by subtle systemic symptoms and signs such as mild fever, general malaise, or pharyngitis. Oral lesions of primary infection are widespread with small vesicles that may form anywhere on the lips and mucosa. Generalized gingivitis may also occur. The vesicles soon coalesce and rupture to form widespread ulcers, often described as primary herpetic gingivostomatitis. The oral lesions resolve in 10 to 14 days without a trace. Stress, strong sunlight exposure, and immune suppression status are some of the triggers that can lead to reactivation of the virus and recurrence of the lesions. Recurrent lesions are usually less severe and the oral lesions only occur on keratinized tissue, such as the paraoral skin, gingiva, and hard palate. The appearance of the lesions is usually preceded by itching, burning and/or tingling at the intraoral site. The vesicles are short-lived and the ulcers are discrete, characteristically smaller than 2 mm. If the patient experiences recurring painful episodes of intraoral herpes infection, antiviral medications may shorten the course.

Candidiasis

Candidiasis is an opportunistic infection of the genus *Candida*, most often *Candida albicans* (eFigure 2.29). These organisms are commensal in the human gastrointestinal tract and lower female reproductive tract. Most healthy individuals have candida-specific innate immunity. Candidiasis occurs only when these innate defense mechanisms are defective, the candida organisms alter their virulence, or environmental factors favor their growth. Predisposing factors include human immunodeficiency virus/acquired immune deficiency syndrome (HIV/AIDS), diabetes mellitus, cancer chemotherapy, systemic or inhaled corticosteroids, an extended course of antibiotics, birth control pills, pregnancy, hyposalivation, tobacco smoking, and aging.

Oral candidiasis has several clinical forms: pseudomembranous, erythematous, central papillary atrophy (median rhomboid glossitis), candida-associated angular cheilitis, and chronic hyperplastic candidiasis. Denture stomatitis is often attributed to Candida infection but the current literature indicates that in many cases this is a reactive lesion and not a form of infection.[2] Identification and correction of the predisposing factors remains the first and most effective management; most lesions can be resolved with this approach. If not, oral lesions can usually be treated effectively with antifungal agents. Persistent or systemic forms of candidiasis should be referred to the primary healthcare provider for further identification and elimination of the predisposing factors or antifungal treatment.

Angular Cheilitis

Angular cheilitis presents as an inflammation at the corner of the mouth (Figure 2.7). Most cases are caused by a mixture of infective organisms such as candida albicans, staphylococcus aureus, and beta-hemolytic streptococcus. The condition occurs most frequently in aged individuals with deep labial folds after loss of occlusal height (decreased vertical dimension of occlusion). The deep labial folds become red, sore, and fissured after constant bathing by saliva. In some cases, habitual licking of the corner of the mouth may also lead to the development of angular cheilitis without deep labial folds. Deficiencies of vitamin B, iron, or folic acid have been reported as predisposing factors. Resolution can usually be achieved with the elimination of the causes. Application of topical antifungal agents can temporarily resolve the lesions.

Verruca Vulgaris/Squamous Papilloma/Condyloma Acuminatum

This is a group of human papillomavirus-related oral mucosal lesions. They share clinical and histologic features that make differentiation difficult for oral healthcare providers. It is important to acknowledge that although these lesions look alike clinically, they differ in location and causative HPV genotypes that may necessitate differences in management.

Verruca vulgaris (Latin for "common wart") is a benign epithelial lesion of the skin and mucous membrane. Caused by human papillomavirus (HPV) types 2 and 4, the lesions usually occur on the skin. When they occur intraorally, the most common sites are vermillion, labial mucosa, palate, and anterior part of the tongue. They appear as pedunculated or sessile papules with a whitish and/or light pink cauliflower-like surface (eFigure 2.30). Management is by excision.

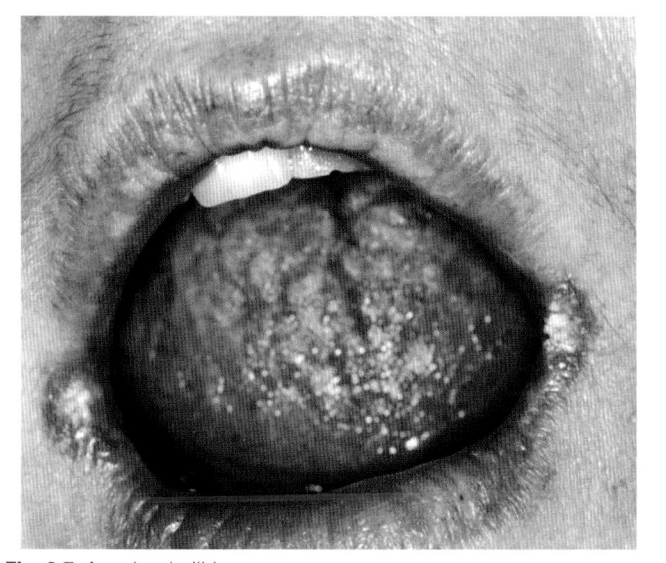

Fig. 2.7 Angular cheilitis.

Squamous papilloma, caused by HPV 6 and 11, commonly occurs on the palate, tongue, and labial mucosa. The lesion is usually pedunculated with a stalk. When it occurs on the gingiva of an individual in late middle age or older, papillary SCCA should be ruled out by biopsy.

Condyloma acuminatum is caused by HPV 6,11,16,and 18. It commonly occurs on the labial mucosa, soft palate, and lingual frenum. The lesion tends to be larger than squamous papilloma and more frequently in multiples. Similar to squamous papilloma, when condyloma acuminatum is detected on gingiva of an older individual, excisional biopsy is warranted to rule out papillary SCCA.

Autoimmune Processes

Aphthous Ulcers

Aphthous ulcers (also known as recurrent aphthous ulcers [RAU], aphthous stomatitis, recurrent aphthous stomatitis [RAS], or canker sores) are a common oral mucosal disease (eFigure 2.31). They are ulcerations with no known cause and a wide spectrum of severity and frequency of recurrence. Clinically, RAU consists of solitary or multiple nonspecific ulcers, usually on nonkeratinized oral mucosa, characterized by a fibrinous center with an erythematous halo. Based on the size of the ulcers, three clinical forms have been identified: major aphthae, minor aphthae, and herpetiform aphthae. The pathogenesis of RAU remains unclear. At one point it was proposed that RAU represents an autoimmune reaction. The lesions may be precipitated by stress or hormonal changes. They can be associated with various systemic conditions such as vitamin deficiencies, iron deficiency, and inflammatory bowel diseases. Severe and painful lesions can be treated with topical steroids.

Lichen Planus

Lichen planus is a chronic inflammatory skin disorder characterized by pruritic, purple eruptions with white streaks (Wickham striae) on the surface (eFigure 2.32). The lesions can persist for months or years. Lichen planus is believed to be a cell-mediated immune response with characteristics of a bandlike, subepidermal lymphocytic infiltration and basement membrane degeneration. The cause is unknown. The oral form of lichen planus (oral lichen planus [OLP]) may occur before, concurrent with, or after the development of skin lesions. In addition to the classic clinical presentation of interlacing white lines, OLP can present as a plaque, erosion, or ulceration of the oral mucosa and may pose diagnostic challenges. The erosive form of lichen planus can be treated effectively with topical steroids or a short course of systemic steroids. Other immunologic treatments, such as intravenous immunoglobulin (IVIG) or monoclonal antibodies have also been used.

Lichenoid Reaction

A **lichenoid reaction** is an oral mucosal condition that is clinically and histologically indistinguishable from OLP. However, with lichenoid reaction the apparent or presumed cause is identifiable. When the cause, such as a metallic restoration or an offending medication, is removed, the lesion will resolve with time.

Atrophic Glossitis (Bald Tongue/Burning Tongue)

Atrophic glossitis refers to papillary atrophy of the tongue, characterized by an absence of filiform and fungiform papillae (eFigure 2.33). Frequently the tongue is also fiery red, edematous, and painful, hence the term "burning tongue." Many systemic conditions have been reported to be associated with this condition including vitamin B deficiency and other avitaminoses, anemia, hyposalivation, Sjögren syndrome, and graft versus host disease. Treatment will vary depending on the cause of the condition.

Cysts/Tumors/Neoplasias of Soft Tissue Origin

Developmental Odontogenic Cysts

(See also Section G, *Abnormalities of the Maxilla and Mandible: Common Radiographic Findings.*) A cyst is a pathologic cavity lined with epithelium and usually contains fluid or semi-solid material in the lumen. Developmental odontogenic cysts arise from the epithelium of the tooth-forming apparatus. They are not inflammatory in nature and thus are to be distinguished from periapical (radicular) cysts. Developmental odontogenic cysts include dentigerous cyst, odontogenic keratocyst, lateral periodontal cyst, and gingival cyst of the adult. The decision to perform a surgical biopsy depends on the lesion size and location, whether there has been a significant change in the radiographic appearance over time, whether there are positive findings from an aspirational biopsy, or if not removing the lesion could lead to tooth loss or a jaw fracture.

Leukoplakia

The term **leukoplakia** is derived from the Greek and means simply "white patch" (eFigure 2.34). It is a clinical diagnosis and has no specific histologic implication. It is a diagnosis of exclusion after other white lesions such as frictional keratosis, hyperplastic candidiasis, white sponge nevus, burns, and smoker's keratosis have been ruled out.[3] Leukoplakia has been applied to a clinically evident white plaque or patch that has malignant potential. When the clinical diagnosis of leukoplakia is made, regardless of the location of the lesion, biopsy should be performed to rule out dysplasia (precancerous), carcinoma in situ (early malignancy), or invasive cancer (malignancy) and to establish the definitive diagnosis.

Erythroplakia

Erythroplakia (eFigure 2.35) is a flat red patch or lesion of unknown etiology on the oral or pharyngeal surfaces with a high risk of cancer or epithelial dysplasia present at the time of discovery.[3] Oral erythroplakia, like oral leukoplakia, is a term that has been used as a clinical but not a histologic diagnosis. Several conditions, such as lichen planus and prosthetic irritations, need to be ruled out before deciding to perform a biopsy.

Erythroleukoplakia

Erythroleukoplakia, also known as speckled leukoplakia or speckled erythroplakia, is a clinical diagnosis of an oral leukoplakia with a red component or an oral erythroplakia intermingled with white plaque (eFigure 2.36). Such lesions should be considered potentially malignant indicating that biopsy is essential.[4]

Squamous Cell Carcinoma

SCCA is by far the most common oral malignancy. The lateral border of the tongue, floor of the mouth, and oropharynx are the most common sites. Clinical presentation can be a white plaque, a red plaque, a lesion with white and red components, ulceration, a papule, or a nodule (eFigure 2.37). The most common contributing factors are tobacco and alcohol. Because early detection and treatment are the keys to survival and because oral health care providers are better qualified than other health care providers to examine oral tissues, any suspicious lesion in a patient with the most common risk factors should raise an alert to the health care provider of the possibility of SCCA. Differentiating SCCA from a benign lesion with similar clinical features can be challenging. In light of the morbidity and mortality associated with an SCCA, it is imperative that any suspicious lesion be biopsied.

Evidence has accumulated over the past two decades that HPV has a causal association with approximately 70% of oropharyngeal cancers in the United States.[5] These cancers arise in the soft palate, posterior pharyngeal wall, palatine tonsils, and base of the tongue. It is currently believed that high risk (oncogenic) types of HPV infection combined with traditional risk factors, such as tobacco and alcohol, cause the development of these cancers. The incidence of this subset of oral cancer is increasing in the United States. Dentists, in addition to being vigilant in oral cancer screening, referring, advocating tobacco cessation, now should encourage early HPV vaccination.

F. SALIVARY GLAND ABNORMALITIES

An abnormality of the salivary glands may be an incidental finding or a clinical correlation made secondary to a symptom reported by the patient. It is important to remember that the major and minor salivary glands must be visually inspected and palpated. The orifices of the Stenson and Wharton ducts must be evaluated and saliva must be expressed bilaterally. Saliva should be clear and thin.

Nonneoplastic Lesions

Mucocele and Ranula

When saliva is retained, it may be located inside the duct or the gland, or it may be in the surrounding tissue spaces. If the saliva has escaped the duct, the term used is **extravasation phenomenon**. The common clinical term used for mucous extravasation phenomenon is mucocele. A **mucocele** is most commonly found on the mucosal surface of the lower lip (Figure. 2.8A).

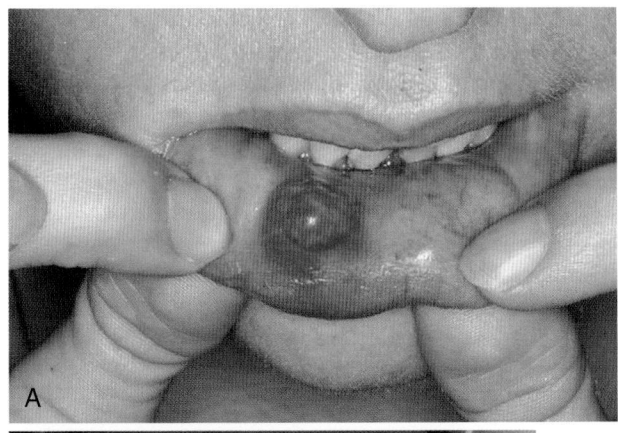

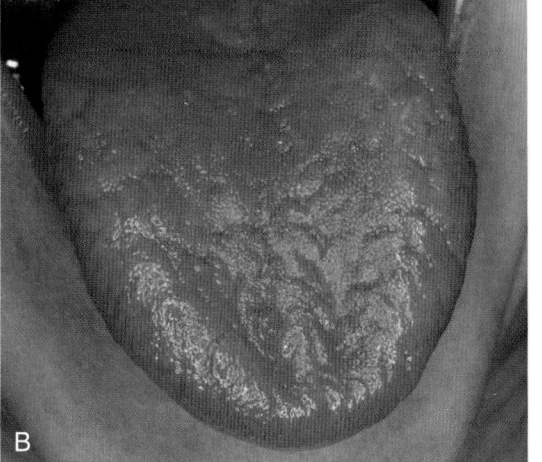

Fig. 2.8 **(A)** Mucocele. **(B)** Sjögren syndrome. (**A**, courtesy Dr. S Hum, Raleigh NC; **B**, from Ibsen OAC, Phelan JA. *Oral Pathology for the Dental Hygienist.* 6th ed. St Louis: Saunders; 2014.)

If the mucous extravasation phenomenon is associated with the submandibular or sublingual glands and is located in the floor of the mouth, it is known as a ranula. A **ranula** that occurs below the mylohyoid muscle is known as a plunging ranula and will be more evident extraorally than intraorally, in contrast to a conventional ranula, which usually is evident in the floor of the mouth and elevates the tongue (eFigure 2.38). A ranula should be surgically removed. The patient may elect to have a mucocele removed if it persists, if it is repeatedly traumatized, or if its presence is annoying. Some mucoceles will scar and form a fibroma.

Sialolithiasis (Salivary Stones)

Salivary stones are most commonly found in the submandibular gland and corresponding duct and less frequently in the parotid gland or parotic duct. They are rarely encountered in the minor salivary or the sublingual glands. Sialoliths can present as any or all of the following: salivary fluid blockage; ductal or glandular swelling that may be symptomatic especially before meals; or as radiopacities visible in radiographs. Radiographic evidence of a sialolith is only obtainable when the stone is sufficiently calcified to prevent the x-rays from reaching the sensor or film. If the patient is unable to pass the stone and continues to exhibit symptoms, surgical removal is necessary.

Hyposalivation

Hyposalivation (hypoptyalism) is defined as a reduced secretion of saliva as demonstrated with diminished salivary flow rates (unstimulated whole salivary flow rate of less than 0.3–0.4 mL per minute during waking hours). The condition may be associated with one of several factors or in combination with more than one. Such factors include dehydration, radiation therapy for the salivary gland regions, anxiety, menopause, use of certain drugs, vitamin deficiency, inflammation or infection of the salivary glands.

Xerostomia

Xerostomia is a clinical condition where the patient experiences oral dryness or dry mouth. It may be caused by a primary degenerative or autoimmune disease that affects the salivary glands or by a secondary condition that inhibits salivary secretion. Secondary xerostomia is frequently a side effect of some medications, dehydration, and hormonal imbalances. Commonly, antihypertensives, antihistamines, antidepressants, antipsychotics, and antiasthmatic medications may cause dry mouth. Xerostomia has many oral consequences, including poor oral lubrication; oral discomfort, increased incidence of caries and oral infections, altered digestion and deglutition, and speech alteration.

The management of dry mouth should focus initially on identifying the cause and eliminating it if possible. If this cannot be accomplished, mitigation with salivary substitutes and oral lubricants will be necessary. Discussion of the management of xerostomia can be found in Chapters 13, 16, and 18.

Sjögren Syndrome

Sjögren syndrome (SS) is an autoimmune disorder that affects the exocrine glands, specifically the lacrimal and salivary glands, causing dry eyes and dry mouth (Figure. 2.8B) (eFigure 2.39). The disorder can be classified as primary or secondary. In primary SS there may also be vaginal or nasal dryness and chronic bronchitis. Secondary SS is associated with other autoimmune diseases such as lupus, scleroderma, sarcoidosis, or rheumatoid arthritis. The diagnosis of SS is based on clinical, laboratory, and sometimes histopathological criteria. Patients with SS have a higher incidence of certain types of lymphoma. They commonly exhibit the same oral complaints and problems as described previously for xerostomia.

Neoplastic Lesions
Pleomorphic Adenoma (PA)

There are many different salivary gland neoplasias in adults and children; the most common is the **pleomorphic adenoma** referred to in the older literature as a "benign mixed tumor." Intraorally, like most salivary gland neoplasms, it is often located on the palate, but any site that contains salivary glands may develop a PA (eFigure 2.40). It presents initially as a dome-shaped mass without ulceration or symptoms. Because it is asymptomatic and slow growing, the patient is often unaware of it and the dentist is the first to recognize the abnormality during a comprehensive or a periodic examination. If the lesion is traumatized, the patient may develop secondary ulceration, swelling, inflammation, and pain—findings that may mislead the clinician to think that the lesion is malignant. PAs are comprised of ductal and myoepithelial cells. The supporting stroma may vary from myxoid to cartilaginous and the texture of the lesion can therefore range from firm to very soft. This tumor is managed with surgical excision.

G. ABNORMALITIES OF THE MAXILLA AND MANDIBLE: COMMON RADIOGRAPHIC FINDINGS

Many abnormalities of the maxilla and mandible have clinical signs and symptoms that make radiographic imaging an integral component to the diagnostic process. The radiographic image can provide additional information that may not be evident in clinical evaluation. In addition, some abnormalities may not have a clinical presentation, especially in the early stages, and will be first identified through radiographic imaging.

Only a few abnormalities are definitively diagnosed based on radiographic imaging alone; therefore, developing a differential diagnosis is essential to the diagnostic process and subsequent management and treatment. An effective method for developing a differential diagnosis involves first identifying key radiographic features and second, analyzing the ways in which those features relate to typical patterns and behaviors of various disease processes. From these, the clinician can select one or more disease categories that seem most likely to represent the abnormality. The differential diagnosis may list the disease category or a more specific entity within the selected category. Table 2.1 provides examples of the basic radiographic features of more common abnormalities located in the dentoalveolar region.

TABLE 2.1 Abnormalities of the Maxilla and Mandible: Common Radiographic Findings					
Category	**Disease Process**	**General Radiographic Features**	**Significance**	**Radiographic Examples of Abnormalities of the Jaws**	**Image Description**
Odontogenic cysts	Remnant epithelial cells proliferate, and cellular debris centrally draws fluid internally from surrounding cells that expand the cavity similar to water filling a balloon.	Uniform round or oval, some scalloped; Corticated border; Unilocular; Slow growth	Usually painless unless secondarily infected. May prevent eruption of a tooth, displace teeth or cause tooth resorption. May displace inferior alveolar canal or paranasal sinus borders. May expand, thin, and erode cortical bony plates.		Odontogenic cyst: dentigerous cyst.
Benign odontogenic tumors	Abnormal growth of cells within the tissue of origin. Although their growth is unlimited, generally these cells do not invade adjacent tissues.	Well-defined; Uniform smooth borders; May or may not be corticated; Radiolucent, radiopaque, mixed; Unilocular or multilocular with septa; Slow growth	May cause pain or paresthesia. May prevent eruption of a tooth; displace or resorb teeth. May displace inferior alveolar canal. May expand, thin, and erode cortical bony plates. May displace the cortical boundary of paranasal sinuses.		Benign odontogenic tumor: multilocular ameloblastoma
Malignant tumors	Abnormal growth of cells that have unlimited growth potential and the ability to invade and destroy any tissue.	Ill-defined; Mostly Radiolucent; Floating teeth; Spiked root resorption; Irregular resorption of cortical borders; Sunburst appearance of bone; Invasive growth	May cause pain or paresthesia. Impacts adjacent structures by destroying cortical bone, teeth. Left untreated the tumor can metastasize to bone or lungs, impacting mortality.		Malignant tumor, squamous cell

Continued

TABLE 2.1	Abnormalities of the Maxilla and Mandible: Common Radiographic Findings—cont'd				
Category	**Disease Process**	**General Radiographic Features**	**Significance**	**Radiographic Examples of Abnormalities of the Jaws**	**Image Description**
Bone Dysplasias	Fibrous connective tissue with calcified components. Replaces normal bone.	Variable, dependent upon process Cemento-osseous dysplasia: defined with internal radiolucent rim and central amorphous radiopaque nidus. Fibrous dysplasia: poorly defined with granular appearance.	Generally growth ceases at skeletal maturity, although hormonal changes may reactivate the lesions. Impacts appearance by deforming affected bone areas.	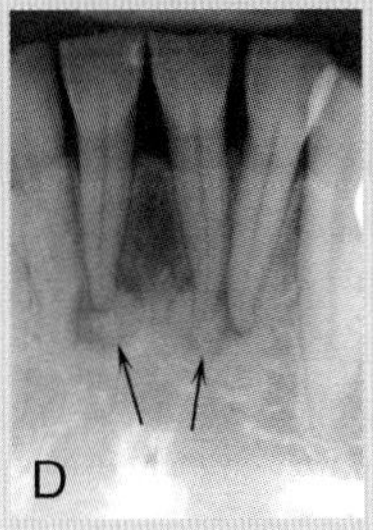	Osseous dysplasia, periapical cemento-osseous dysplasia
Dystrophic calcifications	Damaged soft tissue has influx of calcium; calcification may progress to ossification.	Radiopacity located within soft tissue; May be small round or large irregular; Various locations dependent on anatomy	Impact dependent on location. Ossification of the stylohyoid ligament may present as an incidental finding with no required treatment. Calcification within the carotid arteries reduces blood flow, increasing the risk of a cerebrovascular incident (i.e., stroke).	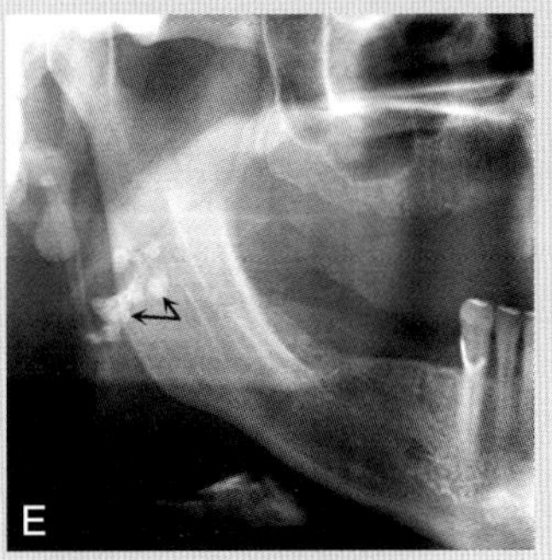	Dystrophic calcification, tonsilloliths, and calcified stylohyoid ligament
Trauma (fractures of teeth and/or jaws)	Traumatic insult is most likely cause.	Radiolucent line Discontinuity of cortical borders Step deformity Increased radiopacity due to overlapping/ displaced structures	May impact adjacent structures, impacting innervation and circulation. Some fractures may heal inappropriately, leading to occlusal and functional problems.		Trauma, fractured tooth Trauma, fractured jaw
Inflammation (e.g., osteomyelitis; sinusitis)	Reaction to injury; involves an imbalance between osteoclastic and osteoblastic processes	Localized or generalized Ill-defined borders Radiolucent and/or radiopaque	May spread to fascial planes, impacting patient's overall health and well-being.	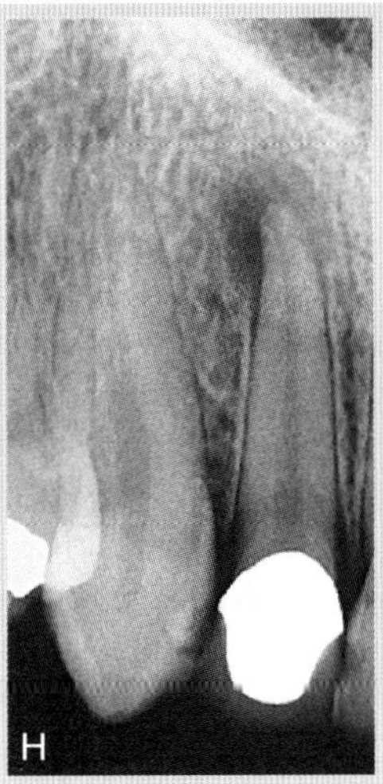	Inflammation, apical rarefying osteitis

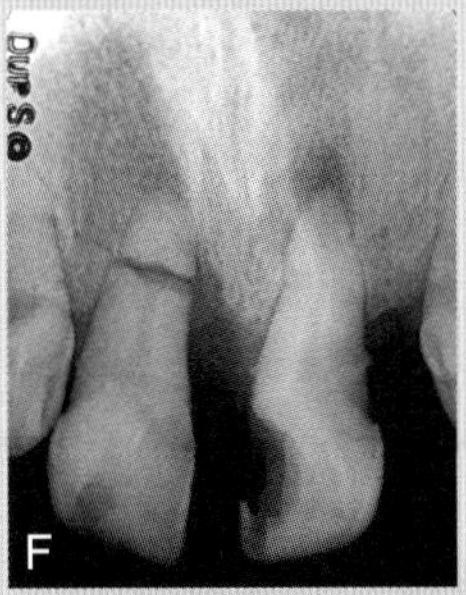

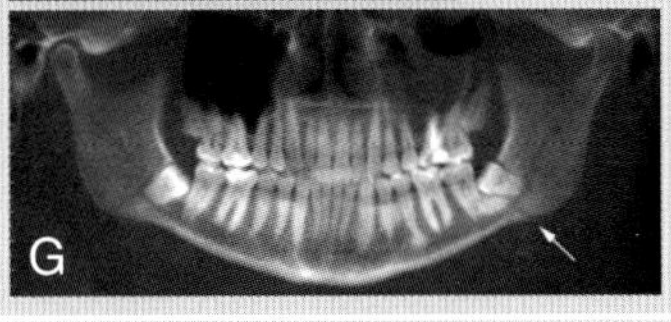

Continued

TABLE 2.1		**Abnormalities of the Maxilla and Mandible: Common Radiographic Findings—cont'd**			
Category	**Disease Process**	**General Radiographic Features**	**Significance**	**Radiographic Examples of Abnormalities of the Jaws**	**Image Description**
Systemic/metabolic (e.g., osteoporosis)	Disturbance of the body's normal physiological processes	Variable, usually generalized to entire regions	Dependent on particular process; may impact patient's overall general health and well-being.	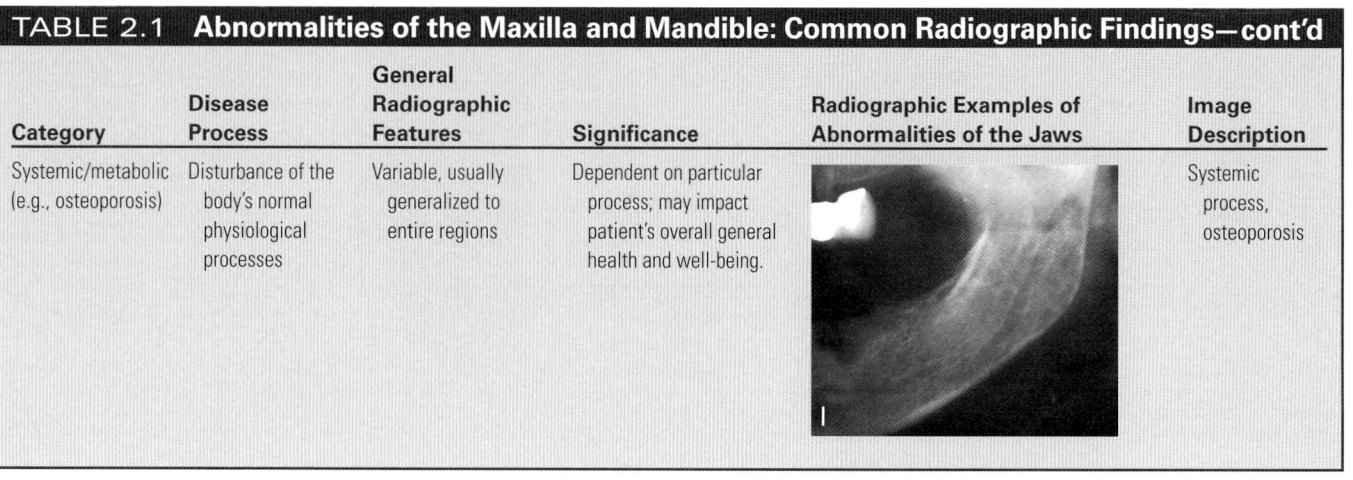	Systemic process, osteoporosis

Images from White SC, Pharoah M. *Oral Radiology: Principles and Interpretation.* 7th ed. St Louis: Mosby; 2014.

Radiographic Abnormalities of the TMJ Complex

Radiographic imaging of the temporomandibular joint complements the diagnostic process when clinical signs and symptoms suggest a history of trauma, a developmental abnormality, or a suspected tumor or other pathologic process. eTable 2.1 illustrates radiographic findings of abnormalities associated with the temporomandibular complex.

H. TEMPOROMANDIBULAR DISORDERS, TRIGEMINAL NEUROPATHIC PAIN AND HEADACHES

Temporomandibular Disorders

Temporomandibular disorders (TMD) are a group of musculoskeletal and neuromuscular conditions affecting the masticatory muscles, the TMJ, and associated structures.[6] These conditions mainly affect women in the reproductive age group. Common symptoms of TMD include TMJ popping/clicking or crepitus during jaw movement, jaw locking, restricted mouth opening, jaw pain, headaches, ear symptoms (e.g., fullness in the ear, earache, and tinnitus), and bruxism. The signs and symptoms of TMD often wax and wane throughout life. The etiopathogenesis of TMD is complex and involves elevated psychological distress (including depression, anxiety disorder, and somatization), increased pain sensitivity, environmental contributing factors, and genetic risk factors.[7] Chronic TMD is highly comorbid with other bodily pain conditions such as fibromyalgia, irritable bowel syndrome, headaches, vulvodynia, spinal pain, and low back pain. TMJ disorders include arthralgia, arthritis, articular disc disorders, hyper- and hypo-mobility disorders, joint diseases, fractures, and congenital/developmental disorders. Masticatory muscle disorders include myalgia, contracture, hypertrophy, neoplasm, movement disorders, and myalgia attributed to systemic/central pain disorders.[8] A useful screener for the presence of TMD is the validated 3Q/TMD.[9] (See Chapter 10 for more information on TMD.)

Trigeminal Neuropathic Pain

Neuropathic pain is defined as pain that arises as a direct consequence of a lesion or disease affecting the peripheral and/or central somatosensory system. Three of the more common types of trigeminal neuropathic pain are described here.

Trigeminal Neuralgia

Trigeminal neuralgia (TN), also known as *tic douloureux*, is characterized by paroxysmal lancinating pain affecting one or more divisions of the trigeminal nerve.[10] The pain may be spontaneous or evoked by nonpainful stimuli such as lightly touching the face, brushing the teeth, or talking. The pain is typically severe, and each pain episode lasts seconds to minutes. TN is characterized by periods of pain remissions and recurrences.

Painful Posttraumatic Trigeminal Neuropathy

Painful posttraumatic trigeminal neuropathy (PPTTN) refers to pain in the distribution of the trigeminal nerve affected by an identifiable nerve trauma with evident nerve dysfunction.[11,12] Trigeminal nerve injuries may occur following surgical removal of third molars, dental implant placement, or local anesthetic injections and may result in pain and interference with eating and speech. The prevalence of PPTTN following endodontic treatment is estimated to be 3.4%. Important clinical considerations include prompt alleviation of preoperative pain, preemptive analgesia, and identification of patients at risk (such as chronic widespread pain and history of orofacial pain).

Burning Mouth Syndrome

Burning mouth syndrome (BMS) is characterized by intraoral burning or dysesthesia in the absence of causative lesions.[11,13] Burning pain secondary to local (e.g., candidiasis) or systemic (e.g., diabetes) causes must be ruled out. BMS is more prevalent in peri- and postmenopausal females and is often associated with xerostomia, dysgeusia, and bodily pain.

Headaches
Orofacial Migraine

Orofacial Migraine is characterized by pain occurring exclusively in the orofacial region, without head pain, with the characteristics and associated features of migraine.[14] The pain is unilateral, pulsatile, of moderate or severe intensity, aggravated by routine physical activity, and associated with nausea and/or photo- and phonophobia. The two subtypes are episodic and chronic orofacial migraine. Migraine is a risk factor for the development of TMD.[15]

Headache Attributed to TMD

Headache Attributed to TMD (TMDH) is a secondary headache disorder with pain in the temple area which is modified by jaw movement, function, or parafunction.[16] It is one of 12 most common types of TMD. Distinguishing TMDH from primary headaches such as migraine and tension-type headache is important due to different treatment implications.

I. SLEEP DISORDERS

Obstructive sleep apnea (OSA) is a sleep disorder that is characterized by repetitive partial or complete collapse of the upper airway and/or arousal from sleep due to increased upper airway resistance. These events result in chronic intermittent hypoxia, oxidative stress, activation of the sympathetic nervous system and systemic inflammation.[17] OSA has been associated with hypertension, cardiovascular and cerebrovascular disease, heart failure, arrhythmias, metabolic syndrome/diabetes, and dementia.[18,19] It has also been associated with temporomandibular disorder,[20] periodontal disease,[21] and sleep bruxism.[20] All individuals with OSA have some degree of unfavorable upper airway anatomy that decreases its patency.[22] Impairments in the airway protective reflexes, particularly those involving the genioglossal muscle of the tongue, and in the neurological control of breathing also contribute to OSA in about two-thirds of adults with the disorder.[22]

It is estimated that 37% of adults in the United Stated (over 50 million) have at least mild OSA.[23] Commonly reported symptoms and signs of OSA include loud snoring, excessive daytime sleepiness (males) or fatigue (females), witnessed cessation of breathing during sleep, and hypertension.[18,19] Many individuals with OSA snore, but snoring (*primary snoring*) can occur in the absence of OSA. Risk factors for OSA include male gender, aging, and weight gain/obesity. These factors are associated with increased collapsibility of the upper airway. In addition, observations made during the intraoral and extraoral examination of the dental patient bear on an increased risk of OSA. Intraoral risk indicators include macroglossia,[24] limited visibility of the soft palate,[24,25] enlarged uvula,[26] enlarged tonsils,[27] lateral pharyngeal narrowing,[27,28] and maxillary constriction with or without posterior dental crossbite.[29] Dental attrition, dental erosion and findings suggestive of GERD and/or sleep bruxism have been associated with OSA, but not without controversy.[30] Extraoral risk indicators include micro- and retro-gnathia,[31] a steep mandibular

plane angle,[32] and an increased neck circumference (>16" in females and >17" in males).[33] Mouth breathing is also a risk indicator for OSA[34]

Dental patients who are at increased risk of OSA are referred to a medical provider for follow-up evaluation and diagnosis. OSA is diagnosed and graded in severity based on the presence of symptoms and the results of sleep apnea testing. The gold standard test is in-laboratory polysomnography (type I PSG) during which sleep, airflow, respiratory effort and cardiovascular variables are measured continuously and monitored by a technologist. A less comprehensive, accurate, expensive and burdensome test (type III or type IV Home Sleep Apnea Test, HSAT) can be conducted in the home for patients who are healthy and have no symptoms of other sleep disorders. In either case the test results must be interpreted by a physician who is certified or board-eligible in sleep medicine. The results substantiate a diagnosis of the presence and severity of the patient's OSA, which in turn bear on the treatment options recommended for the patient (see Chapter 10).

J. PERIODONTAL DISEASES

The supporting periodontal tissues may be affected by a number of different diseases and conditions and common language is needed to support the consistent description and classification of these various clinical presentations. Various workshops have been conducted over the last 50 years or more to help standardize classification. Most recently, an international workshop was jointly sponsored by the American Academy of Periodontology and the European Federation of Periodontology in 2017 to revisit disease classifications due to advancements in knowledge.

The current classification system utilizes four broad categories and various subcategories:[35]

Periodontal health, gingival diseases and conditions
  Periodontal and gingival health
  Gingivitis: dental biofilm-induced
  Gingival Diseases: nondental biofilm-induced
Periodontitis
  Periodontitis
  Necrotizing periodontal diseases
  Periodontitis as a manifestation of systemic disease
  Periodontal abscesses and endodontic-periodontal lesions
Periodontal manifestations of systemic diseases and developmental and acquired conditions
  Systemic diseases or conditions affecting the periodontal supporting tissues
  Mucogingival deformities and conditions
  Traumatic occlusal forces
  Tooth- and prosthesis-related factors
Peri-implant diseases and conditions
  Peri-implant health
  Peri-implant mucositis
  Peri-implantitis
  Peri-implant soft and hard tissue deficiencies
Terminology describing the most common clinical presentations to assist in classification may be found in Table 2.2.

TABLE 2.2 Terminology of Common Periodontal Conditions and Diagnoses

Periodontal Health

Gingival health on an intact periodontium

Gingival health on a reduced periodontium: non-periodontitis patient (gingival recession)

Gingival health on a reduced periodontium: stable/treated periodontitis patient

Gingivitis

Gingivitis on an intact periodontium

Gingivitis on a reduced periodontium – non-periodontitis patient (gingival recession)

Gingivitis on a reduced periodontium in a successfully treated periodontitis patient

Periodontitis

Periodontitis:
- Periodontitis Stage I: mild
- Periodontitis Stage II: moderate
- Periodontitis Stage III: severe
- Periodontitis Stage IV: very severe

Periodontitis distribution:
- Localized (<30% of teeth involved)
- Generalized (≥30% of teeth involved)
- Molar/Incisor Pattern

Periodontitis progression:
- Grade A: Slow
- Grade B: Moderate
- Grade C: Rapid

Implants

Peri-implant health

Peri-implant mucositis

Peri-implantitis

Peri-implant soft and hard tissue deficiencies

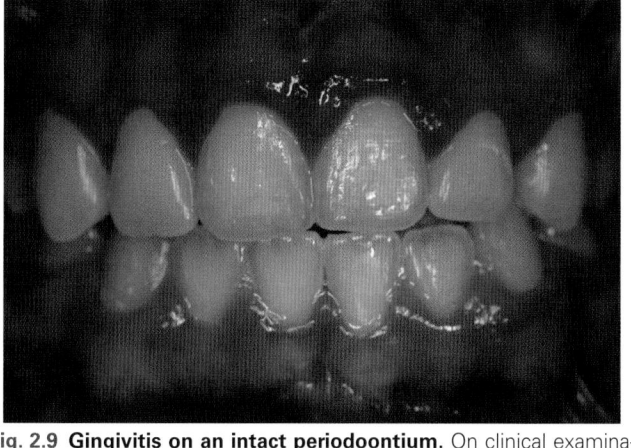

Fig. 2.9 Gingivitis on an intact periodoontium. On clinical examination, this 16-year-old female has notable erythema and edema of the marginal gingival. Generalized light plaque deposits are present, especially on the lingual and interproximal surfaces. Generalized probing depths of 3 mm or less are measured during your clinical examination with bleeding on probing detected along most surfaces of the mandibular anterior teeth. No appreciable attachment loss is identified and ideal crestal bone heights are noted on radiographic examination. Given this patient's age and sex, the impact of fluctuating sex steroid hormones associated with puberty and/or the patient's menstrual cycle must be considered when evaluating her gingival presentation.

Gingivitis

Gingivitis is one of the most common conditions affecting all ages of humankind. Up to 90% of all adults worldwide are affected by gingivitis.[36] Bacterial biofilm is the primary etiology of gingivitis. Clinically, changes in color, volume, and texture can be observed manifesting as reddening and swelling of the marginal gingiva with a loss of stippling and rolling of the margins (Figure. 2.9). Although deeper probing depths may be present, no progressive alveolar bone or attachment loss is detected (i.e., the alveolar bone levels are stable). Upon periodontal probing, bleeding is likely to occur. In addition, the patient may notice bleeding when brushing and flossing. These changes most often occur in the presence of plaque/bacterial biofilm. Calculus may be present. If left untreated, gingivitis may result in damage to the periodontal tissues (i.e., the development of periodontitis). Timely removal of the insulting bacterial biofilm typically results in the resolution of clinical signs of gingivitis with no irreversible damage to the periodontal tissues.

Because of individual differences in immune system response, the rate of disease progression varies between individuals. Some patients show resistance to the development of periodontitis in the longstanding presence of bacterial insult and others experience damage to the periodontium at a more rapid rate. It is important to treat patients with gingivitis for two primary reasons:
1. The difficulty in predicting the rate of progression from gingivitis to periodontitis because of individual differences in immune response; and
2. The possibility of potential systemic effects resulting from the presence of a persistent inflammatory burden.

Periodontitis

Approximately 42% of the dentate US adult population 30 years or older is affected by **periodontitis**, with nearly 8% affected by a severe form of this disease. Further, approximately 60% of all adults aged 65 years and older are affected by periodontitis.[37] In these patients, the clinical signs of gingivitis are present with the addition of progressive attachment and alveolar bone loss (Figures. 2.10 A and B and 2.11 A and B). Increased probing depths are commonly seen. Plaque/bacterial biofilm and calculus are commonly present along the root surface apical to the cementoenamel junction (CEJ). Roughness of the root surfaces may be detected.

The 2017 World Workshop introduced a new classification system for periodontitis based on a multidimensional staging and grading system. Staging is used to classify the severity and extent of a patient's disease and is based on the presence of interdental clinical attachment loss, radiographic bone loss, and/or tooth loss due to periodontitis. The distribution of disease is also included with each stage and describes the extent of destruction. Grading forecasts the rate of disease progression and is based on the evidence of disease progression and various risk factors[38] (see Table 2.3). American Academy of Periodontology STAGING AND GRADING PERIODONTITIS.

Staging and Grading Periodontitis

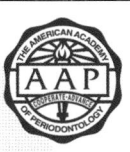

The 2017 World Workshop on the Classification of Periodontal and Peri-Implant Diseases and Conditions resulted in a new classification of periodontitis characterized by a multidimensional staging and grading system. The charts below provide an overview. Please visit **perio.org/2017wwdc** for the complete suite of reviews, case definition papers, and consensus reports.

PERIODONTITIS: STAGING

Staging intends to classify the severity and extent of a patient's disease based on the measurable amount of destroyed and/or damaged tissue as a result of periodontitis and to assess the specific factors that may attribute to the complexity of long-term case management.

Initial stage should be determined using clinical attachment loss (CAL). If CAL is not available, radiographic bone loss (RBL) should be used. Tooth loss due to periodontitis may modify stage definition. One or more complexity factors may shift the stage to a higher level. See **perio.org/2017wwdc** for additional information.

	Periodontitis	Stage I	Stage II	Stage III	Stage IV
Severity	**Interdental CAL** *(at site of greatest loss)*	1 – 2 mm	3 – 4 mm	≥5 mm	≥5 mm
	RBL	Coronal third (<15%)	Coronal third (15% - 33%)	Extending to middle third of root and beyond	Extending to middle third of root and beyond
	Tooth loss *(due to periodontitis)*	No tooth loss		≤4 teeth	≥5 teeth

Complexity	**Local**	• Max. probing depth ≤4 mm
		• Mostly horizontal bone loss
			• Max. probing depth ≤5 mm
			• Mostly horizontal bone loss
				In addition to Stage II complexity:
				• Probing depths ≥6 mm
				• Vertical bone loss ≥3 mm
				• Furcation involvement Class II or III
				• Moderate ridge defects
					In addition to Stage III complexity:
					• Need for complex rehabilitation due to:
					  – Masticatory dysfunction
					  – Secondary occlusal trauma (tooth mobility degree ≥2)
					  – Severe ridge defects
					  – Bite collapse, drifting, flaring
					  – < 20 remaining teeth (10 opposing pairs)

Extent and distribution	**Add to stage as descriptor**	For each stage, describe extent as: • Localized (<30% of teeth involved); • Generalized; or • Molar/incisor pattern			

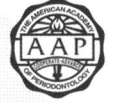

PERIODONTITIS: GRADING

Grading aims to indicate the rate of periodontitis progression, responsiveness to standard therapy, and potential impact on systemic health.

Clinicians should initially assume grade B disease and seek specific evidence to shift to grade A or C.
See **perio.org/2017wwdc** for additional information.

	Progression		Grade A: Slow rate	Grade B: Moderate rate	Grade C: Rapid rate
Primary criteria	Direct evidence of progression	Radiographic bone loss or CAL	No loss over 5 years	<2 mm over 5 years	≥2 mm over 5 years
Whenever available, direct evidence should be used.	Indirect evidence of progression	% bone loss / age	<0.25	0.25 to 1.0	>1.0
		Case phenotype	Heavy biofilm deposits with low levels of destruction	Destruction commensurate with biofilm deposits	Destruction exceeds expectations given biofilm deposits; specific clinical patterns suggestive of periods of rapid progression and/or early onset disease
Grade modifiers	Risk factors	Smoking	Non-smoker	<10 cigarettes/day	≥10 cigarettes/day
		Diabetes	Normoglycemic/no diagnosis of diabetes	HbA1c <7.0% in patients with diabetes	HbA1c ≥7.0% in patients with diabetes

The 2017 World Workshop on the Classification of Periodontal and Peri-Implant Diseases and Conditions was co-presented by the American Academy of Periodontology (AAP) and the European Federation of Periodontology (EFP).

Tables from Tonetti, Greenwell, Kornman. *J Periodontol* 2018;89 (Suppl 1): S159-S172.

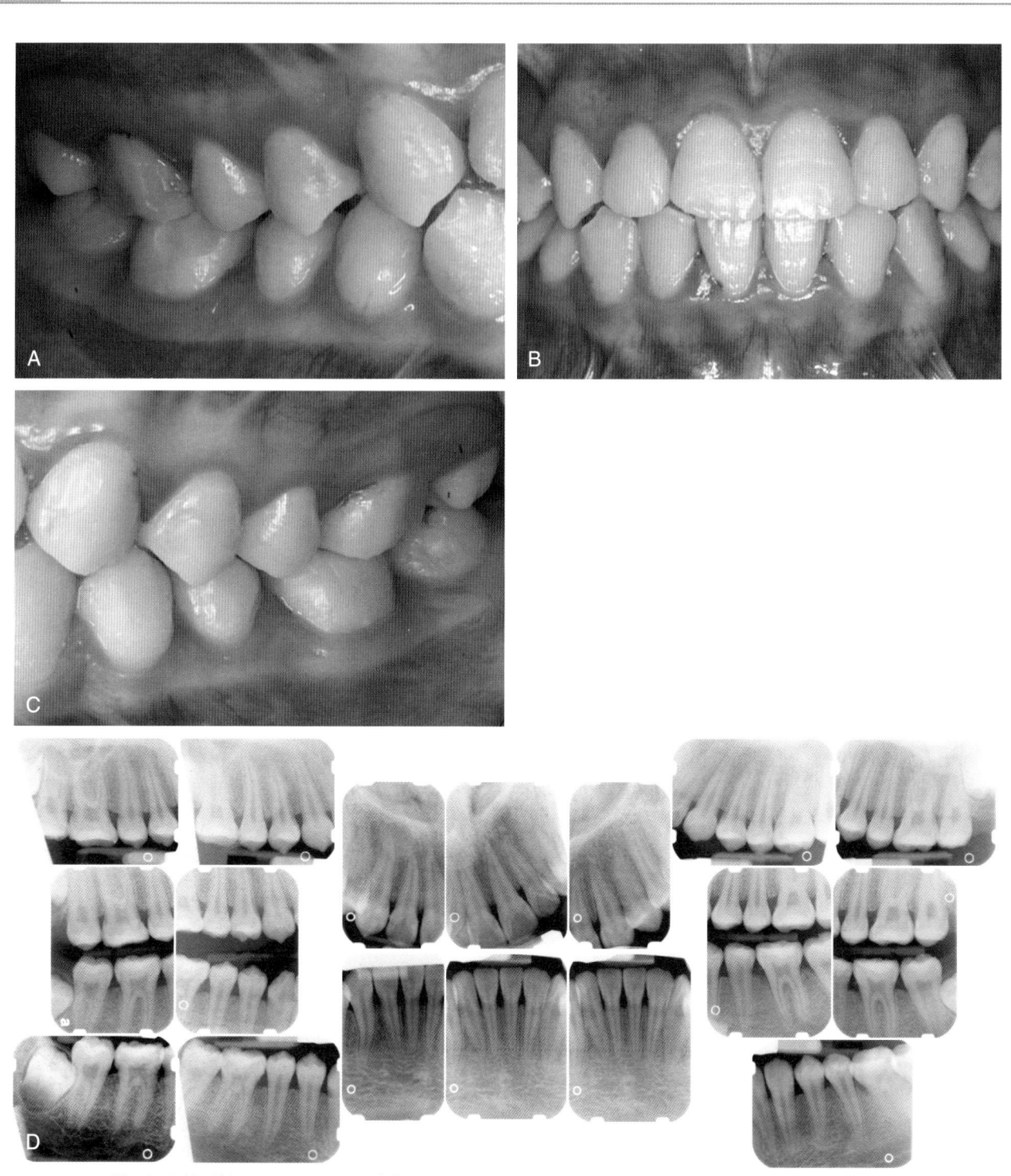

Fig. 2.10 (A–C) Intraoral photos and **(D)** radiographs showing molar-incisor stage 1 grade B **periodontitis**. This 16-year-old female has bleeding on probing and probing depths of 4 mm in the posterior sextants and select anterior teeth. Supragingival and subgingival calculus and plaque are detected clinically on enamel and root surfaces. Heavy subgingival calculus is noted on the palatal/lingual surfaces of the posterior teeth. Concurrent with radiographic signs of localized slight bone loss, attachment loss no greater than 1 to 2 mm affects select molars and incisors. The presence of gingival inflammation, the slight increases in probing depth, the presence of plaque and calculus, and the patterns and degree of attachment loss all justify the diagnosis of molar-incisor stage 1 grade B periodontitis.

Although previous classification systems categorized different forms of periodontitis (e.g., adult vs. juvenile/early-onset periodontitis; chronic vs. aggressive periodontitis), the 2017 Classification condensed all forms of the disease into one entity: periodontitis. This decision was driven by a large body of scientific evidence that failed to support different pathophysiologically-distinct forms of periodontitis. Although periodontitis typically occurs in older adults, it can also occur in children, adolescents, and young adults. The clinician should always assess the periodontal status of *every* patient and classify their

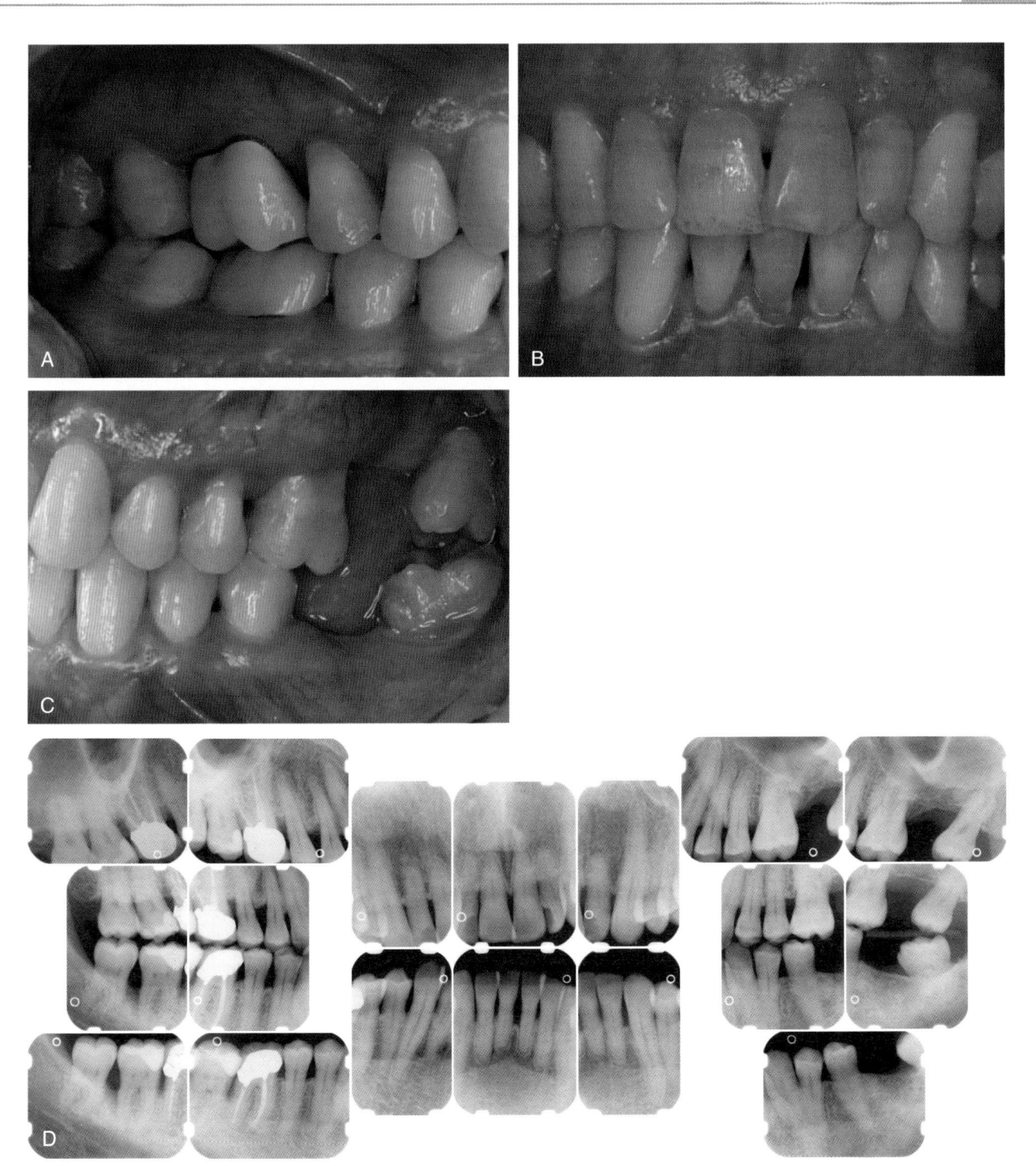

Fig. 2.11 **(A–C)** Intraoral photos and **(D)** radiographs showing generalized stage III, grade C **periodontitis**. This 49-year-old male one pack-per-day cigarette smoker has generalized probing depths of 4 to 6 mm with localized 7-9 mm probing depths in the posterior sextants. Light bleeding on probing is present. Supragingival and subgingival calculus and plaque are detected clinically on enamel and select root surfaces. ≥30% of sites have attachment loss of 5 mm or greater. The percentage of affected teeth justifies the distribution, the extent of attachment and bone loss justifies the stage, and the percentage of radiographic bone loss relative to age and smoking history justify the grade.

clinical presentation accordingly. While the pathophysiology of periodontitis in children and adolescents is similar to what is seen in adults, more aggressive treatment options, such as the use of systemic antibiotics, are typically required.

Untreated periodontitis will result in progressive alveolar bone loss, attachment loss, gingival recession, tooth mobility, furcation involvement, and possible tooth loss. As with gingivitis, this inflammatory burden may affect systemic health. Prompt treatment is necessary not only for arresting disease progression but also for improving the overall health of the patient.

The Concept of the Reduced Periodontium

The clinician may find difficulty in diagnosing a patient with clinically healthy gingiva in the presence of generalized gingival recession (i.e., attachment and alveolar bone loss) (Figure. 2.12 A and B). To understand this presentation, the concept of the **reduced periodontium** becomes important. Attachment loss may occur as a result of periodontitis or other habits and conditions (Box 2.2). Treatment of these diseases/events focuses on restoring health to the periodontal tissues but, in most cases, alveolar bone and attachment loss is irreversible. Despite this, gingival health may be restored and the progression of attachment loss arrested. Based on the previously outlined classification criteria, the novice clinician may erroneously classify these patients as exhibiting periodontitis when they may be exhibiting either periodontal health or gingivitis on a reduced periodontium. This diagnosis suggests that the occurrence or development of attachment and alveolar bone loss is halted. Repeated periodontal examinations over multiple time points are necessary to confirm this diagnosis.

When classifying periodontal health or gingivitis, it is important to note whether the patient has an intact periodontium or a reduced periodontium (i.e., the presence or absence of attachment and alveolar bone loss). If a reduced periodontium is identified, the clinician must further indicate if the patient has a history of treated periodontitis or not.[39]

Peri-Implant Diseases and Conditions

For the first time in a periodontal classification workshop, the 2017 World Workshop includes case definitions and diagnostic considerations for peri-implant diseases and conditions,

---

BOX 2.2   Causes of Attachment Loss

Plaque-induced periodontitis
- Patients with a history of treated periodontitis

Non-plaque-induced periodontitis
- Anatomic variations (thin gingival biotype, tooth malpositioning)
- Iatrogenic defects
- Deleterious habits (traumatic tooth brushing, factitial injuries)
- Advanced age

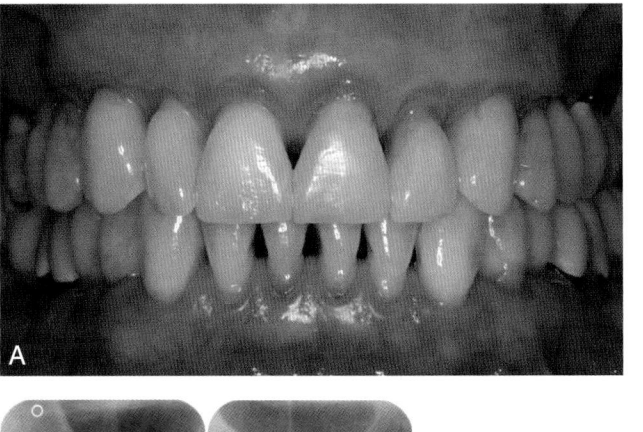

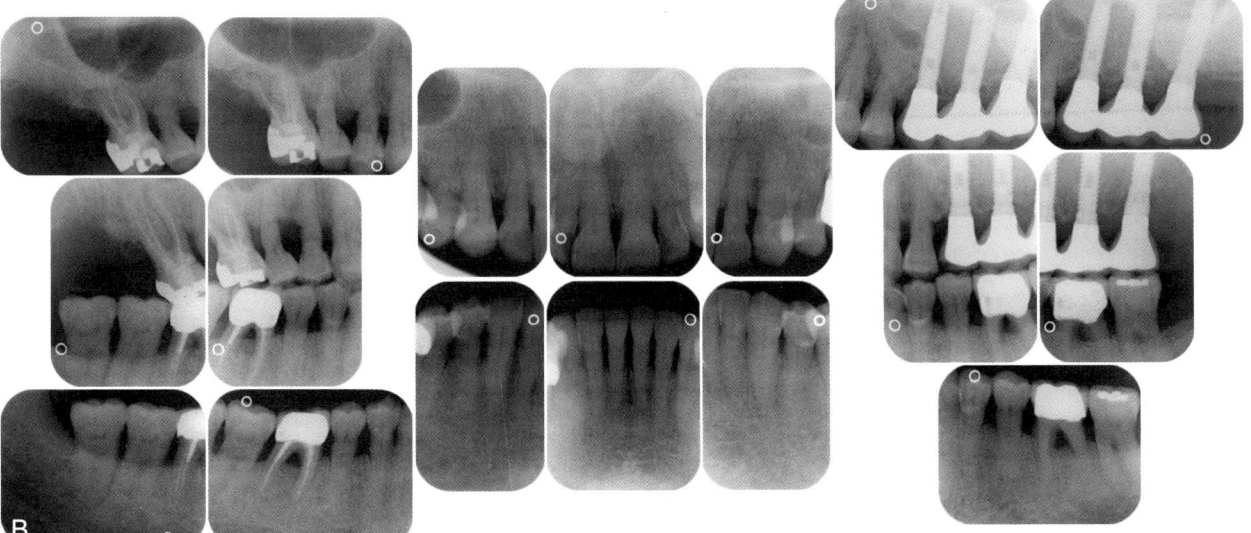

Fig. 2.12 Gingival health on a reduced periodontium. On clinical examination, this 52-year-old female has probing depths of 3 mm or less with no bleeding on probing. Generalized attachment loss and gingival recession are detected. Mobility is present on the mandibular anterior teeth. Through-and-through furcation involvement is noted on some of the molars. The stability of her periodontium has been monitored over the course of the past 3 years.

to include peri-implant health, peri-implant mucositis, peri-implantitis, and soft- and hard-tissue deficiencies. With an increased use of dental implant-supported restorations worldwide, there has been a realization that dental implants can be affected by bacterial biofilm and inflammatory mechanisms resembling those seen around teeth. Therefore, criteria for describing peri-implant health and disease were deemed necessary to standardize diagnosis and classification.

Probing depths and the assessment of radiographic bone levels are critical in evaluating peri-implant health. Peri-implant health exists when an implant is free of any clinical signs of inflammation, to include erythema, edema, bleeding on probing, and/or suppuration. With **peri-implant mucositis**, clinical signs of inflammation and deeper probing depths are now present but radiographic bone levels remain stable. **Peri-implantitis** has similar findings to peri-implant mucositis along with the addition of progressive radiographic bone loss. Routine visual inspection of the peri-implant mucosa is important, as is probing of the peri-implant sulcus. Radiographic assessments should occur routinely following implant restoration to establish baseline peri-implant bone levels and favor the early detection of bone loss.

An accurate periodontal diagnosis and classification will guide the clinician to deliver appropriate treatment and ensure consistent, long-term care and communication among various providers in the patient's care team. Treatment to begin addressing these periodontal conditions will largely be based on the presence or absence of plaque (and other etiologic factors), probing depths, and the extent of attachment or alveolar bone loss. These factors are detailed in Chapter 10.

Correct classification of the patient's periodontal status is critically important because treatment planning is inextricably linked with the diagnosis and an incorrect diagnosis often leads to inappropriate treatment. Overclassifying periodontal disease (incorrectly diagnosing gingivitis as periodontitis) may be seen as insurance fraud. Under diagnosis (failing to identify gingivitis or periodontitis when it is present) has led many patients to pursue litigation when, years later, it becomes apparent that he or she was not informed and/or that the periodontal disease was not effectively managed by the dental team. The careful examination and classification of clinical presentations will help to ensure that patients are receiving the best care.

K. PULPAL AND PERIAPICAL DIAGNOSES

The dentist bases a diagnosis and classification of pulpal disease on patient symptoms and clinical findings. Pain of dental origin may reflect conditions that are reversible or irreversible in nature. **Reversible pulpitis** is a clinical diagnosis based on subjective and objective findings that suggest the inflammation will probably resolve and the pulp return to normal. Reversible pulpitis is usually a temporary condition characterized by pain that is not severe and is associated with a specific stimulus, such as cold. The pain ceases within a short period after removal of the stimulus. In contrast, a constant, severe pain that seems to arise without provocation characterizes **irreversible pulpitis**; the classic presentation for a toothache. Irreversible pulpitis is

a clinical diagnosis based on subjective and objective findings indicating that the vital inflamed pulp is not capable of healing. Common symptoms are lingering thermal pain, spontaneous pain, and referred pain. The pain may awaken the patient from sleep. Frequently the patient will have been taking analgesics that may or may not have been effective in relieving the pain. A clinical diagnosis of **pulpal necrosis** indicates the death of the dental pulp. This diagnosis is made when pulp testing is negative to thermal and electrical testing. Often, pulpal necrosis will be associated with clinical or radiographic signs of apical pathology or changes in tooth color.

When pulpal inflammation extends to the apical periodontium, it can produce clinical symptoms including a painful response to biting and/or percussion or palpation. This clinical diagnosis, called a **symptomatic apical periodontitis**, may or not be associated with an apical radiolucency area. An **asymptomatic apical periodontitis** is associated with radiographically evident inflammation and destruction of the apical tissues secondary to pulp necrosis, but without pain or swelling. An **acute apical abscess** (Figure. 2.13) is an inflammatory reaction to pulpal infection and necrosis characterized by rapid onset, spontaneous pain, tenderness of the tooth to pressure, pus formation, and swelling of the associated area. Mobility of the affected tooth is sometimes seen.

If the infection is not locally contained, it may progress into a **cellulitis** characterized by painful swelling with diffuse borders and invasion into the subperiosteum or facial spaces. Typically, the patient will have signs of elevated temperature, lymphadenopathy, and sometimes malaise. A **chronic apical abscess** is also associated with pulpal necrosis, but is characterized by gradual onset with little or no discomfort and exhibits a usually nonpainful discharge of pus through a sinus tract. **Condensing osteitis** is the clinical designation for a tooth with chronic apical inflammation from a low-grade inflammatory stimulus that will appear on a radiograph as a diffuse opacity (see later section on apical sclerosing osteitis).

Radiographic findings associated with the dental pulp and surrounding tissue may suggest several diagnoses (Table 2.4).

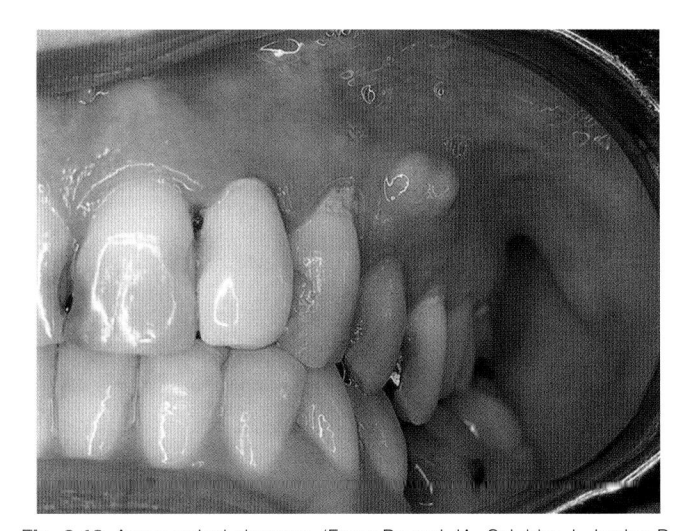

Fig. 2.13 Acute apical abscess. (From Regezi JA, Sciubba J, Jordan R. Oral Pathology. 6th ed. St Louis: Saunders; 2012.)

TABLE 2.4   Pulpal and Periapical Diagnoses/Radiographic Findings

Common Diagnoses	Description	Illustration
Apical rarefying osteitis	<ul><li>Loss of bone density at the apex of the tooth.</li><li>The term encompasses the following entities, which are difficult to differentiate radiographically:</li><li>periapical abscess</li><li>periapical granuloma</li><li>radicular cyst\</li></ul>	
Apical sclerosing osteitis	<ul><li>Increase in bone density in the region of the apex of the tooth in response to inflammation.</li><li>Frequently described as condensing osteitis.</li></ul>	
Combination apical rarefying osteitis and apical sclerosing osteitis	<ul><li>Combination of rarefying and sclerosing osteitis.</li></ul>	
Internal resorption	<ul><li>Uniform localized widening of the internal aspect of the canal, radiolucency.</li><li>Radiolucency confined to internal aspect of the tooth.</li></ul>	

Continued

TABLE 2.4 Pulpal and Periapical Diagnoses/Radiographic Findings—cont'd

Common Diagnoses	Description	Illustration
External resorption	• Uniform localized loss of external root surface, radiolucency • Canal is unaffected. • May occur at apical or lateral aspect of the tooth root. • May affect the adjacent bone.	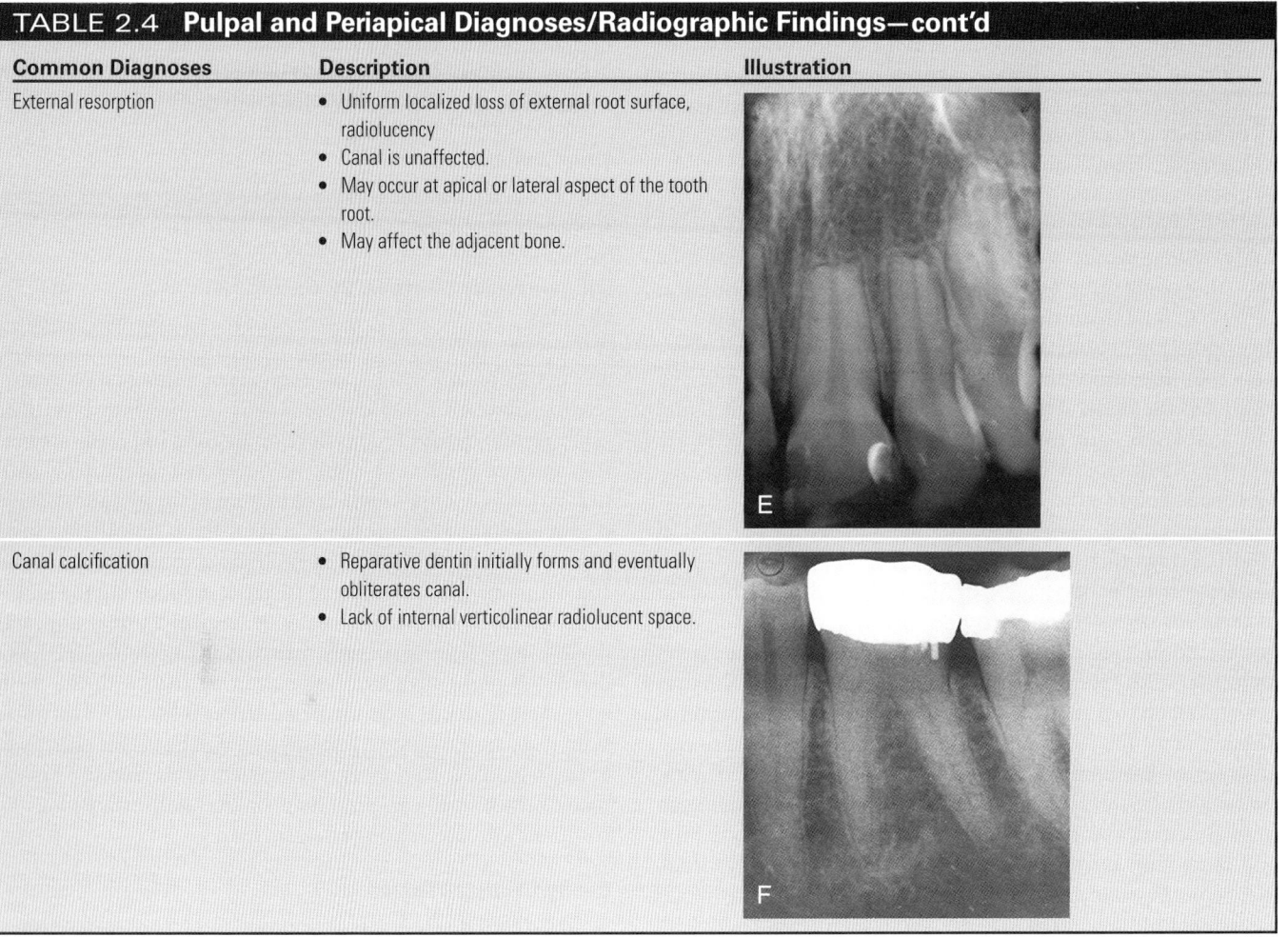
Canal calcification	• Reparative dentin initially forms and eventually obliterates canal. • Lack of internal verticolinear radiolucent space.	

From **(B, D–F)** Torabinejad M, Fouad A, Walton R. *Endodontics: Principles and Practice.* 5th ed. St Louis: Saunders; 2014; **(C)** courtesy Dr. Angie Broome.

The dentist may interpret a missing pulp space as evidence of calcified canals. An irregularly enlarged root canal space suggests **internal resorption**. Resorption of the root from the outside, around the periodontal ligament space, is **external resorption**. Common radiographic periapical diagnoses include **apical rarefying osteitis** (ARO), **apical sclerosing osteitis** (ASO), and **apical rarefying and sclerosing osteitis** (ARSO). Root fractures that occur in conjunction with facial trauma are often seen on radiographs. (See Table 2.1.)

L. DENTAL CARIES

Dental caries is a biofilm-mediated, diet-modulated, multifactorial, noncommunicable, dynamic disease resulting in net mineral loss of dental hard tissues. It is determined by biological, behavioral, psychosocial, and environmental factors. As a consequence of this process, a caries lesion develops.[40] To diagnose dental caries involves not only an objective determination of whether or not lesions or disease are present (i.e., caries *detection*) and, if present, a characterization of its severity (i.e., caries *assessment*) but, most importantly, a summation of all data available for determination of whether the condition is the result of the dental caries process and whether it is active or arrested. This diagnosis should be a guiding factor for caries risk assessment (i.e., the risk of developing new lesions in the future) and management (encompassing restorative and nonrestorative care and prevention). Numerous instruments are available to aid the clinician in caries detection and assessment, including radiographs and other technology-based aids (e.g., fluorescence-based methods, electrical conductance methods; see Chapter 4).

Some Guiding Definitions[41,42]

• **Caries detection:** A process involving recognition of changes in enamel, dentin, and/or cementum, which are consistent with the caries process. In other words, the process involves identifying the signs (consequences) of bacterial destruction of the dynamic caries process. It must be noted, however, that lesion detection, without assessment, is not practical or useful.
• **Caries assessment:** An evaluation of the characteristics of a caries lesion after the lesion has been detected. These characteristics may include visual, physical, chemical, or biochemical parameters, including color, size, surface roughness/harness, and surface integrity or cavitation.

- **Caries diagnosis:** The professional summation of all the signs (following detection and lesion assessment) and symptoms of the caries disease; arrives at a determination of whether or not the caries lesion is active, progressing rapidly or slowly, or is already arrested. Without this information, a logical decision about treatment cannot be made.

Caries Lesion Severity

Caries lesion severity is the stage of lesion progression along the spectrum of net mineral loss, from the initial loss at the molecular level to total tissue destruction. Such an assessment involves determination of both the extent of the lesion in a pulpal direction (i.e., proximity to the dentin-enamel junction and the pulp) and the mineral loss in volume terms. Noncavitated and cavitated lesions are, for example, two specific stages of lesion severity. As discussed in Chapter 1, the ability to detect caries lesions and to differentiate among different levels of severity depends on the caries detection method and/or the clinical criteria being utilized.

Many criteria have been developed for the examination of teeth for caries lesion detection and assessment, including visual and/or tactile-based criteria. The International Caries Detection and Assessment System (ICDAS; www.ICDAS.org) is a representative and generally accepted list of caries criteria. This system is the culmination of an international effort to create a set of harmonized and internationally recognized criteria built on best evidence. To implement this system, the teeth must be clean and dry when examined. The enamel, dentin, and cementum are then evaluated using predominately visual, histologically-validated, clinical criteria. This system allows assessment of both caries severity and level of caries activity.[43] Supporting histological validation for this approach has been reported.[44–46] The ICDAS includes six caries lesion codes (1–6) that can be used individually or collapsed into fewer categories, which are sometimes useful for clinical care—for example, noncavitated lesions (codes 1 and 2) versus cavitated lesions (codes 3-6), or incipient (codes 1 and 2) versus moderate (codes 3 and 4) versus advanced lesions (codes 5 and 6).

Non-Cavitated Lesion

This is a caries/carious lesion whose surface appears macroscopically to be intact (Figure. 2.14). In other words, it is a caries lesion without visual evidence of cavitation. Such a lesion is still potentially reversible by chemical means or arrestable by chemical (e.g., fluoride) or mechanical (e.g., sealant) means.[47] It is sometimes referred to as an incipient lesion, initial lesion, an early lesion or a white spot lesion (a color designation is misleading, however, because these lesions can be white, brown, or other colors). Caries lesions develop in areas of plaque stagnation and may appear as a white/yellow/brown coloration, which may be limited to the confines or bottom of the pits and fissures on occlusal surfaces or extend beyond them into the occlusal planes. On smooth surfaces caries lesions occur cervical to the contact point on interproximal surfaces or following the gingival contour if occurring buccally or lingually. Initial noncavitated "white" lesions are only seen visually when the teeth are dried, but more advanced lesions can be seen with the teeth either wet or dry. If a noncavitated lesion picks up an extrinsic stain (e.g., appears brown), however, it will be visible either wet or dry regardless of whether it is incipient or advanced.[48] In fact, many such stained carious lesions on occlusal surfaces may be confused with noncarious extrinsic stain.

Cavity/Cavitated Lesion

A cavity/cavitated lesion is a carious lesion whose surface is not macroscopically intact, with a distinct discontinuity or break in the surface integrity, as determined utilizing optical or tactile means (Figure 2.15).

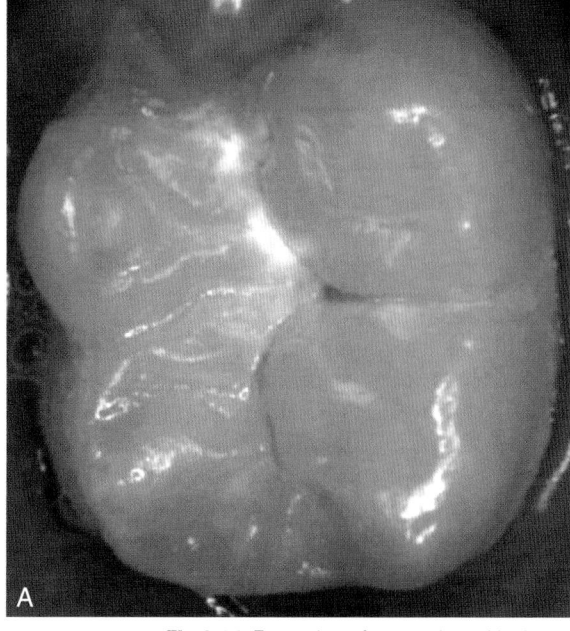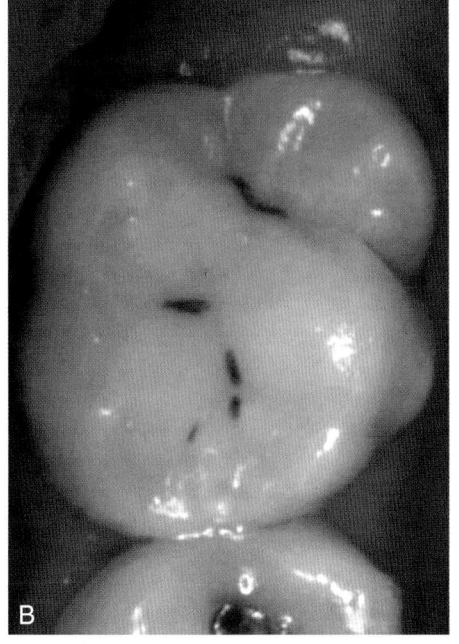

Fig 2.14 Examples of noncavitated lesion. (Courtesy Dr. Margherita Fontana)

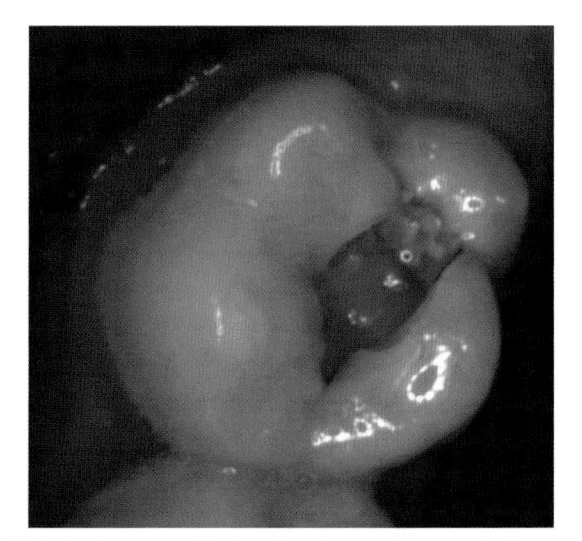

Fig. 2.15 Cavity/cavitated lesion. (Courtesy Dr. Margherita Fontana)

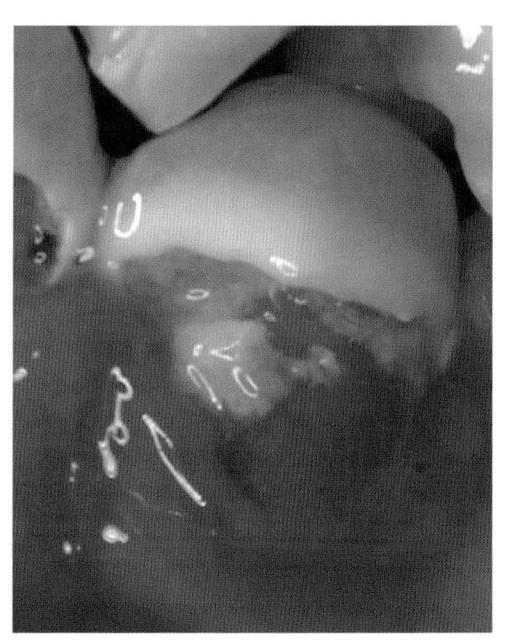

Fig. 2.16 This is an example of a cavitated, active, coronal lesion. Notice plaque within the lesion and associated plaque-induced gingival inflammation. (Courtesy Dr. Margherita Fontana)

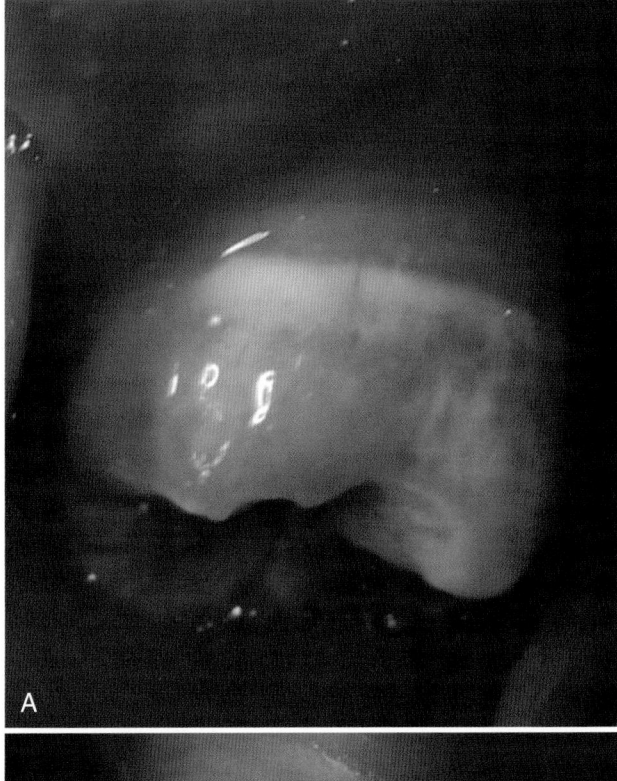

A

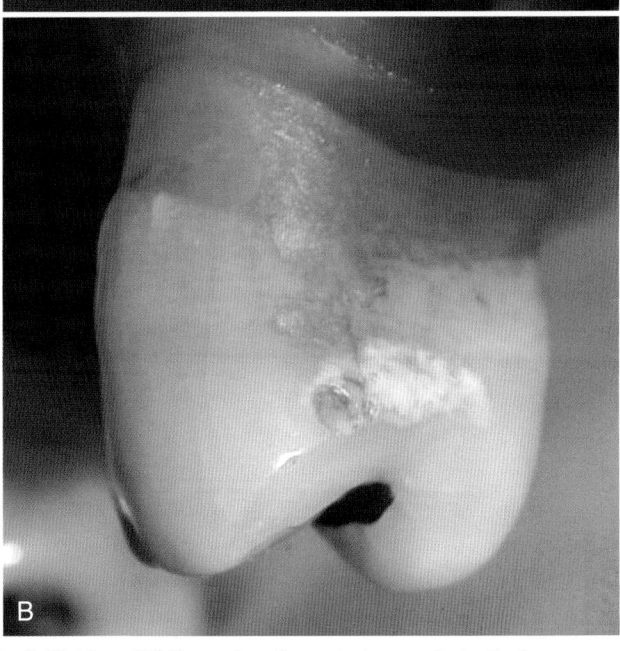

B

Fig. 2.17 (A and B) Examples of arrested noncavitated lesions on coronal smooth surfaces (notice the buccal lesion's distance from the gum line; very shiny and smooth). **(B)** The proximal lesion probably developed when teeth were in contact. When the neighboring tooth was extracted, the proximal lesion arrested. (Notice it is now NOT in a plaque stagnation area). (Courtesy Dr. Margherita Fontana)

Caries Lesion Activity (Net Progression Toward Demineralization)

Caries lesion activity is the summation of the dynamics of the caries process resulting in the net loss, over time, of mineral from the tooth enamel (i.e., active lesion progression).

Active Caries Lesion

An **active caries lesion** is a caries lesion from which, over a specified period of time, there is net mineral loss (i.e., the lesion is progressing) (Figure. 2.16). Clinical observations to be taken into consideration for assessing caries lesion activity include visual appearance, tactile perception, and potential for plaque accumulation. A lesion is likely to be active when the surface of the enamel is whitish/yellowish opaque and chalky (with loss of luster); feels rough when the tip of the probe is moved gently across the surface; is in a plaque stagnation area (i.e., pits and

fissures, near the gingival margin, and interproximal surface cervical to the contact point). In dentin the lesion is probably active when the dentin is soft or leathery on gentle probing.

Arrested or Inactive Caries Lesion

An **arrested or inactive caries lesion** is not undergoing net mineral loss—that is, the caries process is no longer progressing (Figure. 2.17). This lesion represents a "scar" of past disease activity. Clinical observations to be taken into consideration for assessing caries lesion activity will be based on visual appearance, tactile feeling, and potential for plaque accumulation. A lesion is probably inactive when the surface of the enamel is whitish, brownish, or black. The enamel may be shiny and generally feels hard and smooth when the tip of a probe is moved gently across the surface. Caries lesions on smooth surfaces are more likely to be inactive when located in sites without plaque accumulation (i.e., at some distance from the gingival margin following gingival recession). In dentin, the cavity may appear shiny and feel firm on gentle probing.

Classification of Lesions by Anatomical Location[49]
Coronal Primary Caries Lesion

A **coronal primary caries lesion** is produced by direct extension from an external surface in the coronal portion of a tooth (Figure. 2.18). Such lesions develop in areas of plaque stagnation; thus they may be located in the pits and fissures of teeth, on interproximal surfaces (cervical to the contact point), or on smooth surfaces (buccal or lingual, following the gingival contour).

Secondary Caries, Recurrent Caries, or Caries Lesions Associated with Restorations and Sealants (Cars)

Secondary caries are lesions that occur at the margin of, or adjacent to, an existing filling (Figure. 2.19). These lesions have classically been described as occurring in two ways:

an *outer lesion* or a *wall lesion*. The chemical and histological processes involved in outer lesions are the same as with primary caries and they may occur as the result of a new,

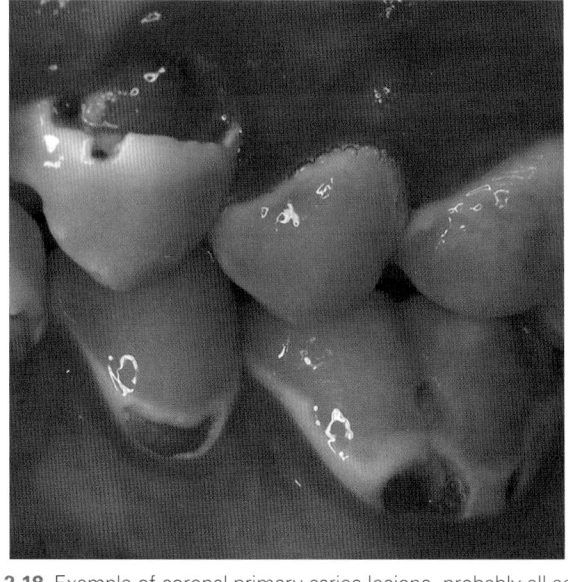

Fig. 2.18 Example of coronal primary caries lesions, probably all active; some are cavitated with exposed dentin and some are noncavitated. (Courtesy Dr. Margherita Fontana)

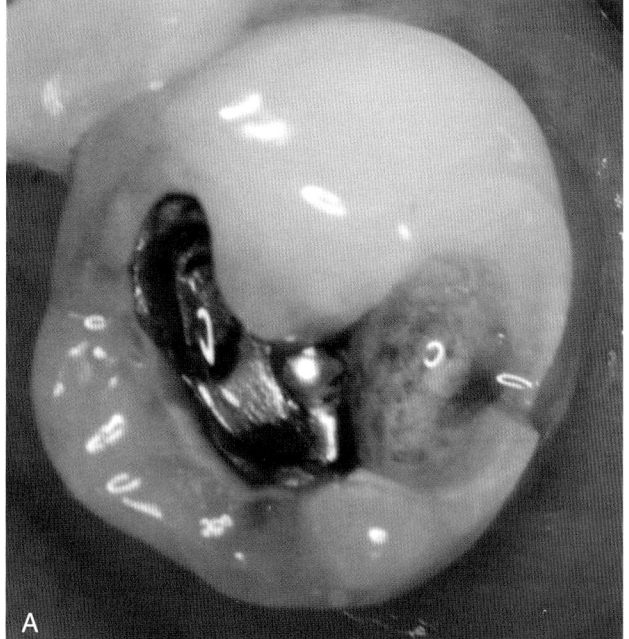

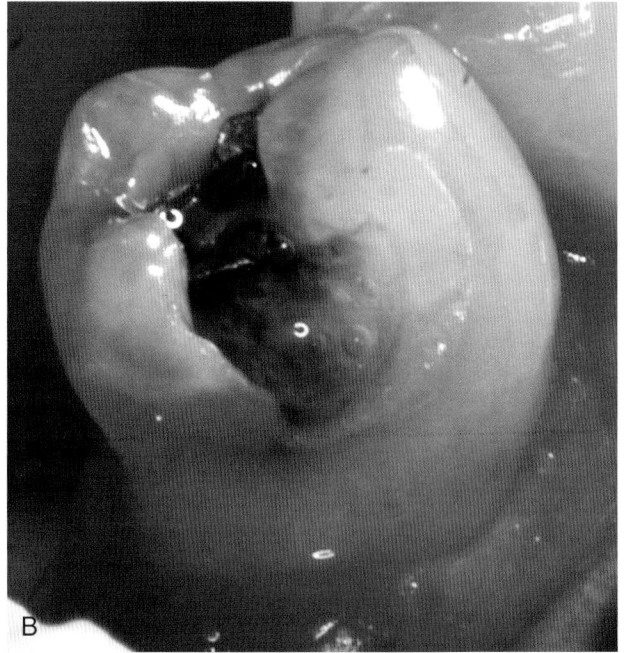

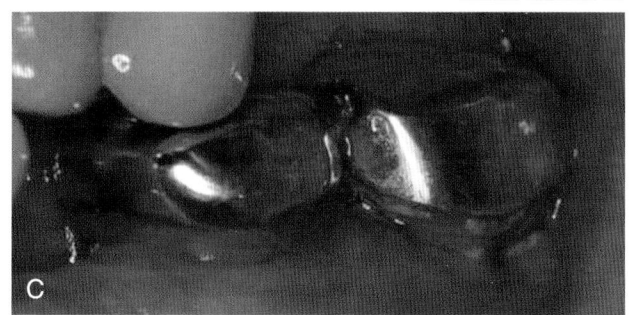

Fig. 2.19 Examples of secondary caries after restoration either broken (**A** and **B** are from the same tooth viewed in different angles) or around the margins of a gold crown (**C**).

primary, attack on the surface of the tooth adjacent to the filling. Several researchers have suggested that caries identified as "secondary" are quite likely to actually be primary caries adjacent to fillings.[50]

Root Surface Caries Lesions. Root surface caries lesions are frequently observed near the CEJ, although they may appear anywhere on the root surface (Figure. 2.20). **Root caries** lesions appear as distinct, clearly demarcated circular or linear discolorations at the CEJ or wholly on the root surface.[41,42]

Caries Risk Assessment (See Also Chapter 3)

Caries risk is the probability that caries lesions will develop or progress if conditions remain the same within a certain period of time. Caries risk status, whether higher or lower risk, can only be validated over time.[40] Risk of dental caries is a proxy for the true outcome, which is development of new caries lesions or progression of existing lesions. In practice, many existing caries risk assessment forms/tools are used not only to aid in prediction, but also to help identify factors that if modified may help decrease risk of future disease. Risk assessment status is also used in practice to inform the frequency of patient recall, with higher caries risk patients likely benefiting from shorter recall periods than lower risk patients, for monitoring, reevaluation, and provision of preventive interventions.[51]

Caries risk indicators are characteristics associated with increased probability or occurrence of caries lesions, which are not causally associated with the disease. Examples include sociodemographic variables and presence of caries lesions or restorations. **Caries risk factors** are environmental, behavioral, or biological factors confirmed by temporal sequence, usually in longitudinal studies, which,

if present, directly increase the probability of caries occurrence. Risk factors are part of the dental caries causal chain.[40] Examples include frequent consumption of a cariogenic diet, stagnant dental plaque and xerostomia. **Protective factors** can decrease the risk of disease when present, such as adequate exposure to fluoride, presence of dental sealants and regular preventive care. The strongest indicator of increased caries risk continues to be recent caries experience. A summary of caries risk factors and caries protective factors is presented in Figure. 3.3.

Validated caries risk assessment tools could be used to target cost-effective interventions to manage the caries disease process and more accurately determine the periodicity of caries diagnostic and management services. Unfortunately, many risk forms are still not adequately validated to the populations in which they are used.[52] In the absence of validated caries risk tools, a patient's risk level is generally derived from an analysis of sociodemographic, medical, behavioral (oral hygiene, diet, etc.) and past caries experience, together with an oral examination to determine presence of active caries lesions. The clinician must then weigh the patient's risk and protective indicators/factors (see Figure 3.3) against each other in order to assess the likely probability of future disease activity. Lower risk status is easy to identify as the absence of both caries risk indicators/factors and absence of active caries lesions.[51] Patients' caries risk must be assessed regularly because risk may change over time, should be documented in the dental record, should be clearly communicated to the patient, and should be used to influence clinical decision-making regarding treatment needs and alternatives, and the provision of other services (e.g., frequency of radiographs, periodicity of recall, etc.).

There are numerous tests designed to aid with caries risk assessment, for example by measuring the quantity of cariogenic bacteria, such as *Streptococcus mutans* and lactobacilli. A sample of the patient's saliva is placed on a special agar medium, which is then incubated. The patient's caries risk is then estimated to be related to the number of bacterial colonies that grow on the plate. However, the accuracy and impact of these tests on risk assessment is still questionable. On the other hand, a low salivary flow rate (<0.7 mL/min of stimulated saliva, <0.1 mL/min unstimulated saliva) is considered a risk factor for increased caries activity (Figure 3.3). The evaluation of other characteristics or components in a patient's saliva have yet to be proven helpful to improve the accuracy of caries risk assessment. They do, however have benefit in the overall management of the caries active and high caries risk patient (see Chapter 10).

Clinical and Radiographic Detection of the Caries Lesion

Visual techniques are the mainstay for detection of pit and fissure and clinically visible smooth surface caries lesions. See Chapter 1 for discussion of visual and tactile caries detection methods and Chapter 4 for discussion of digital caries detection instruments. The use of magnification in caries detection and radiographic discovery of approximal caries lesions is discussed here.

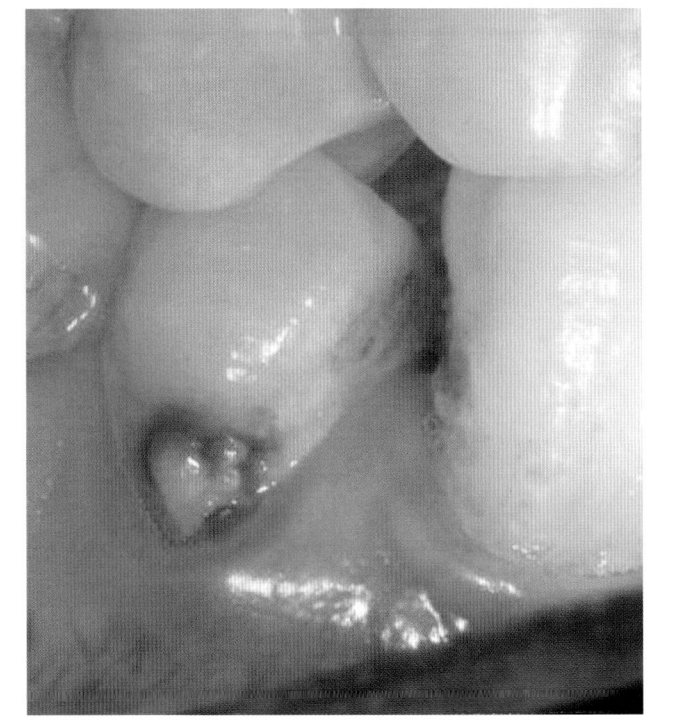

Fig. 2.20 Example of an active cavitated root surface lesion. Notice plaque within the lesion.

Use of Magnification

In recent decades, a concerted effort has been made in dentistry to identify ways to enhance visual examination, including the use of magnification and the adoption of technology-based methods (see Chapter 4) for detecting carious lesions and/or quantifying demineralization in noncavitated lesions.[53,54] Magnification may be useful for tooth examination; however, there is relatively little research on its use for caries detection and assessment. Among the in vitro studies that do exist, comparisons of visual assessment with or without magnification present conflicting results. Some preliminary clinical data suggest that, although use of magnification may not affect the ability of expert clinicians to distinguish between different stages of lesion severity, this technology may lead to more aggressive treatment decisions.[55] Thus, if magnification is to be used for caries detection and assessment, it must be used with caution. For example, it is possible that with increased magnification, noncavitated lesions may actually appear cavitated, thus leading to more aggressive or unnecessary interventions.[56]

Radiographic Interpretation

In clinical practice the diagnosis of caries is made on the basis of clinical signs and symptoms and with the utilization of radiographic imaging aids. Radiographic detection is possible only after sufficient demineralization of the enamel and dentin has occurred. When exposed to the x-rays the demineralized area reduces the beam attenuation in comparison to the sound tooth structure, allowing more x-rays to reach the receptor. The resultant radiographic image displays the demineralization as a dark area or radiolucency that is the result of past caries activity.

Radiographic images are useful in identifying caries lesions that are not visible clinically, such as approximal primary and secondary caries (Table 2.5). Compared with visual detection alone, images are most useful in detecting approximal and occlusal caries lesions past the dentin-enamel junction.[57,58] Radiographic images are also helpful in determining the depth of the lesion and its proximity to the pulp chamber and pulp horns. However, it must be emphasized that a radiographic image of a caries lesion can represent an arrested or active lesion. A single radiographic image cannot be used to determine caries lesion activity.

TABLE 2.5	Dental Caries/Radiographic Findings	
Caries Detection	**Description**	**Illustration**
Occlusal caries	• Dentinal radiolucency appearing below the pits and fissures of the occlusal surface • Mushroom-shaped radiolucency	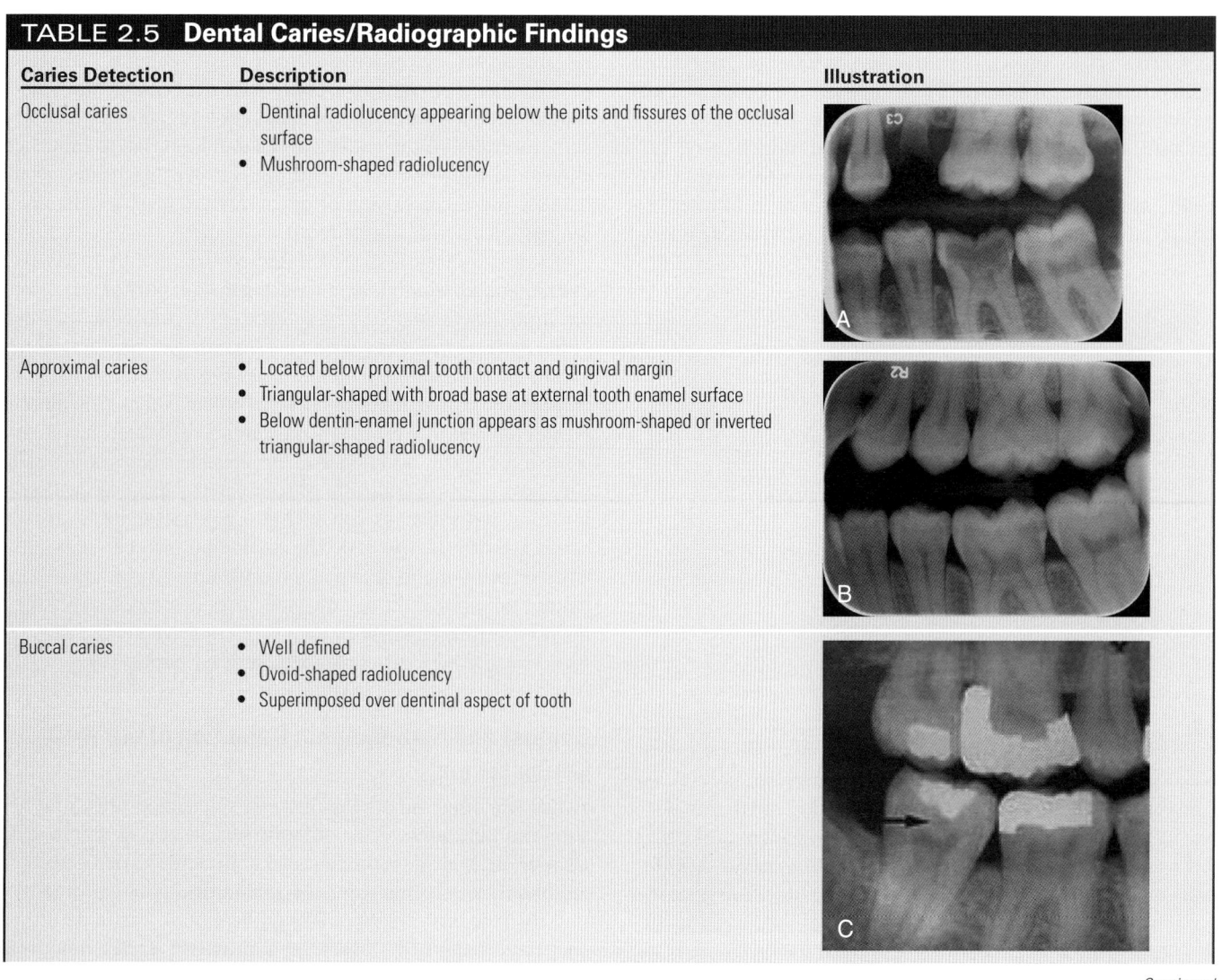
Approximal caries	• Located below proximal tooth contact and gingival margin • Triangular-shaped with broad base at external tooth enamel surface • Below dentin-enamel junction appears as mushroom-shaped or inverted triangular-shaped radiolucency	
Buccal caries	• Well defined • Ovoid-shaped radiolucency • Superimposed over dentinal aspect of tooth	

Continued

TABLE 2.5	Dental Caries/Radiographic Findings—cont'd	
Caries Detection	**Description**	**Illustration**
Root caries	• Associated gingival recession • Located above crestal bone • Radiolucency on root surface is diffuse, rounded internal border	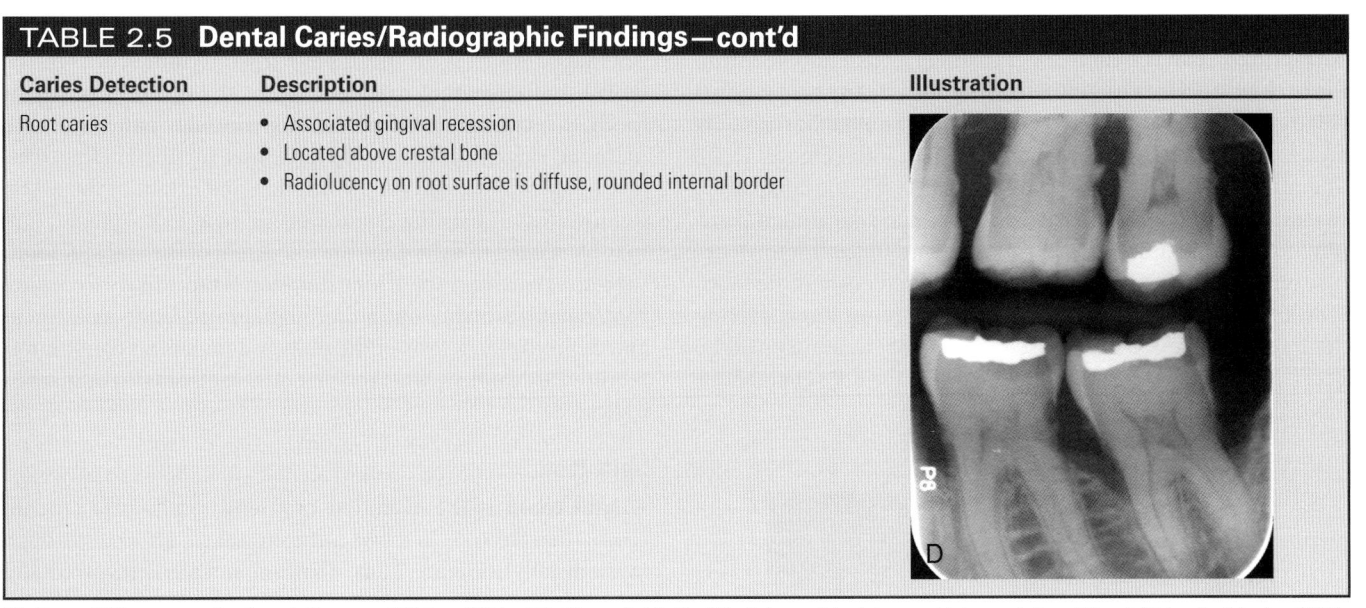

(A, B, and D) courtesy Dr. Angela Broome; **(C)** from White SC, Pharoah M. *Oral Radiology: Principles and Interpretation.* 7th ed. St Louis: Mosby: 2014.

Comparison of radiographs overtime can be used as an indicator of lesion activity if clear change is seen. Lack of change over time is an indication of lesion arrest. Caries lesions radiographically into enamel are predominantly noncavitated lesions and thus, if thought to be active, can be arrested by nonrestorative means.[13] Caries lesions at the DEJ and outer third of dentin are also mostly noncavitated lesions, with the chance of cavitation increasing with dentinal radiographic depth. Thus, a decision on caries lesion management should be made based on a combination of clinical and radiographic information (and change over time if that information is available from past records), lesion severity and activity, and caries risk of the patient.

M. TOOTH CRACKS AND FRACTURES

When the clinician identifies a fracture or crack in a tooth, it will be important to investigate its extent and thereby attempt to discern the prognosis for the tooth in question. Fractures that occur due to blunt force trauma may be horizontal, angular or vertical. Cracks or fractures that result from protracted occlusal trauma from mastication or parafunctional habits commonly cause vertical fractures that may propagate apically over time.

Aside from the risk of a catastrophic fracture that renders the tooth nonrestorable, a major concern is the potential for bacterial penetration, which can lead to inflammation and pulpal, periapical or periodontal disease. A crack may not necessarily require treatment, especially in the short term, but nevertheless the patient needs to be informed of the finding and the attendant risks. When intervention is indicated, the patient and dentist will need to decide between treatment alternatives including extraction vs root canal treatment and/ or restoration (that may have an uncertain or guarded prognosis).

Fractured teeth can present with a variety of symptoms ranging from nonexistent to acute and severe. When the bacteria reach the pulp space of a vital tooth through the fracture line, thermal symptoms will begin. If the fracture line reaches the periodontal ligament, this may cause pain in the "gum" on biting. A displaceable crack in the coronal aspect of the tooth will commonly produce an intermittent pain on biting certain foods when applied in a particular occlusal vector.

The dentist can draw on multiple evaluation techniques to discern the location and extent of the crack. Initially the clinician will proceed with pulp vitality and periapical testing. This should be followed by periodontal probing. A localized deep probing defect is usually indicative of a vertical root fracture. Next a bite test (with a Burlew wheel, cotton-tipped applicator, or Tooth Slooth™ device) can be made on each cusp to determine whether a specific location triggers more symptoms. At this point, if a fracture is visible, previous old restorations will often need to be removed to assess its full extent. Transillumination can be helpful in visualizing the location and extent of fractures. Staining the fracture with methylene blue is another option. The explorer can also be used for a tactile examination. If the fracture is significant, the segments can be sometimes wedged apart and an explorer catch can be perceived. If the fracture line extends below the gingiva, it may be advantageous to raise a gingival flap to visualize the longitudinal apical extent and thereby better assess the treatment options and their viability.

Classifying the Longitudinal Fractures and Cracks
Craze Lines

Many adult teeth exhibit **craze lines**, especially posterior teeth with large direct fill restorations (Figure. 2.21). Craze lines are seen even more frequently with advanced age. Craze lines are usually limited to the enamel and should cause the patient no pain. A craze line can be distinguished from a crack using transillumination. Light will normally penetrate enamel in the presence of a craze line, but will be blocked by a crack line that extends through the enamel to the dentin-enamel junction. No restorative treatment is required.

Fractured Cusp

A **fractured cusp** is a complete fracture of a cusp initiated from the occlusal surface, usually extending apically from a marginal ridge and a buccal or lingual groove, and wrapping horizontally around a cusp in the cervical area of the tooth (Figure. 2.22). The affected cusp may be missing or may be movable while remaining attached to the periodontal tissues. Treatment planning for this condition depends on the amount of tooth structure remaining after removal of the fractured cusp. If the tooth is deemed restorable, a direct or an indirect restoration covering the fractured margin can be used. Root canal treatment will be necessary if the fracture has encroached on the pulp chamber or has caused an irreversible pulpitis.

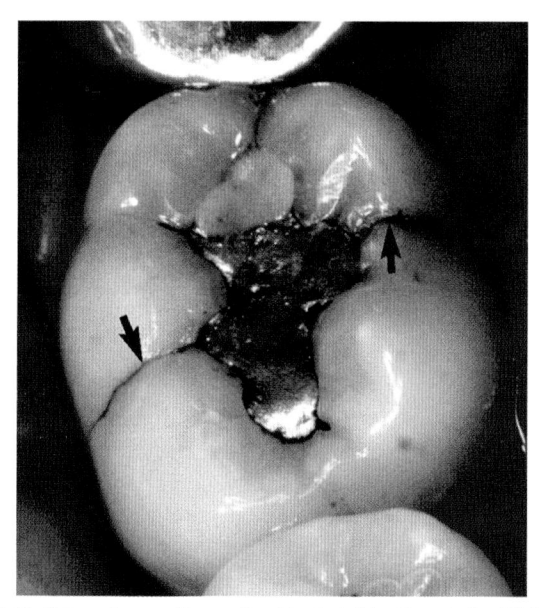

Fig. 2.21 Craze lines. (From Torabinejad M, Fouad A, Walton R. *Endodontics: Principles and Practice*. 6th ed. St Louis: Saunders; 2014.)

Cracked Tooth

A **cracked tooth** is an incomplete fracture initiated from the crown and extending apically (Figure. 2.23). On a posterior tooth the crack commonly extends through either or both marginal ridge(s) and onto the proximal surface(s). The treatment plan will depend on the location and extent of the crack. Removal of an existing restoration or new tooth preparation may be needed to determine the full extent of the crack. A tooth with an extensive crack of long duration is more likely to require root canal treatment, but a thorough and accurate assessment and definitive diagnosis of the pulp and periapical condition is required to confirm whether or not a root canal treatment is indicated.

Split Tooth

A **split tooth** is the evolution (and end result) of a cracked tooth; the fracture is now complete (through and through mesiodistally) (Figure. 2.24). The root surface is involved and the two segments are completely separate. The split may occur suddenly but more often results from deterioration of an incompletely cracked tooth. In most instances a split tooth will require extraction.

Vertical Root Fracture

A true **vertical root fracture** is a complete or incomplete fracture line initiated from the root and running parallel (or slightly oblique) to the long axis of the tooth (Figure. 2.25). It occurs most frequently in teeth that have received root canal treatment and in patients over 40 years of age. If the fracture extends coronally to the cervical periodontal attachment, a localized narrow deep periodontal defect can be detected. The only predictable treatment for a vertical root fracture is removal of the apical fractured segment or extraction of the tooth. In multirooted teeth, removal of the whole fractured root may be performed by root amputation (root resection) or hemisection.

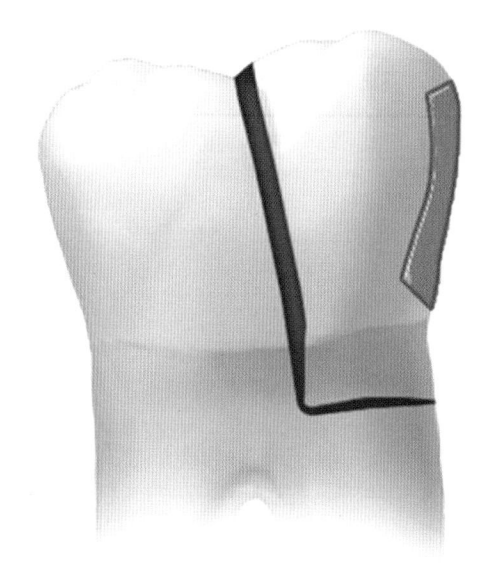 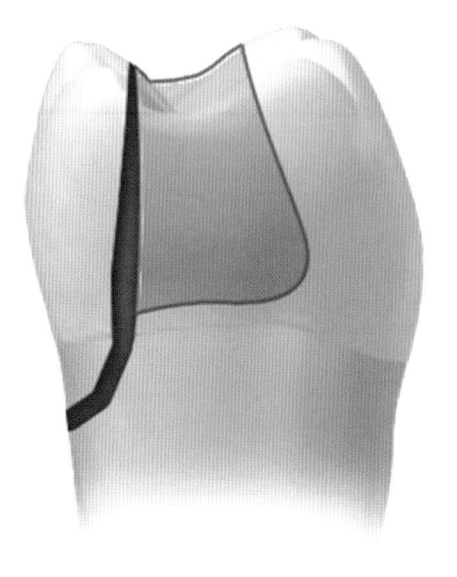

Fig. 2.22 Fractured cusp. (From Torabinejad M, Fouad A, Shabahang S. *Endodontics: Principles and Practice*. 6th ed. St Louis: Saunders; 2020.)

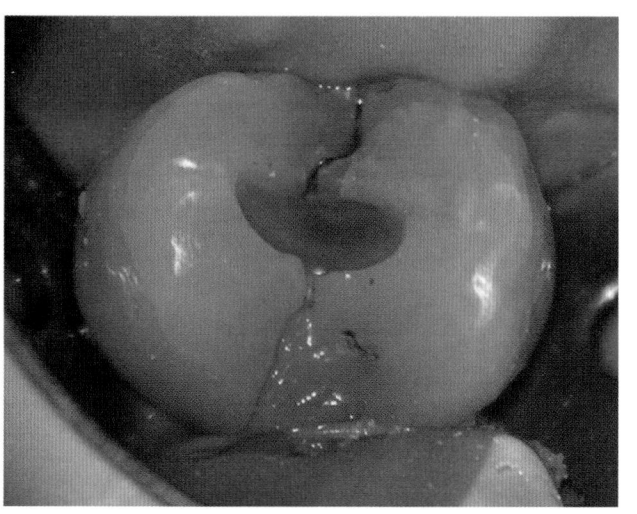

Fig. 2.23 Cracked tooth. (Courtesy Dr. Peter Tawil, Chapel Hill, NC.)

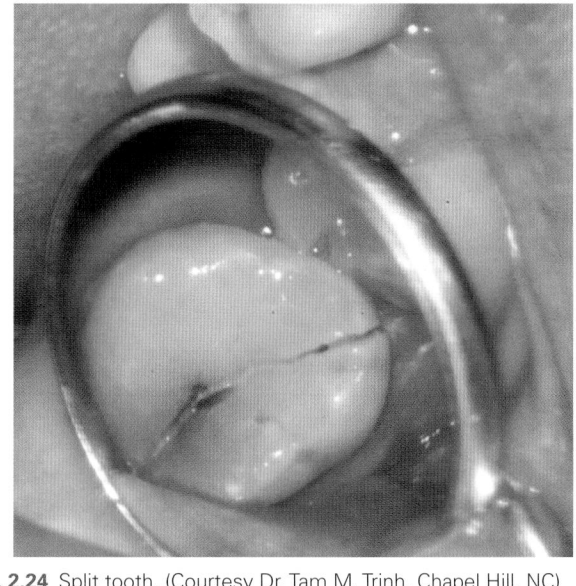

Fig. 2.24 Split tooth. (Courtesy Dr. Tam M. Trinh, Chapel Hill, NC)

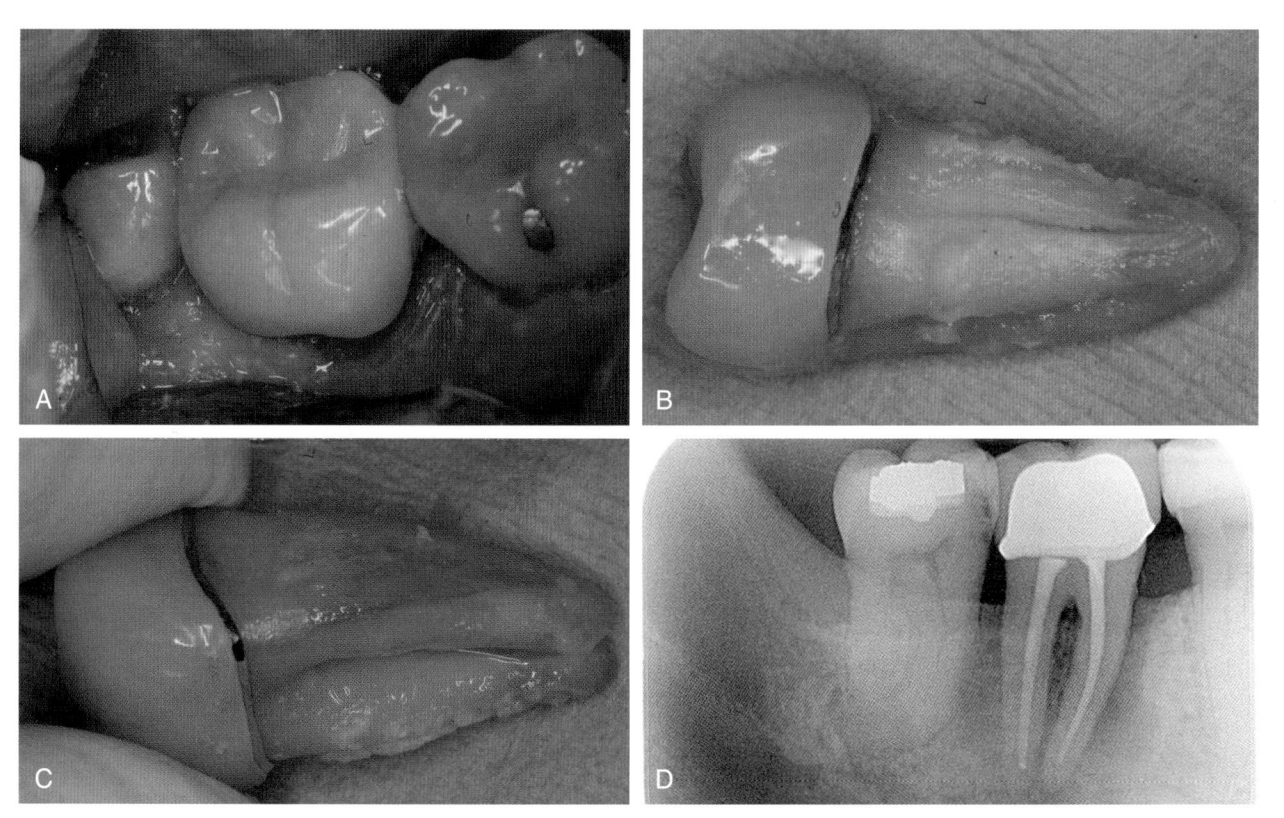

Fig. 2.25 (A–D) Tooth with vertical root fracture—mesial and the distal roots **(B and C)** both exhibit fracture lines. (Courtesy Dr. John Moriarty, Chapel Hill, NC)

N. OTHER NONCARIOUS ABNORMALITIES OF TEETH

There are many common environmentally or functionally induced abnormalities of the teeth (Table 2.6). Dental **erosion**, the loss external tooth structure due to acid exposure, has become commonplace and widespread and may result from both extrinsic and intrinsic sources. Extrinsic sources include widely available acidic drinks such as sodas, energy drinks and sports drinks. The most common intrinsic source is gastroesophageal reflux disease. Patients who suffer from sleep apnea are also at increased risk of intrinsic acid exposure in the oral cavity and the associated dental erosion. **Cervical notching** (noncarious cervical lesion) is often seen in middle aged and older individuals and may be caused by a combination of **abfraction** (occlusal forces), erosion (chemical wear)

TABLE 2.6 Other Noncarious Abnormalities of Teeth

Diagnosis	Description	Illustration	Potential Clinical Problem(s)
Erosion	Chemically induced wear of exposed enamel and/or dentin; appears as glazed thin enamel, or cupped or notched dentin		Tooth sensitivity; loss of tooth volume; darkened tooth enamel; pulpal pathology
Abfraction	Cervical notching induced by chronic traumatic occlusal forces		Tooth sensitivity; pulpal pathology; tooth fracture; caries
Abrasion	Tooth notching or wear caused by mechanical forces (e.g., toothbrush)		Tooth sensitivity; pulpal pathology; tooth fracture; caries
Attrition	Incisal/occlusal wear induced by mastication and/or bruxism		Tooth sensitivity; loss of vertical dimension of occlusion; pulpal pathology
Retained root(s)	Decoronated tooth with root or roots remaining in the jaw		Infection; periodontal disease; caries
Ankylosed tooth	Tooth root fused to bone; characterized by submersion apical to the occlusal plane, immobility, bright sound on percussion		Malocclusion; hypereruption of opposing tooth; surgical challenge if tooth is extracted

Continued

TABLE 2.6 Other Noncarious Abnormalities of Teeth—cont'd

Diagnosis	Description	Illustration	Potential Clinical Problem(s)
Developmental abnormalities (e.g., hypocalcification [pictured], hypoplasia, fever lines, amelogenesis imperfecta, fluorosis, tetracycline stain)	Defects of enamel matrix formation or calcification; commonly appears as mottled, discolored tooth, and/or porous, rough tooth surface	G	Patient has esthetic concerns; caries; risk for tooth fracture and enamel shearing
Impacted tooth	Tooth (commonly a third molar) incompletely erupted and maintained in an abnormal position by adjacent tooth or teeth	H	Surgical complications (sinus perforation, paresthesia); potential postoperative complications (infection, dry socket)
Hypercementosis	Overgrowth of the cementum layer of a tooth (usually at the apex of the tooth)	I	Surgical challenge if tooth is being extracted
Supernumerary tooth	Tooth additional to the normal complement (e.g., paramolar or mesiodens); commonly diminutive in size	J	May displace surrounding tooth or teeth; malposition of teeth; malocclusion
Odontoma	Developmental abnormality of irregular but definable tooth components (compound odontoma), or no defined tooth shape and undifferentiated mass of enamel, dentin, and pulp components (complex odontoma)	K	May impede normal eruption of adjacent teeth

From **(A and G)** Heymann HO, Swift EJ, Ritter AV. *Sturdevant's Art and Science of Operative Dentistry*. 6th ed. St Louis: Mosby; 2013. **(B–D, F, H, J, K)** Ibsen OAC, Phelan JA. *Oral Pathology for the Dental Hygienist*. 6th ed. St Louis: Saunders; 2014. **(E)** Costich ER, White RP Jr. *Fundamentals of Oral Surgery*. Philadelphia: Saunders; 1971. **(I)** Iannucci (PER COURTNEY)

and **abrasion** (mechanical forces such as aggressive frequent horizontal tooth brushing). **Attrition** is common in individuals who consume a coarse and abrasive diet, or those with **parafunctional habits** such as bruxing or clenching.

Common developmental anomalies of the teeth include **hypoplasia** and **hypocalcification**, "fever lines," **fluorosis**, **tetracycline stain**, and **amelogenesis imperfecta**. These conditions are evident clinically. **Odontomas** and **hypercementosis** are developmental processes that will be visible on radiographic imaging.

This category also includes abnormalities of tooth number and position including **supernumerary teeth** (paramolar); **impacted teeth**; **ankylosed**, submerged, or partially erupted teeth; and **ectopic eruption**.

O. OCCLUSAL ABNORMALITIES

Occlusal abnormalities include jaw and skeletal relationships that do not conform to a normal profile such as angle classification II (maxillary protrusion or "buck tooth") or angle classification III (mandibular protrusion or "Dick Tracy"). Other common occlusal abnormalities are malpositioned individual teeth within the dental arch and abnormal relationships between approximating teeth; and abnormalities in the interdigitation of the teeth in **maximum intercuspation (MI)** or during excursive jaw movements. This category also includes **clenching**, **bruxism**, and the ill effects of excessive or otherwise abnormal occlusal forces on the dentition and periodontium. Table 2.7 summarizes the more common occlusal abnormalities.

TABLE 2.7	Occlusal Abnormalities		
Diagnosis	**Description**	**Illustration**	**Potential Clinical Problem(s)**
Tooth malalignment / malpositioning	Crowding, tipping, drifting, rotation		Esthetic, functional, or periodontal problems
Marginal ridge discrepancies	Proximating marginal ridges at differing levels		Food impaction; periodontal problems
Open proximal contacts	Proximating teeth not in contact		Food impaction; periodontal problems
Extrusion/hypereruption	Tooth migrates vertically into space left by missing tooth		Esthetic problem; unfavorable crown-root ratio; tissue impingement
Occlusal plane discrepancies	Irregular or imbalanced occlusal plane (e.g., reverse curve of Spee; extrusion of tooth or bone base)		TMD; may require occlusal adjustment or reconstruction prior to fabrication of prosthesis
Skeletal malalignment	Maxillary and mandibular jaws incorrectly aligned relative to each other		Esthetic or functional problem; may require compre-hensive orthodontics and/ or orthognathic surgery
Reduced vertical dimension of occlusion [VDO]	Reduced interarch space when teeth are occluded in maximum Intercuspation		TMD; impaired function; may require reconstruction prior to fabrication of prosthesis

Continued

TABLE 2.7	Occlusal Abnormalities—cont'd		
Diagnosis	**Description**	**Illustration**	**Potential Clinical Problem(s)**
Primary occlusal trauma	Occlusal forces in excess of what tooth or attachment apparatus can tolerate in otherwise healthy periodontium	NA	Acute symptoms (see Chapter 9); compromised periodontal support; pulpal pathology; tooth fracture; tooth loss
Secondary occlusal trauma	Occlusal forces in excess of attachment apparatus tolerance in presence of compromised periodontium (clinical attachment loss)	NA	Compromised periodontal support; pulpal pathology; tooth loss
Clenching/bruxism/parafunction	Occlusal contact that occurs outside of masticatory function	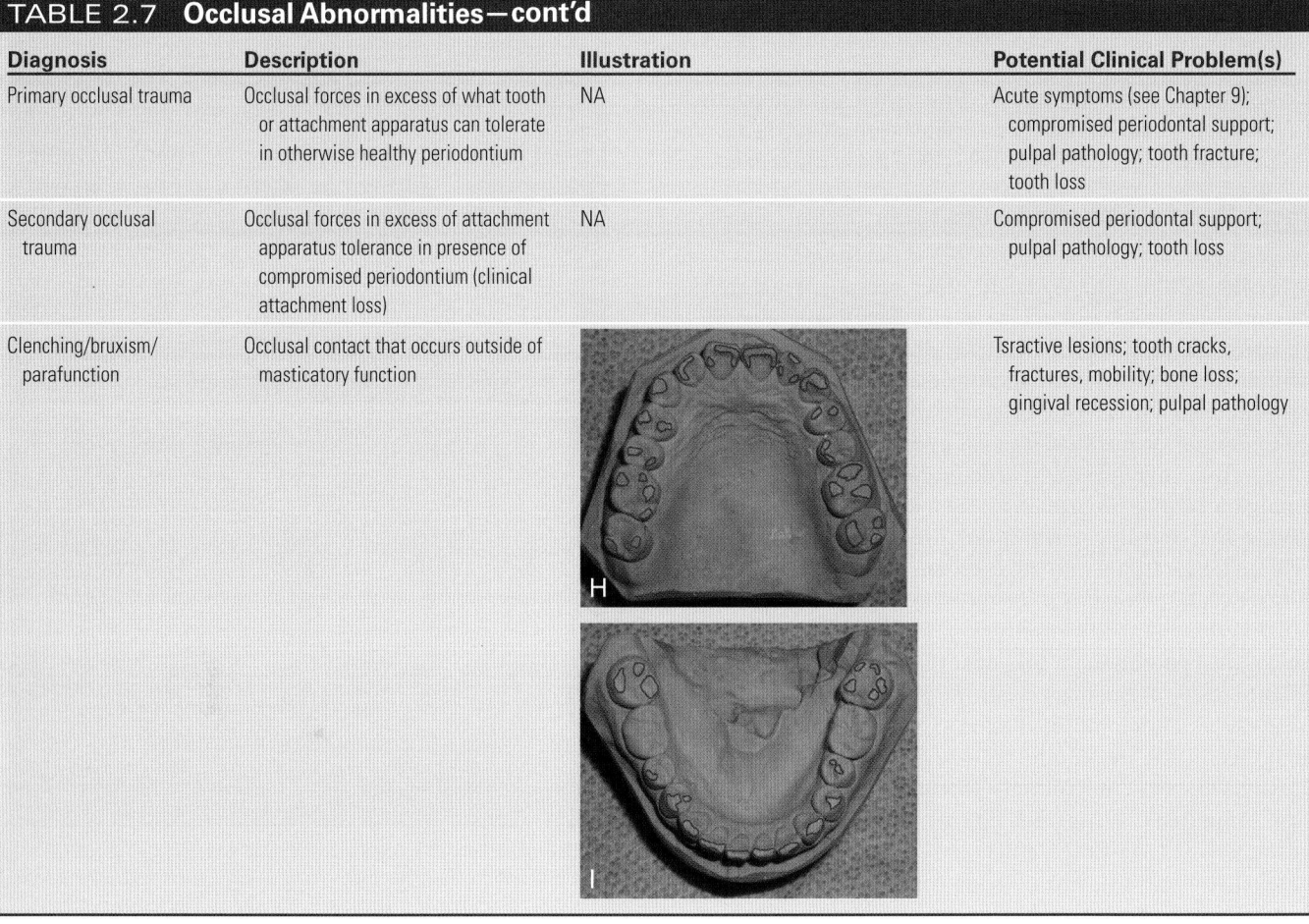	Tsractive lesions; tooth cracks, fractures, mobility; bone loss; gingival recession; pulpal pathology

TMD, Temporomandibular disorders.
Image of skeletal malalignment from Proffit WR, Fields HW, Sarver DM. *Contemporary Orthodontics.* 6th ed. St Louis: Mosby; 2018.

P. ESTHETIC PROBLEMS

Patients sometimes present with concerns relating to the appearance of the face, mouth, smile, teeth, or gums. The dental team must be responsive to those concerns and must be able to discern the underlying cause of the patient's perceived problem. Esthetic problems generally can be classified into one of three categories: (1) problems that emanate from abnormal skeletal structures or relationships; (2) problems relating to tooth position, form, or color; and (3) problems relating to the periodontium and lips. A patient may exhibit problems from one, two, or all three of these categories. The following discussion summarizes common esthetic concerns that may be apparent to the patient and/or the dentist.

Dentofacial Issues

Dentofacial issues are usually esthetic problems caused by abnormal size or contour of the jaw bones or malposition of the maxilla or mandible relative to the face or to the opposing jaw. Often these problems are developmental in origin and in some cases are part of a syndrome or complex of genetically induced abnormalities. Occasionally these skeletal changes are caused by

trauma to the face or as a result of surgical treatment to eliminate cancer of the jaw. Pediatric sleep disorders are now also believed to be the cause of some dentofacial malformations. The following are brief descriptions of the more common problems in this category:

Lateral facial asymmetry: the left and right sides of the jaws or face are not symmetric

Vertical facial asymmetry: middle and inferior thirds of face are out of proportion with each other

Angle classification II relationship: protrusive (or procumbent) maxilla; "buck teeth"; may be the result of a retruded mandible

Angle classification III relationship: protrusive (or prognathic) mandible and/or retrognathic maxilla; may exhibit anterior crossbite

Narrow maxillary arch development: often this is characterized by **excess buccal corridor display**; patient may exhibit a bilateral posterior crossbite

Misaligned dental midline: the dental midline is not coincident with the facial midline (note that this can be caused by a malpositioned tooth and/or by a maxillary arch form abnormality)

Tipped frontal occlusal plane: maxillary anterior incisal edge plane is not parallel to the horizontal plane or the plane of the interpupillary line

Dentoalveolar extrusion and vertical maxillary excess: these bony abnormalities may be associated with altered facial profile, malalignment of teeth, or occlusal plane discrepancies

Tooth-Related Esthetic Issues

The **esthetic zone** is that portion of the dentition that is readily visible to the patient and to other persons. Fractured or missing teeth in the esthetic zone may be a major concern to a patient and may cause personal embarrassment, loss of self-confidence, or limit social and professional activities. Visible caries lesions can also be of concern. Some patients exhibit discoloration or intrinsic stain of a tooth or teeth caused by tetracycline, hypoplasia, decalcification, pulp necrosis, or **amalgam bluing** (Figure. 2.26). Some patients will, in time, decide that metallic restorations are unsightly and tooth-colored restorations may take on an unesthetic appearance (Figure. 2.27). Composite restorations may develop surface roughness or porosity resulting in staining, changes in the hue of the restoration, or loss of surface luster. **Microleakage** (Figure. 2.28) at the margins of the restoration can also lead to areas of discoloration. Patients may become concerned about teeth that are an unusual size or contour; for example, fan-shaped teeth, microdonts (including "peg lateral incisors") (Figure. 2.29), or teeth that are large relative to the size of the jaw or face. Patients may seek correction for teeth or coronal restorations with bulbous contours. Patients may be aware that their teeth appear to be "too high" or "too low," "too far forward" or" too far back," which may or may not reflect an underlying skeletal abnormality. Many patients will be interested in closing spaces between the teeth, **diastemas** (Figure. 2.30), or in straightening teeth that are tipped, rotated, crowded, or otherwise misaligned. It is not unusual for patients to seek correction for age- and function-related changes such as craze lines, attrition, incisal chipping, or altered occlusal plane contours. Some patients will raise concerns relating to a tipped occlusal horizontal plane, in which the maxillary incisal edge line is no longer parallel to the horizontal plane, or the mandibular anterior occlusal plane no longer follows the lower lip line.

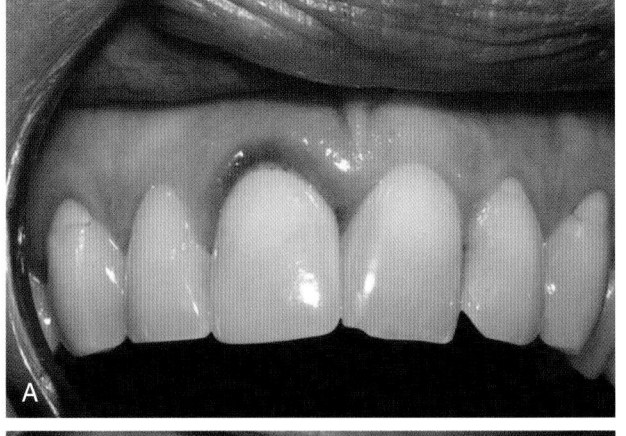

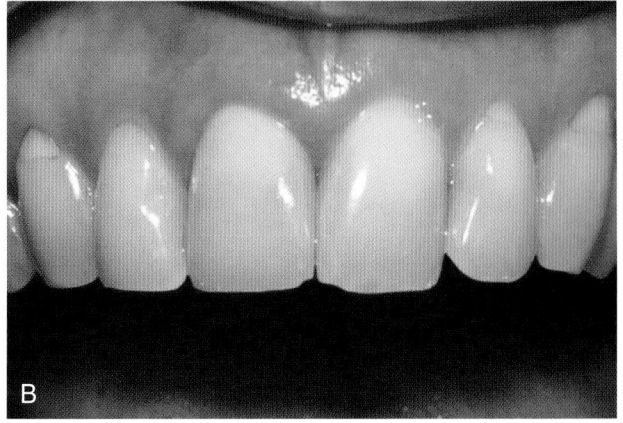

Fig. 2.27 (A) Unesthetic, poorly contoured, and unhygienic full coverage restoration. **(B)** Replacement restoration—note the improved shade, incisal contour, and gingival response. (Courtesy Dr. BE Kanoy, Durham, NC)

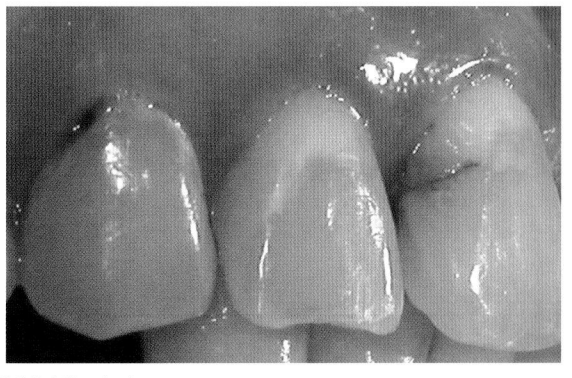

Fig. 2.28 Microleakage.

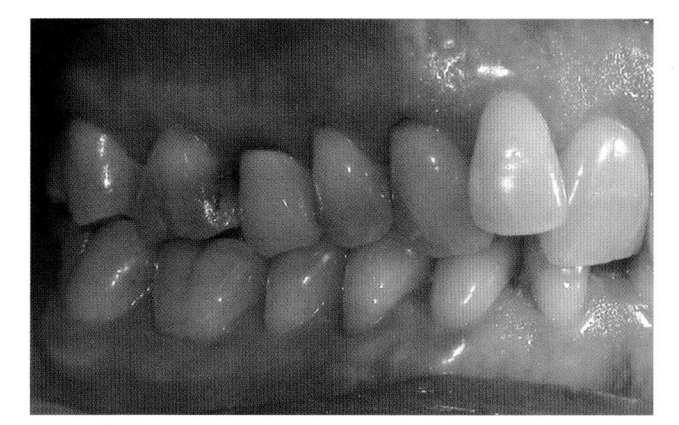

Fig. 2.26 Amalgam bluing.

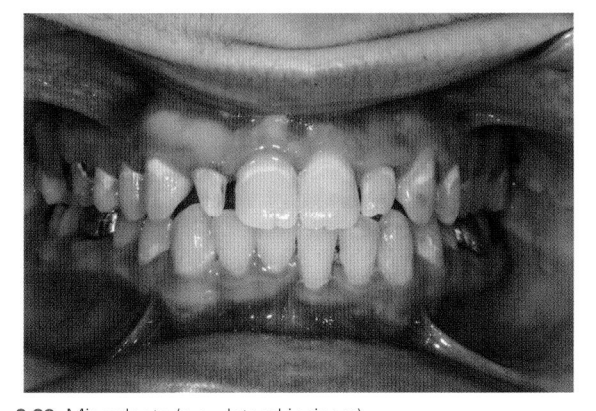

Fig. 2.29 Microdonts (e.g., lateral incisors).

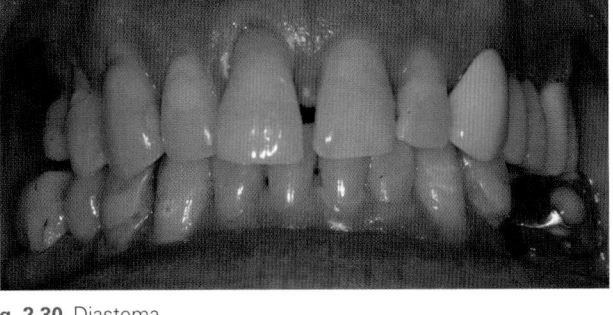

Fig. 2.30 Diastema.

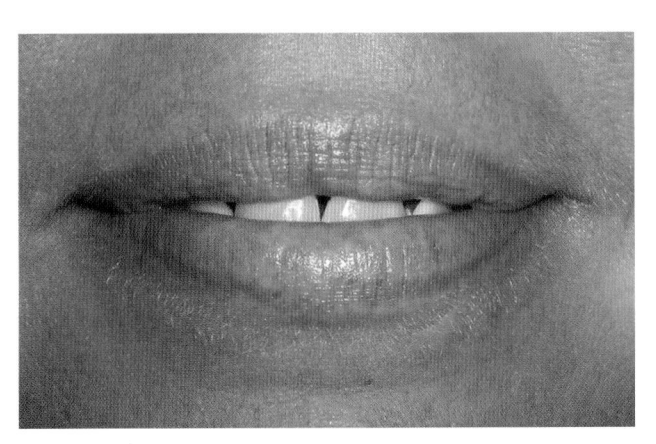

Fig. 2.31 Lip incompetence.

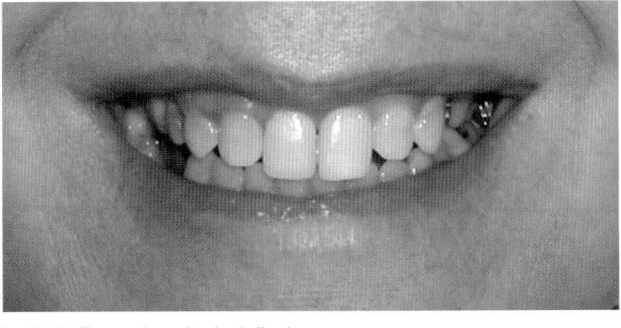

Fig. 2.32 Excessive gingival display.

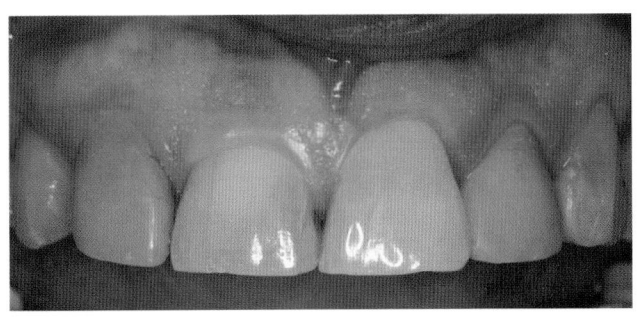

Fig. 2.33 Uneven gingival zeniths.

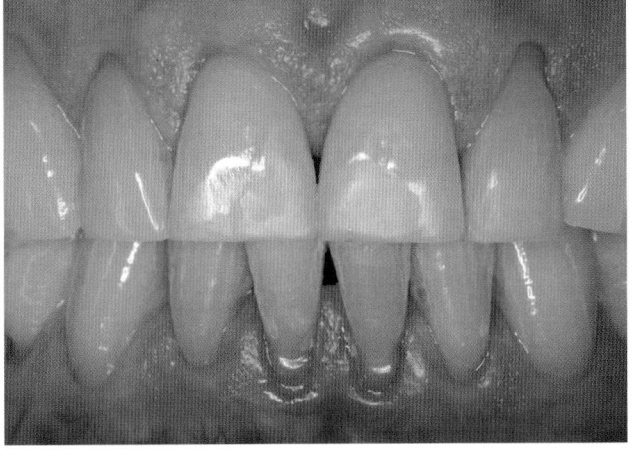

Fig. 2.34 Black triangles.

Lip and Gingival Esthetic Issues

Patients may present with esthetic concerns related to the position of the lips or gingival tissues. Common problems in this category include:

- A short upper lip or over contoured maxillary anterior restorations may lead to a larger than normal display of the facial surfaces of the maxillary anterior teeth when the patient's face is at repose. This condition is known as **lip incompetence** (Figure. 2.31). These patients may develop the self-conscious habit of rolling the lip down over the incisal edges in an effort to disguise the "toothy" appearance.
- Excess lip mobility or **hyperactive lip** is evident when the lip raises above the gingival margins of the maxillary anterior teeth as the patient is speaking or smiling.
- **Excessive gingival display** (Figure. 2.32) of the maxillary anterior teeth can be caused by a prominent maxilla, short

upper lip, hyperactive lip, short clinical crowns, or hypertrophic or hyperplastic gingiva.

- Gingival scalloping or form irregularities include **uneven gingival zeniths** (Figure. 2.33) and other gingival contour disparities with the opposing side of the arch.
- **Black triangles** (Figure. 2.34) are caused by gingival recession and the exposure of interproximal spaces at the cervical portion of the teeth.

Q. SINGLE TOOTH RESTORATION DEFECTS

This section details commonly encountered problems with single tooth restorations (Table 2.8). Some of these issues arise at the time of restoration placement and some will occur years or even decades later. Some are iatrogenic in nature and others are part of the normal life cycle of a restoration.

R. FIXED PROSTHODONTIC PROBLEMS

When a patient has a missing tooth or teeth with remaining teeth on both sides of the edentulous space, that area is referred to as a **bounded edentulous space (BES)**. When the BES is in the **esthetic zone**, the patient will often be self-conscious about it and have a strong desire to replace it. The missing tooth or teeth may result in an altered chewing pattern, loss of lip support, lip

TABLE 2.8   Single Tooth Restoration Defects

Diagnosis	Description	Illustration	Possible Significance
Overhang	Margin of restoration extends outside the confines of the tooth contour		Food impaction; acute or chronic periodontal disease; secondary caries
Underhang	Margin of restoration is closed but under-contoured		Food impaction; acute or chronic periodontal disease; secondary caries
Discoloration (body of restoration)	Restoration shade does not match shade of adjacent tooth structure	Note: MF restoration maxillary right lateral incisor	Patient may elect replacement
Marginal defects (gaps)	Extrinsic stain or microleakage at restoration margin; visual and tactile discontinuity at the tooth-restoration interface	Gingival margin MF maxillary left lateral incisor	May need restoration repair or replacement
Fractured restoration (amalgam/ composite/ ceramic)	Bulk fracture; fractured isthmus; missing sliver of restorative material		May need restoration repair or replacement

Continued

TABLE 2.8   Single Tooth Restoration Defects—cont'd

Diagnosis	Description	Illustration	Possible Significance
		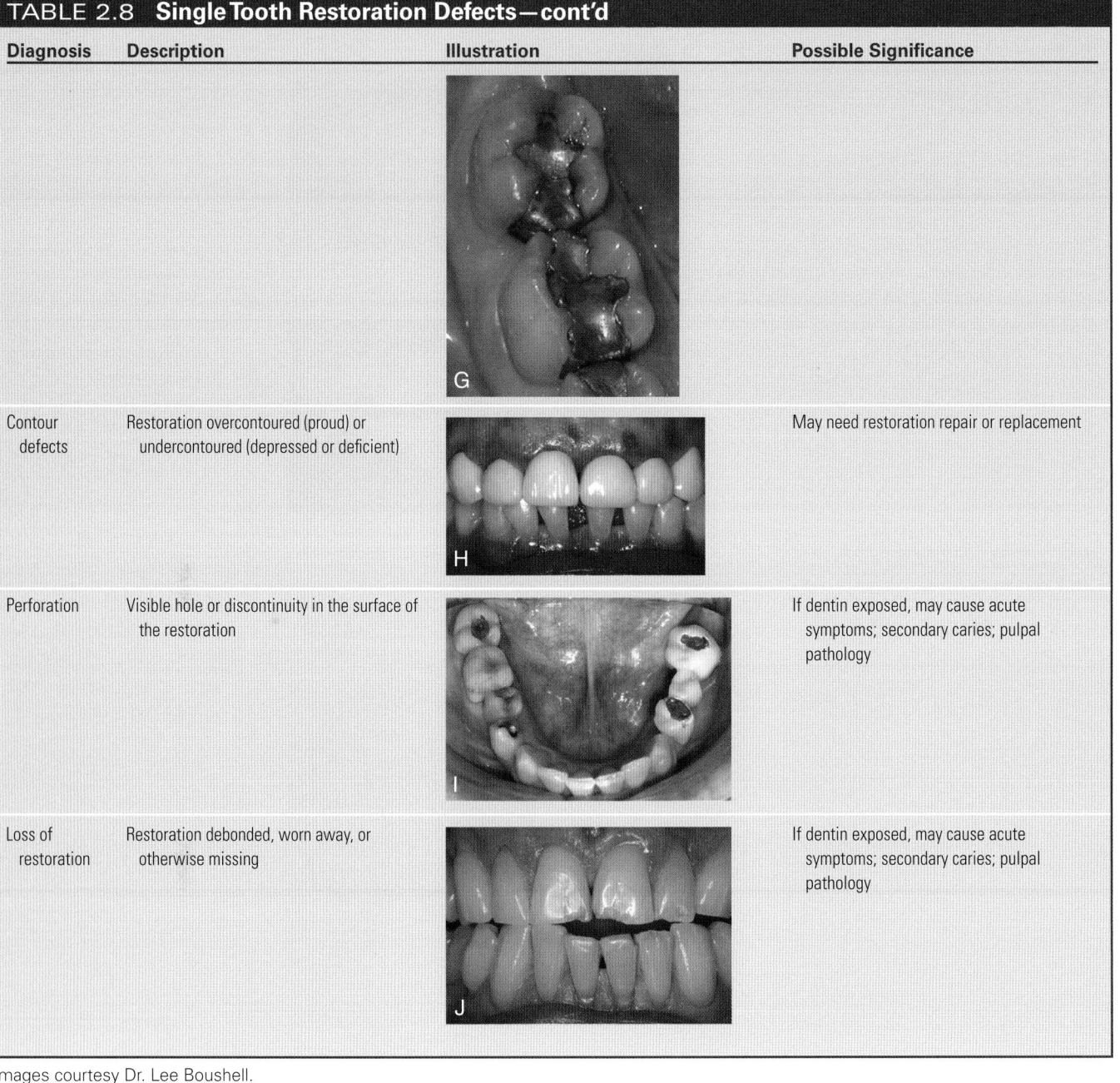	
Contour defects	Restoration overcontoured (proud) or undercontoured (depressed or deficient)		May need restoration repair or replacement
Perforation	Visible hole or discontinuity in the surface of the restoration		If dentin exposed, may cause acute symptoms; secondary caries; pulpal pathology
Loss of restoration	Restoration debonded, worn away, or otherwise missing		If dentin exposed, may cause acute symptoms; secondary caries; pulpal pathology

Images courtesy Dr. Lee Boushell.

or cheek biting, or recurring trauma to the edentulous ridge. In time the BES may result in extrusion of an opposing tooth or tipping of the adjacent teeth. If the patient wishes to replace the missing tooth or teeth, several treatment options are available. These options, and their indications and contraindications, are discussed in detail in Chapter 11.

When the BES has been restored, multiple other problems may arise that the dentist will be called upon to address. If the fixed prosthesis has natural tooth abutments, the abutment teeth are subject to secondary caries, advancing periodontal disease, tooth fracture, pulpal necrosis, occlusal trauma, and fracture of the various materials and components of the prosthesis. The role of the dentist in such cases is to diagnose the nature of the problem or defect, determine the underlying cause, discern the available treatment alternatives, and explain those alternatives to the patient with sufficient detail that he or she is prepared to make an informed treatment decision. Table 2.9 describes common problems associated with fixed dental prostheses.

S. REMOVABLE PROSTHODONTIC PROBLEMS

If there are no remaining natural teeth in the mouth, the patient is categorized as **edentulous** or **edentate**. If a dentate patient has missing teeth with no teeth remaining posterior to the edentulous space, that area is referred to as an *unbounded edentulous*

TABLE 2.9 Fixed Prosthodontic Problems

Diagnosis	Description	Illustration	Possible Significance
Partial edentulism— bounded edentulous space	Tooth or teeth missing with tooth or teeth present on both sides of the edentulous space		Esthetic or functional problem; malposition of adjacent or opposing tooth; trauma to gingiva, lip, or cheek
Fractured abutment tooth	Includes cracked tooth, split tooth, vertical root fracture (see Section L, Tooth Cracks & Fractures)		Extraction usually necessary
Recurrent caries	Secondary caries		Restoration or extraction required; root canal treatment may be necessary; if crown, may need replacement; may cause premature tooth loss
Occlusal trauma	(see Section O, Occlusal Abnormalities)		Attrition, tooth fracture; premature tooth loss
Broken connector/pontic	Material fracture or loss; separation of the FPD components		Loss of prosthesis (repair usually not feasible)
Debonded retainer	Retainer now can be separated from the abutment tooth		Need section and remove retainer; loss of prosthesis
Fractured restorative material	Portion of restoration (usually porcelain) detached from the remainder of the crown restoration or tooth		Esthetic problem; deficient tooth form; trauma to oral tissues; may necessitate repair or replacement restoration
Esthetic issues	Secondary caries, poor shade match, black triangles (see Section P, ESTHETIC PROBLEMS)		May necessitate repair or replacement of prosthesis

(B and G) courtesy Dr. Carlos H. Barrero, Chapel Hill, NC; (C) courtesy Dr. Sompop Bencharit, Chapel Hill, NC; (D-F) courtesy Dr. Elana Celliers, Chapel Hill, NC.

space (**UES**). As with a BES, when the UES is in the esthetic zone, the patient will usually be concerned about it. In addition, an edentate patient or a patient with an UES has the potential for significantly compromised function, reduced chewing ability, and loss of *vertical dimension of occlusion* (VDO), with accompanying changes in facial profile and contour and lip support. The UES patient may also be subject to lip or cheek biting, trauma to the tissues of the edentulous ridge, accelerated ridge resorption, and in time, extrusion of any teeth opposing the space. Treatment options for edentate and partially dentate patients, and their indications and contraindications, are detailed in Chapter 11.

Patients will often present to an initial appointment with an existing denture or removable partial denture. Common problems with a removable prosthesis include: lack of retention; denture sores (traumatic ulcers); excessive occlusal wear or occlusal disharmony; and fractures of the denture base, denture teeth, clasps, or other framework components. If the prosthesis utilizes natural tooth abutments, the abutment teeth are subject to secondary caries, advancing periodontal disease, tooth fracture, pulpal necrosis, occlusal trauma, or fracture of the various materials or components. Table 2.10 outlines common problems associated with removable dental prostheses.

TABLE 2.10 Removable Prosthodontic Issues

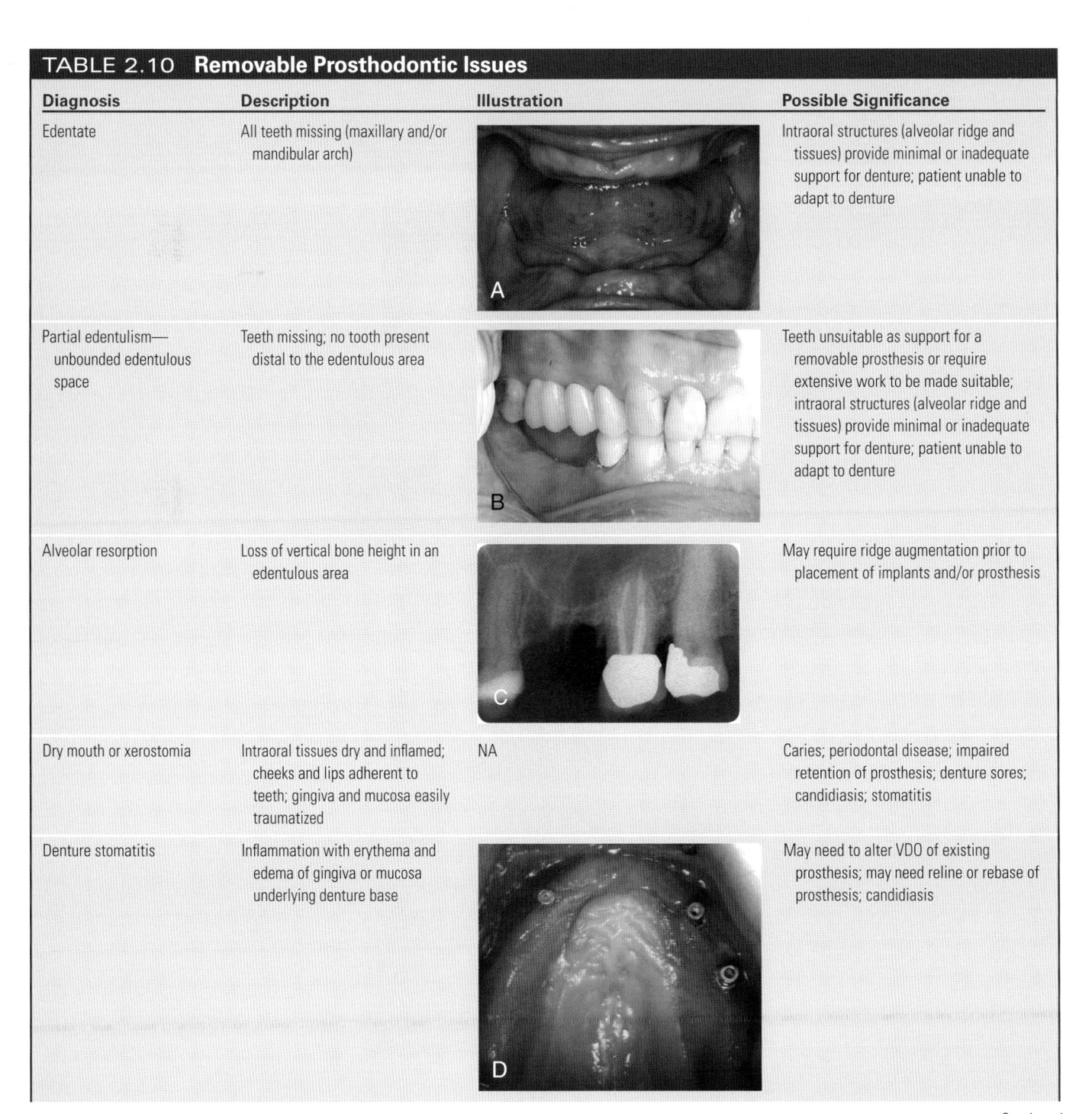

Diagnosis	Description	Illustration	Possible Significance
Edentate	All teeth missing (maxillary and/or mandibular arch)	A	Intraoral structures (alveolar ridge and tissues) provide minimal or inadequate support for denture; patient unable to adapt to denture
Partial edentulism— unbounded edentulous space	Teeth missing; no tooth present distal to the edentulous area	B	Teeth unsuitable as support for a removable prosthesis or require extensive work to be made suitable; intraoral structures (alveolar ridge and tissues) provide minimal or inadequate support for denture; patient unable to adapt to denture
Alveolar resorption	Loss of vertical bone height in an edentulous area	C	May require ridge augmentation prior to placement of implants and/or prosthesis
Dry mouth or xerostomia	Intraoral tissues dry and inflamed; cheeks and lips adherent to teeth; gingiva and mucosa easily traumatized	NA	Caries; periodontal disease; impaired retention of prosthesis; denture sores; candidiasis; stomatitis
Denture stomatitis	Inflammation with erythema and edema of gingiva or mucosa underlying denture base	D	May need to alter VDO of existing prosthesis; may need reline or rebase of prosthesis; candidiasis

Continued

TABLE 2.10 Removable Prosthodontic Issues—cont'd

Diagnosis	Description	Illustration	Possible Significance
Inflammatory fibrous hyperplasia (epulis fissuratum)	Fibrous hyperplasia adjacent to the periphery of a denture flange	E	May require surgical correction
Denture sore (frictional or decubitous ulcer)	Traumatic ulcer under the base or periphery of a denture	F	May need to adjust occlusion and/or denture base
Denture base defects	Visible but nondisplaced crack, fracture with partial separation, or portion of denture base fractured and missing	G	May require repair or replacement
Denture tooth defects	Denture teeth severely worn (attrition), broken, or missing	H	Individual teeth can be replaced; generalized tooth wear often requires new prosthesis
Partial denture clasp defects	Clasp tip does not engage undercut (not retentive); broken clasp	I	Clasp adjustment or repair necessary, or prosthesis replacement
Infraocclusion	Single tooth or multiple teeth not in contact with the opposing tooth or teeth	J	Restoration of natural or denture teeth needed

Continued

TABLE 2.10   Removable Prosthodontic Issues—cont'd

Diagnosis	Description	Illustration	Possible Significance
Complications with abutment teeth	Caries, periodontal disease, pulpal pathology, inadequate crown:root ratio		Extensive treatment may be required to retain tooth; tooth loss
Esthetic issues	Prosthetic tooth shade, alignment and position, midline, occlusal plane)		New prosthesis needed to resolve many of these problems
Maladaptation	Patient inability to accept and effectively use the prosthesis		May be resolved with implant-retained prosthesis
Excessive or deficient vertical dimension of occlusion (VDO)	VDO too great (insufficient freeway space) or VDO diminished (too much freeway space)	NA	New prosthesis necessary to resolve this problem

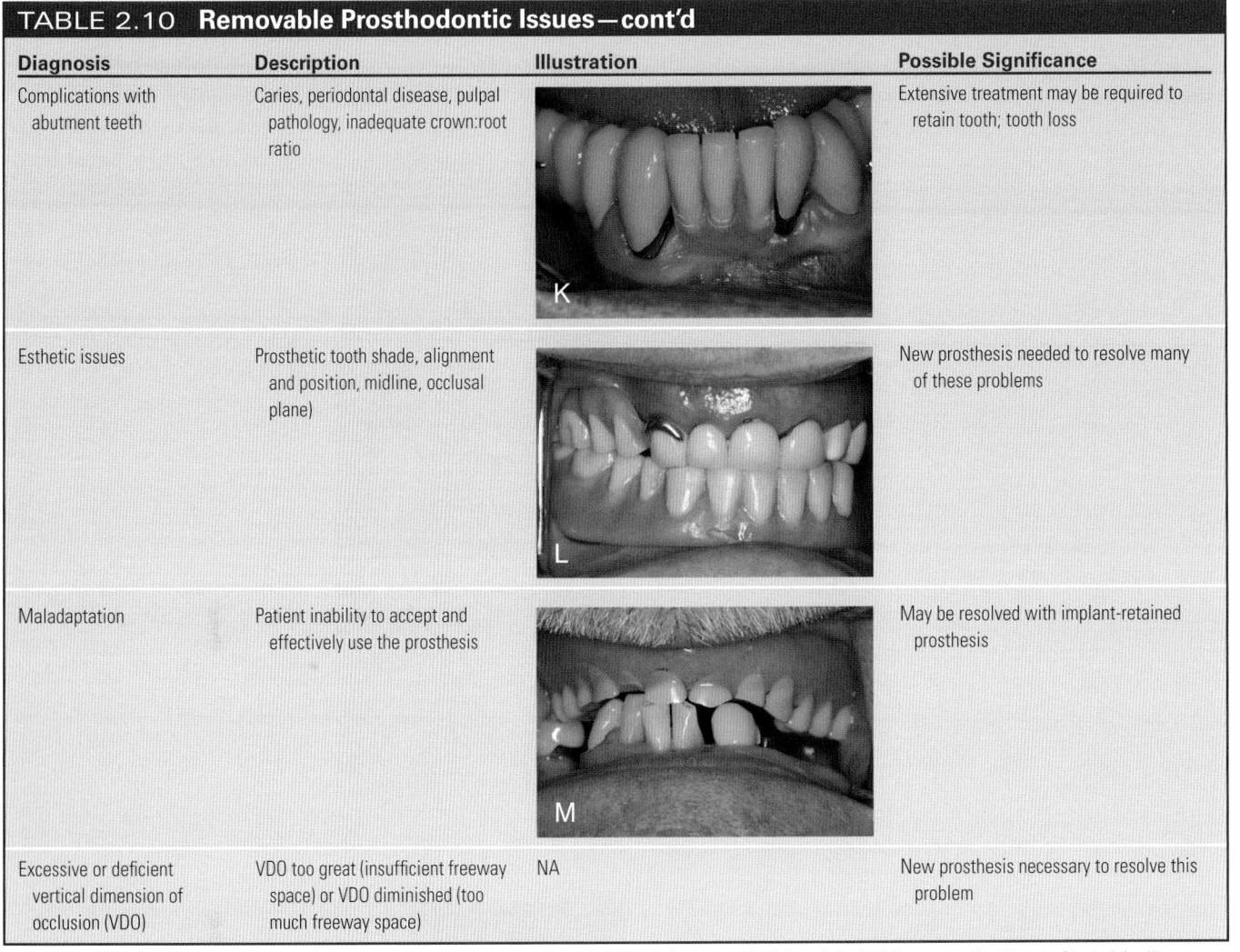

(**A, B, D, F, H, I, K, L**) courtesy Dr. Carlos H. Barrero; (**C**) from Geminiani A, Papadimitriou DEV, Ercoli C; (**G**) Courtesy Dr Wendy Clark. Maxillary sinus augmentation with a sonic handpiece for the osteotomy of the lateral window: a clinical report. *J Prosthet Dent* 2011:106(5):279–283; (**E**) from Sapp JP, Eversole LR. *Contemporary Oral and Maxillofacial Pathology*. 2nd ed. St Louis: Mosby; 2004; (**J**) Giachetti L, Bertini F, Landi D. Morphological and functional rehabilitation of severely infra-occluded primary molars in the presence of aplasia of the permanent premolar: a clinical report. *J Prosthet Dent* 2005:93(2):121–124.

T. IMPLANT-RELATED DIAGNOSES

Common clinical problems may arise as a result of implant placement or may develop with the implant fixture or the implant-retained prosthesis in subsequent months and years. Implant site excavation that invades the mandibular canal space may cause paresthesia. Implant fixture placement may infringe on the floor of the maxillary sinus, necessitating a **transalveolar sinus floor elevation** (aka osteotome sinus lift) or **lateral window sinus floor elevation** (aka lateral window sinus lift) procedure. Postoperative infection may occur. **Augmentation** procedures are not always successful in achieving the desired bone shape and height.

After initial healing and in the years that follow, the implant fixture may be susceptible to **peri-implant mucositis** or **peri-implantitis** (see Section J earlier in this chapter). When peri-implantitis occurs shortly after cementation of an implant crown, the most probable cause is retained excess cement.

When the peri-implantitis affects the **osseointegration** of the embedded portions of an implant fixture, the fixture may become mobile and removal may be necessary. Implant fixtures may fracture and, if the implant is critical to the retention of the prosthesis, the broken implant must be removed and replaced. Alternatively, a substitute implant may be placed in another location.

A variety of problems may occur with implant restorations including debonding of a cemented prosthesis and fracture of ceramic restorative material. Abutments may fracture. The screw on a screw-retained abutment or crown may break or loosen. Proximal contacts may open with teeth adjacent to the implant.[59] Implant-retained removable prostheses are subject to the same problems as described earlier for nonimplant retained dentures and removable partial dentures.

Table 2.11 summarizes common clinical problems associated with implants and implant-retained prostheses and their possible significance.

TABLE 2.11   Implant-Related Diagnoses

Diagnosis	Description	Illustration	Possible Significance
Paresthesia	Iatrogenic damage to nerve during implant placement	NA	Prolonged or permanent paresthesia
Peri-implantitis	Infection of the peri-implant tissues		May require surgical therapy to resolve; loss of the implant
Fractured fixture	Angular or horizontal fracture of the implant fixture; often appears as isolated deep pocket		Loss of implant
Fractured abutment	Angular or horizontal fracture of the implant abutment		Need to replace abutment; if custom abutment, will also need to replace the coronal restoration
Debonded cement-retained crown	Crown separated from the abutment (abutment still attached to implant fixture)	NA	Usually possible to re-cement the crown or retainer
Mobile screw-retained abutment or crown	Crown no longer firmly attached to implant fixture; usually result of loose or broken screw		Occlusal access to screw necessary—if screw is broken, remove remaining portion; re-torque or replace screw; crown or retainer replacement may be necessary; if screw cannot be removed without damaging fixture threads, may need replace implant fixture
Fractured implant-retained crown	Portion of crown restoration (usually porcelain) detached from the remainder of the crown restoration or abutment		Esthetic problem; deficient tooth form; trauma to oral tissues; loss of restoration; usually need to replace crown
Worn or missing retention cap	Compromised denture retention	NA	Need to replace retention cap

From **A**, Ascenzi M, Reilly GC. Bone tissue: hierarchical simulations for clinical applications. *J Biomech.* 2011:44(2):211–212; **B**, Conrad HJ, Schulte JK, Vallee MC. Fractures related to occlusal overload with single posterior implants: a clinical report. *J Prosthet Dent.* 2008:99(4):251–256; **C**, Pow EHN, Wat, PYP. A technique for salvaging an implant-supported crown with a fractured abutment screw. *J Prosthet Dent.* 2006:95(2):169–170; **D**, courtesy Dr. Carlos H. Barrero; **E**, courtesy Dr. Ibrahim Duqum.

REVIEW QUESTIONS

- What are the benefits of creating a diagnosis list?
- What is the relationship between a patient's diagnosis and their treatment plan?
- What should be included in a patient's diagnosis?
- What are common psychosocial issues that will shape a patient's treatment plan?
- What are the categories of jaw abnormalities? Which radiographic signs differentiate the categories?
- What are the signs and symptoms are commonly associated with TMD?
- What are the signs and symptoms are commonly associated with sleep disorders?
- Demonstrate how periodontitis is staged and graded. What is meant by reduced periodontium and how is it related to a periodontal diagnosis?
- Define and describe the diagnoses for pulpal and apical tissues in the American Association of Endodontists (AAE) classification system.
- How are caries lesions identified and classified?

- Identify and describe the common types of tooth cracks and fractures.
- What occlusal problems are commonly encountered in patients? How are each of those problems recognized and diagnosed?
- What dental and facial esthetic problems are commonly encountered in patients? How are each of those problems recognized and diagnosed?
- List single tooth restorative defects commonly found in patients. How might each of these cause problems for the patient?
- What are some common problems that may occur in conjunction with fixed dental prostheses? What impact might each of these have on the patient?
- What are some common problems that can occur in conjunction with removable dental prostheses? What impact might each of these have on the patient?
- List common problems associated with implants. Describe the possible negative outcomes that can arise with each of these problems.

REFERENCES

1. my.clevelandclinic.org
2. Hannah VE, O'Donnell L, Robertson D, Ramage G. Denture Stomatitis: Causes, Cures and Prevention. *Prim Dent J.* 2017
3. Mosby's Dental Dictionary. Amsterdam: Elsevier; 2020. 4th ed.
4. Wetzel SL, Wollenberg J. Oral Potentially Malignant Disorders. *Dent Clin North Am.* 2020;64(1):25–37.
5. Gougousis S, Mouchtaropoulou E, Besli I, Vrochidis P, Skoumpas I, Constantinidis I. HPV-Related Oropharyngeal Cancer and Biomarkers Based on Epigenetics and Microbiome Profile. *Front Cell Dev Biol.* 2021;8:625330.
6. De Leeuw R, KG, ed. *Orofacial Pain: Guidelines for Assessment, Diagnosis, and Management.* 6th ed. : Quintessence Publishing; 2018.
7. Maixner W, Diatchenko L, Dubner R, et al. Orofacial pain prospective evaluation and risk assessment study--the OPPERA study. *J Pain.* 2011;12(11 Suppl). T4-11 e1-2.
8. Peck CC, Goulet J-P, Lobbezoo F, et al. Expanding the taxonomy of the diagnostic criteria for temporomandibular disorders. *J Oral Rehabil.* 2014;41(1):2–23.
9. Lovgren A, Visscher CM, Haggman-Henrikson B, Lobbezoo F, Marklund S, Wanman A, et al. Validity of three screening questions (3Q/TMD) in relation to the DC/TMD. *J Oral Rehabil.* 2016;43(10):729–736.
10. Bendtsen L, Zakrzewska JM, Heinskou TB, et al. Advances in diagnosis, classification, pathophysiology, and management of trigeminal neuralgia. *Lancet Neurol.* 2020;19(9):784–796.
11. Headache Classification Committee of the International Headache Society (IHS) The International Classification of Headache Disorders, 3rd edition. Cephalalgia, 2018. **38**(1): p. 1–211.
12. Baad-Hansen L, Benoliel R. Neuropathic orofacial pain: Facts and fiction. *Cephalalgia.* 2017;37(7):670–679.
13. Imamura Y, Shinozaki T, Okada-Ogawa A, et al. An updated review on pathophysiology and management of burning mouth syndrome with endocrinological, psychological and neuropathic perspectives. *J Oral Rehabil.* 2019;46(6):574–587.
14. International Classification of Orofacial Pain, 1st ed (ICOP). Cephalalgia, 2020. **40**(2): p. 129-221.
15. Tchivileva IE, Ohrbach R, Fillingim RB, Greenspan JD, Maixner W, Slade GD. Temporal change in headache and its contribution to the risk of developing first-onset temporomandibular disorder in the Orofacial Pain: Prospective Evaluation and Risk Assessment (OPPERA) study. *Pain.* 2017;158(1):120–129.
16. Schiffman E, Ohrbach R. Diagnostic Criteria for Temporomandibular Disorders (DC/TMD) for Clinical and Research Applications: recommendations of the International RDC/TMD Consortium Network* and Orofacial Pain Special Interest Groupdagger. *J Oral Facial Pain Headache.* 2014;28(1):6–27.
17. Arnardottir ES, Mackiewicz M, Gislason T, Teff KL, Pack AI. Molecular signatures of obstructive sleep apnea in adults: a review and perspective. *Sleep.* 2009;32(4):447–470.
18. Gharibeh T, Mehra R. Obstructive sleep apnea syndrome: natural history, diagnosis, and emerging treatment options. *Nat Sci Sleep.* 2010 Sep 28;2:233–255.
19. Stansbury RC, Strollo PJ. Clinical manifestations of sleep apnea. *J Thorac Dis.* 2015;7(9):E298–E310.
20. Essick G.K., Di Giosia M., Alonso A., Raphael K.G., Sanders A.E., Lavigne G.J. Temporomandibular Disorders in Relation to Sleep-Disordered Breathing and Sleep Bruxism. Chapter 172 in: Kryger M, Roth T, Dement WC, eds. Principles and Practice of Sleep Medicine, 7th edition.
21. Lembo D, Caroccia F, Lopes C, Moscagiuri F, Sinjari B, D'Attilio M. Obstructive Sleep Apnea and Periodontal Disease: A Systematic Review. *Medicina (Kaunas).* 2021;57(6):640.
22. Eckert DJ. Phenotypic approaches to obstructive sleep apnoea - New pathways for targeted therapy. *Sleep Med Rev.* 2018;37:45–59.
23. Benjafield AV, Ayas NT, Eastwood PR, et al. Estimation of the global prevalence and burden of obstructive sleep apnoea: a literature-based analysis. *Lancet Respir Med.* 2019;7(8):687–698.
24. Schwab RJ, Leinwand SE, Bearn CB, Maislin G, Rao RB, Nagaraja A, Wang S, Keenan BT. Digital Morphometrics: A New Upper Airway Phenotyping Paradigm in OSA. *Chest,* 2017;152(2):330–342.

25. Yu JL, Rosen I. Utility of the modified Mallampati grade and Friedman tongue position in the assessment of obstructive sleep apnea. *J Clin Sleep Med.* 2020;16(2):303–308.

26. Chang ET, Baik G, Torre C, Brietzke SE, Camacho M. The relationship of the uvula with snoring and obstructive sleep apnea: a systematic review. *Sleep Breath.* 2018;22(4):955–961.

27. Schellenberg JB, Maislin G, Schwab RJ. Physical findings and the risk for obstructive sleep apnea. The importance of oropharyngeal structures. *Am J Respir Crit Care Med.* 2000;162(2 Pt 1):740–748.

28. Tsai WH, Remmers JE, Brant R, Flemons WW, Davies J, Macarthur C. A decision rule for diagnostic testing in obstructive sleep apnea. *Am J Respir Crit Care Med.* 2003 15;167(10):1427–1432.

29. Yu C, Ahn HW, Kim SH. Three-dimensional morphological evaluation of the hard palate in Korean adults with mild-to-moderate obstructive sleep apnea. *Korean J Orthod.* 2018;48(3):133–142.

30. Wetselaar P, Manfredini D, Ahlberg J, Johansson A, Aarab G, Papagianni CE, Reyes Sevilla M, Koutris M, Lobbezoo F. Associations between tooth wear and dental sleep disorders: A narrative overview. *J Oral Rehabil.* 2019;46(8):765–775.

31. Lowe AA, Ozbek MM, Miyamoto K, Pae EK, Fleetham JA. Cephalometric and demographic characteristics of obstructive sleep apnea: an evaluation with partial least squares analysis. *Angle Orthod.* 1997;67(2):143–153.

32. Johns FR, Strollo Jr PJ, Buckley M, Constantino J. The influence of craniofacial structure on obstructive sleep apnea in young adults. *J Oral Maxillofac Surg.* 1998;56(5):596–602. discussion 602-3.

33. Hoffstein V, Mateika S. Differences in abdominal and neck circumferences in patients with and without obstructive sleep apnoea. *Eur Respir J.* 1992;5(4):377–381.

34. Koutsourelakis I, Vagiakis E, Roussos C, Zakynthinos S. Obstructive sleep apnoea and oral breathing in patients free of nasal obstruction. *Eur Respir J.* 2006;28(6):1222–1228.

35. Caton JG, Armitage G, Berglundh T, et al. A new classification scheme for periodontal and per-implant diseases and conditions – introduction and key changes from the 1999 classification. *J Periodont.* 2018;89(suppl 1):S1–S8.

36. Pihlstrom BL, Michalowicz BS, Johnson NW. Periodontal diseases. *Lancet.* 2005;366(9499):1809–1820.

37. Eke PI, Thornton-Evans GO, Wei L, Borgnakke WS, Dye BA, Genco RJ. Periodontitis in US adults: national health and nutrition examination survey 2009-2014. *J Am Dent Assoc.* 2018;149(7):576–588.

38. Tonetti MS, Greenwell H, Kornman KS. Staging and Grading of Periodontitis: Framework and proposal of a new classification and case definition. *J Periodont.* 2018;89(suppl 1):S159–S172.

39. Chapple ILC, Mealey BL, Van Dyke TE, et al. Periodontal health and gingival diseases and conditions on an intact and a reduced periodontium – Consensus report 1. *J Periodont.* 2018;89(Suppl 1):S74–S84.

40. Machiulskiene V, Campus G, Carvalho J. Terminology of Dental Caries and Dental Caries Management: Consensus Report of a Workshop Organized by ORCA and Cariology Research Group of IADR. *Caries Res.* 2020;54:7–14.

41. Fontana M, Young D, Wolff M, et al. Defining dental caries for 2010 and beyond. *Dental Clinics of North America.* 2010;54(3):423–440.

42. Longbottom C, Huysmans M-Ch, Pitts N, Fontana M. Glossary of key terms. *Mongr Oral Sci.* 2009;21:209–216.

43. Shivakumar K, Prasad S, Chandu G. International caries detection and assessment system: A new paradigm in detection of dental caries. *J Conserv Dent.* 2009;12(1):10–16.

44. Pitts N. "ICDAS"—an international system for caries detection and assessment being developed to facilitate caries epidemiology, research and appropriate clinical management. *Community Dent Health.* 2004;21:193–198.

45. Jablonski-Momeni A, Stachniss V, Ricketts DN, et al. Reproducibility and Accuracy of the ICDAS-II for Detection of Occlusal Caries in vitro. *Caries Res.* 2008;42:79–87.

46. Shoaib L, Deery C, Ricketts DNJ, Nugent ZJ. Validity and reproducibility of ICDAS II in primary teeth. *Caries Res.* 2009;43:442–448.

47. Slayton RL, Urquhart O, Araujo MWB, et al. Evidence-based clinical practice guideline on nonrestorative treatments for carious lesions: A report from the American Dental Association. *J Am Dent Assoc.* 2018;149(10):837–849.e19.

48. Fontana M, Gonzalez-Cabezas C, Fitzgerald M. Cariology for the 21st century: current caries management concepts for dental practice. *Journal Michigan Dent Association.* 2013:32–40.

49. International Caries Detection & Assessment System Coordinating Committee: The International Caries Detection and Assessment System (ICDAS II), Workshop sponsored by the NIDCR, the ADA, and the International Association for Dental Research. <https://www.icdas.org/> (Criteria Manual for The International Caries Detection and Assessment System [ICDAS II]).

50. Kidd EAM, Beighton D. Prediction of secondary caries around tooth-colored restorations: a clinical and microbiological study. *Journal of Dental Research.* 1996;75(12):1942–1946.

51. Martignon S, Pitts NB, Goffin G, et al. Caries care practice guide: consensus on evidence into practice. *Br Dent J.* 2019;227:353–362.

52. Fontana M, Carrasco-Labra A, Spallek H, Eckert G, Katz B. Improving Caries Risk Prediction Modeling: A Call for Action. *Journal of Dental Research.* 2020;99(11):1215–1220.

53. Stookey GK, Gonzalez Cabezas C. Emerging methods of caries diagnosis. *J Dent Educ.* 2001;65:1001–1006.

54. Fontana M, Gonzalez-Cabezas C. Changing paradigm. A different view of caries lesions. *Compendium.* 2011;32(Special Issue 4):24–27.

55. Stump A, Fontana M, Gonzalez-Cabezas C, et al. The effect of magnification on occlusal carious lesion treatment decisions. *IADR meeting.* 2011:2554 Abstract.

56. Fontana M, Zero D, Beltrán-Aguilar E, Grey SK. Techniques for tooth surface assessments in school-based sealant programs. *J Amer Dent Assoc.* 2010;141(7):854–860.

57. Wenzel A. Current trends in radiographic caries imaging. *Oral Surgery, Oral Medicine, Oral Pathology, Oral Radiology, and Endodontology.* 1995;80(5):527–539.

58. Wenzel A. Bitewing and digital bitewing radiography for detection of caries lesions. *Journal of Dental Research.* 2004;83 (suppl 1):C72–C75.

59. Bento VAA, Gomes JML, Lemos CAA, Limirio JPJO, Rosa CDDRD, Pellizzer EP. Prevalence of proximal contact loss between implant-supported prostheses and adjacent natural teeth: A systematic review and meta-analysis. *Journal of Prosthetic Dentistry.* July 19, 2021 Abstr. Fadi.

SUGGESTED READINGS

D. EXTRAORAL DIAGNOSES

Little JW, Miller C, Rhodus NL. *Dental Management of the Medically Compromised Patient.* ed 9 St Louis: Elsevier; 2018.

Malamed SF. *Medical Emergencies in the Dental Office.* 7th ed. St. Louis: Elsevier; 2014.

Neville BW, Damm DD, Allen CM, Chi A. *Oral and Maxillofacial Pathology.* ed 4 St Louis: Elsevier; 2015.

Regezi JA, Sciubba J, Jordan RC. *Oral Pathology: Clinical-Pathological Correlations.* ed 7 St Louis: Elsevier; 2016.

Scully C. *Oral and Maxillofacial Medicine.* ed 3 St Louis: Elsevier; 2013.

E. INTRAORAL SOFT TISSUE DIAGNOSES

Neville BW, Damm DD, Allen CM, Chi A. *Oral and Maxillofacial Pathology*. ed 4 St Louis: Elsevier; 2015.
Regezi JA, Sciubba J, Jordan RC. *Oral Pathology: Clinical-Pathological Correlations*. ed 7 St Louis: Elsevier; 2016.
Scully C. *Oral and Maxillofacial Medicine*. ed 3 St Louis: Elsevier; 2013.

F. SALIVARY GLAND ABNORMALITIES

Neville BW, Damm DD, Allen CM, Chi A. *Oral and Maxillofacial Pathology*. ed 4 St Louis: Elsevier; 2015.
Regezi JA, Sciubba J, Jordan RC. *Oral Pathology: Clinical-Pathological Correlations*. ed 7 St Louis: Elsevier; 2016.

G. ABNORMALITIES OF THE MAXILLA AND MANDIBLE

Mllya S, Lam E. *White & Pharoah's Oral Radiology: Principles and Interpretation*. ed 8 St Louis: Mosby; 2018.
Neville B, Damm DD, Allen CM, Chi A. *Oral and Maxillofacial Pathology*. ed 4 St Louis: Elsevier; 2015.

H. TEMPOROMANDIBULAR DISORDERS, TRIGEMINAL NEUROPATHIC PAIN AND HEADACHES

De Leeuw R, ed. *American Academy of Orofacial Pain: Orofacial Pain—Guidelines for Assessment, Diagnosis and Management*. ed 6 Chicago: Quintessence; 2018.
Koenig LJ. *Diagnostic Imaging: Oral and Maxillofacial*. ed 2 Salt Lake City: Elsevier; 2017.
Mllya S, Lam E. *White & Pharoah's Oral Radiology: Principles and Interpretation*. ed 8 St Louis: Mosby; 2018.
Okeson J.P.: *Bell's Oral & Facial Pain*, ed 7, Management of temporomandibular disorders and occlusion, ed 7, Chicago, 2014, Quintessence.
Zakrewska JM. *Orofacial Pain*. Oxford: Oxford Press; 2009.

J. PERIODONTAL DISEASES

Caton JG, Armitage G, Berglundh T, Al. A new classification scheme for periodontal and per-implant diseases and conditions – introduction and key changes from the 1999 classification. *Journal of Periodontology*. 2018;89(suppl 1):S1–S8.
Newman MG, Takei HH, Klokkevoid PR, Carranza FA. *Newman and Carranza's Clinical Periodontology*. ed 13 St Louis: Saunders; 2018.

K. PULPAL AND PERIAPICAL DIAGNOSES

A.A.E. Consensus Conference Recommended Diagnostic Terminology Journal of Endodontics 35(12):1634, 2009.
Berman LH, Hargreaves KM. *Cohen's Pathways of the Pulp*. ed 12 St Louis: Mosby; 2021.
Koenig L. *Diagnostic Imaging: Oral and Maxillofacial*. ed 2 Salt Lake City: Elsevier; 2017.
Torabinejab M, Fouad A, Shabahang S. *Endodontics: Principles and Practice*. ed 6 St Louis: Saunders; 2020.

L. DENTAL CARIES

American Dental Association, Evidence-based Clinical Practice Guidelines. https://www.ada.org/resources/research/science-and-research-institute/evidence-based-dental-research
(see the ones related to caries and caries prevention and management)

Cochrane Collaboration. www.cochrane.org/reviews/clibintro.htm/ (see Oral health: caries, and related topics, such as fluorides, sealants, etc.).
Fejerskov O, Kidd E. *Dental Caries: The Disease and Its Clinical Management*. third edition Oxford: Blackwell; 2015.
Ritter AV, Boushell L, Walter R. *Sturdevant's the Art and Science of Operative Dentistry, ed 7*. St Louis. : Mosby; 2018.
Caries Management by Risk Assessment (CAMBRA) group (Doméjean S, White JM, Featherstone JD.) Validation of the CDA CAMBRA caries risk assessment—a six-year retrospective study, *J Calif Dent Assoc*. 39(10):709–715, 2011.

M. TOOTH CRACKS AND FRACTURES

American Association of Endodontists: Endodontics: colleague for excellence. Cracking the cracked tooth code: detection and treatment of various longitudinal tooth fractures, Summer 2008. <http://www.aae.org/uploadedfiles/publications_and_research/endodontics_colleagues_for_excellence_newsletter/ecfesum08.pdf/>, 2008

O. OCCLUSAL ABNORMALITIES

Dawson PE. *Functional Occlusion: From TMJ to Smile Design*. ed 1 St Louis: Mosby; 2006.
Graber N.V.R., Vig K., Huang G. Orthodontics, Current Principles and Techniques. 6th ed 2017.
Okeson J. *Management of Temporomandibular Disorders and Occlusion*. ed 8 St Louis: Mosby; 2019.
Proffit W, Fields H, Larson B, Sarver D, eds. *Contemporary Orthodontics*. ed 6 St Louis: Mosby; 2018.

P. ESTHETIC PROBLEMS

American Academy of Cosmetic Dentistry.
El Askary A E-S. *Fundamentals of Esthetic Implant Dentistry*. ed 2 Oxford: Blackwell; 2008.
Freedman GA. *Contemporary Esthetic Dentistry*. St Louis: Elsevier; 2012.
Geissberger M. *Esthetic Dentistry in Clinical Practice*. Oxford: Blackwell; 2010.
Goldstein R, Chu S, Lee E, Stappert F. ed 3 *Esthetics in Dentistry*. 2 vols Oxford: Wiley; 2018.
Magne P. *Biomimetric Restorative Dentistry*. Chicago: Quintessence; 2022.
Mistry S. Principles of smile demystified. *J Cosmetic Dentistry*. 2012; 28(2):116–124.

T. IMPLANT-RELATED DIAGNOSES

Berglundh T, Giannobile W, Lang N, Sanz M. *Lindhe's Clinical Periodontology and Implant Dentistry*. ed 7 Oxford: Wiley; 2021.
Hughes F, Seymour K, Turner W, eds. *Clinical Problem Solving in Periodontology and Implantology*. St Louis: Elsevier; 2012.

The Treatment Planning Process

3

Evidence-Based Treatment Planning: Assessment of Risk, Prognosis, and Expected Outcomes

Leonardo Marchini and Samuel Nesbit

Visit eBooks.Health.Elsevier.com

OUTLINE

The purpose of this chapter is to explain and demonstrate how **evidence-based dentistry** (EBD) is essential to the treatment planning process. As a profession we have effectively migrated away from an environment where empirical decision making was the norm and "what works best in my hands" was the practitioner's de facto recommendation to the patient. EBD has now become the basis for many of our decisions in oral health care. In recent years, an extensive body of evidence-based literature has been developed. The authors of this chapter have taken a practical approach to this topic and have focused on the central issue of *how EBD is useful to the oral health care practitioner and the patient in the formulation of the patient's treatment plan.*

Some of questions we will try to answer include:
- Which clinical questions are critical to this patient's treatment and how does the evidence enlighten and help resolve those questions?
- How do we efficiently and effectively gather evidence related to seminal clinical questions?

- How do we evaluate the evidence?
- How do we use the evidence to inform and educate and arrive collaboratively at a treatment decision with the patient?

Highlighted in this chapter are the concepts of **Risk Assessment**, **Prognosis Determination**, and **Outcomes Assessment**. All three of these entities are heavily dependent on EBD for their definition and application and they are integral to the treatment planning process and the informed consent discussion with the patient. They have a natural home in this chapter and the definitions and examples presented here will be referenced at multiple junctures in upcoming chapters.

The chapter also includes discussion regarding the limitations of EBD and how to proceed in the absence of compelling evidence, in the presence of weak or conflicting evidence, or when patient preferences and considerations override prevailing evidence.

This chapter provides a foundation for the detailed process of treatment planning, which is discussed in Chapter 5 and then applied throughout the remainder of this textbook.

DEFINITION OF EVIDENCE-BASED DENTISTRY, RISK ASSESSMENT, PROGNOSIS, AND TREATMENT OUTCOMES

Evidence-Based Dentistry

Evidence-based dentistry (EBD) is derived from evidence-based medicine (EBM), which was initially based on what was called "critical appraisal." Critical appraisal was essentially managing patients based on what scientific evidence showed worked rather than what authorities were recommending ("expert-based medicine"). Later, EBM distinguished itself from critical appraisal by combining clinical expertise and the patient's values with the research-derived evidence.[1]

Currently, EBM is defined as "the conscientious, explicit, and judicious use of current best evidence in making decisions about the care of individual patients." Current best evidence is the evidence provided by clinically relevant research. Clinical expertise is understood to be clinical judgement and diagnostic and therapeutic proficiency acquired during years of clinical experience and practice. Those two concepts (clinical expertise and best evidence) should be used in synchrony and neither of them is good enough alone. That is because clinical practice can quickly become obsolete without using the current best evidence and even the best evidence may not be applicable to an individual patient.[2] From the last statement, it is possible to understand the importance of taking the patient values and preferences into the decision-making process.

Evidence-based dentistry uses the same structured process from EBM and can be defined as a systematic approach to integrate the best scientific evidence available with dentists' expertise and patients' values and expectations into a decision-making process for delivering oral health care.

EBD requires a careful assessment of clinically relevant scientific evidence in light of:
- the patient's oral and general health
- the dentist's knowledge, experience and clinical expertise, and
- the patient's preferences and values.

Risk Assessment

Risk assessment is the *determination of the likelihood of a patient developing a specific disease or condition*. Not all patients are equally likely to develop a particular disease. Some patients, because of genetics, environment, diet, personal habits, systemic health, medications, or other factors, are more likely than others to develop and/or continue to be afflicted by certain conditions. Those patients who have **risk factors**, i.e., predisposing conditions, or who engage in behaviors known to promote a particular disease, are described as **at increased risk**. This differs from the epidemiologic definition of "at risk." In epidemiology, anyone who could potentially develop the condition is "at risk" and individuals who could not develop the condition are "not at risk." Edentulous patients, for example, are not at risk of caries development; but everyone who has at least one natural tooth *is* at risk of caries development. This distinction is important in determining the denominator for incidence and prevalence estimates. In both realms, however, clinical and epidemiologic, someone who has a strong probability of developing the condition is "at high risk."

Prognosis

A **prognosis** is a prediction, based on present circumstances, of the patient's future condition. It is usually expressed in such general terms as "excellent," "good," "favorable," "unfavorable," "fair," "poor," "questionable," or "hopeless." A prognosis can be made for an individual tooth, for various oral conditions (e.g., oral cancer, periodontal disease), for the various treatment disciplines, or for the patient's overall prognosis. An essential difference between risk assessment and prognosis is that the former focuses on the propensity to *develop* a disease; the latter predicts the *future course of the disease* (progression or regression) both with and without treatment.

For a specific patient, varying prognoses can be determined for multiple disease processes as well as for recommended treatments. Although the prognosis for the disease and the treatment may be related, they are not necessarily the same. For example, a patient with moderate periodontitis may have a good prognosis for control of the disease, but a poor or questionable prognosis for a long span, fixed partial denture that is anchored on the involved teeth. Conversely a patient with severe periodontitis on the lower teeth may be described as having a poor prognosis for control of the disease, but a good prognosis for an upper complete denture.

Treatment Outcomes

Outcomes, in the context of this discussion, are the specific, tangible results of treatment. The results that a patient and practitioner anticipate receiving as a result of a course of treatment are **outcome expectations**. An outcome expectation will be closely linked to both risk assessment and prognosis determination. For example, if the patient remains at increased risk of new caries and the prognosis for control of the caries is poor, it follows that the outcomes of treatment can be expected to be unfavorable. But the two differ fundamentally in that while prognosis always looks to the patient's future condition; outcomes assessment looks at past performance (both individual and group) and, even when the outcomes measures are used to estimate future success, those expectations are still predictions based on past performance.

Expected outcomes are usually expressed in quantifiable terms based on sound clinical research, such as the *average life expectancy* of a restoration. While outcome measures for the complete range of dental treatment procedures are not yet available, some meaningful work has been published and examples of selected findings are discussed later in this chapter.

It is very important for the practitioner to be aware that patient's expectations about treatment outcomes can differ drastically from the outcomes reported in the literature and/or the outcomes that the practitioner has witnessed in their own experience. This discrepancy between patient's and practitioner's expectations should be addressed early in dental treatment, so that the dentist can explain what the past performance has been and what would be a realistic expectation for the proposed treatment, preferably before starting the treatment. By doing that, the dentist avoids patient's future frustration with the outcomes, which might have a negative impact in the relationship between the patient and the dentist.[3]

EVIDENCE-BASED DECISION MAKING

How to Apply EBD in the Treatment Planning Process

Richards et al.[4] have advocated the use of a five-step process to implement EBD in clinical practice. The first step is ASK, in which the practitioner will translate the clinical problem into a question that encompasses the population, the intervention, other comparable interventions, and which outcomes of the intervention are more important, both for the practitioner and the patient. This type of inquiry is commonly formulated as a PICO question, where P is for population (or problem), I for intervention (or exposure), C for comparison, and O for outcome. The second step is ACQUIRE, which relates to searching and identifying the best research-derived evidence using health sciences databases. The third step, APPRAISE, is the assessment of the quality of the research that was retrieved. Only quality science should be used in the decision-making process. In the fourth step, APPLY, the literature findings must be integrated with the clinical circumstances and patient's values and preferences. ASSESS is the fifth step, in which the dentist should evaluate the outcomes of the treatment with the intention of improving their skills for providing even better dental care for the next patient.[4] For appropriate self-assessment, the dentist must be aware of their own biases.

The EBD approach[5] has several positive aspects, such as helping dentists to make rational, research-backed treatment decisions. It also has the potential to reduce costs by avoiding buying new but ineffective supplies and equipment, it helps dentists to stay updated and to educate their patients, it provides dentists with a self-improvement tool and it helps dentists choose which continuing education courses to take, as dentists may become more familiar with the important authors for each topic by constantly checking the current literature.

EBD is based on scientific principles and treatment regimens that have been tried, tested, and proven worthy by accurate, substantiated, and reproducible studies. Ideally, any treatment method, whether in dentistry or medicine, should be supported by current, controlled, blinded, prospective longitudinal studies. Unfortunately, for many, if not most dental treatments, this type of evidence is not yet available.

Where valid current applicable research exists, it can affirm or disprove the efficacy of various dental treatments and thereby provide compelling guidance to the patient and practitioner on the "treat versus not treat" question. In other situations, when several different viable alternatives are being weighed, it can provide the basis for moving to a specific decision. The strength of the evidence needs to be considered as it is factored into the decision-making. The stronger the evidence, the more seriously it should be weighed. Conversely, the weaker the evidence, the less likely that it will drive or influence decision making.[6]

Although the use of research findings has become an integral component of the treatment planning process, other factors must also be considered. The application of dental research and published studies must be tempered by an understanding of the limitations of these resources:

- Many recent treatments remain to be analyzed, especially in the long term.
- There is insufficient evidence to determine the viability of many treatments.
- Many treatments do not have strong evidentiary support, but may still be viable (especially when compared to other even less attractive alternatives).
- The findings of relevant studies may not be directly applicable to one individual patient circumstances (e.g., general health; immune response; oral disease risk; or condition of the oral cavity, individual tooth, or specific tooth surface).
- Most outcomes used in different studies look exclusively at treatment efficacy and rarely correlate that efficacy with individual patient preferences and desires.
- Most studies do not address patient factors (e.g., patient's prior experience, personal and cultural values) as impact treatment decisions or treatment outcomes.
- Most studies do not investigate patient-centered outcomes, such as patient satisfaction with the treatment received.

How then does the dentist make decisions and recommend treatment when evidence does not exist for a particular situation, or when the evidence is weak or conflicting? To make a treatment planning decision under such circumstances, the dentist and patient may need to rely more heavily on other professional (what has your experience revealed?) or patient driven (what has been the patient's previous experience with a similar procedure?) parameters. The range of treatment options may have to be expanded to accommodate other treatment approaches that may be similarly unproven but that may be viable in this situation. In any case, it is incumbent on the dentist to check the patient's expectations and ensure that the patient is informed about the limits of our evidence-based knowledge. It is essential for the patient to be an informed and active partner in the decision making. When there is limited or conflicted evidence base for treatment planning, the dentist has an obligation for wider, not narrower, disclosure in achieving informed consent.

How to Find the Best Evidence

The expanded section titled *How to Find the Best Evidence* –For Dentists is included in the electronic version of this chapter. *How to Find The Best Evidence* In this section, the reader will be able to find initial guidance about how to search for the best available evidence in the dental literature and how to have access to full text articles when you are not affiliated with a University library.

RISK ASSESSMENT

Risk Assessment in Dentistry

Risk indicators are identifiable conditions that, when present, are known to be associated with a higher probability of the occurrence of a particular disease. **Risk factors** are conditions for which a demonstrable causal link between the factor and the disease has been shown to exist. Risk factors are best confirmed by **longitudinal studies** during which patients with the hypothesized risk factor are evaluated over sufficient time to determine whether they do or do not develop the specific disease or problem in question. Risk indicators may be identified by taking a cross section, or sample, of individuals and looking for instances of the risk indicator and the disease occurring together.[7] Although risk and causality may be linked, they are not the same. For example, a diet that is heavily laden with refined sugars constitutes a risk indicator (and a risk factor) for caries. However, a specific patient who consumes a highly cariogenic diet may never be afflicted with caries.

Another categorization that is particularly useful to keep in mind in the dental setting is the distinction between **modifiable** (mutable) and **nonmodifiable** (immutable) **risk factors** or risk indicators. Modifiable risk indicators, such as diet, oral self-care, smoking, poorly contoured restorations, can be changed, while nonmodifiable risk indicators, such as age, genetics, or fluoride history are factors that cannot be changed. The dental team can and should use all reasonable interventions that have the potential to mitigate or eliminate modifiable risk indicators. In the case of nonmodifiable risk indicators, however, the value of their identification may be limited to risk assessment and guiding the prescription of preventive therapy, which can be useful tools in health promotion and oral disease prevention.

Assessing risk assists the dentist in identifying which patients are more likely to develop a particular disease or condition or to have recurrence of the disease. When that identification has been made, the patient can be informed about the risks and, when feasible, efforts can be made to eliminate or mitigate the specific cause or causes of the disease. When successful, such efforts help the patient preserve their oral health. Elimination of a specific cause or causes of an oral disease early in the progression of the condition can, in some cases, reduce the severity and the duration of the disease (e.g., periodontal disease). Once the disease process is initiated, however, removal of a risk indicator or indicators that are not known to be direct causes of the disease may have no effect on the duration or course of the disease (e.g., oral cancer).

To describe the strength of the relationship between risk and future disease occurrence, it is often helpful to specify the *degree* of risk with terms such as "high," "moderate," or "low." Defining the degree of risk varies with the clinical context or with the parameters of the individual study or protocol. In any setting, it can be assumed that the higher the risk, the more likely the occurrence or recurrence of the disease. In the presence of multiple risk indicators and/or strong risk indicators, the occurrence of disease is also more likely. For example, in general, the patient who has multiple risk indicators for dental caries (e.g., lack of previous and current fluoride exposure, and a cariogenic diet) is more likely to be afflicted by dental caries than a patient with only one or no known risk indicators. Also, as discussed later in this text, an older adult patient with a strong risk indicator, e.g., **dry mouth**, is more likely to develop dental caries than a

similar patient with a less strong risk indicator, such as lack of fluoride exposure as a child.

Eight categories of conditions or behaviors that may be risk indicators for oral disease can be described and are discussed in the following sections. It must be noted that, although the categories and their relevance to treatment planning are presented here as distinct entities, many potential risk indicators do not fit neatly into a single category but may appropriately be placed in two or more.

Heritable Conditions

Heritable oral conditions include specific tooth abnormalities such as amelogenesis imperfecta, dentinogenesis imperfecta or dentinal dysplasia; and extradental abnormalities such as epidermolysis bullosum, a palatal cleft, or a skeletal deformity (Figure 3.1). Recent genome-wide association studies have found potential genetic components to caries, which, heretofore, had not been thought to exist.[8,9] A patient (or their progeny) with a family history of a heritable condition may be at increased risk of developing that same condition.

Systemic Disease as a Risk Indicator for Oral Health Problems

Patients with gastroesophageal reflux disease are at significantly increased risk of developing dental erosion.[10,11] Similarly, patients who are afflicted with bulimia are also much more likely to have dental erosion.[12] Leukemia may cause a wide variety of intraoral soft tissue abnormalities. Advanced liver disease is a risk factor for intraoral ulceration, petechia formation, ecchymosis, and bleeding. Systemic diseases such as diabetes can be risk factors, predisposing the patient to significant oral problems such as oral ulceration, mucositis, infection, and poor wound healing. The poorly controlled diabetic patient is more likely to develop and exhibit progression of periodontitis.[13]

Oral health problems may also be risk indicators for common systemic diseases. For instance, periodontal disease is modestly associated (10%–50% increase in risk) with atherosclerotic vascular disease and clinical events, and this association is independent of other shared risk factors. Some uncertainty remains, however, about the existence of such independent associations between periodontal disease and atherosclerotic vascular disease.[14] A systematic review suggests that treatment of periodontal disease improves endothelial function and reduces biomarkers of atherosclerotic disease, especially in those already suffering from cardiovascular disease and/or diabetes.[15]

Many other general health problems are risk factors for intraoral pathology. When the patient has a systemic disease, the dentist must be aware of any related risks for oral disorders, the possible need for antibiotic premedication, the advisability of modifying or postponing dental treatment, and the need to be prepared for an emergency in the dental office (see Chapter 8).

Dietary and Other Behavioral Risk Indicators

If the patient's behavior, diet, or habits contribute to an increased risk of the development of oral disease, it is appropriate for the dentist to educate the patient about those risks

Patient Name: **Score:**

Birth Date: **Date:**

Age: **Initials:**

		Low Risk (0)	Moderate Risk (1)	High Risk (10)	Patient Risk
	Contributing Conditions				
I.	**Fluoride Exposure** (through drinking water, supplements, professional applications, toothpaste)	Yes	No		
II.	**Sugary Foods or Drinks** (including juice, carbonated or non-carbonated soft drinks, energy drinks, medicinal syrups)	Primarily at mealtimes		Frequent or prolonged between meal exposures/day	
III.	**Caries Experience of Mother, Caregiver** and/or other **Siblings** (for patients ages 6-14)	No carious lesions in last 24 months	Carious lesions in last 7-23 months	Carious lesions in last 6 months	
IV.	**Dental Home**: established patient of record, receiving regular dental care in a dental office	Yes	No		
	General Health Conditions				
I.	**Special Healthcare Needs***	No	Yes (over age 14)	Yes (ages 6-14)	
II.	**Chemo/Radiation Therapy**	No		Yes	
III.	**Eating Disorders**	No	Yes		
IV.	**Medications that Reduce Salivary Flow**	No	Yes		
V.	**Drug/Alcohol Abuse**	No	Yes		
	Clinical Conditions				
I.	**Cavitated or Non-Cavitated** (incipient) **Carious Lesions or Restorations** (visually or radiographically evident)	No new carious lesions or restorations in last 36 months	1 or 2 new carious lesions or restorations in last 36 months	3 or more carious lesions or restorations in last 36 months	
II.	**Teeth Missing Due to Caries in past 36 months**	No		Yes	
III.	**Visible Plaque**	No	Yes		
IV.	**Unusual Tooth Morphology** that compromises oral hygiene	No	Yes		
V.	**Interproximal Restorations - 1 or more**	No	Yes		
VI.	**Exposed Root Surfaces** Present	No	Yes		
VII.	**Restorations with Overhangs** and/or **Open Margins**; **Open Contacts** with Food Impaction	No	Yes		
VIII.	**Dental/Orthodontic Appliances** (fixed or removable)	No	Yes		
IX.	**Severe Dry Mouth (Xerostomia)**	No		Yes	
				TOTAL:	

Patient Instructions:

*Patients with developmental, physical, medical or mental disabilities that prevent or limit performance of adequate oral healthcare by themselves or caregivers.

Fig. 3.1 Caries Management by Risk Assessment (CAMBRA) caries risk assessment form.

and to encourage modification or elimination of the behavior. Use of tobacco products, excessive alcohol consumption, recreational use of drugs, or frequent ingestion of cariogenic foods and beverages are examples of behavior that can be deleterious. On occasion, even seemingly beneficial habits, such as overuse or misuse (e.g., prior to brushing) of low pH and or high alcohol percentage mouth rinses, may be detrimental, especially in patients reporting dry mouth. The dentist has the responsibility to assess this information and to notify the patient of the possible negative consequences of continuance and to remain vigilant for the occurrence of signs suggestive of pathologic developments such as oral cancer or dental erosion.[16,17] An example of a behavioral problem linked to an oral pathologic condition is the patient with obsessive-compulsive disorder who should be monitored for the development of severe dental abrasion and other traumatic or factitious injuries.

Risk Indicators Related to Stress and Anxiety

Patients can be at risk of many forms of oral pathologic conditions because of significant life stresses or other environmental influences. Erosive lichen planus is an example of an oral condition for which stress is a strong risk factor. Stress has also been one of the multiple factors implicated in the etiology of temporomandibular disorders.[18] An all too common problem is the patient whose anxiety about going to the dentist leads to avoidance of needed treatment. As discussed in Chapter 15, the implications for an anxious patient of the development of oral problems and the potential impact on the way dental treatment will be planned and carried out can be enormous. The dentist has the obligation to identify these risk indicators, to inform the patient of their deleterious potential, and to mitigate them whenever possible.

Functional or Trauma-Related Conditions

Functional or trauma-related conditions also incur risk. For example, the patient who bruxes and who has fractured teeth in the past would likely be at risk for additional tooth fractures. If the patient continues to be at risk, appropriate reconstructive and/or preventive measures should be considered. For the patient with severe attrition, large existing amalgam restorations, and a history of fractured teeth, sound recommendations may be crowns and an occlusal guard. If new restorations are warranted, but the patient cannot afford crowns, using a protective cusp design rather than a conventional preparation design for direct fill restorations may be a reasonable alternative. Another example: when a tooth is acutely traumatized, it may develop pulpal necrosis, periapical pathology, and/or tooth or root resorption.

Environmental Risk Indicators

Food service workers, who have constant and unlimited access to sweetened and carbonated beverages, are at increased risk of both dental caries and dental erosion. Frequent swimming in pools with chlorinated water can cause significant dental erosion in susceptible individuals.[19] Patients who are allergic to certain foods, latex, metals, or other environmental agents may develop ulceration, mucositis, hives or, less commonly, an anaphylactic reaction. Obviously, the best strategy in managing these patients is to eliminate exposure to the allergen or allergens. Sometimes this can be difficult. For example, because peanuts and peanut products are ubiquitous in the North American processed food chain, the patient who is very reactive to peanuts may have difficulty in avoiding exposure.

Social Determinants of Health

The validity of **Social Determinants of Health (SDH)** as a risk factor for oral health problems is uncertain and controversial. Although caries, periodontal disease, and tooth loss are more prevalent in individuals from lower income groups,[20] it often remains unclear whether the disease process is the *consequence* of SDHs such as poor nutrition, low self-esteem, lack of health literacy or lack of access to health care or whether the SDHs are comorbid conditions. Even if one accepts that SDHs are risk indicators for certain oral conditions on a population-wide basis, there is little support for the assertion that it is a risk factor for a specific patient's disease state. For a provider to attribute a patient's oral health problems to one or more SDHs risks being insensitive to a patient's humanity and can be reflective of inherent individual provider or societal bias. For individual patients, social determinants of health should be considered as a modifiable rather than a nonmodifiable risk factor. The important take-home message here is that SDHs should not be seen as a limitation to treatment, but rather as a window of opportunity as the dental team works creatively with a patient to help them achieve a more optimal state of oral health within the context of existing SDHs. An open and honest conversation with the patient about their personal challenges and difficulties will often provide an opportunity to build rapport and will help to ensure that the treatment plan will be relevant and appropriate.[21–25] (See Chapter 19 for a more specific discussion of the needs of patients who are motivationally or financially challenged.)

Previous Disease Experience

Previous disease experience can be a strong predictor (in some cases, the single best predictor) of future disease. For many oral conditions, including dental caries, periodontal disease, oral cancer, and tooth fracture, if the patient has experienced the problem in the past, the probability is greater that the same problem will arise again in the future.[26–28]

Because past disease experience is an immutable risk indicator, the best management strategy is to identify other causes of the condition and mitigate or eliminate those whenever possible. Treatment interventions should be recommended and instituted to prevent recurrence. Placement of a cusp protective restoration on a tooth at high risk of fracture is one such example.

To summarize, risk assessment can be a useful adjunct to the dental treatment planning process in the following ways:
- identifying the need for counseling the patient, spouse, or offspring about heritable oral conditions and diseases;
- working to eliminate recognized causes of oral disease when the patient is known to be at risk;
- initiating preventive measures to forestall the occurrence of oral disease when potential causes of oral disease cannot be eliminated;
- providing prophylactic behavioral, chemotherapeutic, and restorative intervention to prevent an undesirable outcome;
- providing early restorative intervention in situations in which delayed treatment would put the patient at risk of requiring more comprehensive treatment in the future.

In theory, with a complete understanding of the patient's risk of oral disease, any oral disease for any patient could be prevented or, at least, managed more effectively. In clinical practice, this is not feasible or practical. Time would not permit such an exhaustive review for every patient and our present scientific base is insufficient to support such an undertaking. Nevertheless, assessing risk provides a valuable resource in treatment planning. In the following discussion, four oral conditions are described in which risk assessment should be critically linked to shaping the patient's plan of care.

Oral Cancer Risk Assessment

Oral cancer is a generic term applied to any malignancy affecting the oral cavity and/or jawbones. The majority of primary malignancies occurring in the mouth derive from the surface stratified squamous epithelium of the oral mucosa. Most common sites include: tongue, tonsils, oropharynx, gums, floor of mouth. (https://www.cancer.net>types of cancer> oral and oropharyngeal cancer:Introduction). Other primary oral cancers include malignant neoplasms of salivary gland origin, sarcomas in soft connective tissue or bone, lymphomas, melanomas, and odontogenic carcinomas. Secondary or metastatic cancers, originating from any distant organ or tissue (breast, prostate, colon, liver, etc.), may also occur in the mouth. The following discussion focuses on oral squamous cell carcinoma because this diagnosis represents over 80% of cases of oral cancer.[29]

Oral squamous cell carcinoma (OSCCA) is the result of the malignant transformation of keratinocytes in the surface epithelium. The epithelium usually undergoes a progressive transformation from normal, to dysplastic, to invasive carcinoma. However, such a progression may be very rapid and the dysplastic changes may not be detected early or are only recognized after invasive carcinoma ensues. Dysplasia or carcinoma may present clinically as a white, red, white-red, ulcerated, verrucous lesion; or as a combination of these characteristics. Sometimes patients will develop more than one lesion with dysplasia.

Several substances and behaviors are known to contribute to the initial formation of OSCCA. Even with eradication of the lesion by surgical excision or other means, the patient remains vulnerable. In particular, if exposure to carcinogens continues, the patient is at risk of cancer recurrence or development of additional lesions in other oral sites (second primary tumors).[30]

Risk Factors for Oral Cancer

Tobacco. Any form of tobacco has the potential to induce carcinogenesis of the oral epithelium.[31] This is a dose-dependent phenomenon. Patients with a history of having used any tobacco products within the preceding 10 years should be considered at elevated risk of OSCCA. The type of tobacco, frequency of use, and duration of use must be documented and monitored. Patients who are exposed to tobacco, including secondhand smoking should be counseled to avoid it.

Alcohol. Ethanol use is known to be a risk factor for OSCCA.[32] Multiple mechanisms may be in effect including increased cell turnover that leads to opportunity for DNA mutation and chromosomal alteration;[33] increased permeability of oral tissues to carcinogenic agents; alteration of the cells of the liver and thereby modifying the systemic processing of carcinogens in the liver and the entire organism;[34,35] and with comorbid nutritional deficiency, reduced effectiveness

of antioxidants to prevent cancer.[36] Moderate drinkers have been shown to be 1.8 times more likely to develop oral and oropharyngeal cancer and heavy drinkers five times more likely.[37] The type, amount, and frequency of alcohol consumption should be documented, monitored, and discouraged if it is determined to be excessive.

High-risk human papillomavirus infection. [38]Recently the association of high-risk subtypes of HPV (for example HPV 16 and HPV 18) has been linked to a small percentage (1%–5%) of OSCCA and approximately 75% of oropharyngeal squamous cell carcinoma. The eighth edition of the American Joint Commission on Cancer (AJCC) now stipulates that the oropharynx includes the soft palate, uvula, tonsillar pillars, tonsils, adenoids, posterior pharyngeal wall, lingual tonsils, and base of tongue.[39] The profile of patients who develop HPV-driven SCC is different from patients with non-HPV cancer in the head and neck region (often nonsmoker, nondrinker, educated, older [median age 61 years],[40] males). The lesions tend to be found in a different location (oropharynx), and these lesions generally respond more favorably to treatment.[41]

Trauma. Although trauma per se does not cause carcinogenesis, it may induce epithelial damage and subsequent repair. The repair of epithelium demands cell duplication and, by increasing the cells that undergo division, the possibility that one of those cells will develop mutations and undergo neoplastic transformation is increased. Lesions that are determined to be of traumatic etiology must be resolved and the source of trauma eliminated to avoid unnecessary cell division and the possible increased risk of neoplastic change.[42,43]

Immune system compromise and immunosuppression. If the immune system of a patient is compromised (as with a debilitating disease) or suppressed (as caused by taking corticosteroid drugs), its ability to destroy transformed neoplastic cells is decreased, allowing tumors to grow unchecked. As a result, patients who are immunocompromised or immunosuppressed are at greater risk of developing oral cancer.[44]

Radiation treatment. Patients undergoing radiation therapy for head and neck malignancies often experience multiple side effects (see Chapter 6). Several of these, including xerostomia, mucositis, tissue atrophy, and hypovascularity, may be contributing factors to new or recurrent cancer development. In some cases, radiation induces malignant transformation or de-differentiation of preexisting tumors. Common neoplasms that develop due to radiation include osteosarcoma and fibrosarcoma.[45] The damage induced by radiation is dose-dependent.

Previous history of oral cancer. Patients with previous histories of oral cancer should be monitored carefully for recurrences or second primaries.[46,47] In patients with a history of cancer at a site other than the oral cavity, the possibility of metastatic disease should always be considered in the differential diagnosis of any oral lesion that cannot be diagnosed clinically. Therefore, in patients with a history of any type of cancer, any and all oral lesions should be biopsied unless the clinician can be certain of its diagnosis based on clinical evaluation alone.

With the identification of risk factors or risk indicators for oral cancer, every effort should be made to eliminate those factors and to educate the patient about oral cancer. Strategies for smoking cessation, elimination of smokeless tobacco, and management of alcohol abuse are discussed in detail in Chapters 10 and 14. When the discovery is made by the dentist at the initial oral examination, it is imperative that the dentist evaluate additional specific areas of vulnerability during the course of the clinical examination (e.g., area of the lip where a cigarette is held, vestibular site where snuff or chew is harbored, site of buccal mucosa adjacent to a sharp tooth fragment or broken restoration, floor of the mouth/ventral tongue in smokers, oropharyngeal area in cases of high-risk types of HPV). Where it is possible to eliminate local sources of tissue trauma (e.g., a defective restoration), it should be accomplished early in the treatment plan. Any lesion that cannot be clinically diagnosed or that cannot be unequivocally associated with trauma must be biopsied for diagnostic pathology. Management of other questionable lesions is discussed in Chapter 1. If the risk indicator(s) for oral cancer cannot be eliminated, then the patient must be carefully monitored as long as the individual remains in the practice. Patient education about oral cancer risk factors should be ongoing and presented in multiple formats and media.

Caries Risk Assessment

Some clinical conditions (such as the presence of plaque) and some behavioral patterns (such as frequent fermentable carbohydrate consumption) have strong associations with the occurrence of dental caries. Nevertheless, the presence of those factors alone has been shown to have limited predictability of current or future caries activity.

Recent caries experience and current disease activity continue to be the most important factors for predicting future caries activity.[48] Past caries experience represents the combination of many risk factors to which an individual has been exposed over a long period of time. Current dental caries activity represents recent exposure to risk factors and, if those factors remain unchanged, suggest a high likelihood of continuing caries activity in the future. It is unfortunate that dentists must rely on the appearance of clinical signs of the disease in order to have a high degree of certainty about future risk determination but, on the positive side, detecting caries lesions is a relatively simple and inexpensive clinical activity and early detection of lesions and the elevation of caries risk can lead to early and effective management of both risk factors and the disease process.

To diagnose, assess the risk level, and effectively manage active dental caries, an array of information must be obtained. Collecting information on risk factors such as presence and location of stagnant plaque, regularity of consumption of fermentable carbohydrates (particularly between meals), and salivary flow levels along with information about protective factors, such as fluoride exposure and the presence of sealants, will provide the dental team and the patient with an understanding of the causes and origins of the caries activity (see Figure 3.3). This information will also be used to develop an individualized management plan for the patient.[49] (See Chapter 10.)

Several dental organizations have developed caries risk assessment modules designed with the primary purpose of determining a patient's level of risk based on identified risk factors, as well as protective factors that are believed to be closely associated with limiting dental caries progression. Several of these instruments are available on dental organization websites or in recent publications. (See *Suggested Readings and Resources* at the end of this chapter). Two notable examples include the Caries Management by Risk Assessment (CAMBRA) group[50] (see Figure 3.1) and the Cariogram software program developed at the University of Malmo (http://www.aapd.org/media/Policies_Guidelines/G_CariesRiskAssessment.pdf; Figure 3.2). These risk assessment modules have been developed primarily based on expert opinion and limited evidence is available on their validity.[51] In addition, the use of the module in adults is based primarily on evidence from younger groups because most of the reported studies have been conducted on younger age groups.[49]

To determine the risk level, the modules combine caries indicators (caries lesion presence in recent years), risk factors, and protective factors. In general, a patient is considered to be at low risk when no active caries lesions have been found in the preceding 3 to 5 years combined with no recent changes in risk and protective factors. Patients considered at moderate or high caries risk are those presenting recent caries lesions and/or detrimental changes in risk or protective factors. The following cases are examples of some of the types of patients who should be considered to be at elevated caries risk:

- A patient with apparently good oral hygiene but with new caries lesions providing clear evidence that current risk factors result in development of lesions.
- A patient with no new detectable caries lesions, but with a recent severe drop in salivary flow due to a new medication.
- A patient who has been using fluoridated toothpaste all their life and with no/minimal caries activity in the last few years but who has recently decided to stop using fluoride. This patient will have a significant diminishing of the protective factors potentially leading to an increase in dental caries activity.

All patients with these characteristics should have individualized management to reduce the risk of developing new lesions.

Although collecting caries risk information regularly is perceived as an extremely time-consuming process for the busy practitioner, most of the needed information is readily available via a well-conducted medical/dental history and exam. In most instances, no additional testing is necessary. In fact, the practitioner's subjective assessment based on clinical experience is a useful determinate of risk.[52] Nevertheless, systematic collection and recording of objective data is important for consistency across multiple members of the dental team, for monitoring progress of the caries management plan, and for legal protection.

Although many of the risk and protective factors associated with development of both root caries and recurrent caries are similar to those for coronal caries, there are a few unique aspects of root caries development and occurrence of which the practitioner should be cognizant. Root surface exposure to the oral environment is a prerequisite for the development of caries lesions on the root surface. The drop in biofilm mineral saturation necessary for demineralization of the dentin/cementum is less than that needed for enamel demineralization suggesting that root caries lesions can be developing but enamel surfaces are unaffected.[53] Nevertheless, there is a clear association

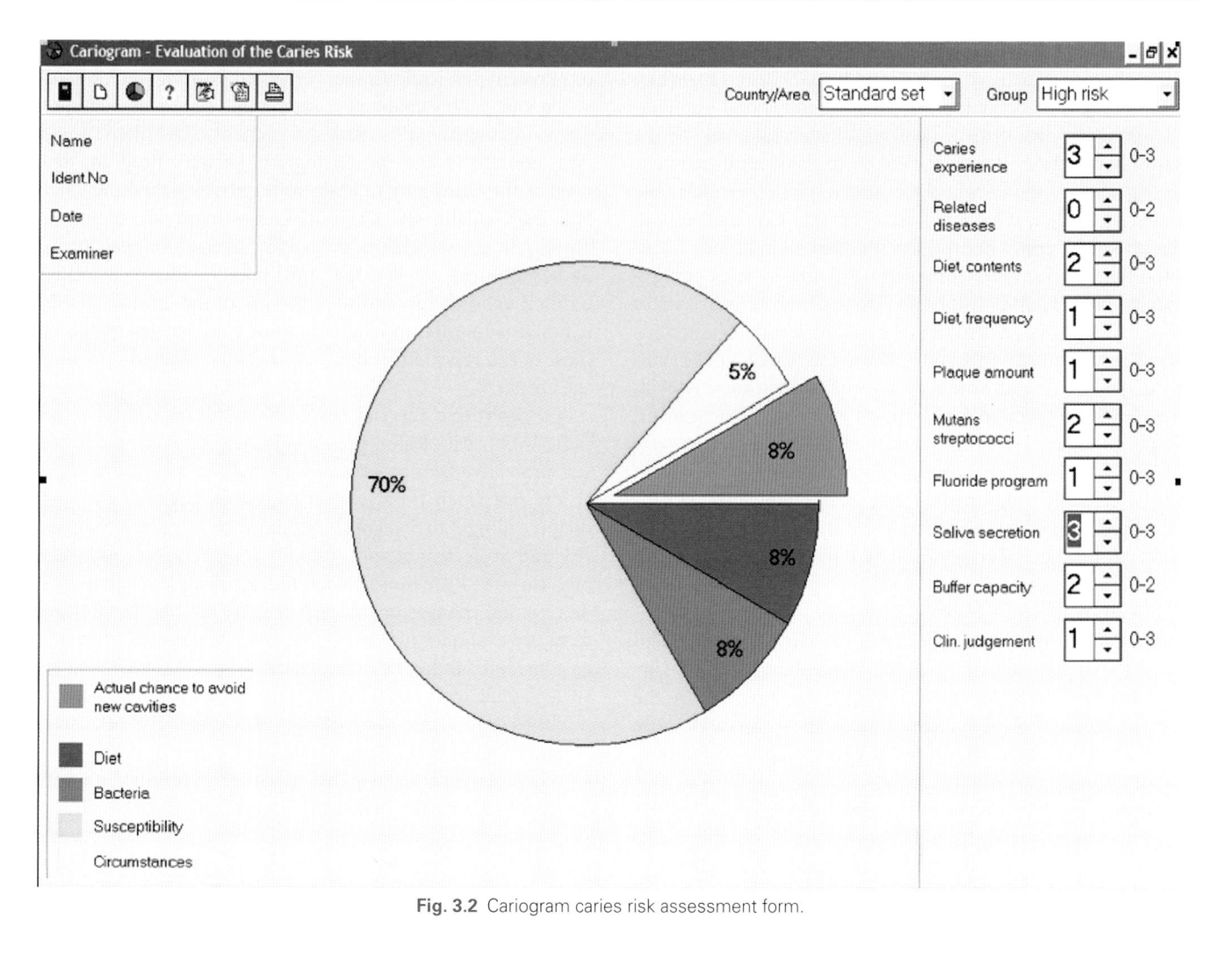

Fig. 3.2 Cariogram caries risk assessment form.

between root caries and active coronal caries.[54] In the United States, males exhibit a higher prevalence and greater severity of root caries. As for coronal caries, individuals with higher income and more education exhibit a lower prevalence of root caries. Importantly, however, most of these differences tend to disappear later in life.[55] It is of particular importance to continue monitoring patients when they enter their later years in life because salivary, dietary, and oral hygiene behaviors frequently change.

For recurrent (i.e., secondary) caries, the quality of the tooth-restoration interface is of particular importance, especially in interproximal areas where most of these lesions develop. Large gaps between the tooth and the restorative material have been associated with increased caries development.[56] Gaps that can be penetrated with the tip of an explorer tend to be wider than 100 μm and should be considered a high-risk location for recurrent (i.e., secondary) caries development.

Once a patient has been determined to be at increased risk of caries, the patient needs to be informed, risk indicators discussed, and an appropriate intervention put in place. The basic caries control protocol and optional interventions to manage the patient with active caries are described in Chapter 10. It is also essential to continue to monitor the patient's caries activity and to reassess caries risk at periodic intervals. Caries risk may diminish, increase, or remain static over time. The dental team must be vigilant to ensure that any increase in caries risk status is recognized and that aggressive intervention can be implemented.

Periodontal Disease Risk Assessment

Periodontal risk assessment gained attention in the dental literature in the early 1990s.[57–59] Efforts have been made to characterize periodontal risk by quantifying clinical and radiographic findings and applying these values to validated algorithms.[60–62] These tools look at a number of parameters which, when input, will generate a summarized report categorizing the risk level and suggesting treatment strategies. Assessed parameters include:

- probing depth
- bleeding on probing
- tooth loss
- extent of radiographic bone loss
- patient age relative to extent of disease
- diabetes mellitus
- genetic factors (IL1 genotype status)
- cigarette smoking
- tooth-related factors (presence of furcation involvement, vertical bone loss, subgingival restorations, and/or calculus deposits)
- treatment history (previous non-surgical and/or surgical periodontal therapy)

CARIES PROTECTIVE FACTORS	CARIES RISK FACTORS
FLUORIDE TOOTHPASTE • Twice daily brushing with fluoridated toothpaste (at least 1000 ppm) **DENTAL CARE** • Regular preventive-oriented dental care, including for example application of topical fluoride **SYSTEMIC FLUORIDE** • Access to fluoridated drinking water or other community fluoride vehicles (where available)	**RISK FACTORS, SOCIAL/MEDICAL/BEHAVIORAL** • Hyposalivation, either drug-, disease-, head/neck-radiation or/and age-induced • High intake (amount/frequency) of free sugars from drinks (including fruit juice/smoothies), snacks and meals • Low socioeconomic level, low health literacy, health access barriers • Inability to comply, low motivation and engagement • Special health care needs, physical disabilities • Symptomatic-driven dental attendance) **RISK FACTORS, CLINICAL** • Recent caries experience and presence of active caries lesion(s) • PRS/prs* • Poor oral hygiene with thick plaque accumulation • Plaque stagnation areas (higher biofilm retention) • Low salivary flow rate **ADDITIONAL RISK FACTORS FOR CHILDREN** • Mother/caregiver with active caries lesions • Bottle/non-spill cup/pacifier containing natural or added sugar used frequently or at night (this includes milk and fruit juices/smoothies) • Non-daily use of at least 1000 ppm fluoride toothpaste • Erupting molar teeth **PARTICULAR RISK FACTORS FOR ELDERLY** • Exposed root surfaces (dentine) • Reduced ability to deliver oral hygiene
AT LOWER RISK: • Protective factors are present • None of the risk factors marked in red are present • Any other risk factors are within 'safe' ranges (e.g. sugary snacks, oral hygiene practice, fluoride exposure)	**AT HIGHER RISK:** • One or more of the risk factors marked in red are present • The level or combination of other risk factors suggests a higher risk status • With protective factors absent

*Pulpal Involvement-Roots-Sepsis Index (modified from PUFA/pufa): clinical consequences of untreated caries. P/p: caries process reached pulp chamber: Roots (R/r): caries process destroyed tooth structures (non-restorable): S/s: pus-releasing tract/tooth-related pus containing swelling.

Note: Risk factors in red/underlined will always classify an individual as high caries risk.

Fig. 3.3 Caries risk factors. (From Martignon S, Pitts NB, Goffin G, et al. CariesCare practice guide: consensus on evidence into practice. Br Dent J 2019;227:353–362.)

Risk factors, listed by the American Academy of Periodontology (http://www.perio.org/consumer/risk-factors), that can exacerbate or otherwise affect periodontal disease progression include:
• age
• smoking/tobacco use
• genetics
• stress
• medications
• clenching/bruxism
• systemic diseases (cardiovascular disease, diabetes, rheumatoid arthritis)
• poor nutrition and obesity

Evidence of linkage between periodontal disease risk and patient outcomes has been reported. Patients who have been determined to be at high risk of periodontal disease have been shown to have higher rates of tooth loss, even when compliant with treatment. Periodontal risk assessments have also been shown to be predictive of treatment outcomes.[63,64]

Periodontal disease risk assessment should be completed as part of any comprehensive or periodic dental examination. Given the slow and often asymptomatic progression of most periodontal diseases, all patients benefit from such an assessment. Assessing periodontal risk gives both the clinician and the patient a framework in which to discuss treatment and prevention strategies. Such an assessment helps to identify those factors that can or cannot be modified that will ultimately guide the long-term management of the patient. Consequently, a comprehensive assessment of a patient's periodontal risk factors is necessary throughout care.

Effective early management strategies should address modifiable risk factors. Possible therapies for patients with risk factors for periodontitis include:

- Oral hygiene instructions to review plaque removal techniques
- Smoking cessation, including referrals to other healthcare professionals as needed
- Referral to a physician for diabetes management
- Replacement of restorations with defective margins to eliminate plaque-retentive factors

Detailed information on the management of periodontal diseases can be found in Chapters 10 and 11.

Occlusal/Functional Risk Assessment

Appropriate assessment of dental occlusion and masticatory system function should be part of the initial comprehensive examination (Chapter 1), when a detailed patient history and careful clinical examination will reveal current occlusal problems, such as signs and symptoms of parafunctional habits, clenching, bruxing, or limitation of jaw movements. This assessment will enable the dentist to ascertain the risk of future occlusal-related problems. Dentists should also be regularly assessing these items during subsequent periodic exams.

When occlusal or functional problems are recognized or new problems anticipated, the dentist should consider implementing preventive or interventional strategies. An example, at the most basic level, is to identify patients involved in contact sports who will benefit from use of a protective mouth guard. At the more advanced level, this assessment would identify patients who are at higher risk of such problems as occlusal trauma, tooth fracture, worn or fractured restorations, bruxism, temporomandibular disorder (TMD), loss of vertical dimension of occlusion, or loss of function caused by occlusal abnormalities or missing teeth.

Unlike caries risk and periodontal risk, there are no standardized instruments to establish a level of occlusal or functional risk. Risk assessment of three common occlusal/functional issues are addressed in the following sections.

Bruxism

Bruxism is a relatively common parafunctional habit and is estimated to be present in up to 20% of dental patients.[65] It has been suggested that bruxism may lead to or exacerbate other conditions such as headaches, TMJ pain, muscle tenderness,

fractured teeth/restorations/implants, loss of tooth structure, premature loss of teeth secondary to fracture, and may be related to sleep apnea.[66] The presence of bruxism is a complicating factor for any planned prosthodontic rehabilitation. Failure to address bruxism prior to extensive restorative dentistry may lead to various unfavorable outcomes including tooth fracture and premature loss of teeth.[67] Box 3.1 lists some suggested risk indicators or risk factors for bruxism.

Since bruxism is believed to be multifactorial in origin and there is rarely an effective means of arresting the process, the target of existing bruxism management strategies is to minimize the consequences of bruxism such as TMD symptoms, excessive tooth wear (attrition), fractures of teeth or restorations, or loss of vertical dimension of occlusion. However, it is important to keep in mind that not all bruxers will become symptomatic or require treatment. Decisions regarding whether treatment is to be implemented and which treatment will be optimal must be made with the full informed consent of the patient. The discussion needs to address not only the potential risks and hazards of bruxism for the patient, but also the probability of negative outcomes with and without treatment given the patient's age, past dental experience and specific oral condition. Common treatment options are presented in Box 3.2.

Tooth Fracture

Tooth fracture may occur when heavy occlusal forces are applied to a vulnerable tooth. Such occurrences may be predicted from the initial comprehensive examination of the patient. Study casts are a useful adjunct to the examination because they usually show the existing wear of teeth more clearly than will direct observation of the teeth. It is generally recognized that heavily

---

BOX 3.1   Risk Indictors or Risk Factors for Bruxism[68,69]

- Family history/genetics
- Emotional stress
- Sleep disorders
- Psychological disorders (depression, psychoses, obsessive compulsive disorder)[70]
- Nighttime alcohol consumption[71]
- Heavy caffeine consumption
- Smoking
- Gastroesophageal reflux disorder
- Obstructive sleep apnea syndrome[72]

BOX 3.2   Possible Management Strategies for Patients Who Are Bruxers (or Patients Who Are at Elevated Risk of Becoming Bruxers)[68,69,73]

- Occlusal splint
- Sleep hygiene
- Patient education
- Botulinum toxin
- Behavioral therapy (behavioral modification)
- Psychological therapy (medications and/or desensitization therapy or other forms of psychotherapy)

restored endodontically-treated teeth that lack cuspal protection are more susceptible to fracture. Other risk indicators or risk factors for tooth fracture include:

- Clenching or bruxism[74]
- History tooth/restoration fractures
- Generalized attrition, wear facets
- Existing large direct fill restorations (compromised cusp integrity)
- Occlusal trauma (primary or secondary)
- Excessive occlusal forces
  Typical strategies to mitigate the risk for fracture include:
- fabrication of an occlusal guard/splint
- placement of cusp protective restorations
- replacement of missing teeth to defray the occlusal load on the existing teeth
- occlusal adjustment in the presence of acute occlusal trauma

As with bruxism, the "no treatment option" deserves serious consideration, especially if the patient is advanced in years, has not had significant problems with fractures in the recent past, has a conservative treatment philosophy, and is willing to accept the consequences and risks of not intervening at this time.

Temporomandibular Disorders. TMDs are typically multifactorial in origin and are identified most commonly in young adult women.[75] Common risk factors for patients with chronic TMDs include: health status and other pain disorders, depression, history of trauma, stress (psychosocial), bruxism, and parafunctional activity.[76]

The question of whether occlusal/functional problems cause or exacerbate TMDs remains controversial. In spite of the long-held truism that such a cause-effect relationship exists, the research evidence has not been definitive on this point. In this situation the *lack* of evidence to support more aggressive and invasive treatment has led to the adoption of more conservative and less costly approaches and in some cases more favorable patient outcomes.[77,78]

A systematic review identified only two significant occlusal risk factors for TMDs, lack of lateral cuspid guidance and Class II malocclusions.[79] Others have reported evidence that "grinding one's teeth" is a significant risk factor for myofascial pain[80] and have demonstrated that self-reported bruxism and variations in dental occlusion are linked to TMJ signs and symptoms.[81]

It is noteworthy that quantitative studies and those discussing specific methods for diagnosing bruxism have found a much lower association with TMD symptoms compared with self-reporting studies.[82] Most of the recent literature does not support the contention that malocclusion *causes* temporomandibular disorders[77] and orthodontic treatment has not been found to be a risk indicator or cause of temporomandibular problems.

It is reasonable to assume, however, that the patient *may* have an elevated risk of developing a TMD when, at the initial or periodic examination, the patient's history is positive for any of the following:

- joint clicking and pain
- clenching or bruxing
- jaw locking
- head/jaw trauma
  and/or upon clinical examination the dentist observes:

> **BOX 3.3 Common Strategies to Prevent and Treat Temporomandibular Disorders[83,84]**
>
> - Patient education (e.g., no gum chewing, change in sleep position, sleep hygiene, etc.)
> - Using heating pads over tender masticatory muscles
> - Jaw relaxation
> - Passive opening stretches
> - Nonsteroidal antiinflammatory drugs (in acute phase)
> - Fabrication of an occlusal guard/splint
> - Behavioral modification therapy
> - Referral to mental healthcare professionals

- severe attrition caused by bruxism
- symptomatic occlusal interferences
- functional limitations in jaw movement
- TMJ noises associated with pain
- masticatory muscles tenderness on palpation

The management and treatment of acute TMDs is discussed in Chapter 9 and other issues relating to TMDs in Chapter 10. When patients are identified as at risk of TMDs, any recommended treatment should be as minimally invasive as will be effective. Common treatment strategies to prevent and treat occlusally related TMJ problems are listed in Box 3.3.

PROGNOSIS [80,81,85–89]

Prognosis can be related to risk. For example, if a patient is at high risk of caries, the prognosis for the desired successful outcome, the control of the caries, may be poor unless the risk factors or indicators are modified or eliminated. It is critical to remember that risk and prognosis are distinctly different concepts. Several issues that may influence the prognosis may not themselves be risk indicators. Examples of such issues include severity of the disease at the onset of treatment, the ability and commitment of the dentist, and the patient's level of motivation to achieve a state of good oral health. Risk factors are used to estimate the probability of the patient acquiring the disease; whereas prognosis is a prediction of the outcome of the disease process or of our ability to manage it, our prediction of the success of associated treatments.

Because prognosis is a prediction of *future* outcomes, there is an inherent potential for inaccuracy. Most oral diseases are multifactorial in nature and, for each patient, the strength of the various causes and their relative impact amidst a dynamic oral condition with often changing social determinants of health, make it difficult to predict the future oral health condition accurately. Another uncertainty is the impact of future initiatives. Samet and Jotkowitz[90] in their seminal work on classification and prognosis for individual teeth described patient categories and treatment-related factors that play a role in determining the prognosis. These include:

- biological risks (e.g., general health conditions that impair immune function or limit oral hygiene)
- environmental risks
- financial and behavioral/personal risks (e.g., finances, motivation, commitment, compromised oral hygiene)

- quality of the dental treatment
- quality of oral health maintenance

Embedded within these categories are both mutable and immutable patient-specific conditions that can be highly variable in their impact and that may change significantly during the course of treatment.

Generally speaking, prognosis is a professional judgment about the outcome of a health condition with or without treatment. In the dental setting, prognosis is established by the dentist. Determination of the prognosis can be used to frame the discussion with the patient about the relative merits of various treatment options and to provide the patient with invaluable information on which to base treatment planning decisions. In sharing the prognosis determination with the patient, the dentist must also be mindful of, and relate to the patient, some sense of the relative certainty (confidence level) held in assessing prognosis.

Descriptors of Prognosis

There are clear benefits to both provider and patient in assigning a prognosis to a patient's condition and treatment plan. Although others have proposed classification systems[90-93] for prognoses in dentistry, there is no universally accepted system. In the context of this book the descriptors used here pertain to the discussion that the practitioner can be expected to have with the patient regarding the *prognosis of the proposed treatment plans or treatment plan alternatives.*

- Excellent = highest level of certainty in achieving treatment goals; provider confidence level greater than 95%; safe to proceed without reservation; recommendations for treatment can be made freely to the patient by the provider; assurances that can be given to the patient after factoring in the dentist's expertise (experience, skill and training) and the dentist's perception of the patient's motivation, expectations, and anticipated level of cooperation.
- Good = high probability of success; provider confidence level greater than 80%; safe to proceed with selected or limited reservations; recommendations can be made by provider with some caution or limitation; limited assurances can be given to the patient in light of limiting factors and given the experience, skill and training of the dentist; and the dentist's perception of the patient's cooperation, motivation, and expectations.
- Fair = reasonable but limited probability of success; usually one or more negative element influences the prognosis determination; provider confidence level is in the 50% to 80% range; must have realistic discussion of the limiting factors with patient; provider can offer only the most restricted (if any) assurance.
- Poor or Guarded = limited chance of success; provider confidence level less than 50%; patient must be fully informed about the risks, hazards, and possible negative outcomes of treatment; patient must provide documented commitment and informed consent before proceeding with treatment; provider can offer only limited assurance of success.
- Hopeless = no reasonable chance of success; confidence level less than 5%; elective treatment should not be undertaken.
- Uncertain/questionable = may mean that not enough information is available to make a determination of prognosis

(e.g., prognosis cannot be determined until completion of disease control phase treatment); or, even in the presence of adequate diagnostic information, the prognosis cannot be determined (e.g., compelling positive *and* negative variables in force); provider and patient must proceed with caution and patient must provide documented commitment and informed consent before proceeding with treatment; provider can offer no assurance of success.

Domains of Prognosis

A determination of prognosis can be useful in the various domains of dentistry and is commonly ascribed to a wide range of oral diseases and conditions. It can be applied to an individual tooth or to the dentition as a whole particularly as pertains to the prospect for retaining the tooth or teeth in the mouth for an extended period of time. Prognosis is also commonly applied to the probability of success for a proposed dental treatment. Each of these applications is described here.

Prognosis for Specific Diseases or Conditions

In this section, a few representative conditions are described, conditions in which the prognosis has unique and important implications for planning the dental treatment of the patient.

Mucositis. Mucositis may have a singular cause or may be multifactorial in origin; may be acute and extremely debilitating; or chronic, low grade, intermittent and only "mildly annoying" to the patient. When the cause can be clearly determined and can be easily mitigated or eliminated, the prognosis is good or excellent. In this case, the impact on the treatment plan is negligible. If, however, the symptoms are severe and persistent, and the cause elusive, the prognosis will usually be uncertain or poor/guarded. In this situation, managing the mucositis will typically override all other treatment priorities, and may abrogate or delay other planned or needed treatment.

Severe mucositis is usually reported as an oral side-effect of cancer therapy (both chemo and head and neck radiation therapies) and it can cause significant oral pain, making oral hygiene difficult and reducing food intake, that may result in nutritional impairment. When accompanied by xerostomia, it can also lead to rapid oral health deterioration. Therefore, properly management of mucositis is key for oral health maintenance and quality of life in oncology patients.[94] Other causes of mucositis include Behçet syndrome, mechanical or chemical irritation, and hypersensitivity to dental products and foods (contact stomatitis).[95,96]

Oral cancer. The patient with oral cancer may have a varied prognosis:

- At the time of the initial diagnosis the prognosis is typically *uncertain*.
- During the course of cancer treatment the prognosis may be *guarded or fair*.
- Following successful treatment (surgical excision with clean margins and no lymph node involvement) the prognosis is usually *good*.
- A 10-year cancer survivor without recurrence is thought to have an *excellent* prognosis.

The patient undergoing surgery, radiation, and/or chemotherapy for an aggressive squamous cell carcinoma with an uncertain prognosis, will require extensive modification to the treatment plan. The cancer and the side-effects of chemotherapy will require unique interventions. Treatment priorities will be altered. The patient will suffer new oral health problems. Changes in the manner in which dental treatment is delivered may be necessary and there may be significant limitations to the range and complexity of dental treatment in both the short term and for years to come. By contrast, the long-term oral cancer survivor with an excellent prognosis will require minimal adjustment to a treatment plan and is a candidate for a complete range of dental treatment.

Periodontal disease. In their landmark commentary article, Kwok and Caton[97] wrote "prognosis is an integral part of the periodontal practice because it directly influences treatment planning." In that article they make the following key points:

- In years past, most periodontal prognostication systems were primarily based on tooth loss, which has not proven to be a good predictor of future outcomes.
- The stability of the periodontal supporting tissues is a more useful basis for determining periodontal prognosis as it is "influenced by more evidence-based factors and may be more useful in patient management."
- "Periodontal stability can be evaluated continually by clinical attachment and radiographic bone measurements."
- There is value in making both short-term and long-term prognosis determinations, while recognizing that the prognosis may change over time and may be altered by patient behavioral changes and by professional intervention and maintenance.
- It is useful to determine prognosis for individual teeth and for the entire dentition.
- Prognosis should be continuously evaluated to account for the chronic, episodic, and dynamic nature of periodontitis.

Kwok and Caton have identified the following factors that may affect periodontal prognosis:

General Factors:
- Patient compliance in an effective maintenance program.
- Cigarette smoking.
- Diabetes mellitus.
- Other systemic factors. *There are a number of medical conditions that may contribute to more rapid periodontal breakdown.*

Local Factors:
- Deep probing depths and attachment loss. *Sites with probing depths >5 mm are more difficult to maintain, leading to greater residual plaque and calculus deposits, and are more prone to future periodontal breakdown.*
- Other anatomic plaque-retentive factors. *Furcation involvement, enamel pearls, cervical enamel projections, root grooves, crowding, open contacts, overhanging dental restorations, etc. may all contribute to an environment that is challenging to maintain adequate plaque control.*
- Trauma from occlusion and parafunctional habits.
- Mobility.

With updates to the recent periodontal classification system endorsed by the American Academy of Periodontology and the European Federation of Periodontology, the importance of periodontal prognosis and risk assessment are underscored through grading. Each patient should be assigned a grade that incorporates the estimation of future periodontitis risk and likely responsiveness to treatment. The presence of various risk factors may also be considered when assigning a grade. For more information, please see Chapter 2 and Table 2.3.

Other factors that have been identified as predictors of periodontal prognosis include level of plaque control and interleukin-1 genotype.[98] The box *In Clinical Practice: Using Periodontal Prognosis in Treatment Planning* illustrates how this information is useful in treatment planning and patient care.

IN CLINICAL PRACTICE

Using Periodontal Prognosis In Treatment Planning

How can the practitioner utilize this information in a practical way? If, for example, a new patient presents to the practice with poorly controlled diabetes, generalized 5–7 mm probing depths, multiple sites with 4–5 mm of attachment loss, furcation involvement, subgingival calculus deposits, a 60% plaque score, bleeding on probing at 35% of sites, and the individual seems poorly motivated to save their teeth, the initial prognosis would be ***questionable*** and it would be prudent to engage the patient in a disease control phase plan of care (see Chapter 10). At the conclusion of the disease control phase, a reassessment of the patient's condition and the prognosis would be implemented. If, at that time, the diabetes is well controlled, plaque control improved, calculus removed, signs of inflammation dissipated, and the patient is now motivated and enthusiastic about retaining the teeth, the prognosis would elevate to ***favorable***, tooth retention would be encouraged, and a full range of restorative (prosthetic) interventions could be favorably be considered. Conversely, if the diabetes remains poorly controlled, if the plaque score remains high (in spite of best efforts to educate the patient), inflammation persists, attachment loss progresses, and/or the patient's motivation languishes, and they have not been compliant with recommendations for therapy and maintenance, the prognosis worsens to ***unfavorable*** and it may be wise to place the patient on a long-term maintenance schedule or to recommend extraction of severely compromised teeth. Embarking on complex restorative procedures should be postponed until the patient's periodontal condition is stabilized and the prognosis improves.

Prognosis for Individual Tooth or Teeth

It is important to assess prognosis for the whole dentition and for individual teeth. This encourages a broader view of the patient while also helping to develop detailed treatment plans to address localized needs. Samet et al. have devised a comprehensive evidence-based prognosis classification system for individual teeth that can be a reliable guide for the novice or experienced practitioner.[99]

For many patients, there is one tooth, or a select few teeth, that is/are worthy of extensive consideration and for which treatment choices are debatable. There are other patients, those with complex problems and needs, for whom there may be one or a very few teeth whose fate is critical to the overall plan of care. The latter have been described in Chapter 5 as "key" teeth. In either scenario, determining the prognosis for the tooth or teeth in question is essential to making a treatment selection.

Important issues to evaluate in making the prognosis determination for the tooth or teeth include:

- restorability
- periodontal support
- occlusal force on the tooth in maximum intercuspation (MI) and excursive movements
- necessity and feasibility of root canal treatment
- potential for future caries or fracture
- patient commitment (time, finances, energy) to doing what will be required to retain the tooth
- practitioner skill in restoring the tooth or teeth in question

Prognosis Determinants for Specific Treatments

A prognosis can be assigned to a complete array of dental treatments. Table 3.1 includes the category of treatment, factors that may influence the prognosis, and selected related evidence. However, there are other notable determinants of prognosis not mentioned in Table 3.1 that apply universally to any treatment. Two important considerations are patient cooperation during the procedure, and the skill and expertise of the provider, the latter becoming more significant as the complexity of the procedure increases.

Prognosis for Overall Treatment

This is the issue that is usually foremost in the patient's mind. Before embarking on a comprehensive plan of care, the patient will usually ask, and rightfully should expect to know, the prognosis for their condition and for the treatment plan. If multiple treatment plans are being offered, it is appropriate to inform the patient about the prognosis and relative merits of each.

Application and Use of Prognosis in Treatment Planning

It is essential for the dentist to assess carefully and accurately the prognosis for the disease with and without treatment before treatment options are suggested to the patient. This step follows the initial oral examination of the patient and the generation of the diagnosis list from which the prognosis is derived. Determining the prognosis for the patient's treatment typically has some degree of uncertainty. The more complicated the patient's disease state and the more complex the treatment plan, the greater will be the opportunity for error.

To illustrate this point, consider a patient who has been diagnosed with severe periodontal disease and given a prognosis for an excellent outcome (elimination of the active disease and associated signs and symptoms) with a particular treatment plan. In spite of the best efforts of both the patient and the dental team, the periodontal disease continues to advance. The discrepancy between what was predicted (the prognosis), and what actually occurs (the outcome) can arise because of many different factors, any one of which may not have been predicted accurately at the time of treatment planning. In spite such limitations, however, establishing a prognosis affords

TABLE 3.1	**Factors Influencing Prognosis for Selected Types of Treatment**

- Orthodontic treatment: accurate assessment and case diagnosis, complexity of the deformity, type of tooth movement (rotation, tipping, bodily movement, extrusion, intrusion), periodontal health status, caries risk, patient motivation, patient expectations, patient compliance with treatment and oral care regimens
- Orthognathic surgery: accurate assessment and case diagnosis, medical limitations or contraindications to surgery; surgical complications, periodontal health status, caries risk, patient motivation, patient expectations, patient compliance with treatment and oral care regimens
- Endodontic treatment: tooth isolation, restorability of the tooth, marginal periodontal health status, risk for caries, risk for fracture due to severe bruxism, risk-taking lifestyle (potential for future trauma to the tooth), complex anatomy (calcified canals, root dilaceration, accessory canals, etc.), quality of the canal obturation (proper length, diameter, density)
- Periodontal treatment: uncontrolled medical conditions, cigarette smoking, caries, restorative condition (iatrogenic defects) of the teeth, patient ability to perform regular and effective plaque control, microbiota pathogenicity, endodontic status, occlusion, tooth mobility, factitious habits
- Individual restoration(s): magnitude of tooth destruction, material selection, tooth preparation, restoration quality (margins/contours/occlusion), disease control (secondary caries), potential for tooth fracture, occlusion, periodontal health status, patient esthetic expectations
- Implant: medical contraindications, immune compromise, bone height, bone contour, bone density, proximity to important anatomic structures, interocclusal space, occlusion, parafunctional habits, implant selection, implant position, function/load of attached prosthesis, periodontal health status, endodontic health of adjacent teeth[99,100]
- Complete denture: xerostomia, ridge form and extent, interarch space, epuli, bony undercuts, bruxism or parafunctional habits, tongue size/position, gagging, opposing arch plane of occlusion, denture retention and stability, patient expectations, patient level of motivation, patient self-perceived level of function and esthetics, patient ability to comply with oral care regimen, patient willingness to return for recare visits[101–105]
- Partial denture: same as for complete denture plus considerations for the abutment and remaining teeth: periodontal health status of abutment teeth, stability, restorability, potential for fracture or premature loss; ability of abutment teeth to withstand occlusal and functional load of prosthesis, risk for caries and/or periodontal disease on remaining teeth; patient ability to insert/remove/clean/maintain the removable partial denture, patient willingness to return for continuing care visits[106]

the dentist with an important, albeit imprecise, approach to evaluating treatment alternatives and ultimately treatment outcomes. Such a discussion provides the dentist with a basis on which to discuss with the patient which plan will have the greatest chance of success. Less promising treatment options with poorer prognoses can be ruled out and alternatives with a better likelihood of success can be included in the choices presented to the patient.

When the patient has a thorough and accurate understanding of the prognosis, they can make an educated, rational choice on how to proceed. This is not to say that prognosis alone determines which alternative to choose but, along with other issues (e.g., time, degree of discomfort, financial cost, esthetic benefits), the concept can be very important in helping the patient decide among the options. Determining a prognosis is indispensable to the dentist and patient in helping frame the treatment choices, making the best treatment selection, and as part of the overall effort to establish meaningful informed consent.

Multiple variables individually or collectively may have an impact on the prognosis for an oral condition or for the treatment to be provided. These variables may be beneficial, detrimental, or both. The information in Table 3.1 is representative of the kind of evaluation that the practitioner should make for a treatment option before recommending it to a patient.

Following such an analysis, the prognosis for each of the appropriate options (as framed by the dentist) will need to be communicated in a way that is understandable to the patient. Usually this is accomplished seamlessly as part of the larger informed consent discussion. Along with other issues, including financial cost, time and number of visits required for the treatment, and anticipated discomfort, inconvenience, or esthetic limitations during treatment, an understanding of the prognosis for each treatment option can be extremely helpful in assisting the patient to make a definitive treatment selection.

OUTCOMES AND OUTCOMES MEASURES

The Role of Outcomes Measures

Outcome measures are important in direct management of individual patient care as well as for the opportunity they afford the dental profession collectively to compare types of care and to evaluate the effectiveness of various treatments. Many treatment decisions are facilitated by knowledge of the likely outcome for each of the proposed alternatives. Such predictions can help the dentist select the best options, refine the list of realistic choices, and act as an important adjunct to the presentation of the treatment plan to the patient. This information could be even more important to the patient who attempts to weigh the pros and cons of the various treatment options. The most valuable outcome information for the patient would be the success rate for a specific procedure when performed by the practitioner who is proposing the treatment. Unfortunately, these data are usually not formally tracked in the community-based private dental practice and therefore are not readily available for dentists (or patients) to use. When outcome measures are generated in institutional settings (e.g., hospitals, military/veterans affairs dentistry, dental schools/colleges), and when they are used to make quality improvements for those populations, they may have relevance to other practice settings. The American Dental Association has endorsed the position that "to assure that we are providing the highest quality patient-centered dental care, dentistry must measure what works and what doesn't and make changes needed to improve health."[107]

The Guidebook states that a good measure is one that:
1. Covers an important clinical area,
2. Is scientifically acceptable,
3. Is useable, and
4. Is feasible. [108]

When selecting a measure of outcomes the Agency for Healthcare Research and Quality (AHRQ) suggests key questions that should be considered. (https://www.ahrq.gov/talkingquality/keyquestionsaboutmeasures>KeyQuestionsWhenChoosingHealthCareQualityMeasures).

Are the Measures Good?

- Standardization: The measures are standardized at the national level, which means that all health care providers will be reporting the same kind of data in the same way.
- Comparability: If appropriate, the results are adjusted for external factors that could make a health care organization's performance appear better or worse than it really is; such factors include age, education, gender, income, and health status.
- Availability: Data will be available for the majority of health care organizations that you are profiling.
- Timeliness: The results will be available in time for you to produce and distribute a report when it is most needed by consumers.
- Relevance: The measures address the concerns of your audience.
- Validity: The measures have been adequately tested to ensure that they consistently and accurately reflect the performance of health care organizations
- Experience: Health care organizations have experience with these measures, so that you can be confident that the measure reflects actual performance and not shortcomings in information systems. Stability: The measures are not scheduled to be "retired," e.g., removed from a measurement data set to make room for better measures.
- Evaluability: The results can be evaluated as either better or worse than other results, in contrast to descriptive information that merely shows how health care organizations may be different from each other. For example, a complication rate is an evaluable measure because we know that a lower rate is always better; in contrast, a Caesarian-section rate is not evaluable because we don't necessarily know whether a higher rate or a lower rate is desirable.
- Distinguishable: The measures reveal significant differences among health care organizations.
- Credibility: The measures are either audited or do not require an audit.

Are the Measures Appropriate for Your Audience?

- Does the measure support your goal?
- Do consumers view the measure as important?
- Is the measure relevant to your intended audience?

The AHRQ system includes several dozen dental-specific outcome measure. (see https://www.ahrq.gov/talkingquality/measures/index/dental>DentalCare)

Using Outcomes Information in the Treatment Planning Process

A common question that many patients will think of, but may be reluctant to ask, is "How long can I expect my filling, crown, bridge, or denture to last?" This, of course, is a question that is difficult for a practitioner to answer with certainty as there are many patient and professional factors; in addition to specific oral, tooth and surface conditions; that can impact on the longevity of the restoration or prosthesis, But this is a fair and reasonable question and the patient deserves a considered response. Even if the patient does not ask the question, the expected longevity of the restorative treatment options is an important issue to include in consent discussion. In an effort to provide a context for that discussion, the authors have provided a summary of existing evidence in the box **How Long Do Restorations and Prostheses Last** and a more detailed rendition in the e-version of this text. The discussion with the patient will then need to be framed by an explanation of how the specifics of the patient's general and oral health condition will impact on the expected outcome.

Some common clinical situations for which sufficient outcomes information does exist can help to structure the treatment planning discussion. The following clinical problems illustrate the ways in which the dentist can use outcomes information in the treatment planning process and ways the patient can use the information to make a treatment decision.

Can Caries Be Left Under a Permanent Restoration?

A long-held truism in dentistry was that all carious tooth structure needs to be removed from the lesion prior to placement of a definitive restoration. There is now a significant body of evidence demonstrating that this truism is false. In fact, outcome studies have shown that selective caries removal in symptomless teeth is advantageous compared with complete excavation, especially when close to the pulp, because doing so reduces the risk of pulpal exposure.[109–114] Studies show that leaving some caries at the deepest extent of a defect is not detrimental with regard to posttreatment symptoms, tooth vitality, or restoration longevity and results in lower long-term costs.[12,115,116]

Factors when considering selective caries removal are:
* preoperative pulpal symptoms
* radiographic and/or clinical signs of pulpal or periapical disease
* restorability of the tooth

There are two methods for selective caries removal: (1) two-step method in which the tooth is temporarily restored and then reentered and restored definitively at a subsequent appointment (called stepwise excavation) and (2) a one-step method in which the tooth receives its definitive restoration at one appointment.[117] Both approaches have been shown to be effective.[117,118] Proponents of the two-step procedure suggest that it is necessary to remove the temporary base/cement and reexamine the remaining dentin to ensure the presence of healthy tissue (as would be demonstrated by the presence of a dentin bridge, which is formed by dentine that presents hard and dry). The drawback to this step is that it increases the chance of a pulpal exposure.[117,119] The one-step approach has the obvious advantage of lower cost[115] and less time. Outcomes studies suggest that the one-step technique is associated with longer tooth retention and vitality and should therefore be the default procedure.[114,113,119] Other variables (such as fewer involved tooth surfaces) also contribute to higher success rates.[116] Given this evidence, selective caries removal in one step by selective removal to soft dentine should be the standard operating procedure.

When Should a Defective Restoration Be Replaced?[120,121]

Re-restoration is not an innocuous procedure. Research demonstrates that when old restorations are replaced with new ones, the new restorations tend to be larger and more expensive than their predecessors.[122] As intracoronal restorations become successively larger, it is increasingly likely that a protective cusp restoration (usually a crown) will be recommended and that, in a predictable percentage of the cases, undesirable sequelae will occur, such as an irreversible pulpitis and the need for root canal therapy. Outcomes studies provide some guidance[123]:
* Teeth with obvious recurrent caries should be restored.
* Restorations with small marginal discrepancies (ditching) and no overt caries do not need to be replaced.
* Teeth with isolated recurrent caries may be successfully repaired or patched.[124–126]

When faced with the decision whether a restoration should be replaced, a review of the relevant outcomes literature provides the practitioner with additional guidance for the decision, an understanding of the consequences of the available options, and some broad treatment parameters. Such a review will not, however, provide answers to such diagnostic questions whether active caries exist under an old restoration with open or stained margins. If all the information revealed by careful evaluation and inspection of the tooth fails to resolve that question, an exploratory repair preparation may be in order. The decision whether to re-restore the tooth must ultimately be an informed decision made by the patient. The expected outcome of each of the treatment options, including no treatment, is an important piece of information that the patient must have to make a wise choice.

Patients often present with an existing crown that has a marginal gap and/or secondary caries. In this situation the practitioner needs to discern whether replacement of the crown is warranted. The cost of replacing a crown is usually significantly higher when compared with those of direct restorations and it also more time consuming and riskier to the remaining tooth structure. However, practitioners commonly disagree regarding the diagnosis (caries/defective margin) and when it is necessary to replace a crown.[127] More orthodox practitioners are often less tolerant of marginal defects and are more likely to recommend crown replacement. On the other hand, many practitioners might choose to do crown margin repairs using glass-ionomer cements, composite resin, or amalgam. Another option is to apply silver diamine fluoride (SDF) to arrest and prevent caries around defective margins, monitor the site at regular intervals, and reapply SDF as needed. In a recent 18-month clinical trial,[128] caries lesions adjacent to crowns were successfully arrested in 90% of the time using SDF. The latter approaches (crown margin repairs and/or SDF application) have the obvious benefit of reduced costs and risks to the patient, but may be unacceptable in esthetic areas.

Currently, there are no outcome studies showing the long-term results of either approach. For this reason, the "crown margin repair versus crown replacement" situation is a good example of a clinical situation where research-based evidence is not determinative. In such circumstances the practitioner should use a situation analysis approach where the practitioner presents the pros and cons of each option in the context of the specific clinical circumstances including, but not limited to, the patient's health, SDHs, and caries risk; the tooth/surfaces involved; characteristics of the defective area; and the practitioner's clinical judgment regarding the probable outcome, and the possible complications of the treatment alternatives — and allow the patient to make an autonomous decision how to proceed.

When Should a Heavily Restored Tooth Be Crowned?

This is another common clinical scenario that takes on particular importance in the present context because it is one of the most common opportunities for overtreatment in dentistry. To be sure, there are compelling reasons for fabricating a crown on an otherwise heavily restored tooth. A tooth that exhibits pain on biting and has a crack line is one such example. But in the absence of symptoms, new or recurrent caries, restoration defect, or fracture line in the tooth, the question must be asked: *is the mere presence of a large direct fill restoration sufficient indication to recommend a crown to a patient?*

To answer this question, the dentist will need to evaluate several parameters:

- What is the stability and viability of the current restoration? Past history of the tooth and restoration in question is most often a good predictor of future longevity and success. In other words, if the current restoration has been there for many years and there have been no negative outcomes, it is more likely that there will be a continuing track record of success if the restoration is retained.
- Are there excessive occlusal forces on the tooth? Severe attrition indicating possible bruxism, loss of vertical dimension, and heavy lateral or incline forces on the tooth all increase the probability of tooth fracture and therefore increase the probable benefit of crowning the tooth.
- What has been the patient's past experience with tooth fracture? Has it happened frequently, seldom, or not at all? Certainly a patient with a recent history of multiple tooth fractures is at greater risk of future fractures.
- If there is a high risk of fracture on the tooth in question, can the risk be mitigated by other means, such as eliminating all incline contacts on the tooth or fabricating an occlusal guard? Is placement of a crown really the best way to prevent future fracture?
- What is the probability that the process of fabricating the crown will necessitate additional procedures, such as prophylactic or prosthetically-required root canal therapy,

forced eruption, crown lengthening procedure, or placement of a new foundation or a post and core?
- With either treatment option, what is the probability of future negative sequelae such as pulpal necrosis, recurrent caries, coronal amputation, or crown debonding. What would be the consequences of these sequelae?
- What is the prognosis for the tooth with or without the crown?

Ultimately the treat versus no treat decision must be made by the patient after an informative consent discussion. In most situations, when the patient presents with a disease-free and asymptomatic tooth that has a large direct fill restoration, there will not be a compelling argument for placing a crown, but the patient should nevertheless be made aware of the treatment options and the benefits and deficits of those options—including any negative sequelae that may arise with either choice—and the *probability* of those negative sequelae. Here is an instance in which good outcome data can be helpful to the patient who is trying to weigh the options whether to proceed with a crown at this time. A recent systematic review and metanalysis has shown that gold and porcelain-fused to metal crowns have the lowest annual failure rates (less than 1%) compared with other indirect restorations (indirect composite resin 1.8% and zirconia 2.9%) and direct restorations (amalgam 2.7% and composite resin 2.2%) for large posterior restorations.[129]

When Should a Missing Posterior Tooth Be Replaced?

Conventional wisdom has encouraged the replacement of missing teeth when posterior tooth loss has created a bounded edentulous space (BES) (see Figure 3.4). The time-honored assumption has been that unless the space is filled, tipping or extrusion of remaining teeth leading to arch collapse will likely occur, and there will be a significantly increased potential for localized marginal bone loss and periodontal disease, pathologic temporomandibular condition, and occlusal trauma. It has been held that delaying reconstruction may necessitate more complex procedures, such as crown lengthening, root canal therapy, and/

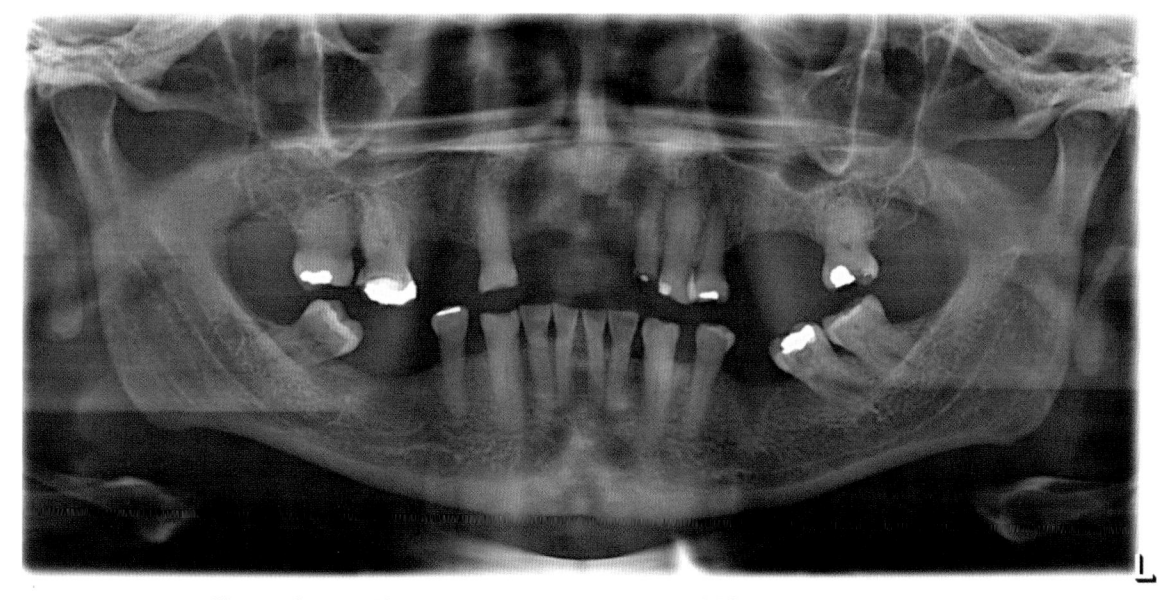

Fig. 3.4 Stable BES's in the maxillary arch; collapsed BES's in the mandibular arch.

or crown placement on an opposing hyper-erupted tooth.[130] Studies suggest that these concerns may be inflated[131] and that replacement with a fixed partial denture has significant limitations.[132] Replacement with an implant-retained crown has a predictably favorable outcome but will typically incur greater cost to the patient. It has been shown that, although some teeth bounding an edentulous space may drift or tip, many do not. Of those that do move, most do so immediately after the extraction.[133]

Given this information (and in the absence of a compelling esthetic or psychological concern), it is reasonable to suggest the option of closely monitoring the space with intervention only if notable change (e.g., >2 mm) begins to occur. Even if intervention becomes necessary, limited treatment, such as a fixed or removable orthodontic device or an occlusal guard, may be all that is necessary to prevent tipping of an adjacent tooth and/ or extrusion of an opposing tooth.

For this situation, outcomes studies have been instrumental in challenging the profession to reconsider conventional wisdom, as long-term follow-up studies have shown unimpaired oral-health related quality of life for people with shortened dental arches.[134,135] Outcomes information allows patient and practitioner to define a wider and more practical range of treatment options and provides research-based information on which to evaluate treatment options. It may still be prudent for the patient to proceed with tooth replacement, but the choice can be made with more knowledge and a clearer understanding of the risks and benefits of the various options.

Should a Tooth With an Unsuccessful Root Canal Treatment Be Re-Treated?[136]

Cumulative statistics from several studies suggest that the overall success rate (lesion healing and tooth retention) for initial root canal therapy is 80% to 85% for nonvital teeth and 90% to 92% for vital teeth under controlled conditions.[137–141] The presence of a periapical lesion before treatment, obturation beyond the radiographic apex, or obturation with silver points, all tend to diminish success. When failure does occur, it is usually the result of bacterial invasion or persistence of bacteria in the root canal system through root fracture, inadequate coronal seal, incomplete obturation, or the presence of lateral canals or other anatomic anomalies. If the initial conventional root canal treatment is not successful, many patients are reluctant to invest additional time, effort, and/or financial resources in the tooth, and may prefer to extract.

Nevertheless, many studies support the benefits of retreatment. As long as the root is not overtly fractured, the success rate averages 80%.[142] Subsequent retreatments show diminished success, however. If retreatment by conventional means is not feasible or has a poor prognosis, or if time constraints weigh in favor of a surgical approach, apicoectomy with retrograde fill may be another alternative. A surgical approach is often recommended when the tooth has an adequate coronal restoration (i.e., good coronal seal with no leakage or recurrent decay) and a previous root canal within the standard of care. Traditional surgical techniques with severe bevels and the use of amalgam retrofills has had a success rate of about 60%. With modern microsurgical techniques, apical microsurgery

has been shown to be successful in 90% of the cases.[143–145] In a direct comparison between endodontic retreatment and dental implants for teeth with an uncertain endodontic prognosis, a 3-year follow-up study showed no significant differences for treatment failure or complications and number of patient visits, but it took more days for the implant treatment to be completed albeit with less chair time. However, implant treatment was significantly more expensive.[146]

In this situation, information obtained from outcomes research provides patient and provider with the resources required to make a rational and informed treatment decision. Based on this information, the patient can make a reasoned choice about whether the benefit (likelihood of retaining the tooth) is worth the cost of conventional or surgical endodontic retreatment. Knowledge about the expected outcome of the common alternative treatment—extraction and placement of a single implant-retained crown—has further aided this process (see *In Clinical Practice: A Common Dilemma—Deciding Between Extraction or Placement of an Implant-Retained Crown Versus Restoration With a Root Canal Treatment, Foundation, and Crown*). Now the patient is in the ideal position of being able to weigh options. *How Long Do Restorations and Prostheses Last*

IN CLINICAL PRACTICE

A Common Dilemma—Deciding Between Extraction or Placement of an Implant-Retained Crown Versus Restoration With a Root Canal Treatment, Foundation, and Crown

Before the development of the osseointegrated implant-retained crown, it was not unusual for the dentist to go to extraordinary lengths to save a badly broken-down tooth. If the tooth was lost, the common replacement alternative had been a fixed or removable partial denture (see Chapter 11 for details). Dentists and patients alike generally sought to avoid those alternatives if reasonably possible. In recent years, replacement of a badly compromised tooth with an implant-retained crown has become a predictable and financially viable alternative, but there are still many situations in which it is preferable to retain a compromised tooth rather than to extract it. The treatment dilemma of when to restore and when to extract a severely decayed or fractured tooth continues to be a common and relevant treatment planning question in the contemporary practice of general dentistry. It is also a good example of how the evolving body of evidence in dentistry can help both dentist and patient make rational and appropriate treatment decisions.

For the dentist, the starting point in this analysis is to determine the prognosis if the tooth were to be restored. What treatment will be required? What is the expected survival rate? If failure occurs, what are the other possible negative outcomes? How can each of those negative outcomes be addressed? What additional treatments could be required at that time? Typically, the patient will be interested in the same questions. They may also seek information on the prognosis, expected outcomes, and the possible discomfort and inconvenience attendant on the alternative treatment of implant placement and restoration. The patient will need to be informed about the financial costs, the time required, and the expected number of visits necessary to accomplish either alternative.

The following information summarizes many of the tooth-specific and patient-specific factors that may have a bearing on this decision-making process:

Factors that favor retention and restoration
- Poor general health contraindicates implant surgery
- Patient aversion to oral surgical procedures
- Root canal treatment has favorable long-term prognosis

- Tooth and restoration have favorable long-term prognosis
- Sufficient biologic width is present (crown lengthening procedure or forced eruption not indicated)
- Low caries risk
- Low risk for tooth fracture

Factors that favor extraction and implant and crown placement

- No general health contraindications to extraction and implant placement
- Patient willing to undergo oral surgical procedures
- Adequate bone for implant fixture retention
- Inadequate biologic width (crown lengthening procedure or forced eruption needed if the tooth is to be retained)
- High caries risk/high risk for tooth fracture
- Patient exhibits significant occlusal trauma

Ultimately the treatment decision must be made as part of an extended conversation with the patient in which these issues are covered in depth. Typically, the immediate situation will have some factors that may weigh in favor of tooth retention and others that will weigh in favor of extraction and implant placement. Many other intangibles, such as a patient's previous personal experience with root canal therapy, often weigh heavily in the patient's mind and will influence the decision. Whenever possible, the dentist should share relevant information from the dental literature and should also augment that information with specific outcomes measures from their own practice. When the decision remains in the balance even after an extended options and consent discussion, the scale is usually tipped in the patient's mind as to whether additional surgical intervention is anticipated, i.e., a crown lengthening procedure in the case of saving the tooth, or augmentation or sinus lift in the case of implant placement. If the prognosis is deemed favorable in both cases, the ultimate cost of the two alternatives may be the determining factor in the decision. At the present time, in most cases, it is still less expensive to restore the tooth with a root canal treatment, foundation (or post and core), and crown than to extract the tooth and then place and restore an implant. Certainly, if a crown lengthening procedure or orthodontic forced eruption is necessary to save the tooth, the total costs for the two options become more equitable.

These examples suggest the ways in which outcomes research can support clinical treatment decisions. Because further research reveals quantified outcomes for additional treatments under various conditions, the practitioner has the responsibility to remain current with the scientific literature and to relate that information to the individual patient's situation. Where reliable longitudinal studies about the specific type of treatment are lacking, the dentist will need to keep updated and critically appraise other, even if less reliable, available literature when making clinical decisions. The dentist may rely in part on their own experience to make a treatment recommendation, but that must be supplemented by guidance from the published literature whenever such evidence is available.

Additional basis for decision making will be available when the dentist has developed individual or practice-based treatment outcome data for a full range of procedures in their own setting. Certainly this information will be helpful to patients as they make treatment choices and the process should help the individual dentist to better assess their own practice techniques. An additional potential benefit of this process is providing the impetus for constant quality improvement in the procedures, materials, and techniques in the practice.

THE EVOLVING USE OF EVIDENCE-BASED DENTISTRY IN TREATMENT PLANNING

Over the past decades, the dental patient population has become larger, more mobile, and more culturally and ethnically diverse. Increasingly, most general dentistry practices are also managing patients who are older, who have more complex health histories, and retain most of their natural teeth albeit in a heavily restored state. Concurrently, the needs of patients and their expectations with respect to treatment outcomes has also grown. Patients are asking more questions and have higher standards for their oral appearance and their ability to chew and function. Before coming to a dental appointment, most patients will seek additional information about their dental issues on the Internet and sometimes seek advice from friends and relatives. Most patients will no longer rely solely on their dentist to provide information regarding the diagnosis and treatment of their oral health care problems.

Today's patient should expect to have autonomy when making treatment-planning decisions and this requires an open and informed conversation with their dental provider. As discussed earlier in this chapter, the further development of an evidence-based body of knowledge about risk assessment, prognosis, and treatment outcomes supports both patient and dentist as they work through the clinical decision-making process. However, in order to reach consensus regarding the optimal plan of care, patients and dentists will need to communicate effectively, which requires mutual understanding and trust. By being acquainted with the existing evidence, the clinical circumstances and knowing the patient as a person, the dentist is much better positioned to achieve this consensus.

In addition, there is a continuous need for reliable and comprehensive research to substantiate which treatment methods are most effective in varying clinical circumstances. From the dentist's perspective, there will be the sustained need to question current practices-—most especially conventional wisdom that lacks any evidence-based support. A constant, thorough, and dedicated reassessment of procedures, techniques, and materials, with a foundation in the emerging body of evidence, is an important tool to help dentists guide their patients through the changing array of treatment options with clarity, candor, and accuracy.

Artificial Intelligence as a Tool to Assist Treatment Planning

In earlier editions of this book, decision pathways and decision trees were discussed in detail. Decision pathways provide direction in identifying the range of treatment options and indicating some of the key decision nodes leading to appropriate treatment decisions. Decision trees not only specify key decision nodes and treatment options, but also include research-based success rates for each of these options. These rates can be based on outcomes of clinical conditions (e.g., effect of tooth loss) or on outcomes of treatment (e.g., success of various therapies for tooth replacement). Decision trees may also be influenced by patient-related variables, such as the patient's preferences, expectations, and financial resources. However, as evidence-based research data became more abundant, decision trees and pathways became too cumbersome for clinical use. Basically, the

WHAT'S THE EVIDENCE?

How Long Do Restorations and Prostheses Last?

The table presents a summarized version of the "What's the Evidence" box about how long do restoration and prostheses last, which you can find in the e-version of this chapter. On Evolve, you will find all the references and accompanying explanations, as well as more details regarding different survival rates times and annual failure rates, where this information was available. In the summarized version presented here, we will present only the survival rates in approximately 5-year intervals.

It is important to highlight that methodological differences among different studies can explain the seemingly incongruent results that are presented in the table. Elements that often differ from study to study include number of patients, dental care setting, number of years of follow-up, number and types of clinicians, number of restorations per patient, type and size of restorations, materials used, parameters for placing a restoration or prosthesis, statistical methods, and most importantly the definition of failure and survival. Therefore, the provider should exercise caution when presenting evidence from longevity studies to the patients because these average results may not apply to the patient's specific circumstances.

Type of Restoration	Years in Place	Survival Rates (%)
Direct resin-based composites	5	50
	10	65–82
	16	50
	29	71.4
Indirect resin-based composites	10	81
	20	57
Amalgam	5	50–90
	10	20–80
	15	10
	20	10–23

Type of Restoration	Years in Place	Survival Rates (%)
Large cuspal amalgam	5	65–78
	10	36–67
	15	36–73
	20	19
Cast gold	5	93
	10	42–96
	15	92
	20	72–87
	30	74
Crowns	5	84–100
	10	68–97
	26	50
Traditional fixed partial dentures	5	79–80
	10	93–98
	15	68
	20	65
Resin-bonded fixed partial dentures	5	64-99
	11	61–90
	15	61
Removable partial dentures	5	90–96
	10	89.8%
Single tooth implant/crown	5	91–99
	10	89
	15	

amount of information outpaced the regular processing capacity for these simple algorithms. But they have paved the way for the development of more sophisticated algorithms and more powerful machines to utilize evidence-based research data in clinical decision making.

The development of large patient databases connected through the Internet in association with growing processing ability and reduced latency time due to advances in information technology infrastructure has allowed a growing utilization of artificial intelligence tools to help healthcare professionals and patients to make clinical decisions in a variety of health care settings.

For example, deep learning tools can be used to recognize dental images and compare them with huge image databases. leading to more accurate and timely diagnosis, and improved prognosis In addition, machine-learning algorithms can use large electronic health records containing diagnosis, laboratory exams, images, genetic information, patient preferences, and demographic data to inform providers and suggesting the best treatment approaches. This information might also be used by robotic devices to perform minimally invasive procedures and/or fabricate diagnostic and therapeutic prostheses.

With the reduced latency rate expected with the advent of 5 G technology, these modalities are expected to become more and more accessible, and they will likely become standard practice in the future.

Clinical Recommendations and Guidelines

"Clinical Practice Guidelines are systematically developed statements to assist practitioners and patient decisions about appropriate health care for specific clinical circumstances".[164] Hallmarks of guidelines include: they are informed by a rigorous systematic analysis of evidence, carefully reviewed and vetted by a panel of experts, and include an assessment of the risks and benefits of alternative care options. Guidelines are not fixed protocols to be followed, but are intended to identify generally accepted courses of action to be considered for a given clinical situation. "They are not presented as a substitute for the advice of a knowledgeable health care professional or provider" (NIH National Center for Complementary and Integrative Health); https://www.nccih.nih.gov/health/providers/clinicalpractice).

The electronic version of this text includes some examples of Guidelines that have been developed for dentistry. *Clinical Recommendations and Guidelines*

Dentists have traditionally resisted any intrusion into the one-on-one doctor-patient discussion of the treatment plan.

Even though managed care plans and insurance carriers have had an impact on how treatment plans are formulated and the timing of treatment delivery, this should not be confused with following practice guidelines. Dental insurance and managed care programs are driven by financial parameters, whereas practice guidelines are driven by the desire to improve patient health and treatment outcomes. Although these are not necessarily mutually exclusive, in practice they often work at cross purposes.

Because of their resistance to relinquish their independence in treatment planning, private dental practitioners in the United States have generally been reluctant to embrace broad guidelines. Where guidelines have been accepted and implemented has usually been in a hospital or community-based health care system. Few studies have investigated adherence to guidelines in dentistry, and these have predominantly been in Europe (especially in the UK) and in the United States. Dental practices have presented some of the lowest compliance to guidelines in the healthcare sector. The most promising strategies to improve compliance in dentistry seems to be pay for performance, education, reminders, and multifaceted interventions (which comprised an association of two or more strategies including audit and feedback, education, fee-for-service or decision support). There is a lack of information about adherence to guidelines in dental care for other areas of the world.[146]

With the advent of Value Based Care initiatives there has been a renewed focus on how to improve quality of care and patient treatment outcomes. This trend is expected to lead to a resurgence and expansion of clinical recommendations and guidelines in the profession.

Practice-Based Networks[148]

Although worldwide the majority of dental patients receive care in private or public dental practices, most dental research happens in academic settings. It is widely understood that the circumstances surrounding care in an academic institution are quite different from those in private and public dental practices and this discrepancy raises questions about the external validity of the studies.

In recent decades many dental practice-based research networks have been developed. Their aim is to generate research outcomes that are relevant to both patients and clinicians in settings that are more representative of the usual dental care. A recent scoping review revealed 24 dental practice-based research networks around the globe, the majority being US-based and 8 being housed in Europe. These dental practice-based research networks were responsible for 202 publications on a wide variety of clinical issues. The majority of these publications occurred after 2010. The most common topics were private practice care habits and patterns (27.7%),

prosthodontics (8.4%), and endodontics (7.4%). The growth of dental practice-based research networks and consequently the scholarship produced by them, albeit significant, is still modest and more funding is needed to improve their capacity.

Providing Evidence and Information for Patients

Finding appropriate sources of research-based evidence might be challenging for the lay person, and it is useful for the practitioner to have some trusted sources of dental information that can be helpful in educating their patients about oral health-related issues. In the online version of this chapter *Oral Health Information for Patients* the reader will find a list of reliable websites that provide oral health-related information in lay language and appropriate for the public. Access to this information can help patients understand their oral health issues and problems, inform their choices about treatment alternatives, and enlighten them about what to expect before, during and after different types of dental treatment.

CONCLUSION

Using research-based evidence, risk analysis, prognosis determination, and outcomes assessment in the treatment plan presentation and discussion, the profession is moving from empirically based to evidenced-based treatment planning. The growing body of reliable scientific evidence is helping practitioners to make recommendations to patients that are increasingly predictable, supportable and professionally appropriate. Patients can expect to have more substantive and accurate information, to be better able to compare and weigh treatment alternatives, and to be prepared to make more informed judgments about what is in their individual best interests. They will also be better prepared for the possibility of adverse outcomes, should they occur. Artificial intelligence tools are expected to help inform patients and providers alike about the treatment alternatives after considering the large array of data available from research and patient-derived sources, such as electronic health records and wearables.

As this paradigm shift is taking place, the dentist's role is changing. On one hand, some control in the decision-making process is being passed from practitioner to patient. At the same time, the dental team's role is expanding as the need to collect, filter, focus, and transmit information to the patient increases. In short, the role of the dentist in presenting the treatment plan is changing from that of singular resource and authority for treatment recommendations to that of a content expert, educator, and advisor to the patient. This shift toward evidence-based person centered care will ultimately be to the advantage of patients, dentists, and the profession.

REVIEW QUESTIONS

- What is evidence-based dentistry? How is it useful to the dentist and to the patient in the formulation of the patient's treatment plan?
- How can risk assessment be a useful adjunct to the dental treatment planning process?

- How does the prognosis for a disease differ from the prognosis for treatment? Give examples of how the prognosis for a treatment can alter the treatment plan presentation to a patient.
- How does outcomes research support clinical treatment decision-making? Give examples.

REFERENCES

1. Richard Smith, Drummond Rennie. Evidence based medicine—an oral history. *BMJ.* 2014;348:g371.
2. Sackett David L, Rosenberg William MC, Gray JAMuir, Haynes RBrian, Richardson WScott. Evidence based medicine: what it is and what it isn't. *BMJ.* 1996;312:71.
3. Colvin J, Dawson DV, Gu H, Marchini L. Patient expectation and satisfaction with different prosthetic treatment modalities. *J Prosthodont.* 2019 Mar;28(3):264–270.
4. Richards D, Clarkson J, Matthews D, Niederman R. *Evidence-Based Dentistry: Managing Information for Better Practice.* London: Quintessence Publishing Co. Ltd; 2008.
5. Simon J. The EBD approach. *J Am Dent Assoc.* 2004 May;135(5):560 562; author reply 562, 564, 566.
6. Ismail AI, Bader JD. Evidence-based dentistry in clinical practice. *J Am Dent Assoc.* 2004;135:78–83.
7. Beck JD. Commentary: risk revisited. *Comm Dent Oral Epidemiol.* 1998;26(4):220–225.
8. Vieira AR, Marazita ML, Goldstein-McHenry T. Genome-wide scan finds suggestive caries loci. *J Dental Res.* 2008;87(5):435–439.
9. Wright JTim. Defining the contribution of genetics in the etiology of dental caries. *J dental Res.* 2010;89(11):1173–1174.
10. Alavi Golsa, et al. Dental erosion in patients with gastro esophageal reflux disease (GERD). *J Dent.* 2013;5(7):62–67.
11. Tantbirojn D, Pintado M, Versluis A, Dunn C, Delong R. Quantitative analysis of tooth surface loss associated with gastroesophageal reflux disease A longitudinal clinical study. *J Am Dental Assoc.* 2012;143(3):278–285.
12. Ganss Carolina, Lussi Adrian, Schlueter Nadine. Dental erosion as oral disease. Insights in etiological factors and pathomechanisms, and current strategies for prevention and therapy. *Am J Dent.* 2012;25(6):351–364.
13. Borgnakke Wenche S, et al. Effect of periodontal disease on diabetes: systematic review of epidemiologic observational evidence. *J periodontology.* 2013;84(4-s):S135–S152.
14. Lockhart Peter B, et al. Periodontal disease and atherosclerotic vascular disease: does the evidence support an independent association? A scientific statement from the American Heart Association. *Circulation.* 2012;125(20):2520–2544.
15. Teeuw Wijnand J, et al. Treatment of periodontitis improves the atherosclerotic profile: a systematic review and meta-analysis. *J Clin periodontology.* 2014;41(1):70–79.
16. Pontefract H, et al. The erosive effects of some mouth rinses on enamel. *J Clin periodontology.* 2001;28(4):319–324.
17. Hellwig E. Oral hygiene products and acidic medicines. *Monogr Oral Sci.* 2006;20:112–118.
18. Ohrbach R, Michelotti A. The Role of Stress in the Etiology of Oral Parafunction and Myofascial Pain. *Oral Maxillofac Surg Clin North Am.* 2018 Aug;30(3):369–379.
19. Buczkowska-Radlińska J, et al. Prevalence of dental erosion in adolescent competitive swimmers exposed to gas-chlorinated swimming pool water. *Clin oral investigations.* 2013;17(2):579–583.
20. Peres MA, Macpherson LMD, Weyant RJ, et al. Oral diseases: a global public health challenge. *Lancet.* 2019 Jul 20;394(10194):249–260.
21. Tanaka Keiko, et al. Socioeconomic status and risk of dental caries in Japanese preschool children: the Osaka Maternal and Child Health Study. *J public health Dent.* 2013;73(3):217–223.
22. Watt Richard G, Aubrey Sheiham. Integrating the common risk factor approach into a social determinants framework. *Community Dent oral Epidemiol.* 2012;40(4):289–296.
23. Jiang Yongwen, et al. Peer reviewed: sociodemographic and health-related risk factors associated with tooth loss among adults in Rhode Island. *Preventing chronic Dis.* 2013;10
24. Costa Simone M, et al. A systematic review of socioeconomic indicators and dental caries in adults. *Int J Environ Res public health.* 2012;9(10):3540–3574.
25. Ferro R, et al. Caries experience in 14-year-olds from Northeast Italy. Is socioeconomic-status (SES) still a risk factor? *Eur J paediatric dentistry: Off J Eur Acad Paediatric Dent.* 2012;13(1):46.
26. Bratthall D, Hansel Peterson G. Cariogram—a multifactorial risk assessment model for a multifactorial disease. *Comm Dent Oral Epidemiol.* 2005;33(4):256–264.
27. Graves R, Disney J, Stamm J, et al. Physical and Environmental Risk Factors in Dental Caries. In: Bader J, ed. *Risk Assessment in Dentistry.* Chapel Hill: University of North Carolina Dental Ecology; 1989.
28. MejÀre I, et al. Caries risk assessment. A systematic review. *Acta Odontologica Scandinavica* 0 (2013):1–11.
29. Neville BW, et al. *Oral and Maxillofacial Pathology.* 3rd Edition : Saunders Elsevier; 2009:409–421.
30. Gan SJ, Dahlstrom KR, Peck BW, et al. Incidence and pattern of second primary malignancies in patients with index oropharyngeal cancers versus index nonoropharyngeal head and neck cancers. *Cancer.* 2013 Jul 15;119(14):2593–2601.
31. Znaor A, Brennan P, Gajalakshmi V, et al. Independent and combined effects of tobacco smoking, chewing and alcohol drinking on the risk of oral, pharyngeal and esophageal cancers in Indian men. *Int J Cancer.* 2003 Jul 10;105(5):681–686.
32. https://www.fdiworlddental.org lancet report ties alcohol use to oral cancer – even moderate consumption is not without risk. 2018.
33. López-Lázaro M. A local mechanism by which alcohol consumption causes cancer. *Oral Oncol.* 2016 Nov;62:149–152.
34. Madani AH, Dikshit M, Bhaduri D, Aghamolaei T, Moosavy SH, Azarpaykan A. Interaction of alcohol use and specific types of smoking on the development of oral cancer. *Int J High Risk Behav Addict.* 2014 Mar 11;3(1):e12120.
35. Maasland DH, van den Brandt PA, Kremer B, Goldbohm RA, Schouten LJ. Alcohol consumption, cigarette smoking and the risk of subtypes of head-neck cancer: results from the Netherlands Cohort Study. *BMC Cancer.* 2014 Mar 14;14:187.
36. Ogden G Alcohol and oral cancer. *Alcohol.* 2005 Apr 35(3):169–73.
37. https://www.cancer.gov Alcohol and Cancer Risk Fact Sheet; updated July 14, 2021.
38. Rosenberg AJ, Agrawal N, Pearson A, et al. Risk and response adapted de-intensified treatment for HPV-associated oropharyngeal cancer: Optima paradigm expanded experience. *Oral Oncol.* 2021 Oct 15;122:105566.
39. Sathish N, Wang X, Yuan Y. Human papillomavirus (HPV)-associated oral cancers and treatment strategies. *J Dent Res.* 2014 Mar 24;93(7 suppl):29S–36S.
40. https://www.cdc.gov/cancer/hpv/basic_info/hpv_oropharyngeal.htm
41. Lingen MW, Xiao W, Schmitt A, et al. Low etiologic fraction for high-risk human papillomavirus in oral cavity squamous cell carcinomas. *Oral Oncol.* 2013 Jan;49(1):1–8.
42. Piemonte E, Lazos J, Belardinelli P, Secchi D, Brunotto M, Lanfranchi-Tizeira H. Oral cancer associated with chronic mechanical irritation of the oral mucosa. *Med Oral Patol Oral Cir Bucal.* 2018 Mar 1;23(2):e151–e160.

43. Gilligan GM, Panico RL, Di Tada C, Piemonte ED, Brunotto MN. Clinical and Immunohistochemical epithelial profile of non-healing chronic traumatic ulcers. *Med Oral Patol Oral Cir Bucal.* 2020 Sep 1;25(5):e706–e713.

44. de Araújo RL, Lyko Kde F, Funke VA, Torres-Pereira CC. Oral cancer after prolonged immunosuppression for multiorgan chronic graft-versus-host disease. *Rev Bras Hematol Hemoter.* 2014;36(1):65–68.

45. Ganesan S, Iype EM, Kapali AS SR. Radiation induced sarcoma of oral cavity-a rare case report and a short review. *J Clin Diagn Res.* 2013 Nov;7(11):2598–2599.

46. Turati F, Edefonti V, Bosetti C, et al. Family history of cancer and the risk of cancer: a network of case-control studies. *Ann Oncol.* 2013 Oct;24(10):2651.

47. Digonnet A, Hamoir M, Andry G, et al. Post-therapeutic surveillance strategies in head and neck squamous cell carcinoma. *Eur Arch Otorhinolaryngol.* 2013 May;270(5):1569–1580.

48. Zero D, Fontana M, Lennon AM. Clinical applications and outcomes of using indicators of risk in caries management. *J dental Educ.* 2001;65(10):1126–1132.

49. Fontana Gonzalez-Cabezas. Minimal intervention dentistry part 2. Caries risk assessment in adults. *Br Dental J.* 2012;213:447–451.

50. Doméjean S, White JM, Featherstone JD. Validation of the CDA CAMBRA caries risk assessment—a six-year retrospective study. *J Calif Dent Assoc.* 2011

51. Tellez M, Gomez J, Pretty I, Ellwood R, Ismail AI. Evidence on existing caries risk assessment systems: are they predictive of future caries? *Community Dent Oral Epidemiol.* 2013;41:67–78.

52. Disney JA, Graves RC, Stamm JW, Bohannan HM, Abernathy JR, Zack D. The University of North Carolina caries risk assessment study: further developments in caries risk prediction. *Community Dent Oral Epidemiol.* 1992;20:64–75.

53. González-Cabezas C. The chemistry of caries: remineralization and demineralization events with direct clinical relevance. *Dent Clin North Am.* 2010 Jul;54(3):469–478.

54. Pappas A, Koski A, Guinta J. Prevalence and intraoral distribution of coronal and root caries in middle-aged and older adults. *Caries Res.* 1992;26:459–465.

55. Dye BA, Tan S, Smith V, et al. National Center for Health Statistics. Trends in oral health status: United States, 1988–1994 and 1999–2004. *Vital Health Stat.* 2007;11(248):1–92.

56. Totiam P, González-Cabezas C, Fontana MR, Zero DT. A new in vitro model to study the relationship of gap size and secondary caries. *Caries Res.* 2007;41:467–473.

57. Grossi SG, Zambon JJ, Ho AW, et al. Assessment of risk for periodontal disease. I. Risk indicators for attachment loss. *J Periodontol.* 1994;65(3):260–267.

58. Grossi SG, Genco RJ, Machtei EE, et al. Assessment of risk for periodontal disease. II. Risk indicators for alveolar bone loss. *J Periodontol.* 1995;66(1):23–29.

59. Locker D, Leake JL. Risk indicators and risk markers for periodontal disease experience in older adults living independently in Ontario, Canada. *J Dent Res.* 1993;72 (1):9–17.

60. Lang NP, Tonetti MS. Periodontal risk assessment (PRA) for patients in supportive periodontal therapy (SPT). *Oral Health Prev Dent.* 2003;1(1):7–16.

61. Page RC, Martin JA, Loeb CF. The oral health information suite (OHIS): its use in the management of periodontal disease. *J Dent Educ.* 2005;69(5):509–520.

62. Page RC, Martin J, Krall EA, Mancl L, Garcia R. Longitudinal validation of a risk calculator for periodontal disease. *J Clin Periodontol.* 2003;30(9):819–827.

63. Matuliene G, et al. Significance of periodontal risk assessment in the recurrence of periodontitis and tooth loss. *J Clin periodontology.* 2010;37(2):191–199. and *J Clin Periodontol.* 2010 May;37(5):427-35.

64. Leininger, Matthieu, Henri Tenenbaum, and Jean-Luc Davideau. Modified periodontal risk assessment score: long-term predictive value of treatment outcomes. A retrospective study. *J Clin periodontology.* 2010;37(5):427–435.

65. Glaros Alan G. Incidence of diurnal and nocturnal bruxism. *J Prosthet Dent.* 1981;45(5):545–549.

66. Ohayon Maurice M, Li Kasey K, Guilleminault Christian. Risk factors for sleep bruxism in the general population. *Chest J.* 2001;119(1):53–61.

67. Johansson Anders, Omar Ridwaan, Carlsson Gunnar E. Bruxism and prosthetic treatment: a critical review. *J prosthodontic Res.* 2011;55(3):127–136.

68. Klasser GD, Rei N, Lavigne GJ. Sleep bruxism etiology: the evolution of a changing paradigm. *J Can Dent Assoc.* 2015;81:f2 PMID: 25633110.

69. Beddis H, Pemberton M, Davies S. Sleep bruxism: an overview for clinicians. *Br Dent J.* 2018 Sep 28;225(6):497–501.

70. Alajbeg IZ, Zuvela A, Tarle Zrinka. Risk factors for bruxism among Croatian navy employees. *J oral rehabilitation.* 2012;39(9): 668–676.

71. Rintakoski Katariina, Kaprio J. Legal Psychoactive Substances as Risk Factors for Sleep-Related Bruxism: A Nationwide Finnish Twin Cohort Study. *Alcohol Alcohol.* 2013;48(4):487–494.

72. Hosoya H, Kitaura H, Hashimoto T, et al. Between sleep bruxism and sleep respiratory events in patients with obstructive sleep apnea syndrome. *Sleep Breath.* 2014 Feb 14

73. Bussadori SK, Motta LJ, Horliana ACRT, Santos EM, Martimbianco ALC. The current trend in management of bruxism and chronic pain: an overview of systematic reviews. *J Pain Res.* 2020 Sep 30;13:2413–2421.

74. van de Sande FH, et al. Patient risk factors' influence on survival of posterior composites. *J dental Res.* 2013;92(7 suppl):S78–S83.

75. Johansson Anders, et al. Gender difference in symptoms related to temporomandibular disorders in a population of 50-year-old subjects. *J Orofac pain.* 2003;17:1.

76. Ohrbach Richard, et al. Clinical findings and pain symptoms as potential risk factors for chronic TMD: descriptive data and empirically identified domains from the OPPERA case-control study. *J Pain.* 2011;12(11):T27–T45. 0.

77. Manfredini D, Lombardo L, Siciliani G. Temporomandibular disorders and dental occlusion. A systematic review of association studies: end of an era? *J Oral Rehabil.* 2017 Nov;44(11):908–923.

78. de Kanter RJAM, Battistuzzi PGFCM, Truin GJ. Temporomandibular disorders: "occlusion" matters! *Pain Res Manag.* 2018 May 15;2018:8746858.

79. Selaimen Caio MP, et al. Occlusal risk factors for temporomandibular disorders. *Angle Orthod.* 2007;77(3):471–477.

80. Kiriakou J, Pandis N, Fleming P, Madianos P, Polychronopoulou A. Reporting quality of systematic review abstracts in leading oral implantology journals. *J Dent.* 2013;41(12):1181–1187.

81. Lang LA, Teich ST. A critical appraisal of evidence-based dentistry: The best available evidence. *J Prosthet Dent.* 2014;111(6):485–492

82. Manfredini D, Lobbezoo F. "Relationship between bruxism and temporomandibular disorders: a systematic review of literature from 1998 to 2008." *Oral Surgery, Oral Medicine, Oral Pathology, Oral Radiology, Endodontology.* 2010;109(6):e26–e50.

83. Costa YM, Porporatti AL, Stuginski-Barbosa J, Bonjardim LR, Speciali JG, Rodrigues Conti PC. Headache attributed to masticatory myofascial pain: clinical features and management outcomes. *J Oral Facial Pain Headache.* 2015 Fall;29(4):323–330.

84. Truelove E, Huggins KH, Mancl L, Dworkin SF. The efficacy of traditional, low-cost and nonsplint therapies for temporomandibular disorder: a randomized controlled trial. *J Am Dent Assoc.* 2006 Aug;137(8):1099–1107; quiz 1169.

85. Tada S, Ikebe K, Matsuda K, Maeda Y. Multifactorial risk assessment for survival of abutments of removable partial dentures based on practice-based longitudinal study. *J Dent.* 2013;41(12):1175–1180.

86. Kalsi JS, Hemmings KW. The influence of patients' decisions on treatment planning in restorative dentistry. *Dent Update.* 2013;40(9):698–710.

87. Faggion C, Giannakopoulos N. Critical appraisal of systematic reviews on the effect of a history of periodontitis on dental implant loss. *J Clin Periodontology.* 2013;40(5):542–552.

88. Ballini A, Capodiferro S, Toia M, et al. Evidence-based dentistry: What's new? *Int J Med Sci.* 2007;4(3):174–178.

89. Thomason JM, Heydecke G, Feine JS, Ellis JS. How do patients perceive the benefit of reconstructive dentistry with regard to oral health-related quality of life and patient satisfaction? A systematic review. *Clin Oral Implant Res.* 2007;18(Suppl 3):168–188.

90. Becker W, Berg BE. Periodontal treatment without maintenance. A retrospective study in 44 patients. *J Periodontol.* 1984;55:505–509.

91. Becker W, Berg BE. The long-term evaluation of periodontal treatment and maintenance in 95 patients. *Int J Periodontics Restor Dent.* 1984;4:54–71.

92. McGuire Michael K. Prognosis versus actual outcome: a long-term survey of 100 treated periodontal patients under maintenance care. *J periodontology.* 1991;62(1):51–58.

93. McGuire Michael K, Martha ENunn. Prognosis versus actual outcome. II. The effectiveness of clinical parameters in developing an accurate prognosis. *J periodontology.* 1996;67(7):658–665.

94. Lalla RV, Brennan MT, Gordon SM, Sonis ST, Rosenthal DI, Keefe DM. Oral mucositis due to high-dose chemotherapy and/or head and neck radiation therapy. *J Natl Cancer Inst Monogr.* 2019 Aug 1;2019(53). lgz011.

95. Akdeniz N, Elmas ÖF, Karadağ AS. Behçet syndrome: A great imitator. *Clin Dermatol.* 2019 May-Jun;37(3):227–239.

96. Cifuentes M, Davari P, Rogers 3rd RS. Contact stomatitis. *Clin Dermatol.* 2017 Sep-Oct;35(5):435–440.

97. Kwok V, Caton JG. Commentary: prognosis revisited: a system for assigning periodontal prognosis. *J Periodontology.* 2007;78:2063–2071.

98. McGuire Michael K, Nunn Martha E. Prognosis versus actual outcome. IV. The effectiveness of clinical parameters and IL-1 genotype in accurately predicting prognoses and tooth survival. *J periodontology.* 1999;70(1):49–56.

99. Samet, Nachum, and Anna Jotkowitz. Classification and prognosis evaluation of individual teeth-A comprehensive approach. *Quintessence International* 40.5 (2009): 377–387.

100. Sbaraini A, Carter SM, Evans RW, Blinkhorn A. Experiences of dental care: what do patients value? *BMC Health Serv Res.* 2012;12:177.

101. de Lima EA, Fernandes dos Santos MB, Marchini L. Patients' expectations of and satisfaction with implant-supported fixed partial dentures and single crowns. *Int J Prosthodontics.* 2012;25(5):484–490.

102. Carlsson GE. Critical review of some dogmas in prosthodontics. *J Prosthodont Res.* 2009;53(1):3–10.

103. Critchlow SB, Ellis JS. Prognostic indicators for conventional complete denture therapy: a review of the literature. *J Dent.* 2010;38(1):2–9.

104. Fenlon MR, Sherriff M, Newton JT. The influence of personality on patients' satisfaction with existing and new complete dentures. *J Dent.* 2007;35(9):744–748.

105. Huumonen S, Haikola B, Oikarinen K, Söderholm AL, Remes-Lyly T, Sipilä K. Residual ridge resorption, lower denture stability and subjective complaints among edentulous individuals. *J Oral Rehabil.* 2012;39(5):384–390.

106. John MT, Micheelis W, Steele JG. Depression as a risk factor for denture dissatisfaction. *J Dent Res.* 2007;86(9):852–856.

107. de Siqueira GP, dos Santos MB, dos Santos JF, Marchini L. Patients' expectation and satisfaction with removable dental prosthesis therapy and correlation with patients' evaluation of the dentists. *Acta Odontol Scand.* 2013;71(1):210–214.

108. https://www.ada.org/~/media/ADA/DQA/2019_Guidebook.pdf?la=en

109. http://www.qualitymeasures.ahrq.gov/tutorial/HealthOutcomeMeasure.aspx (accessed June 2014)

110. Schwendicke F1, Dörfer CE, Paris S. Incomplete caries removal: a systematic review and meta-analysis. *J Dent Res.* 2013 Apr;92(4):306–314.

111. Ricketts DN1, Kidd EA, Innes N, Clarkson J. Complete or ultraconservative removal of decayed tissue in unfilled teeth. *Cochrane Database Syst Rev.* 2006 Jul 19;(3).

112. Maltz M1, Henz SL, de Oliveira EF, Jardim JJ. Conventional caries removal and sealed caries in permanent teeth: a microbiological evaluation. *J Dent.* 2012 Sep;40(9):776–782.

113. Maltz M1, Jardim JJ, Mestrinho HD, et al. Partial removal of carious dentine: a multicenter randomized controlled trial and 18-month follow-up results. *Caries Res.* 2013;47(2):103–109.

114. Schwendicke F1, Stolpe M, Meyer-Lueckel H, Paris S, Dörfer CE. Cost-effectiveness of one- and two-step incomplete and complete excavations. *J Dent Res.* 2013 Oct;92(10):880–887.

115. Maltz M1, Alves LS, Jardim JJ, Moura Mdos S, de Oliveira EF. Incomplete caries removal in deep lesions: a 10-year prospective study. *Am J Dent.* 2011 Aug;24(4):211–214.

116. Giacaman RA, Muñoz-Sandoval C, Neuhaus KW, Fontana M, Chałas R. Evidence-based strategies for the minimally invasive treatment of carious lesions: Review of the literature. *Adv Clin Exp Med.* 2018 Jul;27(7):1009–1016.

117. Orhan AI1 Oz FT, Orhan K. Pulp exposure occurrence and outcomes after 1- or 2-visit indirect pulp therapy vs complete caries removal in primary and permanent molars. *Pediatr Dent.* 2010 Jul-Aug;32(4):347–355.

118. Schwendickea F, Meyer-Lueckelb H, Dörfera C, Parisa S. Failure of incompletely excavated teeth—A systematic review. *J Dent.* July 2013;Volume 41(Issue 7):569–580.

119. Arvanitis G. Criteria for the replacement of defective restorations. *Dent Today.* 2004;23(4):78–81.

120. Reasons for replacement of restorations, Oper Dent 30(4):409–416, 2005.

121. Brantley CF, et al. Does the cycle of rerestoration lead to larger restorations? *J Am Dent Assoc.* 1995;126(10):1407–1412.

122. Anusavice KJ, ed. *Quality Evaluation of Dental Restorations: Criteria for Placement and Replacement.* Chicago: Quintessence Publishing; 1989.

123. Frencken Jo E, et al. Minimal intervention dentistry for managing dental caries–a review. *Int dental J.* 2012;62(5):223–243.

124. Martin Javier, et al. Management of Class I and Class II amalgam restorations with localized defects: five-year results. *Int J Dent.* 2013;2013.

125. Hempel MC, Mjör IA, Gordan VV. Sealing, refurbishment and repair of Class I and Class II defective restorations: a three-year clinical trial. *J Am Dent Assoc.* 2009 Apr;140(4):425–432.

126. Miller DB. A new protocol and standard of care for managing open crown margins. *Gen Dent.* 2019 Mar-Apr;67(2):19–22.

127. Mitchell C, Gross AJ, Milgrom P, Mancl L, Prince DB. Silver diamine fluoride treatment of active root caries lesions in older adults: A case series. *J Dent.* 2021 Feb;105:103561.

128. Vetromilla BM, Opdam NJ, Leida FL, et al. Treatment options for large posterior restorations: a systematic review and network meta-analysis. *J Am Dent Assoc.* 2020 Aug;151(8):614–624.e18.

129. Rosenstiel SF, Land MF, Fujimoto J. *Contemporary Fixed Prosthodontics.* ed 3 St Louis: Mosby; 2000.

130. Shugars DA, et al. Survival rates of teeth adjacent to treated and untreated posterior bounded edentulous spaces. *J Am Dent Assoc.* 1998;129(Aug):1084–1094.

131. Scurria MS, Bader JD, Shugars DA. Meta-analysis of fixed partial denture survival: prostheses and abutments. *J Prosthet Dent.* 1998;79:459–464.

132. Lindskog-Stokland B, Hakeberg M, Hansen K. Molar position associated with a missing opposed and/or adjacent tooth: a follow up study in women. *Swedish Dent J* 2013; 37 97–104.

133. Gerritsen AE, Witter DJ, Creugers NHJ. Long-term follow-up indicates unimpaired oral health-related quality of life for people having shortened dental arches. *J Dent.* 2017 Oct;65:41–44.

134. Fueki K, Baba K. Shortened dental arch and prosthetic effect on oral health-related quality of life: a systematic review and meta-analysis. *J Oral Rehabil.* 2017 Jul;44(7):563–572.

135. Sigurdsson A. Evaluating success and failure. In: Walton RE, Torabinejad M, eds. *Principles and Practice of Endodontics.* ed 3 Philadelphia: WB Saunders; 2001.

136. Kerekes K, Tronstad L. Long-term results of endodontic treatment performed with a standardized technique. *J Endod.* 1979;5(3):83–90.

137. Seltzer S, et al. Factors effecting successful repair after root canal therapy. *J Am Dent Assoc.* 1963;67:651–662.

138. Sjogren U, et al. Influence of infection at the time of root filling in the outcome of endodontic treatment of teeth with apical periodontitis. *Int Endod J.* 1997;30(5):297–306.

139. Friedman S. Success and failure of initial endodontic therapy, Ontario. *Dentist.* 1997;74(1):35–38.

140. Friedman S, Mor C. The success of endodontic therapy—healing and functionality. *J Calif Dent Assoc.* 2004;32(6):493–503.

141. Torabinejad M, Corr R, Handysides R, Shabahang S. Outcomes of nonsurgical retreatment and endodontic surgery: a systematic review. *J Endod.* 2009 Jul;35(7):930–937.

142. Rubinstein RA1, Kim S. Long-term follow-up of cases considered healed one year after apical microsurgery. *J Endod.* 2002 May;28(5):378–383.

143. Tsesis I, Faivishevsky V, Kfir A, Rosen E. Outcome of surgical endodontic treatment performed by a modern technique: a meta-analysis of literature. *J Endod.* 2009 Nov;35(11):1505–1511.

144. Setzer FC1, Shah SB, Kohli MR, Karabucak B, Kim S. Outcome of endodontic surgery: a meta-analysis of the literature—part 1: Comparison of traditional root-end surgery and endodontic microsurgery. *J Endod.* 2010 Nov;36(11):1757–1765.

145. Esposito M, Trullenque-Eriksson A, Tallarico M. Endodontic retreatment versus dental implants of teeth with an uncertain endodontic prognosis: 3-year results from a randomised controlled trial. *Eur J Oral Implantol.* 2018;11(4):423–438.

146. Villarosa AR, Maneze D, Ramjan LM, et al. The effectiveness of guideline implementation strategies in the dental setting: a systematic review. *Implement Sci.* 2019;14:106.

147. Canceill T, Monsarrat P, Faure-Clement E, Tohme M, Vergnes JN, Grosgogeat B. Dental practice-based research networks (D-PBRN) worldwide: A scoping review. *J Dent.* 2021 Jan;104: 103523.

148. Montagner AF, Sande FHV, Müller C, Cenci MS, Susin AH. Survival, reasons for failure and clinical characteristics of anterior/posterior composites: 8-year findings. *Braz Dent J.* 2018;29(6):547–554.

149. Wong C, Blum IR, Louca C, Sparrius M, Wanyonyi K. A retrospective clinical study on the survival of posterior composite restorations in a primary care dental outreach setting over 11years. *J Dent.* 2021;106:103586.

150. Montag R, Dietz W, Nietzsche S, et al. Clinical and micromorphologic 29-year results of posterior composite restorations. *J Dent Res.* 2018;97(13):1431–1437.

151. Frankenberger R, Reinelt C, Glatthöfer C, Krämer N. Clinical performance and SEM marginal quality of extended posterior resin composite restorations after 12 years. *Dent Mater.* 2020;36(7):e217–e228.

152. Ravasini F, Bellussi D, Pedrazzoni M, et al. Treatment outcome of posterior composite indirect restorations: a retrospective 20-year analysis of 525 cases with a mean follow-up of 87 months. *Int J Periodontics Restor Dent.* 2018;38(5):655–663.

153. Collares K, Opdam NJM, Laske M, et al. Longevity of anterior composite restorations in a general dental practice-based network. *J Dent Res.* 2017;96(10):1092–1099.

154. Laske M, Opdam NJM, Bronkhorst EM, Braspenning JCC. Huysmans MCDNJM Ten-year survival of class II restorations placed by general practitioners. *JDR Clin Trans Res.* 2016;1(3):292–299.

155. Laske M, Opdam NJM, Bronkhorst EM, Braspenning JCC. Huysmans MCDNJM Risk factors for dental restoration survival: a practice-based study. *J Dent Res.* 2019;98(4):414–422.

156. Laske M, Opdam NJ, Bronkhorst EM, Braspenning JC, Huysmans MC. Longevity of direct restorations in Dutch dental practices. Descriptive study out of a practice based research network. *J Dent.* 2016;46:12–17.

157. Garling A, Sasse M, Becker MEE, Kern M. Fifteen-year outcome of three-unit fixed dental prostheses made from monolithic lithium disilicate ceramic. *J Dent.* 2019;89:103178.

158. Morimoto S, Rebello de Sampaio FB, Braga MM, Sesma N, Özcan M. Survival rate of resin and ceramic Inlays, Onlays, and overlays: a systematic review and meta-analysis. *J Dent Res.* 2016;95(9):985–994.

159. Becker M, Chaar MS, Garling A, Kern M. Fifteen-year outcome of posterior all-ceramic inlay-retained fixed dental prostheses. *J Dent.* 2019;89:103174.

160. Rinke S, Wehle J, Schulz X, Bürgers R, Rödiger M. Prospective evaluation of posterior fixed zirconia dental prostheses: 10-year clinical results. *Int J Prosthodont.* 2018;31(1):35–42.

161. Sailer I, Balmer M, Hüsler J, Hämmerle CHF, Känel S, Thoma DS. 10-year randomized trial (RCT) of zirconia-ceramic and metal-ceramic fixed dental prostheses. *J Dent.* 2018;76: 32–39.

162. Balasubramaniam GR. Predictability of resin bonded bridges - a systematic review. *Br Dent J.* 2017;222(11):849–858.

163. Mangano F, Lucchina AG, Brucoli M, Migliario M, Mortellaro C, Mangano C. Prosthetic complications affecting single-tooth morse-taper connection implants. *J Craniofac Surg.* 2018;29(8):2255–2262.

164. Institute of Medicine (US) Committee to Advise the Public Health Service on Clinical Practice Guidelines. Clinical Practice Guidelines: Directions for a New Program. Field MJ, Lohr KN, editors. Washington (DC): National Academies Press (US); 1990. PMID: 25144032.

SUGGESTED READINGS AND RESOURCES

EVIDENCE-BASED DENTISTRY

Abt E, Bader JD, Bonetti D. A practitioner's guide to developing critical appraisal skills: translating research into clinical practice. *J Am Dent Assoc.* 2012;143(4):386–390.

ADA Center for Evidence-based Dentistry: http://ebd.ada.org/en/

Kwok V, Caton JG, Polson AM, Hunter PG. Application of evidence-based dentistry: from research to clinical periodontal practice. *Periodontol.* 2012;59(1):61–74. 2000.

Pitts N. Understanding the jigsaw of evidence-based dentistry: 1. *Introduction, Res synthesis, Evidence-Based Dent.* 2004;5:2–4.

Pitts N. Understanding the jigsaw of evidence-based dentistry: 3. *Implement Res Find Clpractice, Evidence-Based Dent.* 2004;5:60–64.

Richards D, Clarkson J, Matthews D, Niederman R. *Evidence-Based Dentistry: Managing Information for Better Practice.* London: Quintessence Publishing Co. Ltd; 2008.

Richard Smith, Drummond Rennie. Evidence based medicine—an oral history. *BMJ.* 2014;348:g371.

Video tutorials on EBD: http://ebd.ada.org/en/education/tutorials

RISK ASSESSMENT

A.D.A. Caries Risk Assessment Form 6 years old: http://www.ada.org/~/media/ADA/Public%20Programs/Files/topics_caries_educational_over6.ashx

A.D.A. Caries Risk Assessment Form Completion Instructions: http://www.ada.org/~/media/ADA/Public%20Programs/Files/topics_caries_instructions_GKAS.ashx

American Academy of Pediatric Dentistry: http://www.aapd.org/media/Policies_Guidelines/G_CariesRiskAssessment.pdf.

American Academy of Periodontology Disease Risk Form: http://service.previser.com/aap/default.aspx

Bussadori SK, Motta LJ, Horliana ACRT, Santos EM, Martimbianco ALC. The current trend in management of bruxism and chronic pain: an overview of systematic reviews. *J Pain Res.* 2020 Sep 30;13:2413–2421.

Caries Management by Risk Assessment (CAMBRA) group Doméjean S, White JM, Featherstone JD. Validation of the CDA CAMBRA caries risk assessment—a six-year retrospective study. *J Calif Dent Assoc.* 2011

Cariogram from the University of Malmo: http://www.mah.se/fakulteter-och-omraden/Odontologiska-fakulteten/Avdelning-och-kansli/Cariologi/Cariogram/

Klasser GD, Rei N, Lavigne GJ. Sleep bruxism etiology: the evolution of a changing paradigm. *J Can Dent Assoc.* 2015;81:f2.

Matuliene G, et al. Significance of periodontal risk assessment in the recurrence of periodontitis and tooth loss. *J Clin Periodontology.* 2010;37(2):191–199.

Peres MA, Macpherson LMD, Weyant RJ, et al. Oral diseases: a global public health challenge. *Lancet.* 2019;394(10194):249–260. Erratum in: Lancet. 2019;394(10203):1010.

PROGNOSIS

Lalla RV, Brennan MT, Gordon SM, Sonis ST, Rosenthal DI, Keefe DM. oral mucositis due to high-dose chemotherapy and/or head and neck radiation therapy. *J Natl Cancer Inst Monogr.* 2019;2019(53):lgz011.

OUTCOMES AND OUTCOMES MEASURES

Bader JD, Shugars DA. Cost implications of differences in dentists' restorative treatment decisions. *J Public Health Dent.* 1996;56:219–222.

Giacaman RA, Muñoz-Sandoval C, Neuhaus KW, Fontana M, Chałas R. Evidence-based strategies for the minimally invasive treatment of carious lesions: Review of the literature. *Adv Clin Exp Med.* 2018;27(7):1009–1016.

Matthews DC. Decision making in periodontics: a review of outcome measures. *J Dent Educ.* 1994;58(8):641–647.

Miller DB. A new protocol and standard of care for managing open crown margins. *Gen Dent.* 2019;67(2):19–22.

Quality Measurement in Dentistry: A Guidebook: https://www.ada.org/~/media/ADA/DQA/2019_Guidebook.pdf?la=en

Vernazza C, Heasman P, Gaunt F, Pennington M. How to measure the cost-effectiveness of periodontal treatments. *Periodontol.* 2012;60(1):138–146. 2000.

Vetromilla BM, Opdam NJ, Leida FL, et al. Treatment options for large posterior restorations: a systematic review and network meta-analysis. *J Am Dent Assoc.* 2020;151(8):614–624. c18.

4

Digital Tools for Diagnosis and Treatment Planning

Stephen J. Stefanac, Erika Benavides, Cassandra Callaghan, Margherita Fontana, Furat George, Lynn Johnson, and Domenica Sweier

 Visit eBooks.Health.Elsevier.com

INTRODUCTION

Although the mirror and explorer are still important tools for diagnosis and treatment planning, they are rapidly being augmented by new digital tools. For dentists, most of these tools are enhancements to traditional diagnostic methods. For example, search engines and databases are replacing books and other reference materials. Images recorded on film are being replaced with digital radiographs and still and video images. Digital scans can replace impressions and plaster models. These advancements are not just helpful for dentists but also for patients who can more easily transfer dental records and radiographic images from one dentist to another. Patients can also share information with their dentist from their electronic health records (EHRs), such as medical diagnoses and a list of medications often with a couple of clicks from their smartphone.

This chapter will cover three broad categories: patient evaluation and diagnosis, communication, and treatment planning tools. Some of the tools may be considered in more than one category. Many of the tools can be used together to create new ways to improve patient care and help clinicians be more efficient and accurate.

Terminology

It is useful to understand several terms that are used when learning how different digital processes work. The basic building blocks for digital systems are **algorithms**. Algorithms are a series of definable processes or instructions that can be implemented by a computer. One common example is the calculation of a patient's body mass index (BMI). A clinician can calculate a patient's BMI by inserting the patient's height and weight into this formula:

$$BMI = \frac{mass_{kg}}{height_m{}^2} = \frac{mass_{lb}}{height_{in}{}^2} \times 703$$

. Alternatively, and more easily, the clinician could use an online calculator to input the values and obtain the same number.[1] **Artificial intelligence (AI)** is possible when many algorithms are used together to simulate human thought and activities. Examples include self-driving cars and industrial robots. Examples in medicine and dentistry include risk calculators prior to surgical care[2] and determining the need to premedicate to prevent infection of an artificial joint.[3] **Machine learning (ML)** is a subcategory of AI and is based on the idea that systems can learn from data, identify patterns, and make decisions with minimal human intervention. **Deep learning (DL)** is a type of ML that applies algorithms in a layered fashion to extract higher-level data from the original raw data. Some examples include facial recognition systems, language translation, and automatic spell checking and correction. In dentistry, for example, ML using DL can be used to analyze radiographs and suggest areas of caries and periodontal bone loss.[4] **Clinical decision support (CDS)**[5] includes tools that provide the clinician with information tailored to an individual patient to enhance patient care and are often coupled with an EHR.

Although it is impossible to remain current and cover all the digital tools available in a textbook, the authors' goal is to provide a structure for the reader to evaluate how these modalities are affecting the practice of dentistry in the realms of diagnosis and treatment planning. The focus will be on software (programs, websites, applications, online resources) more than hardware (e.g., computer-aided design and manufacturing [CAD-CAM] machines). Another focus is on using digital tools for diagnosis and treatment planning and not treatment delivery.

PATIENT EVALUATION AND DIAGNOSIS

Digital Information Resources

Forty years ago, when a recently graduated dentist had questions regarding diagnosis and treatment planning, they referred to textbooks and class notes or spoke with colleagues on the phone or in person. Dentists now can access an array of digital informational resources to help them answer clinical questions and provide information they can then share with their patients. These resources can be divided into two broad categories, which have some measure of overlap: (1) search engines and (2) databases.

Search engines, such as Google and Yahoo, are used to find content available on the Internet. Search engines use proprietary algorithms to rate results for relevance. They are easily accessible, fast, and very popular with over 70,000 searches performed per second (or 5.4 billion per day) in 2020. Using a search engine can provide a large amount of information that must then be evaluated by the clinician and for the patient with regard to the source, level of objectivity, and content (Box 4.1).[6] Using search engines is excellent to obtain data from popular websites, governments, organizations, and individuals.[7] For example, a dentist can find the prevalence of non–insulin-dependent diabetes or alcohol abuse in a US state by reviewing data provided by a local agency. In addition to web pages, search engines are useful for locating images. This can be helpful for the dentist who suspects a lesion in a patient and wants to see examples for comparison before they make a diagnosis. The user should be prepared for a long list of search results unless the search terms are highly specific. Because search results are web pages, they may be presented in a rank order that is influenced by advertising and search engine scoring algorithms as well as the user's location.[8]

Databases, like search engines, provide the user access to information. Databases are best for storing and searching structured data. For example, an electronic record is a very structured database. Search engines, on the other hand, are best for searching unstructured data like web pages.[9] In addition to the EHR, the practicing clinician may search for information from commercial and public databases. For instance, the dentist can use an application on their mobile device that links to a database to review patient medications including their uses and any side effects that may have implications for dentistry. Other databases, especially those accessed using a library, can contain articles from magazines, journals, and newspapers.

There are three advantages when using databases such as Medline (PubMed is the search engine) to answer scientific or clinical questions, or search for scholarly articles.[10] One, the results are usually reliable. Articles are often peer reviewed and the authors and their affiliations are clearly identified in the citations. Two, the most relevant articles can be found by creating a custom search query and limiting the search to recent articles. Many articles can be grouped and interpreted by selecting articles that provide a **systematic review** or a **meta-analysis**. Finally, the information can be accessible as the user can often obtain the full text of an article without having to physically visit a library.

The following demonstrates how a clinician might approach answering several clinical questions about a patient. For this example, a patient has presented with a chief concern of a "sore mouth." You review the patient's health history and see the patient is being treated for breast cancer and is also seeing a dermatologist for a chronic skin condition. The patient shows you the lesions on their arms and legs. You

---

> ### BOX 4.1 Criteria for Evaluating Digital Resources
>
> **Currency:** *The timeliness of the information.*
> - When was the information published or posted? Has the information been revised or updated?
> - Is the information current or out of date for your topic?
> - Are the web links functional?
>
> **Relevance:** *The importance of the information for your needs.*
> - Does the information relate to your topic or answer your question?
> - Who is the intended audience?
> - Is the information at an appropriate level (i.e., not too elementary or advanced)?
> - Have you looked at a variety of sources before determining this is the one you will use?
> - Would you be comfortable citing this source for a research paper?
>
> **Authority:** *The source of the information.*
> - Who is the author/publisher/source/sponsor?
> - Are the author's credentials or organizational affiliations given and what are they?
> - What are the author's qualifications to write on the topic?
> - Is there contact information, such as a publisher or email address?
> - Does the URL reveal anything about the author or source? Examples:
>   - .com (commercial), .edu (educational), .gov (US government), .org (nonprofit organization), .net (network)
>
> **Accuracy:** *The reliability, truthfulness, and correctness of the content.*
> - Where does the information come from?
> - Is the information supported by evidence?
> - Has the information been reviewed or refereed?
> - Can you verify any of the information in another source or from personal knowledge?
> - Does the language or tone seem biased and free of emotion?
> - Are there spelling, grammar, or typographical errors?
>
> **Purpose:** *The reason the information exists.*
> - What is the purpose of the information? It is to inform, teach, sell, entertain, or persuade?
> - Do the authors/sponsors make their intentions or purpose clear?
> - Is the information fact, opinion or propaganda?
> - Does the point of view appear objective and impartial?
> - Are there political, ideological, cultural, religious, institutional, or personal biases?

From Meriam Library - CSU, Chico. Evaluating information – applying the CRAAP Test. 2010. https://library.csuchico.edu/sites/default/files/craap-test.pdf.

look up each of the patient's medications for indications and side effects in a database on your mobile device. Several of the medications being used to treat the cancer have the side effect of causing lichenoid reactions, similar in appearance to lichen planus. You perform a Google search on lichenoid reactions and view many images of the condition in the mouth and on the skin. Both the lesions in the mouth and on the skin look like the images from Google. Armed with a preliminary diagnosis, you wonder how best to treat the patient. You decide to search the literature for a relevant article or two. The initial search produces over 1800 citations. You refine the search term from "lichenoid reaction" to "treating lichenoid reactions in the mouth," then select to view only review articles, and find 21 citations. After examining several articles, you feel confident prescribing a steroid gel for the patient to apply to the sore areas in the mouth after meals and at bedtime. Finally, you find patient information about lichen planus on the American Academy of Oral Medicine's website, which you feel is very reputable, and print a copy for the patient.

Electronic Patient Records

Two hundred years ago, when dentists primarily treated patients with acute dental needs, there was little need for keeping dental records for each patient. With the advent of dental radiology, radiographs were often stored in small envelopes and attached to paper cards and ledgers that recorded patient financial transactions. In the 1960s and 1970s, US academic medical centers and the government (the US Veterans Administration) began developing electronic medical records to store patient information in an accessible format.[11] Early functions of electronic records in dentistry were to just maintain patient demographic and financial information and support other practice management activities such as creating appointment schedules and printing patient recall reminders. In the 1990s this began to change as patient health histories and other forms, in addition to digital radiographs, began to be added. Electronic medical and dental records have merged in many clinical locations, and the term **electronic health record (EHR)** is used to describe an electronic record that can be accessed by different types of clinicians and even the patients themselves.[12]

Electronic patient records today can store many items including forms, treatment notes, radiographic and photographic images, patient financial information, and other data in a format that is accessible and dynamic to review. Some of the advantages and disadvantages of EHRs are shown in Box 4.2. Since dental records can be very inclusive of different data, clinicians should be aware of what information they are required to share from an EHR with a patient. In the United States, this information is referred to as the **designated record set**.[13] This information is typically used to make decisions about an individual patient. Common items in this category include treatment notes, radiographs, forms, and financial information. Information pertaining less to the individual and more for a business or a management function usually does

---

BOX 4.2 Advantages and Disadvantages of Electronic Patient Records as Compared With Paper Records

Advantages
- Very legible
- Easier to copy and share the record with patients and other healthcare providers
- Can serve as one comprehensive container for paper, images, and forms
- Accessible offsite
- Easier for measuring quality assessment and assurance activities
- Can integrate with other tools—appointment reminders, billing, prescriptions, etc.
- Automatic alerts
- Portals to push updates to patients and allow them to review their records
- "Smart" records can analyze data and suggest treatment options
- Clinicians get paid faster, reduces paper for claims and the need to attach physical radiographs
- Possibility exists for integration with medical records
- Standardization of data, e.g., diagnostic codes, health history, etc.
- Greater auditing and reporting capability
- Updates with regulations or insurers can be woven into the logic and feedback from the system

Disadvantages
- Security and privacy protocols are more complex and are needed to prevent hacking. A hacked system might impact patient care, incur fines, and impact the reputation of the practice
- Hardware and software malfunctions
- Transferring records to another software system
- Initial cost of hardware and software, recurring cost, and a consultant may be needed
- Retention of records when closing a practice
- Legal issues when everything is in one place—what do you share?
- Data storage costs
- Interconnections and interoperability of different software systems
- Ongoing training of staff on how to use the system

---

not have to be shared with patients. Examples include information regarding quality assessment or improvement, patient safety, peer review, and provider performance evaluation.

Electronic records are evolving in capability and sophistication. Most all can highlight, or flag, patient conditions that could affect or be affected by dental treatment. For example, if a patient is allergic to penicillin, the EHR would prominently display this fact on the screen to alert the clinician. Some systems may strongly warn, or even prevent, the practitioner from writing a prescription for a drug that the patient is allergic to. Still, other systems may be linked to a medication database that can automatically inform the practitioner when a patient, who takes multiple medications, may have significant side effects that can affect dental treatment or the patient's overall health. The information contained in electronic dental records coupled with AI systems has been shown to be able to assist dentists to make radiographic and clinical diagnoses. This capability can only be expected to grow and improve in the coming years.[14–16]

Imaging

Digital Photography and Videography

Dentists have used film-based camera systems for many years in their practices. Since 1989 when digital cameras were introduced, dentists began to incorporate this technology into their practices.[17] Many clinicians use cameras as a tool to show patients large and clear images of certain dental conditions that otherwise would be difficult for patients to see in the mouth. In one study, patients who saw images of their teeth were more likely, than those who did not, to choose a full coverage (crown) restoration.[18] A major advantage of digital images over photographs and 35-mm slides is that they can be stored on a computer or in an EHR for easy retrieval and sharing with dental laboratories or colleagues.

Extraoral cameras traditionally have consisted of a single lens reflex (SLR) camera body, a macro lens, and either a point or ring flash (Figure 4.1). It is possible with the high resolution of smartphone cameras and additional lighting to take excellent photos.[19] Extraoral cameras are best used to document larger areas like full and partial face views and images of many teeth together such as a whole or partial arch of teeth. Obtaining images of the inside of the mouth often requires the use of cheek retractors and mirrors to be able to expose structures clearly. Image files are then transferred from the camera or storage medium to a computer or EHR for future access. Some clinicians use an inexpensive digital camera to add patient recognition photos to their electronic records.[20]

Intraoral cameras are wand-like devices that can be connected directly to a computer (Figure 4.2). With the use of a computer monitor, it is possible for the dentist and patient to view images in real time. With high-resolution intraoral cameras, some dentists review findings from the dental examination directly on a computer monitor and can record images for their own documentation or for presentation to the patient.[21,22] The latter is very useful for patient education. It is possible to attach images, along with radiographs, to a third-party payment claim to better document the need for treatment.

Both intraoral and extraoral cameras can also record video. There are some very small video cameras that can be mounted on a dental operatory light or the dentist's magnification loupes.[23] The cameras are often connected to a foot pedal to control the on/off function. Clinicians can create videos for educational purposes as they provide treatment or speak with patients. The latter function is used by some dental practices to record consent often for surgical and implant procedures. Having a video of the patient smiling and talking can assist the clinician and laboratory technician evaluate a patient's smile prior to esthetic rehabilitation.[24]

Digital still and video images can be stored in a computer or in an EHR. Cameras, storage media, and intraoral cameras must be compatible with the EHR software to transfer the files successfully. High-resolution video files can be large and require more storage space than still and radiographic images. Images with identifiable patient information on mobile devices should be stored securely and deleted once uploaded to the EHR.

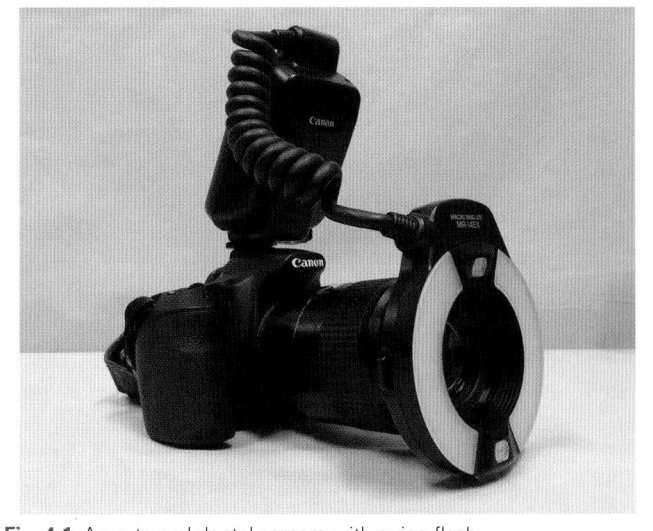

Fig. 4.1 An extraoral dental camera with a ring flash.

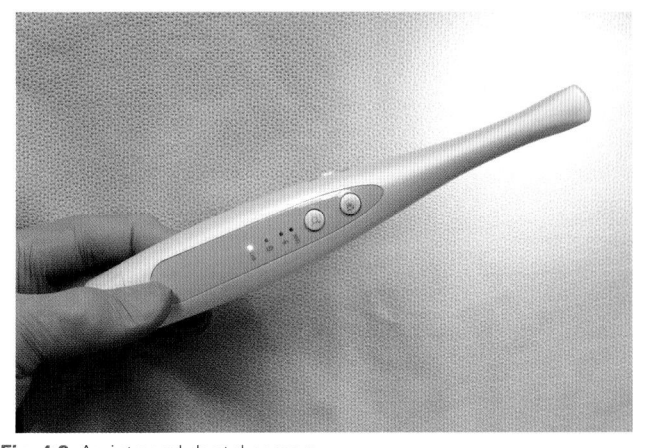

Fig. 4.2 An intraoral dental camera.

Digital Radiography

Dental radiography has advanced significantly since the discovery of x-rays by Dr. Wilhelm Roentgen in 1895 and the first digital radiography system that was introduced in 1987. Some of the advantages of digital radiography over conventional, film-based radiography include the speed of image processing and display, the decreased radiation dose required to obtain a diagnostic quality image, the ability to enhance the image quality postexposure, and the ease of integration with the EHR. Digital images can be easily stored, retrieved, and transferred for consultation and referral without loss of image quality. In addition, digital radiography does not require processing equipment and chemical solutions. However, direct digital imaging has some disadvantages. These include the increased up-front cost for computers and radiology equipment. The rigidity and thickness of intraoral sensors and presence of the sensor cord that can be uncomfortable for patients. There is also a smaller area of coverage compared with conventional film. Table 4.1 provides a comparison of the different digital imaging modalities that will be discussed in this section.

TABLE 4.1	Comparison of MRI, Ultrasound, CBCT, and Digital Intraoral Radiography				
Imaging Modality	Primary Indicated for	Resolution	Exposure/Scan time	Radiation Dose	Examination Cost
Intraoral	Hard tissues	~15–50 μm	<1 s	<1 μSv	$
Panoramic	Hard tissues	~60–200 μm	20 s	~7 μSv	$
CBCT	Hard tissues	~75–400 μm	20 s	~5–1073 μSV	$$
Ultrasound	Soft tissues	~1 mm	<5 min	N/A	$$
MRI	Hard and soft tissues	~0.5–1 mm	30–60 min	N/A	$$$

CBCT, cone-beam computed tomography; *MRI*, magnetic resonance imaging.

Digital intraoral radiography. Digital radiographs are composed of units called **pixels** that are arranged to form a grid. Each pixel displays a different brightness level that depends on the amount of radiant energy received. Brighter areas have received more energy; however, the image intensity is inverted in digital imaging to make it comparable to conventional film, which is a "negative image." There are two types of receptors used to record the images: digital sensors and photostimulable phosphor plates (PSP).

Digital sensors. Digital sensors are similar to the sensors used in cell phones but with an additional layer that allows the conversion of x-rays into visible light. To accommodate and protect all the internal components, sensors are thick and rigid. To allow for instant availability of the image after exposure, sensors are attached to the computer via a cord. The sensor rigidity, thickness, and cord may pose challenges mainly related to patient discomfort during image acquisition. Sensors are also somewhat fragile and can be damaged when dropped on the floor.

Photostimulable phosphor plates (PSPs). PSPs absorb and store the energy from x-rays and are then scanned with a laser light to release this energy. A scanner is then required to process the plates before the image can be displayed on the computer screen, which may be a disadvantage for some clinicians. The advantages of PSP plates are their flexibility and similarity to conventional film and the fact that they are wireless and more comfortable for the patient. However, the plates can get scratched after being reused many times resulting in image artifacts. The plates also degrade after a certain number of exposures losing their ability to capture images of diagnostic quality.

X-ray generation. There are two types of intraoral x-ray machines: alternating current (AC) and direct current (DC). Most modern x-ray machines use direct current, which is the recommended type of x-ray machine for digital radiography because of the constant flow of x-ray photons that helps optimize the efficiency of the digital sensors, which then require less exposure time when compared with conventional film and even plates.

Portable, handheld x-ray machines (Figure 4.3) are also available and extremely convenient for special circumstances where a wall-mounted x-ray machine is not available such as in care facilities, undeveloped areas without a dental office, and hospital operating rooms. Operating a handheld unit requires consistent adherence to the manufacturer's recommendations to avoid unnecessary radiation exposure to the operator as well as minimizing motion artifacts.

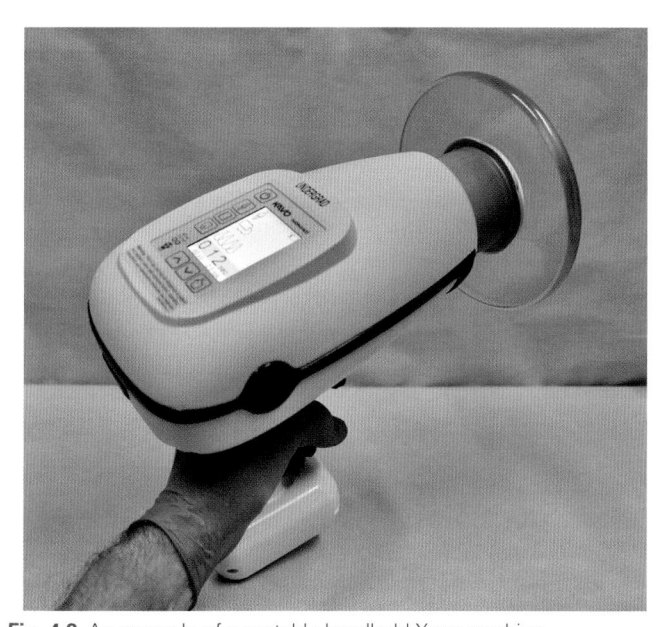

Fig. 4.3 An example of a portable handheld X-ray machine.

Image enhancement tools. The appearance of a digital radiograph displayed on a computer screen can be easily modified by software algorithms, some of which facilitate diagnosis by enhancing certain image characteristics. There is a risk, however, of creating artifacts that may lead to inaccurate diagnosis. One of the most common causes of poor radiographic quality in digital imaging is insufficient exposure, which is usually compensated for by auto-brightness adjustment during image processing.[25] However, because automatic brightness adjustments may mask incorrect exposure settings (too low or too high) this could lead unknowingly to overexposure of the patient. To prevent this, the image acquisition software settings should be calibrated by an information technology expert or the manufacturer's technical support representative.

When the brightness is adjusted by the clinician, there may be a decrease in the overall contrast, making the perception of subtle radiolucencies, like small carious lesions, difficult. Changing the brightness and contrast can be done dynamically for different diagnostic tasks but the adjustments always degrade the data; therefore they should not be made permanent. Retaining the original image is always recommended.

Sharpening filters are often used because they help decrease the perceived blurry or soft appearance of digital radiographs;

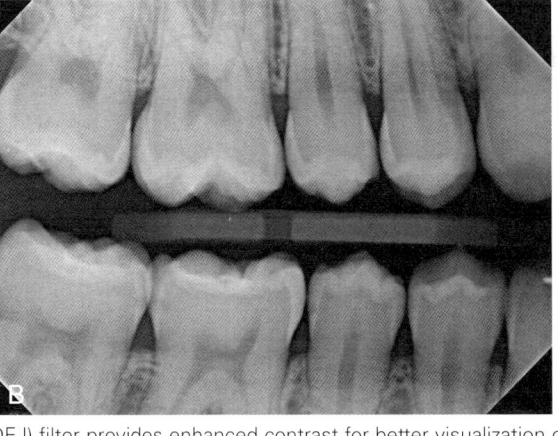
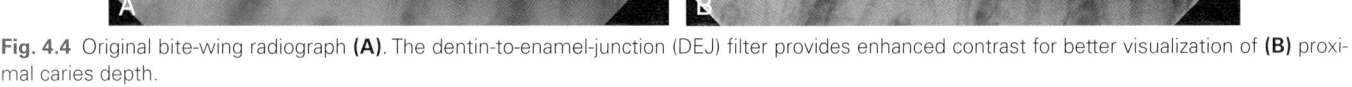

Fig. 4.4 Original bite-wing radiograph **(A)**. The dentin-to-enamel-junction (DEJ) filter provides enhanced contrast for better visualization of **(B)** proximal caries depth.

however, when overused, these filters can produce a shadow effect around bright restorations creating the false appearance of recurrent caries[26] or may increase gray intensity variations resulting in a grainy appearance[27] (Figure 4.4). Noise reduction filters spread out the intensity of a pixel to its surrounding neighbors.

The clinician should avoid diagnosis based on enhanced images only as the use of these filters can introduce artifacts or cause loss of diagnostic detail. Comparison to the original image to confirm findings is always recommended; therefore the enhanced image should be saved as a duplicate and never replace the original image.

Use of artificial intelligence to interpret radiographs. AI uses algorithms to automatically detect and quantify certain image features and patterns that are characteristic of a disease or abnormality. These algorithms have the potential for decreasing the subjectivity during interpretation and can help improve the reliability and validity of dental image analysis. One of the most common algorithms is DL, which is a type of ML that uses **convolutional neural networks** (CNNs). CNNs are trained to discriminate certain features using large data sets. The learning process involves labeling an image and providing both the image and the label to the CNN, which iteratively adjusts itself to eventually be able to predict the presence of the labeled entity, a carious lesion for instance, on unseen data.[28] Notably, using a CNN has shown significantly higher sensitivity than that by dentists, especially for detecting early lesions. The diagnostic process could be optimized by using imaging software that could automatically detect caries lesions and assist in the confirmation of lesion depth using AI algorithms.[29]

Beside caries detection, other dental applications of AI include cephalometric analysis,[30] automatic assessment of the mandibular cortical index, fractal analysis of trabecular bone pattern for bone pathology detection and systemic conditions such as osteoporosis, as well as prescreening for identification of soft tissue calcifications on panoramic radiographs[31] and cone-beam computed tomography (CBCT) scans.[32]

Digital panoramic radiographs. Digital panoramic radiographs provide better visualization of soft tissues and cartilages compared with conventional, film-based panoramic

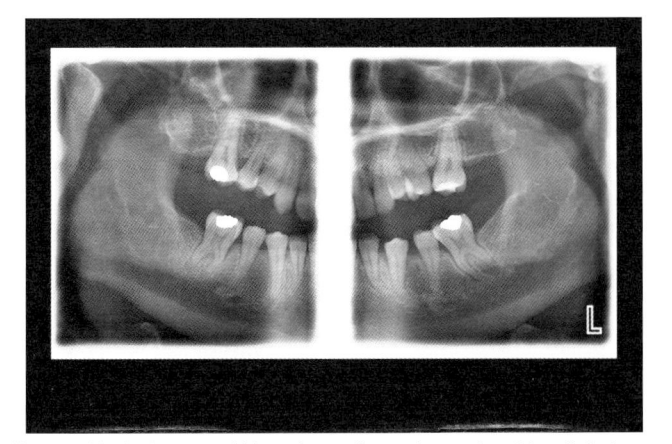

Fig. 4.5 Vertical extraoral bite-wing radiographs made with a digital panoramic machine.

radiographs. This improved soft tissue contrast can help detect soft tissue calcifications and other incidental findings on panoramic radiographs. Image enhancement tools can be particularly helpful in the detection of soft tissue calcifications including calcified carotid atheromas, calcified ligaments, tonsilloliths, and sialoliths, which are highly prevalent in particular among older adults.[33] Adjusting the brightness and contrast can improve visualization of the usually dark neck region on digital panoramic radiographs to differentiate calcified carotid atheromas from normal cartilages in that region.[34]

Another advantage of some digital panoramic machines is the ability to obtain extraoral bite-wings by adjusting the shape and location of the focal trough and limiting the region scanned (Figure 4.5). Extraoral bite-wings are particularly useful when positioning an intraoral sensor or plate is challenging because of limited mouth opening, complex anatomy, increased gag reflex, or severe soft tissue sensitivity. Also, in addition to the crowns and bone levels of maxillary and mandibular teeth, extraoral bite-wings capture the entire root and periapical bone of posterior teeth, better than vertical bite-wings. However, intraoral bite-wings are still preferred for their higher resolution and better reproducibility to open proximal contacts compared with extraoral bite-wings.

Cone-beam computed tomography (CBCT). CBCT is a three-dimensional (3D) imaging system that uses a conically shaped x-ray beam that rotates in one direction and a flat panel detector that rotates in the opposite side. In a single 360-degree rotation around the patient's head, the CBCT machine produces a stack of hundreds of projection images that are reconstructed by the computer using a series of mathematical algorithms. The main advantage of CBCT over intraoral and panoramic radiographs is the ability to see the buccolingual dimension of the jaws and the relation of the teeth to surrounding vital structures without distortion, superimposition of other structures, or magnification. Some of the most important dental applications of CBCT include:

- The evaluation of potential implant sites to determine the amount of ridge atrophy, the need for implant site development, the relative bone density, the degree of ridge inclination, the presence of buccal or lingual concavities, and the proximity to vital structures.
- The assessment of impacted teeth prior to surgical extraction including their exact location, their proximity to other teeth and vital structures, and the presence of external root resorption.
- The evaluation of periapical and other jaw lesions including their extent and effects on surrounding structures.
- The assessment of the osseous components of the temporomandibular joints for the presence of degenerative changes and other abnormalities.

Part of the process of interpreting a CBCT scan includes scrolling through stacks of hundreds of images in the axial (horizontal), coronal, and sagittal planes. Each of these images will display the cross-sectional anatomy as thin slices through the volume. The CBCT data can also be used to reconstruct a panoramic view and cross-sectional images perpendicular to the long axis of the maxilla and mandible to visualize the buccolingual dimension of the bone and can be viewed as a 3D volume that can be rotated in any direction.

There are several factors that affect the image quality of a CBCT scan including, but not limited to, the field of view or region scanned, the **voxel** size, and the type of detector. In general terms, the smaller the region included in the scan the higher the image quality due to less scattering of the x-ray beam. Similarly, the smaller the voxel size the higher the resolution.

There are many different types of CBCT machines that vary significantly in terms of technical specifications, image quality, and radiation dose. Some CBCT machines can only acquire either small or large field of view scans whereas other machines offer a wide range of fields of view that can be as small as a couple of teeth and as large as the entire head. As mentioned earlier, smaller field-of-view scans offer higher spatial resolution that may be needed for dental applications such as endodontic therapy including localization of accessory canals, asymptomatic periapical pathology, and root fractures. Larger field-of-view scans are usually needed for presurgical assessment prior to orthognathic surgery and evaluation of craniofacial anomalies. Some general practitioners may benefit from dual-purpose CBCT machines that can acquire digital panoramic radiographs

and CBCT scans. It is important to select the appropriate imaging protocol depending on the specific dental application. A general rule is to use the smallest field of view applicable to the specific diagnostic task as it increases the image quality, decreases the radiation dose, and decreases the interpretation time and the interpreter's liability for detecting incidental findings.

The main limitations of CBCT are the accentuated artifacts produced by metal restorations and implants and the limited soft tissue contrast. Potential ways to reduce metal artifacts include decreasing the field of view to avoid including the metal restoration in the scan or changing the patient position to change the angle in which artifacts are spread. For example, by having the occlusal plane parallel to the floor, metal artifacts from restorations will not affect the appearance of the bone as they spread horizontally in the same plane where the restoration is present. The limited soft tissue contrast of CBCT scans is mainly because of the divergence of the x-ray beam, the relatively high number of scattered x-ray photons, and artifacts that are inherent to flat panel detectors.

In terms of radiation dose, a meta-analysis of the most CBCT machines available in the market found that the radiation dose from a small CBCT scan can be as low as 5 μSv (which is less than that of a panoramic radiograph) whereas that of a large field-of-view scan can be as high as 1073 μSv[35] (which is similar to that of a multislice/medical computed tomography [CT] scan).

Dental Applications of Intraoral Ultrasound

One of the main advantages of using ultrasound for diagnosis is that this imaging modality does not utilize ionizing radiation. Instead, it uses sound waves that are emitted by a transducer, which travel through the patient's tissues and are reflected back to the transducer when they meet an interface between two tissues that have different acoustic impedance (e.g., gingival tissues and bone). The computer uses the reflected sound waves to form an image based on the amount of energy reflected back. Smaller probes and transducers have been recently developed for intraoral use and some of the applications of ultrasound include the evaluation of the gingival thickness, soft tissue evaluation including the tongue and salivary glands, periimplant defects, and tissue and bone recession.[36,37] The images are dynamic, acquired in real time, and provide an accurate representation of the tissues. However, one of the limitations of ultrasound is that it cannot penetrate bone or the hard tissues of a tooth; therefore it is not indicated for assessment of caries or bone pathology.

Dental Applications of Magnetic Resonance Imaging

Magnetic resonance imaging (MRI) is a hospital-based imaging modality that does not use ionizing radiation. MRI is currently the state-of-art imaging modality to evaluate the soft tissues, including the temporomandibular joint disk and soft tissue lesions such as salivary gland tumors and tongue cancer. More recently, research efforts have focused on dental applications of MRI including detection of caries, periapical lesions, and implant evaluation.[38,39]

COMMUNICATION

Methods of Communication

The revolution in technology and the reliance on the Internet was never more prominent than during the COVID-19 pandemic. Businesses had to shift overnight to communicating online and employees began working remotely. Although clinical dentistry is not something that can be done virtually (outside of a telehealth consult) the impact of technology was still felt. In terms of communication, dental clinics are transitioning from postal mail and phone calls to using online tools such as email, texting, patient portals, websites, and social media. This transition in communication has been unequally adopted by some groups of patients. For instance, Internet access may be difficult for patients in rural areas with limited or no access to Internet providers and for patients who lack the knowledge or financial resources to use new technologies. The purpose of this chapter is to describe the various patient communication channels, how they are leveraged, and an overview of information privacy and security.

Electronic communication can be thought of as being either synchronous or asynchronous in delivery (Figure 4.6). **Synchronous communication** is when two or more people interact in real time to exchange information. **Asynchronous communication** is when two or more people exchange information but not in real time. Some types of communication can be viewed as both. For example, texting is inherently asynchronous. One person sends a message and waits for a response. There is no indication that someone has seen the message and when they will respond. On the other hand, there are some messaging systems with a live chatting feature that enables users to know if someone has read the message and is in the process of

typing a response. Synchronous communication methods are preferred when discussing a patient's protected health information and when privacy is important. This would include discussing personal health information, diagnoses, treatment plans, and treatment options. Asynchronous communication is best when an immediate response is not required. An example would be a dental clinic that sends their patients appointment reminders or posttreatment satisfaction surveys using text messages or email.

Text and Email Messaging

Text and email messaging have become the preferred method of communication for many individuals and several messaging systems are available. Many patients carry a mobile device with them that is used to send and receive text messages, check email, and interact with various applications. For some, the phone may be used rarely for an actual phone call. Text messages are intended to be short quick communications where a simple 'yes' or 'no' response will usually suffice. Text messaging is primarily asynchronous, therefore an immediate response is not expected. According to Pew Research, 97% of US adults use text messaging every day. Specifically, the short message service (SMS) format. There are three other formats for text messages: multimedia message services (MMS), iMessage which can simulate synchronous "live" texting, and rich communication services (RCS). SMS and MMS do not require an Internet or data connection to send and receive messages, whereas iMessage and RCS require an Internet connection and data plan do so.

For most electronic patient records, patients can choose to have appointment reminders sent via text message. Reminders can be sent a few days before the appointment and allow time for the patient to respond back when they have time. Patients can also confirm their appointment with a simple Yes/No response. Some sophisticated text message systems can remind patients to take antibiotic premedication before their appointment or bring a responsible adult to the appointment when sedation is planned. A study[40] in 2020 compared the response time to a text message versus email and showed that texting was more efficient than email.

Email is considered more formal than a text message and can contain more information. Using email allows the clinician to attach files or web links that can be easily sent to multiple people at once. Accessing email requires the user to have a specific application and these applications will require a username and password. Text messages that come to a mobile device usually do not require a username and password to access them. Because of this, email is usually considered more secure than a text message.

What methods are best for communicating with patients? When discussing diagnoses and treatment plans, a synchronous method (face-to-face or via telehealth) is best. The provider can explain why the treatment options are being recommended, share images, and discuss the pros and cons of the proposed treatment plan. The patient can also ask questions and get answers in real time. Using email and text messages for this function can be problematic. See the *In Clinical Practice* box.

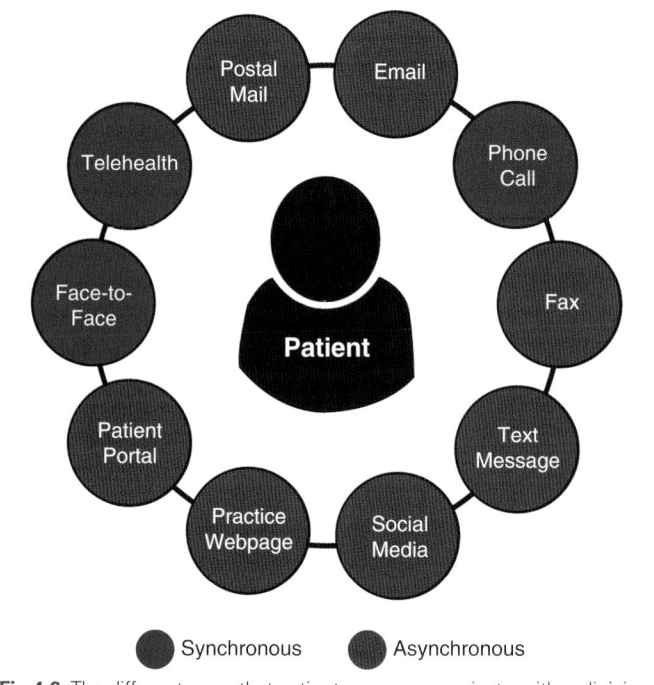

Fig 4.6 The different ways that patients can communicate with a clinician.

IN CLINICAL PRACTICE

Should clinicians use text and email messaging to communicate with patients?

That depends on what you are communicating and if you have consent from the patient. In the United States, as in many other countries, there are laws that guide businesses on the use of electronic communication with its citizens.[41] Although healthcare providers may be exempt from some of these rules, they do state that messages should only convey generic healthcare information such as appointment reminders and scheduling requests, prescription pick-up reminders, etc. Patients usually have to opt in to receive automated messages.

In general, text messages are best used for short quick notifications. An example would be texting a patient a reminder a few days in advance of their appointment and requesting a confirmation response. The message should not include protected health information or other sensitive information such as what the patient is being seen for (cleaning, crown, tooth extraction) or information about the patient's dental or medical health. Email is best when the message is lengthy or when attachments or multiple links are included. Examples include directions to the clinic and attachments such as blank registration and health history forms.

Sometimes a patient may email a clinician or clinic with questions about treatment or that they are having problems after treatment. In such situations it is best to redirect the conversation to a synchronous medium such as a phone call or seeing the patient in person. This helps avoid lengthy back-and-forth exchanges and misunderstandings that can often occur with asynchronous text and email messages.

Social Media and Websites

Social media platforms are a newer form of communication and now the dominant medium for how a significant portion of the world communicates. Some platforms have stopped being used whereas others have increased in the last few years (Figure 4.7). Across the world, wherever Internet connectivity is available, social media is now a part of everyday life for one-third of the world's population. The use of these platforms spans across generations, however, the use among younger generations is much more prevalent.[42]

Social media can affect the way the dental providers diagnose and treat their patients and the services they offer. Most dental clinics now have a website and social media site. These sites provide information about the services such as cosmetic dentistry and implants. Some social media platforms and websites provide user ratings on providers and treatment plan options. Patients can query individuals within their social media network or search websites to research their own specific problems.[43] On some websites the patient can ask questions about the diagnoses and treatment options the provider has given and seek out information about financial costs and practice philosophy. Although friends, family, and social networks can provide their personal perspective or experience with a specific type of treatment, each patient is different. The clinician should

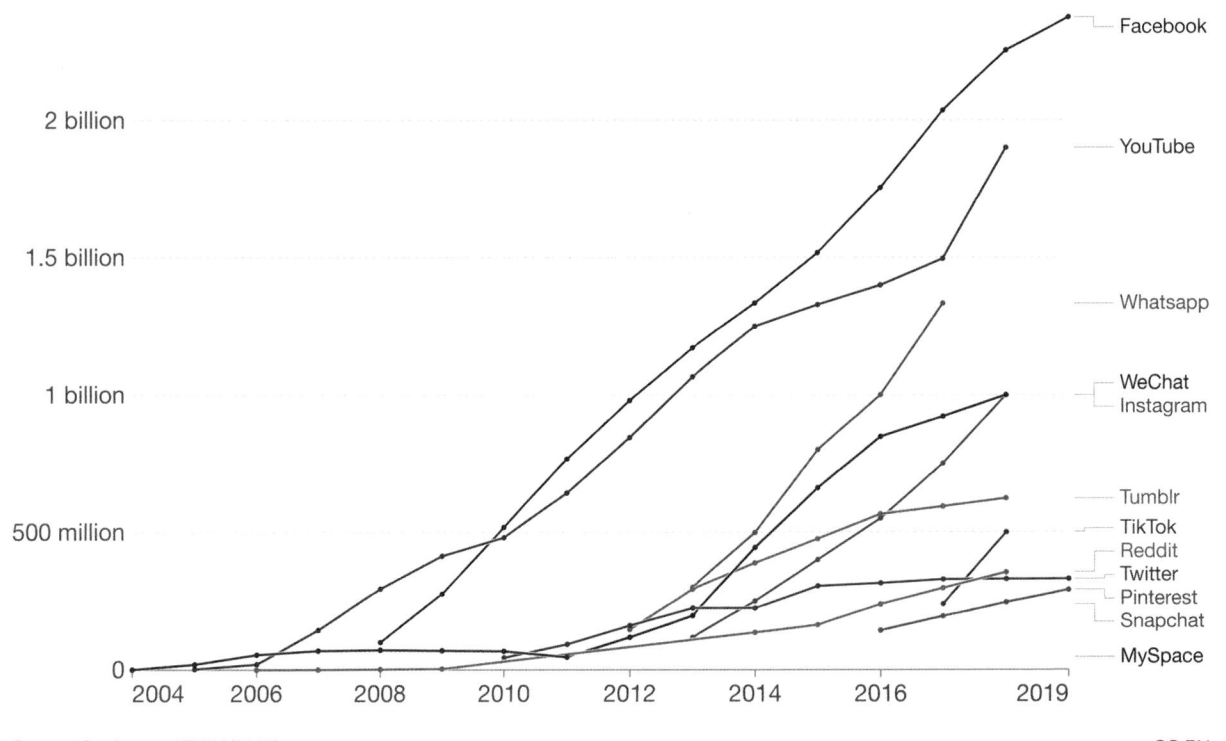

Number of people using social media platforms, 2004 to 2019

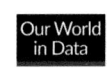

Estimates correspond to monthly active users (MAUs). Facebook, for example, measures MAUs as users that have logged in during the past 30 days. See source for more details.

Source: Statista and TNW (2019)

Fig. 4.7 Number of people using social media platforms over time. Statista: https://ourworldindata.org/rise-of-social-media, https://www.statista.com/statistics/272014/global-social-networks-ranked-by-number-of-users/ and TNW: https://thenextweb.com/tech/2019/06/11/most-popular-social-media-networks-year-animated/

be aware of different sources of information that a patient may be receiving and be prepared to have a thorough discussion about any diagnoses and treatment plans. The clinician should also provide the patient with evidence-based information from reputable sources to review for comparison (see eTables 4.1 and 4.2 on ebooks+).

Patient Portals

Many patients have the capability to communicate with their electronic medical records. These **patient portals** enable patients to review their medical records and include seeing a list of health problems and medications; viewing laboratory results and payment information; requesting an appointment and securely communicating with their providers.[44] The portals also provide a mechanism for patients to supply information before health visits. For example, patients can complete or update health history forms or answer additional questionnaires. They can even review consent forms.[45] Patients can also be sent information based on their unique health needs. Presently, most electronic dental records do not have this capability unless they are part of an EHR system. Some dental clinics have portal-like activities on their websites such as being able to ask questions, make appointments, or pay a bill.

Privacy and Security of Patient Health Information

Privacy is important when a patient and provider are communicating, as sensitive and confidential information is often being shared. Building and maintaining trust within the patient-provider relationship impacts how much information the patient will share regarding the details about their health. Privacy[46] is defined as a framework for deciding who should have the capability to access and alter information, whereas **security**[47] refers to the protection against unauthorized access to the data and what controls are in place to limit who can access the information. In 1996, the United States enacted the *Health Insurance Portability and Accountability Act (HIPAA)* that included privacy and security rules. It provides[48] a patient with rights over their own health information and how it is shared, regardless of the form it is in, and requires specific safeguards to be in place for electronic health information. See Box 4.3 for security best practices for using applications with sensitive information.

The clinician faces several decisions when deciding how best to communicate with a patient. Often this relates to what type of information is being shared and which will be the most secure method. Postal mail is addressed to a specific individual and sent to their preferred address. It is usually in a sealed envelope that protects someone else from seeing any sensitive information contained within. Email is sent to an online address. Although the address is usually for one individual, sometimes several people share an email address or share their username and password information with each other. Unlike a physical envelope that is sealed, an email message may not be secure, or **encrypted**, when sent and therefore would not have the same privacy that the sealed envelope provides.

> ### BOX 4.3   Security Best Practices
>
> Use strong passwords (e.g., at least 10 characters include numbers, capital, and lowercase letters)
> Have different passwords for each website or system
> Use a password manager and change passwords at least annually
> Limit access to patient information
> Install security updates (software, web browsers, and operating systems)
> Enable two-factor authentication
> Install antivirus and malware security software
> Avoid using pop-ups and opening unknown emails, messages, and web links

---

A phone call is usually intended for a specific person in order to have a one-on-one conversation. However, because the clinician cannot see the person, someone else could answer the phone and claim to be that person. If the clinician or staff member is establishing a new relationship with the patient, the sound of the other person's voice may not be recognizable enough to confirm their identity.

Sending a fax is used primarily between healthcare providers than between a provider and patient. The office personnel should be the only ones able to access the fax machine, which itself should be in a secure location. If a fax is sent toward the end of the day and not retrieved by office staff, there is a risk that others who work after hours could potentially see the information on the fax machine. Also, fax machines may not encrypt the information when it is sent electronically and, like email, does not provide the same privacy a sealed envelope would.

When sending a text message, little to no personal information needs to be included. Usually, a text message is used to remind the patient of their appointment day and time and asks them to confirm. There is no need to include private information about treatments that will be taking place or fees to be paid.

A patient's protected health information should never be shared via social media, even if the patient is asking, as it is not private. Generic responses about the types of services provided, the types of insurance accepted, or general educational information for all patients (e.g., brushing and flossing impacts your health in this way) would be appropriate to provide. Even better, asking to speak directly with the patient would be best.

A patient portal is a complex application for access to a significant amount of sensitive data. This enables dialog between a patient and the provider regarding the patient's sensitive health information. The portal application therefore requires the highest level of security to ensure the privacy of the communication. Portals encrypt messages and provide a secure and private digital envelope for messages sent between the patient and the provider.

Telehealth has added another dimension. This simulates an in-person, face-to-face interaction. Because the patient is not physically in the clinical setting, the level of privacy may not be the same, especially if the patient is in a busy work or home environment. It is a good practice to ask patients to find a private location for the video call.

Teledentistry

The term **telemedicine** was first introduced by an American, Thomas Bird, in 1970[49] and is broadly defined as the use of information and communication technologies for healthcare.[50] The synchronous technologies used include phone calls and video calls or conferences. There is also asynchronous remote patient monitoring software and devices, patient self-assessment software, and the recording and forwarding of data via encrypted email. Telemedicine use varies among the medical specialties in the frequency and type of technology used. Radiology, psychology, and cardiology are the specialties that most use telemedicine with patients. Radiology and pathology clinicians record findings and send them asynchronously whereas cardiology and nephrology most frequently use telemedicine for patient monitoring. Emergency physicians use videoconferencing extensively to consult with other healthcare providers.[51]

Teledentistry, the application of telemedicine to the field of dentistry, has been adopted by the dental profession only recently in the history of telemedicine services. The first documented application of teledentistry was by the US Department of Defense in their *Total Dental Access* (TDA) program in 1994.[52] Teledentistry expands dental care options by providing electronic and virtual dental health visits and patient education services. Over the last five decades the technologies have evolved to allow the application of various stored and live electronic systems to the practice of teledentistry. These systems include EHRs (with and without patient portals), electronic referrals, electronic consultations, and electronic prescribing.

Elder care facilities, schools, remote clinics, and rural areas are some of the primary locations where isolated populations can benefit from teledentistry services. The ability to electronically connect patients and providers can improve access to care and provide a virtual dental home.[53] Remote clinics can connect virtually with specialists to review findings and determine whether patients need to travel to be evaluated in person. For example, a person residing in an assisted living facility may be interested in establishing a dental home so they can have a broken tooth removed and their teeth cleaned. A virtual initial evaluation by the dentist might reveal a need to have a medical consultation prior to the first in-person visit to the dentist.

In 2020, the COVID-19 pandemic created a situation where the use of teledentistry rapidly increased. This was in response to the restrictions in shared space and personal contact among healthcare providers and patients, most notably in the practice of dentistry, which requires proximity to the patient and can produce aerosol, splash, and splatter containing patient fluids. The ability to interview and evaluate a patient virtually became the vital connection to maintaining patient care when physical presence was not possible. Using teledentistry is important not only during situations like a pandemic but in other circumstances when a patient's physical presence is not possible such as in catastrophic events like war and natural disasters.[54]

Patient Evaluation

Triage for emergency. One of the best applications of teledentistry is to triage dental emergencies. Dental emergencies do not predictably occur at convenient times or convenient places so the ability to contact a dental provider becomes important. The patient, or another individual helping, can be instructed via video or phone to administer basic first aid to a patient with a dental emergency, including instructions as to when and by whom the patient should be examined in person. A common example is a consultation by a dental provider in a large dental office or dental school who is available after hours via a paging system to contact those patients with urgent concerns by using the phone, video, or text messaging.

In some circumstances, a patient can self-triage using software that evaluates a patient's response to a series of specific and targeted questions about the dental emergency and the patient's general health. Using such self-triage software was shown to have a sensitivity of 87.5% in accurately categorizing the patient's status as emergent or urgent.[55] Guided self-diagnosis using computer software is not new to dentistry and teledentistry software for self-triage is also available.[56] For example, a patient with a parulis and tooth pain can use self-triage software to rule out emergent need for care by the dentist and be scheduled at more convenient time for both the dentist and the patient.

Initial patient evaluation. Teledentistry is useful to evaluate a new patient's medical and dental health histories as well as their chief concerns before they are seen in person. Although this is not a comprehensive examination, the clinician can obtain enough data to decide how best to treat the patient. The primary goal is to gather enough information to make the first in-person visit more efficient and secondarily to help the evaluator decide whether a general dentist or specialist should see the patient. Patients who live in remote locations or who have transportation challenges can benefit from virtual initial patient evaluations. For example, consider a patient residing in a remote location who is interested in establishing a dental home. A virtual initial evaluation with the patient can determine what options are best to address the patient's oral healthcare needs to minimize trips to the dentist and make best use of time while at the dentist.

Unfortunately, making definitive diagnoses virtually is very limited. Inherent in a virtual examination is the inability to examine the patient in 3D, perform a tactile and physical examination, and perform diagnostic tests. Most likely the dental provider will create a list of differential diagnoses from the data collected during a teledentistry visit and decide whether there is a need for emergency care. The patient usually requires a subsequent visit for an in-person comprehensive examination before the clinician can provide definitive treatment recommendations.

Remote patient monitoring. Using teledentistry to monitor a patient remotely requires that a diagnosis has been made and some form of treatment has been or is being administered. The examination of the patient at some predetermined frequency for improvement, or change, constitutes monitoring until the patient is healed, in remission, or there is a decision to consider other treatment options. Therefore monitoring is best done synchronously using live video. For instance, a patient may have a herpetic lip lesion and the dentist can advise the patient when it is safe to be seen for treatment.

Use of applications on mobile devices can be used for asynchronous monitoring of chronic dental conditions as well, such as temporomandibular dysfunction. For example, a patient with a chronic pain condition can use an application to document when the pain occurs, the frequency, location, and intensity[57] (Figure 4.8). This information is recorded and can be shared remotely with other practitioners including dentists, physicians, physical therapists, and researchers. These applications also remind patients when to record their pain and can provide patient education on how to manage the pain.

Teledentistry can be used for postoperative evaluation of patients (see the *In Clinical Practice* box). This is similar to monitoring but for a shorter period of time as complete healing or resolution is expected after the dental procedure. For instance, the dentist can assess a patient's healing after the extraction of multiple teeth to assess postoperative pain, control of bleeding, and any signs of infection.

Electronic consultation. Consulting other providers is valuable when a medical or multidisciplinary assessment of the dental patient is needed prior to providing dental care. Generally, the dentist will request a professional assessment of a specific concern that will impact the safe delivery of dental care. The consultant can address the provider's concerns in the context of the patient's dental needs and systemic health and respond back with recommendations. This may subsequently require an in-person evaluation of the patient by the consultant; however, a phone call, facsimile, or video visit with the consultant beforehand is often informative and sufficient. This is enhanced when provider and consultant can communicate using a common EHR to have access to lab values, systemic diagnoses, medications, and other information. Teledentistry can facilitate communication and consultation among a variety of healthcare providers by connecting the dentist with family physicians, social workers, pediatricians, dermatologists, otolaryngology specialists, emergency medicine physicians, and others as the need arises. For example, a consultation might be sent from a dentist to a physician to confirm a patient's reported medical and medication history and request recent lab values to be able to treat the dental needs of a patient receiving cancer chemotherapy.

Electronic referral. Specialty dental care for patients depends on the availability of specialists, access by the patient, and communication with the primary dental provider. Using virtual tools for referring patients for specialty dental care can eliminate the need for paper referral forms, physical x-rays, and delivery by postal mail. Additionally, a virtual assessment of the patient by the specialty provider can best inform and prepare the specialty provider, as well as the patient, for the specialty care. Radiographic images, photographs, and diagnostic test results are examples of some of the data that can be stored and forwarded to the specialist for consideration prior to the patient's in-person visit. For example, a patient has been referred to an oral surgeon for extraction of third molars with intravenous sedation. The patient may have a virtual visit with the oral surgeon to review the surgical procedure and pain control options, as well as presurgical instructions specific to the patient and procedures.

Patient and Dentist Education and Communication

Both general and customized patient education can be provided using personal electronic devices. This communication is

usually asynchronous, which is convenient for both the patient and the practitioner. The dentist or staff can refer the patient to instructional videos, quick reference sheets (document files or online links), and links to scientific evidence. For example, videos or images that demonstrate proper flossing technique can be sent to a patient after a recent prophylaxis and examination appointment. In addition, patients can participate in virtual health fairs to obtain information about healthcare resources as well as available local dental providers.

Virtual continuing education courses, synchronous or asynchronous, are vital for clinicians serving patients in rural and remote areas. These courses are typically provided by educational institutions, medical and dental professional affiliations, and private companies. For example, a remote medical and dental clinic can participate in a conference about Sjögren's syndrome, an autoimmune disorder with significant oral and systemic manifestations.

The provision of a language interpreter may be a legal requirement for patients who are nonnative speakers. However, the cost to provide an in-person interpreter for a patient on a recurring basis may be prohibitive and language interpreters may not be readily available for a specific language. Clinicians can use synchronous phone or video interpretation of a language while the patient is in the office or on the phone. Providing translation services allows the patient to understand the dental terminology, treatment recommendations, costs, risks, benefits, and other treatment options. Providing language interpretation improves patient care through better communication with the dental provider.

The provision of interpretative services for deaf and hard of hearing patients presents a unique problem for the patient and dentist, particularly if a practice does not have access to a sign language interpreter. National or regional laws may require the dental provider to have a sign language interpreter available for their patients. However, a new patient may not have alerted the office to their need for sign language services, or an in-person interpreter might not be available. Teledentistry can help to alleviate these problems by allowing a sign language interpreter to become involved in real time via video.

Benefits and Limitations

There are cost savings for both patient and provider that may not be immediately realized but occur after the implementation of teledentistry.[52] After the initial investment in equipment, software, and Internet connectivity, the cost savings are realized by the decrease in travel time for the patient and appointment time for the dentist.

Technical limitations are most likely the greatest barriers to fully implementing teledentistry using video. Inherent in its success is the need for infrastructure, equipment, knowledge, and acceptance by both patients and providers. Infrastructure refers to the availability of high-speed Internet for both the patient and the provider. There are remote areas of the United States and other countries without consistent high-speed Internet service. Additionally, the equipment needed for a successful teledentistry encounter may not be available or affordable to the patient. Educating the patient, and anyone assisting the patient,

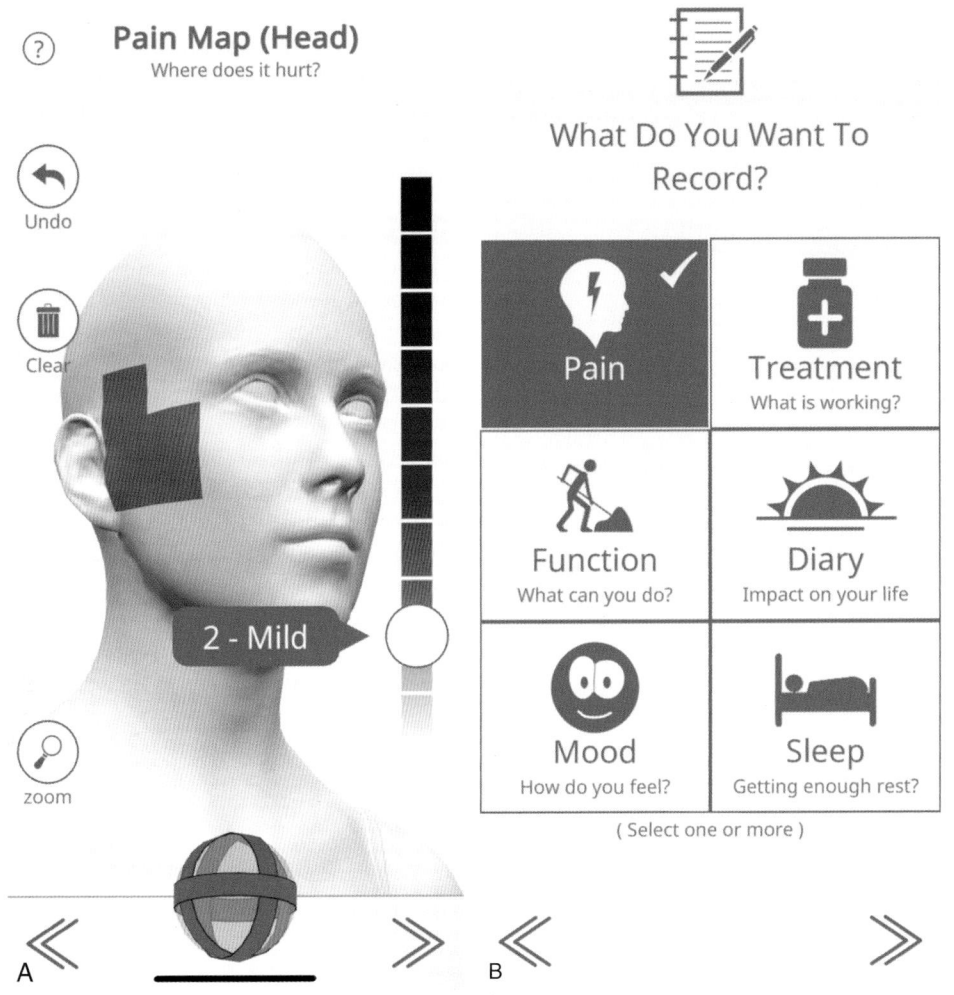

Fig. 4.8 (A) and (B) Mobile application for tracking pain and other conditions over time. (Courtesy Dr. Alexandre DaSilva and Geopain.com.)

about the technology and equipment is imperative for the most successful outcome. Data can be acquired live using cameras on personal devices or may be sent asynchronously as images. Poor image quality and Internet connectivity will affect the ability to fully evaluate the patient. There are commercially developed software systems that provide both private and secure video communication with patients. Most communication software cannot be integrated within a dental EHR, however, there are medical EHR platforms that do have the capability to offer appointments for video visits with patients.

Patients may be apprehensive and even suspicious of teledentistry visits, particularly if the patient is unfamiliar with the technology and equipment. Additionally, although patients are accepting of certain types of teledentistry services in specific circumstances, there are conditions in which those same patients prefer an in-person visit.[58] As an example, a patient may not hesitate to consult a dentist via teledentistry with questions on tooth whitening but will insist on an in-person visit for a broken cusp on a tooth.

There are challenges to overcome in the documentation of teledentistry visits. The practitioner will need to develop their own guidelines for how a video visit is documented. Recording

video visits can create large data files that require additional storage. This can be significant when used regularly for hundreds, perhaps thousands, of patients. Having a screenshot or photo image attached to the written documentation can represent that the patient encounter was performed virtually. Written documentation should include that the patient consented to the virtual visit and to being photographed. The documentation should also include the location of patient and the provider and indicate if the visit was held at a time and place that maintained privacy for the patient's personal information.

The laws governing the practice of dentistry must be carefully reviewed prior to incorporating teledentistry into any practice. There may be teledentistry rules and regulations regarding insurance, billing, the location of licensed provider, the location of patient, scope of practice, and the ability to prescribe medications based on a just a virtual visit. Legal documentation of teledentistry services in the patient's chart must be made as well as documentation of informed consent. The health record is a legal document and must reflect any evaluations, examinations, acquisition of data such as patient images, referrals/consults, and advice/prescriptions provided using teledentistry. Transferring patient information electronically must abide by local laws regarding privacy and by using a secure email messaging system.

DIGITAL HARDWARE AND SOFTWARE FOR TREATMENT PLANNING

Hardware

The use of digital technology for diagnosis and treatment planning has grown tremendously in the past 30 years. As discussed earlier in the chapter, dentists have used digital photography for many years to document dental conditions, show these conditions to patients to improve the communication and patient understanding of their dental conditions, and to communicate with the dental laboratory any information that is difficult to see on dental casts or impressions. Dentists have also used videos of their patients smiling, talking, and chewing to better design restorations for ultimate esthetic results during these functions. All this information is gathered by the dental laboratory and used to fabricate restorations that meet all the patient functional and esthetic needs.

With the introduction of desktop 3D scanners, dental laboratories are able to scan dental impressions or casts to design and produce dental restorations digitally with minimal hands-on procedures. However, a full digital workflow is not possible when using a desktop scanner as it requires a physical impression or model. Intraoral scanners (IOSs) support a full digital workflow. The digital impression is acquired and sent electronically to the design software. After the restoration is designed, it is manufactured using a milling machine or a 3D printer. IOSs have improved significantly in the last 10 years both in accuracy and speed. They are capable of producing digital impressions whose quality and accuracy are comparable to conventional impressions.

Other digital equipment used in dentistry include caries detection devices, shade selection scanners, and oral cancer detection equipment. These devices are continuously improving and helping clinicians in providing the best care to their patients.

Oral Cancer Detection

In the United States in 2022, it is estimated that 54,000 patients will be diagnosed with oral cancer and over 11,000 patients will have died from the disease.[59] Most oral cancers are squamous cell carcinomas[60] and early detection and treatment improve the short- and long-term prognoses for the patient. Clinicians should regularly perform a head and neck examination to detect early signs of disease. Dentists evaluate suspicious soft tissue lesions by reviewing the patient's history and visually examining and palpating the affected areas. For those lesions that are deemed suspicious, a definitive diagnosis is confirmed by obtaining a biopsy specimen with subsequent histopathologic evaluation.

Several new devices use either autofluorescence or tissue reflectance to identify and evaluate suspicious areas intraorally. One device, the VELscope[61] (visually enhanced lesion scope) is used to inspect the oral tissues for areas that might be dysplastic or cancerous and potentially identify cancer in its early stages. The device emits a blue light that excites normal intraoral tissues to fluoresce green. Suspicious areas do not fluoresce and appear dark when viewed through the device. Some clinicians use the device to either examine all the intraoral tissues or just those areas that are of concern after performing a conventional intraoral examination.

The VELscope is a good example of a digital tool that does not replace conventional intraoral examination and palpation. The main concern with these supplemental aids is the false-positive results than that can create undue anxiety for the patient and clinician.[62] False-positive results can come from normal structures such as a linea alba or chronic conditions like lichen planus, that like dysplastic lesions, do not fluoresce (Figure 4.9). False-negative results have also been noted, potentially leading the clinician to not biopsy a lesion that is cancerous.[63] The tool can be used by oral medicine and surgical specialties who are not screening for potential lesions but further evaluating suspicious lesions and establishing the lesion's extent (margins) prior to biopsy.

Caries Detection

Intraoral radiography is considered the standard technique for diagnosing proximal caries. However, many patients refuse routine radiographs to avoid the radiation exposure. New developments in digital technology have led to the introduction of caries detection equipment that use a variety of technologies, including fluorescence, transillumination, and electrical conductance to detect areas of hypomineralization without exposing the patient to radiation.

Although there are many technology-based instruments available to assist the clinician with the detection and

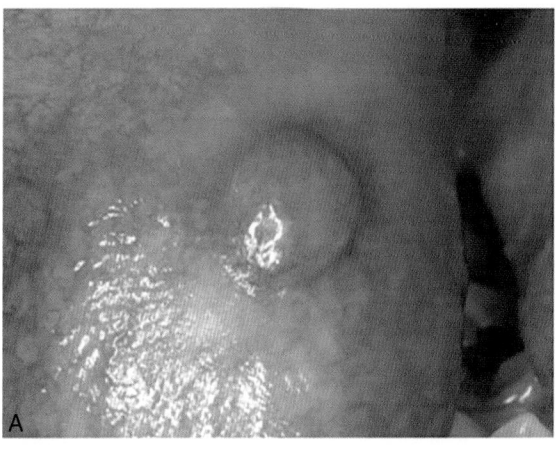

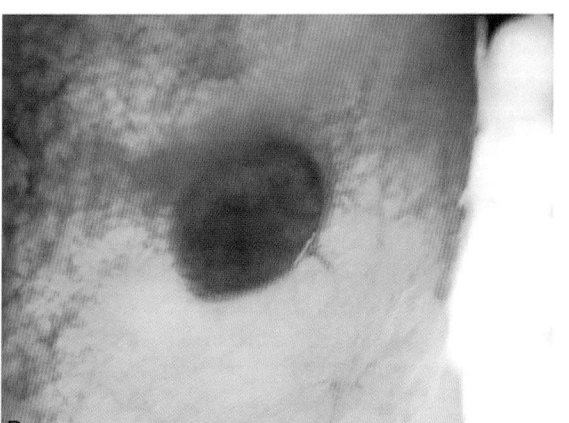

Fig. 4.9 Appearance of a benign lesion, an irritation fibroma, **(A)** clinically and **(B)** through the VELscope.

monitoring of noncavitated lesions, these are not "stand-alone" diagnostic methods that can be used as a substitute for the dentist's clinical judgment.[64,65] These methods serve as aids to visual examination and clinical decision-making. Examples include the use of fiber-optic transillumination (FOTI); digital fiber-optic transillumination (DiFOTI); fluorescence: near-infrared (NIR), red, green, and blue light fluorescence (e.g., DIAGNOdent, quantitative light-induced fluorescence—Figure 4.10); electrical conductance/resistance; and optical coherence tomography (OCT), among many others. In general, when used correctly, these technologies can play an important role in caries lesion detection and, if they allow for quantification, they may additionally help stage the severity of a carious lesion and assist in the diagnosis of caries lesion activity by monitoring lesion changes over time and thus helping to select the most appropriate treatment choice/regimen for a particular patient in a private practice setting.[66] Furthermore, systematic reviews suggest that these instruments have higher sensitivity but lower specificity than traditional visual caries detection methods at the earlier, noncavitated stages in the caries process.[65] This means that in populations for whom caries rates have fallen and caries progression rates have slowed, or in which caries rates are not high, the indiscriminate use of these technologies is likely to result in a high number of false-positive caries diagnoses, which could then, depending on how the instrument's "caries" call is interpreted by the clinician, decrease the number of teeth that could benefit from nonrestorative caries management interventions and/or increase the number of unnecessary restorations.[67] Thus although these technologies can be valuable aids to allow more objective caries detection, assessment, and monitoring

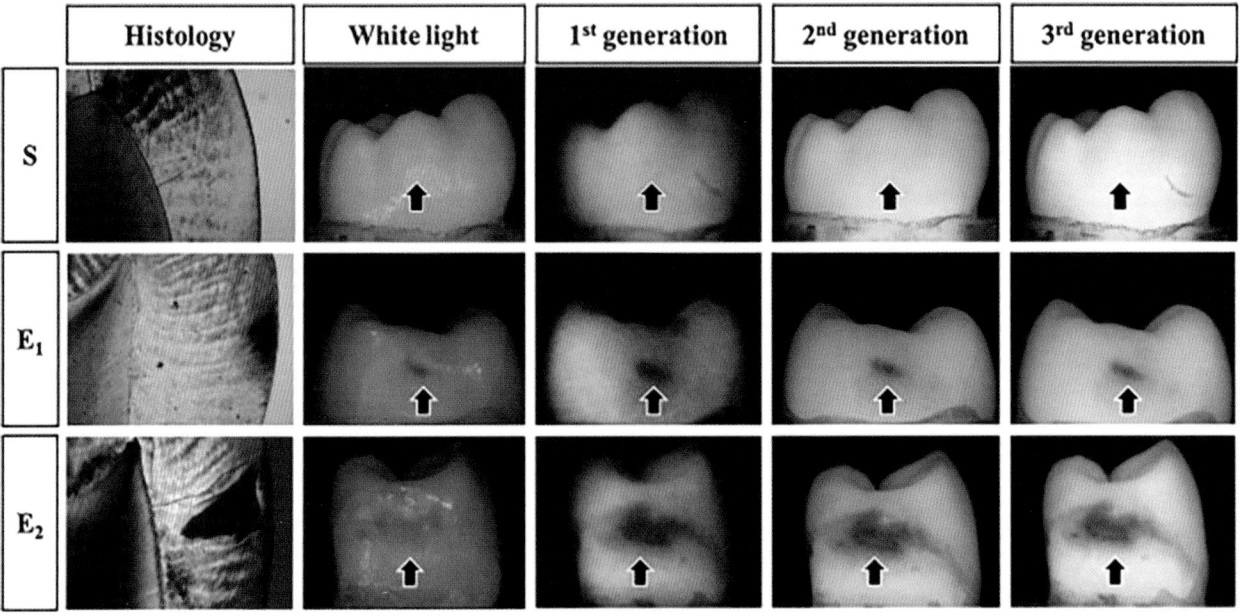

Fig. 4.10 Representative images of 3 teeth. The first row represents a tooth with a surface that is sound *(S)*, the second row represents a tooth with a surface that has demineralization limited to the outer half of the enamel *(E1)*, and the third row shows an image of a tooth with a surface that has demineralization involving the inner half of the enamel *(E2)*. The columns represent views of that surface using different technologies, from left to right: polarized light microscope histology image (PLM, magnified 100×), white light image, and fluorescence images obtained using three generations of quantitative light-induced fluorescence (QLF) devices. *Black arrows* indicate the area of interest (AOI) for QLF image analysis. (From Park SW, Kim SK, Lee HS, Lee ES, de Josselin de Jong E, Kim BI. Comparison of fluorescence parameters between three generations of QLF devices for detecting enamel caries in vitro and on smooth surfaces. Photodiagnosis Photodyn Ther. 2019;25:142-147.)

(especially if a quantitative scale is provided), they require expertise and training for their correct use and for interpretation of the data they produce.

Among available technologies, a recent systematic review concluded[68] that OCT, which is not yet available to the general practitioner, shows the greatest potential, with superior sensitivity (i.e., less false-negative results) compared with NIR and FOTI devices. However, as with all these technologies, its benefit is as an additional tool to support conventional clinical examination, to confirm borderline cases in cases of clinical uncertainty. Although FOTI and NIR are more readily available and easy to use, they show limitations in their ability to detect caries lesions into enamel (low sensitivity) but may be considered successful in the identification of sound teeth (high specificity). This is also the case for fluorescence-based devices, which show a considerable variation in performance.[69] The current evidence base to support the detection and diagnosis of caries with electrical conductance devices is still sparse.[70]

For root surfaces, a recent systematic review concluded that because of limited quantity and quality of existing evidence, it was unclear if there was any benefit of adjunctive technology-based instruments for the detection and diagnosis of root caries lesions. Thus visual-tactile examination remains the recommended method to use detection and diagnosis of root caries.[71]

As these methods are rapidly evolving, and new ones are constantly appearing on the market, the competent user of any technology-based caries detection method should always understand the strength of the supporting evidence and be able to interpret the data obtained, as well as to follow the manufacturer's indications, contraindications, and instructions regarding proper use of the instrument.[72]

Some IOS are equipped with technology to allow caries detection while performing routine intraoral scans. Carious lesions that are discovered using this equipment can be confirmed with radiographs. This can reduce the amount of radiation that patients are subjected to as well as reduce the cost to patient.

Intraoral Optical Scanners

Since its introduction in 1985, intraoral scanning has improved over the years in both speed and accuracy. IOSs either use still images or videos to collect the data and a special software digitizes the data to produce 3D representations of the scanned objects (Figure 4.11). Current IOSs have additional capabilities including taking intraoral photos, caries detection, and shade detection and matching. The accuracy of IOSs has been studied and has been shown to produce very accurate 3D scans that are clinically acceptable and comparable to conventional impressions.[73,74] However, conventional impressions are still recommended for full-arch or long span restorations where IOSs might not produce the same accuracy as conventional impressions.[75] IOSs can also be used to document the progression of certain oral conditions such as occlusal wear, gingival recession, and tooth shifting.

Some of the advantages of IOSs compared with conventional impressions include:

1. Using IOS is easier for most patients, particularly for those who have severe gag reflexes. Many patients cannot tolerate having dental impressions taken, especially when taking impressions of a full arch with a material that can take several minutes to set. Intraoral scanning is better tolerated because the scanner has minimal contact with the tissues during the scan and the scan can be stopped at any time and continued where the last segment of the arch was scanned in case the patient started gagging.

2. Intraoral scanning produces instant digital models without the need for any additional laboratory procedures. Conventional impressions need to be poured with dental stone that require time to set and the models need to be trimmed before they are ready to be used.

3. Obtaining intraoral scans can be faster than conventional impressions. When taking conventional impressions, selecting the proper impression tray, and applying adhesive can take a few minutes before the tray is ready for the impressions. Impression material setting time can vary from one material to another and it can be as long as 5 minutes for

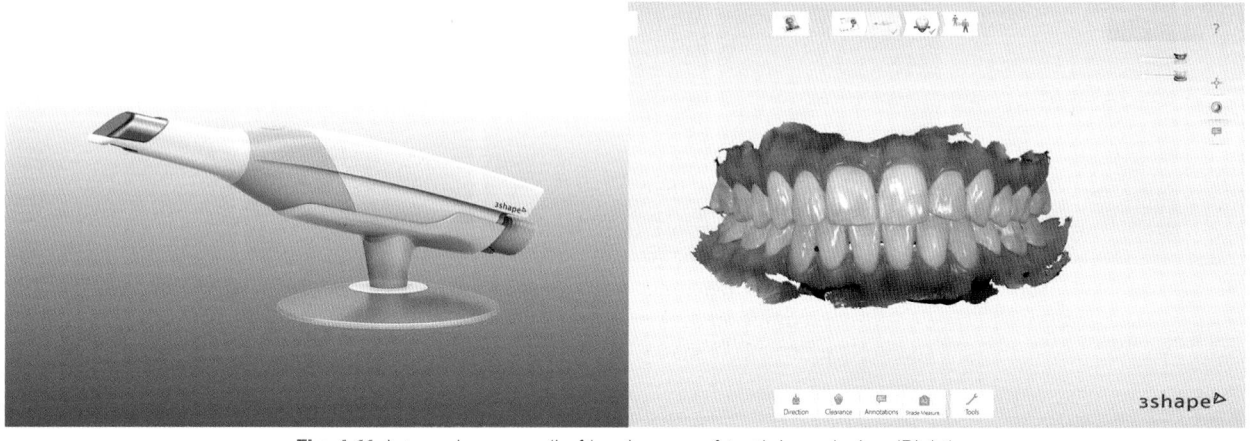

Fig. 4.11 Intraoral scanner *(Left)* and a scan of teeth in occlusion *(Right)*.

some materials. In the hands of an experienced operator, intraoral scanning of a full arch can be completed in about 3 minutes.[76]

4. It is easier to rescan areas missed in the original scan. When taking a conventional impression, it is important to capture all the required details. If an area is missed, a new impression is necessary as it is difficult to capture the missed area using the same impression. In intraoral scanning, if a small area of the scan is not captured properly, rescanning just that area is possible and does not require rescanning the entire arch.

5. Sending a digital scan to the commercial laboratory is instant as compared with conventional impressions that need to be poured into gypsum models and shipped to the commercial laboratory.

Desktop Laboratory Scanners

Desktop scanners are used by dental laboratories to scan conventional impressions or models. The accuracy of desktop scanners is shown to be superior to that of IOSs.[77] However, using a desktop scanner requires taking a conventional impression, which is an extra step in the digital workflow that can introduce inaccuracies. Desktop scanners are also used to scan old models so they can be stored digitally. This saves physical space and makes it easy to retrieve digital models as needed. These digital models can be 3D printed at any time if a physical model is needed.

In dental practices where an IOS is not available, scanning the impression or model using desktop scanners allows the clinician to have periodic digital models that can be used to monitor dental conditions over time. These conditions include, but are not limited to, tooth shifting, occlusal wear, and gingival recession. One of the disadvantages of using desktop scanners for this type of documentation as compared with most IOSs is the lack of oral tissue colors that can be scanned with an IOS. Desktop scanners cannot produce colored scans because they are used to scan impressions or dental models.

Shade Matching Equipment

Shade matching is extremely important when restoring teeth in areas that can be seen when smiling or talking, also referred to as the **esthetic zone**. Most dentists rely on conventional methods for shade matching with results that vary depending on room lighting. Several shade matching systems are available using different technologies. Some have been found to be more reliable than others and they can provide additional data to the commercial laboratory in terms of shade mapping to improve the esthetic outcomes of the restorations.

Physical shade tabs are commonly used to find the closest shade match and instruct the laboratory to fabricate the restoration in that specific shade. It is also common practice that digital photographs of the teeth with the shade tab(s) held next to the teeth are sent to the laboratory to help achieve a shade match when natural teeth shades are complex. Shade matching scanners are also used but can have varying accuracy and reliability in finding the correct tooth shade (Figure 4.12).[78] Shade scanners are used as an aid in the process of shade selection as conventional shade selection methods are still the standard procedure. Some shade matching scanners give one shade for

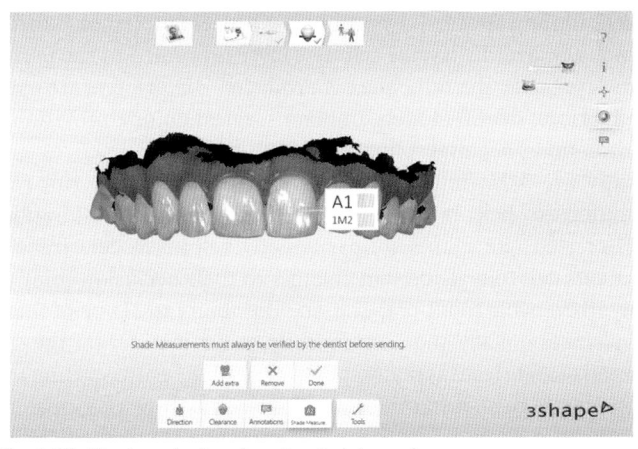
Fig. 4.12 Shade selection function in intraoral scanners.

the entire tooth, which is the average shade read by the scanner. Others can give a complete map of the tooth with the different shades from one area of the tooth to the other as well as information on the hue, chroma, value, translucency, and opacity of each area. This information is helpful to the laboratory especially when fabricating restorations to match natural teeth. Some IOSs have shade selection capabilities but are not shown to be highly accurate. However, it can be a starting point in the shade selection process.

Computer-Aided Design and Manufacturing

Computer-aided design (CAD) is the use of computer software to create and analyze a design of an object whereas **computer-aided manufacturing (CAM)** is the use of computer software to control machinery in the manufacturing of the designed object. Major developments to CAD/CAM in dentistry arose in the 1980s. These major developments are mostly attributed to three dentists: Drs. F. Duret, W.H. Mormann, and M. Andersson.[79]

CAD/CAM technology was initially developed to address a few challenges: to produce restorations with clinically acceptable strength especially in the posterior area; to produce restorations that have satisfactory esthetic characteristics; and to fabricate accurate restorations faster and easier.[80] Since then, CAD/CAM technology has been routinely applied to most aspects of dentistry including diagnosis, treatment planning, treatment, as well as maintenance and treatment follow-up.

Dental CAD/CAM systems include an acquisition device (scanner) that is either intraoral or extraoral, a data collection and storage software, design software, and manufacturing equipment. Many digital workflows have been utilized and investigated in order to develop workflows that can produce successful treatment outcomes while making the patient experience easier.

The process of CAM is either additive or subtractive. Additive manufacturing is a process of adding multiple layers to produce an object as in 3D printing. Subtractive manufacturing involves removing or machining material from a block of material to produce an object as in milling.

The use of 3D printers in dentistry has been increasing in the last few years because of the advancements in 3D printing accuracy and speed. 3D printing is a process of manufacturing an object layer by layer. Each new layer is bonded to the previous layer until the full object is produced. 3D printers are used to fabricate dental models, implant surgical guides, provisional restorations, occlusal splints, and dentures. Many practices currently use 3D printers to fabricate diagnostic or interim restorations to help in determining the proper final restoration. 3D-created bite splints are particularly helpful to determine if patients can tolerate certain changes to their occlusion prior to any irreversible tooth preparation. The ability to 3D print these appliances quickly and economically makes it easier for the clinicians to fabricate as many splints as needed before starting the actual treatment. Interim restorations such as crowns, fixed dental prostheses, and dentures are commonly 3D printed. These interim restorations can be used to help determine if they fulfill the esthetic, functional, and occlusal needs prior to fabricating the final restorations. The ease and speed of 3D printing can also help produce multiple sets of these interim restorations in case the patient fractures or loses their current restorations. As these interim restorations are used for a period and changes are made as needed to satisfy all the esthetic and functional requirements, they can be scanned and copied into the final restoration.

Software

Diagnostic Wax-Up and Restoration Design

Digital diagnostic wax-up has advanced with the advancement in digital scanning and manufacturing. With the use of digital wax-up, an accurate intraoral mock-up is produced to help the clinician design the final restoration as well as to get the patient's approval to proceed with treatment. The software allows the operator to design and complete the virtual wax-up on the digital scan. The software has a library of different teeth molds to select the mold that best fits the patient. The virtual teeth are overlayed over the digital scan and the resulting model can be 3D printed. A vinyl polysiloxane putty matrix or a clear stent is then made on the printed model. Resin material such as bis-acryl provisional resin material is injected into the putty matrix or clear stent and seated over the teeth to complete the intraoral mock-up. The result is an intraoral resin mock-up of the digital design that is helpful for the patient to see a simulation of the final intraoral restoration. The use of digital technology to complete diagnostic wax-ups has many advantages over the conventional wax-up using gypsum models and wax. It can be faster and result in a more predictable outcome especially when establishing symmetry between the right and left side. The software also keeps the original outline of the natural dentition and stretches it to satisfy the new tooth design. Waxing up using gypsum models and wax requires experience and hand skills in shaping the wax and creating the proper tooth outline and anatomy. This can be done by the software digitally and the operator only needs to position and size the teeth to create the proper tooth arrangement.

After the intraoral mock-up is approved by the patient, the same design can be used in the final restoration fabrication. Digital scans of the mock-up or the provisional restoration or the digital wax-up are used during the design of the final restoration to duplicate the design that the patient approved. This process allows clinicians to achieve predictable results that have been tried in the mouth and approved by the patient.

Implant Planning

Dental implants are an important part of prosthodontic rehabilitations. Prosthetically driven implant placement means that implant placement should be guided by the type, position, and angulation of the final restoration. Improper implant placement has adverse effects on the long-term success of the implant and the restoration.[81,82] The merging of data from CBCT, intraoral scans, and implant planning software can allow the clinician to complete a virtual wax-up of the final restoration and position the implant according to that restoration (Figure 4.13).

This process allows the clinician to visualize the bone in the proposed implant position and identify any need for bone grafting procedure to ensure a better chance of success. This plan will also help achieve an ideal implant position and angulation in respect to the adjacent teeth and vital structures (Figure 4.14). Multiple implant planning software systems are available. These systems can be used to visualize and study the bone quantity and quality, the adjacent teeth, as well as virtually place the implant. The clinician can use all that information for better positioning of the implant during freehand implant placement surgery. However, most clinicians take advantage of the capabilities of the software to fabricate a surgical guide that is used during implant surgery to position the implant as it was virtually planned (Figure 4.15). Some of these programs are open system whereas others are closed system programs. Open system programs generate an open STL (Standard Tessellation Language) format file of the surgical guide that can be sent to a 3D printer to fabricate the surgical guide. Closed system programs are less common and only allow clinicians to send the encrypted surgical guide file to the software manufacturer for fabrication of the surgical guide. Using the surgical guide during implant placement has been shown to result in more accurate implant placement than freehand placement.[83] Implant planning software can also serve as a communication tool between the restorative clinician and the surgeon placing the implants. Treatment planning sessions with both the surgeon and the restorative dentist are common practice to help plan the implant position and angulation to satisfy all surgical and restorative needs.

Smile Mock-Up

Many patients seek dental treatment to improve the appearance of their smile. Some of the common restorative dental procedures performed to improve esthetics are bonded composite restorations, ceramic veneers, and crowns. These procedures require tooth preparation that is irreversible. Many patients hesitate to start such comprehensive treatment without seeing what the result can look like. Some dentists show their patients photos of before and after treatment of previous patients to demonstrate the transformation achieved by the type of restoration recommended. However, many of these patients prefer to see a mock-up of the restoration on themselves prior to starting any irreversible tooth preparation.

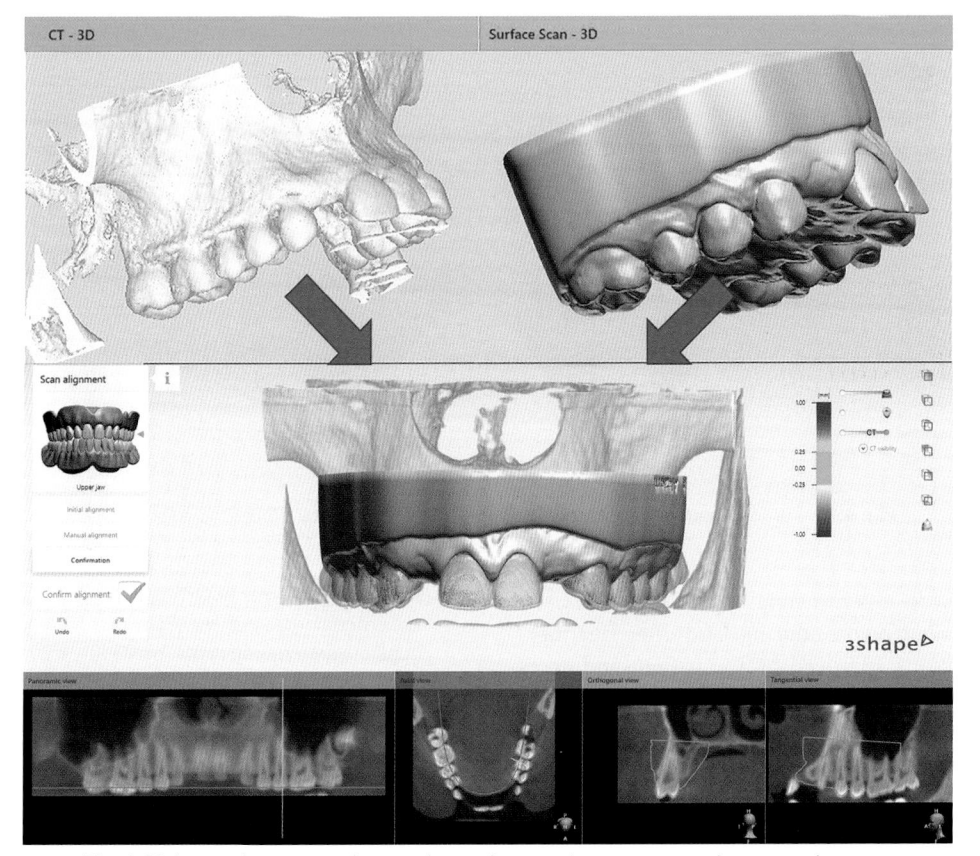

Fig. 4.13 Intraoral scan superimposed over the cone-beam computed tomography scan.

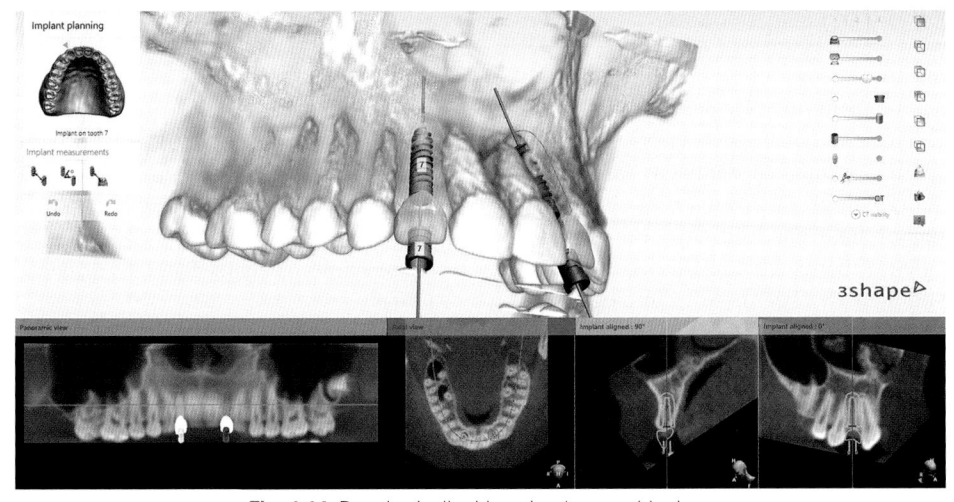

Fig. 4.14 Prosthetically driven implant positioning.

As discussed earlier, wax-ups and intraoral mock-ups using resin material are common practice to show patients a simulation of final restoration. However, many programs and applications have made this process easier and faster by overlaying the restoration digitally over patient's photos or 3D scans. This process allows the patient to give input on the shape, size, and shade of the teeth and changes can be instantly made to compare the results of before and after, before the patient makes any decision to start treatment. Some of these applications are available on smartphones or tablets, which makes it easier and more economic for the clinician and patient. They can provide still images as well as videos with the virtual restorations to give the patient a look at the smile from different angles. Other programs require digital intraoral scans as well as photos to provide the digital mock-ups.

There are many factors that influence which program is used such as ease of use, the ability to record and document the case, cost of the program, time needed to perform the smile simulation, digital workflow, and compatibility with other digital and CAD/CAM systems.[84,85] These virtual mock-ups are very useful to act as a communication tool between the clinician and the patient as well as the clinician and dental laboratory personnel.

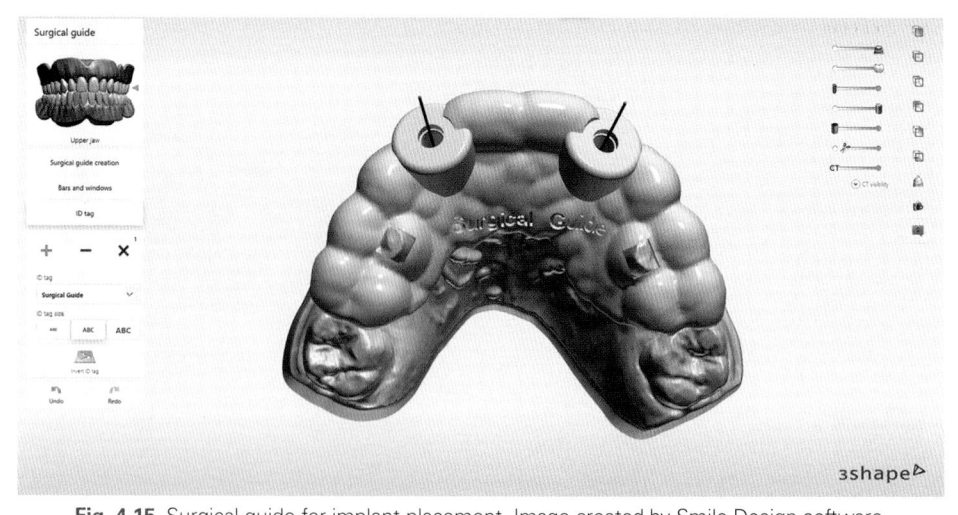

Fig. 4.15 Surgical guide for implant placement. Image created by Smile Design software.

Most dentists work with a commercial dental laboratory that does not see the patient before, during, and after treatment. Virtual smile simulations approved by the patient and accessible by the laboratory make it easier to design the final restoration based on the virtual design. Sometimes, a virtual smile design shows the limitation of what conventional restorations can achieve and can help plan additional prerestorative procedure such as orthodontics to achieve the results expected by the patient and clinician.

CONCLUSION

In this chapter we have touched on a number of technologies, some of them you may be using in your personal life such as text messages and social media, that are increasingly being used in patient care. Others are specific to dentistry, for example, CAD/CAM and digital radiology. One thing is clear, dentistry is becoming increasingly reliant on communication, imaging, treatment planning, digital manufacturing, and record keeping technologies.[86] Although each of these technologies individually will continue to improve, the greatest improvements to healthcare will occur as these technologies come together in integrated systems. No longer will you need to move files from your IOS to your health record; you will just select the scan and it will be in the record. No longer will you take an image from a telehealth session and move it to the record; it will automatically be stored. Technology will improve communication between health professionals and, in turn, make it easier for all healthcare providers to understand a patient's health and thus lead to improved dental and overall health.

REFERENCES

1. Centers for Disease Control and Prevention. Adult BMI calculator. https://www.cdc.gov/healthyweight/assessing/bmi/adult_bmi/english_bmi_calculator/bmi_calculator.html. Published November, 2021. Accessed January 11, 2022.
2. American College of Surgeons. Surgical risk calculator. https://riskcalculator.facs.org/RiskCalculator/PatientInfo.jsp. Accessed January 11, 2022
3. American Academy of Orthopaedic Surgeons. Appropriate use criteria: management of patients with orthopaedic implants undergoing dental procedures, 2016. https://www.orthoguidelines.org/go/auc/auc.cfm?auc_id=224995. Accessed January 11, 2022
4. Schwendicke F, Samek W, Krois J. Artificial intelligence in dentistry: chances and challenges. *J Dent Res.* 2020;99(7):769–774.
5. HeatlhIT.gov. Clinical decision support. https://www.healthit.gov/topic/safety/clinical-decision-support. Published April 2018. Accessed January 11, 2022
6. Meriam Library - CSU, Chico. Evaluating information – applying the CRAAP Test. https://library.csuchico.edu/sites/default/files/craap-test.pdf. Published 2010. Accessed November 29, 2021.
7. Bethel College Library. Evaluating internet-based information: library databases vs. search engines. https://bethelks.libguides.com/c.php?g=11565&p=61196. Published February 2021. Accessed January 13, 2022.
8. McEvoy M. Reasons Google search results vary dramatically (updated and expanded). Web Presence Solutions. https://www.webpresencesolutions.net/7-reasons-google-search-results-vary-dramatically/. Published June 29, 2020. Accessed January 13, 2022.
9. GeeksforGeeks. Difference between database and search engine. https://www.geeksforgeeks.org/difference-between-database-and-search-engine/. Updated July 6, 2022. Accessed January 13, 2022.
10. Illinois Library. Compare databases and search engines. https://www.library.illinois.edu/ugl/howdoi/compare1/. Accessed January 13, 2022.
11. Atherton J. Development of the electronic health record. *Virtual Mentor.* 2011;13(3):186–189.
12. Garrett P, Seidman J. EMR vs EHR – what is the difference? HeatlhITBuzz. https://www.healthit.gov/buzz-blog/electronic-health-and-medical-records/emr-vs-ehr-difference. Published January 2011. Accessed January 13, 2022.
13. U.S. Department of Health & Human Services. What personal health information do individuals have a right under HIPAA to access from their health care providers and health plans? Office for Civil Rights. https://www.hhs.gov/hipaa/for-professionals/faq/2042/what-personal-health-information-do-individuals/index.html. Published June 2016. Accessed January 13, 2022.
14. Chen YW, Stanley K, Att W. Artificial intelligence in dentistry: current applications and future perspectives. *Quintessence Int.* 2020;51(3):248–257.

15. Corbella S, Srinivas S, Cabitza F. Applications of deep learning in dentistry. *Oral Surg Oral Med Oral Pathol Oral Radiol.* 2021;132(2):225–238.

16. Cui Q, Chen Q, Liu P, Liu D, Wen Z. Clinical decision support model for tooth extraction therapy derived from electronic dental records. *J Prosthet Dent.* 2021;126(1):83–90.

17. Lensiora. The history of intraoral cameras. https://www.lensiora.com/the-history-of-intraoral-cameras/. Accessed January 13, 2022.

18. Murrell M, Marchini L, Blanchette D, Ashida S. Intraoral camera use in a dental school clinic: evaluations by faculty, students, and patients. *J Dent Educ.* 2019;83(11):1339–1344.

19. Hardan LS, Moussa C. Mobile dental photography: a simple technique for documentation and communication. *Quintessence Int.* 2020;51(6):510–518.

20. Dental Economics. Should I buy a digital or intraoral camera or both? https://www.dentaleconomics.com/practice/article/16391278/should-i-buy-a-digital-or-intraoral-camera-or-both. Published May 2006. Accessed November 30, 2021

21. Pentapati KC, Siddiq H. Clinical applications of intraoral camera to increase patient compliance - current perspectives. *Clin Cosmet Investig Dent.* 2019;11:267–278.

22. Signori C, Collares K, Cumerlato CBF, Correa MB, Opdam NJM, Cenci MS. Validation of assessment of intraoral digital photography for evaluation of dental restorations in clinical research. *J Dent.* 2018;71:54–60.

23. Futudent. https://www.futudent.com/. Accessed January 15, 2022.

24. Coachman C, Calamita MA, Sesma N. Dynamic documentation of the smile and the 2D/3D digital smile design process. *Int J Periodontics Restorative Dent.* 2017;37(2):183–193.

25. Yoon DC, Mol A, Benn DK, Benavides E. Digital radiographic image processing and analysis. *Dent Clin North Am.* 2018;62(3):341–359.

26. Schweitzer DM, Berg RW. A digital radiographic artifact: a clinical report. *J Prosthet Dent.* 2010;103(6):326–329.

27. Clark LJ, Wadhwani CP, Abramovitch K, Rice DD, Kattadiyil MT. Effect of image sharpening on radiographic image quality. *J Prosthet Dent.* 2018;120(6):927–933.

28. Krois J, Cantu AG, Chaurasia A, et al. Generalizability of deep learning models for dental image analysis. *Sci Rep.* 2021;11(1):6102.

29. Schwendicke F, Rossi JG, Göstemeyer G, et al. Cost-effectiveness of artificial intelligence for proximal caries detection. *J Dent Res.* 2021;100(4):369–376.

30. Kim H, Shim E, Park J, Kim Y-J, Lee U, Kim Y. Web-based fully automated cephalometric analysis by deep learning. *Computer Methods Programs Biomed.* 2020;194:105513.

31. Kats L, Vered M, Zlotogorski-Hurvitz A, Harpaz I. Atherosclerotic carotid plaque on panoramic radiographs: neural network detection. *Int J Comput Dent.* 2019;22(2):163–169.

32. Hung K, Yeung AWK, Tanaka R, Bornstein MM. Current applications, opportunities, and limitations of AI for 3D imaging in dental research and practice. *Int J Environ Res Public Health.* 2020;17(12):4424.

33. Maia PRL, Tomaz AFG, Maia EFT, Lima KC, de Oliveira PT. Prevalence of soft tissue calcifications in panoramic radiographs of the maxillofacial region of older adults [published online ahead of print June 24, 2021]. *Gerontology.* https://doi.org/10.1111/ger.12578.

34. Moreira-Souza L, Michels M, de Melo LPL, Oliveira ML, Asprino L, Freitas DQ. Brightness and contrast adjustments influence the radiographic detection of soft tissue calcification. *Oral Dis.* 2019;25(7):1809–1814.

35. Ludlow JB, Timothy R, Walker C, et al. Effective dose of dental CBCT-a meta-analysis of published data and additional data for nine CBCT units. *Dentomaxillofac Radiol.* 2015;44(1):20140197.

36. Bulbul MG, Tarabichi O, Parikh AS, et al. The utility of intra-oral ultrasound in improving deep margin clearance of oral tongue cancer resections. *Oral Oncol.* 2021;122:105512.

37. Kripfgans OD, Chan HL. Volumetric ultrasound and related dental applications. In: Chan HL, Kripfgans OD, eds. *Dental Ultrasound in Periodontology and Implantology.* Cham: Springer; 2021. https://doi.org/10.1007/978-3-030-51288-0_12.

38. Noorlag R, Nulent TJWK, Delwel VEJ, et al. Assessment of tumour depth in early tongue cancer: accuracy of MRI and intraoral ultrasound. *Oral Oncol.* 2020;110:104895.

39. Kocasarac HD, Geha H, Gaalaas LR, Nixdorf DR. MRI for dental applications. *Dent Clin North Am.* 2018;62(3):467–480.

40. Poblete P, Nieto E. Does time matter? WhatsApp vs electronic mail for dental education. A pilot study. *Eur J Dent Educ.* 2020;24(1):121–125.

41. Telephone Consumer Protection Act 47 U.S.C. § 227. https://www.fcc.gov/sites/default/files/tcpa-rules.pdf. Accessed January 15, 2022

42. Estenban Ortiz-Ospina. The rise of social media. Our World in Data. https://ourworldindata.org/rise-of-social-media. Published September 18, 2019. Accessed November 3, 2021.

43. Examples. http://www.ratemydentist.org/; https://www.healthgrades.com/dentistry-general-directory; http://www.healthcarereviews.com/Ratings/DentistRatings.php; http://www.rankmydentist.com/

44. HealthIT.Gov. What is a patient portal? https://www.healthit.gov/faq/what-patient-portal. Accessed November 3, 2021.

45. EPIC Health. EPIC Health patient portal. https://www.epichs.org/patient-resources/patient-portal/. Accessed November 22, 2021.

46. Bambauer DE. Privacy versus security. *J Crim L Criminology.* 2013;103(3):667–684.

47. HIV.Gov. The difference between security and privacy and why it matters to your program. https://www.hiv.gov/blog/difference-between-security-and-privacy-and-why-it-matters-your-program. Published April 26, 2018. Accessed November 2, 2021.

48. HHS.Gov. Privacy, security, and electronic health records. https://www.hhs.gov/sites/default/files/ocr/privacy/hipaa/understanding/consumers/privacy-security-electronic-records.pdf. Accessed November 2, 2021.

49. Strehle EM, Shabde N. One hundred years of telemedicine: does this new technology have a place in paediatrics. *Arch Dis Child.* 2006;91(12):956–959.

50. Hoogenbosch B, Postma J, de Man-van Ginkel J, Tiemessen N, van Delden J, van Os-Medendorp H. Use and the users of a patient portal: cross-sectional study. *J Med Internet Res.* 2018;20(9):e262.

51. Robeznieks A. Which medical specialties use telemedicine the most? https://www.ama-assn.org/practice-management/digital/which-medical-specialties-use-telemedicine-most. Published January 11, 2019. Accessed November 01, 2021.

52. Rocca MA, Kudryk VL, Pajak JC, Morris T. The evolution of a teledentistry system within the Department of Defense. *Proc AMIA Symp.* 1999;1:921–924.

53. Glassman P, Tellier R. The virtual dental home. VirtualDentalHome_PolicyBrief_Aug_2014_HD_ForPrintOnly.pdf. Accessed November 10, 2021.

54. Keshvardoost S, Bahaadinbeigy K, Fatehi F. Role of telehealth in the management of COVID-19: lessons learned from previous SARS, MERS, and Ebola outbreaks. *Telemed JE Health.* 2020;26(7):850–852.

55. Jusdon TJ, Odisho AY, Neinstein AB, et al. Rapid design and implementation of an integrated patient self-triage and self-scheduling tool for COVID-19. *J Am Med Inform Assoc.* 2020;27(6):860–866.

56. OperaDDS. https://operadds.com/covid-19-screening-form-for-dentists/. Accessed January 15, 2022.

57. GeoPain. https://geopain.com. Accessed January 15, 2022.

58. Noguchi Y. Patients say telehealth is OK, but most prefer to see their doctor in person. NPR.org. https://www.npr.org/sections/health-shots/2021/10/18/1044358309/patients-say-telehealth-ok-but-doctor-visits-in-person-better Published October 18, 2021. Accessed October 22, 2021.

59. American Cancer Society. Key statistics for oral cavity and oropharyngeal cancers. https://www.cancer.org/cancer/oral-cavity-and-oropharyngeal-cancer/about/key-statistics.html. Published January 2022. Accessed January 15, 2022.

60. American Cancer Society. What are oral cavity and oropharyngeal cancers?. https://www.cancer.org/cancer/oral-cavity-and-oropharyngeal-cancer/about/what-is-oral-cavity-cancer.html. Published March 2021. Accessed January 15, 2022.

61. VELscope. https://velscope.com

62. Lingen MW, Tampi MP, Urquhart O, et al. Adjuncts for the evaluation of potentially malignant disorders in the oral cavity: diagnostic test accuracy systematic review and meta-analysis-a report of the American Dental Association. *J Am Dent Assoc.* 2017;148(11):797–813. e752.

63. McNamara KK, Martin BD, Evans EW, Kalmar JR. The role of direct visual fluorescent examination (VELscope) in routine screening for potentially malignant oral mucosal lesions. *Oral Surg Oral Med Oral Pathol Oral Radiol.* 2012;114(5):636–643.

64. Stookey GK, Gonzalez Cabezas C. Emerging methods of caries diagnosis. *J Dent Educ.* 2001;65:1001–1006.

65. Bader JD, Shugars DA. A systematic review of the performance of a laser fluorescence device for detecting caries. *J Am Dent Assoc.* 2004;135:1413–1426.

66. Fontana M, Gonzalez-Cabezas C. Changing paradigm. A different view of caries lesions. *Compendium.* 2011;32(Spec No 4):24–27.

67. Fontana M, Zero D, Beltrán-Aguilar E, Grey SK. Techniques for tooth surface assessments in school-based sealant programs. *J Am Dent Assoc.* 2010;141(7):854–860.

68. Macey R, Walsh T, Riley P, et al. Transillumination and optical coherence tomography for the detection and diagnosis of enamel caries. *Cochrane Database Syst Rev.* 2021;1(1). CD013855.

69. Macey R, Walsh T, Riley P, et al. Fluorescence devices for the detection of dental caries. *Cochrane Database Syst Rev.* 2020;12(12). CD013811.

70. Macey R, Walsh T, Riley P, et al. Electrical conductance for the detection of dental caries. *Cochrane Database Syst Rev.* 2021;3(3). CD014547.

71. Fee PA, Macey R, Walsh T, Clarkson JE, Ricketts D. Tests to detect and inform the diagnosis of root caries. *Cochrane Database Syst Rev.* 2020;12(12). CD013806.

72. Fontana M, Gonzalez-Cabezas C, Fitzgerald M. Cardiology for the 21st century-current caries management concepts for dental practice. *J Mich Dent Assoc.* 2013;95(4):32–40.

73. Mehl A, Ender A, Mörmann W, Attin T. Accuracy testing of a new intraoral 3D camera. *Int J Comput Dent.* 2009;12(1):11–28.

74. Chochlidakis KM, Papaspyridakos P, Geminiani A, Chen CJ, Feng IJ. Digital versus conventional impressions for fixed prosthodontics: a systematic review and meta-analysis. *J Prosthet Dent.* 2016;116:184–190.

75. Zhang YJ, Shi JY, Qian SJ, Qiao SC, Lai HC. Accuracy of full-arch digital implant impressions taken using intraoral scanners and related variables: a systematic review. *Int J Oral Implantol (Berl).* 2021;14(2):157–179.

76. Resende CCD, Barbosa TAQ, Moura GF, et al. Influence of operator experience, scanner type, and scan size on 3D scans. *J Prosthet Dent.* 2021;125(2):294–299.

77. Kang B-h, Son K, Lee K-b. Accuracy of five intraoral scanners and two laboratory scanners for a complete arch: a comparative in vitro study. *Appl Sci.* 2020;10(1):74.

78. Kim-Pusateri S, Brewer JD, Davis EL, Wee AG. Reliability and accuracy of four dental shade-matching devices. *J Prosthet Dent.* 2009;101(3):193–199.

79. Miyazaki T. A review of dental CAD/CAM: current status and future perspectives from 20 years of experience. *Dent Mater J.* 2009;28(1):44–56.

80. Davidowitz G, Kotick PG. The use of CAD/CAM in dentistry. *Dent Clin North Am.* 2011;55(3):559–570. ix.

81. Goodacre CJ, Bernal G, Rungcharassaeng K, Kan JY. Clinical complications with implants and implant prostheses. *J Prosthet Dent.* 2003;90:121–132.

82. Yilmaz B, Ozcelik BT, Sarantopoulos DM, McGlumphy E. Importance of CT scans in diagnosing symptoms from misplaced implants. *Implant Dent.* 2012;21:108–111.

83. Tan PLB, Layton DM, Wise SL. In vitro comparison of guided versus freehand implant placement: use of a new combined TRIOS surface scanning, Implant Studio, CBCT, and stereolithographic virtually planned and guided technique. *Int J Comput Dent.* 2018;21(2):87–95.

84. Omar D, Duarte C. The application of parameters for comprehensive smile aesthetics by digital smile design programs: a review of literature. *Saudi Dent J.* 2018;30(1):7–11.

85. Jafri Z, Ahmad N, Sawai M, Sultan N, Bhardwaj A. Digital smile design-an innovative tool in aesthetic dentistry. *J Oral Biol Craniofac Res.* 2020;10(2):194–198.

86. National Institutes of Health, National Institute for Dental and Craniofacial Research. Oral health in America: advances and challenges. https://www.nidcr.nih.gov/oralhealthinamerica. Published December 2021. Accessed January 15, 2022.

5

Developing the Treatment Plan

Stephen J. Stefanac

 Visit eBooks.Health.Elsevier.com

OUTLINE

Having established the patient's comprehensive diagnosis list, the dentist is prepared to begin developing a treatment plan. This process can be rather simple for patients with few problems and relatively good oral health. Treatment can commence quickly, especially when the patient is knowledgeable about dentistry, harbors little anxiety toward dental treatment, and has the necessary financial resources available. More commonly, though, the patient has many diagnoses and problems, often interrelated and complex, which will require analysis before treatment can begin. The dentist may wonder whether an individual problem can or should be addressed, and what treatment options are available. Would a crown, for instance, be better than a large direct restoration to restore a carious lesion? Would an implant be a more satisfactory option than a fixed partial denture to replace a missing tooth? Which treatment should be provided first, and which procedures can be postponed until later? What role should the patient have in any of these decisions? Are they even fully aware of the specific dental problems? Finally, how successful, overall, will the planned treatment be?

Although all dentists struggle with these questions, experienced practitioners know when to address each issue individually and when to step back and look at all elements of the case as a whole. The experienced dentist is also aware that treatment

planning cannot occur in a vacuum and must involve the patient. This means educating patients about their problems and making them partners in determining both the general direction and the specific elements of a proposed treatment plan.

The purpose of this chapter is to provide the reader with the fundamental skills necessary to begin creating treatment plans for patients. This includes developing treatment objectives, separating treatment into phases, presenting the treatment plan to the patient, sequencing procedures, consulting with other practitioners, obtaining informed consent, and documenting the treatment plan. Much of the material is presented as guidelines, which must be modified by the circumstances of each patient. Few, if any, rules are ironclad when treatment planning, and like many other aspects of dentistry, clinical decisions will improve with experience.

DEVELOPING TREATMENT OBJECTIVES

As discussed in Chapters 1 and 2, the practitioner examines the patient, determines which patient findings are significant, and then creates a comprehensive diagnosis list that will formally document why treatment is necessary. After assessing the patient's risk for ongoing and future disease (discussed in

Chapter 3), the next step in preparing to devise a treatment plan is to articulate, with the patient's assistance, several **treatment objectives** (Figure 5.1). These objectives represent the intent, or rationale, for the final treatment plan. Treatment objectives are usually expressed as short statements and can incorporate several activities aimed at solving the patient's problems. Effectively expressed treatment objectives articulate clear goals from both the dentist's and the patient's perspectives. Objectives will evolve from an understanding of the current diagnoses and problems integrated with the knowledge of what dental procedures are possible. Treatment objectives link to and strongly influence actual treatment (Table 5.1).

Patient Goals and Desires

Before creating any treatment plan, the dentist must first determine the patient's own treatment desires and motivation to receive care. Patients usually have several expectations, or **goals**, that can be both immediate and long term in nature. The

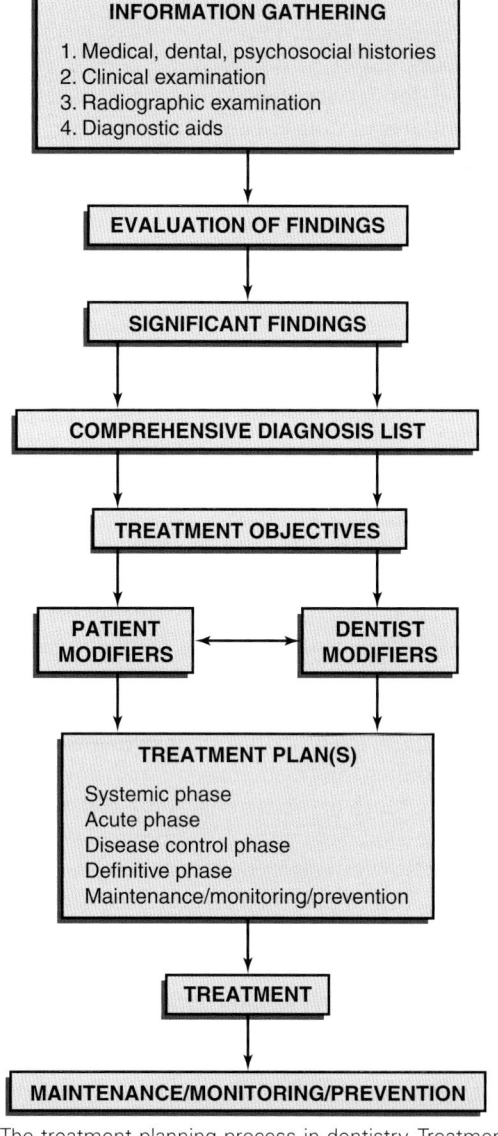

Fig. 5.1 The treatment planning process in dentistry. Treatment objectives contain clear goals that link a patient's diagnoses to the most appropriate plan for treatment.

most common short-term goal will be resolution of the chief complaint or concern—for instance, relieving pain or repairing broken teeth. Long-term goals are usually more global and can be more difficult to identify and articulate, especially if the dentist only focuses on their own preconceived ideas of what the patient desires. For example, an understandable long-term goal would be maintaining oral health and keeping the teeth for a lifetime. Most dentists would extol this expectation, as would many patients, especially those who come to the dentist with good oral health. But for patients with a history of sporadic dental care, poor systemic health, or extensive (and potentially *expensive*) dental needs, individual goals may be quite different. The patient with less than a year to live may only wish to stay free of pain or to replace missing teeth to enable eating more comfortably. On the other hand, a physically healthy patient with recurrent caries around many large restorations may be frustrated with past dental treatment and want any remaining teeth extracted and full dentures constructed. Some patients may have goals that are completely unrealistic. For example, the patient may want to preserve nonrestorable or periodontally hopeless teeth.

Determination of the patient's goals begins during the initial interview and may continue throughout the examination process. Careful probing of the patient's dental history may provide an indication of both past and future treatment goals. The prudent practitioner will avoid asking leading questions about treatment expectations. Such questions may instead convey the dentist's own personal goals, opinions, and biases and inhibit the patient from expressing their own goals and views. Some examples of such biased questions are

"Do you want to keep your teeth for a lifetime?"
"Isn't it worth the time and money to chew better?"
"Wouldn't you like whiter teeth and a prettier smile?"

It will be more effective to use open questions that may elicit the patient's thoughts and feelings and encourage the sharing of genuine concerns, especially regarding the chief complaint:
"Can you describe any problems you're having in your mouth?"
"How well are you able to eat with the teeth you have?"
"How do you feel about the appearance of your teeth?"

The dentist can participate in shaping the patient's treatment goals. This may need to occur when the patient has expectations that are difficult or even impossible to achieve, considering the condition of the mouth. For instance, the patient may wish to retain their natural teeth but be unaware of severe periodontal attachment loss. Ultimately, the dentist needs to educate the patient about the dental problems and, at the same time, begin to suggest possible treatment outcomes.

Patient Modifiers

Treatment goals are frequently influenced by patient attributes, often referred to as **patient modifiers**. Positive modifiers include an interest in oral health, the ability to afford treatment, and a history of regular dental care. Commonly encountered negative modifiers include time or financial constraints, a fear of dental treatment, lack of motivation, poor oral or general health, and destructive oral habits. Many patients are understandably concerned about the potential cost of care, especially when they

TABLE 5.1 The Relationship Between Diagnoses, Problems, Treatment Objectives, and Treatment

Signs and symptoms: Ms. Smith, a 45-year-old patient, requests an examination. She has been diagnosed with Sjögren's syndrome. Her last visit to a dentist was 2 years ago for teeth cleaning. She reports symptoms of sore hands and wrist joints and a dry mouth. Her gingiva is red, and extensive plaque covers the necks of the teeth. Several teeth have small, dark areas on the facial enamel near the gingival margin, which are soft when evaluated with an explorer. The patient works in a convenience store and consumes an average of 1 L of naturally sweetened carbonated beverage per day. Her chief concern is a painful maxillary right molar.

Diagnosis	Problems	At Risk for	Treatment Objectives	Treatment
Sjögren's syndrome	Reduced salivary flow, symptoms of xerostomia (dry mouth)	Caries, poor prosthesis retention, discomfort	Investigate ways to increase salivary flow and/or reduce symptoms	Consider prescribing medications to promote saliva production; saliva substitute products
Rheumatoid arthritis affecting the hands	Unable to use a manual toothbrush	Poor oral hygiene, gingival and periodontal disease	Look for aids to improve oral hygiene	Suggest an electric toothbrush
Gingivitis	Poor plaque control and oral hygiene	Periodontal disease	Restore gingival health	Prophylaxis and oral hygiene instruction
Caries on seven teeth	Increased caries susceptibility resulting from a high-sucrose diet	Pain, tooth loss	Reduce refined carbohydrates in the patient's diet	Diet analysis and counseling; begin a caries control program; topical fluoride
Acute apical abscess	Constant pain in upper right first molar	Infection, swelling	Relieve pain	Emergency endodontic therapy or tooth extraction

recognize that they have many dental problems. Whether the fees for services will function as a barrier to treatment depends on several variables, including the patient's financial resources, the level of immediate care necessary, the types of procedures proposed (i.e., large intracoronal restorations versus crowns or fixed versus removable partial dentures), the feasibility of postponing care, and the availability of third-party assistance with the cost. For more information about caring for patients with limited financial means see Chapter 19.

Poor motivation, poor oral hygiene, or a diet high in refined carbohydrates can significantly affect the prognosis for any treatment plan. Nevertheless, occasionally, such patients may still want treatment involving complex restorations, implants, and fixed or removable partial dentures. Before treatment is provided, the dentist must inform the patient of the high risk for failure and record this discussion in the patient record.

Dentist Goals and Desires

The dentist's goals also influence treatment plan development. Several goals are obvious, such as removing or arresting dental disease and eliminating pain. Others may be less apparent, especially to the patient, but are just as important nonetheless. Examples include determining the correct treatment for each problem, ensuring that the most severe problems are treated first, selecting the best material for a particular restoration, and making efficient use of the patient's and the provider's time.

In gathering these altruistic goals, the dentist will likely wish to create an **ideal treatment plan**. Simply put, such a plan would provide the best, or most preferred, type of treatment for each of the patient's problems. Thus if a tooth has a large composite restoration that requires replacement, placing a crown might be considered the ideal treatment. If the patient has missing teeth, then the dentist might recommend replacing them.

The goal of ideal treatment planning provides a useful starting point for planning care. Unfortunately, such a plan may not take into account important patient modifiers or may fail to meet the patient's *own* treatment objectives. In addition, one dentist's ideal treatment plan may differ significantly from another's, depending on personal preference, experience, and knowledge (*In Clinical Practice: Evaluating Treatment Plans From Other Dentists* box).

Creating a **modified treatment plan** balances the patient's treatment objectives with those of the dentist's. For example, a patient with financial limitations may not be able to afford replacement of missing posterior teeth. The dentist needs to explain (and document) the possible outcomes of failing to implement ideal treatment (i.e., in some instances, tipping and extrusion of the remaining teeth). Or the dentist may need to justify to the patient removal of several periodontally involved teeth, even though the teeth are not excessively mobile or symptomatic at the present time. In this situation, an appropriate treatment objective might be for the dentist to suggest observing or splinting the teeth for the present, with the plan to extract them if mobility increases or the patient reports other symptoms.

At times, incorporating the patient's wishes into a treatment plan can be difficult to implement. A classic example is the patient with rampant dental caries involving both anterior and posterior teeth. For esthetic reasons, the patient may be interested in restoring the anterior teeth first, but the dentist, after interpreting the radiographs, may detect more serious problems with the posterior teeth, such as caries nearing the pulp, and wish to treat these teeth first. Another example is the patient with poor oral hygiene and severe periodontal disease who wishes to have extensive fixed prosthodontics treatment begun immediately.

IN CLINICAL PRACTICE

Evaluating Treatment Plans from Other Dentists

Occasionally, a dentist may be asked to evaluate a treatment plan created by another dentist. This can result from litigation or peer review, but more commonly, such an evaluation is initiated by a patient who wishes a second opinion. The patient may have reservations about some or all of a proposed treatment plan or simply want a second opinion to confirm the adequacy of what the first dentist has recommended. In some instances, the fees for service quoted by the first dentist are the primary reason the patient seeks the advice of a second dentist. No matter the reason, the second dentist must consider several factors before rendering an opinion.

Diagnostic information and documentation: Sometimes, such a patient will present without a written treatment plan and be able only to generally recall what the other provider has proposed. "The dentist told me I need three crowns and six fillings. I am not sure I want all that treatment." Without documentation, it is difficult to corroborate or refute this information, and it is possible that the patient may be incorrectly stating the first dentist's recommendations. Without diagnostic materials, such as radiographs and models, rendering a second opinion is further complicated, particularly for a comprehensive treatment plan involving multiple procedures. Some patients may consent to additional radiographs by the second dentist or may request that copies of radiographs be sent from the original dentist.

Patient examination: The second dentist will need to examine the patient to validate findings, diagnoses, and treatment recommendations from the first dentist. This may be a problem-focused examination, in which a single tooth or area has been treatment planned. If the original treatment plan contains more procedures, however, the dentist will need to perform a comprehensive examination. The clinician should avoid rendering opinions based on hasty analysis. The patient must be informed in advance of the time required and fee for examination before a second opinion can be offered.

Reasons for differences in treatment plans: There are several reasons that treatment plans will differ from one dentist to another. Errors when making a diagnosis or in assessing the severity of a diagnosis can lead to inappropriate treatment selection. The first dentist may have relied on empirical versus evidence-based decision making or have failed to offer the patient a range of treatment options. The first dentist may not have adequately evaluated the effect of the patient's treatment objectives and modifiers when developing the treatment plan. The patient who is particularly concerned about cost and desires a conservative, incremental treatment approach may conclude that an all-encompassing treatment plan with many definitive phase procedures represents overtreatment. Finally, the patient may not fully understand or be willing to accept the extent of their dental problems and the rationale for the treatment procedures that have been recommended. The second dentist must clearly and objectively communicate to the patient any differences of opinion with the first practitioner and allow the patient to decide how to proceed.

All dentists should be mindful that other professionals may review the treatment plans they develop for their patients. When this occurs, the reviewed dentist should avoid feeling defensive and should facilitate sharing diagnostic information. Often, the patient who receives a second opinion returns and is more confident in pursuing treatment.

Dentist Modifiers

Every dentist brings factors to the treatment planning task that can influence the goals for patient care and ultimately the sort of treatment plans that they develop. The astute dentist is aware of these modifiers, especially when they limit their ability to devise the most appropriate treatment plan to satisfy the patient's dental needs and personal desires.

Knowledge

The dentist's level of knowledge and experience can influence the selection of goals and objectives for patient care. At one extreme is the beginning dental student, with a limited knowledge base and little experience in treating patients. Such early practitioners may not recognize the patient's treatment desires and modifying factors. As a result, they may create only "ideal" treatment plans, overlooking more appropriate solutions. At the other extreme is the complacent dentist who has been in practice for many years and has substantial clinical experience, but a knowledge base that has changed little since graduation. Such dentists may lack information about new treatment modalities that could be offered to patients, preferring instead to limit what they do. For these clinicians, the adage, "If all you have is a hammer, then everything is a nail," unfortunately may be true. The conscientious practitioner will be a lifelong student who is never complacent and learns not only from their own experiences but from those of others as well. This dentist keeps up with current developments in the profession by attending continuing education courses, interacting with peers, and critically reading the professional literature, searching for evidence-based care.

Technical Skills

In addition to a sound knowledge base, the dentist must also have the technical ability to provide treatment. Many dentists choose not to provide certain procedures, such as implant placement, extraction of impacted third molars, or endodontic treatment for multirooted teeth. This is not necessarily a limiting factor per se when treatment planning, but it can be if the dentist does not refer the patient to another dentist who has the expertise to provide the treatment.

Treatment Planning Philosophy

Finally, each dentist develops an individual treatment planning philosophy that will continue to evolve over years of treating patients. Philosophies relating to treatment planning may vary considerably among individual dentists as a result of differences in their knowledge bases, technical skills, clinical experience, and judgment (*In Clinical Practice: Treatment Planning a Patient Versus Just a Tooth*). Treatment planning in a dental school environment can be different from treatment planning in a private practice. Students are often frustrated when instructors differ among themselves in treatment philosophies because of differing educational backgrounds. Dental schools and dental practices may also control or recommend which treatment options practitioners can provide to patients. The recent graduate, starting out in practice, is often motivated to incorporate new techniques and materials different from those used in dental school. Dentists who have been in practice several years strive to keep up with new developments in the profession, which, in theory, can influence the ways in which they develop treatment plans for patients. Patients often benefit from the practitioner's use of new materials and techniques. Patient care suffers however, when experienced or inexperienced practitioners adopt treatment philosophies for which there is little supporting evidence. For example, the unwarranted removal of sound amalgam restorations and their replacement with composite resin under the premise that amalgam affects the patient's systemic health, is such a procedure. Such treatment can be unethical and may represent a disservice to the patient by exposing teeth to the risk of pulpal damage, fracture, or unnecessary removal of additional tooth structure.

IN CLINICAL PRACTICE

Treatment Planning a Patient Versus Just a Tooth

Traditionally, US dental students have been taught that other than emergency/urgent dental treatment, every patient must have a comprehensive treatment plan. This plan is developed following a stepwise process: first, a thorough evaluation and examination of the patient is conducted; next, diagnoses are made and/or a problem list is developed; and finally, a series of treatments is constructed and presented by the dentist and agreed to by the patient.[1] This model is the basis for the treatment planning process described throughout this text.

In practice, however, many dentists do not follow the stepwise model when treatment planning for their patients. Often, each individual tooth condition or other oral problem is evaluated, and the dentist makes an immediate recommendation to the patient about what should be done to resolve the problem.[2] This may be an expedient way for the practitioner to gain some level of consent from the patient to begin treatment. However, a clearly articulated diagnosis and prognosis list is often *not* made, and even in those cases in which the dentist makes a mental judgment about the rationale for treatment, the diagnosis may not be explicitly *stated* to the patient. Thus the patient may remain relatively uninformed about the nature of the problem and the rationale for a particular treatment.

The patient who remains relatively uninformed about diagnoses and treatment options, however, is ill prepared to provide meaningful informed consent for treatment. This can be both unwise and hazardous from a risk management perspective (see Chapter 7). The need to achieve fully informed consent is a central theme of this text.

Another concern associated with focusing on individual tooth problems and failing to follow a stepwise comprehensive approach to treatment planning is that the dentist does not have the opportunity to factor in where that problem fits in the overall context of the patient's oral condition. For instance, a severely decayed tooth may require endodontic therapy, a post and core and an extracoronal restoration. Although the expense for treating this one tooth may be reasonable to a patient, when confronted with other problems they have, the overall cost for treatment may be prohibitive. The patient might decide to have the tooth extracted so they can preserve financial resources to treat other problems. It is better to develop a comprehensive treatment plan with an emphasis on disease control and inform the patient about all problems, treatment options, and prognosis for treatment.

ESTABLISHING THE NATURE AND SCOPE OF THE TREATMENT PLAN

With the examination finished and the dentist confident that they have gained an awareness of the patient's treatment desires, it is time to develop the treatment plan. The dentist has the responsibility to determine what treatment is possible, realistic, and practical for the patient. In many instances, this is a relatively straightforward process, especially for those patients with few problems and the resources for and interest in preserving oral health. At the other end of the spectrum, the process is more complex. Patients with many interrelated oral problems and a high degree of unpredictability regarding the final treatment outcome present planning challenges. For such cases, the dentist has at their disposal several useful techniques for developing a treatment plan: these include visioning, identification of key teeth, and phasing procedures.

Visioning

Dentists naturally contemplate treatment options while examining patients. The experienced practitioner will also develop a **vision** of what the patient's final condition will be when the course of treatment is completed. The concept of having a vision of the final result could be described as analogous to deciding on the destination before starting a journey. Imagining one or more end points for the completed case is beneficial when evaluating different treatment approaches. For the patient with many severely decayed teeth in both arches, the dentist might see the individual ultimately wearing complete dentures or, alternatively, might consider retaining some teeth and placing a removable partial denture, or even restoring more teeth and using implants to support fixed or removable prostheses (Figure 5.2).

Further exploration of each option requires the dentist to identify the steps that will be necessary to reach the treatment goals. Experienced dentists commonly use this technique of "deconstructive" thinking to explore each option. In the first example, the dentures can only be fabricated after the remaining teeth have been extracted. Will all the teeth be extracted at the same time? The patient will need time to heal and might

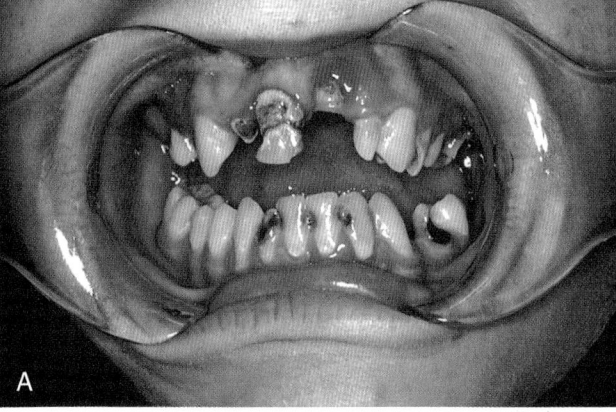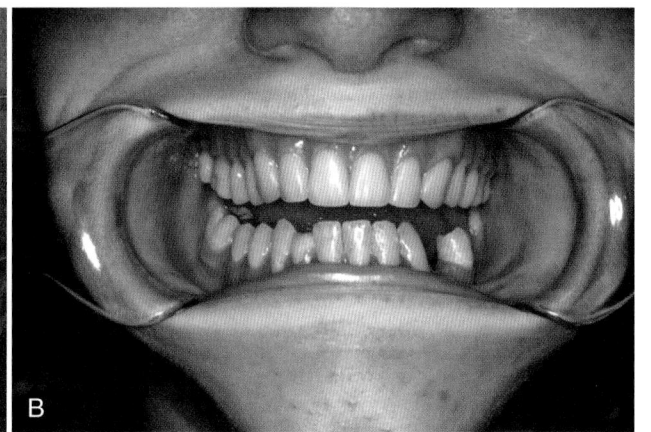

Fig. 5.2 Visioning skills are useful when trying to arrive at treatment options for the patient with many problems. **(A)** This 20-year-old patient had extensive dental caries, nonrestorable teeth, and limited financial resources. **(B)** Of the several options presented, the patient chose to have the maxillary teeth removed and mandibular teeth restored.

be without teeth for several weeks. On the other hand, possibly only the posterior teeth should be removed at first and the anterior teeth retained to maintain a good appearance. After healing, dentures could be constructed for immediate placement after extraction of the remaining anterior teeth. Thinking ahead again, the dentist takes into account the fact that immediate dentures often require relining 6 to 12 months after placement. Is the patient prepared to accept this additional cost?

Considering the second option, the dentist might envision the patient with removable partial dentures and again begin the process of deconstructing the final result. Which teeth will serve as abutments for the removable partial denture? A surveyed crown may be necessary on some or all of the teeth to achieve adequate retention of the prosthesis. For the teeth needing such crowns, insufficient tooth structure may remain, and a foundation restoration or post and core will need to be provided. Endodontic therapy must first be performed before a post and core can be placed. The dentist may determine that the periodontal condition of several abutment teeth is poor, calling for a new treatment plan designed around different abutment teeth. Can a suitable partial denture be made using these alternative abutment teeth?

Experienced dentists perform this mental dance of forward and backward thinking almost automatically, constructing and deconstructing various treatment plans. Such practitioners can simultaneously envision proposed changes in the treatment plan at three levels: the individual tooth, the arch, and the overall patient. Dental students and recent graduates who lack experience and visioning skills need to work harder at coming up with various options and testing their clinical validity. Even for straightforward cases, it may be advantageous to construct mounted study casts and make diagnostic waxings to aid in the evaluation of possible options. Being part of a network of experienced dentists with whom casts and radiographs can be shared and cases discussed can be helpful. The dentist who practices alone may need to join a study club or develop relationships with experienced general and specialist dentists.

Key Teeth

A first step in developing a treatment plan for the patient with a variety of tooth-related problems, such as periodontal disease, caries, and failing large restorations, may be to identify the important or **key teeth** that can be salvaged. Such teeth may often serve as abutments for fixed and removable partial dentures, and their position in an arch will add stability to a dental prosthesis. Retaining key teeth also often improves the prognosis for other teeth or the case as a whole. Conversely, the loss of a key tooth can limit the number of treatment options available to the patient.

Key teeth can be characterized as having several qualities. If enough of these qualities are present, the tooth or teeth may be important enough to make an extra effort to retain them.

- Key teeth should be periodontally stable. Although some loss of bone or periodontal attachment may be evident from radiographs and during periodontal probing, the tooth usually should exhibit little mobility. Of the anterior teeth, the canines have the most favorable crown-to-root ratios and are

particularly valuable as abutments. Similarly, posterior key teeth, such as multirooted first molars, have a better prognosis as abutments—especially if the roots are divergent—than do single-rooted teeth or those with tapered or fused roots.

- Key teeth are usually favorably positioned in the arch. For example, imagine the patient who has many missing or nonrestorable maxillary teeth. The dentist would like to identify several key teeth, ideally spread throughout the arch, to secure a fixed or removable prosthesis, or to be used as overdenture abutments. Hopefully, the maxillary canines and at least one posterior molar can be retained for stability of the prosthesis. In addition to being favorably located in the arch, key teeth should not be excessively extruded from the occlusal plane (supraerupted), tipped into edentulous spaces, rotated, or located in an extreme buccal or lingual position. Third molars and often some second molars are not suitable to serve as key teeth because of their position in the arch and the difficulties involved in restoring them. The dentist can evaluate the positions of individual teeth directly during the examination, with mounted casts and by surveying study casts.

- Key teeth that are decayed or broken must be restorable. Teeth that have caries extending below the level of the alveolar crest may be poor candidates for restorative treatment and subsequent use as an abutment. In situations with less tooth destruction but with the margin of the final restoration approaching the alveolar crest, the periodontal health of the tooth may be compromised. Orthodontic extrusion of the tooth or clinical crown-lengthening surgery can improve the situation, although the loss of periodontal attachment may lead to increased mobility and decreased suitability as a key tooth.

Phasing

When preparing to treat a patient with complex needs, the dentist may find it advantageous to break the treatment plan into segments, or phases. Sorting treatment into **phases** helps the clinician organize the plan and can improve the overall prognosis of the case. In addition, patients often comprehend a complicated treatment plan more easily when it is separated into segments. The five general categories of phasing are systemic phase, acute phase, disease control phase, definitive treatment phase, and maintenance care phase.

Systemic Phase

The systemic phase of treatment involves a thorough evaluation of the patient's current and past health histories and any procedures necessary to manage the patient's general and psychological health before or during dental treatment. This may include consultation with other health providers, antibiotic prophylaxis, stress and fear management, avoidance of certain medications and products (e.g., latex), and any other precautions necessary to deliver treatment safely to patients with serious general health problems.

Acute Phase

The purpose of an acute phase of treatment is to resolve any symptomatic problems with which a patient may present. Any number of patient problems may require attention during this phase. Common complaints include pain, swelling, infection, broken teeth, and missing restorations. Possible acute phase treatments include extractions, endodontic therapy, initial periodontal therapy, placement of **provisional** (temporary) or permanent restorations, and repair of prostheses. The dentist may also choose to prescribe medications to control pain and infection. Acute phase procedures are often provided before a comprehensive treatment plan is created.

Disease Control Phase

The goal of the disease control phase is to control active oral disease and infection, stop occlusal and esthetic deterioration, and manage any risk factors that cause oral problems. For many patients, this means controlling dental caries and periodontal disease before deciding how to rebuild or replace teeth. Common procedures during the disease control phase include oral hygiene instruction and procedures such as prophylaxis, application of fluorides, scaling and root planing, caries risk assessment and prevention, endodontic therapy, extraction of hopeless teeth, and operative treatment to eradicate dental caries and replace or repair defective restorations.[3]

A disease control–only phase can be valuable when the dentist is uncertain about disease severity, available treatment options, or patient commitment to treatment (Figure 5.3). The outcomes of the disease control phase are evaluated with a **posttreatment assessment examination** before proceeding with definitive treatment procedures. If the patient's dental disease is not controlled, or if the patient wishes to limit treatment, they may enter a holding period and not proceed to definitive treatment.

Definitive Treatment Phase

Definitive treatment aims to rehabilitate the patient's oral condition and includes procedures that improve appearance and function. Depending on the patient and the dentist's level of experience, several procedures in the various disciplines of dentistry, such as prosthodontics, periodontics, and endodontics,

may be required. Examples of definitive treatment procedures include the following:

- Additional periodontal treatment, including periodontal surgery
- Orthodontic treatment and occlusal therapy
- Oral surgery (elective extractions, preprosthetic surgery, and orthognathic surgery)
- Elective (nonacute) endodontic procedures
- Single tooth restorations
- Replacement of missing teeth with fixed or removable prosthodontics, including implants
- Cosmetic or esthetic procedures (composite bonding, veneers, bleaching)

The accompanying *In Clinical Practice* box examines how comprehensive a treatment plan should be.

IN CLINICAL PRACTICE

How Comprehensive Should a Patient's Treatment Plan Be?

When a patient has extensive dental problems, it may be difficult, if not impossible, to develop a comprehensive treatment plan incorporating both disease control and definitive phases. This is especially true when the patient has significant periodontal disease or many carious, missing, or broken-down teeth.

Patients often want to know as soon as possible all that will be involved in rehabilitating their oral condition, and the dentist may feel pressured at an early stage to create a comprehensive treatment plan. Unfortunately, with the level of unpredictability that extensive problems involve, this may be impossible. In this situation, the clinician has two treatment planning options available, depending on the complexity of the case.

Designing a disease control–only plan. Such a plan improves predictability by controlling variables, such as rampant dental caries or active periodontal disease, and simplifies the situation by removing hopeless teeth. During this time, it may be necessary to fabricate provisional replacements for missing teeth to satisfy the patient's esthetic and functional needs.

At the conclusion of the disease control phase, the dentist performs a posttreatment assessment. Depending on the level of disease resolution, patient compliance, and desire for further care, the dentist may decide to simply maintain the patient or alternatively may begin designing a definitive phase treatment plan.

Designing a disease control and tentative definitive treatment plan. For patients with greater predictability, it may be possible to control disease while developing a vision for the definitive treatment to follow. For example, by identifying key teeth and planning for a removable partial denture, the dentist might opt to perform endodontic therapy when a carious exposure occurs during disease control, instead of placing a liner and restoring the tooth. It may be necessary to prepare mounted study casts and perform some preliminary surveying or diagnostic wax-ups to arrive at a tentative plan. The dentist may also need to consult with specialists, such as orthodontists or prosthodontists, regarding treatment options.

Having a tentative treatment plan in mind enables the dentist to discuss a possible end point with the patient while retaining the flexibility to change directions if necessary. As with the disease control–only plan alternative, however, it is imperative to have a posttreatment assessment examination to evaluate that the patient is stable before beginning further definitive care.

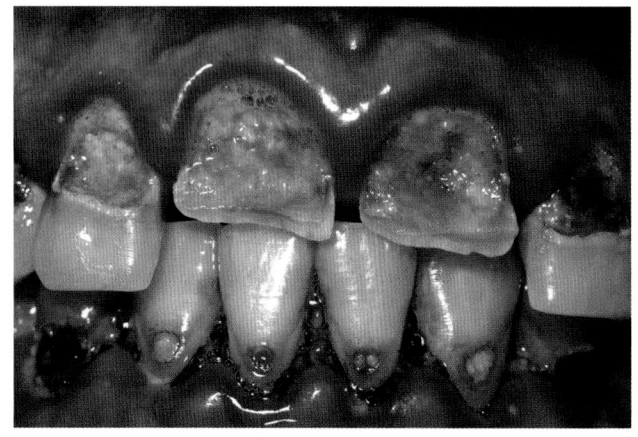

Fig. 5.3 This patient had ignored their teeth for many years and has rampant caries and periodontal disease. A disease control–only phase of care is indicated before any definitive care, such as crowns, can be planned.

Maintenance Care Phase

Unfortunately, many dentists fail to specify a maintenance phase of care to follow after completion of other treatment. Without a plan to periodically reevaluate the patient and provide supportive care, the patient's oral condition may relapse and disease may recur. The maintenance phase is more than simply a "check-up every 6 months"; rather, it constitutes a highly personalized plan that strives to maintain the patient in optimum oral health. Unlike the acute care, disease control, and definitive phases of care that end after completing a "work order" of procedures, a systemic and maintenance phase treatment plan is ongoing and continuous. Maintenance phase procedures may include periodic hard and soft tissue examinations, radiographic examination, periodontal maintenance treatment, application of fluoride, and oral hygiene instruction.

PRESENTING TREATMENT PLANS AND REACHING CONSENSUS WITH THE PATIENT

During the examination process, the dentist has had a chance to listen to the patient's concerns, evaluate their oral and systemic condition, assess the risk for progressive or future disease, and begin mentally envisioning ways to achieve sustainable oral health, function, and appearance. As discussed earlier, effective treatment plans attempt to address all patient problems and still accommodate the treatment goals of both dentist and patient. Once the dentist has begun to build a relationship of trust and rapport with the patient, they must now use communication skills to reach consensus on the final treatment plan. If handled properly, the practitioner will be viewed in a respected, professional manner. If handled poorly, the patient may perceive the dentist as uncertain, lacking confidence, self-serving, arrogant, or even incompetent. The dentist must be prepared to discuss all aspects of the case and remain open to any questions or concerns the patient may have. (See Video 5.1 Presenting a Treatment Plan on ebooks+.)

The presentation begins by educating the patient about their problems and diagnoses. Careful attention should be paid to any

chief complaints and other symptoms so that the patient understands *why* treatment is necessary. The clinician should also emphasize the importance of eliminating disease and achieving and maintaining oral health. It is important to use terminology that the patient can understand and to present information in a simple and organized manner. For example, the patient may better understand the intricacies of a three-wall infrabony pocket if described as "a loss of bone around the teeth." Rather than pointing out each carious lesion in the mouth, the condition might be summarized as "decay on six teeth." Extraoral and intraoral images, mounted casts (Figure 5.4), radiographs, clinical images, diagnostic wax-ups, drawings, and informational pamphlets may be used to educate patients and help them visualize their own problems. Throughout this discussion, the dentist should encourage questions and periodically verify that the patient understands what is being said.

Next, the dentist can begin discussing treatment options. Before presenting this information, the dentist should have evaluated all possible treatment alternatives available to meet the patient's needs. Thinking in general terms facilitates this approach (i.e., large fillings versus crowns, fixed versus removable prosthetics, replacing or not replacing teeth). Once the patient has decided on a general direction for care, the advantages and disadvantages of the individual options should be discussed. The dentist should clearly describe the short- and long-term prognosis for each type of treatment and for the plan as a whole, as well as describing what can be expected if no treatment is provided at all. The importance of the patient's cooperation in plaque control, smoking cessation, reducing parafunctional habits, and returning for maintenance therapy should be emphasized, including the effect of that cooperation (or lack of it) on the overall prognosis for treatment. Again, the patient should be prompted for questions.

About this time, many patients are beginning to think about the cost for services, the number of appointments, and the

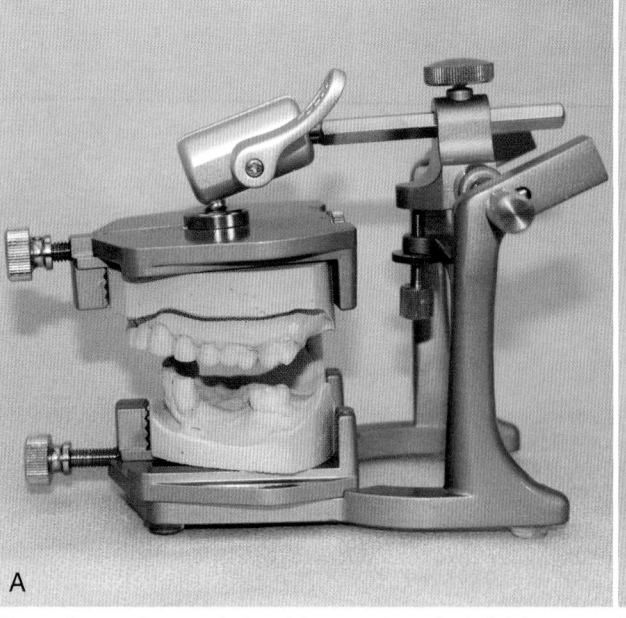 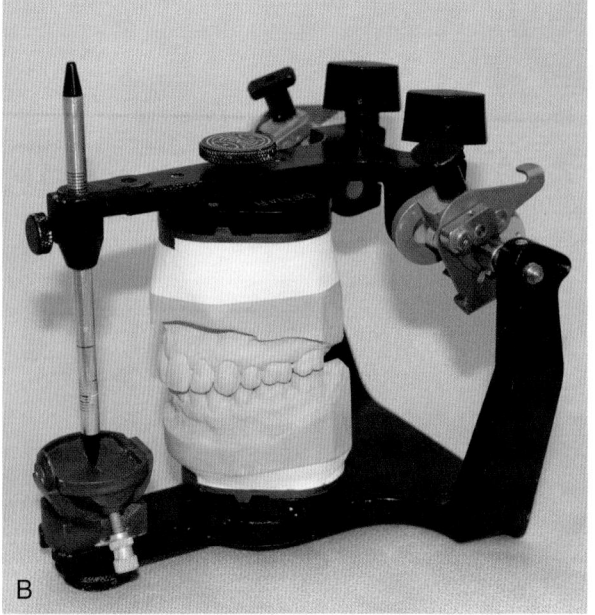

Fig. 5.4 Depending on the complexity of the case, it can be helpful to use patient models with either **(A)** a plasterless or **(B)** a conventional articulator.

length of time involved for treatment. The *What's the Evidence? Improving Patient Acceptance of Treatment Plans* and *In Clinical Practice: Suggestions for Presenting Treatment Plans to Patients* boxes offer additional information about presenting treatment plans. The dentist should be prepared to discuss some general time and fee ranges, letting the patient know that a more precise estimate will be available before beginning treatment. Many practitioners have chosen to delegate much of this discussion to a business manager or other office staff. If so, the dentist should be available to answer questions if the plan changes.

WHAT'S THE EVIDENCE?

Improving Patient Acceptance of Treatment Plans

Confronting the patient's health beliefs is a useful technique for gaining acceptance of your treatment plans or understanding why a patient is reluctant to proceed with treatment. Developed to investigate the widespread failure of patients to accept preventive treatment for diseases, **the health belief model**[4] argues that patients must hold four beliefs before they will accept treatment for a particular disease. According to the model, patients must believe

1. That they are susceptible to the specific disease to be treated.
2. That contracting the disease has serious consequences for them.
3. That the disease can be prevented or limited if the patient engages in certain activities or receives treatment.
4. That engaging in these preventive or disease-limiting activities is preferable to suffering from the disease.

Medical and dental researchers have used the health belief model to better understand why patients accept or reject treatment.[5-7] Although its ability to predict health behaviors has not been proven, the model does provide a useful framework for explaining why people do or do not engage in health-related activities. Practitioners can improve case acceptance by addressing each aspect of the model during the treatment plan presentation.

- **Perceived susceptibility**. This comes from a thorough discussion of the list of the patient's problems. The patient must understand and accept the dentist's diagnoses before treatment will be agreed to. This is usually not an obstacle if the patient believes the dentist is competent and a complete and thorough examination has been performed. The practitioner may wish to use educational aids, models, images, and radiographs to help instruct the patient about their problems.
- **Perceived severity**. The patient must recognize that there is some level of severity in their oral condition before treatment will be considered. This is especially important if the patient does not have symptoms and has been unaware of a particular dental problem. For instance, the dentist may interpret a large, asymptomatic, periapical radiolucency as very serious, but the patient may not share that perception until the dentist characterizes its significance. Again, patient education is the key, especially discussion of what the consequences may be if the patient chooses *not* to have the problem treated.
- **Perceived benefits**. A patient must believe that the proposed treatment plan will help solve their problems. This usually is achieved by spending time discussing the prognosis with the patient. Photographs of completed cases can be a helpful adjunct to this discussion.
- **Perceived barriers**. Surprisingly, it may be necessary to convince the patient that accepting the treatment plan is better than living with their dental problems. Patients often have—or perceive that they have—barriers to receiving treatment. The most common barriers are cost, time, and fear of pain. The dentist should make it a point to always address these three issues when presenting a treatment plan.

In addition to the individual's health beliefs and lack of oral health education, the patient may choose not to follow professional recommendations because of poor dentist-patient communication. Communication is an interaction that involves the patient and the dentist. Good patient-provider communication in dentistry includes creating a pleasant interpersonal relationship, exchanging information, and making cooperative treatment-related decisions. A pleasant interpersonal relationship is created when the dentist carefully explains procedures with a calm demeanor and encourages the patient to ask questions. Most patients prefer to receive information in an interaction in which they do not feel that the dentist is attempting to dominate them and in which they can comfortably provide information about themselves. When the patient is calm, trustful, and free of anxiety, they are more likely to comply with the dentist's recommendations.

Exchanging information allows the dentist to make the diagnosis and create the treatment plan with an understanding of the patient's preferences and expectations. During this time, the dentist not only educates the patient about what good oral health practices involve but also motivates the patient to incorporate good oral health practices into their daily life. When treatment-related decision making is shared with the patient, the patient is more likely to perceive that they have a vested interest in the process and will be motivated to comply with the proposed treatment. Although the dentist is the professional in the relationship and may perform services of the highest quality, if the patient has a negative perception of the relationship, the treatment outcome may be compromised. Because patient-provider communication requires mutual participation, the interpersonal skills of the dentist are as important as the personality and motivation of the patient.

IN CLINICAL PRACTICE

Suggestions for Presenting Treatment Plans to Patients

- Have the patient sitting upright; never present a treatment plan with the patient in a reclining position.
- Sit facing the patient at eye level while presenting the plan.
- Use language that the patient can understand and consider using an interpreter when English is not the patient's first language.
- Avoid using threatening or anxiety-producing terms.
- Talk *with* the patient; do not lecture or preach. Be aware of your body language.
- Do not overwhelm the patient with the minute details.
- Use casts, wax-ups, images, and radiographs to emphasize key points.
- Ask the patient to repeat information back to you to confirm understanding of the treatment plan.

GUIDELINES FOR SEQUENCING DENTAL TREATMENT

Once the patient's problems have been identified and a general course of therapy proposed, the dentist's next major responsibility is sequencing the individual treatment procedures. This process can be particularly challenging when the patient has many interrelated problems and treatment needs. Modifiers, such as patient finances, insurance coverage, time availability, and the need to resolve the chief complaint, may also influence the sequence of treatment.

Although the order in which treatment should proceed will vary, some general guidelines can be followed initially to sequence procedures (Box 5.1). In general, these guidelines parallel the recommendations for phasing treatment. The practitioner begins by assigning procedures to each phase and then sequences the procedures within each phase according to the level of problem severity. The resulting list of procedures addresses the patient's most severe problems first and concludes with those of less consequence.

Because it may be difficult to create a linear, step-by-step prescription for addressing all of the patient's problems, the dentist must remain flexible throughout this process. In some situations, it may be helpful to group treatments together or to create a cluster within a phase and not specify a specific order. For instance, a patient may need a number of teeth restored to control caries. By clustering the planned restorations into groups labeled as "treat early" and "treat later," sequencing is achieved, yet the practitioner retains some flexibility to decide later which restoration to do first, second, etc. As discussed earlier, although the dentist can follow certain guidelines when sequencing treatment, exceptions can and will arise. Many of the challenges in sequencing are associated with the issues described in the following sections.

Resolution of Chief Complaint

New patients usually have specific concerns or complaints. To help build rapport, the dentist should sequence the treatment for these complaints early in the treatment plan when feasible. Obviously, it makes sense to provide treatment immediately when the patient has pain or swelling, but occasionally the solution to the patient's problems is complicated and, from the dentist's point of view, should be addressed later in the plan. For example, although a patient may request that missing teeth be replaced so that they can function better, it may be inappropriate to fabricate a fixed partial denture if the patient has active periodontal disease or more immediate restorative needs. When this situation occurs, the dentist must carefully explain the significance of the disease control phase and its relationship to the success of future treatment. One solution may be to provide a provisional removable partial denture. Another example is the patient with rampant caries who, for esthetic reasons, wants the anterior teeth restored before treating the often more severely decayed posterior teeth. Again, the dentist will need to discuss the situation with the patient and reach some consensus. Perhaps treating the most severe posterior tooth and one or two anterior teeth at the next appointment will be an acceptable compromise. Occasionally, as discussed in *In Clinical Practice: Referring Patients to Dental Specialists* box, the dentist will refer a patient to a specialist to resolve certain problems.

BOX 5.1   Guidelines for Sequencing Dental Treatment

I. Systemic treatment
  A. Consultation with patient's healthcare provider
  B. Premedication
  C. Stress and fear management
  D. Special positioning of the patient
  E. Any necessary treatment considerations for systemic disease
II. Acute treatment
  A. Emergency treatment for pain or infection
  B. Treatment of the urgent chief complaint when possible
III. Disease control
  A. Caries removal to determine restorability of questionable teeth
  B. Extraction of hopeless or problematic teeth
    1. Possible provisional replacement of teeth
  C. Periodontal disease control
    1. Oral hygiene instruction
    2. Initial therapy
      a. Scaling and root planing, prophylaxis
      b. Controlling other contributing factors
        (1) Replace defective restorations, remove caries
        (2) Reduce or eliminate parafunctional habits, smoking
  D. Caries control
    1. Caries risk assessment
    2. Provisional (temporary) restorations
    3. Definitive restorations (i.e., amalgam, composite, glass ionomers)
  E. Replace or repair defective restorations
  F. Endodontic therapy for pathologic pulpal or periapical conditions
  G. Stabilization of teeth with provisional or foundation restorations
  H. Posttreatment assessment
IV. Definitive treatment
  A. Advanced periodontal therapy
  B. Stabilize occlusion (vertical dimension of occlusion, anterior guidance, and plane of occlusion)
  C. Orthodontic and/or orthognathic surgical treatment
  D. Occlusal adjustment
  E. Esthetic dentistry (i.e., tooth whitening, esthetic restorations)
  F. Definitive restoration of individual teeth
    1. For endodontically treated teeth
    2. For key teeth
    3. Other teeth
  G. Elective extraction of asymptomatic teeth
  H. Replacement of missing teeth
    1. Fixed partial dentures, implants
    2. Removable partial dentures
    3. Complete dentures
  I. Posttreatment assessment
V. Maintenance therapy
  A. Periodic visits

IN CLINICAL PRACTICE

Referring Patients to Dental Specialists

General dentists refer patients to specialists for several reasons. Most commonly, the practitioner wants the specialist's assistance in diagnosing or treating a patient's problem. Many general dentists choose not to provide certain types of treatment procedures or do not possess the skills necessary to perform them. Treatment complexity may also be a concern. Occasionally, the generalist's treatment of the patient's problem is not progressing well or has resulted in an unfavorable outcome. Examples of the second situation might include the inability to extract an impacted third molar or complaints of pain by a patient 6 months after completion of root canal therapy.

The patient's well-being should be first and foremost when deciding whether to refer for treatment. Most patients look favorably on the dentist who seeks assistance for their problems. The referral process flows more smoothly if the dentist observes the following guidelines:

- Inform the patient of the reason for the referral, including any pertinent diagnoses or problems from prior treatment rendered. Make sure the patient understands the consequences of *not* seeking specialty treatment.
- Familiarize the patient with the specialist's area of expertise and, in general, what types of treatment will be provided.

- Assist the patient in making contact with appropriate specialists by providing names and telephone numbers. Some practices choose to make the first appointment for the patient.
- Provide the specialist with copies of any radiographs, photographic images, casts, or other diagnostic aids before the patient's first appointment.
- Communicate the particulars of the case to the specialist, especially the reason for referral, a summary of the overall treatment plan, and any special concerns regarding patient management. Many specialists provide dentists with referral pads for conveying this information, but often a short letter is better. Some specialty practices have online referral forms. In the event of an emergency referral, the dentist should speak first with the specialist on the telephone before arranging the patient's visit.
- Maintain a referral log to assist with follow-up of referred patients. Specialists often send an acknowledgment after their examination or completion of treatment. If the general dentist recommends and makes a referral but the patient does not follow-up by contacting the recommended clinician, this should be documented in the patient record. In certain circumstances, such referral for evaluation of possible cancerous lesion, the dentist will want to contact the patient and even send a letter if they do not see the specialist.

The general dentist is responsible for coordinating overall patient care between specialists and the general dental practice. On occasion, the dentist may need to consult with the patient when specialty opinions or changes to the treatment plan conflict. The general dentist must also confirm with the specialist any need for future treatment or reevaluation. A classic example is the orchestration of periodontal maintenance treatment between the periodontist and the general dentist. Other examples include periodic evaluation of implant therapy and treatment for pathologic oral conditions.

Periodontal Therapy

In a dental school environment, initial periodontal therapy often is sequenced first in a treatment plan. Although this may be appropriate for the individual with few additional treatment needs, it may not be appropriate for others, especially those who are experiencing some discomfort. To ensure appropriate care, periodontal therapy should occur as early as possible in the plan, but it can be delayed for several reasons. One frequently encountered justification is the decision to first resolve a simple complaint, such as replacing a lost restoration or extracting symptomatic impacted third molars. Another example is the patient with large carious lesions, especially those located subgingivally. Restoring such teeth with a permanent or provisional filling should make periodontal treatment more comfortable for the patient and begin to resolve the gingivitis that accompanies subgingival lesions. Lastly, teeth that are nonrestorable or periodontally hopeless are often extracted before beginning scaling and root planing procedures.

Occasionally, it may be appropriate to begin periodontal treatment *before* completing the patient's dental examination. This typically occurs when the patient has not seen a dentist for many years, and the dentition is covered with plaque and calculus. The dentist may decide to begin gross scaling or plaque debridement of the teeth to permit examination of the teeth.

Caries Control

For the patient with many carious lesions, treatment consists of restoring lost or decayed tooth structure and implementing preventive strategies designed to prevent caries from occurring

in the future. Strategies such as controlling refined carbohydrate consumption, improving the patient's plaque removal technique, and applying fluorides, should commence immediately and be regularly reinforced, ideally at every appointment.

The following guidelines should be followed when sequencing treatment for caries:

- Address any symptomatic teeth first. Extract those that should not be retained for obvious periodontal or restorative reasons. For other symptomatic teeth, remove all caries, begin endodontic therapy if necessary, and place a permanent or provisional restoration.
- Treat any asymptomatic carious lesions that may be nearing the pulp as determined clinically or interpreted on radiographs. The goal is to prevent symptoms for the patient and avoid irreversible injury to the pulp.
- Remove caries to determine restorability. For teeth with caries at or below the alveolar crest radiographically, remove the caries and decide whether the tooth can be restored (Figure 5.5). Endodontic therapy should not be provided until the tooth is deemed periodontally sound and restorable.
- Finally, remove caries from asymptomatic teeth and, when possible, restore with a definitive restoration, such as composite resin or amalgam. For efficiency, sequence first by severity and then by quadrant.

Endodontic Therapy

Endodontic therapy consists of a series of treatments, including removing pulpal tissue, filing and shaping root canals, obturating the root canal space, and placing a permanent restoration for the tooth. For some patients, it may be appropriate to do each step in succession, especially when no other problems have been identified. For patients with many deep carious lesions or pulpal pain, simply removing the caries and pulpal tissue, followed by rudimentary filing and shaping, and placement of a temporary **provisional restoration** is preferred. After establishing some level of disease control, endodontic therapy can then be completed. Permanent restorations for endodontically treated teeth should be sequenced before those for vital teeth if at all possible.[8]

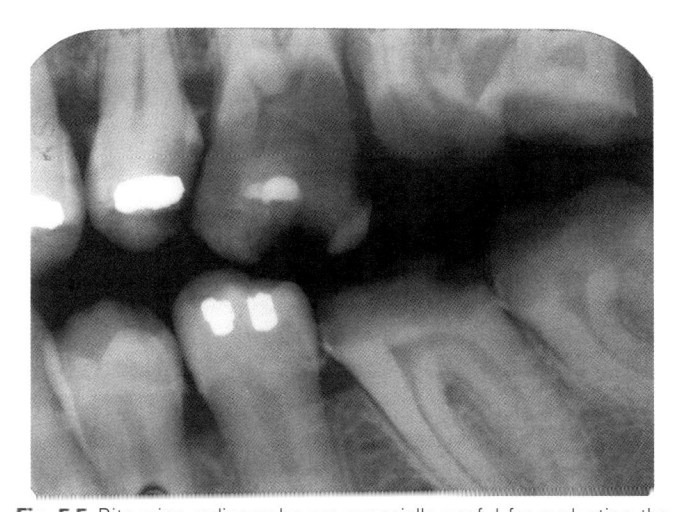

Fig. 5.5 Bite-wing radiographs are especially useful for evaluating the extent of caries in relation to the alveolar crest. In this patient, the maxillary and mandibular molars are probably not restorable.

Extraction

When possible, tooth extractions should be sequenced early in the treatment plan to permit healing to take place, especially before tooth replacements are fabricated. The dentist should attempt to limit the number of surgical appointments and extract all hopeless or nonrestorable teeth at the same time. It may be necessary to delay the extraction of asymptomatic teeth for short periods of time so that provisional replacements can be fabricated to preserve appearance or to maintain the position of opposing and adjacent teeth. The classic example of this concept involves planning to place immediate dentures. The process begins by removing the posterior teeth, leaving the anterior teeth for esthetic reasons. Impressions for the dentures are taken 6 to 8 weeks later, after some healing of the posterior segments has occurred. Dentures can be fabricated using altered casts and delivered when the anterior teeth are extracted.

Sequencing removal of third molars may vary in a treatment plan. When symptomatic, they should be removed immediately. Asymptomatic or impacted teeth may be removed at the end of the disease control phase or during the definitive treatment. If the treatment plan includes extracting a third molar and fabricating a crown or placing an implant for the second molar anterior to it, the third molar should be removed first because of the potential to damage adjacent teeth during the oral surgery and to obtain better access.

Occlusion

Achieving a stable occlusal relationship represents an important goal when developing a comprehensive treatment plan. During the examination, the dentist will have identified any occlusal problems, such as malocclusion, tooth mobility, loss of vertical dimension, malposed teeth, or signs of parafunctional habits, such as bruxism. Mounted study casts are essential for evaluating and planning occlusal relationships, especially if multiple crown and bridge restorations are planned.

The practitioner should have a clear vision of the final occlusion before beginning definitive care, especially when the plan involves prosthodontics treatment. Treatment for occlusal problems normally begins after the disease control phase and may involve orthodontic treatment, occlusal adjustment, or altering the vertical dimension. In some instances, occlusal therapy, such as a limited occlusal adjustment, may be part of the initial therapy. When restoring or replacing teeth with crowns or a fixed or removable prosthodontic prosthesis, procedures should be sequenced to develop the anterior occlusion first, followed by development of the posterior occlusion.[9]

Replacements for Teeth

Patients who eventually will need to have teeth replaced with implants, fixed and removable partial dentures typically have several dental problems. Controlling caries and periodontal disease should begin immediately. It may also be necessary to fabricate provisional partial dentures to satisfy the patient's esthetic and functional needs during this interval. The practitioner should also begin identifying key teeth during the disease control phase, particularly those that will serve as abutments

for fixed and removable partial dentures. It may be necessary to do a preliminary removable partial denture design on study casts with the help of a **dental surveyor**. At the same time, the dentist should be evaluating the potential need for preprosthetic surgery, especially torus removal and maxillary tuberosity reduction.

Key teeth should receive special attention during the posttreatment assessment, especially in terms of their response to disease control procedures and their suitability as abutments. The partial denture design should be finalized before beginning definitive care. This is particularly important in enabling the dentist to incorporate occlusal rests, guide planes, and retentive areas into the restoration design as needed. Preprosthetic surgery, endodontic therapy, post and cores, survey crowns, and fixed partial dentures will precede fabrication of the removable partial denture.

Third Parties

The most fundamental dental relationship involves just two parties, the dentist and the patient. Ideally, in such a relationship, outside interference with treatment planning decisions is minimal because all aspects of the plan will be decided on by the dentist and patient. Frequently, however, **third parties** participate in treatment planning decisions and affect how dentistry is practiced. Although dental insurance companies are generally seen as the major third-party influence on dental care, it is important to remember that other individuals—for example, a patient's parent or guardian, may modify the dentist-patient relationship and function as a third party (Figure 5.6).

Public Assistance Plans

This type of insurance plan, commonly associated with such programs as Medicaid in the United States, is often restrictive. Here, the third party exerts limits on both the *type* of treatment covered and the *level of payment* for particular dental procedures. If the dentist's regular fee is higher than what the program pays, the dentist cannot charge the patient the difference. Medicaid programs are controlled at the state level, with coverage varying from state to state. Although the programs provide many individuals with some access to dental care, they often do not pay for the ideal or most appropriate type of treatment. For example, if the patient has an ill-fitting maxillary partial denture, the program may only pay for extractions in preparation for a complete denture, regardless of the condition of the abutment teeth. The program may set an upper limit on the number of posterior teeth in occlusion before authorizing removable tooth replacements.

When the program dictates an extremely limited treatment plan that, in the dentist's judgment, constitutes irrational or poor dental care, the dentist is faced with an ethical dilemma. To render the optimal treatment at no charge may not be economically feasible, yet to perform the "approved" treatment may constitute substandard care. The dentist and patient must decide on a course of treatment that represents the best available option under the circumstances. In some cases, the dentist may decide not to accept the patient for treatment under the third-party restrictions. More often, however, at least minimal disease

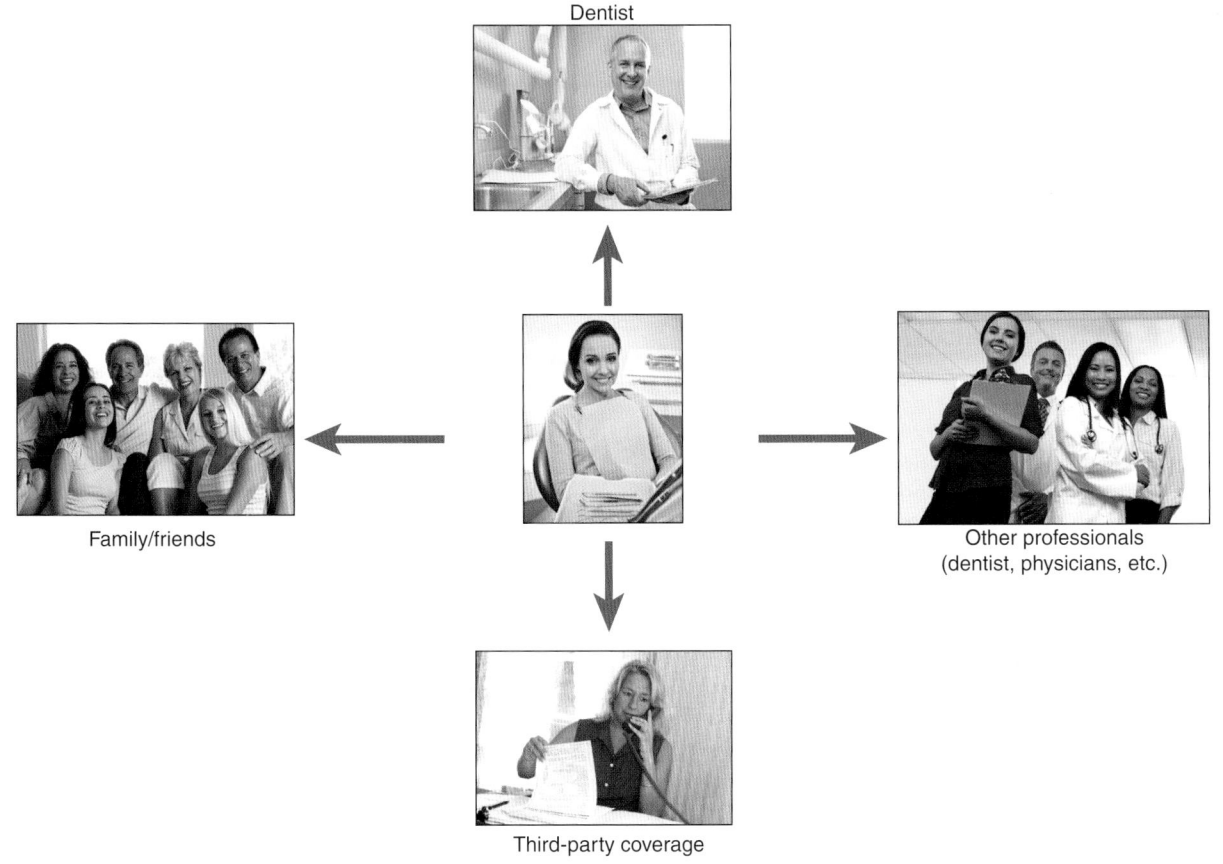

Fig. 5.6 A number of relationships may need to be considered when treating a patient. (Photos courtesy iStock.)

control can be carried out within the limitations of the program. Patients may later choose to pay for further treatment on their own. Providing informed consent concerning what public assistance will and will not cover is critical before beginning treatment. The dentist also needs to inform the patient of the existence of treatment procedures that could be performed—for example, implants versus a removable prosthesis—but are not paid for by the public assistance program. For more information about managing patients with financial limitations and government-sponsored and public assistance programs, see Chapter 19.

Private Fee-for-Service Dental Insurance Policies

With private fee-for-service insurance, the third party is usually more generous with treatment covered and levels of payment, compared with public assistance programs. The insurance companies control reimbursement for services by
- Limiting the types of treatment covered
- Setting a maximum allowable fee
- Paying only a fixed amount or a percentage of the dentist's fee for each service, with patients often expected to pay the difference
- Setting yearly or lifetime maximum benefit limits

For the patient with limited treatment needs, this type of third party may cover all of the proposed treatment at a high level of payment. When there are extensive oral health needs, the patient may ask the dentist to provide treatment in stages

to coincide with annual benefit limitations. Sometimes, treatment can be begun at the end of one policy year and concluded into the next, thus taking advantage of two benefit years. The dentist will often wish, and may be required, to request authorization from the third party before beginning treatment so as to determine the patient's benefit levels, particularly for treatments involving tooth replacement.

Occasionally, an extensive treatment plan may be extended over 3, 4, or even 5 years to take maximum advantage of the insurance benefits. Such long-term treatment planning is challenging and assumes a stable dentist-patient-third party relationship. For such a plan to work, the current insurance coverage must remain in effect during the entire treatment period and the patient must remain eligible for benefits and must not move or change dentists during the course of treatment. If any of these conditions is likely to change, this type of extended treatment planning is inadvisable.

The dentist must also consider whether delivery of treatment can be safely extended over several years without jeopardizing the final result. Typically, with an extended treatment plan, the dentist performs disease control therapy first, placing interim restorations and building up teeth while postponing more costly rehabilitation of the dentition. This may be impossible in some cases—for example, when restoring several endodontically treated teeth that should have full crowns placed for protection. Although repairing large, defective amalgams or composites instead of providing full-coverage restorations, such as crowns or onlays, may save the patient money, such a strategy may only postpone the inevitable. When teeth need to be replaced, transitional removable prostheses may be attempted to preserve appearance in lieu of definitive removable or fixed partial dentures. Unfortunately, many patients cannot or will not tolerate these interim prostheses for an extended period, and the prostheses may damage remaining teeth and underlying tissues.

OBTAINING INFORMED CONSENT AND DOCUMENTING THE TREATMENT PLAN

Informed Consent

The treatment plan presentation appointment is the appropriate time to discuss the risks of the planned procedures, a discussion that can serve as the basis for obtaining informed consent from the patient to begin treatment. This type of discussion not only helps reduce the risk of malpractice claims but also serves to better educate patients and prepare them for treatment. The topic of informed consent is discussed in greater detail in Chapter 7, but a brief review is presented here.

In general, for the patient to make an informed decision regarding treatment, the dentist must have described and discussed all diagnoses and problems, treatment alternatives, and the advantages and disadvantages of each alternative. The consenting individual must be mentally competent and of majority age (in the United States, usually 18 years of age or older). The consent must not have been obtained by fraudulent means or under a situation of duress. It may be necessary to have interpretation services available if the patient has a limited ability to speak and understand English or they are deaf or hard of hearing.

Specifically, the dentist must disclose

- The nature of the condition being treated (i.e., the diagnosis and problem list)
- The proposed treatment
- Any risks involved in undergoing the proposed treatment
- Any potential complications or side effects
- Any consequences or risks of *not* undergoing the proposed treatment
- Any alternative procedures that might be used
- The prognosis for the treatment

When obtaining informed consent, the dentist should use lay terms to the extent possible. In addition, the patient must be given the opportunity to ask, and have answered to their satisfaction, any questions regarding the intended treatment. It may be helpful to draw sketches or use casts, images, and radiographs to assist in the explanation and to add these to the patient record. Although often not a legal requirement, patients should also be provided with information about the cost for treatment. (See Video 5.2 Obtaining Informed Consent for a Treatment Plan on ebooks+.)

Treatment Plan Documentation

In addition to examination findings (see Chapter 1), and patient diagnoses (see Chapter 2), the dentist must also document the proposed treatment plan. Besides the obvious risk management benefits, a clearly written treatment plan is a useful practice management tool. With such a plan, the dentist, staff, and patient will all be aware of the procedures to be performed, the sequence of care, and the fees that will be charged. It is a good idea to include treatment *objectives* in the documented plan, especially for disease control and limited treatment patients. Supplying the patient with information about their diagnoses and problems, and treatment objectives, can be useful in educating the individual in preparation for obtaining informed consent for the overall treatment plan. A disease control–only treatment plan should include a clearly written statement articulating the need for reevaluation and further definitive care.

Depending on the patient's needs, treatment plans may be simple or extremely complex documents. For patients requiring only one or two procedures, a short entry in the record, often in the progress notes, will provide sufficient information. For more complex treatment plans, particularly those with multiple options, the dentist may choose to give the patient hard copies of several alternative treatment plans to review later, independently or with others.

Once a plan is agreed on and informed consent established, the patient affirms acceptance with their signature.

Usually, two types of treatment plans must be documented. Much of the discussion in this chapter has focused on the **active treatment plan** (Figure 5.7). The active treatment plan is typically a list of disease control and definitive procedures sequenced in the order in which they will be provided. Most patient information systems include software functions for creating active treatment plans and for integrating such plans into the appointing and billing systems. Although the listing of fees is optional from a legal standpoint, they are often included to provide the patient with an estimate of cost. Active treatment plans will have an end point, often a posttreatment evaluation (see Chapters 10 and 11). In contrast, the perpetual treatment plan has no end point. The perpetual plan addresses patient concerns, issues, and needs that will remain relevant beyond the completion of the active plan—and that may continue for the life of the patient. **Perpetual treatment plans** commonly include specific systemic and maintenance procedures and actions. Examples of perpetual plan items are listed in Box 5.2. A detailed discussion of how such actions can be incorporated into the patient's plan of care will be found in Chapter 12. Although tracking the need for periodontal maintenance intervals is commonly found in patient information systems, other perpetual plan items can be more challenging for systems to record, follow, and inform the clinician when an action is required.

Finally, an **appointment plan or plan for treatment** lists the activities and procedures that will occur at each appointment. This will be a separate document from the active treatment plan (Box 5.3). An appointment plan is useful for providing an estimate of the number of appointments that will be necessary and the overall time that will be required to complete the treatment plan. A well-thought-out appointment plan enables the dentist and staff to be prepared and efficient at each appointment as they work with the patient to complete the active plan.

UNIVERSITY SCHOOL OF DENTISTRY

Draft Treatment Plan

Patient: lior lior (781952)

Phase	Tooth	Surface	Code	Provider	Description	Patient	Insurance	Total Estimate
Disease Control Treatment								
1:0	30	MO	D2150	Stefanac, Stephen	Amal 2Surf Prim or Perm	0.00	0.00	0.00
1:0	31	MO	D2150	Stefanac, Stephen	Amal 2Surf Prim or Perm	0.00	0.00	0.00
1:1			D1110	Stefanac, Stephen	Adult Prophy	0.00	0.00	0.00
1:2	3	MOL	D2160	Stefanac, Stephen	Amal 3Surf Prim or Perm	0.00	0.00	0.00
1:2	13	MOD	D2160	Stefanac, Stephen	Amal 3Surf Prim or Perm	0.00	0.00	0.00
1:2	18	MO	D2150	Stefanac, Stephen	Amal 2Surf Prim or Perm	0.00	0.00	0.00
					Estimated Fee for this Phase:	$0.00	0.00	$0.00
Corrective Treatment								
2:1	FM		D5986C	Stefanac, Stephen	Home Bleaching (2arches)	0.00	0.00	0.00
2:2	7	F	D2962	Stefanac, Stephen	VenrPorcLamntLab	0.00	0.00	0.00
2:2	8	F	D2962	Stefanac, Stephen	VenrPorcLamntLab	0.00	0.00	0.00
2:2	9	F	D2962	Stefanac, Stephen	VenrPorcLamntLab	0.00	0.00	0.00
2:2	10	F	D2962	Stefanac, Stephen	VenrPorcLamntLab	0.00	0.00	0.00
2:3	H	F	D2330	Stefanac, Stephen	Anterior Resin 1	0.00	0.00	0.00
					Estimated Fee for this Phase:	$0.00	0.00	$0.00
Maintenance Treatment								
3:1	19	D	D0170WS	Stefanac, Stephen	Observe Tooth Surface N/C	0.00	0.00	0.00
					Estimated Fee for this Phase:	$0.00	0.00	$0.00
					Estimated Total Fee:	$0.00	0.00	$0.00

I consent to begin the procedures listed above. I have had an opportunity to have the proposed procedures and alternative treatments explained to me, including risks and potential complications. Any questions I have concerning the proposed treatment have been answered to my satisfaction.

I understand that the fees listed on this treatment plan are only an estimate of my costs. Additional charges will be made for unforeseen changes in the treatment plan. I understand that the School of Dentistry fees change annually and I will be charged current fees at the time service is rendered. I understand that some services as indicated above may not be covered or may require pre-authorization by my dental plan. If I or my dependent choose to obtain any non-covered services, I agree to be personally responsible for paying the School of Dentistry's charges for these services.

Fig. 5.7 An example of an active treatment plan.

BOX 5.2 Examples of Perpetual Plan Items

- Systemic actions and actions necessary for improving patient comfort
- Evaluation for use/refill of medications
  - Premedication and other medications
- Active warnings
  - Examples: "Avoid penicillin," "Take BP at every appt."
- Anxiety management
- Special chair positioning
- Preventive and periodontal maintenance procedures
- Periodontal evaluation
- Oral hygiene recommendations
  - Fluoride and other product recommendations
- Evaluation for new radiographs
- Periodic examination
- Head and neck, soft tissue, and oral cancer evaluation

- Dental conditions
  - Caries evaluation
  - Evaluation of current restorations
  - Evaluation of occlusion
- Reevaluations
- Periodic evaluation of pathologic lesions detected clinically and radiographically
- Endodontic posttreatment evaluation
- Preventive actions and reevaluation
- Diet analysis
- Smoking cessation
- Other habits
- Review of treatment declined by the patient (e.g., third molar removal, full-coverage restorations, replacement of missing teeth)

BOX 5.3   A Treatment Plan Versus an Appointment Plan

Clinical Summary

A patient presents for a new patient examination. It has been 5 years since the individual's last visit to a dentist. The patient complains of a loose maxillary denture, a broken lower molar, and a dark area on a lower canine tooth. After examination, the dentist diagnoses a poorly fitting denture, a broken cusp on a lower left molar, caries on the distal surface of the right mandibular canine, and generalized marginal gingivitis.

Treatment Plan
- Comprehensive examination
- Prophylaxis
- Porcelain crown, left mandibular first molar
- Composite restoration, distal right mandibular canine
- Maxillary denture
- Reevaluation

Appointment Plan
Appointment 1 (60 minutes)
- Examination
- Radiographs
- Preliminary denture impression

Appointment 2 (60 minutes)
- Prophylaxis, oral hygiene instructions

Appointment 3 (90 minutes)
- Composite restoration, distal lower right canine
- Prepare porcelain crown
  - Two-week laboratory turnaround for crown fabrication

Appointment 4 (90 minutes)
- Adjust and cement crown
- Final impression for the maxillary denture, lower alginate impression
  - Two-week laboratory turnaround to pour impression and fabricate wax rim

Appointment 5 (60 minutes)
- Wax rim adjustment, occlusal records, and tooth selection
  - Two-week laboratory turnaround to fabricate wax try-in

Appointment 6 (30 minutes)
- Wax try-in and patient approval
  - Two-week laboratory turnaround to process denture

Appointment 7 (30 minutes)
- Deliver maxillary denture
  - Reevaluate in 1 week

Appointment 8 (30 minutes)
- Reevaluate denture
- Periodontal reevaluation

CONCLUSION

The well-constructed treatment plan provides a foundation for the long-term relationship between dentist and patient. A functional treatment plan is dynamic, not static, evolving in response to changes in the patient's oral or general health. A sound and flexible treatment plan facilitates communication and strengthens the doctor-patient relationship. Its contribution to good patient care and effective practice building makes it well worth the time and thought required for its development.

REVIEW QUESTIONS

- How are treatment objectives developed with and for a patient?
- What role does "visioning" play in establishing the nature and scope of the treatment plan?
- What are the five treatment plan phases? What is the purpose of each?
- Identify "dos" and "don'ts" when presenting treatment plan options to a patient.
- What is the importance of sequencing in dental treatment planning? Create a list of sequencing guidelines.
- What constitutes informed consent, and how is it achieved?
- What is the difference between an active and perpetual treatment plans?

REFERENCES

1. Hook CR, Comer RW, Trombly RM, Guinn 3rd JW, Shrout MK. Treatment planning processes in dental schools. *J Dent Educ.* 2002;66(1):68–74.
2. Bader JD, Shugars DA. Understanding dentists' restorative treatment decisions. *J Public Health Dent.* 1992;52(2):102–110.
3. da Costa JB, Frazier K, Duong ML, Khajotia S, Kumar P, Urquhart O. Defective restoration repair or replacement: an American Dental Association Clinical Evaluators Panel survey. *J Am Dent Assoc.* 2021;152(4):329–330. e322.
4. Becker MH. The health belief model and personal health behavior. *Health Educ Monogr.* 1974;2:324–508.
5. Simbar M, Ghazanfarpour M, Abdolahian S. Effects of training based on the health belief model on Iranian women's performance about cervical screening: a systematic review and meta-analysis. *J Educ Health Promot.* 2020;9:179.
6. Ritchie D, Van den Broucke S, Van Hal G. The health belief model and theory of planned behavior applied to mammography screening: a systematic review and meta-analysis. *Public Health Nurs.* 2020
7. Lau J, Lim TZ, Jianlin Wong G, Tan KK. The health belief model and colorectal cancer screening in the general population: a systematic review. *Prev Med Rep.* 2020;20:101223.
8. Schwartz RS. A new look at the endo-restorative interface. *J Endod.* 2020;2.
9. Dawson PE. *Functional Occlusion: From TMJ to Smile Design.* Elsevier; 2006. [e-book].

Interprofessional Treatment Planning

Stephanie M. Munz and Carol Anne Murdoch-Kinch

 Visit eBooks.Health.Elsevier.com

DEFINITION OF INTERPROFESSIONAL CARE

The general dentist has a central role in oral healthcare delivery. Every day, general dentists treat patients with increasingly complex dental, medical, and behavioral conditions and needs. In addition to providing comprehensive oral healthcare and planning and coordinating multidisciplinary dental treatment (*intra*professional collaboration), the dentist must also work collaboratively with other health professionals, as well as with family members, advocates, and patient caregivers, to develop a mutually acceptable dental treatment plan focused on the patient's needs and values. Some patients, especially the frail elderly and individuals with craniofacial anomalies, cancer, or chronic illnesses, receive ongoing care from a wide variety of healthcare providers, including dentists. An interdisciplinary model of care and coordinated treatment planning is essential for such patients.

Interprofessional care (IPC) is defined as the provision of comprehensive health services to patients by multiple healthcare providers in various fields working collaboratively to deliver quality care within and across settings. IPC has great potential to improve patient safety and quality of care. Global health agencies, including the World Health Organization (WHO), the

US Institute of Medicine (IOM), and a variety of national health authorities[1] now advocate interprofessional (IP) education and collaborative care as a way to achieve the following four aims[2]:

1. Improve how patients experience care in terms of quality, efficiency, and overall patient satisfaction.
2. Improve the health of populations.
3. Reduce the per capita cost of healthcare.
4. Improve the work life and satisfaction of healthcare providers.

Although a thorough understanding of the whole patient and their healthcare needs is always necessary to provide optimal dental care, in certain specific circumstances, some of which will be described throughout this chapter, it is essential the dentist collaborate with other members of the healthcare team to develop a dental treatment plan with goals that are *aligned* with the overall treatment goals of the patient, and that ensure treatment delivery is *coordinated* with the overall management of the patient's diverse health problems. In the following sections we will illustrate how, in these situations, the presence of complex and competing patient needs requires effective communication and coordination to optimize patient safety and quality of care. In these circumstances, the dentist may need to adjust an otherwise ideal dental treatment plan to accommodate more urgent needs that must be addressed by other members of the healthcare team. Ideally, in a truly integrated care model, the patient's dental treatment plan is integrated into an overall treatment plan that has been developed in partnership with the patient and the other members of the healthcare team.

The most urgent health problems confronting the world's populations are increasingly complex and reflect the interdependent nature of chronic illnesses. Collaborative care models engage a collaborative practice-ready healthcare workforce trained to take on complex or emergent problems and solve them together. These healthcare workers have gained the skills needed to collaborate with colleagues from other professions and put their IP knowledge into action, doing so with respect for and in concert with the expertise and skills of their colleagues.

Notable benefits of IP collaborative care include the following:

1. Benefits to patients: Collaborative practice can improve access to and coordination of health services, improve health outcomes for people with chronic diseases, and enhance patient care and safety. This includes avoiding medication errors and adverse events, such as bleeding, infection, and other medical emergencies that could have been prevented with proper precautions.
2. Benefits to healthcare providers and payers: Collaborative practice can decrease the total number of patient complications, length of hospital stays, tension and conflict among caregivers, staff turnover, hospital admissions and readmissions, clinical error rates, mortality rates, and medicolegal risk.
3. Benefits to society: Collaborative practice can reduce the costs of care, as well as improve the overall health of the population.
4. Benefits to the work life and satisfaction of healthcare providers: Collaborative practice can increase the resiliency of providers as part of a team, support each other, and provide better care through increased efforts toward health equity through support, empowerment, and mutual respect.

Collaborative care models will increasingly include dentistry as an essential component of primary care, while retaining elements of our current oral healthcare delivery systems. Even though most oral healthcare today is delivered in a uniprofessional practice model (private practice dental offices, large group dental practices), the complex healthcare needs of a global population will require dentists to practice collaboratively with other members of the healthcare team to provide the best treatment outcomes for patients.[3] For example, as a consequence of the COVID-19 pandemic, care coordination with diligent sequencing for procedures that generate aerosols has become increasingly important to reduce the number of visits as well as the need for additional preprocedural COVID testing.

An emphasis on the role of *intra*professional collaboration in dentistry can already be observed. Oral health professionals recognize the importance of collaboration among the various kinds of clinician within dentistry: general dentists, dental specialists, dental hygienists, dental assistants, and, in some settings, midlevel providers, such as expanded function dental hygienists and dental therapists. Extending this collaboration to other members of the healthcare team requires the same competencies: a basic knowledge of each other's roles and responsibilities, an

IN CLINICAL PRACTICE

The Fully Integrated Interprofessional Practice: A Developing Model

An example of a single location, collaborative practice approach can be seen in a community-based primary care facility that houses medical and dental primary care under one roof. In such an environment, care providers from multiple disciplines can readily review the medical and dental records of patients scheduled for the day during a morning huddle, planning care for patients identified as needing a coordinated approach. This strategy allows the dentist to work collaboratively with the other healthcare providers in the facility to provide optimal care for individual patients. The dentist can provide patient education and treatment recommendations for patients with chronic conditions such as diabetes, hypertension, obesity, smoking, and asthma while other healthcare providers reinforce the value of oral health and appropriate oral healthcare to general health and wellness. This type of management is associated with reductions in barriers to care (often supported by the aid of social workers), increases in active patient involvement in their own care and quality of life, and reductions in total care cost.

This type of treatment setting can pose some challenges. For example, patient autonomy and right to privacy can be more difficult to manage. The patient must understand how the team collaborates and provide explicit consent for interclinician communication. Also, a collaborative approach to patient care emphasizes the value of a shared understanding of all the patient's problems and chief concerns, communication between team members to prioritize problems and treatment options, and coordination of care, all with "the whole patient" at the center of care. For this approach to work, these values must be embraced and practiced by all healthcare providers.

In a community health clinic, *coordination* of care is essential for team-based comprehensive treatment. *Coordinated* care requires the dentists to collaborate with other healthcare professionals to develop *shared treatment goals and priorities*, and a treatment plan aligned with these goals and priorities, and optimally sequenced for efficiency and effectiveness of care. The dental treatment plan is integrated into and sequenced within this overall treatment plan. Team-based collaboration requires professionals to understand each other's roles and responsibilities, respect each other's expertise, and work effectively to share the decision making for the patient who requires multidisciplinary care. Ultimately, the rewards of improved treatment outcomes and cost reductions are worth the challenges, and this construct may be considered an emerging model for future general practice.

attitude of mutual understanding, respect, and patient-centeredness, and well-developed communication and teamwork skills. *Shared decision making* is a hallmark of collaborative care and emphasized by the Interprofessional Education Collaborative (IPEC) as a founding principle of a team-oriented healthcare provider.[4] One example of how the healthcare system may better remove barriers for collaboration is the growing trend of linking electronic dental and medical records for the benefit of sharing information that is accessible to multiple providers.[5]

Depending on the patient population, this IP team may include primary care physicians (PCPs), nurses, physician assistants (PAs), medical specialists, pharmacists, psychologists and mental health counselors, physical therapists, occupational therapists, speech and language pathologists, dietitians, and other allied health professionals, as well as the patient's family and social support. The team may actually work together in one location or, more commonly, as a "virtual team," connected through electronic communications, such as an electronic health record, or by telephone, email, or video communications. In this environment, it is essential to respect the patient's autonomy and right to privacy. The patient must consent to communication with other healthcare providers, as well as with family members and caregivers.

REQUIREMENTS FOR SHARED DECISION MAKING

Shared decision making is a hallmark of IP team-based collaborative care. Organizations such as the Center for Interprofessional Education (IPE) at University of Toronto and the IPEC have identified *core competencies* for collaborative care.[4,6] These competencies can be organized into four domains:
- Values and professionalism
- Teams and teamwork
- Communication and collaboration
- Roles and responsibilities

To ensure that patients receive the *right care at the right time* from the *right providers* is dependent on adherence to the following principles that are reflected in the core competencies for collaborative care:
1. Practitioners need to recognize that they are part of a diverse team. Collegiality in a setting involving competing interests and varying perspectives is essential for continuity and effectiveness in delivering care.
2. Practitioners must communicate effectively with the patient and family, as well as with other members of the team. Identification of what questions to ask is essential, and a willingness to address gaps in information requires openness among providers.
3. To limit duplication and avoid gaps in care, it is important for each team member to have some understanding of the other team members' specialties.
4. Practitioners must be prepared to work with each other to optimize care so that the patient's journey from one healthcare setting to the next is experienced as a seamless transition. Such coordination should eliminate inefficiencies and avoid gaps in optimization of care and missed opportunities for early and ordered intervention.[4]

MEMBERS OF AN INTERPROFESSIONAL TEAM

The Patient and Their Social Support

The patient is both the central focus and an integral member of the team. In many cases, the family and caregivers will also be part of the team. For example, an older man with Alzheimer's disease may depend on his spouse to assist him with most **activities of daily living** (ADL), as well as serving as his advocate, making decisions relating to his medical treatment. The spouse would need to be involved in any decision making related to treatment priorities and the patient's needs and desires, and to have a realistic understanding of the situation when faced with an urgent decision, such as to whether or not to restore a tooth or extract it.

If the patient has other urgent healthcare needs (e.g., a pending surgical procedure), then extensive dental treatment may not be in his best interest. The spouse's own healthcare needs may play a role as well. As a couple, what is the best decision for both?

The community may also play an important role in the team, as when public health approaches to disease prevention and health promotion are considered as part of the context of care. For example, a dentist working in an urban community with underserved patients may encounter many children with extensive dental caries. In this setting, many patients will have a variety of health problems related to poverty, lack of access to healthy food choices because there are no grocery stores within the neighborhood, and an unfluoridated municipal water supply. In such cases, a public health approach will include community engagement to develop urban farming, legislation to fluoridate the water, school-based oral health programs, and tax incentives to businesses that provide healthy food choices to the community. The dentist treats the patient but must also partner with other health professionals and the community to modify the environmental risk factors for dental and systemic disease. The patient's dental treatment plan will include consideration of all of these activities and goals.

Dental Team Members

Depending on the context of care and patient population, the oral healthcare team may include some or all of the following:
- General or primary care dentist, dental assistant, and dental hygienist
- Midlevel provider, dental therapist, expanded duty hygienist
- Dental laboratory technician
- Denturists
- Dental specialists

Other Health Professionals

Depending on the patient, other health professionals may include the providers listed in Box 6.1, as well as others not listed here. Also, the descriptions that follow depict US health professionals and may be different in other countries.

Primary Care Physician/Family Practice Physician

The PCP or family practice physician provides general medical care, including assessment and identification of previously

---

> **BOX 6.1   Other Providers That Dentists or Patients May Seek**
>
> Athletic trainer
> Clinical geneticist/genetic counselor
> Clinical psychologist
> Doctor of chiropractic
> Ethicist
> Occupational therapist
> Optometrist
> Orthotist/prosthetist
> Podiatrist
> Religious/spiritual counsellor
> Social worker

undiagnosed medical conditions, health maintenance, and management of medical conditions. They provide detailed histories of positive responses to the health questionnaire and contribute to decisions relating to preoperative risk assessment and evaluation of severity and stability of medical diagnoses, and offer insights related to long-term prognosis, treatment compliance, and mutual treatment goals. Similar to the role of the general dentist, the PCP can serve as a coordinator of care and provide referrals to other healthcare providers, as described in the following sections. The PCP is the default primary resource for most medical consultations.

Physician—Medical Specialties

Dental professionals may also interact with medical specialists in neurology, dermatology, radiation oncology, medical oncology, hematology oncology, psychiatry, pain medicine, and infectious disease, as well as with emergency physicians. For example, when treating a patient with dental pain that triggers trigeminal neuralgia, the dentist will need to collaborate with a neurologist. The dentist will treat the acute dental problem and coordinate care with the neurologist who treats the neuralgia, which is typically a chronic condition requiring long-term medical treatment. A neurosurgeon may be involved if the patient has a neurologic problem that has not responded to medical therapy.

Physician—Surgical Specialties

In addition to working with oral and maxillofacial surgeons (many of whom have also earned a medical degree), dental professionals may interact with specialists in otolaryngology, plastic surgery, transplant medicine, or cardiac surgery. Consider a patient who suffers from injuries resulting from maxillofacial trauma received in a motor vehicle crash. The dentist assesses and manages traumatic injuries to the teeth and alveolus. To restore the occlusion in setting a mandibular or maxillary fracture, the clinician may coordinate dental treatment with a surgeon (otolaryngology, plastic and reconstructive surgery, or oral and maxillofacial surgery), who will reduce and immobilize the jaw fracture with rigid fixation.

Physician Assistant or Associate

The PA or physician associate is licensed to practice medicine under the direct supervision of a physician, and their role overlaps significantly with that of the physician (doctor of medicine [MD] or doctor of osteopathic medicine [DO]). PAs are involved in primary care medicine, as well as in the medical and surgical specialties; their responsibilities depend on the setting in which they work, their level of experience and training, and regional laws. Similar to a physician, the PA compiles histories and conducts physical assessments, provides detailed medical information, orders and interprets diagnostic tests, and diagnoses and treats illnesses, including prescribing medications. PAs (usually medical, not surgical PAs) frequently provide direct patient care in such facilities as nursing homes or group homes.

Nurse/Registered Nurse/Licensed Practical Nurse

The registered nurse (RN) is responsible for the daily care tasks and administration of medications, often in an inpatient setting, but also in outpatient and home care settings. The nurse is trained to closely assess patient needs and detect small, yet significant, changes in function and status, which can be critical for any necessary treatment modifications. A licensed practical nurse (LPN) has been trained to provide home health or nursing care under the supervision of an RN or a medical doctor. These individuals, along with nurse's aides, provide direct patient care, such as oral cleansing. An LPN provides regular reminders and support services, reinforces exercise and good nutrition regimens, and may provide daily oral home care. Hospice nurses provide palliative care, including emotional and spiritual support, for individuals with chronic or terminal illnesses.

Nurse's Aide or Nursing Assistant

The nursing assistant works directly with patients, providing assistance with activities of daily living (ADL), including oral home care, eating, drinking, dressing, toileting, and bathing.

Advanced Practice Nurse, Including Nurse Practitioner

The advanced practice nurse or nurse practitioner (NP) has completed advanced training beyond the RN and is trained for expanded practice capabilities, including independent practice, depending on training and jurisdiction.

Certified Registered Nurse Anesthetist or Anesthetist

The certified registered nurse anesthetist (CRNA) has completed advanced training beyond the RN with a focus on administration of anesthesia, sedation, and control of pain and anxiety. Nurse anesthetists work in collaboration with surgeons, anesthesiologists, dentists, podiatrists, and other qualified health professionals.[7] They may be the primary providers of anesthesia care in rural settings and often provide general anesthesia (GA) in an operating room or outpatient treatment setting for patients unable to tolerate dental care in a standard clinic setting.

Pharmacist

The pharmacist is a health professional who is trained to provide a broad spectrum of services, including conducting health and wellness testing, managing chronic diseases, performing medication management, and administering immunizations. Pharmacists are medication experts within the healthcare team and have the ability to recognize drug interactions, disease-specific drug contraindications, and barriers to medication compliance. Some pharmacists specialize in compounding medications when commercial drug products are either not available or when custom-made formulations will better suit the patient's needs. In an inpatient setting, the pharmacist may administer daily medications and titrate to appropriate doses; provide expertise on drug combinations, interactions, and efficacy; identify patient allergies to medications; and make recommendations regarding discontinuation or alteration of anticoagulants or chemotherapy agents when acute side effects are noted. In an outpatient or retail setting, the pharmacist provides patients with access to prescription and over-the-counter (OTC) medications, administers some immunizations, performs health screenings, monitors drug combinations and interactions, and educates patients and other health professionals about drug side effects and frequency of administration. The pharmacist can be an excellent resource to the dental team, suggesting strategies for improving patient compliance in taking the medications and enhancing drug efficacy. The dental team may contact a patient's pharmacist to obtain a list of the patient's medications.

Social Worker/Case Worker

These professionals can provide essential emotional and social support for the patient, their caregiver, and family. Through biopsychosocial assessments and evaluating the factors that impact health, social workers can be helpful in a large range of supportive services. Information of the individual's strengths and barriers from these assessments can be shared with the dental team to develop a treatment plan that is best for the patient. Emotional support can include short-term counseling for periods of adjustment, as well as referral to services for ongoing mental health needs or substance use interventions, and to address safety concerns. A social worker can team with patients to address barriers to adherence to a treatment plan, assist patients with calming strategies, as well as communicate with family members who may question the plan. Social support can include identifying needs and providing referral to community-based funding sources for housing, clothing, food, and transportation. A social worker can guide patients in applying for healthcare insurance and assist patients in identifying medical providers, which will increase access to healthcare. If patients have difficulty providing for their ADL, the social worker can engage with family, friends, providers, and their community, which may include a guardian, and work together to determine safe living conditions, decisional capacity, durable power of attorney (DPOA) and guardianship needs. Social workers can also help secure informed consent and understanding for the treatment recommendations of oral healthcare needs. Often, the social worker will implement discharge planning for an admitted hospital patient and can similarly coordinate care for patients in outpatient clinics. With a focus on improving patient's overall quality of life, social workers can provide valuable medical, social, and financial information about the patient to the dental team for consideration in developing treatment options.

Mental Healthcare Professional

This provider routinely works to develop strategies and plans to enhance patient well-being, cooperation, and compliance for individuals with special challenges or distractions, specifically those who may have cognitive impairment or mental illness, or exhibit unhealthy behaviors or self-destructive habits. Collaborative efforts with oral health professionals can aid in facilitating care. For example, patients with dental fear are often treated in a team-based clinical setting. The mental healthcare professional can provide cognitive behavioral therapy or biofeedback to help the patient manage fear and anxiety, so that they can receive dental treatment with less discomfort. The dentist may augment this therapy with pain or anxiolytic medications as well. In some situations, the patient may also be receiving treatment from a psychiatrist for underlying mental illness. All of the team members work together with the patient to determine the best treatment plan for the individual.

Speech and Language Pathologist

The speech and language pathologist can provide evaluation and rehabilitation for the patient who has suffered a stroke or received head trauma or for the patient with head and neck cancer who has undergone surgical and/or radiation therapy. A speech and language pathologist will have expertise in the evaluation of such patients and in therapies for treating difficulty in swallowing (dysphagia), aspiration, or voice and articulation, all of which affect quality of life. Therapists in these areas also care for patients with neurologic disorders and craniofacial anomalies affecting speech and swallowing, as well as assessing patients for functional swallowing capacity before tracheostomy or feeding tube removal. Working with a speech and language pathologist may assist the patient in achieving improved, mitigated, or corrected communication function. An improved ability to communicate with the dentist can have multiple benefits for the dental team and will help to make the provision of oral healthcare services more efficient and effective.

Audiologist

The audiologist may contribute to the care of the patient with a suspected hearing deficit. This provider assesses hearing function and communication skills and the ways in which these problems may affect social interactions and relationships in various environments, including school and workplace. Audiologists are a critical component of the craniofacial and cleft lip/palate team.

Physical Therapist

This professional provides therapy, stretching, and exercises to address muscle-associated temporomandibular disorders (TMDs), as well as **trismus** (defined as any restriction to mouth or interarch opening, including restrictions caused by trauma, surgery, or radiation) and **microstomia** (a congenital or acquired reduction in the size of the oral opening that is severe enough to compromise physical appearance, nutrition, and quality of life). Although the dentist and other healthcare providers have some strategies to address these issues, the physical therapist has specific training and expertise that will be essential for the optimal and comprehensive management of such problems.

Dietitian

This licensed healthcare professional assists and advises patients about healthy diets and dietary alternatives, especially individuals with metabolic diseases, such as diabetes or hypercholesterolemia, and those with hypertension, vitamin deficiencies, or food allergies. They have expertise in determining nutrient/caloric recommendations for patients undergoing head and

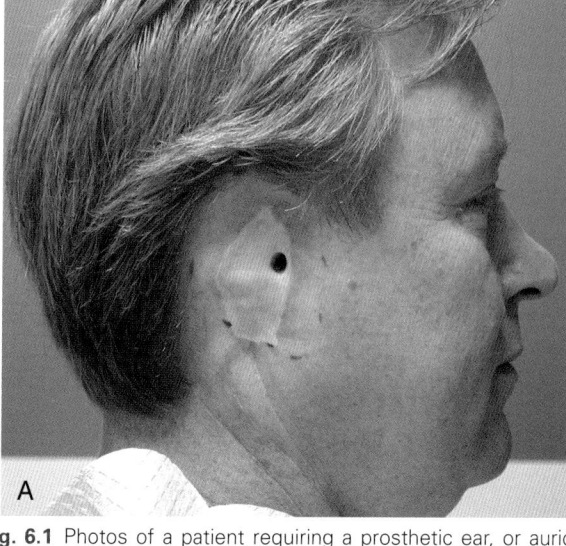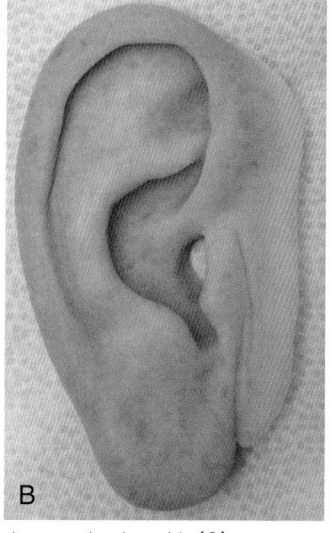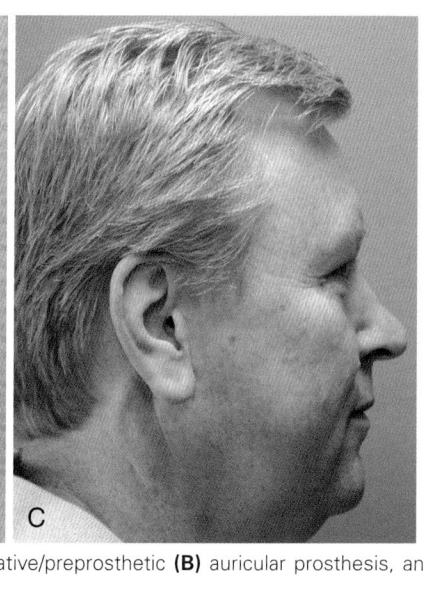

Fig. 6.1 Photos of a patient requiring a prosthetic ear, or auricular prosthesis, with **(A)** postoperative/preprosthetic **(B)** auricular prosthesis, and **(C)** postprosthetic photographs. (Courtesy Stephanie Kline, MSE, MS, Ann Arbor, MI)

neck cancer treatment or who suffer from protracted forms of stomatitis, hyposalivation, or dysphagia. The dietitian can prescribe medical therapeutic nutrition[8] as well as provide counsel for dietary considerations for caries control in the patient presenting with a high caries rate and compounding risk factors and dietary habits.

Anaplastologist/Maxillofacial Prosthetist and Technologist

This provider focuses on the prosthetic rehabilitation of an absent, disfigured, or malformed anatomically critical segment of the face or body. These providers can work in collaboration with a maxillofacial prosthodontist and/or ocularist to customize the fabrication of a facial prosthesis, including ocular within orbital, nasal, and auricular prostheses. See Figure. 6.1 for treatment photographs of a patient with a maxillofacial prosthesis.

COMMUNICATION OR REFERRALS TO OTHER HEALTH PROFESSIONALS

At several points throughout the course of patient assessment, diagnosis, treatment, and continuing care can be identified at which the dentist may need to communicate with or refer the patient to other health professionals. The following section will illustrate when and how collaboration should occur in those cases in which the complexity of the patient's problems requires collaboration to provide safe and effective treatment. In some situations, it may not be *feasible* for dental treatment to proceed because of lack of key information or there are barriers to care that cannot be overcome without teamwork and the participation of all team members. The extent to which dental care and care provided by other health professionals is integrated into a cohesive treatment plan depends on a *shared understanding* of all the patient's problems and chief concerns, the *prioritization* of problems and treatment options, and the *coordination* of care.

> **BOX 6.2   Decision-Making Checklist**
>
> - Do I need to modify my treatment to prevent a medical emergency or other complications?
>   - Does my patient have any significant allergies?
>   - What is the risk of medical emergency, adverse event, or error during dental treatment?
>   - Is there an increased risk of bleeding?
>   - What techniques could be used to mitigate this risk?
>   - Is there an increased risk of perioperative infection?
>   - What techniques could be used to mitigate this risk?
>   - Medications?
>   - Any interactions with drugs I will prescribe/recommend/administer?
>   - Any oral side effects?
> - Do I need information from the physician or another healthcare collaborator? How will this alter my treatment plan or intervention?
> - Does the patient's medical condition, psychosocial factors, or compliance affect oral disease risk or vice versa?

The oral health provider must consider several factors when coordinating care or consulting with other health professionals (Box 6.2). A **consultation** involves referring a patient to another clinician for an opinion and/or treatment for a specific problem or communicating with the patient's current healthcare providers to obtain specific information about the patient's condition, history, treatment, or prognosis.[9] The process for creating and obtaining a consultation with another healthcare provider is discussed in Chapter 8.

When determining the need for a consultation request, the dentist should consider the following questions:
1. Is a consultation needed, and with whom?
2. How could this help the patient?
3. When (timing) would the consultation be requested?
4. What focused questions will be asked?
5. How will the response impact the next step in management?

The following section illustrates how collaboration with a physician and other members of the healthcare team may be needed at various times during the course of patient care, including in relation to initial patient evaluation, treatment planning, and active treatment, and during maintenance care.

Patient Evaluation

At the time of examination and assessment, the dentist screens the patient for signs and symptoms of systemic conditions that may affect oral health or dental treatment, as well as conditions that could have an effect on systemic health and the management of medical conditions (see Chapter 8). The dentist may observe and recognize the need to manage oral manifestations of systemic diseases or oral reactions to systemic medications, such as dry mouth and taste disorders. Collaboration with other members of the healthcare team will be necessary to ensure that oral problems are appropriately addressed. Some common reasons for requesting an evaluation or consultation with a nondental care provider include the following.

Screening for and Optimal Management of Systemic Conditions

For example, the dentist routinely obtains blood pressure readings for each patient at the time of initial or recall examination. Repeated elevated blood pressure readings may indicate undiagnosed or poorly controlled hypertension. Similarly, a patient seeking dental care for recurrent oral fungal infections or a recurrent periodontal abscess may exhibit elevated blood glucose readings and elevated $HbA1_c$, indicators of possible undiagnosed diabetes. In such cases, it is appropriate for the dentist to consult with the patient's primary medical care provider for further evaluation of the patient.

Systemic Conditions Contributing to an Oral Health Problem

A patient with posttraumatic stress disorder, anxiety, or depression may be taking psychoactive medications, many of which can cause dry mouth. As the number of such medications increases, the likelihood of xerostomia greatly increases. Consider the situation in which such a patient presents to the dentist with multiple carious lesions and toothaches, secondary to dry mouth and dietary factors. Eliminating current pain is an urgent priority. After this, however, optimal control of the mental illness and its symptoms is the highest priority for the patient, although preventing long-term dental disease and its associated pain and costs of care are also high priorities. To treat the active caries and reduce the long-term risk of recurrence, the dentist must collaborate with the primary prescriber to consider selection of alternative medications that will be less likely to cause dry mouth while accomplishing the higher-priority goal of managing the patient's mental illness. The pharmacist, with deep expertise in pharmacotherapeutics, can be involved to help solve this difficult problem and offer solutions that will achieve the competing goals for treatment. The dietitian may assist with diet counseling to minimize long-term caries risk. This type of teamwork should be active at the time of the patient's initial evaluation, as expert input is necessary to prioritize treatment goals that will affect the prognosis as well as the dental treatment options available.

Oral Manifestations of Systemic Conditions

Often, the early signs of Sjögren's syndrome or other autoimmune diseases include dry mouth and increased caries activity. The dentist may sometimes be the first healthcare provider to recognize this problem. The dentist then refers the patient to either the primary care medical provider or a medical specialist in rheumatology for evaluation and diagnosis. It will be important to have information about the diagnosis before beginning dental treatment because such information may significantly alter the patient's dental prognosis and the development of an appropriate treatment plan. A team approach allows the dentist to design and prioritize treatment so as to manage all of the relevant complications associated with this disease. The team will probably include an ophthalmologist to treat eye symptoms, a speech and language pathologist to manage swallowing problems, a dietitian to determine an appropriate diet, a rheumatologist to diagnosis and treat the Sjögren's disease itself, and a pharmacist to help select medications and products, such as saliva substitutes, that will optimize salivary function.

Oral Health Problems Associated With Medical Treatment

An example can be seen in the patient who develops mouth pain and ulceration during the course of cancer chemotherapy. With the rest of the oncology team, the dentist helps to identify the source, rule out or treat active dental or other oral disease, and assist the patient in oral hygiene practices and pain management to restore and maintain oral health and facilitate adequate nutritional intake.

Quality of Life and Life Expectancy Concerns

Oral health-related quality of life in patients with cancer can have a major effect on long-term prognosis. Similarly, dysgeusia and other taste disorders are associated with a significant reduction in the quality of life. A persistent bad taste in the mouth often requires a team approach to diagnosis and management. The first step is to determine whether there is an intraoral cause of the bad taste, such as dental caries or periodontal disease. The patient may be convinced that the cause is in the oral cavity—for example, that dental restorations need to be replaced—but in the absence of positive oral findings, the dentist must comprehensively assess the patient, in collaboration with others—for example, otolaryngologists, neurologists, or psychiatrists. The team-based taste disorders clinic includes all of these disciplines, along with dentistry. In another example, patients with a reduced life expectancy may need simplification or modification of the dental treatment plan and a realistic assessment of the effect of dental treatment on their quality of life. This patient may benefit from the psychosocial support of a social worker, mental health worker, religious or spiritual counselor, or psychologist. When death is imminent, hospice care may be appropriate, and the dental treatment plan may be modified to provide urgent treatment of pain and manage other sources of discomfort, such as dry mouth; treatment of active disease not likely to cause pain or infection becomes a low priority.

Treatment Planning

During the course of treatment planning, the dentist may consult with other members of the healthcare team. For example, dental care for the patient with head and neck cancer will be planned in concert with a head and neck tumor board. The dentist plays an integral role in the shared treatment planning, for such a patient and the treatment options and prognosis will often determine what dental treatment will be optimal. For example, the patient who will be treated by resection of a portion of the mandible will have very different dental treatment options than a patient whose primary curative therapy is radiation therapy. The dentist must present the concerns about oral health and their management in a way that can be well understood by other team members to ensure the best treatment plan for the patient can be designed.

For example, the otolaryngologist/head and neck surgeon may recommend surgical treatment of a tumor in the floor of mouth or lateral sides of the tongue to be followed by soft tissue reconstruction that will result in limited tongue mobility and/or a reduction in the depth of the floor of mouth. These treatment side effects can be expected to impede oral hygiene practices and compromise the prognosis of any retained teeth. The dentist and the rest of the healthcare team need this information before any treatment is provided, as extraction of teeth near the surgical site may be necessary to avoid complications. Postsurgical radiation therapy may also be recommended. In this case, any mandibular posterior teeth in the field may need to be extracted because of dental caries, extensive restorations, or periodontal disease, as these conditions increase the risk for postradiation complications, and the affected teeth should be extracted before the radiation for optimal results. The dentist must ensure that the other team members understand the need to extract these teeth before radiation therapy, and ideally these extractions should be planned to be done at the time of the tongue surgery, to ensure adequate surgical access for the extractions. Otherwise, the tumor resection, oral reconstruction, and dental extractions are potentially compromised and the patient's overall prognosis is negatively affected. As much as the rest of the team must understand the dental diagnosis and recommended treatment, the dentist also must not proceed with treatment until all aspects of the patient's overall treatment plan, sequence of care, and overall treatment goals are well defined and understood.

Active Treatment

Through the course of active dental treatment, the dentist may collaborate with other members of the healthcare team to provide an evaluation of the patient's response to treatment—for example, in the case of a diabetic patient, to evaluate response to treatment for periodontal therapy. During treatment, the dentist may also need to consult with other healthcare team members for patients requiring additional medical care. For example, a patient receiving comprehensive dental treatment who suffers from oral-facial pain may need to be referred to other specialists (physical therapist, counseling psychologist, neurologist) or oral health specialists (oral and maxillofacial radiologist, orofacial pain specialist) for management of persistent facial pain before initiation of the rehabilitative phase of the dental treatment.

IN CLINICAL PRACTICE

Interprofessional Collaboration in a Hospital

The most integrated example of IP collaboration in oral healthcare occurs in the hospital dentistry practice setting (although collaborative care involving oral healthcare professionals can and should also occur outside the hospital setting). Dental professionals working in a hospital contribute to team-based decisions in daily practice, in addition to providing care in an environment similar to a private dental practice.

Dental professionals in a hospital setting integrate their practice within the larger scope of collaborative care in several ways. This includes not only inpatient care of admitted patients with a focus on urgent care but also comprehensive outpatient and operating room care of patients with special healthcare needs, head and neck cancer, or congenital anomalies of the head and neck. Hospital dentists have ready access to the use of operating rooms and general anesthesia (GA) experts for those patients unable to tolerate care in a routine outpatient clinic setting. With the use of an electronic health record, they can readily access patient medical data and make thorough medical assessments, as well as communicate with other medical providers. They can rapidly consult with other specialists or emergency services for patients with medical complexity and special healthcare needs, including collaborative services for patients requiring emergency treatment around the clock. Examples of such emergency treatment include significant odontogenic infection, maxillofacial trauma, and posttreatment complications, such as bleeding. Blood products can be ordered, coordinated, and administered relative to the timing of invasive dental procedures. Advanced imaging modalities are accessible for diagnosis and treatment planning. Dental professionals in a hospital setting provide medically necessary dental care and constitute a significant element in collaborative care. The scope of hospital-based dental care is further depicted in eFigure 6.1 found in the expanded chapter on ebooks+.

In the United States, practitioners must obtain clinical privileges for the hospital in which they wish to work. In most instances, postdoctoral training is required to become such a provider. In the United States, this training is typically achieved by participating in a general practice residency (GPR) program. A GPR program not only provides an advanced general dental education but also includes additional training in anesthesiology, pharmacology, operating room procedures, and treatment of medically complex patients. In the hospital setting, verification of healthcare practitioners' credentials and approval of the procedures they are allowed to perform based on these credentials are required to increase patient safety, reduce medical errors, and ensure high-quality healthcare services. **Credentialing** is the process of assessing and confirming the qualifications of a healthcare practitioner. This complex process includes collecting and verifying information about a practitioner, assessing and interpreting the information, and making decisions as to the individual's qualifications. **Privileging** is the process healthcare organizations use in authorizing practitioners to provide specific services to patients. A health center must verify that its licensed or certified healthcare practitioners possess the requisite skills and expertise to manage and treat patients and to perform the procedures that are required to implement the authorized services.[9] Oral health professionals can request hospital privileges in their surrounding practice communities to serve the local populations who would otherwise encounter challenges accessing dental care ranging from those with emergency dental treatment needs such as facial swelling and dentoalveolar trauma to those who cannot tolerate dental care in a routine setting due to medical and/ or behavioral diagnoses.

Maintenance Care

During the maintenance phase of dental treatment, the dentist will collaborate with other healthcare providers to (1) help minimize the risk for recurrent or relapse of oral diseases and (2) minimize the side effects and complications of treatment. In the case of an oral cancer survivor, for example, the dentist shares responsibility for recurrence surveillance with the head and neck surgeon, the medical oncologist, and the radiation oncologist through periodic oral and head and neck examinations and reinforcement of tobacco cessation. A patient who resumes smoking will need to be referred back to a behaviorist and/or pharmacist for tobacco cessation counseling and to the head and neck surgeon for additional biopsies and other diagnostic tests if new oral lesions are detected. Consultation with the pharmacist and other prescribing providers to reduce xerostomia associated with medications and other cancer therapies may also be necessary to ensure continued oral health.

DENTISTRY AS PART OF THE MEDICAL TEAM

A dentist may work with other healthcare providers as part of a collaborative healthcare team that has been assembled to treat patients with complex problems—for example, individuals with craniofacial anomalies. A team assembled to support a cancer clinical trial to treat head and neck cancer with a new agent or technique is another example. In these settings, all patients are assessed and managed by all team members, often with coordinated appointments and regular team meetings, to discuss diagnosis, treatment planning, and outcomes.

The three major reasons that the dentist may be consulted or asked to collaborate in the care of a patient who is being managed primarily by another health professional are as follows:

- Oral disease is contributing to or has the potential to contribute to a general health problem or compromise its treatment.
- During examination, dental issues are detected that raise concerns to a healthcare provider who is not a dentist.
- Specific referrals are made to the dental team for assessment, diagnosis, and treatment.

Oral Disease Contributing to a General Health Problem

The link between oral health and systemic health has been described in great detail in the literature.[10–17] Several systemic diseases may be associated with periodontal disease, for example, including adverse pregnancy outcomes (preterm birth or low birth weight); increased risk of heart attack, stroke, and other cardiovascular events; increased risk of kidney disease; and increased risk of dementia. Oral infection, as occurs with a dental abscess or active periodontal disease, can contribute to systemic infection in an immunocompromised patient who is about to undergo surgery (e.g., cardiac valve replacement) and increase the risk of infective endocarditis. Other healthcare professionals may refer the patient to a dentist to assess whether an oral health problem is contributing to a patient's general health problems. An obstetrician may consult with a dentist concerning a pregnant patient to help ensure an optimal pregnancy outcome, as well as the optimal health of the child after delivery. Halitosis or dysgeusia (bad breath and/or bad taste) can be associated with dental disease but may also be associated with conditions such as sinus infections or digestive problems. After the dentist

has ruled out oral problems, they will need to consult with the patient's primary healthcare provider, who may refer the patient to an otolaryngologist or gastroenterologist for examination and treatment.

Dental Issues That Arise During Examination by a Nondental Healthcare Provider

Oral health is important to overall health. Increasingly, dentistry is included in the primary care setting, and this regular interaction has afforded other health professionals the opportunity to learn more about oral health and its importance. Also, some patients may seek care from another healthcare provider, such as the emergency physician or primary medical provider, for dental complaints, because they have limited access to dental care. Dental problems may also be detected during the course of evaluation for nondental problems—for example, during an annual health maintenance examination.

Common oral conditions that nondental providers will recognize and refer to the dental team include caries, signs and symptoms of periodontal disease, fractured or missing teeth, broken or defective restorations, and limited chewing function or inability to chew properly. Through collaboration with dental team members, other healthcare professionals can be sensitized to recognize that oral health problems contribute to more general issues, such as social isolation and anxiety and poor school performance due to oral pain and oral pathology that may cause an altered facial appearance—for example, facial asymmetry or swelling.

Specific Referrals to the Dental Team

There are many contexts in which referrals are routinely made to the dental team. These include referrals for comprehensive evaluation and treatment—for example, preprocedural oral evaluation or dental clearance, and oral healthcare for patients in supportive care facilities, as well as for management of a specific problem (e.g., evaluation for a potential oral source of systemic infection or oral evaluation in an emergency clinic). These are further described in the following sections.

Preprocedural Oral Evaluation

Providing **dental evaluation and clearance** is a routine practice in areas such as transplant medicine, head and neck oncology, and cardiac surgery to ensure provision of any necessary dental treatment that could minimize the risk of infection and oral complications before such procedures. Whether a patient presents before systemic chemotherapy, bone marrow transplant, full organ transplant, cardiac surgical procedures, or head and neck cancer therapy, dentistry is an integral part of the overall management of the patient. Untreated dental infection or periodontal disease has the potential to compromise the patient's overall health by increasing the risk of systemic or localized infection and sepsis, rejection of grafted organs/tissues, and complications such as **osteoradionecrosis** (ORN) or medication-related osteonecrosis of the jaw (MRONJ). Dental treatment goals and planned treatment must be aligned with the overall treatment goals, as well as the timing and sequencing of the proposed medical treatments. Dental treatment options will depend on the patient's prognosis and the natural history of the disease.

Clear and Timely Communication and Collaboration

Clear and timely communication and collaboration between all of the medical specialties involved is essential in situations in which the potential for morbidity and mortality is high. It is not always possible to execute the disease control phase to completion before medical intervention is necessary and prioritized; however, the dentist is responsible for contributing to the prioritized care needs that may impact the outcome of the medical intervention and the patient's overall health status. The dentist must have a clear understanding of the patient's health status, prognosis, and medical treatment plan before initiating any dental treatment. For example, the patient with end-stage liver disease who is a candidate for liver transplant will be scored using the Model for End-Stage Liver Disease (MELD) score. This score, a predictor of the patient's mortality risk, is used to prioritize care for such individuals. The dentist who is treating such a patient must know the MELD score to understand how much time is available for provision of the necessary dental treatment and the likelihood of the patient's receiving an organ transplant within the next few months. Extensive restorative treatment may not be appropriate for a patient with a high MELD score. Before any invasive dental care, laboratory studies are needed to assess and manage risks, such as the excessive oral bleeding and infection associated with end-stage liver disease. Necessary dental care to treat pain, infection, and active disease must be completed before the medical procedures for the transplant. For example, any oral conditions that pose a risk for infection must be treated before a patient's official listing for organ transplantation.

(NOTE: Refer to eFigure 6.2 for further details regarding the considerations and ordered logistics of providing dental clearance. Healthcare providers may use a specified format to communicate dental clearance status, as well as planned medical treatment decisions. See eFigures 6.2–6.4 for examples in the expanded chapter on ebooks+.)

MRONJ is a possible complication related primarily to the use of intravenous bisphosphonates. The long-term use of oral bisphosphonates poses a risk, as do newer antiresorptive agents.[18] Appropriate patient education and aggressive management of dental disease with invasive dental treatment provided before the start of the medication can help prevent this devastating complication. The entire healthcare team must collaborate to ensure that dental treatment is provided before the initiation of therapy and also that regular oral examination and follow-up are provided to optimize oral health and prevent long-term complications. Decisions to modify medical therapy must be shared by the team that includes the patient, the dentist and/or oral surgeon, and the medical oncologist or endocrinologist.

Oral Health Status in Supportive Care Facilities

Patients who reside in assisted living, nursing home, or group home facilities require a special degree of monitoring and continued assessment of oral health. Collaborative efforts with staff in these facilities, including caregivers, nurses, and physicians who provide care routinely, can improve the oral health status of these patients through preventive education in daily oral hygiene strategies and monitoring for signs and symptoms of pain and infection.

A staff member or health professional may be the most accessible individual and the person most familiar with the patient available to provide screening for oral health problems. The dental team can play a significant role in advocating for appropriate oral health assessments through education and calibration of the direct care staff in these facilities. When a patient has a known oral health diagnosis, a collaborative effort among the dental team, care facility staff, and the patient or their caregiver will be essential. The treatment plan may involve improved oral hygiene, use of a daily fluoride rinse, treatment of oral ulcerations or trauma, monitoring for signs and symptoms of pain after recent dental treatment, and even maintenance of removable prostheses.

These patients may express concerns relating to esthetics, function, or other problems; they may be unable to communicate that they have oral pain or tolerate routine daily oral care owing to cognitive or physical limitations; or they may exhibit uncooperative or combative behavior. (See Chapters 13, 16 and 18 for further details on this topic.)

Evaluation for Possible Oral Source of Infection

This type of evaluation may most often occur in a hospital setting, and as a result of the severity and urgency of the patient's condition, the oral health professional may be consulted regarding a possible source of infection in the oral cavity. A patient may present with a fever of unknown origin or an altered mental status, and an oral cause of infection may become the identified source. Similarly, a patient may present with a serious, life-threatening sepsis of unknown source, and culture of blood-borne bacteria may suggest an oral origin of the infection—for example, *Streptococcus*. In this situation, the medical team, including infectious disease specialists and critical care medicine providers, will rely on the dental team to identify the source of the infection and treat it appropriately. This process will require ongoing dialogue between the dentist, infectious disease specialist, and pharmacist to determine an optimal antibiotic therapy. If the patient has other medical and/or social problems, each of the healthcare professionals responsible for their care may be involved in the long-term management of these problems.

Oral Evaluation in an Emergency Medicine Setting

Patients may present to a hospital emergency department (ED) with a chief concern related to the teeth, periodontium, jaws, or other oral structures or tissues. Common concerns include pain, infection, dentoalveolar trauma, and bleeding. The perspective and accessibility of a dentist can aid in the evaluation and treatment of a patient with emergency oral treatment needs. Procedures that are commonly carried out by the dental team in a hospital emergency setting include the following:

- Identification of an oral source of infection and management with intravenous or oral antibiotic therapy.
- Incision and drainage of an oral abscess.
- Splinting or stabilization of traumatized teeth.
- Pulpal management of fractured teeth.
- Achieving hemostasis in a patient with oral bleeding.

It is important to recognize that patients may have avoided seeking treatment in a dental office because of lack of funds or fear and anxiety. It may not be possible, or even appropriate, to execute definitive dental treatment in the ED. Nevertheless, the oral health professional can play a pivotal role in the assessment and diagnosis of the patient's oral problems and make treatment recommendations regarding both acute phase (see Chapter 9) and long-term (see Chapter 11) definitive treatment. If the ED has a dental component, some urgent care dental treatment, such as pulp extirpation, simple extraction, or a provisional restoration, can be provided on site by the dentist or dental team. This lessens the burden on medical colleagues who may not have the expertise to provide these services.

CONDITIONS BEST MANAGED BY AN INTERPROFESSIONAL TEAM THAT INCLUDES DENTISTRY

This section discusses six conditions that are best managed by an IP team that includes dentistry. The first two are often administratively organized around all-inclusive regular IP team meetings (e.g., the head and neck oncology tumor board or the craniofacial and cleft lip/palate team). Typical members of these teams are listed in Box 6.3.

Head and Neck Cancer

The dental team plays an essential role in recognizing, diagnosing, treating, and managing follow-up for patients with oral cancer and is solely responsible for managing and treating any dental problems for the patient throughout this process. The following discussion delineates the sequential roles of the general dentist and dental specialists and highlights the ways in which those roles are integrated with those of other IP team members.

BOX 6.3   Examples of Specialties Involved in Organized Collaborative Team Care

Example 1: Head and Neck Tumor Board
Oral and maxillofacial surgery
Otolaryngology
General dentistry
Maxillofacial prosthodontics
Radiology
Radiation oncology
Medical oncology
Speech and language pathology
Social work

Example 2: Craniofacial, Cleft Lip/Palate Multidisciplinary Team
Oral and maxillofacial surgery
Plastic surgery
Pediatric/general dentistry/orthodontics
Maxillofacial prosthodontics
Audiology
Nutrition
Speech and language pathology
Social work

Initial Recognition of Oral Cancer

The American Dental Association reports that 60% of the US population sees a dentist once a year. These visits provide an excellent opportunity for a thorough head and neck cancer screening. According to the National Cancer Institute, as of 2011 there were an estimated 281,591 people living with oral cavity and pharyngeal cancer in the United States. There were an estimated 42,440 new diagnoses of oral cavity and pharyngeal cancer in 2014, which represents 2.5% of all new cancer cases. This represents 11 new cases per 100,000 men and women per year. Head and neck cancers have an approximate 5-year survival rate of 62.7%. These survival rates are contingent on the cancer stage at diagnosis, a categorization that refers to the extent of a cancer in the body. Extent may be described as localized, regional, distant, or unknown. Early diagnosis, especially at the local stage, can lead to survival rates of up to 82.6%.[19]

Referral for Definitive Diagnosis and Treatment of Oral Cancer

The dental team should arrange for appropriate referrals when head and neck cancer is suspected. With many intraoral and perioral cancers, the oral and maxillofacial surgeon is often the first resource when a biopsy of a suspicious lesion is necessary. Lesions found on the skin of the face, neck, or scalp may be referred to a dermatologist or plastic surgeon for evaluation and treatment. Suspicious lesions in the pharynx or changes in the voice may be referred directly to an otolaryngologist (ear, nose, throat [ENT] surgeon) or to the patient's primary healthcare provider. The written referral should describe the appearance and location of the lesion, the length of time the patient has been aware of it, and any other symptoms. The results of any tests or treatment performed by the dental team should also be included.

The dental professional should notify the PCP of the cancer diagnosis and any specialist referrals that have been and are being made. The referring dentist should follow-up with the specialist to confirm the diagnosis and proposed plan of care. The general dentist will need to be available to answer patient questions. Patients will often ask the dental team about what to expect if the lesion is found to be malignant. Although the dentist will not be providing definitive cancer treatment, they will play a supportive role during the course of therapy. If a complete management team is not already in place, the dentist may appropriately provide additional referrals to a psychologist, medical social worker, or other health professionals and support groups. For the distraught, anxious patient facing a potentially life-threatening event, the compassionate professionalism provided by the dental team can be invaluable.

Treatment for cancer often involves a multidisciplinary team. Such teams, usually found at major teaching hospitals or academic health centers, are often called a **tumor board** and typically include a medical oncologist, radiation oncologist, and surgical specialist. For head and neck cancer patients, the team would include an oral and maxillofacial surgeon or an ENT surgeon. Often, a maxillofacial prosthodontist or general dentist is also included. Team-based decision making provides the foundation for developing the next steps in a patient's head and neck cancer care.

Planning Dental Treatment After Diagnosis of Head and Neck Cancer

Once the diagnosis of head and neck cancer has been made, the dental team, in collaboration with the other health professionals, will need to treat the cancer and provide long-term rehabilitative and preventive care for the patient. These patients present unique challenges for the dental team from the time of the initial visit through the diagnosis and treatment planning phases, and continuing through the remaining years of life. Throughout the process of treatment, rehabilitation, and maintenance, the dental team fills a pivotal role. Both the patient and dentist must be knowledgeable about the short- and long-term effects of the cancer and its treatments. Often, there are difficult treatment choices to be made—selecting from among multiple options, all with serious potential hazards and complications. Helping the patient to select from among several challenging treatment choices can be intellectually taxing and emotionally wrenching, but is also an integral part of being a holistic healthcare provider.

The dental patient diagnosed with head and neck cancer should have a complete dental assessment in preparation for treatment. A comprehensive dental examination, including radiographs and periodontal assessment, will be necessary to determine the extent of dental care necessary before the start of cancer therapy.[20-24] The presence of untreated oral disease can increase the risk of adverse effects from the cancer therapy.

As part of the dental treatment planning process, even the patient without dental disease must be informed of the transient and residual adverse effects of cancer therapies on both the hard and soft oral tissues. The edentulous patient should receive a dental examination before cancer therapies, including panoramic radiographs to identify any residual roots, impacted teeth, or cysts. Precancer treatment concerns, such as denture sores, candidiasis, bony exostoses, and tori, may be identified in the edentulous patient.[22,25,26] After a comprehensive assessment of the patient's oral condition has been made, treatment planning for pre- and postcancer therapy can be addressed. Factors to be considered in planning urgent dental treatment for a patient with oral cancer must include the dental examination findings, head and neck cancer prognosis, head and neck cancer treatment plan and potential adverse effects, and individual characteristics of the patient.

The patient's dental history and motivation are important factors to consider when planning dental treatment. A patient's financial situation may also affect dental treatment decisions because it will affect the individual's ability to maintain their teeth after cancer therapy.[20,22,23] Even the patient who is normally diligent with oral hygiene measures and regularly seeks routine dental care can be expected to be less diligent with personal oral care during this difficult time of cancer therapy. After successful cancer treatment, some long-term adverse effects, such as limited mouth opening and discomfort, may make oral hygiene a challenge. In addition, the change in the quantity and composition of saliva greatly increases susceptibility to dental caries. This is especially critical for the patient who has a history of dental caries and multiple restorations and/or endodontic therapy. Even a patient who has previously had a low incidence of dental caries may develop radiation caries after cancer therapy.

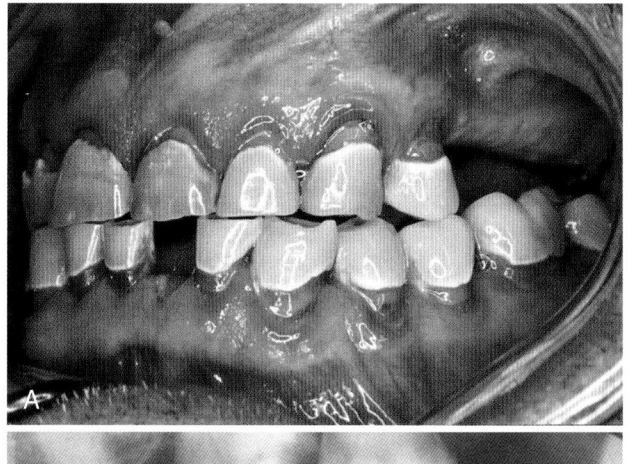
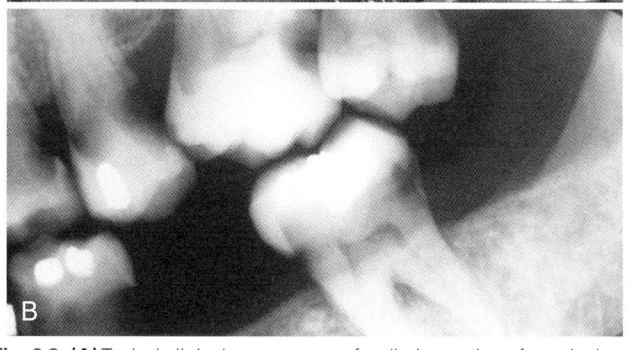

Fig. 6.2 **(A)** Typical clinical appearance of radiation caries of cervical and incisal surfaces. **(B)** Typical radiographic appearance of radiation caries. (From Hupp JR, Ellis E, Tucker MR. Contemporary Oral and Maxillofacial Surgery. St. Louis: Mosby; 2014.)

Carious lesions may be found encircling the cervical surfaces of the teeth and on the incisal edges, as seen in Figure 6.2. These rapidly progressing carious lesions affect all remaining teeth, not just those in the field of radiation. This condition is attributed to an alteration of the saliva's buffering capacity, resulting in an acidic change in the patient's saliva.[20]

The type and location of the head and neck cancer are also important for dental treatment planning. The cell type and stage of the cancer will determine what therapies will be necessary and adverse effects that can be expected. Some head and neck cancers are treated with only local surgical excision, whereas others may require a combination of modalities (surgery, chemotherapy, and/or radiation therapy). The location and extent of the cancer will determine the dose and area of exposure to radiation therapy. The dentist needs to know which, if any, teeth will be in the field of radiation and whether the salivary glands will be affected. This must be communicated before initiation of radiation therapy. For example, a total radiation dose of less than 5500 cGy to the mandible is not associated with the same high risk of ORN as would be found with doses higher than 6500 cGy to the same area. In advanced stages of head and neck cancer, the prognosis for the patient's survival should be considered. In very advanced cancers, the treatment may be planned only to palliate symptoms. In these patients, the dental treatment plan may be primarily focused on pain management and the treatment of infection rather than on future oral rehabilitation.

The potential adverse effects of each type of cancer therapy must be taken into account in planning dental care. This is especially important for potentially permanent changes that will affect future dental treatment. Examples of adverse effects from cancer surgery or radiation therapy that may limit future prosthetic treatment options include oral structural changes caused by loss of hard or soft tissues or limited ability to open the mouth. Severe xerostomia may also follow surgery or radiation therapy and can lead to the development of caries and difficulty wearing dental prostheses. See eFigure 6.4C, Radiation Therapy Template, in the expanded chapter on ebooks+.

Coordinating Dental Care in Patients Before Cancer Therapy

Any urgent dental treatment should be provided without delaying the onset of therapy for the cancer. It is critical that any invasive dental treatment be performed as soon as possible because the oral cavity must be given time to heal after dental treatment and before initiation of chemotherapy or radiation therapy. Early involvement of the dental team ensures optimal planning and timing of dental treatment before cancer treatment, so as to prevent debilitating complications, such as pain and oral infections.

An essential goal of dental treatment before any cancer therapy is to eliminate oral sources of bacteria and dental infection, such as periodontal disease, pericoronitis, and periapical pathosis.[20,23,24] If chemotherapy is planned to treat the head and neck cancer, infection should be eliminated before the onset of chemotherapy because the agents used can cause the patient to become immunocompromised. In some cases, the patient may only need a dental prophylaxis, but any teeth with significant periodontal disease involvement should be extracted. This would include teeth at risk for an acute periodontal infection—for example, teeth with periodontal pockets 6 mm or larger, and those that are grossly mobile or have alveolar bone loss involving the furcation. Carious teeth need to be restored or removed. If there is a question of the caries involving the pulp, the tooth should be extracted to minimize the risk of continued or recurrent pulpal infection. Teeth with periapical pathology should be more strongly considered for extraction rather than performing initial or retreatment root canal therapy.[24] There are, however, exceptions to this recommendation. These include the patient who may not require chemoradiation therapy, the patient who is highly motivated to retain and maintain their dentition and demonstrates excellent oral hygiene, and the patient with abutment teeth that are or will be important for retention of a current or future prosthesis.

If the cancer therapy plan includes radiation therapy with or without surgery and/or chemotherapy, the dental treatment may need to be more aggressive, especially for a patient who has a history of poor oral hygiene practices and sporadic dental care. In areas of irradiated bone, a significantly increased risk is associated with the development of dental infection or complications after the extraction of teeth—most notably, ORN can be anticipated. In addition to extractions for caries, pulpal disease, or periodontal disease, as described previously, any other teeth with questionable long-term prognoses in the areas affected by radiation should be removed. In determining prognosis, the dentist must remember that even a patient with very good hygiene and regular dental visits will have great difficulty preventing radiation caries. Patient motivation is crucial, as is the patient's dental history. A significant change in the patient's habits is highly unlikely. Current dietary sugar intake, effectiveness of personal oral hygiene practices, and frequency of visits to the dental office must all be taken into account. Ideally, atraumatic extractions, alveoloplasty, and removal of exostoses should be performed using primary surgical closure. It is advisable to prescribe an antibiotic for patients with an acute infection at the time of oral surgery or at risk for infection during healing.[20,27] Patients who have an implant-supported dental prosthesis at the time of cancer diagnosis will need to have the metal components of the prosthesis removed before radiation therapy to prevent increasing the radiation dose to adjacent tissues as a result of radiation scatter. Healing caps may be placed on the osseointegrated implant fixture.[20] Often, the onset of radiation therapy is planned to begin within 6 weeks after cancer surgery. A delay in beginning this therapy can reduce the chances for cure and survival. Oral surgery must be completed at least 14 to 21 days before onset of radiation therapy to allow adequate time for soft tissue healing.[20,23,24,27] If at all possible, any oral infection should be eliminated before the onset of radiation therapy. Unfortunately, such a patient may be severely debilitated, have a poor prognosis or rapidly progressive disease, and require an immediate start of radiotherapy.

If any teeth are retained, the patient needs to be aware of the critical importance of maintaining oral health during and after cancer therapy. Before initiation of radiation therapy, radiation guards or a tongue-depressing stent should be provided to patients with metal restorations and must be coordinated to be delivered before the planning session for radiation therapy. As with any highly caries-prone dental patient, the fabrication of fluoride trays and initiation of daily home fluoride treatment is indicated. Patients are instructed to apply a 1.1% neutral pH sodium fluoride gel for 5 minutes daily. Fluoride treatment should be begun before cancer therapy, continued throughout cancer therapy, and considered for maintenance as well. Study casts may be necessary for constructing surgical stents or obturators, or for planning of future prosthetic rehabilitation.[20,25]

Supportive Dental Care During Cancer Therapy

Maintaining oral hygiene and monitoring for adverse effects are two of the more important tasks to be implemented during cancer therapy. Side effects such as **mucositis** (the development of painful mouth sores), trismus, and xerostomia may develop during treatment. Many patients will be uncomfortable performing their usual oral hygiene regimens. Normal oral hygiene routines may cause excessive gingival bleeding, and the patient may only be able to tolerate oral rinses during this time. Encourage the patient to continue with the regimen for oral care using a soft toothbrush, antimicrobial oral rinses, and fluoride trays. An alternative to toothbrushing is to use wet gauze or sponge-tipped swabs to gently wipe plaque and debris from the teeth and gums. Dietary counseling is also important during this phase of treatment. Caloric and protein intake must be monitored and maintained during cancer therapy.

Many prescribed dietary supplements have high concentrations of sucrose in a thick liquid that adheres to teeth. Patient education in oral hygiene is critical so as not to increase risk of dental disease.

Symptomatic care is continued as necessary. In the absence of infection, mucositis usually resolves within 2 to 4 weeks after completion of cancer therapy. Healing of oral tissue after radiation treatment may take as long as 6 weeks. Periodic oral examinations to evaluate the condition of the mucosa are needed. Any complication, such as an exposed bone spicule, should be treated promptly. It is helpful to review the potential signs and symptoms of adverse effects with the patient and their caregiver.

Coordinating Dental Care After Cancer Therapy

After cancer therapy, the dentist continues to serve in an essential, often central, role, helping the patient to maintain optimal oral health, managing any oral complications or problems that arise, alerting other members of the healthcare team to any medical complications or recurrence of the cancer, and providing (or supporting the provision of) long-term prosthodontic reconstruction and oral rehabilitation. Treated successfully, these patients will value and appreciate a return to oral health, masticatory function, and an improved quality of life. Reconstruction of an esthetically problematic facial disfigurement can allow the individual to return to a more normal routine with an improved self-image and renewed purpose for living.

Prosthetic Rehabilitation

Replacement of teeth may be indicated for patients who have received therapy for head and neck cancer. Prosthetic devices replacing both hard and soft tissue may be used to restore function and improve esthetics. This may include medically necessary maxillofacial prosthetics, such as a maxillary obturator, a mandibular resection prosthesis, and/or a palatal augmentation prosthesis, which may be retained or supported by natural teeth, the residual edentulous alveolus, or, in certain scenarios, dental implants. In planning prosthetic rehabilitation, the overall oral condition must first be evaluated, and the prosthesis should be specifically designed and maintained to minimize mucosal trauma and irritation while optimizing speech, chewing, and swallowing functions. Such prosthetic rehabilitation can restore both form as well as function, improving nutrition, and restoring a sense of normalcy (see Figure. 6.3 for an example of a maxillary obturator prosthesis).

Long-Term Follow-Up: Maintenance and Surveillance

Scheduling regular dental appointments with the dental team is extremely important for patients who have been diagnosed and treated for head and neck cancer. The reasons include maintaining oral health, preventing oral disease, and monitoring for complications or recurrence of the cancer. A close follow-up of head and neck cancer patients is crucial to ensure diagnosis of a recurrence at an early stage (Figure. 6.4). The patient and dental team must keep this in mind at each recall visit. Head and neck cancer recurrences have a much less favorable prognosis than the original disease and require more aggressive treatment. The patient may need additional surgery, chemotherapy, or radiation

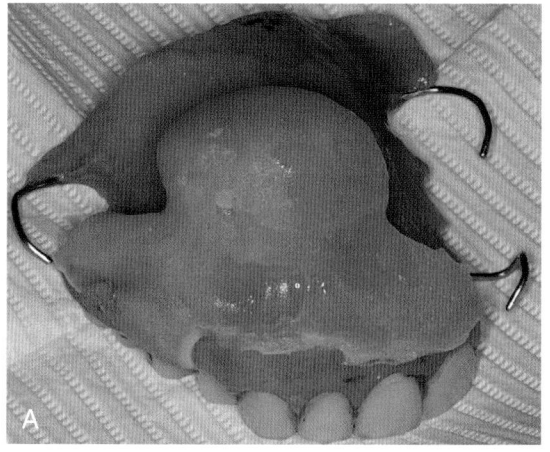
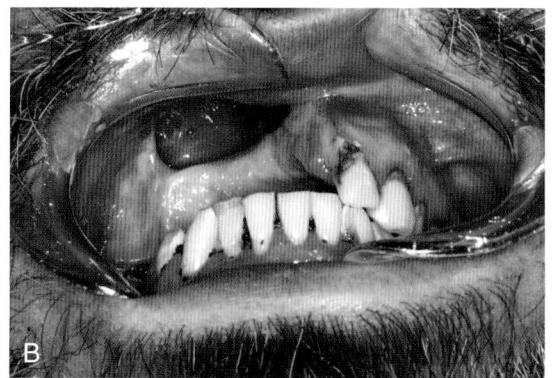
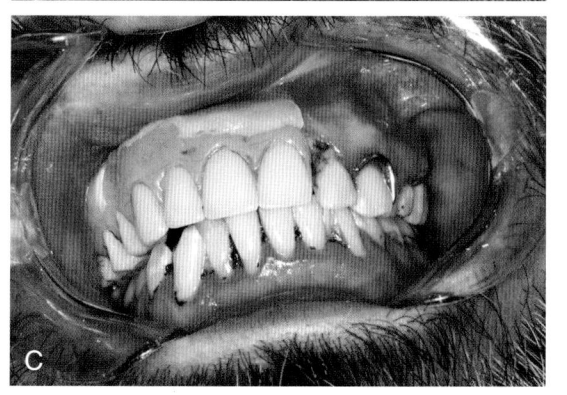

Fig. 6.3 An example of an obturator used to restore a maxillary defect in a patient after cancer surgery. **(A)** Partial denture with obturator bulb. **(B)** Postsurgical defect. **(C)** Obturator in place, restoring appearance, speech, and masticatory function. (Courtesy Dr. Samuel Zwetchkenbaum.)

therapy, or a combination of these therapies. The dental team should be vigilant to ensure provision of an early diagnosis and to prepare the patient for any additional cancer therapy if recurrence occurs. Edentulous patients, in particular, must be seen for regular oral examinations to evaluate the condition of the soft tissue and monitor for disease or complications of previous therapy. Patients wearing removable prosthetics may have an increased risk of ulcerations caused by decreased quality and quantity of saliva. Without adequate saliva, the friction of the denture base against the mucosa increases; soft liners, therefore, are to be avoided, and special attention should be given to the fit of the denture, especially in undercut areas.

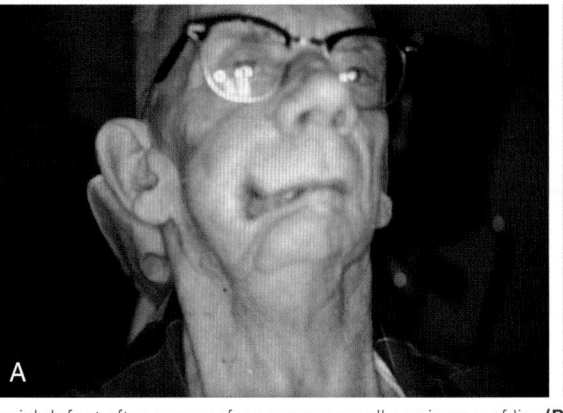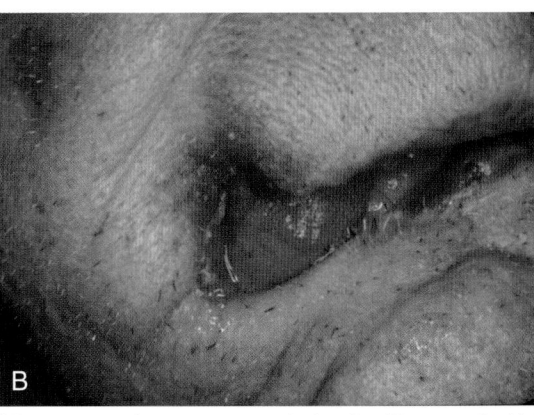

Fig. 6.4 **(A)** Facial defect after surgery for squamous cell carcinoma of lip. **(B)** Recurrence of cancer on anterior border. (Courtesy Dr. H. Dean Millard, Ann Arbor, MI)

It is also the standard of care that the treating nondental care provider will also perform routine surveillance evaluations to monitor for recurrence and manage any associated medical complications that may emerge. There may be other health professionals who can help the patient cope with issues of facial disfigurement, changes in personal relationships, ability to function in society, and financial consequences of the cancer and its treatment. In these cases, the dentist plays a particular role on the team with the other health professionals who contribute to the patient's cancer care.

Cleft Palate/Craniofacial Anomalies

The cleft palate/craniofacial (CP/CF) team provides expert, coordinated, collaborative, and comprehensive care for patients with congenital and acquired craniofacial anomalies and also collaborates with the patient's community-based healthcare providers, including the family dentist. Because these problems are less common and are complex and often unique, the healthcare providers' experience and special expertise greatly affect patient outcomes. Furthermore, coordinated care is essential to maximize patient safety and quality of care. Most CP/CF teams are located in tertiary care children's hospitals, often in larger cities or university communities, where the team can provide the care necessary to reconstruct the anatomic defects and coordinate plastic and reconstructive surgery, otolaryngology, and oral surgical care with dentistry, nursing and dietetics, and the anesthesiology team.

There are two primary roles for the CP/CF team:
- *Provide expert coordinated care for complex problems.* Most surgical and surgical/orthodontic treatment, prosthodontic rehabilitation, and subspecialty medical care is provided by the team at the children's hospital. Social workers and psychologists/mental health professionals play an important role in providing support to the patient and their family during the treatment and recovery period and between surgeries. To reduce the risks associated with general anesthesia, efforts are made to perform several necessary surgical procedures during a single operation (e.g., ear tube placements, dental extractions, and lip revision surgery).
- *Provide shared treatment plan recommendations for providers* who will treat the child in the community—for example,

pediatric or general dentistry, orthodontics, school-based speech and language pathology, and primary pediatrics. The CP/CF team typically sees the patient once yearly for a periodic assessment. During this visit, which may require several hours, the various team members assess the patient, perform diagnostic imaging and other tests, and then meet to share their findings and recommendations and negotiate a final treatment plan. This plan is communicated to the patient and the patient's family and to the patient's primary healthcare providers—for example, the general dentist, pediatrician or family doctor, and school speech and language pathologist.

The child with cleft lip/palate will typically undergo several surgeries, sometimes beginning in the first 3 postnatal months, to support feeding and parental bonding with the infant, and then periodically throughout childhood and adolescence. Surgery is planned to coincide with critical stages of growth and development to repair the lip, close the palate, place bone grafts in the site of the cleft, place dental implants to replace missing teeth, and, in some cases, perform orthognathic surgery to facilitate proper function and esthetics, as well as soft tissue surgical revisions to the lip and nose. The orthodontist teams with the oral and maxillofacial surgeon and plastic and reconstructive surgeon to coordinate tooth movement and jaw surgery. Clinical psychologists and developmental pediatrics specialists work with the families to prepare the individual and their family for these difficult surgeries and postoperative challenges, and to provide support for the child's overall growth and development. At each step of the way, good oral health will be critical to the long-term success of the treatment.

Oral health must be established and maintained to support complete rehabilitation of these anomalies. Dental infections and active disease must be controlled before surgery to minimize postoperative complications. Dental care may be provided by a pediatric dentist or a general dentist who is a member of the team, but in many cases this care is provided by a dentist in the community, under the guidance and recommendations of the CP/CF team. Recall and routine dental care can be safely provided by the patient's own community dentist, but they must know when to contact the CP/CF team to better understand the long-term plan for the patient or discuss problems detected that must be addressed by the team.

Temporomandibular Joint Disorders/Orofacial Pain

Orofacial pain and headaches are often diagnosed and managed by a team, including a general dentist or orofacial pain specialist, neurologist, physiatrist (a specialist in rehabilitative medicine), physical therapist, and clinical or behavioral psychologist. Patients with chronic facial pain, either posttrauma or as a component of a complex chronic pain syndrome such as fibromyalgia, will often benefit from a multidisciplinary approach to pain management and rehabilitation. For example, a patient who presents with a chief concern of jaw pain and headache after a motor vehicle accident (MVA) may require treatment by the dentist, physical therapist, and counseling psychologist/behaviorist. Once neurologic pathology is ruled out by the neurologist, the dentist will rule out or treat dental causes for the pain and diagnose the source of the jaw pain through a comprehensive assessment of the patient, including diagnostic imaging of the temporomandibular joints (TMJs) and associated structures provided by an oral and maxillofacial radiologist. The physical therapist can help the patient improve range of motion and reduce pain through a combination of therapies that may include spray and stretch exercise, massage, and postural education. The counseling psychologist can identify coexisting mental health conditions that may contribute to the patient's pain experience or interfere with recovery and provide cognitive behavioral therapy and stress management to help the patient cope with the pain, as appropriate, or recommend referral to a psychiatrist for diagnosis and medical management of underlying depression or anxiety. If medication is needed to help manage pain, and the patient is already being treated for chronic pain and/or a mental health disorder, it will be desirable for one prescriber to provide the pharmacotherapy required to manage all of the patient's pain complaints to avoid complications associated with drug interactions or the development of dependence/abuse of opiate analgesics. The dentist must work with this provider if acute dental problems and treatment require short-term opiate analgesics. The dentist or a prosthodontist may provide occlusal appliance therapy. In some cases, the dentist may lead the team in the assessment and management of such patients; in other cases, the neurologist or general physician may lead and coordinate care. Some dental schools and medical centers have established facial pain clinics that provide IP team-based care for patients with complex orofacial pain conditions. The comprehensive diagnosis and shared treatment plan, developed with the patient at the center, anchor the care of patients with chronic and/or complex facial pain conditions.

Obstructive Sleep Apnea

Multiple risk factors associated with obstructive sleep apnea (OSA) may be identified by an oral health provider, including body mass index (BMI) and/or neck circumference that is larger than normal, irritability and difficulty concentrating on tasks, daytime sleepiness, snoring, cardiovascular disease, and retrognathia. The oral health provider may identify these signs and symptoms and recommend consultation with a sleep specialist to establish a diagnosis. The diagnosis can be determined with a sleep study that records the number and extent of apneic or hypoxic events, measured in terms of an apneic hypoxic index (AHI). Standard treatment includes the use of a nocturnal continuous positive airway pressure (CPAP) device, but surgical intervention may also be considered. For patients who may be unable to tolerate a CPAP device or who would prefer to avoid an invasive surgery, an oral appliance may be an alternative treatment. In that case, the sleep specialist or primary physician may also refer the patient to a dentist with advanced expertise in sleep dentistry for this therapy. The efficacy of the appliance is tested with a posttreatment sleep study, and further modifications may be necessary (eFigure 6.5). Long-term surveillance by the dentist is recommended to monitor the patient for changes in efficacy of the prosthesis, alterations of the patient's occlusion due to regular mandibular protrusion and need for adjustment or eventual replacement.

Head and Neck Trauma (Gunshot, Explosion, Motor Vehicle Crash)

Multidisciplinary care of the head and neck trauma patient is essential in optimizing and achieving a stable and functional result. A surgical service with specialization in the head and neck, such as oral and maxillofacial surgery, otolaryngology, or plastic surgery, is essential if the patient has sustained facial trauma, skull or jaw fractures, lacerations, or compromised airway. Neurology may also be critical if the patient has sustained neurologic or brain damage. The dental professional may not be consulted early in critical care but has an important role to play in assessment of the dentition and occlusion. Stabilization of a fractured maxilla or mandible requires the expertise of a dentist to determine a stable and functional occlusion for fixation. Nonrestorable teeth may pose the risk of aspiration in the traumatized patient and should be extracted as soon as possible. Such extraction will also minimize the risk for infection in the fixated patient. Traumatized patients requiring significant and urgent reconstruction will benefit from the dentist's specialized knowledge of the maxilla-mandibular relationship of the jaws if no other anatomic landmarks are available owing to the extent of the trauma. After stabilization of the patient's trauma status, rehabilitation often requires intraoral and extraoral maxillofacial prosthodontic treatment to optimize form and function. Specialists involved may also include a maxillofacial prosthodontist, an anaplastologist, and an ocularist.

Combined Treatment in an Operating Room Setting

General anesthesia in an operating room setting can provide safe and predictable treatment of patients who are unable to tolerate care in a routine clinic setting or who require complicated or invasive procedures. Medically complex patients may require a general anesthetic if a systemic disease condition is unstable or if the provision of blood products may be necessary. Although surgical repair of a cleft lip and wide local excision of an oral cancer are obvious examples, comprehensive dental treatment in an operating room setting is also possible, especially for those patients with cognitive or physical impairments, mental illness, severe anxiety, or trismus.

GA is associated with medical risk, even for healthy patients. Performing multiple procedures at the same operation under

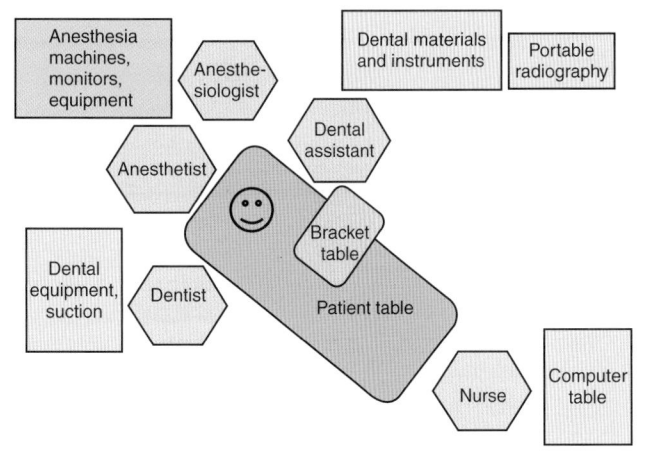

Fig. 6.5 The arrangement of a typical operating room theater for dental treatment.

GA can help minimize these risks by limiting the number of episodes of GA. Since the onset of the COVID-19 pandemic, combining procedures has become essential to reduce necessary time spent in the healthcare setting as well as decrease the need for duplicate preoperative preparations, including preoperative viral tests. Additional infection control procedures, including high-level personal protective equipment is often required for intubation and extubation procedures by an anesthesiology clinician like dental care that involves aerosols. Some medical procedures can be safely performed along with oral surgery and dental treatment. Examples of coordinated care include placement of ear tubes, performing a gynecologic examination, obtaining advanced imaging, and even trimming finger and toenails. The operating room theater for a typical dental case is exhibited in Figure 6.5.

CONCLUSION

This chapter has described ways in which dental treatment planning and delivery of care are performed in the context of an IP team-based collaborative approach. Around the world and in the United States and Canada, integrated collaborative care models are emerging that include dentistry as an essential component. In addition to providing comprehensive oral healthcare and coordinating multidisciplinary dental treatment (*intra*professional collaboration), the dentist must work collaboratively with other health professionals, family members, and caregivers to develop a mutually acceptable dental treatment plan centered on the patient's needs and values. Some patients, especially the frail elderly and those with craniofacial anomalies, cancer, or complex chronic illnesses, receive ongoing care from a wide variety of healthcare providers, including dentists. These patients are particularly well served by an IP model of care and coordinated treatment planning.

IP education and IPC aim to improve healthcare systematically through improved outcomes, improved patient experiences, reduced costs, and enhanced satisfaction of healthcare workers ("Quadruple Aim" for healthcare improvement).[3] In the past, dental care has been provided primarily in a delivery system external to the medical healthcare system. New and emerging public health models include dentistry as an integral branch of healthcare teams responsible for the health of an increasingly medically complex patient population. All health professionals on the team must recognize and value the role and responsibilities of each provider. Team-based care requires this interdependence and a certain essential openness and flexibility to meet the challenge of synchronizing varying perspectives on the patient's healthcare needs and requirements.

REFERENCES

1. Government of Canada Publications. Building on values: the future of health care in Canada. https://publications.gc.ca/site/eng/237274/publication.html. Accessed August 12, 2021.
2. Institute for Healthcare Improvement. The Triple Aim or the Quadruple Aim? Four points to help set your strategy. http://www.ihi.org/communities/blogs/the-triple-aim-or-the-quadruple-aim-four-points-to-help-set-your-strategy. Accessed August 12, 2021.
3. Craig C, Eby D, Whittington J. *Care coordination model: better care at lower cost for people with multiple health and social needs*. *IHI Innovation Series*. Cambridge, MA: Institute for Healthcare Improvement; 2011. http://www.ihi.org/resources/Pages/IHIWhitePapers/IHICareCoordinationModelWhitePaper.aspx. Accessed August 12, 2021.
4. Interprofessional Education Collaborative. *Core Competencies for Interprofessional Collaborative Practice: 2016 Update*. Washington, DC: Interprofessional Education Collaborative; 2016. https://ipec.memberclicks.net/assets/2016-Update.pdf. Accessed August 12, 2021..
5. Rudman W, Hart-Hester S, Jones W, Caputo N, Madison M. Integrating medical and dental records. A new frontier in health information management. *J AHIMA*. 2010;81(10):36–39.
6. Nelson S, Tassone M, Hodges B. *Creating the Healthcare Team of the Future: The Toronto Model of Interprofessional Education and Practice*. Ithaca, NY: Cornell University Press; 2014.
7. American Association of Nurse Anesthetists (AANA). Certified registered nurse anesthetists fact sheet. https://www.aana.com/membership/become-a-crna/crna-fact-sheet. Accessed August 12, 2021.
8. Academy of Nutrition and Dietetics. Certified registered nurse anesthetists fact sheet. http://www.eatrightpro.org/resources/about-us/what-is-an-rdn-and-dtr/what-is-a-registered-dietitian-nutritionist. Accessed August 12, 2021.
9. Lockhart PB. *Oral Medicine and Medically Complex Patients*. 6th ed. Ames, IA: Wiley-Blackwell; 2013.
10. Chapter 5: clinical staffing—HRSA program requirements. https://bphc.hrsa.gov/programrequirements/compliancemanual/chapter-5.html. Accessed October 10, 2021.
11. Otomo-Corgel J, Pucher JJ, Rethamn MP, Reynolds MA. State of the science: chronic periodontitis and systemic health. *J Evid Based Dent Pract*. 2012;12(suppl 3):20–28.
12. Teles R, Wang C-Y. Mechanisms involved in the association between periodontal disease and cardiovascular disease. *Oral Dis*. 2011;17(5):450–461.
13. De Souza CM, Braosi AP, Luczyszyn SM, et al. Association among oral health parameters, periodontitis and its treatment and mortality in patients undergoing hemodialysis. *J Periodontol*. 2014;85(6):169–178.
14. Lee CF, Lin CL, Lin MC, Lin SY, et al. Surgical treatment for periodontal disease reduces risk of end-stage renal disease: a

nationwide population-based retrospective cohort study. *J Periodontol.* 2014;85(1):50–56.

15. Sanz M, Kornman K. working group 3 of the joint EFP/AAP workshop. Periodontitis and adverse pregnancy outcomes: consensus report of the Joint EFP/AAP Workshop on Periodontitis and Systemic Diseases. *J Periodontol.* 2013;84 (suppl 4):S164–S169.

16. Holtfreyer B, Empen K, Glaser S, et al. Periodontitis is associated with endothelial dysfunction in a general population: a cross-sectional study. *PLoS One.* 2013;8(12):e84603.

17. Mawardi HH, Elbadawi LS, Sonis ST. Current understanding of the relationship between periodontal and systemic diseases. *Saudi Med J.* 2015;36(2):150–158.

18. Ruggiero SL, Dodson TB, Fantasia J, et al. Medication-related osteonecrosis of the jaw—2022 update. American Association of Oral and Maxillofacial Surgeons: Special Committee on Medication-Related Osteonecrosis of the Jaws. https://www. aaoms.org/docs/govt_affairs/advocacy_white_papers/mronj_ position_paper.pdf. Accessed October 19, 2022.

19. National Cancer Institute. Surveillance, Epidemiology, and End Results Program (SEER) stats fact sheets: oral cavity and pharynx cancer. http://seer.cancer.gov/statfacts/html/oralcav.html. Accessed August 12, 2021.

20. Silverman S. *American Cancer Society Atlas of Clinical Oncology: Oral Cancer.* 5th ed. Hamilton, ON: BC Decker; 2003.

21. DeWitt KD, Lee N. Benign and malignant lesions of the oral cavity, oropharynx, and nasopharynx. In: Lalwani AK, ed. *Current Diagnosis and Treatment in Otolaryngology—Head and Neck Surgery.* New York: Lange Medical Books/McGraw-Hill; 2004.

22. Lockhart PB, Clark J. Pretherapy dental status of patients with malignant conditions of the head and neck. *Oral Surg Oral Med Oral Pathol.* 1994;77(3):236–241.

23. Bruins HH, Jolly DE, Koole R. Preradiation dental extraction decisions in patients with head and neck cancer. *Oral Surg Oral Med Oral Pathol Oral Radiol Endod.* 1999;88(4):406–412.

24. Bruins HH, Koole R, Jolly DE. Preradiation dental decisions in patients with head and neck cancer: a proposed model for dental decision support. *Oral Surg Oral Med Oral Pathol Oral Radiol Endod.* 1998;86(3):256–267.

25. Beamer J, Marunick M, Esposito S. *Maxillofacial Rehabilitation: Prosthodontic and Surgical Management of Cancer-Related, Acquired, and Congenital Defects of the Head and Neck.* Hanover Park, IL: Quintessence Publishing CO, Inc; 2011.

26. Beumer J, Curtis T, Morrish LR. Radiation complications in edentulous patients. *J Prosthet Dent.* 1976;36:193–203.

27. Sulaiman F, Huryn JM, Zlotolow IM. Dental extractions in the irradiated head and neck patient: a retrospective analysis of Memorial Sloan-Kettering Cancer Center protocols, criteria, and end results. *J Oral Maxillofac Surg.* 2003;61(10):1123–1131.

7

Ethical and Legal Considerations When Treatment Planning

*Pamela Zarkowski, Helen Sharp, and Robert Barsley**

⬢ Visit eBooks.Health.Elsevier.com

OUTLINE

An oral health professional is educated to deliver evidence-based, quality care in a competent manner adhering to the profession's standards. In addition to critical thinking skills and technical proficiency, knowledge of and applying ethical principles in all aspects of care is a hallmark of a professional. A legal foundation compliments the ethical principles integrated into patient care and guides today's practitioners. This chapter explores how treatment planning is shaped by the higher aspirations of the profession and the ethical and legal foundations that guide modern dental practice.

The successful practice of dentistry involves more than simply the delivery of technically excellent treatment. To be skilled in the art and science of dentistry, the dentist must assess each patient's condition, help the patient understand the risks and benefitss associated with various treatment options, achieve agreement about a plan of care, and then deliver oral healthcare at a level that meets or exceeds the **standard of care**. Underlying each of these aspects of successful practice are the ethical principles that apply to all healthcare professions. The dentist–patient relationship is built on a foundation of trust fostered by the dentist, who is skilled, empathetic, and invested in working with each patient to determine what is in their best interest.

This chapter introduces the ethical aspects of treatment planning in dentistry and introduces legal considerations that affect how oral healthcare is delivered. The chapter highlights the importance of building a relationship of trust with patients through excellent communication and adherence to the core principles of biomedical ethics. The importance of confidentiality in the provider/patient relationship is emphasized. Practitioners must be aware of critical legal constructs to guide their patient assessment, treatment planning, and record keeping. Strategies for minimizing legal risk in treatment planning and the practice of dentistry are also introduced.

It is important to recognize at the outset that simply meeting minimal legal requirements will not fully satisfy the expectations held by individual patients, the profession, or society at large. The successful professional is aware of relevant laws and professional standards and can characterize the moral and ethical rationale for each law or rule; and practices in a manner that is consistent with the highest aspirational goals of the

*Deceased 9/28/2019.

profession rather than merely meeting minimum requirements. The accomplished dentist is also prepared to apply systematic and critical thinking to reach a rational resolution when rules, laws, or ethics appear to be in conflict.

ETHICAL FOUNDATIONS OF DENTISTRY

Societal Expectations of Health-Related Professions

The selflessness that grounds all healthcare professions is an ancient expectation expressed in the Hippocratic Oath. That oath formalizes the expectation that physicians are obligated to act for the benefit of the patient, demonstrate skill and good judgment, and maintain confidentiality. The core values expressed in the oath form the foundation for contemporary societal expectations of all healthcare professionals, including dentists.

Dental students frequently participate in the public statement of a professional oath. The oaths may be specific to a discipline such as dentistry, or modified by a particular institution to address their mission or specific healthcare discipline. In most instances the themes repeated in the oath parallel those found in the Hippocratic Oath (Box 7.1). Many educational programs hold a specific "white coat" ceremony to mark entry into the profession, the transition to clinical work, or graduation, and these ceremonies exemplify the personal and public commitment dentists make with or without such ceremonies to fulfill the expectations of the profession.

Principles of Biomedical Ethics

Ethics is a branch of philosophy dealing with values of human conduct. Professional ethics assists in distinguishing between acceptable and unacceptable conduct and provides a perspective on how to act or address complex problems. Five core principles form the basis for the "The Principles of Ethics and Code of Professional Responsibility" published by the American Dental Association.[1] Respect for **patient autonomy** asserts that dentists "have a duty to treat the patient according to the patient's desires, within the bounds of accepted treatment, and to protect the patient's confidentiality".[1] **Nonmaleficence** or "do no harm" *(primum non nocere)* requires that dentists act to avoid harm or risk to patients. This responsibility requires that the dentist recognize their limitations. The principle of **beneficence** requires that dentists act to maximize the patient's welfare at all times. **Justice** asserts that dentists "have a duty to be fair in their dealings with patients, colleagues and society."[1] Justice prohibits dentists from discrimination against individual patients (or groups of people) and obligates dentists to assure access to oral health services for all members of society. The fifth principle, **veracity**, stipulates that dentists maintain truthfulness in all professional relationships. Each of these core principles of ethics is shared among the health professions. The ethical principles of integrity, trust, and confidentiality impact the provider/patient relationship. Patients expect their dentist to be competent and have their best interests in mind. Patients

---

BOX 7.1 Sample Oaths

Hippocratic Oath for Dentistry

- I swear to fulfill, to the best of my ability and judgment, this covenant:
- I will respect the hard-won scientific gains of those dental professionals in whose steps, I walk, and gladly share such knowledge as is mine with those who are to follow.
- I will apply, for the benefit of the sick, all measures which are required, avoiding those twin traps of overtreatment and therapeutic nihilism.
- I will remember that there is art to dentistry as well as science, and that warmth, sympathy, and understanding may outweigh the surgeon's knife or the chemist's drug.
- I will not be ashamed to say "I know not"; nor will I fail to call in my colleagues when the skills of another are needed for a patient's well-being.
- I will respect the privacy of my patients, for their problems are not disclosed to me that the world may know. Most especially must I tread with care in matters of life and death. If it is given me to save a life, all thanks. But it may also be within my power to take a life; this awesome responsibility must be faced with great humility and awareness of my own frailty. Above all, I must not play at God.
- I will remember that I do not treat a fever chart or a cancerous growth, but a sick human being, whose illness may affect the person's family and economic stability. My responsibility includes these related problems, if I am to care adequately for the sick.
- I will prevent disease whenever I can, for prevention is preferable to cure.
- I will remember that I remain a member of society, with special obligations to all my fellow human beings, those sound of mind and body as well as the infirm.
- If I do not violate this oath, may I enjoy life and art, respected while I live and re-membered with affection thereafter. May I always act so as to preserve the finest traditions of my calling and may I long experience the joy of healing those who seek my help.

From Edelstein, L. The Hippocratic Oath: Text, Translation and Interpretation. Baltimore: John Hopkins Press; 1943

Modified for use by dentists by Professor Lakshman Samaranaya based on the Hippocratic Oath, the Prayer of Maimonides and the 1947 Declaration of Geneva.

Oath Taken by Students at the UNLV School of Dental Medicine (https://www.unlv.edu/dental/pledge)

As a student of dentistry and as a dentist, I will conduct myself with competence and integrity, with candor and compassion, and with personal commitment to the best interests of my patients.

I shall care for my patients, as I would be cared for. The health and well-being of my patients will be my first consideration. I shall obtain consultation when it is appropriate. I shall include my patients in all important decisions about their care.

I shall accept all patients in a non-judgmental manner, and use my skills to serve those in need. I shall respect the full human dignity of each individual regardless of their race, economic status or religion. I will provide absolute discretion and confidentiality for those who entrust me with their care.

The high regard of my profession is born of society's trust in its practitioners. I will strive to merit that trust. I shall at all times and in all places conduct myself with honor and integrity.

I will strive to advance my profession by seeking new knowledge and by re-examining the ideas and practices of the past. I will attend to my own physical, mental, spiritual, intellectual and professional development in the best interest of serving others.

I pledge myself to the service of humanity, my patients, my community and my profession.

I promise to uphold UNLV School of Dental Medicine's Student Code of Honor and Professional Responsibility.

I promise to observe the code of ethics for the profession of dentistry from this day forward.

also recognize that the relationship with their provider, whether taking a health history or sharing health information with a dental colleague as part of a treatment plan is held to appropriate confidentiality requirements.

Codes of conduct or ethics are found within dental specialties, dental hygiene, and student groups, including the Student Code of Conduct of the American Student Dental Association (ASDA), which is based on the ADA *Principles of Ethics and Code of Professional Conduct*, and applies to students throughout their training.[2] The American Dental Education Association (ADEA) has a statement on professionalism and identifies six values defining professionalism: competence, fairness, integrity, responsibility, respect and service-mindedness.[3]

Students may also be held to specific codes of conduct within their academic program or university.

RELATIONSHIP BETWEEN ETHICS AND LAW

Types of Law

In the United States, three main areas of law relate to dentistry: civil law, criminal law, and administrative law. **Civil law** governs the private legal relationships between two or more parties. The two types of civil law that impact patient care are **contracts and torts**. Dentists and patients create a contractual relationship when there is an agreement between a provider and the patient. This agreement can be in writing, such as a written treatment plan signed by both parties and is referred to as an **express contract**. An **implied contract** is created by the actions of the dentist and the patient. Similar to any contractual relationship, there are obligations for both parties. For example, the dentist must provide competent and timely care, use qualified and licensed staff when appropriate and work within the accepted norms of the profession. The patient also has responsibilities, including providing accurate health information, cooperating in care and paying the fees for their care. If either party fails to meet their obligation, there is a breach of contract that may result in monetary damages. Dentists may take a patient to court to collect unpaid fees, for example, if a patient fails to pay their balance.

Tort is the second category of civil law. Tort law includes both intentional and unintentional actions. Intentional tort occurs when an individual intentionally commits a wrongful act causing harm to another individual. There is a requirement to demonstrate that the person committing the tort did so on purpose. Dentists can be accused of intentional torts (Box 7.2) and malpractice insurance may not cover the damages that would be paid if the dentist is found liable.

Unintentional Torts occur when there is unintended harm to a person and a failure to exercise a reasonable standard of care.

Dentists must practice in a manner that meets or exceeds the **standard of care**, defined as *delivery of a level of care that a reasonably prudent dentist would provide in the same or similar circumstances, time, and place.* If a dentist does not meet the standard of care, they may be guilty of negligence.

BOX 7.2	**Brief Summary of Intentional Torts With Examples**	
Specific Tort	**Description**	**Example**
Assault	The threat of bodily harm to another; there does not have to be physical contact	Waving a syringe in a threatening manner
Battery	Bodily harm without permission	Extracting a tooth without the consent of the patient
False imprisonment	Violation of personal liberty through unlawful restraint	Refusing to allow a patient to leave the operator/office
Mental distress	Purposeful cause of anguish	False diagnosis of oral cancer
Defamation of character	Damage caused to a person's reputation either in writing, (libel) or spoken (slander)	Making an untrue negative statement about a dental peer
Misrepresentation	Incorrect or false representation	Falsely promising a cure for an oral health problem

Dentists may be accused of violating duties associated with the provision of care resulting in an allegation of dental negligence. Examples of these duties include patient assessment and diagnosis of oral diseases, treatment planning to maintain or restore oral health, obtaining informed consent, use of accepted dental materials, safe administration of anesthetics and appropriate referral. To prove the dentist was negligent, a patient's attorney must show a duty existed, that the dentist failed to meet that duty, and that the failure resulted in the patient being harmed. A judge or jury hears the evidence of the plaintiff (patient) and the defendant (the dentist) and determines guilt or innocence. The legal standard used in dental negligence cases is preponderance of evidence. In a jury trial, for example, the jury would return a judgment in favor of the plaintiff if the plaintiff showed that a particular fact or event was "more likely than not" to have occurred or, put another way, that the jury perceives a greater than 50% chance that the claim made by the plaintiff is true.

Criminal law is invoked when an individual commits a wrongful act against society or the public, as, for example, driving while under the influence of alcohol. Criminal charges of assault may be brought against a dentist when there is unwanted touching (breast fondling or instruments placed on the chest of a female patient). Drug diversion and fraudulent billing are chargeable offenses when they occur in conjunction with the practice of dentistry. Criminal charges may also be brought against a dentist when there is alleged wrongful death as a result of a dental procedure. In criminal law the legal standard is "beyond a reasonable doubt". In the US legal system, attorneys typically represent clients in any civil or criminal case. Criminal or civil cases may be decided by a jury or by a judge alone.

The third type of law in the United States is **administrative law**, a smaller division of law governing state and federal regulatory areas relevant to the practice of dentistry—for example, coverage and billing rules applicable to US Medicare and Medicaid programs. In addition, states typically have an administrative code or set of laws that define the qualifications required to practice a specified profession, requirements for licensure, and state-specific regulations relating to the practice of that profession. For dentistry, the laws governing the practice of dentistry may be called the Dental Practice Act or Administrative Rules for the Practice of Dentistry. The dental practice act includes important guidelines for record keeping, record retention, the legally accepted functions for dental assistants, dental hygienists and other licensed providers, continuing education requirements and other legally mandated responsibilities such as reporting adult and child abuse or human trafficking. Dental professionals are expected to be knowledgeable about the administrative rules governing the practice of dentistry in their state.

The Intersection of Law and Ethics

Ethics governs why and how one ought to act. Law is more structured and sets minimum expected requirements. The law's function is to decide when to act and to apply sanctions when an individual has committed a particular act. Ethical principles serve as a foundation for many laws. For example, to support patient autonomy, a patient's right to make decisions about their healthcare, there is a parallel legal obligation to obtain informed consent for care. The ethical obligation of nonmaleficence, doing no harm, supports the Occupational Safety and Health Administration (OSHA) requirements for patient and provider safety in the workplace. Dental providers must recognize that an activity may be unethical, such as unprofessional conduct although the behavior may be legal. An action may also be considered ethical, such as prescribing medical marijuana, but considered illegal. Dentists are challenged when either the law or an ethical principle is debatable in its guidance. Law and ethical standards have many parallels and often provide similar conclusions in "gray" areas of practice. As a result, it is tempting to look first to the legal system to provide clear direction. In practice, however, professionals must be capable of applying ethical principles and critical thinking when faced with uncertainty. In many clinical situations, there are no specific laws or previous case law on which to rely. Where case law exists, patterns of legal response can prove helpful but may also provide conflicting outcomes because of variations in specific cases. Some administrative laws simply state acceptable or unacceptable actions but do not provide clear guidance on how to weigh, or decide between, alternatives. For example, the law may *allow* a clinician to disclose information about infectious diseases but not *require* such disclosure. Although it is helpful for the professional to understand that the law permits either disclosure or nondisclosure, the dentist is left to make a reasoned decision between the two alternatives. Therefore, the dentists' decision and justification for the decision are best grounded in ethically based decision-making.

DENTIST–PATIENT RELATIONSHIP

The dentist–patient relationship is founded on the assumption that patients and the public can trust the dentist to uphold the best interests of those served. Any relationship grounded in assumed trust is referred to as a **fiduciary relationship**. The dentist's duty in a fiduciary role is to offer every patient oral healthcare informed by the skills and judgment consistent with those held by any "reasonable" dentist. In legal terms, a "reasonable" dentist is expected to adhere to established standards of care. Standard of care is described as what a reasonable, prudent dentist would do under the same or similar circumstances, time and place, when applying scientific evidence-based concepts. It is clear from case law that educational program standards, readily available continuing education, and access to the evidence base found in the professional literature serve as the foundation for broadly accepted standards of care. Most malpractice cases allege that the dentist, through either an act of omission or commission, failed to provide appropriate quality care or failed to take reasonable precautions when providing care. It is left to the judge or jury to listen to the facts to determine what they believe to be the standard of care. An ethically-based standard of care is described as the conscientious applications of up-to-date knowledge, competent skill, and reasoned judgment in the best interest of the patient, while honoring the autonomy of the patient.[4]

Dentists are expected to maintain their skills and update their knowledge through reading the literature and participating in continuing education. Academic institutions, regional and local dental societies, specialty academies, the Academy of General Dentistry, and the American Dental Association provide guidance for dentists to access current evidence and obtain continuing education so that dentists can meet national or state licensure requirements, and the ethical imperative to be a knowledgeable and competent practitioner.[5]

Confidentiality

Confidentiality is the expectation that disclosures made to healthcare professionals will be protected. Confidentiality is a long-recognized duty of the members of any healthcare profession and is described in the Hippocratic Oath. Confidentiality builds trust within professional–patient relationships. Without it, patients may be reluctant to share details about their health that could be relevant to the overall outcome of care.

Aspects of the patient's history that are particularly sensitive, such as a history of substance abuse or mental health problems, often require additional protection by health professionals. For example, US federal law and the Health Insurance Portability and Accountability Act (HIPAA) uphold the right to nondisclosure of certain aspects of healthcare, such as mental health records. State-specific administrative laws may place a higher burden of confidentiality on healthcare providers and the records they maintain. The expectation of confidentiality extends to all dental practice employees, all of whom must also honor the confidential nature of the contents of the dental record and other healthcare information related to the patient. This includes statements by the patient that are not recorded in the chart or information gathered through the normal course of business in the office. Under the legal theory of **respondeat superior**, the dentist, as employer and master under the law, can be found liable for damage to a patient resulting from breach of confidence by any employee in the dental practice. Therefore, dentists are responsible for training their staff and should have specific written policies related to confidentiality (see *Confidentiality Case* on ebooks+).

For both legal and ethical reasons, any disclosure of personal, financial, or health-related information within a treatment facility should be limited to those individuals who have a need to know the information to perform their official duties. Under HIPAA, monetary fines can be assessed for breaches of patient privacy, even unintentional or accidental ones. The law specifies that knowledge of private healthcare information must not be shared among staff who have no need to receive the information and that other private non-health-related information, such as financial data, must also be given the same protection.

Ethical and legal exceptions to the health professional's requirement to maintain confidentiality include identification of abuse and neglect, and specific health-related findings, such as certain infectious diseases. In the United States, every state requires licensed health professionals to report suspected physical abuse and neglect of a child, domestic partner, or older adult. Some infectious diseases or conditions, including sexually transmitted infections, may require disclosure to the state health department. However, there is considerable variability in these reporting obligations and the requirements may also change over time. For example, in the United States, some states require disclosure of human immunodeficiency virus (HIV) infection, whereas others specifically forbid it. Recent reporting obligations included mumps, Zika virus, and Lyme disease in some jurisdictions. State requirements for health professionals, or specific language in a dental practice act, may obligate a dentist to report other issues. For example, some states require dentists to report suspected human trafficking.

Because confidentiality is not absolute, clinicians may encounter dilemmas relating to the disclosure of health-related information. For example, should an individual patient's infectious disease status be shared with parents, guardians, partners, or other family members? In many states, disclosure guidelines are permissive, meaning that the dentist *may* disclose to another party without fear of repercussion, but is not required to do so. When the law is not conclusive and there are competing ethical considerations, the dentist will have to make a systematic and reasoned decision. Various guides for making ethical decisions are available in the literature (see, for example, *American College of Dentists' ACD Test for Ethical Decisions*; https://dentalethics. org>Ethics Handbook for Dentists>the ACD Test for Ethical Decisions *, and a Model for Ethical Decision-making adapted from Dental Ethics at Chairside*).

These stepwise approaches to ethical decision-making can be applied when the dentist is faced with any ethical dilemma. If the dentist perceives that the patient or patient's family may pursue litigation, it is also appropriate for the dentist to seek legal counsel.

Accepting Patients into Dental Practice

Although the dentist has no legal obligation to accept all prospective patients into the practice, caution must be exercised in this area. The principle of justice is highlighted in the ADA's Principles of Ethics and Code of Professional Conduct: "the dentist's primary obligations include dealing with people justly and delivering dental care without prejudice."[1] The refusal to appoint, examine, or treat a patient cannot be based on a legally impermissible reason. For example, in the United States, it is illegal for a dentist to refuse to treat a patient if the refusal can be shown to be based on the race, creed, gender, or any other constitutionally protected class. Laws such as the Americans with Disabilities Act have broadened the list of persons with legally protected status to include, among others, persons with acquired immunodeficiency syndrome (AIDS) or those who are HIV positive.

After the initial oral evaluation, there may be patients whom the dentist may decline to treat. Examples include patients who require treatment beyond the dentist's skill level or capability, patients who are known to be overtly litigious, or patients with unrealistic expectations. It is expected that a general dentist would act to provide relief of pain or treatment of acute infection to a patient who is new to the practice, but it is not required that the dentist accept such a patient into the practice for comprehensive care.

When Does the Dentist–Patient Relationship Begin?

Although not always subject to precise definition, treatment begins when the dentist moves beyond the examination stage and implements treatment. The definition implies the understanding that the dentist who initiates treatment has entered into the **dentist–patient relationship**. The establishment of such a relationship creates specific ethical and legal responsibilities for the dentist. Creation of a treatment plan that the patient has signed is clear confirmation of an established relationship.

In certain circumstances, a dentist may limit the clinical relationship to consultative services only. This might include an examination conducted to give a second opinion. Similarly, when a specialist accepts a referral for a particular procedure, the clinical relationship is usually limited to the procedure needed in that phase of treatment. However, when multiple dentists are involved, there may be questions about which professional is responsible for immediate and long-term follow-up care. Similar difficulties may arise in cases in which treatment must be interrupted: How, when, and at whose direction should treatment be restarted? Any limited-care arrangement should be expressly discussed between dentist and patient, agreed to, and documented in the record beforehand.

Who Must Be Treated?

The dentist has an obligation to relieve pain and treat acute infection when possible. Therefore, a patient must be thoroughly examined to diagnose the cause of the pain or infection. Consultation with the patient should include a discussion of the proposed treatment and overall prognosis and consider the dentist's skills and ability to provide the treatment in question.

Through the proper disclosure in advance of the examination, it is possible to limit the patient's care to the examination only or to specify that only necessary urgent care will be provided or to provide a limited-scope treatment plan.

Terminating the Dentist–Patient Relationship

If personal issues interfere with the dentist's ability to care adequately for the patient at any stage in treatment, treatment may be terminated. In such cases, the dentist must document the circumstances in the health record. The entry should be factual and nonjudgmental, noting the problem (e.g., failed appointments, the patient's repeated noncompliance with clear and agreed-on instructions, failure to honor financial commitments), and any attempts that have been made to rectify it.

It is advisable to establish clear, documented practice policies related to patient behaviors, such as repeatedly failing to keep appointments or nonpayment of charges. These policies should be given and explained to patients at the time of enrollment in the practice and again in the event of a missed appointment or payment, and must be readily available in paper or digital form when requested by a patient.

In those cases, in which ongoing treatment is interrupted or suspended, a letter should be mailed to the patient. The letter should outline the facts and any related practice policy, specify the intent to sever the relationship with a specific date, and should offer the provision of emergency care only, access to records, and a recommendation to seek another dental provider. The dentist should usually offer to complete treatment already started. In cases involving multi-visit definitive prostheses, the patient should be provided with a foundation or stable provisional restoration at a minimum. It is customary (and required in some jurisdictions) to provide emergency services for 30 days after notification of intent to terminate the relationship. If the patient's oral status is not negatively affected by a reasonable delay in accessing continued care, this judgment should be documented in the patient's record. A copy of the letter sent to the patient should be retained in the patient record (Box 7.3).

Referring Patients

When referring a patient, whether to a dental specialist, general dentist, or other healthcare provider, it is particularly important that the referral and reasons for it are noted in the patient record. In most situations, the referral to another professional should be made in digital or written ommunication. A copy of the communication should be kept in the patient's record. In addition, the dentist should note in the record any follow-up phone calls or other communications with the other professional, and with the patient (see additional discussion of referral letters in Chapters 6, 8, and 13).

Designed to protect patients' confidential health information, HIPAA makes important exceptions for the exchange of health information among providers, most notably the Treatment, Payment, and Operations (TPO) exceptions. A practice (a covered entity under HIPAA) may exchange clinical information with other providers to further the treatment of a patient. The information exchanged between the providers should adhere to the "need to know" guideline previously described for

---

> ### BOX 7.3 The Four-Paragraph Dismissal Letter
>
> *First paragraph:* Establish the facts—describe the diagnosis and the agreed-on treatment, stressing the role the patient was to play. State that the patient's active participation (e.g., cooperation or attendance for appointments) was vital to the success of the treatment. If dismissal is for a non-clinically based reason, e.g., staff harassment, failure to pay fees, indicate that the termination is based on the patients lack of willingness to adhere to office policies or protocols. It is not necessary to list the behavior as the patient may allege it is an allegation or accusation that needs to be defended. Include reference to any relevant policies and include copies of the policies as attachments.
>
> *Second paragraph:* Describe and document how the patient has failed to uphold their part of the doctor-patient relationship. State that this failure has negatively affected the prognosis for care and created a situation in which the dentist can no longer continue treatment.
>
> *Third paragraph:* State the intent to sever the relationship. Indicate that emergency care will be provided on an appointment basis for a period of time, e.g., 30 days from the date of this notification. Point out the need for action on the patient's part, such as scheduling an appointment with another dentist.
>
> *Fourth paragraph:* Discuss the availability of records and willingness to forward records (duplicates only) with signed permission of the patient. Close politely and include contact information.

---

confidential health information. But the receiving professional must have all necessary historical and clinical information to be able to make an accurate diagnosis and treatment recommendation. Because the purpose of referral and consultation is to benefit the patient, these communications generally fall under the TPO exception. Nevertheless, it is good practice to inform the patient before communicating or sharing protected health information.

The TPO exception is consistent with the ethical principle of beneficence if the goal of the communication is to enhance the patient's well-being. In practice, it is wise to maintain respect for patient autonomy and to uphold the principle of beneficence by notifying the patient before making a referral. Should the patient object, the referral should not be made to that particular specialist and other options should be explored in consultation with the patient. The referral, the patient's agreement to the referral, and the patient's follow-up should all be documented in the patient record. Typically, the referred-to practitioner will communicate with the referring dentist to confirm the acceptance of the referral and again at the completion of specialty treatment. If no communication is received, the primary dentist is responsible for contacting the patient to resume care. All follow-up communication with the referred-to specialist should be noted in the patient's record.

Nonreferral of Patients

The dentist must also be aware of issues surrounding failure to consult or make appropriate referrals to specialists. Cases in some jurisdictions have attributed negligence to a dentist for failure to refer a patient if expert testimony can demonstrate that a specialist would have likely had a better result or even that the patient might have had a better chance at a positive result if the referral had been made. Negligence may also be found in cases in which referral to another practitioner was appropriate, but the referring dentist knew or should have known that the referred-to dentist was not capable of successfully treating the patient.

APPLYING ETHICS AND LAW TO DIAGNOSIS AND TREATMENT PLANNING

The principle of respect for patient autonomy underlies the necessity for the dentist to work with each patient to reach an agreed-on plan of care. The patient is not expected to know and understand all of the factors a professional considers in developing a treatment plan, so it is the dentist's responsibility to educate the patient so that they can make an informed choice. This process is often referred to as **shared decision-making**. In the United States, the courts have long recognized the right of a legally competent adult to decide what may happen to their own body. In 1914 in *Schloendorff v. Society of New York Hospital* Justice Cardozo wrote, "every human being of adult years and sound mind has a right to determine what shall be done with his own body; …"[6] This right applies in all healthcare settings, including dentistry, and in practice requires that dentists obtain informed consent before engaging in any evaluation or treatment procedures.

Informed Consent

Informed consent is the process of shared decision-making that allows a patient to make a voluntary decision based on an understanding of the clinical problem, options available, and risks and benefits of each option.

The Process of Informed Consent

The patient gives informed consent through a process that requires the dentist to explain the treatment plan, potential complications, alternatives, and any anticipated consequences of nontreatment in a way that the patient is likely to understand. During the conversation, the dentist must allow the patient an opportunity to ask questions and discuss options. The dentist must provide clear, understandable answers to any questions posed by the patient. The dentist should make every effort to observe and respond to both verbal and nonverbal signs of concern and convey genuine interest in ensuring that the patient understands the options and is not feeling pressured to make a decision. This process helps dentist and patient arrive at a shared understanding before the patient freely commits to what may be an irreversible course of treatment. Meaningful informed consent cannot be obtained when a patient is in acute pain, is highly anxious, or after they have been sedated for surgery, because under such circumstances the individual is unable to ask meaningful questions, understand the choices, or use clear reasoning to make decisions.

Capacity to make decisions is a critical aspect of informed consent. Dentists should verify capacity to consent by assessing the patient's understanding of the proposed course of evaluation or treatment in the context of obtaining consent. In any situation where a provider observes signs that psychiatric illness, trauma, sedation, confusion, or intoxication impair a patient's cognitive abilities, dentists should determine capacity for consent and document the steps taken to do so.

Dentists should identify any administrative laws in their jurisdiction that address additional requirements for consent. Some statutes require disclosures associated with specific procedures or may specify when written consent is required.

Who Can Give Informed Consent? Competence and Decision-Making Capacity

In most countries, the right to make independent medical and financial decisions and other legally binding commitments, is granted to adults when they have reached the legally defined age of majority. In the United States, this construct is called **legal competence** and is assumed on the 18th birthday for any individual who has not been declared incompetent through a legal hearing. Thus, most adults are considered legally competent to make health-related decisions. However, changes in cognitive capacity may occur among adult populations in association with medications, anxiety, injury, illness, or degenerative conditions. As a result, an adult may lack the cognitive capacity to provide voluntary, informed consent in a clinical setting.

Through the process of obtaining informed consent, the dentist should assess the extent to which the patient exhibits evidence of understanding the proposed treatment, including its risks and benefits, other options available, and the consequences of nontreatment. In addition, the patient must exhibit rationality in weighing the options and must communicate a choice. If all these criteria are met, the patient is considered to have decision-making capacity.[7] Capacity for informed decision-making is not static. Patients may temporarily lose capacity after taking a sedative but regain it again when the effects of the medication diminish. Capacity is considered a sliding scale, which means that patients may have capacity for some decisions, yet lack sufficient decision-making skills for more significant or irreversible decisions (e.g., orthognathic surgery). Because capacity can vary over time and with the seriousness of the decision, dentists should not assume that patients have capacity and should assess patients' capacity to consent for each evaluation and treatment decision presented.[2]

When a Patient Lacks Decision-Making Capacity

Adults with developmental, acute, or chronic cognitive disorders may lack the capacity to make their own dental and other healthcare decisions. In cases in which a judge has deemed a patient to be incompetent for healthcare decisions, a legal guardian is appointed by the court to serve as the patient's surrogate, and permission to evaluate or treat should be obtained from the legal guardian. In many cases, no legal ruling on the patient's competence will be available, therefore the clinical professional or team of professionals must determine whether an individual lacks the capacity to give consent. When a patient is unable to make an informed choice, the dentist must identify another person to serve as the patient's representative. The dentist is not empowered to make decisions on the patient's behalf. The person who speaks for the patient is referred to as a **surrogate decision maker** or proxy.

Under such circumstances, the dentist should establish whether the patient has identified an individual to serve as a surrogate decision maker for healthcare decisions. In the United States, this role can be formalized using a Durable Power of Attorney for Healthcare (DPAHC) document. If the patient has not identified a DPAHC, the surrogate will most often be someone in the "next of kin" hierarchy: spouse, adult child, parent, adult sibling, adult grandchild, close friend, or guardian of the estate.[3]

Patients who are deemed legally incompetent or lack the capacity for informed consent should still be provided with an explanation of assessment and treatment plans and have an opportunity to ask questions, much like the model for obtaining **assent** used in pediatric and adolescent care (see Chapter 17). Most dental care requires patient cooperation, and including the individual with confusion, dementia, or developmental delay in the discussion may strengthen the clinical relationship and facilitate cooperation.

When the patient's cognitive capacity is unclear, the dentist should seek further guidance from the patient's physician or other health professionals involved in the patient's care, such as a social worker or nurse, before accepting the patient's consent to receive treatment. If the cause of uncertainty about capacity appears to be temporary—for example, self-medication before the appointment—the appointment should be suspended and the consent process conducted at a later time when the patient is capable of giving informed, voluntary consent.

Emancipated and Mature Minors

Most adolescents do not have the legal authority to give fully informed consent. However, there are some exceptions for adolescents and these exceptions vary considerably by state in the United States and by country around the world. Minors may have decision-making capacity and should always be engaged in a process of assent, even when an adult caregiver gives consent. Some jurisdictions recognize exceptions that give minors the authority to consent to medical intervention.

Emancipation is a legal status granted to some minors. States vary in their guidelines, however, and marriage or divorce, active duty in the US armed forces, or declaration of emancipation from the courts provides such status. Emancipation typically requires that the individual is financially independent and living separately from their parent or guardian. An emancipated minor may consent to dental treatment. A state may also have guidelines defining "mature minors" that provide adolescents with limited authority to consent to diagnosis and treatment for specific types of conditions including drug and alcohol abuse, pregnancy, sexual assault and infectious and communicable diseases, reproductive health including birth control, and outpatient mental health services.

Informed Refusal

The process of shared decision-making includes the possibility that the patient will make an informed decision to refuse the dentist's recommended plan. As with informed consent, the dentist should ensure that the patient is fully informed, the refusal is voluntary, and the patient demonstrates decision-making capacity. In some instances, the decision by the patient to refuse treatment will require more explicit evaluation of their decision-making capacity with careful documentation because the patient is electing to elevate their level of risk. For example, if the patient's refusal poses an overall health risk, the dentist should ensure that the patient understands the risk. The associated discussion and decision should be carefully documented.

When a patient refuses treatment, the dentist should seek to understand the reason or reasons for the refusal but avoid trying to coerce the patient into accepting treatment, because such efforts obviate the voluntary nature of informed consent. If the reason for refusal can be addressed (e.g., cost), the dentist should make every effort to do so. The dentist should make a clear treatment recommendation, discuss the risks and benefits of secondary options or nontreatment with the patient, and convey a level of concern about the patient's health appropriate to the situation. The discussion should be carefully documented and include:

- The information provided to the patient including oral and general health risks,
- The patient's reason for refusal,
- Examples of the patient's statements that document comprehension of the risk.

Obtaining the patient's signature and the dentist's and that of a witness is useful documentation. It is preferable to leave open the possibility of the patient returning for treatment at a later date.

The dentist is not obligated to provide the patient's requested treatment if the dentist believes the treatment would be professionally unsound or pose a danger to the patient. Similarly, the dentist is not obligated to continue to provide care for a patient when the patient is refusing treatment that the dentist believes to be critical for the health and safety of the patient. The *In Clinical Practice: An Ethical Dilemma* box illustrates this point.

Documenting Informed Consent or Informed Refusal

The essential element in generating informed consent is open dialogue between the dentist and patient. The routine use of written consent forms has significant benefits and, when used appropriately, provides prima facie evidence that informed consent has been achieved. Nevertheless, consent documented with a written and signed consent form should be viewed as an adjunct to, but not a replacement for, the consent conversation between dentist and patient. Informed consent is an interactive process that must include discussion with the patient. It is advisable to supplement the consent form with progress notes, detailing the treatment alternatives discussed, the questions asked by the patient and the answers provided, and including the reasons (if given) that a particular treatment recommendation was accepted or declined. These notes provide more patient-specific verification of the process of consent than does a signed standardized form alone, particularly if the patient does not or cannot read the form before signing it.

Although written evidence of consent is preferred, the court may *attribute* consent in some instances. The lowest level of agreement or minimal consent (also called assent) is often sufficient when patients are new to the practice and seek an initial examination. However, the practice of explaining examination

---

IN CLINICAL PRACTICE

An Ethical Dilemma

After graduation from dental school more than 20 years ago, some classmates kept in close touch as our practices were beginning. One classmate called during the first winter to discuss a new patient. When the patient had presented for his first examination, my friend noticed a lesion on the upper lip that he suspected might be cancerous. He called the lesion to the attention of the patient and suggested a biopsy. The patient declined; he only wanted his teeth restored. When the patient returned 2 weeks later, the lesion had increased in size and my friend's clinical impression was that this was a melanoma—a frightening prospect. He again pointed out the extreme urgency of seeking prompt and thorough intervention. He even considered removing the lesion without the patient's consent while the area was anesthetized for a nearby restoration. He felt strongly that he should intervene, but the patient was adamant in refusing the recommended treatment, even though it might be lifesaving. After the second visit, my friend wondered if he could ethically continue to treat this individual. One could argue that refusing to provide further care could only make matters worse, because by the time the patient had found a new dentist, the melanoma might be too advanced for effective treatment should the patient change his mind. The outcome? Unknown. The patient never returned for that third visit. He was, as is so often noted in our professional journals, "lost to follow-up."

When you have completed your study of this chapter, ask yourself the following questions. What were the alternatives the dentist could have considered to manage the dilemma presented.? How could he have encouraged the patient to seek evaluation? Were there other management options that the dentist could offer short of dismissing the patient? What ethical principles could have guided the dentist's analysis of the situation? What will you do if faced with a similar circumstance?

Robert Barsley

IN CLINICAL PRACTICE

Informed Consent When the Plan is Changing

The patient's formal written consent for treatment is based on the information the practitioner provides to the patient about the diagnosis, prognosis, and treatment options. In some situations, the practitioner may be uncertain at the outset about what complications may arise, or what eventualities may occur. For example, during a planned restorative procedure, the dentist may discover that caries is more extensive than had been anticipated at the treatment planning stage. Now, faced with a carious exposure, the dentist recommended treatment is to do a root canal treatment and a foundation and crown on the tooth.

If the treatment plan is to be changed during active treatment, the dentist has several options for obtaining the patient's consent to proceed. Although it may be tempting to simply explain the problem to the patient and continue with little or no discussion, most patients cannot give truly informed consent while reclined in the dental chair with a rubber dam in place. The patient should be given the opportunity to ask questions and consider additional options, such as extraction. This interaction can be best achieved by removing the rubber dam and allowing the patient to sit up for a face-to-face discussion with the dentist. The revised treatment plan should be documented.

When it is necessary for the dentist to enter into a treatment plan with some uncertainty, questions about informed consent may be avoided by a thorough discussion of the possibilities before initiating treatment. If the dentist obtains consent for a straightforward restoration but, before beginning, explains that the decay may be more extensive, the patient's preferences for further discussion or proceeding immediately with more extensive treatment can be established before treatment is begun.

---

procedures contributes to building trust between dentist and patient. Assent may also apply to patients who are established in a practice and undergo a routine procedure, such as a periodic examination and oral prophylaxis. This informal agreement is acceptable if the dentist ensures that the patient has an ongoing understanding of the purpose of the procedure, has previously experienced the same or similar procedures, and has previously been informed about and understands the benefits, risks, and alternatives. Changes in the patient's oral or general health status may necessitate a return to verbal and/or written consent(See Box *In Clinical Practice: Informed Consent When the Plan Is Changing*).

When the dentist chooses not to use a signed consent form—for instance, with a "simple" restorative treatment plan and no notable alternatives to the treatment proposed—it is required that the dentist document in the dental record that the procedure was discussed, the elements of consent were covered, and the patient gave verbal agreement to the proposed treatment. With or without the completion of an informed consent document, the process of informed consent should be recorded in the progress notes. One format for such notes is to document the following points: Procedure, Alternatives, Risks, and Questions (PARQ). A **PARQ note** should include the following:

Procedure: A summary of the proposed treatment plan or procedures and why the plan or procedures are necessary.

Alternatives: A list of possible alternative treatments.

Risks: The adverse outcomes possible as a result of the treatment plan or procedures, and the risks of *not* receiving treatment.

Questions: Any questions raised by the patient and the responses given. If the patient had no questions, that must also be documented. (See Example *Informed Consent PARQ Note*).

Informed Consent in the Eyes of the Law

Proceeding with treatment in the absence of patient consent is considered an assault or battery, a form of unprivileged touching. As such, it may be actionable as an intentional tort under US law.

Verification that informed consent was obtained can be a crucial factor in a malpractice allegation. It is important to recognize that a signed consent form does not inherently demonstrate that valid and voluntary informed consent was obtained. If the validity of the consent is questioned, the patient may allege that insufficient information was provided and that if the facts at issue had been known, consent for the treatment would not have been given. Consent forms should include required elements, such as a clear location for reporting the date, patient's name, provider's name, diagnosis, treatment plan, options, known risks, space for specific details to be written in, clear acknowledgment of understanding and satisfactory opportunity to have questions answered, and agreement to the described treatment (Box 7.4).

Blanket consent to an unspecified course of dental treatment is not considered valid. For that reason, in addition to a general consent for dental assessment and treatment, it is advantageous to have specific consent forms for use in conjunction with

---

EXAMPLE INFORMED CONSENT *PARQ* NOTE

Procedure:

Maxillary left first premolar with vertical root fracture – tooth non-restorable. Patient elects extraction with site preservat and after 3 months healing placement of an implant, and after an additional 3 months healing placement of an implant retained crown. Patient declined the option of an immediate provisional removable partial denture.

Alternatives:

- No treatment
- Extraction and defer replacement
- Extraction and removable partial denture
- Extraction and fixed partial denture

Risks & Benefits:

Discussed the risks, benefits, and costs of the proposed treatment as well as the alternatives. Placement of the implant and implant crown while time consuming and costly in the short run, will provide the best prognosis and the best overall esthetic and functional result. Specific risks and limitations of the alternative treatment options that were explained to the patient:
- No treatment – significant risk of pain, swelling, and infection
- Extraction and defer replacement – in the absence of a tooth replacement the patient may have drifting or tipping of adjacent tooth, diminished function, and will have an obvious "tooth gap"
- Extraction and removable partial denture – removable RPD can provide a modicum of function and esthetics, but is less convenient, must be removed at night, and required special cleaning and maintenance
- Extraction and fixed partial denture – would require removal and replacement of the existing crown on the adjacent second premolar, and significant removal of healthy tooth structure on the adjacent canine tooth

Questions:

Mrs. Smith was given the opportunity and encouraged to ask questions. She declined to do so and expressed appreciation for the thorough explanation of the treatment options. *Note:* Patient's spouse was present for the consent discussion and he expressed concurrence with the proposed plan.

---

various specialty and higher-risk procedures that are performed in the practice. Special consideration should be given to endodontic procedures, extractions, implant placement, periodontal surgery, orthodontic treatment, and procedures to be provided under sedation or general anesthesia. Patients must be advised of changes in the status of their disease and of any modifications that might be advisable or undertaken. A long, continuing course of treatment may require periodic renewals of consent.

It is important to note that obtaining informed consent is not protective of the dentist when the treatment does not meet the standard of care or is considered negligent. A patient cannot give valid consent to a course of "maltreatment" or malpractice.

Can Informed Consent Be Obtained by Another Staff Member?

Usually the provider cannot delegate this duty to a less-qualified employee, because the provider alone has the full intimate knowledge of the case and treatment objectives and must be ultimately responsible for ensuring that the patient has decision-making capacity and has given fully informed consent.

Is Informed Consent Always Necessary?

The only exception to the necessity of obtaining consent is the existence of a life-threatening emergency, an event that is relatively rare in dental practice.

Patient Health Record

What Is Included in the Patient Health Record?

The patient record should include a comprehensive patient history (see Chapter 1), oral health findings, diagnoses and tests, radiographs and photographs, a well thought-out and clearly recorded treatment plan, and written informed consent forms signed by the patient. Progress notes are added as treatment is provided and should include summaries of any discussions with the patient relating to evaluation, treatment, or post-treatment care, such as PARQ notes described previously. The patient's questions, concerns, or complaints should be documented in the progress note, together with the ways in which these were addressed. Telephone conversations with the patient or other health professionals related to the patient's care should be included in the progress notes. Communication via email should also be included or scanned into the record. Notes relating to patient noncompliance and missed appointments, and records of follow-up and periodic visits, should be maintained.

Any written communications to or from the patient should be retained as part of the record. For example, copies of written postoperative instructions should be included either by reference or by the insertion of the document(s). Copies of letters of referral or formal notifications of dismissal from the practice should also be included in the record.

BOX 7.4 Designing a Consent Form

Although the elements of consent remain generally the same across all disciplines of dentistry, certain procedures (perhaps entire disciplines) are better served with more detailed consent forms. To demonstrate that the consent is freely given and informed, every consent form must include the following:

Demographics: The date, patient name, dentist's name, and office location or location of proposed treatment

Diagnosis: The diagnosis, disease, or condition that led to the proposed procedure's being undertaken

The Plan: The procedure itself explained in straightforward nontechnical language (e.g., "cutting" rather than "incision" and "stitches" rather than "sutures").

The Goal: State the anticipated benefit or purpose of the procedures and expected outcomes.

The Risks: List the oral and general health risks and possible complications associated with the treatment (including the risks associated with no treatment); alternatives to treatment, including no treatment; and the types of medications, materials, and anesthetics that may be used during the treatment, along with their associated risks.

Acknowledgment: A statement that the patient acknowledges that all of the above sections of the consent form have been explained clearly, the patient has read the consent form, has had an opportunity to ask questions and these questions have been answered, the patient understands that results cannot be guaranteed, and authorization for the treatment is given to the named dentist and that the person agreeing to the treatment does so willingly.

Signature: The patient, appropriate surrogate, or legal guardian must sign the document.

Although much of the form can be preprinted, the areas for listing the disease, treatment/procedures, risks, and alternatives should consist of blank lines to be filled in as necessary and reviewed with the patient before the patient reads and signs the consent.

In addition to the above required components of a consent form, supplemental areas include listing the possibility that the dentist will be assisted by staff or students; consultation with other healthcare providers may occur; the disease or deformity may be greater or lesser in scope than originally recognized, requiring more or less treatment; contingencies that may arise; the prognosis for the disease with and without treatment: what will happen with removed tissues; postoperative instructions and duties for the patient; and, if relevant, a release to use photographic images.

One area of record keeping deserves special mention—the prescribing and dispensing of medications. In the United States, specific federal requirements for documentation must be followed when controlled substances are prescribed. State laws may also affect these requirements.

Finally, agreements with health or dental insurance companies and/or with Medicare/Medicaid agencies often impose additional record-keeping requirements on the dental office in terms of documenting treatment claimed for reimbursement.

Office management documents, such as the appointment book and telephone log, are also considered to be valid and legal documents and should be preserved even if the patient leaves the practice.

How Should Information Be Recorded in the Patient Record?

The progress (or treatment) note is generally considered to be among the most valuable of the many parts of the record.

A common format for progress notes, particularly in the acute care patient, is to document the **S**ubjective findings, **O**bjective findings, **A**ssessment, and **P**lan (SOAP) a format described in Chapter 9. Documenting treatment for the patient undergoing active care is described in Chapter 1 (see Figure 1.20). Progress notes for the periodic recall visit are described in Chapter 12.

If the practice is using a handwritten (hard copy) record, all entries must be legible, dated, and should be in ink (black or blue are generally preferred; blue ink has an advantage because copies can easily be distinguished from the original), and should be organized in chronologic order. Explanations for any out-of-sequence entries should be included. Any incorrect entries should be struck through with a single line so that they remain decipherable and should be dated and initialed by the person making the change. The correct entry, including the reason for the change, should be made in the next available space. These notes do not need to be handwritten by the dentist; however, if written by office personnel, the note should be initialed by the writer, and the office should have some method for later identification of the initials should the need arise. If notes are dictated and transcribed, the dates of dictation and transcription should be made a part of the record and the dentist should review, correct, and sign the final note.

Electronic Patient Records

Electronic health records (EHR) are increasingly used in all healthcare settings. Dental practice management software integrates all aspects of the dental practice into a single, digital file containing all of the types of entries that were commonly found in written patient records.

There are many significant benefits to use of an EHR system. Laboratory test results, photographs, radiographs, and other images, and all consultation and progress notes, are all housed within a single record. From a legal perspective, the EHR has some clear advantages because the record is optimally organized and the notes are more legible. Progress notes are generally more structured, with fewer recording errors and missed components. In addition, electronic systems encourage timely completion of notes, and the availability of rapid information retrieval promotes more efficient delivery of patient care. Additional quality assurance benefits include the following:

- Errors related to misreading handwritten notes are reduced.
- Prescription writing errors are reduced.
- Authorship of each note is clearly indicated.
- Changes in the notes are readily identifiable.

On the other hand, the EHR complicates some processes that were once relatively simple. For example, a signed informed consent document was simply added to the paper chart in the past but is now either an electronic document signed via signature pad, or it must be scanned and attached to the patient's file. Many EHRs adopt a "menu" system for the entry of notes and other information. Although the physical act of entering the note may be delegated, the dentist remains responsible for ensuring that a complete and accurate note is entered. If changes are made to an electronic progress note, it is imperative that the date of the original entry and the original text be recorded and archived. Although there is no relevant dental case law as yet, it is clear from business and criminal cases in other areas that forgeries and alterations to electronic documents remain detectable.

Electronic records should comply with all the record-keeping principles and requirements outlined in traditional (hard copy) dental records. All staff should receive appropriate training for use of the electronic management system used by a dental office. Federal and state laws that apply to paper records also apply to electronic records.

Who Owns the Patient Record?

Although the dental record is owned by and made for the benefit of the dentist, patients (or their legal representatives) may request copies of their own records and these must be provided at a nominal (or no) fee. Because financial records and accounting records serve different purposes, unrelated to healthcare per se, such records should be maintained separately from the clinical patient record. Similarly, the dentist has a legal right to maintain an "incident report" as a separate file in case a litigious or potentially litigious situation should arise. Such a report or file can include personal reflections or judgments that would not be appropriate to include in the patient record but that may be valuable to the dentist or the dentist's insurance carrier and/or attorney. As long as such notes are not attached to the patient record or referenced in it, they are **nondiscoverable** and are, therefore, subject to the confidentiality maintained between attorney and client (dentist).

If the patient requests that their dental records be forwarded to another dentist, the dentist must comply with this request. Dentists should be aware of administrative law concerning any protected parts of the record (such as HIV status) that may only be forwarded with the patient's explicit permission. When records are to be transferred with the sale of a practice, the patient must be given the opportunity to object to the transfer of the record to the new owner. In that circumstance, the patient may request that their records be transferred to a dentist of the patient's choosing rather than to the new owner.

A dentist has a legal right to the original patient record and a patient has a legal right to a copy of the record. The patient's ownership rights apply even if the patient owes a balance to the dentist. The ADA Principles of Ethics and Code of Professional Conduct specifically addresses the dentists' obligation to provide a copy of the patient record in accordance with applicable law that will be beneficial for the future treatment of the patient. The ADA Code notes this obligation exists whether or not the patient's account is paid in full.[1]

Legal Value of the Patient Record

The importance of a well-organized patient record cannot be overemphasized because this record serves as core evidence of professional competence. It is the repository of the patient's history and all clinical findings identified at the initial examination (see Chapter 1), the diagnoses, evidence of informed consent, plan of care, and all treatment rendered to the patient. It therefore provides the best evidence as to whether the dentist has

performed due diligence in providing professional care for the patient. When questions arise as to whether the dentist has provided appropriate and safe treatment that meets the standard of care, the patient record becomes the focal point of the analysis. In addition, successful defense of malpractice claims often rely on the clinician's ability to produce all original radiographs, documented clinical findings, and progress notes pertaining to the case. Juries tend to rule against dentists who cannot produce records, whose record keeping is sloppy or lax, or who have been shown to have altered the patient record.

Patient records also have important economic value as part of the "goodwill" on the sale of a practice. If the practice and records are sold, however, the seller should arrange a mechanism that will ensure continued access to the records of prior treatment if necessary—for example, to assist in the defense of a malpractice claim filed after the sale is final.

How Long Should Patient Records Be Kept?

It is advisable to retain patient records as long as is practical. It is generally easier to store and maintain electronic rather than paper patient records, but the dentist must continue to back up the EHR to a secure remote site. Many jurisdictions specify a minimum number of years for which healthcare records must be retained and dentists are obligated to meet these minimum requirements. Additional requirements concerning record retention may be imposed by contracts with insurance carriers or by employment or affiliation contracts. For example, Medicaid regulations require that records be kept a minimum of 3 years from the date a claim is filed for reimbursement. Because federal income tax issues can arise up to 6 years after taxes are paid, many experts advise keeping records a minimum of 7 years. Many jurisdictions suspend the typical statute of limitations for children until they reach the age of majority because a case of alleged negligence involving a very young patient may arise as many as 16 to 18 years after treatment.

MALPRACTICE AND PROFESSIONAL LIABILITY

To be successful, a malpractice claim must fulfill four elements: (1) a duty owed to the plaintiff, (2) a breach of that duty, (3) the breach of the owed duty must result in damage to the plaintiff, and (4) the breach of duty must be shown to be the proximate cause of the damages. Each of these four components is explained in the following text.

Malpractice claims usually allege that the breach of duty was negligence or fault by the dentist. The negligent act may arise as a result of either something the dentist did (commission) or something they failed to do (omission) during evaluation or treatment. In malpractice cases, the patient, known as the plaintiff, bears the "burden of proof" and must provide a preponderance of credible evidence that addresses each of the four elements. Failure to address and prove each element can result in dismissal of the case in the defendant's favor.

Duty

The dentist owes each patient the degree of skill, care, and judgment possessed by a "reasonable" dentist. This is the benchmark against which an alleged negligent act is judged and is most often established by expert testimony. Courts have cited the significantly increased opportunities for professional communication and education as the foundation for a prevailing standard of care in dentistry. In many jurisdictions, however, a plaintiff cannot use the testimony of a *specialist* to establish the standard of care for a *general* dentist. However, general dentists who hold themselves out as specialists (and in some jurisdictions, even those who do not) are held to the national standard when performing treatment that falls within the realm of the specialist. In essence, the courts require all dentists to diagnose properly and treat disease appropriately.

The **duty** to treat arises from the doctor–patient relationship. This relationship may be either an expressed or tacit agreement. A patient may unilaterally sever the dentist–patient relationship or it can be terminated by mutual consent, but the dentist may not sever the relationship arbitrarily. To sever the relationship, a dentist must adhere to certain guidelines (see *Terminating the Dentist–Patient Relationship*, earlier in this chapter). An improper termination of the dentist–patient relationship may constitute patient abandonment leaving the dentist open to liability for damages.

In most instances, a patient enters the dental office expecting treatment and does not differentiate between the examination, presentation of the treatment plan, and actual treatment. If the treatment plan is not agreed to for any reason, both the dentist and patient must clearly understand the next steps to be taken. It is important to realize that even if the relationship is properly severed, the dentist may still owe a duty to arrange for the opportunity of continuing treatment, including providing referrals and making copies of records available.

Breach of Duty

A **breach of duty** owed to a patient is a negligent action defined as doing or failing to do something that the ordinary, prudent, or "reasonable" dentist would do or not do in the same or similar circumstances. A less-than-optimal result or unforeseen result does not constitute negligence per se.

Negligence is established by one of two general methods. The first and perhaps the simplest is through the doctrine known as *res ipsa loquitur*, in which the deviation from the standard of care is so obvious that expert testimony does not need to be offered to prove the departure. For example, a patient who sustained injury as a result of a radiographic unit toppling over or because a dental instrument was dropped in the patient's eye need only show that the injury occurred. It is commonly understood that such injuries are not the normal expected results of a dental visit. The extraction of the wrong tooth would also fall into this category of claims, although the services of a dental expert may be required to provide comment on the extent of the injury sustained.

The majority of malpractice cases require a demonstration of the standard of care from which the defendant is alleged to have deviated negligently. The degree of skill, care, or judgment required of the defendant dentist is that of the reasonable and prudent practitioner. As pointed out previously, another qualified dentist must testify as to exactly what that means in each

case. The standard of care testified to by the expert should not be "what in my opinion I would have done," but rather whether the treatment (or lack thereof) is one that the reasonable (average) dentist might have provided under similar circumstances. Because errors associated with diagnosis have the potential to deprive a patient of the future opportunity for proper treatment, courts have often held that the highest standard of care applies in the area of diagnosis. (See in *In Clinical Practice: Breach of Duty* for case illustration on ebooks+.)

Damages

It is important to differentiate between a negative outcome associated with the known risks of a procedure that are explained through the consent process and damages associated with negligence. The breach of duty and finding of negligence must be shown to have resulted in **damage** to the patient (in legal terms, the plaintiff). The nature of the damage is usually, but not necessarily, in the form of a physical injury. This undesired result must be shown to be directly related to the breach of duty. The

---

IN CLINICAL PRACTICE

Breach of Duty

Some years ago, the author was asked to review, before trial, a case of alleged dental negligence from a neighboring state. A woman in her early twenties faced the imminent loss of several molar teeth because of severe periodontal bone loss. At her request, her dentist had furnished his complete dental record documenting the treatment that she had received from age 10 years through the prior year. The record consisted of a single-page form combining an odontogram and progress notes. Numerous bite-wing and periapical radiographs were included in the chart folder. According to the notes, she had been seen every 6 to 8 months throughout the period in question. The notes mentioned that approximately seven teeth had been restored with Class II amalgams during this time. Additionally, she had received "prophy, BWX, P.A. × 2" at nearly every visit. The record included no charting of or mention of periodontal probing or any other diagnostic testing, nor was there a treatment plan or any updated health history beyond the one completed by her mother at her first visit.

The bite-wing radiographs revealed no calculus, but when viewed sequentially, showed a clear progression over time of generalized periodontal destruction. Bone loss was greatest in the areas between the teeth that had been restored, apparently because nearly every interproximal box restored by this dentist had resulted in overfills with large overhangs. Corresponding maxillary and mandibular periapical views of the incisor teeth were included for each of the bite-wing sets. When questioned at deposition, the dentist maintained that his abbreviation "P.A." actually stood for "periodontal assessment" rather than "periapical." Of course, this case settled before trial. This patient may have had a systemic condition that accelerated her response to the local irritants or she may have been the victim of an aggressive form of early-onset periodontitis. Nevertheless, this dentist's failure to recognize the progress of the disease, or if he had recognized it, to inform her of her deteriorating oral condition, cost her several teeth and his insurer tens of thousands of dollars.

This case illustrates the importance of assessing and recording the findings from current diagnostic aids in the light of previous tests and aids and of regularly updating the patient's health history. I suspect that this dentist viewed each session's radiographs in a vacuum as it were, never comparing them with any others beyond the most recent and thereby missing the insidious, but relentless, progress of her disease.

Robert Barsley

facts must show that the event must also have been avoidable by the dentist. Although it is not necessary that the dentist anticipate the exact type or extent of damage, at a minimum, the facts must show that some type of damage was foreseeable under the circumstances.

Damages must also be quantifiable, not speculative. Commonly, a monetary amount is established that the court may award to a successful plaintiff as compensatory damages. The awarded amount is designed "to make the plaintiff whole" or to restore plaintiffs to the condition they were in before the negligent act. Compensatory damages include amounts for actual damages, such as past and future medical or dental expenses, loss of earnings, loss of consortium (e.g., love and affection), and any other damages proven during a trial. Compensatory damages may also include nonmonetary damages, such as pain and suffering. In certain jurisdictions, an additional award, known as punitive damages, may be assessed to punish the wrongdoer or hold that individual up as an example to others to deter similar occurrences in the future.

Proximate Cause

The patient with a malpractice claim must demonstrate that the damages claimed flow directly from the negligent action of the dentist without another intervening cause and that the injuries would not have occurred but for that negligent act. This is referred to as **proximate cause**. Even in instances where the dentist (defendant) deviated from the standard of care, if the patient (plaintiff) did not sustain any injury, then the case will fail the proximate cause test. Similarly, even if the plaintiff sustains an injury, the results may not be any different from the result that would have been likely to occur in the absence of negligence. For example, the extraction of a hopelessly periodontally involved tooth without the patient's informed consent may not result in actual damages.

Two notable actions that the courts have upheld as proximate cause include failure to refer and referral to a specialist shown to be incompetent.

Common Causes for Litigation

Dentists who build a practice based on strong dentist–patient relationships with a foundation of trust and mutual respect tend to reduce the likelihood of malpractice litigation. Nevertheless, even excellent dentists may be sued for malpractice by a patient. It will be useful to understand the most common reasons for litigation. This knowledge allows dentists to design practice and documentation patterns to avoid common pitfalls in practice.

Statistics relating to the types of legal cases filed are difficult to obtain, because many cases are resolved or settled privately and these data are not widely shared. One large national liability insurer points to the "failure to diagnose, treat, or refer" as the three most frequent causes of litigation. Some of the largest monetary awards have been made for failure to diagnose conditions, such as abscesses and other infections that in some cases led to death. Recently, an increasing number of claims have alleged that the dentist failed to diagnose oral cancer. Because modern treatment modalities offer an increasingly good prognosis for this condition when coupled with early detection, the question then becomes at which point should the reasonable dentist have included cancer in a differential diagnosis and referred the patient for a biopsy or other definitive evaluation? Failure to diagnose periodontal disease remains a common claim by patients who have lost teeth or undergone extensive periodontal therapy. Recent advances in periodontal therapy treatment modalities have increased the likelihood that what once may have been only a weak claim could be judged meritorious today. Additional examples of litigation include medication errors and procedural errors that occur during a procedure such as implants or endodontic treatment.

Another category of lawsuits involves the failure of dentists to obtain the relevant health history of the patient. *In Clinical Practice: Health Questionnaires* illustrates a rare but serious consequence of failing to obtain information about the patient's health history. Prescribing the wrong medication, prescribing incorrect dose or frequency, or not informing the patient about known deleterious side effects of a medication can be fertile ground for litigation, especially if the systemic effects of such errors can include long-term disability or death.

Areas of dentistry that most often generate litigation include difficult extractions, treatment for TMJ problems, and treatment involving implants. An increasing number of cases have involved orthodontic treatment, including orthodontic relapse, root resorption, and a lack of informed consent on the part of an adolescent patient. Other lawsuits involve misdiagnosis or late diagnosis, failure to refer to a specialist, and adverse drug reactions.

The dentist has an ethical and legal obligation to disclose any mistakes or untoward events during treatment, for example, a broken endodontic file or reamer. Failure to disclose can lead to several undesirable results. First, when the patient discovers that the file separation occurred, they will naturally think that the dentist was less than honest and raise the question, "What

IN CLINICAL PRACTICE

Health Questionnaires

A briefly described but truly frightening case involves a dentist who commonly made "one-stop painless" dentures—inviting prospective patients to come in with natural teeth and leave with dentures. The dentist made an unbelievable blunder. He failed to take a health history on a patient who in fact had myriad systemic complications, including untreated hypertension. As was the dentist's normal procedure, he sedated the patient for the many extractions needed. Before the extractions could be begun, however, the patient had to be rushed to the hospital with a suspected heart attack. He was released the next day. Unbelievably, the patient returned to the dentist the following week and, even more unbelievably, the dentist again did not ask him to complete a health questionnaire or query him orally about his general health. Again the dentist began to sedate the patient for the requisite extractions. Again the patient coded, but this time he did not survive. The civil law implications of failing to take an adequate history, apparently failing to secure an informed consent, and performing admittedly risky procedures in an office setting paled next to the criminal implications—this dentist was charged with negligent homicide.

Robert Barsley

else was the dentist dishonest about?" The patient may feel betrayed, be more likely to blame any problems on the dentist, and be more likely to seek legal redress. The law in many states views the purposeful nondisclosure of such acts as a form of fraud. Alleging fraud may lessen the patient's burden of proof in litigation (i.e., the patient would not need to prove violation of the standard of care) and may also lengthen the time available in which to file a claim (statute of limitations and/or repose).

Clinical errors must be fully documented in the patient record and the patient should be informed as soon as is practical. If appropriate informed consent was obtained, the discussion of risks will have envisioned many of the complications in dental treatment. In any case, the dentist should be forthright about what has occurred and explain what can and will be done to mitigate the situation. The dentist needs to maintain contact with the patient and be available to respond to questions or concerns of the patient or patient's family. (Discussing the case with the family may need patient permission.) It is necessary to follow through with appropriate recommendations or offers for additional treatment or referral (often at reduced or no fee) and to do so in a timely way. Throughout the process, the dentist should demonstrate genuine concern for the patient's welfare and remain committed to resolving the patient's problems. It is important to note that many jurisdictions now have a codified "apology clause" that gives sanction to the healthcare provider to apologize to the patient without automatically incurring the legal implication of negligence.

Suit-Prone Patients

What are the chances that a particular dentist will be involved in a lawsuit alleging professional misconduct? Patients have become more consumer-oriented in their approach to healthcare and, at the same time, the practice of dentistry may seem more remote and impersonal to many. The solo practice, or practice with a single associate, is being replaced with large group, corporate, and institutionally based practice models. Practice management consultants commonly advocate administrative "improvements," such as multipatient scheduling, to reduce the effect of cost centers (i.e., operatories) on the financial bottom line. With these changes, the time and the quality of the interaction between patient and dentist has often diminished. As dentistry has become depersonalized, the risk of malpractice litigation has increased.

Although the overall risk of lawsuits has increased, not all practitioners are similarly affected. Primarily at risk are practitioners who may be technically competent in dentistry, but who lack competence in interpersonal skills or "chairside manner."[4] Mastery of the ability to interact effectively with patients also includes the ability to recognize quickly those individuals with whom the dentist may develop a substantive personality conflict. Certain individuals act or react in a manner that provides a clue they may be more prone to litigious behavior. One cardinal warning sign is the patient who immediately complains about the care, price, attitude, office condition, and so on of their previous dentist or who encourages the dentist to find fault with previous treatment. Many lawsuits have been initiated and many

---

IN CLINICAL PRACTICE

Courtroom Issues

The three situations in which a dentist may face the necessity of testifying in court or being deposed by counsel in a malpractice suit include:

- appearing as a defendant,
- appearing as an expert witness for either the plaintiff or defendant, or
- appearing as a treating (either previous or subsequent) dentist.

The first and last situations are most often not of the dentist's choosing. Only the expert witness has offered to testify and is typically compensated for case review, preparation, and testifying during the court proceedings.

Whatever the reason for an appearance in court or at a deposition, the dentist should heed certain maxims.

- First, review and ensure current knowledge about laws governing the practice of dentistry, e.g., dental practice act as well as other applicable legal information pertinent to the case. The dentist should be clear about the specific complaints or violations that are being alleged.
- Second, be aware that the law and operates subject to rules and processes that may be unfamiliar to a practicing dentist. Legal procedures move at their own pace, with the final outcome often not readily apparent during the process.
- Third, the dentist must be able to trust their attorney fully. This implies full and complete communication in both directions. As a defendant, it is difficult for the attorney to present the dentist's strongest case if communication is lacking.
- Fourth, the dentist should accept the advice of counsel, who will be responsible for providing guidance through the labyrinth of the law. Often, counsel will advise the client to avoid answering hastily, sometimes to not answer at all, and never to volunteer information—advice that may be difficult for the dentist to comply with.
- Fifth, remember that, as a witness, the dentist seeks to educate the judge or jury. To do so successfully, the dentist should strive to be certain that communication is clear and technical jargon is avoided.
- Finally, resist the temptation to engage in arguments or verbal jousting with the attorneys, particularly with opposing counsel.

---

dentists have found themselves unwilling witnesses because of a hastily uttered comment about another dentist while examining or treating the patient. A dentist clearly has a duty to disclose failed or failing dentistry but should do so in a factual, nonjudgmental fashion. Often the full story is not known at the point of initial discovery—the patient may have been noncompliant or may have refused a recommended, optimal treatment. A telephone call should be made to the previous dentist to understand more fully the situation before a dentist makes a hasty proclamation alleging substandard care. However, if the dentist becomes aware of egregious or a pattern of recurring, unprofessional or unethical behavior by another dentist, they have a professional responsibility to report the finding to the appropriate dental licensing agency.

If the dentist feels stressed, anxious, or tense while treating a patient, the chance of saying or doing something inappropriate or of being left with a less positive outcome, increases. When these pitfalls are recognized, the dentist can act quickly to refer the patient prior to entering a dentist–patient relationship or to develop a thoughtful, professional strategy for managing the patient. In the latter situation it is usually helpful and effective if the entire dental team is informed about, and engaged in, this effort.

RISK MANAGEMENT

Risk management goals are to increase patient safety, to reduce exposure to a malpractice claims, and to minimize financial loss if a claim occurs. In broad terms, this means upholding the core ethical principles, building relationships of trust with patients and maintaining excellent documentation. A body of literature containing practical "dos and don'ts" to guide dentists and healthcare professionals in this effort can be found in the Suggested Readings at the end of this chapter. Although it is beyond the scope of this text to explore risk management in detail, some overarching concepts are worthy of consideration.

- Know your state Dental Practice Acts or equivalent. State laws are available online and may be found under "Administrative Code," "Legislative Code", or other similar terms. The information assists in record keeping, delegation of responsibilities to staff, reporting obligations and requirements for continuing dental education.
- Maintain a good (and appropriate) patient/provider relationship. Practice shared decision-making that demonstrates respect for autonomy and the patient's best interests. Patients who like their dentist are less likely to pursue litigation.
- Adhere to excellent record keeping practices. Documentation in the patient record should be complete and reflect the events that are chronicled. Never include derogatory comments about a patient in their own chart.
- Meet the standard of care.
- Adhere to the fundamental principles of ethics and professionalism. Reasoned decision-making and adherence to the ethical principles discussed earlier in this chapter provide a basis for appropriate professional conduct. In the vast majority of situations in which a dentist or other health professional is sued, a professional who consistently acts on those grounds will find that a prospective plaintiff elects not to pursue litigation, a frivolous claim is dismissed, awarded damages are minimized, or a judgment is found in favor of the dentist.
- The dentist and all of the office staff should adhere to contemporary standards of care and systematically reevaluate and seek to improve policies and procedures. It is important to assess all aspects of care delivery from the patient's point of view and to assess each patient's treatment experience. These efforts will provide several important risk management benefits, including better patient care, improved patient satisfaction, better treatment outcomes, and reduced risk of malpractice litigation. When difficult situations arise, the entire practice staff should develop policies or procedures to prevent similar problems from recurring in future. Policy and procedure manuals should be updated and followed by all staff, including the dentist.

Social Media

The use of social media and other electronic forms of communication brings opportunities and challenges. Advertising materials, including the office website, should never offer guarantees for treatment outcomes. Electronic or paper publication of recognizable images or attributed patient statements requires explicit permission from the patient and may be subject to specific federal or state laws, which vary by jurisdiction and over time. The law concerning web "rating" services is currently unclear regarding which remedies the dentist may have relative to negative comments posted by members of the public and options for their removal. Some websites (such as *Angie*) have established procedures for resolving such disputes and arriving at a conclusion deemed satisfactory by all concerned.

A dentist should create a social media policy for the dental staff outlining what is permitted and what is prohibited. Dental practices should provide explicit training for all staff about the inherent risk of breach of confidentiality and inappropriate remarks about the practice, patients or other breaches of professionalism associated with the ease of posting to various web and social media sites. Laws regarding discrimination, privacy or employment policies apply to the social media world.

The American Dental Association suggests five rules of engagement:[8]

- Do not post copyrighted or trademarked content without permission from the content owner or a citation, as appropriate.
- Do not disclose any of the practice's confidential or proprietary information.
- Do not post information about a patient, employee, or another individual, including a testimonial, photograph, radiograph, or even a name, without the appropriate written consent, authorization, waiver and release signed by the patient (or the patient's guardian).
- All postings on your social media sites should be monitored for compliance by a designated individual in your practice. Keep in mind that if your practice has a policy to monitor media sites and fails to do so (or fails to act on information discovered through monitoring), it could be exposed to liability. Inappropriate, derogatory, or disparaging postings should be removed at your discretion—err on the side of caution.
- Maintain final approval on postings, even if you designate an employee to monitor and manage social media. Employees should not speak on the practice's behalf unless you have authorized them to do so.

Liability Insurance

Although a dentist may believe that the primary reason for purchasing professional liability insurance is to cover the payment of any judgment of liability, in fact, by far the most important benefit of such coverage is access to legal counsel and the payment of legal defense fees should a claim be brought. Very few claims ever reach trial and, of those, in only a small percentage is the dentist ruled liable. The failure to file a timely answer to a legal claim of negligence, however, represents an admission of liability, and the services of an attorney are vital to crafting the answer to the claim. In that light, the costs of even the "simplest" defense continue to escalate annually and may exceed the "value" of many claims. These costs include direct expenses, such as attorney fees and expert witness costs, along with nonmonetary costs, such as the necessity to be absent from the practice to attend to matters associated with the case. Enormous personal and professional costs can also accrue, including the potential for negative publicity that may surround the case if tried in court or the local press. Psychological costs may also accrue and no professional enjoys having a patient or patient's lawyer call into question the quality of their services.

The professional liability insurer also serves as a valuable resource in the prevention of liability claims. A forthright discussion with the agent about actual, potential, and hypothetical cases can help point out shortcomings in the office setting, which may then be corrected in advance of formal complaints. Many professional liability insurers offer courses and materials on risk reduction and may reduce the cost of policies to complete such a course successfully. It is essential to recognize that the insurance carrier should be contacted at the first hint of the possibility of a suit or even the suspicion that an unusual office occurrence may lead to a suit. Advice concerning documentation of the incident, communication with the patient, and instructions to staff could have a substantial effect on the final resolution of the matter.

Other Considerations

Malpractice reform has resulted in a wide variance among the states concerning professional liability. For example, some states (e.g., Louisiana) *require* that a dentist participate in a professional liability insurance coverage plan (or else provide a bond) for legally imposed limits on liability to apply. Some states impose limits on the amount of damages that can be awarded and some require that before a lawsuit claiming negligence against a healthcare provider can be filed, the potential plaintiff must meet certain procedural standards.

It is the responsibility of the dentist to be knowledgeable about the relevant law in the state in which the practice is located.

CONCLUSION

In this era of rapid advances in dental materials, technology, and techniques, and changing patient expectations for dental treatment, it is increasingly important for the dental team to keep its attention on the primary mission of any oral healthcare provider: to serve patients, partner with the patient in shared decision-making, and do the utmost to promote the patient's oral and general health in both the short and long term. The knowledge and skills dentists bring to ensure proper diagnosis and treatment planning are the foundation for excellence in dental practice and must be coupled with a relationship of trust between dentist and patient.

Trust is achieved through excellence in treatment, high standards of confidentiality, and a policy of engaging each patient in a meaningful informed consent process. Careful and accurate documentation of the patient's condition, diagnoses, plan of care, and the treatment rendered provides the main benchmark by which the quality of the care provided to the patient is judged. The dentist is expected to provide every patient with a thorough and careful diagnosis and a well-founded treatment plan, whether the treatment is limited or comprehensive in scope. The dentist who builds patient care around ethical principles and practices is more likely to provide better care, achieve better relationships with patients, develop a stable and successful practice, and avoid legal problems.

This chapter is not intended by the author, editors, or publisher to serve as legal advice. In the event a legal claim is made or if you are concerned about the possibility that a claim may be brought in the future, you are encouraged to contact your liability insurance carrier and obtain legal counsel.

REVIEW QUESTIONS

- Define each of the core principles of ethics: respect for autonomy, beneficence, nonmaleficence, justice, and veracity.
- Fiduciary relationships are built on trust. What are three things a dentist can do to build trust within the dentist-patient relationship?
- Must the dentist accept every patient into the practice? What are the patient's rights? What are the dentist's rights?
- What are the required components of informed consent?
- What steps must a dentist take to obtain and document informed consent?
- What is informed refusal? When is it used? How is documented?

- Under what circumstances does a patient lack capacity to make their own oral healthcare decisions?
- What are some limitations of relying on consent forms as evidence of informed consent? What can the dentist do to minimize these limitations?
- To be successful, malpractice claims must satisfy four elements. List and define each element.
- What are the uses of the dental record? Whose property is it? How should information be recorded in it?
- List some of the "dos and don'ts" in dealing with a potentially litigious patient.
- List two suggestions for dentists using social media.
- What are common causes of dental malpractice litigation?

PRACTICE ENHANCEMENT

Develop a Risk Reduction Plan for Your Practice

Assess your practice for legal risk and vulnerability. Set realistic, stepwise, measurable goals. Develop an action plan and assign individual staff team responsibilities. Assess progress at selected intervals (start/ stop/ continue). Take corrective action as needed. Document efforts, progress, setbacks and plan adjustments. Comprehensively reassess the plan at scheduled (quarterly/ semi-annual/ annual) intervals.

REFERENCES

1. American Dental Association: Principles of ethics and code of professional conduct, 2020. https://www.ada.org/~/media/ADA/Member%20Center/Ethics/ADA_Code_Of_Ethics_November_2020.pdf?la=en.
2. American Student Dental Association Student Code of Ethics. https://www.asdanet.org/about-asda/leaders-and-governance/current-statements-of-position-or-policy/dental-education-administration/statement-on-policy/E-8. Accessed May 1, 2021.
3. ADEA Statement on Professionalism in Dental Education. https://www.adea.org/pages/professionalism.aspx. Accessed May 14, 2021.
4. Peltier, B, Jenson, L. Dental Ethics Primer, American College of Dentists, 2017. https://www.acd.org/wp-content/uploads/Dental-Ethics-Primer-2017_Peltier-and-Jensen.pdf.
5. The Standard of Care in Dentistry. American Dental Association. https://success.ada.org/en/practice-management/guidelines-for-practice-success/gps-managing-professional-risks/the-standard-of-care-in-dentistry. Accessed May 1, 2021.
6. Schloendorff v. Society of New York Hospital (1914). 211 N.Y. 125; 105 N.E. 92 (Lexis 1028). Court of Appeals of New York. http://academic.udayton.edu/LawrenceUlrich/schloendorff.htm.
7. Appelbaum PS, Grisso T. Assessing patients' capacities to consent to treatment. *N Engl J Med*. 1988;319:1635–1638.
8. Social Media Policies for Dentists. American Dental Association. https://success.ada.org/en/practice-management/marketing/social-media-policies-for-dentists.

SUGGESTED READINGS

American College of Dentists Practice Ethics Assessment and Development (PEAD). https://www.dentalethics.org/pead/. Accessed May 1, 2021.

American College of Dentists Ethical Dilemmas. https://www.dentalethics.org/resources/. Accessed May 1, 2021.

American College of Dentists: Ethics courses online. https://www.dentalethics.org/code/courses/. Accessed May 10, 2021.

American College of Dentists: Ethics Resources. https://www.dentalethics.org/resources/. Accessed May 15, 2021.

American Dental Association. *A Dentists' Guide to the Law. 246 Things Every Dentist Should Know*. 2021.

American Dental Association. The Standard of Care in Dentistry. https://success.ada.org/en/practice-management/guidelines-for-practice-success/gps-managing-professional-risks/the-standard-of-care-in-dentistry. Accessed May 31, 2021.

Beauchamp TL, Childress JT. *Principles of Biomedical Ethics*. 8th ed. Oxford: Oxford Press; 2019.

Graskemper JP. A new perspective on dental malpractice. *JADA*. 2002; 133:752–757.

Graskemper JP. *Professional Responsibility in Dentistry: A Practical Guide to Law and Ethics*. : Wiley-Blackwell; 2011.

Graskemper JP. The standard of care in dentistry. *JADA*. 2004;135: 1449–1455.

Ozar DT, Sokol DJ, Patthoff DE. *Dental Ethics at Chairside: Professional Obligations and Practical Applications*. 3rd ed. Washington, DC: Georgetown University Press; 2018.

Pollack BR. *Law and Risk Management in Dental Practice*. Chicago: Quintessence; 2002.

Rule JT, Veatch RM. *Ethical Questions in Dentistry*. 2nd ed. Chicago: Quintessence; 2004.

Phases of the Treatment Plan

8

The Systemic Phase of Treatment

Stephen J. Stefanac

Visit eBooks.Health.Elsevier.com

INTRODUCTION

Before engaging in active therapy, the dentist must assess the patient's overall general health and what, if any, effect any health conditions present may have on the delivery of dental care and outcome of treatment. Characterized as the **systemic phase** of treatment, this phase provides an opportunity for the dentist to influence and ensure the best possible state of physical health for the patient before, during, and after treatment. To accomplish this, the dentist must be aware of the pathophysiology of all the patient's health problems and the implications that each alone, and in combination, will have for the delivery of dental care. Based on this knowledge, the dentist must devise a strategy for managing comprehensive dental treatment in the context of the patient's general health. The best and safest method to resolve any dental problems must be determined in light of the patient's overall condition.

Each patient has their own unique set of health issues and dental needs. Thus, a core function of the systemic phase is to evaluate the severity and complexity of this set of health issues and assess how those issues may affect dental treatment. Through this analysis, the dentist determines whether altering, limiting, or even postponing dental treatment will be necessary. At one

end of the spectrum is the patient with few, if any, health problems, who takes no medications and requires only preventive services and no invasive dental treatment. For such a patient, the systemic phase may consist simply of evaluating vital signs followed by updating the health history at regular intervals. At the opposite end of the spectrum is the person with multiple health problems, for whom many medications have been prescribed and who presents with both urgent and complex dental needs. This patient may require a multifaceted systemic phase of care that includes consultation with the patient's healthcare provider an evaluation of medications, laboratory testing, possible modification of dental treatment, and careful monitoring of the patient's health before, during, and after each dental visit. In addition, and of at least equal importance, the dentist needs to discover, investigate, and document any previously *undiagnosed* health problems.

Systemic issues are highly variable in their relevance to and effect on the dental treatment plan. Some conditions will trigger certain automatic modifications to the way dental care is delivered: for example, a prosthetic heart valve will require antibiotic prophylaxis to prevent bacterial endocarditis. Conditions such as arthritis or asthma, on the other hand, may or may not have a significant effect on dental treatment, depending on their nature and severity.

A comprehensive survey of the relationship to dental treatment planning of all major systemic disorders is beyond the scope of this book. Instead, the purpose of this chapter is to give the reader an overview of the effect that systemic disease may have on treatment planning and suggest guidelines for evaluating the patient's systemic health and for appropriate adaptation of the provision of treatment when the patient has significant health problems. An assessment of the patient's general health and capacity to withstand the rigors of dental treatment physically and psychologically *should be performed at every appointment*.

IMPORTANCE OF THE SYSTEMIC PHASE OF TREATMENT

In the United States, 51.8% of adult patients had at least one chronic condition such as arthritis, cancer, chronic obstructive pulmonary disease, coronary heart disease, current asthma, diabetes, hepatitis, hypertension, stroke, and weak or failing kidneys, and 27.2% had multiple conditions.[1] Systemic health has significant relevance for dental treatment planning because (1) the population of elderly persons, many of them retaining their teeth into old age, continues to increase, and (2) as a result of recent advances in healthcare, people of all ages who suffer from serious illnesses are more likely to remain active and ambulatory and to have increased life expectancies. In the recent past, individuals with severe systemic illnesses such as liver, kidney, or cardiac failure did not seek dental services unless they had an acute dental problem. Nor did the medical profession always appreciate the interrelationships between oral health and overall physical health. Unfortunately, the poor prognosis for many systemic conditions provided a rational excuse for patients, physicians, and dentists to place a low priority on achieving and maintaining optimal oral health.

Because the medical and surgical management of patients with serious systemic problems has improved immensely, greater numbers of persons with serious general health problems can be expected to present to dentists' offices requiring a broad spectrum of treatments. As a result, dentists must be proficient in obtaining and evaluating each patient's health history and in determining how to provide dental care in a safe and efficacious manner.

Many physicians, especially those involved with treating patients with cancer or failing organs that require replacement, now appreciate the effect that preventing dental problems can have on the overall prognosis for their patients. For those patients who are immunocompromised because of systemic disease or immunosuppressive drugs, untreated periodontal disease, deep carious lesions, or pathologic periapical conditions represent potential sources for serious, even life-threatening, infections. Standard medical protocols usually require the patient who will be receiving an organ transplant, radiation treatment, chemotherapy, or heart valve replacement to receive a dental evaluation and to have any oral disease controlled before undergoing treatment, although there is some controversy in this recommendation.[2,3] Additional information about dentistry and interprofessional teams can be found in Chapter 6.

The patient's systemic health is a critical issue for the increasing numbers of dentists practicing in hospital settings. Current trends in US healthcare reflect increasing use of outpatient care for chronic conditions and increased use of ambulatory surgical care facilities. As a result, those patients who are hospitalized are generally individuals suffering from more serious conditions and with more complex medical treatment requirements.[4] For these patients, dental pain and infection can be life threatening. Treatment of dental problems for this group can be challenging, however, because hospitalized patients are often significantly debilitated, bedridden, and unable to receive treatment in a traditional dental setting. Fortunately, practitioners do have ready access to the patient's medical record and can more easily request and view laboratory tests and consult with the patient's physician and other healthcare providers.

RATIONALE FOR SYSTEMIC THERAPY

The need for systemic therapy must be assessed when the patient first presents for treatment and at every appointment thereafter. Performing this service is important for the well-being of the patient and for overall risk management in the dental practice. The service also discharges a professional responsibility that is inherent in the practice of dentistry as a healthcare profession.

The patient's general health must be considered when planning dental treatment for the following reasons:
1. To recognize symptoms and signs of undiagnosed systemic disease and refer the patient to their healthcare provider for medical evaluation
2. To limit or modify dental treatment based on systemic findings
3. To prevent emergencies in the dental office
4. To prevent serious postoperative complications in conjunction with dental treatment

The clinician should perform a systemic phase review for all patients before beginning treatment (Box 8.1).

BOX 8.1   Systemic Phase Checklist

✓ Do I need to modify my treatment to prevent a medical emergency or other complications?
 • Does the patient have any significant allergies?
 • Is there a risk of a medical emergency during dental treatment?
 • Is there an increased risk of bleeding?
 • Is there an increased risk of perioperative infection?
 • Medications
  • Are there significant oral and systemic side effects to be aware of?
  • Are there any interactions with drugs that are prescribed, recommended, or administered by a dentist?
✓ Do I need information from the patient's healthcare provider? How will this alter my treatment plan?
✓ Does the patient's medical condition affect their risk for oral disease?

Courtesy Dr. Carol Anne Murdoch-Kinch.

Recognition of Systemic Disease and Patient Referral for Appropriate Treatment

Because many patients visit the dental office for maintenance care more frequently than they see a physician for evaluation, all dentists, as healthcare providers, have the responsibility to be alert for signs of undetected systemic diseases in individual patients. Occasionally, findings from the patient's vital signs, general appearance, or oral examination are suggestive of a potentially serious physical problem. If, for example, the patient has signs or symptoms suggestive of hypertension, diabetes, hyperthyroidism, or cancer, further investigation is warranted. Once the symptoms or signs of systemic disease are recognized in the individual patient, the dentist is then responsible for making a timely referral to an appropriate medical colleague so that treatment can be undertaken. Screening dental patients for diabetes, high blood pressure, and high cholesterol could save the US health system between $42 and $102 million a year in additional medical costs and is accepted by patients.[5]

Modifying or Limiting Dental Treatment

A number of health problems require the dentist to modify or limit dental treatment for patients. For example, warfarin sodium, a vitamin K antagonist more commonly known by its trade name, Coumadin, is a frequently prescribed oral anticoagulant for patients with circulatory and cardiac conditions. The dentist may need to delay procedures that cause bleeding such as oral and periodontal surgery until the patient's physician can be contacted regarding the level of anticoagulation. This is usually reported in units referred to as the **international normalized ratio (INR)**. The INR for a patient with normal coagulation is 1. Most patients taking anticoagulants are maintained in the INR range of 2 to 3, except for those conditions (e.g., patients with mechanical prosthetic heart valves) that require higher INR values from 2.5 to 3.5. The risk of postoperative bleeding after extraction can be reduced with modifications such as using a hemostatic dressing and careful suturing of the extraction site. Multiple extraction appointments (e.g., three teeth at a time) can be planned to minimize bleeding when full mouth extractions are planned. Scaling and root planing is performed in an organized fashion, one tooth at a time, to evaluate the bleeding response. Applying pressure at the site with moist gauze for several minutes may reduce bleeding. Certain medications for pain control, particularly aspirin, must be avoided and the dentist will also want to confer with the physician regarding which medications they recommend. Many other examples of modifying or limiting treatment for individuals with chronic illness or the potential for greater risk can be found in the chapters discussing elderly patients and patients with special needs (Chapters 13 and 18).

Prevention of Medical Emergencies During Dental Treatment

Although uncommon, life-threatening emergencies do sometimes occur in the dental office. Patients who appear to be in relatively good health may have systemic problems that can be aggravated by seemingly routine dental treatment. Medical emergencies occur with greater frequency in patients with multiple systemic illnesses. A careful review of each patient's medical and dental health history may suggest ways to alter treatment delivery and prevent problems. When adequate precautions are taken, most dental procedures can be provided safely in a general dentistry setting.

Two medical emergencies that dentists may encounter occur when a patient faints, usually from vasodepressor syncope, or when a patient experiences chest pain. Vasodepressor syncope may be caused by the stress and fear associated with receiving dental treatment or simply by rapid positional changes, such as sitting or standing up quickly. Careful questioning of all new patients to assess the individual's level of dental anxiety and determine any prior history of syncope may indicate that the practitioner needs to manage the patient's anxiety and pay close attention to the positioning in the dental chair. Patients who have a history of low blood flow to the heart (referred to as *angina*) may feel chest pain. Other types of medical emergencies seen in dentistry include allergic reactions to drugs and dental materials, seizures, and breathing difficulties including swallowing and even aspirating dental materials and devices. In most instances, the dentist can prevent these problems from occurring by carefully reviewing each patient's health history and modifying dental treatment appropriately. It may be necessary to delay treating a patient with uncontrolled medical conditions until the dentist can be certain the individual is medically stable.

Prevention of Postoperative Complications

Most patients expect some minor discomfort after receiving dental treatment. Some procedures, especially those involving oral surgery, routinely have postoperative sequelae such as bleeding, pain, and swelling. After restorative or endodontic treatment, individual teeth may be sensitive to heat, cold, or chewing pressure. For healthy patients, most of these symptoms can be relieved with nonnarcotic analgesics and resolve in a short time.

When the patient's health is seriously compromised, however, more severe problems can follow dental treatment. Patients with compromised immune systems, poorly controlled diabetes, or kidney failure may be more susceptible to postoperative infection and, consequently, will experience more severe pain and swelling. After consultation with a physician, it may be appropriate to provide these patients with antibiotic coverage before and for a short time after treatment.[6] Blood loss can be significant if the patient does not have normal clotting mechanisms because of the use of anticoagulant medications or because of failing liver function, such as may occur with long-term alcohol use. Mild levels of pain and discomfort are normally not a problem in a healthy individual but can create increased stress in the individual who has poor health, exacerbating the consequences of other diseases and conditions.

The practitioner can prevent severe complications in patients such as these by being knowledgeable about each individual's general health and the potential for more significant postoperative problems to occur. The patient should be given instructions describing the kinds of discomfort that may occur after treatment and in what kinds of situations the office should be contacted. The dentist may also wish to call the patient at home in the early evening. The use of stress reduction procedures, including prescribing medications to alleviate anxiety, may have additional preventive value. Several of these systemic therapies are discussed in the next section.

EVALUATING THE PATIENT'S CURRENT HEALTH STATUS

To ensure the safe delivery of dental treatment and to minimize postoperative problems, dentists must be able to recognize when a patient needs or will benefit from systemic phase treatment. The practitioner has two tools available to assist in this endeavor: (1) a thorough review of the general health history and (2) an examination of the patient for signs of systemic disease. Several elements in a medical history can point to concerns that may affect the delivery of dental care. Other significant findings can be drawn from the practitioner's review of the health questionnaire, including information about any medications that the patient uses regularly. The dentist may detect signs of disease through a systematic evaluation of the patient's vital signs and overall appearance, including a careful examination of the orofacial structures. *At a minimum, this evaluation should always occur at the initial oral examination and at the periodic examination.* The competent practitioner will be attentive to changes in the patient's appearance or general health at each dental visit.

Reviewing General Health History

Planning for the systemic phase of treatment begins with a thorough analysis of the patient's health history. As discussed in Chapter 1, patients complete a health questionnaire when they first visit a dental office and at regular intervals thereafter. The dentist, dental hygienist, or dental assistant then interviews the patient regarding any positive findings or new health-related information. In addition to providing important information, reviewing the health history with the patient is an important rapport-building exercise. The practitioner must exercise some interviewing skills, asking the patient both open and closed questions, remain objective, and be a good listener. Failure to discover important health information can occur for two reasons. First, the patient may accidentally or intentionally fail to report a significant health problem when completing the health questionnaire. The following *In Clinical Practice* box addresses how to improve the accuracy of health questionnaires. Second, some problems, such as mental disorders, recreational drug use, or sexually transmitted diseases carry a social stigma making patients reluctant to reveal them to the dentist. Some individuals may believe that information about their general health has no relevance to dental treatment or that the questionnaire takes too much time to complete. Others may not fully understand a health question, answering it incorrectly. For some patients, English is a second language and the questions may not be understood. Finally, the patient who completely refuses to complete the form may actually be functionally illiterate or not fluent enough in English to read or understand the questionnaire. For all these reasons, using an interpreter or an oral interview of the patient may be necessary.

IN CLINICAL PRACTICE

Improving the Accuracy and Reliability of the Health Questionnaire

Dentists use positive findings from the health questionnaire to indicate whether special precautions may be necessary when providing dental treatment for a particular patient. Several actions can be taken to ensure gathering good information about the patient's health.

1. Include a short statement at the beginning of the health questionnaire, stressing the importance of providing accurate information.
2. Written and oral instructions to the patient should indicate that any information provided about general health is necessary and important for treatment purposes and will remain confidential.
3. Ensure that all members of the dental team understand that all patient information is personal and confidential.
4. Make sure new patients arrive early enough to have time to complete the health questionnaire and other forms.
5. Consider mailing or emailing the health questionnaire and forms to the patient before the first appointment. A day or two before the appointment, the office staff should call and remind the patient to bring in the forms.
6. Consider having forms in other languages.

Health History

The patient's health history will reveal diseases and conditions that may or may not be significant to the dentist when providing treatment. The clinician must evaluate both the *severity* of the problem and *how recently* it occurred. The patient who reports a heart attack less than 1 month ago is at greater risk of having a second attack or a significant episode of cardiac arrhythmia during a stressful dental visit than an individual who had an attack 3 years ago. The dentist should also be concerned if a patient reports a history of systemic disease that has now reappeared or is worsening.

Any past problems that have led to damage to a major organ system are highly significant. For instance, a patient who contracted rheumatic fever as a child may have residual heart damage, predisposing the individual to an infection of the heart, **infective endocarditis**, after certain types of dental treatment. On the other hand, a healthy patient who had syphilis 30 years ago and was treated promptly with antibiotics is probably not at risk of systemic complications during dental treatment.

The practitioner should take particular note of any past hospitalizations, including outpatient surgery. Important examples include treatment for cancer, cardiovascular surgery, or placement of prosthetic joints or other prostheses. If medical or surgical procedures are part of a patient's history, the dentist will want to know whether complications such as excessive pain, bleeding, infection, poor healing, or adverse reactions to drugs occurred during the treatment. A history of such events suggests the possibility that similar occurrences may occur in association with dental treatment. At every appointment the dentist should ask the patient if any medications have changed because of new surgical or medical treatments.

When a potentially life-limiting disease, such as cancer or severe congestive heart failure, has been diagnosed, the patient's long-term prognosis should be determined, because that information may influence decisions regarding which treatment options are most appropriate. For instance, a patient who is being treated for pancreatic cancer may wish to have missing teeth replaced to be able to chew food better or to improve esthetics. Although dental implants may be an ideal long-term solution, a less expensive and more immediate solution, such as a provisional removable partial denture, may be more appropriate. It is important to note, however, that the dentist has a professional responsibility to share all reasonable treatment options with any patient, regardless of age, physical condition, or financial status.

Current Health Information

In addition to identifying past health problems, the dentist needs to investigate findings related to current health conditions. The systemic health problems of many ambulatory patients relate directly or indirectly to chronic conditions such arthritis, pulmonary diseases, heart disease, asthma, cancer, diabetes, hepatitis, hypertension, stroke, and weak or failing kidneys.[1] Other problems, more episodic in nature, may not be associated with a chronic disease. Examples include seizure disorders, fainting, and seasonal allergies. Certain habits, such as tobacco use, excessive alcohol consumption, or substance abuse, can influence both systemic and oral health.

An important source of information about the patient's current health is an evaluation of the prescription and over-the-counter drugs taken on a regular basis. All medications should be carefully documented and monitored, including prescription drugs, over-the-counter products, health and nutritional supplements, herbal medicines, and illicit substances. When all the patient's medications have been identified, the dentist should determine the indications for each, consulting a drug reference book or online resource, if necessary. This information should corroborate findings from the health questionnaire and provide some insight into the severity of a particular disease. Occasionally, the patient may be taking medications for conditions not originally identified on the health questionnaire. For example, an elderly patient may report taking furosemide (Lasix) and digoxin (Lanoxin) for a blood pressure problem. The astute dentist will recognize that these drugs are commonly used to treat congestive heart failure, a much more serious condition. Patients with chronic conditions such as hypertension or diabetes may need to be questioned about their level

of compliance taking medications if these conditions are not under control.

In addition to recognizing or determining the indications for each of the patient's medications, the dentist must be aware of possible side effects. Of particular concern will be those side effects that adversely affect oral health or could cause problems for the patient while receiving dental treatment. For example, aspirin or anticoagulant drugs may promote excessive bleeding during periodontal or oral surgical procedures. Many medications affect the quantity and quality of saliva produced, predisposing the patient to increased risk of caries, periodontal disease, and mucosal diseases.

After examining the health questionnaire and medication list, the dentist interviews the patient. How severe are the reported health problems? Does the patient see a physician or other heath professional regularly? Is the patient taking the prescribed medications as directed and are they effective in treating the conditions they were prescribed for? When this information has been gathered, the dentist needs to evaluate whether the patent's systemic problems present a risk to providing dental care or could adversely affect the prognosis for the proposed dental treatment. The American Society of Anesthesiologists (ASA) has adopted a widely used classification system for estimating patient risk status (Table 8.1).[7] The dentist may require an ASA category III or IV patient to seek medical consultation before treatment. For example, a patient who cannot climb a flight of stairs without resting and complains of occasional chest pain on exertion may be referred to a physician to evaluate for ischemic heart disease.

Patients should be asked about allergies or reactions to drugs or other substances. The dentist will be most interested in avoiding reactions to materials commonly used in dentistry. These include allergies or reactions to drugs such as penicillin, erythromycin, aspirin, nonsteroidal antiinflammatory drugs (NSAIDs), codeine, and other narcotics. Some patients are sensitive to latex products and others to certain metals in dental restorations. Patients may report problems with local and topical anesthetics or flavorings used in dentistry. The dentist needs to discern whether the patient has a true allergy, has experienced a side effect or toxic reaction, or simply does not care for

TABLE 8.1	American Society of Anesthesiologists (ASA) Physical Status Classification With Examples	
Category	Definition	Examples
ASA I	A normal healthy patient with no evidence of systemic disease	
ASA II	A patient with mild systemic disease or a significant health risk factor; the patient is able to walk up a flight of stairs or two level city blocks without difficulty	Well-controlled diabetes, controlled hypertension, history of asthma, mild obesity, pregnancy, smoker, extreme anxiety or fear toward dentistry
ASA III	A patient with moderate to severe systemic disease that limits activity but is not incapacitating; the patient can walk up one flight of stairs or two level city blocks, but stops at times because of distress	Stable angina, postmyocardial infarction, poorly controlled hypertension, symptomatic respiratory disease, massive obesity
ASA IV	A patient with severe systemic disease that is life threatening; the patient is unable to walk up a flight of stairs or two level city blocks; patient is in distress at rest	Unstable angina, liver failure, severe congestive heart failure, or end-stage renal disease

the product. If it is determined that the patient has a true allergy, a medical alert label or warning message should be prominently displayed in the record. Frequently seen medical alert warnings in dentistry include allergies to latex and certain antibiotics such as penicillin or erythromycin, bleeding and blood pressure problems, and the need for antibiotic premedication.

In some institutional settings, or healthcare clinics providing both medical and dental services, the dentist may be able to review the patient's electronic medical record. This can be helpful to study the patient's medical problem list, current medications and allergies and laboratory test results. The patient may also have access to their own medical records via a **patient portal** (see Chapter 4). In such instances, the patient, and not just their primary care practitioner, may be able to provide important information using their mobile phone or another electronic device.

Findings From Physical Evaluation

Vital Signs

One of the most commonly detected vital sign abnormalities is high blood pressure or hypertension. The value, significance, and methods for obtaining a patient's vital signs are discussed in Chapter 1. Blood pressure measurements should be taken and recorded at every patient appointment. Most patients with hypertension can receive dental treatment but may also need a referral to the healthcare provider for evaluation and treatment (Table 8.2). Systemic phase treatment for patients with hypertension may include medical consultation, reducing anxiety and stress, and careful attention to rapid changes in chair position. Moderate amounts of local anesthesia with epinephrine may be used in hypertensive patients.

Visual Inspection and Oral Examination

Evaluation of the patient's general appearance may suggest the presence of one or more systemic diseases. Abnormalities in appearance alone are usually not sufficient to support a definitive diagnosis, but they may corroborate other findings from the health history. Because the dental profession encourages regular maintenance visits and many patients comply with this standard, the dentist has the opportunity to evaluate the patient at regular intervals and, as a result, may sometimes be the first healthcare provider to identify a systemic problem (Figure 8.1). Signs of

such problems might be increased weight caused by water retention resulting from cardiopulmonary problems or changes in skin color and fingernail beds. Changes in gait or posture may indicate neurologic or musculoskeletal problems, such as arthritis of the hip or knee, a stroke, or Parkinson's disease.

Examination of the head and neck region may reveal other findings indicative of systemic disease. Skin color may vary from red and ruddy, suggestive of alcohol abuse, to a pale yellow seen with liver damage associated with hepatitis. Malodors from the mouth may be a sign of excessive alcohol consumption or, when a fruity smell is detected, poorly controlled diabetes. The clinician should pay close attention to the condition of eyes and other facial structures. For example, thinning hair and eyebrows accompanied by dry skin may be a sign of a thyroid disorder. The dentist should also rule out systemic disease as a cause of abnormalities detected during palpation and examination of the head, neck, and oral cavity (Table 8.3). The dentist may choose to refer the patient for a medical consultation or laboratory test when abnormal findings are detected during the physical examination. Some patients can access their medical records electronically and may share information about health problems, medications, and blood test values.

EVALUATING RELATIONSHIP BETWEEN SYSTEMIC HEALTH AND DENTAL TREATMENT

When the need for systemic treatment for a general health condition has been identified, the dentist must weigh the risk of aggravating health problems by providing treatment for dental disease against the risk of delaying treatment. For example, a patient with frequent chest pain, suggestive of unstable angina, may best be referred to a physician for evaluation and treatment before a potentially stressful dental treatment, such as the extraction of several teeth. On the other hand, a new patient who has a blood pressure measurement of 150/95 mm Hg and no other health concerns may also need to be referred to a physician to be evaluated for hypertension, but the dentist will probably feel comfortable providing such services as an examination or prophylaxis.

For the patient with serious health problems, the dentist must consider several questions. How critical would a particular treatment be to the overall oral health of the patient? For example, removing an asymptomatic, impacted third molar even in

TABLE 8.2 Dental Management and Follow-Up Recommendations Based on Blood Pressure

Blood Pressure (mmHg)	Dental Treatment Recommendations	Follow-Up Recommendations
≤120/80	Any required	No physician referral necessary
≥120/80 but <140/90	Any required	Encourage patient to see physician
≥140/90 but <160/100	Any required	Encourage patient to see physician
≥160/100 but <180/110	Any required; consider intraoperative monitoring of blood pressure for upper-level stage 2 hypertension	Refer patient to physician promptly (within 1 month)
≥180/110	Defer elective treatment	Refer to physician as soon as possible; if patient is symptomatic, refer immediately

From Little JW, Miller CS, Rhodus NL. *Little and Falace's Dental Management of the Medically Compromised Patient*. 9th ed. St. Louis: Elsevier; 2018.

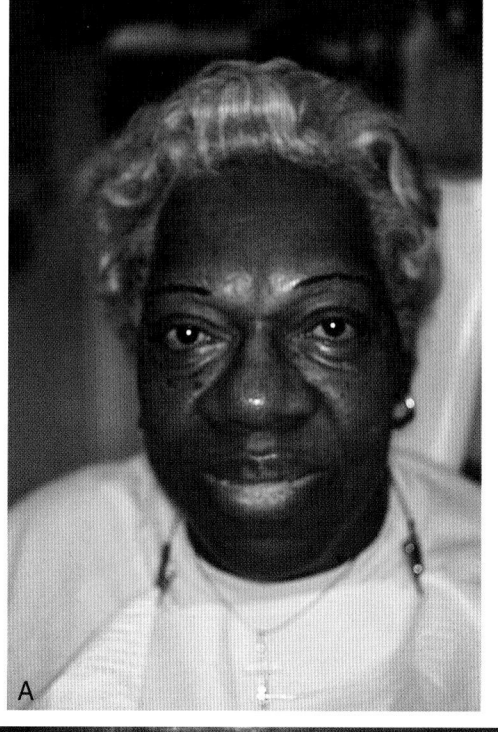

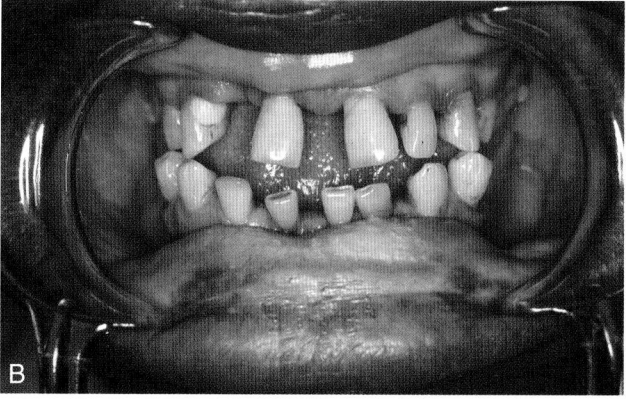

Fig. 8.1 When viewed alone, this patient's full lips and thick nose do not suggest a systemic problem. The patient came to the dentist complaining of the growing spaces between her teeth and an inability to wear her removable partial dentures. She also reported that her hands seemed larger and her rings and gloves no longer fit. The dentist suspected a systemic problem and referred the patient to a physician. The patient was diagnosed with acromegaly, a condition in adults in which excessive growth hormone is produced. A benign tumor on her pituitary gland was discovered and removed.

a healthy 60-year-old woman may not be indicated. Additional questions to consider when evaluating the patient with serious health problems include the following:

- Is the patient in pain or do they have an infection?
- Does the patient want comprehensive care or are they interested only in having a specific procedure done?
- Are there other dental problems that need immediate attention?
- Does the patient have a physician? Are they willing to seek medical evaluation if it is warranted? How severe are the individual's health problems?
- What would be the ramifications of providing no treatment at this time?

TABLE 8.3	**Examples of Oral Signs of Systemic Conditions**
Finding	**Possible Problem**
Erosion of the teeth, especially anterior teeth	Gastroesophageal reflux disease, bulimia
Oral yeast infection	Decreased immunity associated with poorly controlled diabetes, AIDS, chemotherapy, or severely debilitated patients
Reduced saliva production, caries	Medication side effect, autoimmune disease such as Sjögren's syndrome, dehydration, bulimia
Gingival hyperplasia	Local reaction to cancer chemotherapy, seizure control drugs, or some cardiac medications

TABLE 8.4	**Risk Categories for Selected Dental Procedures**
Dental Procedures	**Risk of Systemic Complications**
Oral examination, radiographs, study models	Little to none
Local anesthesia, simple restorative treatment, prophylaxis, asymptomatic endodontic therapy, straightforward extractions, orthodontic treatment	Low
Symptomatic endodontic therapy, multiple extractions, single implant placement, deep scaling, and root planing	Medium
Extensive surgical procedures, multiple implant placement, general anesthesia	High

The clinician is most cautious about providing services that would be particularly stressful for the patient. To be sure, much of the stress may be caused by the patient's level of anxiety, but some procedures, such as extractions and periodontal surgery, are inherently invasive and more challenging for patients to tolerate. Any outpatient treatment requiring long appointment times or during which excessive bleeding might occur should be provided only to relatively healthy patients, those in ASA categories I and II. Patients in ASA category III or IV who are in pain as a result of dental or periodontal conditions may best be managed with analgesics and possibly antibiotic medication and consultation with or referral to a physician. Table 8.4 lists the risk of systemic complications associated with some common dental procedures.

SYSTEMIC PROCEDURES

Most of the therapies discussed throughout this book pertain specifically to treatment of the teeth and surrounding structures. Systemic therapy, in contrast, focuses on the entire patient, with the goal of ensuring that dental care is delivered safely and comfortably. Some systemic procedures address the patient's physical concerns directly, such as postponing care and consulting a physician, prescribing drugs for pain and infection, and making the patient comfortable in the dental chair. Other techniques are instituted to effect behavioral changes—for example, instruction in smoking cessation or diet modification. Some techniques serve to reduce patient stress and anxiety. In addition, the dentist provides an important service by reviewing and updating the patient's health history on a regular basis. Although none of these therapies is technically difficult to provide, the challenge for dental practitioners is recognizing when, why, and how to provide them in support of the patient's systemic health and overall well-being. The dentist must assess the patient before, during, and after treatment to determine whether any of these therapies is indicated and reassess the patient at future appointments.

Regularly Reviewing and Updating the General Health History

The practitioner should review each patient's health history before beginning dental treatment. In busy dental offices, this routine can easily be overlooked, leading to common mistakes, such as using latex gloves with a latex-sensitive patient or prescribing the wrong type of antibiotic or other medication. Most electronic health records display prominent alerts regarding allergies, significant systemic conditions, or the need to premedicate or take other preparatory actions with the patient. For practices that use a paper health questionnaire, it should be in a conspicuous location at the start of each appointment (possibly paper-clipped to the outside of the patient's record) to serve as a reminder of this important task.

Every practitioner should have procedures in place for a regular review and updating of the health questionnaire, recording any changes in the patient's health. This procedure may need to be implemented at every appointment for patients with serious systemic conditions, whereas the dental hygienist can interview other patients during regular maintenance visits.

Questions that may rouse the patient's memory regarding changes in health status include:

- "Are you being treated by a physician for any new disease or condition? These are the conditions currently we have listed in your record. When was your last visit to your physician? For what reason?"
- "Has there been any change in the medications you are taking? Here is what I have listed in your record."
- "Have you developed any new allergies or sensitivities to drugs?"

For a more thorough review of changes, the patient should complete a new health questionnaire every 2 to 3 years or after a specified number of updates.

Postponing or Limiting Treatment

Deciding whether it is in the best interests of the patient to limit or postpone dental care is always a difficult decision. The determination is usually made after a review of the patient's physical and psychological condition with respect to the level of invasiveness of the dental treatment to be provided. Sometimes the decision is straightforward. Consider, for example, the patient scheduled for periodontal surgery whose blood pressure registers at 180/110 mm Hg. Such a finding would be a clear indication

for postponing the procedure so that the patient can seek medical consultation. It may not be necessary to cancel treatment for a patient with elevated blood pressure, particularly if the patient is taking medication, is being monitored by a healthcare provider and does not demonstrate signs of angina pectoris or congestive heart failure.[8] Other situations for which it may be advisable to delay treatment include those involving the patient who is not feeling well, is extremely anxious, demonstrates signs of intoxication from alcohol or other substances, or has a health condition that requires immediate medical attention.

Managing the patient with significant systemic problems or abnormal vital signs and an acute dental problem, such as severe pain associated with an irreversible pulpitis, presents particular difficulties. It may be necessary to provide limited therapy, such as initiating root canal therapy or prescribing an antibiotic, and analgesic drugs for pain control. The dentist can also use a long-acting local anesthetic, such as bupivacaine HCl (Marcaine), to provide immediate relief while conducting a more detailed examination, contacting a physician by phone, or reevaluating the patient's vital signs.

Consultation With a Physician or Other Healthcare Provider

All dentists should feel comfortable contacting other health professionals to discuss a patient's condition. Three common reasons for contacting a patient's physician can be described. First, a physician may be contacted to request physical evaluation and treatment for the patient when signs of systemic disease are initially discovered in the dental office. In this situation, a written consult is most useful, particularly if the patient does not have a regular physician currently (see *In Clinical Practice: Writing a Medical Consultation Letter* box). For example, a patient might be referred for treatment of hypertension with a letter that contains the most recent blood pressure measurements, a summary of the dental treatment planned, and a request to evaluate and treat the hypertension.

Second, the dentist may wish to request additional information about or clarification of the patient's current physical condition. This might include confirming systemic diagnoses, such as the patient's cardiac condition after a heart attack, obtaining laboratory values (blood tests), or reviewing current medication regimens. As discussed in the *In Clinical Practice: Consulting a Another Healthcare Provider by Telephone* box, contact by phone is typical. Any new information should be documented in the patient's record.

Finally, the dentist may need input from the physician to help determine whether providing dental treatment for the patient would be a prudent course of action. For example, consider the patient with many health concerns, who is under treatment by several medical specialists. Unless one physician is coordinating care, the dentist may need to discuss the situation with several physicians, gathering information and opinions to help determine which course should be taken. This does not involve asking permission to provide dental care, but is rather a collegial discussion of the proposed treatment plan and the risks and benefits it brings to the patient. The desired outcome of such conversations is a mutual decision as to which treatment can

Writing a Medical Consultation Letter

A medical consultation letter to another healthcare provider must contain the following five items:

1. Patient identifying information. At a minimum, the full patient name and birthdate should be listed in the consultation letter. Some dentists include a release of health information statement that is signed by the patient.
2. The patient's history and/or the findings that indicated the consultation letter; the patient's medication history with dosages may also be included.
3. The proposed dental treatment, including some indication of how physically stressful the treatment may be; a listing of drugs (anesthetics/analgesics) proposed to be used during and after the treatment also may be included. Avoid unnecessary detail and technical terminology when describing proposed treatment. "Mesial occlusal composite resin on a lower left premolar and removal of impacted third molar" might be better stated as "one dental filling and surgical removal of a tooth."
4. A specific request for information or action. Examples include requests for physical evaluation and management of hypertension or diabetes, sharing blood test results, or rendering an opinion as to whether the patient should be premedicated.
5. The dentist's name, address, telephone, email address and fax phone number.

Remember that the dental treatment of the patient is your responsibility. You should not expect the healthcare provider to accept that responsibility or dictate treatment. You are asking the provider, in light of their knowledge and understanding of the patient's condition, to assist you in making an appropriate decision about what level of treatment the patient can tolerate. The following is an example of such a letter to a physician:

October 13, 2023

From: Stephen J Stefanac, DDS, MS

To: John Smith, MD

RE: Rebecca Roe (DOB: March 28,1954)

Dear Doctor Smith:

When Rebecca Roe presented for a new patient examination, blood pressure measurements from her right arm while sitting were 160/95, 162/93, and 160/96 mm Hg. The only medication she reports taking is metformin for type 2 diabetes.

Ms. Roe will require deep cleaning of her teeth, four fillings, and a crown. All procedures can be accomplished with minimal stress using local anesthetic containing 2% lidocaine and 1:100,000 epinephrine.

Please evaluate and treat Ms. Roe's hypertension and inform me when her blood pressure is optimized with acceptable risk to proceed. If there are any other health considerations of which I should be aware, please let me know and also make any recommendations you see fit.

Should you require any additional information, please do not hesitate to contact me.

Sincerely,

Stephen J Stefanac, DDS, MS

1011 N, University St,

Ann Arbor, MI 48109-1078

stefanac@umich.edu

734.555.1212 734.555.1213 fax

Consulting Another Healthcare Provider by Telephone

Often, the most expeditious method for consulting with a physician or other healthcare provider, especially when the patient has both significant health problems and urgent dental needs, is a telephone call. Because patients may receive care from a number of physicians, the dentist must first confirm who is the best physician to call. Is it the primary care physician or a specialist? It may be necessary first to fax or email a form signed by the patient permitting the physician to discuss their health information.

Ideally, the dentist should place the call, although some practitioners delegate straightforward consultations to other staff members. During the call, the patient's record should be available for reference, including identifying information, such as date of birth and home address. Writing specific questions out beforehand helps ensure that all necessary information is obtained.

When the receptionist in the physician's office answers the phone, the dentist should clearly state the patient's name and the general purpose of the call, and request to speak with the physician. In situations involving simple requests, laboratory values, or test results, it may be appropriate to speak with a nurse or the physician's assistant.

When the physician is on the line, the dentist should again confirm the patient's name and birthdate and state the reason for the telephone call. All significant systemic diagnoses and any medications the patient may be taking should be verified. Although unnecessary detail concerning the proposed dental treatment should be avoided, the physician should be informed of the urgency of the procedure (i.e., elective, urgent, emergency) and the anticipated levels of stress, blood loss, and possible postoperative problems. Any drugs that will be used before, during, and after treatment should be discussed. With questions to the physician that are clear and to the point, the dentist should gain sufficient information to reshape plans for treatment appropriately. Copies of any laboratory results in the physician's record for the patient may be requested and can be sent by secure email or fax for incorporation into the patient's dental record. All other new information should be documented in the patient record immediately after the telephone call.

and should be provided, and how the care can be delivered to minimize patient health risks.

Several problems can occur when consulting a physician. If there is no answer to a written consultation request, the dentist will want to confirm, usually by telephone, that the physician did indeed receive it. The dentist may first wish to determine whether a correct mailing address was used or, if the request was to be hand-carried by the patient, confirm that the patient actually visited the physician. Occasionally, a physician will return a written request with an unclear response or one that the dentist may not agree with. When this occurs, the dentist will want to contact the physician by phone for additional clarification or further discussion of the patient's health problems.

Stress Management

Many patients find visiting the dentist to be an anxiety-provoking experience. A detailed discussion of the manifestations, implications, and management of fear and anxiety is presented in Chapter 15. Anxiety frequently manifests itself as **stress**, a disturbance in the individual's normal homeostasis resulting from events that may be physical, mental, or emotional in nature. Helping the patient cope with stress represents one of the most beneficial systemic treatments a dentist can provide. This will be particularly important for patients with such systemic problems as cardiac disease, diabetes, and adrenocortical insufficiency.

Stressful events have a physiologic effect on the body, primarily because of the release of a class of substances called *catecholamines*, which include epinephrine and norepinephrine. These chemicals tend to speed up the body's metabolism, in particular making the heart work harder by increasing heart rate and creating an increased need for more oxygen in the cardiac muscle. Imagine, for a moment, how an anxious but physically healthy patient is affected by stress. The stressful experience often begins with a loss of sleep for one or more days before the dental appointment. The stress builds during the day as the patient worries about seeing the dentist and continues as they sit in the reception area, anticipating the dreaded appointment. Once in the dental chair, the patient may experience an increase in blood pressure and heart rate and may breathe rapidly, or even excessively, a condition referred to as **hyperventilation**. Such a patient will have a heightened awareness to pain that may persist even with sufficient amounts of local anesthetic. Under these circumstances, the appointment will be an unpleasant experience for both the patient and the dentist.

Patients whose health is severely compromised may experience even more severe reactions to stress than those described for a healthy patient. Patients with poor blood flow to the heart muscle may have chest pain or **angina**. Individuals with congestive heart failure can retain fluid in the lungs, developing **acute pulmonary edema**. Patients with asthma may have problems breathing. During a stressful event, the insulin-dependent diabetic patient may have altered glucose metabolism and develop symptoms from low blood sugar levels. Patients who have been taking corticosteroid medication for extended periods may be unable to tolerate high levels of stress, suffering an **adrenocortical crisis**.

Managing stress for the patient with severe systemic conditions involves several procedures, summarized in Box 8.2. As always, the clinician begins with a careful review of the health history, followed by a sympathetic discussion of the patient's level of anxiety. The patient should be encouraged to freely express any fears, including describing any past unpleasant experiences in the dental chair. Discussing the details of the treatment plan so that the patient is familiar with the planned procedures and can ask questions about them may help alleviate the anxiety. For some patients, it may be advantageous to prescribe a medication in advance of the appointment to improve sleep the night before and help reduce anxiety.

For patients whose health is severely compromised, additional measures to control stress may be necessary.

BOX 8.2 Managing Stress for the Patient With Serious Health Problems

1. Review the health history and interview the patient regarding their level of stress.
2. Discuss the treatment plan, options for pain management, and possible postoperative complications.
3. Consider contacting the patient's primary care provider about prescribing medication to reduce anxiety and improve sleep before appointments.
4. Schedule short appointments. If longer appointments are required, give the patient time for breaks.
5. Minimize the time the patient spends waiting for the appointment to begin by scheduling them as the first patient in the morning or afternoon.
6. Consider using nitrous oxide, antianxiety medication, or conscious sedation.
7. Obtain good local anesthesia.
8. Plan for postoperative pain and complications; prescribe analgesics and antibiotic medication if necessary.
9. Contact the patient at home after treatment; be available should complications or questions arise after hours.

Shorter appointments when the patient is feeling physically and psychologically well can be arranged. The patient should not have to wait long to be seen after arriving for the appointment. The dentist may wish to consider using relaxation techniques or medications to help reduce anxiety and stress. These include hypnosis, guided imagery, nitrous oxide analgesia, oral antianxiety drugs, and intravenous sedation. It will be critical to control the patient's pain with adequate amounts of local anesthetic. At the conclusion of treatment, possible postoperative problems, especially the potential for pain and infection, should be explained to the patient. For some compromised individuals, it may be appropriate to prescribe analgesic medications and antibiotics to prevent infection. Finally, the dentist should assure the patient that they can be contacted by phone after the appointment if the patient has questions or postoperative complications. Some dentists regularly make early evening phone calls to patients who have had stressful procedures performed earlier in the day.

Prescribing or Altering Patient Medication

Several medication options are available for the treatment of both systemic and dental problems. The medications most commonly prescribed by general dentists are antibiotics and medications used to control pain and anxiety. Less frequently, dentists may recommend corticosteroid drugs to control inflammation or need to administer epinephrine and oxygen in the event of a patient emergency.

Antibiotics

Antibiotic drugs may be prescribed to treat or to prevent infection. The usual sources of oral infection stem from problems with the teeth and periodontal tissues—for example, apical or periodontal abscesses. These conditions are best treated by eliminating the cause of the problem by performing endodontic therapy, extracting the offending tooth, or debriding an area with periodontal inflammation. When the infection has spread beyond the original source, causing extensive swelling or lymphadenitis, or when signs of systemic infection appear, such as an elevated temperature, fever, and malaise, antibiotic drugs may be indicated.

A particular concern for the dentist is to prevent the occurrence of heart infections. Some patients have cardiac conditions that put them at risk of developing **infective endocarditis** several weeks after receiving dental treatment. To prevent this infection, dentists in the United States prescribe a single oral dose of antibiotic medication to be taken by the patient 1 hour before the procedure. Boxes 8.3 and 8.4 list the dental procedures and cardiac abnormalities for which the American Heart Association has recommended antibiotic prophylaxis. Table 8.5 lists the various oral antibiotic regimens currently available. A discussion of the issues associated with administering antibiotics for the prevention of prosthetic joint infection is presented in Chapter 18.

Pain Medications

As discussed earlier, controlling pain is a crucial objective when managing stress. A wide variety of medications can be used to

BOX 8.3 Dental Procedures for Which Endocarditis Prophylaxis Is Recommended for Patients

All dental procedures that involve manipulation of gingival tissue or the periapical region of teeth or perforation of the oral mucosa.

The following procedures and events **do not require** prophylaxis: Anesthetic injections through noninfected tissue, taking dental radiographs, placement of removable prosthodontic or orthodontic appliances, adjustment of orthodontic appliances, placement of orthodontic brackets, shedding of primary teeth, and bleeding from trauma to the lips or oral mucosa

From Wilson WR, Gewitz M, Lockhart PB, et al.; American Heart Association Young Hearts Rheumatic Fever, Endocarditis and Kawasaki Disease Committee of the Council on Lifelong Congenital Heart Disease and Heart Health in the Young; Council on Cardiovascular and Stroke Nursing; Council on Quality of Care and Outcomes Research. Prevention of viridans group streptococcal infective endocarditis: a scientific statement from the American Heart Association. *Circulation.* 2021;143(20):e963-e978.

BOX 8.4 Underlying Conditions for Which Antibiotic Prophylaxis Is Suggested

Prosthetic cardiac valve or material
- Presence of cardiac prosthetic valve
- Transcatheter implantation of prosthetic valves
- Cardiac valve repair with devices, including annuloplasty, rings, or clips
- Left ventricular assist devices or implantable heart

Previous, relapse, or recurrent infective endocarditis

Congenital heart disease (CHD)
- Unrepaired cyanotic congenital CHD, including palliative shunts and conduits
- Completely repaired congenital heart defect with prosthetic material or device, whether placed by surgery or by transcatheter during the first 6 months after the procedure
- Repaired CHD with residual defects at the site or adjacent to the site of or adjacent to the site of a prosthetic patch or prosthetic device

Cardiac transplantation recipients who develop cardiac valvulopathy

Procedure for which antibiotic prophylaxis is **not suggested:**
- Implantable electronic devices such as a pacemaker or similar devices
- Septal defect closure device when complete closure is achieved
- Peripheral vascular grafts and patches including those used for hemodialysis
- Coronary artery stents or other vascular stents
- CNS ventricular shunts
- Vena cava filter
- Pledgets

From Wilson WR, Gewitz M, Lockhart PB, et al.; American Heart Association Young Hearts Rheumatic Fever, Endocarditis and Kawasaki Disease Committee of the Council on Lifelong Congenital Heart Disease and Heart Health in the Young; Council on Cardiovascular and Stroke Nursing; Council on Quality of Care and Outcomes Research. Prevention of Viridans Group Streptococcal Infective Endocarditis: A Scientific Statement From the American Heart Association. Circulation. 2021;143(20):e963-e978.

TABLE 8.5 Adult Oral Antibiotic Regimens for the Prevention of Bacterial Endocarditis

Situation	Agent	Regimen: Single dose 30–60 min before procedure
Not allergic to penicillin	Amoxicillin	2 g
Allergic to penicillin	Cephalexin[a]	2 g
	Or	
	Azithromycin or clarithromycin	500 mg
	Or	
	Doxycycline	100 mg

[a]Cephalosporins should not be used in an individual with a history of anaphylaxis, angioedema, or urticaria after taking penicillin or ampicillin.

From Wilson WR, Gewitz M, Lockhart PB, et al.; American Heart Association Young Hearts Rheumatic Fever, Endocarditis and Kawasaki Disease Committee of the Council on Lifelong Congenital Heart Disease and Heart Health in the Young; Council on Cardiovascular and Stroke Nursing; and the Council on Quality of Care and Outcomes Research. Prevention of viridans group streptococcal infective endocarditis: a scientific statement from the American Heart Association. *Circulation.* 2021;143(20):e963-e978.

example, a patient who takes the blood thinning (anticoagulant) medication warfarin sodium (Coumadin) must avoid aspirin and many other medications. Most narcotics depress respiratory function and should therefore be very cautiously used in patients with pulmonary diseases, such as emphysema. Antianxiety and sedative drugs are frequently used to manage stress in the patient with compromised health and are discussed in more detail in Chapter 15. Consultation with the patient's physician may be necessary to resolve these questions and, in some instances, may facilitate a temporary alteration in the patient's medication regimen to accommodate dental treatment requirements. For example, the diabetic patient may adjust the insulin dose taken before a lengthy appointment or the dose of an anticoagulant drug may be reduced before a surgical procedure although this practice may not be necessary for most dental extractions.[9-11]

Positioning Patient in Dental Chair

Some patients may be unable to tolerate being placed in certain positions in the dental chair. Conditions such as congestive heart failure or emphysema can be aggravated when the patient is reclined for even a short period. Before beginning treatment, the practitioner should query the patient about what reclining angle is comfortable. Patients with arthritis or back problems appreciate being offered a pillow or folded towel to use for additional neck and back support. Women in the last trimester of pregnancy often feel more comfortable turned slightly to the side in the chair. During treatment, patients with serious health problems should be asked how they are doing at regular intervals and should be allowed to take a break occasionally and sit up. The patient who feels cold in the dental chair will appreciate being offered a blanket for warmth.

To prevent inducing faintness by a rapid change in position, raise the chair slowly after an extended dental procedure.

help control pain. Such nonprescription analgesic drugs as aspirin, ibuprofen, and acetaminophen can be effective. Prescription medications include narcotic and nonnarcotic pain relievers, many with both analgesic and antiinflammatory properties. Some patients with serious health problems cannot tolerate or should not be given certain types of analgesic medications, often because they will interact with other drugs the patient is taking. For

Faintness after a change from a reclining to a sitting position or from sitting to standing, caused by **orthostatic hypotension**, may happen with any patient but is seen more frequently in individuals with poor circulatory reflexes from heart problems or as an effect of certain medications prescribed to treat high blood pressure. To prevent this problem, the chair should be raised in two to three increments, pausing for 10 to 20 seconds at each stop.

HOW SYSTEMIC CONDITIONS CAN AFFECT TREATMENT PLANNING

Although it is beyond the scope of this textbook to provide a comprehensive discussion of all systemic health conditions that could affect the delivery of dental care, the following three examples describe situations that occur with some frequency in a dental office. The examples illustrate the fact that simple rules alone cannot always provide sufficient guidance on how to treat such patients. Every dentist has a professional duty to be aware of treatment modifications that may be required when managing patients with significant systemic conditions. The core of this knowledge is first gained in dental school and must be supplemented regularly by experience, reading journal articles and textbooks, participating in continuing education programs, and consulting with other health professionals.

Both dentistry and medicine have entered an era of rapid change in the ways in which diseases are diagnosed and treated. Some studies have proposed that certain oral diseases may be predictive of, or cause, diseases such as preterm birth, diabetes, cardiovascular disease, stroke, and cancer.[12] Unfortunately, there is a lack of high-quality evidence and the association of an oral condition with a systemic disease does not prove causation.[13] Conversely, there are also strong associations between certain systemic conditions, such as diabetes and cardiovascular disease, and oral health.[14] Although definitive evidence may be lacking at this time, helping patients achieve and maintain oral health is nevertheless important to maintaining overall health.

Chronic Renal Failure

The kidneys provide a number of functions for healthy individuals. These include removing waste and drugs from the body, secretion of hormones, and maintenance of overall metabolic functions. Chronic kidney disease (CKD) affects approximately 15% of adults in the United States, most commonly over 65 years of age. As many as 9 in 10 adults are unaware they have the condition.[15] Common causes of kidney failure include congenital abnormalities and poorly managed diabetes and hypertension.

Kidney function is measured by evaluating the urinary level of albumin, the glomerular filtration rate and creatinine clearance. Blood serum values most used to evaluate kidney disease include creatine and blood urea nitrogen levels (see Table 8.6) for the range of values). Patients with early signs of kidney disease are managed with diet modification and control of diabetes or hypertension when present. Patients with severe kidney disease and renal failure are referred to as having end-stage renal disease (ESRD) and must have their kidney function replaced by receiving regular dialysis treatments (71% of patients) or by receiving a kidney transplant (29%).[15] Patients receiving kidney transplants can be treated in a similar manner as patients without kidney disease although treatment modifications may be necessary because of antirejection drugs such as cyclosporine.[16]

CKD is a good example of a systemic condition that can affect many other organ systems (Figure 8.2). The disorders of most concern to the dentist are hypertension, drug intolerance, and abnormal bleeding. The dentist should regularly review the patient's medications and measure the patient's blood pressure before, during, and after treatment. If the patient has a dialysis shunt in their forearm, blood pressure measurements should be

TABLE 8.6	**Laboratory Values for the Assessment of Renal Function and Failure**		
Laboratory Test	**Reference Value**	**Indicator[a] of Renal Insufficiency (Stages II-IV)**	**Indicator of Renal Failure (Stage V)**
URINE			
Albuminuria	<30 mg/g	30–300 mg /g	>300 mg/g
Creatinine clearance	85–125 mL/min (women)	50–90 mL/ min	Moderate: 10–50 mL/ min; severe: <10 mL/ min
	97–140 mL/min[c]		
Glomerular filtration rate (GFR)[b]	100–150 mL/min	15–89 mL/ min	Moderate: <15 mL/ min; severe: <10 mL/ min
SERUM			
Blood urea nitrogen	8–18 mg/dL (3–6.5 mmol/L)	20–30 mg/dL	Moderate: 30–50 mg/dL; severe: >50 mg /dL
Creatinine	0.6–1.20 mg/dL	2–3 mg/dL	Moderate: 3–6 mg/dL; severe: >6 mg /dL

[a]Secondary indicators of renal function. Normal reference values: calcium, 8.2–11.2 mg/dL; chloride, 95–103 mmol/L; inorganic phosphorus, 2.7–4.5 mg/dL; potassium, 3.8–5 mmol/L; sodium, 136–142 mmol/L; total carbon dioxide for venous blood, 22–26 mmoUL; and uric acid, 2.4–7.0 mg/dL.
[b]GFR is often calculated using the Cockcroft-Gault equation, the Modification of Diet in Renal Disease Study equation, or the Chronic Kidney Disease Epidemiology Collaboration equation.
[c]Gavalda C, Bagan J, Scully C, et al. Renal hemodialysis patients: oral, salivary, dental and periodontal findings in 105 adult cases. Oral Dis. 1999;5(4):299–302.
From Little JW, Miller CS, Rhodus NL. *Little and Falace's Dental Management of the Medically Compromised Patient.* 9th ed. [Table 12.2] St. Louis: Elsevier; 2018.

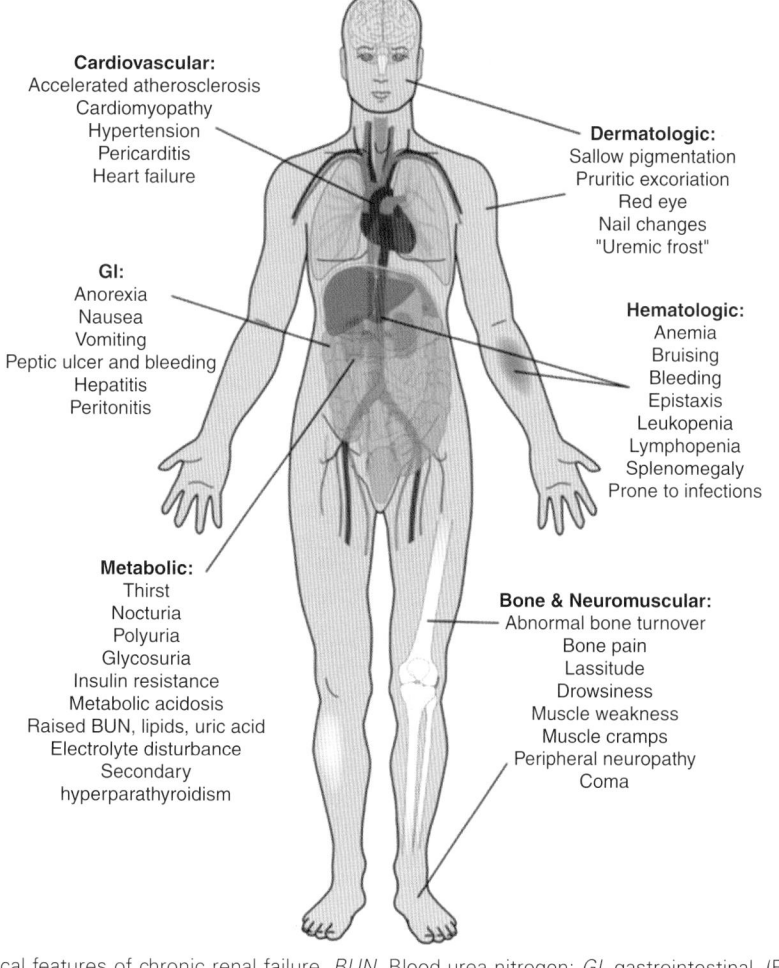

Cardiovascular:
Accelerated atherosclerosis
Cardiomyopathy
Hypertension
Pericarditis
Heart failure

Dermatologic:
Sallow pigmentation
Pruritic excoriation
Red eye
Nail changes
"Uremic frost"

GI:
Anorexia
Nausea
Vomiting
Peptic ulcer and bleeding
Hepatitis
Peritonitis

Hematologic:
Anemia
Bruising
Bleeding
Epistaxis
Leukopenia
Lymphopenia
Splenomegaly
Prone to infections

Metabolic:
Thirst
Nocturia
Polyuria
Glycosuria
Insulin resistance
Metabolic acidosis
Raised BUN, lipids, uric acid
Electrolyte disturbance
Secondary
hyperparathyroidism

Bone & Neuromuscular:
Abnormal bone turnover
Bone pain
Lassitude
Drowsiness
Muscle weakness
Muscle cramps
Peripheral neuropathy
Coma

Fig. 8.2 Clinical features of chronic renal failure. *BUN*, Blood urea nitrogen; *GI*, gastrointestinal. (From Little JW, Miller CS, Rhodus NL. *Little and Falace's Dental Management of the Medically Compromised Patient.* 9th ed. [Fig. 12.5] St. Louis: Elsevier; 2018.)

obtained from the other arm. Oral signs and symptoms of kidney failure include pallor of the oral tissues secondary to anemia, xerostomia caused by reduced liquid intake, disorders of taste, halitosis, periodontitis, and oral mucositis.[17]

Systemic considerations

Most systemic phase procedures are necessary for patients with CKD, especially those with ESRD. It's important to remember that CKD patients often present with other systemic conditions such as anemia, diabetes, hypertension, and increased risk of bleeding and infection.[17]

Consultation with physician. For patients with moderate to severe kidney disease the dentist will want to contact the patient's primary healthcare provider and possibly their nephrologist, especially if the patient is receiving dialysis treatments. It is important to inquire about the stage of kidney disease and the patient's overall prognosis, any medications that are being prescribed and obtain recent laboratory test results. The consultation request should also include a short description of planned dental treatment and any medications that will be given to the patient. The dentist should also ask the physician to suggest which antibiotic and/or pain medications can be given should they be required. The dentist should ask the

physician whether there is a need for antibiotic prophylaxis before treatment.

Postponing treatment. Patients with ESRD may be receiving regular dialysis treatments and it may be necessary to postpone treatment. Peritoneal dialysis can be used for moderate to severe kidney failure and involves introducing 1–2 liters of fluid via an indwelling catheter into the peritoneum for several hours and then removing the fluid. Hemodialysis treatment is more common and requires the patient to be connected to a dialysis machine for 3–4 hours, three or four times a week. During this time the patient's blood flows through the machine and is processed so that waste can be removed. Patients are given the anticoagulant heparin just before treatment to prevent blood clotting in the dialysis machine. As a result, patients should not be treated on the same day they receive hemodialysis treatment. Since heparin is relatively short-acting, dental treatment can be provided the day after a dialysis treatment.

Limiting treatment. As mentioned earlier, patients with ESRD frequently have many associated medical conditions such as anemia, hypertension, and diabetes. Depending on the patient's prognosis, it may be appropriate to create only a disease control treatment plan and reevaluate later for any definitive phase procedures. Having the patient's dental disease under control may be required if the patient is preparing for a kidney transplant.

Prescribing or altering patient medication. Dentists frequently use drugs to provide local anesthesia, pain control, or to prevent and treat infection. In addition to the liver, some drugs are metabolized in the kidneys and their concentration levels can increase if the kidneys are damaged. Other drugs are toxic to the kidney and should be avoided. Other drugs are removed during hemodialysis and their dosages adjusted to compensate for the loss. Selection of antibiotic and pain control medication should be done in consultation with the patient's physician. With regard to local anesthesia drugs, they are relatively safe because they are metabolized in the liver.

Stress reduction. Some renal patients are taking steroid medication on a regular basis to help treat their CKD. As a result, the potential exists for an adrenal insufficiency during stressful dental procedures such as oral or periodontal surgery.[18] The patient should continue their regular dose of the drug and be carefully monitored during and after treatment. Supplemental steroid medication may be required before and after treatment. Again, the dentist should consult with the patient's physician.

Patient positioning. Finally, patients with CKD are often taking medications to treat hypertension. Any changes in chair position should be done gradually to avoid orthostatic hypotension.

Pregnant Patients

With more than 3.5 million births each year in the United States, the chances are strong that a general dentist will be evaluating pregnant patients.[19] When planning treatment for the pregnant patient, the dentist is, in essence, planning care for two individuals—the expectant mother and the developing fetus. A dilemma arises when appropriate care for one may not be in the best interest of the other. A significant number of dentists are hesitant to provide treatment for pregnant patients.[20] Although the decision to defer treatment until after the baby is born may sometimes seem most prudent, deferral may not be realistic in the presence of serious oral problems. The challenge to the dentist is to weigh the benefit of providing dental treatment against the potential for harm to the fetus.

The history-taking stage is particularly important with this patient both for developing rapport and for gathering information that will help determine how care should be delivered. Women of childbearing age should be asked regularly if they could be pregnant before exposing them to diagnostic radiation or prescribing medications. For new patients who are pregnant, the health history must be reviewed for evidence of systemic diseases, such as diabetes or hypertension, which could complicate the pregnancy. Several physiologic changes may accompany pregnancy and certain systemic diseases may develop or be aggravated by these changes (Box 8.5). The patient's blood pressure and pulse rate should be taken and recorded along with the expected date of delivery. The decision to contact the patient's physician or obstetrician may be indicated when conditions such as diabetes, hypertension, pulmonary or cardiac disease, or bleeding disorders are present.[21]

> ### BOX 8.5 Changes and Conditions Associated With Pregnancy
>
> **Physiologic Changes**
> - Weight gain
> - Increased need to urinate
> - Restricted breathing
> - Increase in clotting factors
>
> **Conditions That Occur With Increased Frequency**
> - Anemia
> - Postural hypotension
> - Hypoglycemia
> - Hyperglycemia
> - Systolic ejection murmurs

A 2012 experts' consensus statement concluded that providing dental care to a pregnant patient throughout all trimesters of pregnancy is safe and effective and that dental care should not be withheld because of pregnancy. Although dental procedures can be safely performed during the last months of pregnancy, concern for the mother's comfort may limit the extent of treatment. When the patient is in the third trimester, short appointments, allowing the patient to adjust her position periodically and avoiding putting her in an extreme supine position will help make the patient more comfortable during treatment. The 2012 consensus statement also concluded that routine preventive, periodontal, diagnostic, and restorative treatments during pregnancy do not increase adverse pregnancy outcomes.[21]

Radiographs

Although the use of ionizing radiation during pregnancy might appear to be a concern, current scientific evidence suggests that radiographic imaging is not contraindicated during pregnancy.[22,23] As with all patients, the clinician should take the minimum number of images needed for diagnosis and treatment and provide the patient with a protective thyroid collar and abdominal apron. The pregnant patient may refuse radiographs, but the clinician should remember that an accusation of providing substandard care could be made if restorative treatment, extractions, or endodontic therapy is done without making appropriate radiographs. It may be necessary, in such cases, not to treat the patient unless they agree to have radiographs taken.

Medications

The prudent dentist minimizes the use of medications when treating the pregnant patient. At the same time, however, local anesthetics may be necessary to make treatment comfortable and reduce the patient's stress. No drug has been proven absolutely safe for a patient who is pregnant, but research suggests that when necessary, most local anesthetic agents with vasoconstrictors can be used safely.[23]

If an antibiotic is indicated, as in the presence of swelling or an elevated temperature accompanying an oral infection, penicillin, amoxicillin, cephalosporins, clindamycin, and metronidazole are the medications of choice.[23] The tetracyclines should be avoided because of the potential for causing intrinsic staining of the child's developing teeth.

If pain control medication is necessary after treatment, it is advisable to contact the patient's obstetrician. The patient's obstetrician should be also consulted before the use of nitrous oxide, intravenous sedation, or general anesthesia.

Managing Dental Emergencies During Pregnancy

A pregnant patient with dental pain should receive the necessary radiographs to permit a diagnosis. The decision to treat depends on the source of the problem, its severity, the patient's symptoms, and the stage of pregnancy. For example, a patient in the late third trimester with an occasional mild intermittent pain from four impacted third molars could be treated with conservative, nonsurgical measures. On the other hand, if a patient reports the inability to sleep because of an irreversible pulpitis, root canal therapy or an extraction would be indicated even during the first trimester. In either situation, the patient should be informed about the consequences of treatment or no treatment.

Disease Control and Definitive Care

The most common oral problem experienced during pregnancy is gingival inflammation and hypertrophy, often referred to as **pregnancy gingivitis** (Figure 8.3). The condition may arise from hormonal changes leading to an increased blood flow to the gingival tissues, coupled with the presence of local irritants, such as plaque and calculus. The bleeding typically increases as the pregnancy progresses, usually beginning to subside in the eighth month. Many patients who have not previously received regular dental care will seek treatment when the condition becomes painful or if they are concerned about "bleeding gums." Often these patients will have entered pregnancy with poor oral hygiene and marginal gingivitis. The dentist or hygienist should debride affected areas to remove plaque and calculus. If necessary, local anesthetic can be used to make the patient more comfortable during this process. All pregnant patients should receive oral hygiene instruction.

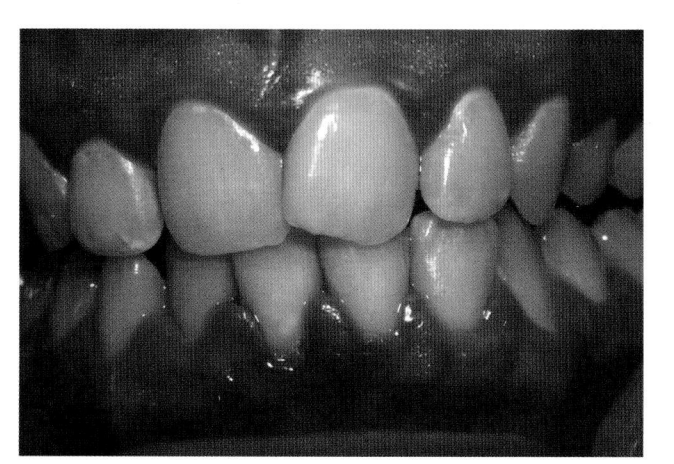

Fig. 8.3 This 20-year-old woman complained of sore gums, was 3 months pregnant, and had pregnancy gingivitis. The patient had poor oral hygiene and the gingiva was inflamed, especially in the mandibular arch. With improved oral hygiene and periodontal treatment, the condition improved and eventually disappeared.

Other disease control procedures, such as restorations to control caries and endodontic therapy, can be provided during pregnancy. The clinician should be observant for signs of tooth erosion that can follow nausea and vomiting, usually during the first trimester. The patient and dentist may decide to postpone extensive definitive care, such as multiple crowns, fixed partial dentures, implants, and periprosthetic surgery, until after the baby is born.

Diabetes

Diabetes is a relatively common disease affecting 422 million people worldwide in 2014 (up from 108 million in 1980) and has been rising faster in mid- to low-income countries than in high-income countries.[24] In the United States in 2018, diabetes affected 34.2 million people, 10.5% of the population with 2.8% undiagnosed as having the condition.[25] Type 1 diabetes, previously referred to as *insulin-dependent diabetes*, accounts for 5% of all diagnosed cases of diabetes and is most frequently discovered in the mid-teens or before. Type 2 diabetes usually occurs later in life and accounts for 90% to 95% of all diagnosed cases. Two to ten percent of women with no history of the disease can develop gestational diabetes during the second and third trimester of pregnancy and 50% of these patients develop Type 2 diabetes after the baby is born.[26]

Identification of a diabetic patient in the dental practice usually occurs after reviewing the patient's responses on the health questionnaire. For a patient with undiagnosed disease, the dentist may suspect diabetes if the patient has symptoms of high blood sugar, **hyperglycemia**, such as increased thirst or frequent urination, or if the patient is overweight and/or hypertensive and not regularly seeing a health care provider. In such instances, the dentist may choose to measure the patient's blood glucose level with a blood glycosometer. The diagnostic criteria for diagnosing diabetes mellitus are presented in Table 8.7.

For a patient with a diagnosis of diabetes, the dentist should make note of any medications the patient is taking and be aware of any side effects, because several oral hypoglycemic medications can have an effect on the oral cavity such as taste disorders and xerostomia. The level of metabolic control attained by the patient should be assessed from both an overall and a same-day perspective. Most diabetics can accurately

TABLE 8.7	**Diagnostic Criteria for Diabetes Mellitus**	
Test	**Prediabetes**	**Overt Diabetes Mellitus**
Hb A$_{1c}$ (glycolated hemoglobin)	5.7%–6.4%	≥6.5%
Fasting plasma glucose test	100–126 mg/dL	≥126
Random (nonfasting) glucose with signs of hyperglycemia[a]	Not applicable	≥200

[a]Increased thirst, headaches, frequent urination, fatigue, blurred vision.

assess their level of control on a long- and short-term basis. At the beginning of each appointment, the dentist should ask the diabetic patient how they are feeling, when and what type of food was eaten before the appointment, and whether insulin or oral hypoglycemic medication has been taken as prescribed by the individual's physician. Routinely taking blood glucose measurements before nonsurgical treatment for patients taking medication and under regular care by a physician is usually not necessary.

All diabetic patients should make regular visits to the physician and have periodic monitoring of blood sugar levels. An insulin-dependent patient should be questioned about the usual levels of blood glucose maintained and the frequency of blood testing for glucose. Any reported emergency visits for hyperglycemia or hypoglycemia should be documented. Last, when reviewing the health questionnaire with the patient, the practitioner should learn whether the patient suffers from any of the other conditions frequently seen in the diabetic patient, such as kidney, cardiovascular, or peripheral vascular and neurologic diseases.

Treatment Implications

If the patient's diabetes is poorly controlled or the patient has many of the complications seen with diabetes, such as severe cardiovascular disease, it may be necessary to consult the patient's physician before beginning treatment. Well-controlled diabetics should be advised to eat normal meals before appointments and ideally should be scheduled mid-morning for treatment. The dentist should be alert for signs that the patient is becoming **hypoglycemic**. Early signs and symptoms of hypoglycemia include hunger, weakness, trembling, pallor, and a rapid heart rate (**tachycardia**). Because eating regular meals is an important part of glycemic control, especially for the insulin-dependent diabetic, the patient may need to adjust the insulin dosage if they are unable to return to a regular eating schedule immediately after a dental procedure.

Several oral problems may be more common in the diabetic patient and should be taken into consideration when planning the disease control phase. Some diabetic patients may have a greater incidence of periodontal disease, dental caries, missing teeth, xerostomia, and fungal infections.[27] In addition, they may be more likely to suffer adverse outcomes after treatment such as delayed healing or infection. Diabetic patients may need more frequent periodontal maintenance visits and should be encouraged to maintain a noncariogenic diet and a high level of oral hygiene.

DOCUMENTATION OF SYSTEMIC CONCERNS

Like findings from other parts of the patient's examination, information regarding the systemic health of the patient must be documented clearly in the patient's physical or electronic record. Significant medical diagnoses and other health concerns should be gathered and summarized in one area of the record so that the dentist can easily review this information before each appointment. A running list of all medications taken by the patient should be updated regularly. Most electronic record systems have conspicuous medical alert notifications. Colored stickers and ink stamps can be applied to a prominent place on a physical record to flag those patients with potentially life-threatening conditions, such as allergies to latex or penicillin, or the need for antibiotic premedication before treatment.

Although for most patients, attention to systemic concerns continues throughout the entire treatment, for some it may be useful to document a discrete systemic phase plan at the start of therapy. For example, if the patient has severe health problems (ASA III or IV) and the dentist has to consider limiting the nature and scope of the treatment plan, a written systemic phase of care is warranted. Consider the following example of a plan for a lymphatic cancer patient, who is preparing for radiation and chemotherapy to treat tumors in the head and neck region:

Systemic phase:
1. Consult with physician:
   a. To determine patient's upcoming radiation and chemotherapy schedule.
   b. To discuss plans to remove all hopeless teeth now and consider replacement at the conclusion of chemotherapy.
2. Obtain a complete blood count before removing remaining teeth.
3. Provide palliative treatment for xerostomia and radiation mucositis during radiation therapy.

If a patient has significant dental and periodontal disease, it is often best to remove all the teeth before head and neck radiation, even when a few teeth may be salvageable. The systemic treatment plan presented supports this decision and clearly states what the dentist must do to deliver care safely and help the patient during radiation therapy. More information on this subject can be found in Chapter 6. Many dentists and dental schools find it useful to document all types of systemic therapy at the beginning of the patient's treatment plan.

CONCLUSION

Dentistry, as a profession, evolved significantly as a result of research into the causes of oral diseases, the development of new research-based therapies, and a stronger emphasis on preventing oral problems. The relationship between oral health and general health is now more widely recognized by both the dental and medical professions. It has become increasingly important for dentists to be knowledgeable about human physiology, pathology, and pharmacology, and about the effect of dental treatment on the general health of each patient. This broad knowledge base becomes even more significant as more patients who are elderly or have serious systemic illness seek our services. Only through careful inquiry and attention to each patient's general and oral health do dentists earn the privilege of the title *doctor*.

REVIEW QUESTIONS

- What are the objectives of the systemic phase?
- Why has systemic phase treatment become increasingly important in the practice of dentistry?
- What is the ASA classification for a patient with severe congestive heart failure who is incapable of walking one block without rest?
- Describe common problems, usually identified in the patient history, that suggest the need for a systemic phase of care.

- Describe common problems, usually identified in the physical evaluation of the patient, that suggest the need for a systemic phase of care.
- Under what circumstances would it be advisable to postpone treatment or limit treatment for a dental patient?
- Describe some situations in which it would be appropriate to prescribe medications for a patient.

REFERENCES

1. Boersma P, Black LI, Ward BW. Prevalence of multiple chronic conditions among us adults, 2018. *Prev Chronic Dis.* 2020;17:E106.
2. Casale MJ, Lurie JM, Khromava M, Silvay G. Dental clearance and postoperative heart infections: Observations from a preoperative evaluation clinic for day-admission surgery. *J Periop Pract.* 2020;30(4):97–101.
3. Frey C, Navarro SM, Blackwell T, Lidner C, Del Schutte Jr. H. Impact of dental clearance on total joint arthroplasty: A systematic review. *World J Orthop.* 2019;10(12):416–423.
4. Association AH. Sicker, More complex patients are driving up intensity of ED care. 2013; https://www.healthcaredive.com/news/fewer-but-sicker-patients-visit-ascension-hospitals-in-its-latest-fiscal/589605/.
5. Nasseh K, Greenberg B, Vujicic M, Glick M. The effect of chairside chronic disease screenings by oral health professionals on health care costs. *Am J Public Health.* 2014;104(4):744–750.
6. Stein K, Farmer J, Singhal S, Marra F, Sutherland S, Quiñonez C. The use and misuse of antibiotics in dentistry: A scoping review. *J Am Dent Assoc.* 2018;149(10):869–884.e865.
7. American Society of Anesthesiologists (ASA) Physical Status Classification System. 2020; https://www.asahq.org/standards-and-guidelines/asa-physical-status-classification-system.
8. Yarows SA, Vornovitsky O, Eber RM, Bisognano JD, Basile J. Canceling dental procedures due to elevated blood pressure: Is it appropriate? *J Am Dent Assoc.* 2020;151(4):239–244.
9. Serrano-Sánchez V, Ripollés-de Ramón J, Collado-Yurrita L, et al. New horizons in anticoagulation: Direct oral anticoagulants and their implications in oral surgery. *Med Oral Patol Oral Cir Bucal.* 2017;22(5):e601–e608.
10. Lupi SM, Rodriguez YBA. Patients taking direct oral anticoagulants (DOAC) undergoing oral surgery: a review of the literature and a proposal of a peri-operative management protocol. *Healthcare (Basel).* 2020(3):8.
11. Caliskan M, Tükel HC, Benlidayi ME, Deniz A. Is it necessary to alter anticoagulation therapy for tooth extraction in patients taking direct oral anticoagulants? *Med Oral Patol Oral Cir Bucal.* 2017;22(6):e767–e773.
12. Teng YT, Taylor GW, Scannapieco F, et al. Periodontal health and systemic disorders. *J Can Dent Assoc.* 2002;68(3):188–192.
13. Pihlstrom BL, Hodges JS, Michalowicz B, Wohlfahrt JC, Garcia RI. Promoting oral health care because of its possible effect on systemic disease is premature and may be misleading. *J Am Dent Assoc.* 2018;149(6):401–403.
14. Tavares M, Lindefjeld Calabi KA, San Martin L. Systemic diseases and oral health. *Dent Clin North Am.* 2014;58(4):797–814.
15. Centers for Disease Control and Prevention. Chronic kidney disease in the United States 2021. In: Prevention CfDCa, ed. *US Department of Health and Human Services*: US Department of Health and Human Services.
16. Caliento R, Sarmento DJS, Kobayashi-Velasco S, de Sá SNC, Shibutani PP, Gallotini M. Clinical outcome of dental procedures among renal transplant recipients. *Spec Care Dentist.* 2018;38(3):146–149.
17. Costantinides F, Castronovo G, Vettori E, et al. Dental care for patients with end-stage renal disease and undergoing hemodialysis. *Int J Dent.* 2018;2018:9610892.
18. Little JW, Miller CS, Rhodus NL. *Little and Falace's Dental Management of the Medically Compromised Patient.* 9th ed St Louis: Elsevier; 2018.
19. Martin JA, Hamilton BE, Osterman MJK, Driscoll AK. Births: final data for 2019. *Natl Vital Stat Rep.* 2021;70(2):1–51.
20. Favero V, Bacci C, Volpato A, Bandiera M, Favero L, Zanette G. Pregnancy and dentistry: a literature review on risk management during dental surgical procedures. *Dent J (Basel).* 2021;9(4).
21. Oral Health Care During Pregnancy Expert Workgroup: Oral health care during pregnancy: a national consensus statement. 2021; https://www.mchoralhealth.org/PDFs/OralHealthPregnancyConsensus.pdf.
22. Mayberry ME. Is dental treatment safe for pregnant women? *J Mich Dent Assoc.* 2020;102(8):24–27.
23. American Dental Association. Oral Health Topics - Pregnancy. Oral Health Topics 2021; https://www.ada.org/en/member-center/oral-health-topics/pregnancy.
24. World Health Organization (WHO). Diabetes. 2021; https://www.who.int/news-room/fact-sheets/detail/diabetes.
25. Centers for Disease Control and Prevention. National Diabetes Statistics Report, 2020. 2020; https://www.cdc.gov/diabetes/data/statistics-report/index.html?CDC_AA_refVal=https%3A%2F%2Fwww.cdc.gov%2Fdiabetes%2Fdata%2Fstatistics%2Fstatistics-report.html.
26. Centers for Disease Control and Prevention. Gestational Diabetes. 2021; https://www.cdc.gov/diabetes/basics/gestational.html.
27. Rohani B. Oral manifestations in patients with diabetes mellitus. *World J Diabetes.* 2019;10(9):485–489.

9

The Acute Phase of Treatment

Stephen J. Stefanac

 Visit eBooks.Health.Elsevier.com

The **acute phase** of care incorporates diagnostic and treatment procedures aimed at solving urgent oral problems. Acute care can involve a myriad of services, from controlling pain and swelling to just replacing a broken tooth on a denture. All types of patients may need acute care, including those under active treatment or on maintenance recall, new to a dental practice, or returning to a practice after a lengthy absence. There are no consistent professional guidelines in the United States regarding the responsibility of a dentist to provide emergency dental care.[1] That said, most people expect a dentist to be available to treat any immediate problems and are drawn to offices that provide such services. Good practice management and professional responsibility require that every dentist effectively and efficiently manage patients with immediate treatment needs without unnecessary disruption to the flow of the practice. The dentist is also responsible for managing their patients when they have acute problems outside of normal office hours.

The purpose of this chapter is to provide information about how to design, record, and execute the acute phase of a dental treatment plan. In the course of this discussion, the reader will become acquainted with the unique challenges of providing acute dental care. The profile of the acute patient's typical problems is described. Guidance is given for evaluating, diagnosing, treating, and providing follow-up care for such a patient. In addition, suggestions for documenting all aspects of acute care are presented.

The reader will encounter two important and related distinctions throughout this chapter. An **emergency problem** is one that incapacitates the patient and has the potential to become a life-threatening condition. In such cases, immediate attention is required. Examples include severe dental pain, swelling, bleeding, systemic infection, or trauma to the face or jaws. In most instances, the dentist will see the patient with emergency needs on the same day that contact is made. In contrast, an **urgent problem** does not require immediate attention but is a problem that the dentist—or, more commonly, the patient—thinks should be attended to "now" or "soon" (Figure 9.1). Examples include mild to moderate pain without active infection, asymptomatic broken teeth, lost restorations, and other purely esthetic problems. Treatment of urgent problems may, theoretically, be postponed without causing the patient unnecessary pain or the risk of systemic illness. Often, these problems can be managed with **palliative care** (for example, by treating the pain, but not the underlying problem), until the patient can be conveniently worked into the office schedule.

Making the distinction between emergency and urgent problems is important to both the dentist and patient to ensure that no true emergency problem goes unattended. On another level, the experienced dental practitioner recognizes that this distinction may seem irrelevant to an anxious, distraught patient. From a practice management perspective, it is important that the office be prepared to accommodate patients with acute

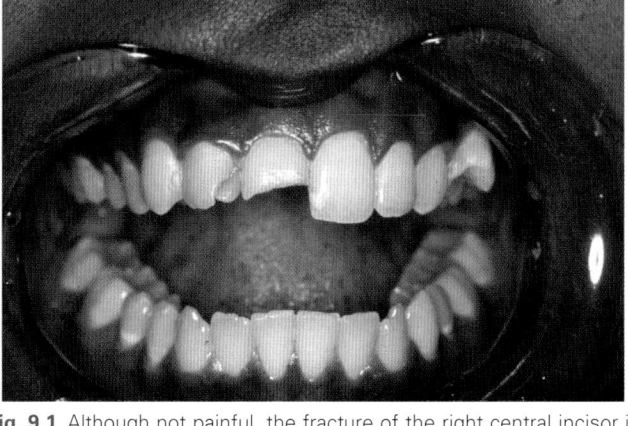

Fig. 9.1 Although not painful, the fracture of the right central incisor is an urgent problem that needs prompt attention.

needs in a timely and attentive manner, regardless of whether a potentially serious health issue exists.

Not infrequently, patients have questions about "new" findings in the oral cavity they believe may need immediate attention. Examples include sore areas that are thought to be cancer or esthetic problems that affect their personal appearance and self-esteem. These concerns, although not true emergencies, do require the dentist's recognition, if only to reassure the patient and to reschedule for more definitive care.

CHALLENGES

Treating patients with acute care needs can be challenging in many ways. Initially, the practitioner must determine whether the patient's complaint is a true emergency requiring immediate attention or an urgent problem that can be treated at a more convenient time. Usually, this discussion occurs over the telephone and may be resolved by an office staff member without the dentist's direct involvement. On the other hand, the dentist usually manages after-hours emergencies. Once the decision to see the patient has been made, sufficient time must be available in the dentist's schedule to diagnose and treat the patient's problem. This can be difficult when the practitioner's day is tightly scheduled. Some busy practices reserve time in the dentist's schedule or book segments of the schedule lightly to accommodate occasional add-on appointments. Patients are becoming more adept as using personal electronic devices to send images to a dental office. Some practices are using teledentistry (see Chapter 4) to speak directly with patients about their problems before they are seen in person.[2]

Arriving at a diagnosis and an acute care treatment plan can be time consuming. This problem is compounded significantly when the acute needs patient is new to the practice. Many patients with emergency problems have a history of irregular dental visits.[3] In the absence of an existing health and dental history and an established relationship with the patient, the dentist must work without many of the usual clues or cues that would otherwise guide the process. The dentist needs to assess for the first time the patient's health history, perform a limited oral examination and diagnostic tests, obtain radiographs if necessary, decide on the appropriate treatment, obtain informed

consent from the patient, and execute some level of care to alleviate symptoms. Difficult enough for the patient of record, this task can be extremely challenging when it involves an anxious and emotionally labile patient whom the dentist has not met.

During an initial emergency appointment, the amount of time available to develop rapport will probably be limited. If the patient is in significant pain or has been awake all night, they may not be thinking rationally. Some patients will be fearful or irritable or may not be respectful of staff members. As a result, communicating the nature of the problem and the treatment options to the patient may be difficult. The patient may have difficulty making a treatment decision or providing informed consent, especially for irreversible procedures, such as extractions or endodontic therapy.

Furthermore, it is common for some patients, especially those who have never been seen in the practice before, to expect to have an acute need managed immediately and simply. These individuals may have experienced a lifetime of episodic dental care, may not understand the nature of the problem, and may be unrealistic about the scope or complexity of the needed treatment. This can be frustrating for some practitioners, who may see such patients as demanding, intrusive, and unappreciative of the value of comprehensive dental care. Nevertheless, the dentist has the obligation, insofar as is possible, to educate the patient about their overall oral condition and to describe how the prospective emergency or urgent care treatment will fit into the context of the person's overall oral health. To help the patient understand and accept this vision, the dentist must be a good listener, take the time to explore all reasonable treatment options with the patient, and thoroughly discuss any barriers to treatment that the patient might perceive, especially with regard to time, financial cost, and pain. To accomplish this quickly, efficiently, and professionally—and to do so with a personalized and caring delivery—can be difficult for even the most experienced practitioner.

REWARDS

Efficiently managing the patient with acute problems is essential to attracting new patients and serving the needs of patients already in the practice. Dentists who are prepared to treat emergency and urgent problems promptly will retain patient loyalty and see their practices grow. Relieving pain or restoring a broken tooth can also provide great personal satisfaction to the dentist. Often, patients with such problems will arrive fearful and unsure of what treatment will be required. A kind, empathetic approach to care and the prompt resolution of the dental problem may encourage some patients who originally presented for episodic treatment only to become comprehensive care patients.

PROFILE OF THE PATIENT REQUESTING IMMEDIATE TREATMENT

Comprehensive Care Patient

Patients expect that their regular dentist will see them promptly if they are in pain, break a tooth or prosthesis, or lose a temporary restoration. Such problems can sometimes be anticipated or they may come as a surprise to both patient and provider. Even when the problem is anticipated, however, the timing of the event cannot be predicted with certainty.

Patients who are new to the practice and request comprehensive care for many dental problems may require immediate treatment, often to control or prevent dental pain and infection. When planning treatment, it is possible to identify those urgent problems that, if untreated, are likely to become dental emergencies and to sequence them early in the treatment plan. For example, the patient whose tooth has significant decay and is experiencing prolonged sensitivity to heat may require immediate caries removal and a pulpectomy to avoid the possibility of increased pain and development of an apical infection. Other common urgent care procedures include repairing prostheses or replacing restorations, especially in esthetic locations or when a tooth is sensitive.

Acute care may also become unexpectedly necessary while a patient is undergoing regular active treatment. Many procedures in dentistry may have associated postoperative complications, such as pain, bleeding, or swelling. Experienced dentists are aware of the potential for complications associated with the procedures they perform and will discuss the chances for postoperative problems with the patient. If a problem arises, the dentist may only need to speak with the patient on the telephone; however, if the problem is more serious, the person may need to return for evaluation.

Patients on periodic recall may also develop urgent treatment needs. The problem may be related to prior treatment (e.g., pain from a tooth that had received a restoration near the pulp) or to a chronic condition, such as a deep periodontal pocket that has developed a periodontal abscess. Common complaints include sensitive or chipped teeth, lost or fractured restorations, broken prostheses, oral infections, and traumatic injuries. These issues require prompt attention to satisfy patient expectations.

Patients of record who have not been seen for some time require special consideration during an examination for acute care problems. The dentist should determine whether other dentists have provided treatment since the patient was last seen and whether the patient has been receiving maintenance care on a regular basis. The patient's health questionnaire will need to be updated or redone to discover any new or continued health and dental problems.

Limited Care Patient

Depending on household income, 20% to 51% of patients actually visited a dentist in the United States last year.[4] Included in this group are those individuals who receive at least an annual oral evaluation and maintenance procedures for the teeth and prostheses. For the remainder of the population, dental care is usually both episodic in nature and limited in scope. There are several reasons for this. Many individuals are afraid of receiving dental services, often because of unpleasant past experiences with a dentist and fears that treatment will be painful or costly, or both. Understanding the reasons for this anxiety and treating the fearful patient are discussed further in Chapter 15. For many individuals, a real or perceived lack of financial resources to pay for dental treatment represents a significant barrier.[4]

In the United States, low-income patients without dental insurance may seek dental care in a hospital emergency department.[2,5] For elderly people or individuals with severe health problems, dental treatment may not be accessible or may be considered a low priority compared with more life-threatening concerns. For some persons, dental care and good oral health are simply low priorities (see Chapter 19). These patients may appear apathetic, be reluctant to commit to a comprehensive treatment approach, miss appointments, and ultimately disappear from the practice altogether. Last, some young persons may have had regular care in their youth but have not yet taken responsibility for maintaining oral health as an adult. Often, for these individuals, making the time or even remembering to see a dentist regularly constitutes the biggest barrier to care.

Although the persons just described may not be regular visitors to a dental office, it is probable that they will need treatment *sometime* in their lives. Most often, a particular event has provoked the patient to action. For example, a molar tooth, sensitive to hot and cold for several months, has now become a constant throbbing problem. For others, especially those who believe they are in reasonably good dental health, the symptoms may be less acute but disturbing all the same. Common complaints include loose teeth, bleeding gums, sensitivity to heat or cold, fractured teeth or restorations, food impaction, and broken prosthodontic work. Fear of worsening pain or the anticipation of additional dental problems may also motivate these persons to seek dental treatment.

Culturally, the population of the United States places a high value on personal appearance. For many, self-esteem can be greatly affected—positively or negatively—by the appearance of their teeth and smile. As a result, many limited care patients seek dental services because of esthetic concerns. Often, encouraged by friends and family to see a dentist, the patient may believe that they need to look better to improve social and business opportunities. For such patients, a dark or missing anterior tooth may be perceived as a more severe problem than the broken down or chronically infected posterior teeth also identified during examination (Figure 9.2). This can be of concern to the dentist who would rather first treat the more serious problems than address an esthetic concern.

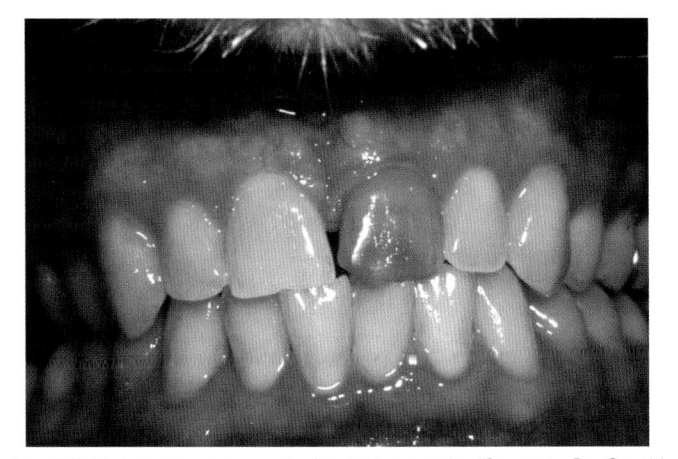

Fig. 9.2 Dark tooth as a result of pulpal necrosis. (Courtesy Dr. Gerald Scott.)

PATIENT EVALUATION

Although the evaluation of the acute care patient requires the same components as an evaluation of a patient seeking comprehensive care—a patient history, physical and clinical examination, and radiographs or any other necessary special diagnostic tests—each component is handled differently with the acute care patient. Of necessity, the acute care evaluation will often be more abbreviated, although in some cases additional diagnostic procedures are performed. Having accurate documentation of the acute care visit is critical, even under time constraints, to prevent medicolegal complication.[6] The practitioner may find it helpful to develop a checklist to avoid omitting any component of the evaluation process.[7] With any acute care patient, the findings, both positive and negative, take on a different and often increased level of importance because of the urgency of the situation.

Patient History

Methods and techniques for obtaining a comprehensive patient history are described in Chapter 1. The content of the acute care patient's history will focus on issues that affect the diagnosis and management of the immediate problem or problems for which the patient has sought treatment. Acute care patients usually complete the same health history questionnaire as the comprehensive care patient, but a detailed investigation of positive findings, particularly in the dental history, may be more selective and associated with the chief concern (see Chapter 1 for a discussion of the inquiry process used to review the health history information with the patient.) The clinician realizes that many new patients who are in pain at the first visit are also anxious and may not be thinking or communicating clearly. Many of the issues discussed in Chapter 15 relating to the evaluation and treatment planning for an anxious patient will also apply to a patient with acute care needs.

Chief Concern and History of the Concern

The term **chief concern** (also referred to as the **chief complaint**) designates the immediate reason the patient seeks treatment. Recording the concern in the patient's own words not only identifies the issue that needs attention, but also provides important information about the patient's *perception* of the problem. The way in which the patient phrases the concern may provide important insight into the patient's dental knowledge and awareness. As illustrated in the *In Clinical Practice: Value of Listening to the Patient's Concerns* box, the patient's words may also give the dentist a glimpse of the patient's unexpressed fears. As the starting point for investigating the patient's problem, articulation of the chief concern is critical to making an accurate diagnosis of an acute problem. A clear, concisely stated chief concern helps the patient and the dentist focus on the important issues and saves considerable time in the evaluation process. Even a vague or poorly focused chief concern, however, can trigger questions that will enable the dentist to begin the process of establishing possible diagnoses. (See Video 9.1 Interview of a Patient in Pain on ebooks+.)

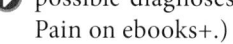

Value of Listening to the Patient's Concerns

The following encounter provided one dentist with a valuable lesson about the importance of open communication and complete informed consent while managing the acute care patient.

A middle-aged man in apparent good health presented to the emergency service at a school of dentistry. His chief concern was the "swelling in my jaw" adjacent to an upper molar. The history of the chief concern revealed that the man recently had seen his private dentist in his hometown, an hour's car drive away. His dentist had referred him to a local endodontist for root canal treatment. The root canal had been initiated and the patient reported no postoperative discomfort. Based on the conversation and the patient's reported outcome, it appeared that the diagnosis had been correct and that all treatment had been performed according to the standard of care.

Further discussion revealed the patient's real concern. The swelling that had begun as a diffuse, poorly localized tenderness had now localized and was indurated with smooth, well-defined borders. From the clinician's perspective, this was attributable to a normal progression in the natural history of a dental abscess. But the patient was convinced he had oral cancer.

Apparently, neither the general dentist nor the endodontist had taken the time to inform the patient fully about the diagnosis, the nature of the treatment, the expected outcome, and possible sequelae. Had that been done, the patient could have been spared considerable time and unnecessary worry. A few minutes of open and candid conversation at an earlier stage might have given this patient some desperately needed information, allayed his unwarranted fears, and provided him with a more positive experience with the profession.

The history of the chief concern enriches the dentist's understanding of the primary problem and the way in which it arose (Box 9.1). More important, the history helps the dentist to develop a short list of possible diagnoses and discern which specific areas should be examined, which radiographic images should be taken, and which clinical tests should be performed to identify the problem's source.

The careful and astute practitioner can make a tentative diagnosis for most acute care problems on the basis of the chief concern as expressed by the patient and the related history. A dilemma may arise, however, if the patient is allowed to ramble, raising multiple complaints and symptoms. The dentist may become distracted and have difficulty arriving at the essential

---

BOX 9.1   Typical Questions to Ask Acute Care Patients

- What brings you in today?
- How long have you had the pain or problem (days, weeks, months)?
- Is it getting better, worse, or staying the same?
- On a scale of 1 to 10, how severe is the pain?
- What makes the pain worse (hot, cold, sweets, pressure)?
- How long does the pain last (seconds, minutes, hours)?
- Does the pain follow some pattern, such as worse at night or when lying flat?
- Have you been using any medication for the problem? Does the medication help?
- Do you have swelling or drainage?
- Have you been examined or treated elsewhere for this problem?

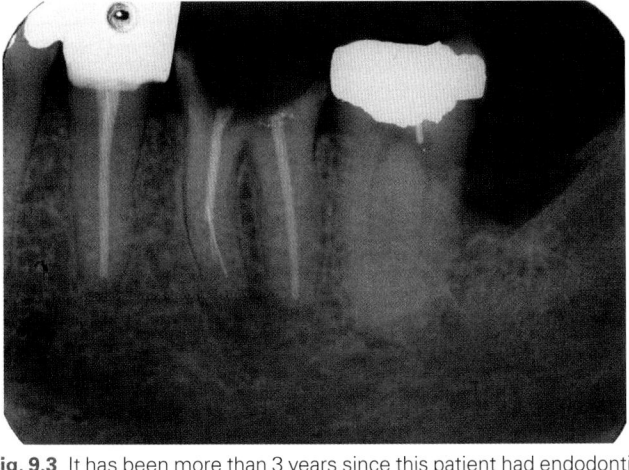

Fig. 9.3 It has been more than 3 years since this patient had endodontic treatment of the first molar and the tooth still has not received a final restoration. It may now be unrestorable.

working diagnosis, and, more important, treatment for the primary problem may be delayed as a result. On occasion, however, the patient's seemingly unrelated concerns may provide important clues, helping the dentist to make a diagnosis and treatment recommendation more quickly and accurately. Discerning when these other issues may be important and when they are a distraction takes considerable experience, sensitivity, and skill.

Health and Medication Histories

Although the health history for the acute care patient can be abbreviated, it cannot be overlooked. The minimal questions necessary to include in an acute care health history are listed in Box 9.2. As with the health history for the nonacute comprehensive care patient, the health history for the acute patient may be gathered through an oral interview, a health questionnaire, or a combination of both. For the patient of record who presents with an acute problem, an update of the existing health history is usually sufficient.

The dentist must investigate any positive patient responses and document significant additional findings in the patient's record. Some patients who do not visit the dentist regularly may not see a physician either. The dentist is responsible for determining that there are no systemic health limitations or contraindications to dental treatment before performing any invasive examination procedures or before performing treatment on the patient. If the dentist cannot make that determination, it may be necessary to consult with the patient's physician before proceeding.

Past Dental History

It is not necessary to complete a comprehensive dental history for the acute care patient. On occasion, however, pertinent findings from a brief dental history may augment the information derived from the chief concern and its history and assist in making a diagnosis. More commonly, a few questions related to the patient's past dental treatment can provide the dentist with important insights into which previous treatments have been successful or unsuccessful and help determine which treatment options will be most appropriate in the present situation.

For example, the patient who has had root canal therapy initiated on one or more teeth but has never returned to have the treatment completed or the tooth restored, is unlikely to be a good candidate for heroic efforts to save a newly fractured or severely decayed tooth (Figure 9.3).

Social History

In most instances, a formal social history is not recorded for an acute care patient. Some issues, however, particularly the patient's ability to pay for a particular procedure, may have a bearing on the treatment selection. For instance, a patient with limited income who uses all discretionary monies to cover the cost of prescription medications would probably not be a candidate for extensive endodontic, periodontal, and restorative therapy to save a tooth.

Clinical Examination

Examination of the acute care patient must, of necessity, include a detailed assessment of the area of chief concern. This is not the only important part of the clinical evaluation, however, and the dentist should consider including at least the five components in the acute care examination (Box 9.3).

Diagnostic Tests and Techniques

The rationale for and use of diagnostic tests and techniques is discussed in Chapter 1. Some of these techniques are used frequently with the acute care patient and have particular importance in that setting. Although, with some exceptions, the dentist may carry out these tests and techniques at the same time as the examination process previously described, they are discussed separately here for purposes of clarity.

The following list includes some of the evaluation methods most frequently used when diagnosing the acute care patient, along with a brief description of how each might be used:

- ***Inspection*** is the first and most used technique in the dentist's arsenal. In many cases, carious lesions, fractures of teeth, defective restorations, periodontal disease, or soft tissue infections may be detected by visual inspection alone

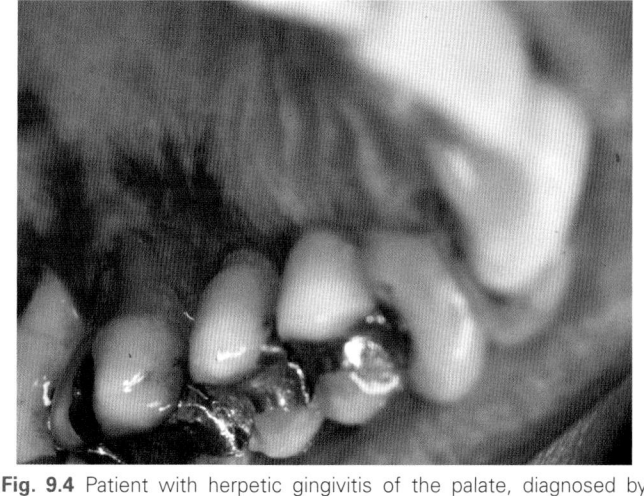

Fig. 9.4 Patient with herpetic gingivitis of the palate, diagnosed by recent onset and the characteristic appearance.

inflammation or in delineating the borders and relative firmness of an abscess. It is often the sole means of detecting **lymphadenopathy** or **lymphadenitis**. With noninflammatory swelling, palpation can be a critical tool for ruling in or out cancer from the differential diagnosis. Palpation can also be used to evaluate the muscles of mastication for pain and tenderness.

- **Percussion** is the primary technique used to determine the presence of periapical inflammation. This issue is crucial to both patient and provider, because positive findings often determine whether treatment for an irreversible pulpitis is necessary, such as an extraction or root canal therapy. In the absence of pulpal involvement, it is important to rule out a periodontal source of pain to percussion.
- **Periodontal probing** is indispensable as a means of detecting periodontal disease and measuring attachment loss. In the presence of bleeding on probing, active infection can usually be assumed. Marked sensitivity on probing often confirms that the patient's concern is periodontal in origin and that the problem is not simply an incidental finding. An isolated narrow pocket that traverses to the apex of the tooth may indicate a primary endodontic lesion, a combined periodontal/endodontic lesion, or a sign of a vertical root fracture. In a patient with an otherwise healthy periodontal condition, an isolated deep pocket may indicate a vertical tooth fracture, which has a poor prognosis (Figure 9.5).
- **Tooth mobility**, although in itself not a clear diagnostic indicator, may, in conjunction with other tests and findings, confirm the presence and severity of occlusal trauma, periodontal disease, or a dental or periodontal abscess. The degree of mobility, especially compared with the other teeth, can be an important determinant in estimating the tooth's prognosis and usability as a future abutment for a prosthesis.
- **Pulp vitality testing** is essential to determining the state of health of the pulp in an offending tooth. Along with evaluation of the patient's symptoms, vitality testing is an important diagnostic indicator in determining whether root canal treatment is definitely indicated or may be indicated in the

(Figure 9.4). When the problem is not readily apparent, exploration, transillumination, and the use of various dyes in conjunction with visual inspection may detect more subtle carious lesions, tooth defects, or fractures.

- **Palpation** is particularly useful for identifying subperiosteal swelling that may have arisen in conjunction with periapical

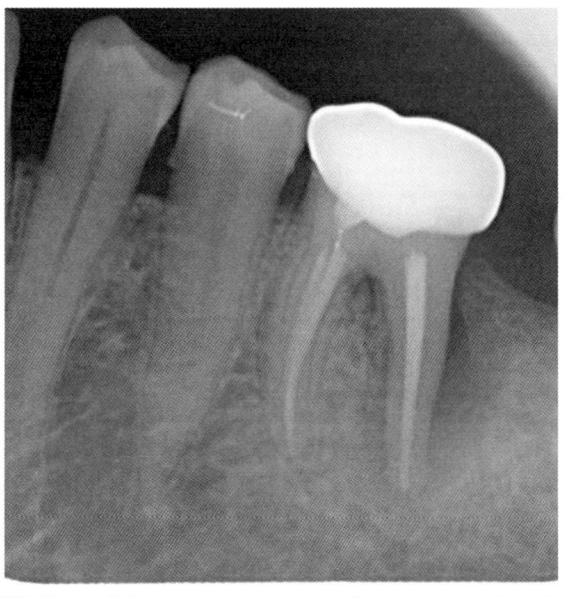

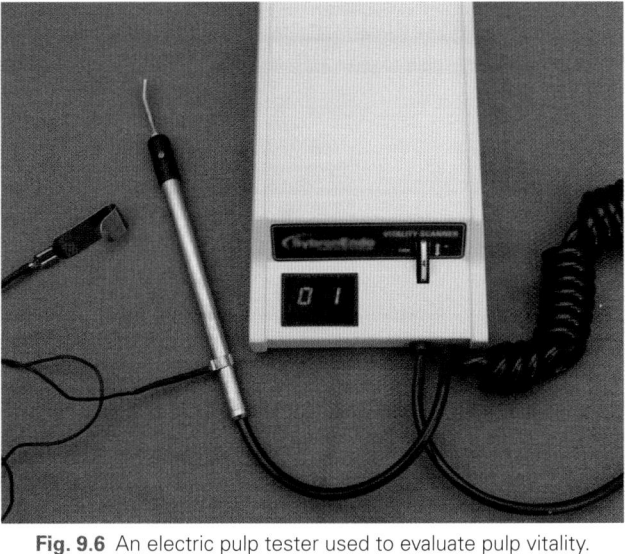

Fig. 9.6 An electric pulp tester used to evaluate pulp vitality.

Fig. 9.5 The radiolucent appearance and deep periodontal pocket on the distal root of this molar are highly suggestive of a vertical fracture of the tooth.

Potential Common Interpretation Errors of Responses Obtained From Electric Pulp Testing

False-positive responses

    Partial pulp necrosis
    Patient's high anxiety
    Ineffective tooth isolation
    Contact with metal restorations

False-negative responses

    Calcific obliterations in the root canals
    Recently traumatized teeth
    Immature apex
    Drugs that increase patient's threshold for pain
    Poor contact of pulp tester to tooth

Fig. 9.7 There are number of reasons for inaccurate results from electric pulp testing. (BOX 1.14 from Cohen's Pathways of the Pulp, 12th Edition)

future. Cold testing is the easiest and quickest way to evaluate pulpal vitality. An electric pulp tester (Figure 9.6) is helpful but the results can be misinterpreted (Figure 9.7).[8] In the absence of vitality tests, the dentist cannot make sound treatment recommendations and the patient cannot make informed choices about which treatment option will provide an optimal outcome. (See Video 9.2 Tooth Vitality Testing on ebooks+.)

Radiographic Examination

To meet the standard of care, a radiograph should be taken of any tooth before extraction or root canal treatment. Table 9.1 includes guidelines that can be used to select images for some of the more common acute dental conditions. In managing the acute care patient, multiple projections of the tooth or the area in question may be necessary.

COMMON ACUTE PROBLEMS AND DIAGNOSES

After evaluation of the chief concern, the dentist must define the problem or problems—usually, in terms of a diagnosis. In some cases, the diagnosis is definitive, but in many others, it is a working or tentative diagnosis, to be confirmed later by additional testing or by observing the response to therapy or how the chief concern changes over time with no treatment.

The following section reviews selected problems that are likely to require acute care. Common conditions for which a patient may seek immediate attention are described, including key features that will assist the dentist in making a diagnosis. In instances in which a differential diagnosis is particularly problematic, advice on how to make those distinctions is provided. The issues discussed here are intentionally selective and exclude chronic complaints and milder concerns that usually

TABLE 9.1 Radiographic Image Selection for Common Acute Dental Problems

Presenting Condition	Recommended Images
Isolated periodontal problem, pockets <5 mm	Periapical and conventional bite-wing radiographs
Isolated periodontal problem, pockets >5 mm	Periapical and vertical bite-wing radiographs
Symptomatic tooth, restorability in question	Periapical and bite-wing radiographs
Symptomatic tooth, restorability *not* in question	Periapical radiographs
Nonrestorable tooth	Panoramic or periapical radiograph showing the entire root and nearby anatomic structures, such as the sinus floor or the mandibular canal
Eruption pain or pericoronitis	Panoramic or periapical radiograph
Possible jaw fracture	Panoramic radiograph (plus 3D imaging as indicated)
Blunt trauma to tooth or teeth	3D imaging and periapical radiographs, often from multiple angles, of traumatized tooth or teeth and any opposing teeth
Acute symptoms of temporomandibular dysfunction	Panoramic radiograph (plus other imaging modalities as needed)

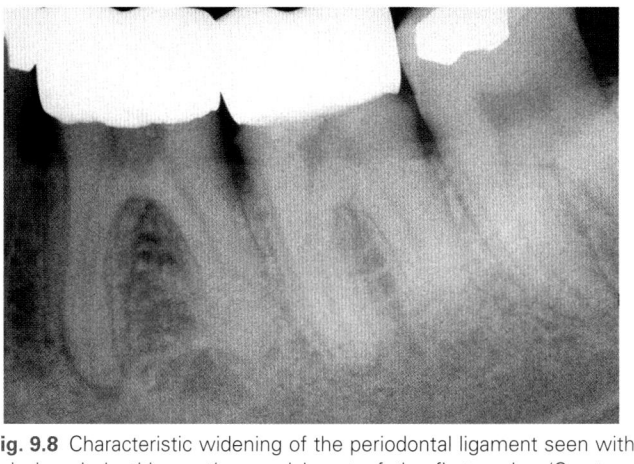

Fig. 9.8 Characteristic widening of the periodontal ligament seen with apical periodontitis on the mesial root of the first molar. (Courtesy Dr. Gerald Scott.)

do not require *immediate* attention. The reader should also be aware that the classification of acute problems by their origin and primary characteristic, although convenient, is artificial. Frequently, these problems do not exist in isolation. Patients may have multiple related or unrelated complaints. Over time, the complaint may change and what has been primarily a concern relating to pain may become a concern relating to swelling. Furthermore, at any given time, several clinical features for the same problem may be present.

Complaint of Pain

Pain is a common concern leading an individual to seek immediate care from the dentist.[4] Pain has many possible sources. Here, they are classified as pulpal or periapical pain, periodontal pain, pain associated with tooth eruption, pain associated with previous dental treatment, or other types of oral, head, and neck pain.

Pain of Pulpal or Periapical Origin

An acute or symptomatic **reversible** pulpitis is a clinical diagnosis based on subjective and objective findings indicating that the inflammation should resolve and the pulp tissue return to normal.[9] This condition is characterized by intermittent, brief (few seconds) discomfort initiated by cold or air, without lingering or spontaneous pain. Usually, the discomfort has not resulted in loss of sleep and no analgesics have been tried (or are necessary). Pulp vitality tests are positive (vital) with no prolonged response on removal of the stimulus. **Percussion** and **palpation** tests are negative. Usually, no apical change is evident on the radiograph.

An acute or symptomatic **irreversible pulpitis** is a clinical diagnosis based on subjective and objective findings indicating that the vital inflamed pulp is incapable of healing. The patient may complain of lingering thermal pain, spontaneous pain (minutes or hours in duration) or referred pain. The tooth may be sensitive to cold, air, or heat. Analgesics often will have been tried and have not been effective. The patient may report that the pain interferes with sleep. Pulp vitality tests often reveal no response or a heightened response and a lingering pain on stimulus removal. There may be a delayed response to cold. Palpation is negative, and percussion often is negative as well. In multirooted teeth, some pulpal tissue may remain vital and responsive to vitality tests, whereas other areas demonstrate pulpal necrosis, develop apical periodontitis, and show a corresponding positive response to percussion.

An acute or symptomatic **apical periodontitis** results from necrotic or partially necrotic pulp tissue. The inflammation causing the symptoms is usually located in the apical periodontium (rather than in the tooth itself) and produces clinical symptoms including a painful response to biting and/or percussion or palpation. The pain is often described as a prolonged dull ache. Analgesic medication usually will have been tried with moderate success, depending on the patient's pain threshold, the dose taken, whether a therapeutic blood level has been maintained, and other factors. Often, the patient reports loss of sleep. The radiograph may reveal a widening of the periodontal ligament space at the apex of the tooth (Figure 9.8). Vitality tests are generally negative. Percussion is positive as the inflammatory process progresses from root canal to periapical tissue. Palpation is usually negative at this stage.

An apical periodontitis with abscess formation is called an **acute apical abscess**. An acute apical abscess is an inflammatory reaction to pulpal infection and necrosis characterized by rapid onset, spontaneous pain, tenderness of the tooth to pressure, pus formation, and swelling of associated tissues. An acute apical abscess has a profile similar to apical periodontitis, but subperiosteal or intraoral swelling is now present and palpation sensitivity is significantly more pronounced. The radiograph demonstrates the same radiolucent periapical changes seen with an apical periodontitis or apical rarefying osteitis. A diffuse swelling with poorly defined borders occurring along with fever, malaise, or other constitutional symptoms suggests **cellulitis**. A localized, pointing abscess or "gum boil" clearly visible on the surface is referred to as a **parulis**. A tooth with a chronic or persistent abscess that drains purulent exudate is said to have a **sinus tract** (often less painful) and a diagnosis of **chronic apical periodontitis**. If the source of infection cannot be identified, inserting a gutta-percha cone into the tract and then taking a radiograph may facilitate location of the problematic tooth.

Patients with a nondisplaced tooth fracture will often have a specific set of clinical findings and symptoms. A classic offender is a posterior tooth with a large existing restoration. The patient reports a sharp, sometimes lingering pain on biting specific foods. The pain may be aggravated by cold or air and, less commonly, by heat. Percussion and palpation are negative, as are radiographic findings. Careful clinical inspection of the dry tooth (which can be aided by dye solution and/or transillumination) often reveals a hairline fracture through a marginal ridge or adjacent to an existing restoration. In some cases, a horizontal fracture line may be visible surrounding one or more cusps on the tooth. A good clinical test is to put lateral pressure on each individual cusp, one at a time. This can be done with a mirror handle, a Burlew wheel, or a specific device designed for this purpose (Tooth Slooth) (Figure 9.9). If the test recreates the symptoms, either when biting down or on release, a fracture is suspected. If the pain lingers, this is an additional indication of cracked tooth syndrome. Cracked teeth may mimic an irreversible pulpitis, especially when the patient clenches or bruxes. The fracture may also involve the pulp of the tooth. Fractures and **craze lines** in teeth may also be visually seen using a focused light source. This process is referred to as **transillumination** (Figure 9.10).

Occasionally, a patient may have a periapical lesion from a pulpal infection drain by forming a pathway along the root to the gingival margin. The condition is referred to as a **periodontal/endodontic lesion**. Patients often experience the acute symptoms of an irreversible pulpitis and must be managed with both periodontal and endodontic therapies.

Pain Associated With Periodontal Tissues

Most periodontal problems are chronic in nature and rarely reach acute exacerbation. Some are acute, however, and may cause the patient to seek immediate care.

Patients with gingivitis may have tender gingival tissues in the absence of detectable periodontal pockets. The patient complains of "sore gums." Typically, this problem is characterized by

notable inflammation with edema and hemorrhage on manipulation of the tissues, although these features may be absent in an immunocompromised host. Local factors, most notably calculus, are present and are the primary cause of the patient's discomfort.

Patients with chronic periodontitis may also become symptomatic. The patient typically describes itching or burning soft tissue with persistent pain. Mild temporary relief may be achieved using various rinses or by massaging the soft tissue. Although annoying and disruptive to activities of daily living, the pain is usually not intense and typically does not disrupt sleep. Common clinical findings include periodontal pockets with bleeding on probing. Subgingival deposits are almost invariably present. Probing the pockets recreates the primary complaint. Although the patient may have difficulty differentiating between pain of pulpal origin and periodontal pain, probing pockets will usually be discriminatory. Confirmation of pulp vitality also helps make the distinction.

A **periodontal abscess** has symptoms and features similar to the previously described apical periodontitis with abscess formation (Figure 9.11). In this case, however, the exudate more commonly drains through the periodontal pocket rather than through the facial or lingual bone and soft tissue.

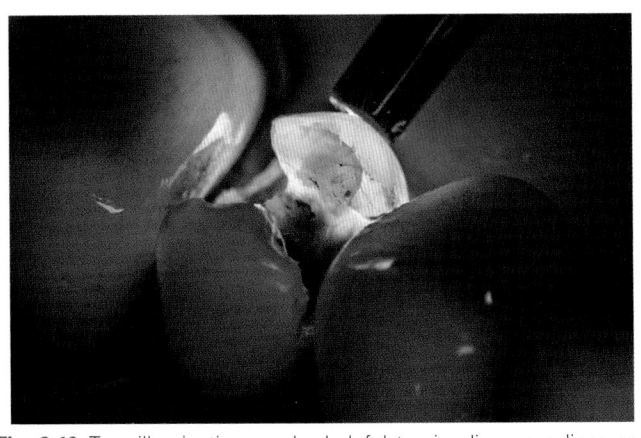

Fig. 9.10 Transillumination can be helpful to visualize craze lines and fracture lines in teeth. (Courtesy Dr. Lee Boushell)

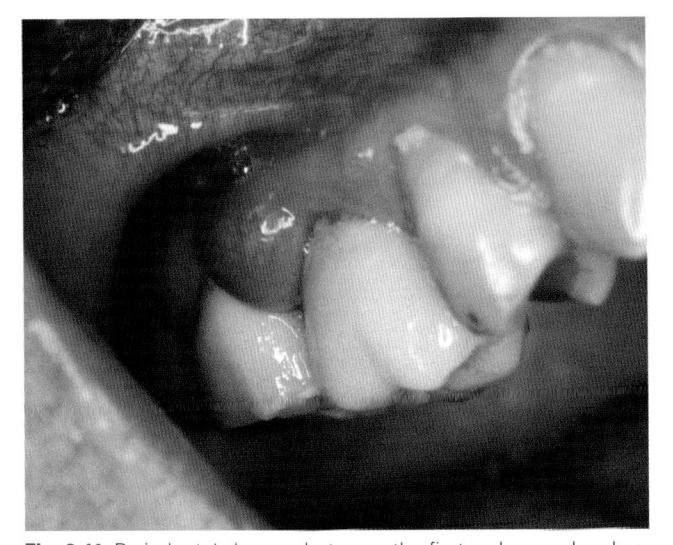

Fig. 9.11 Periodontal abscess between the first and second molars.

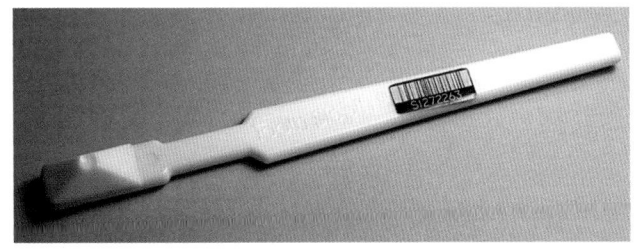

Fig. 9.9 Tooth Slooth instrument used to evaluate for cracked tooth syndrome. The apex of the instrument tip is placed on each cusp of the tooth sequentially and the patient is instructed to bite down. If biting down is painful, the tooth may be fractured.

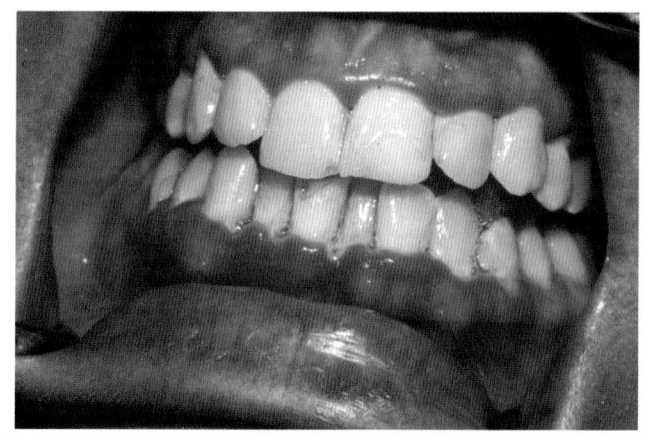

Fig. 9.12 Patient with necrotizing ulcerative gingivitis (NUG). Note the loss of interdental papillae, especially around the mandibular incisors. (Courtesy Ms. Nancy Slach.)

Exceptions occur, however, because calculus or other foreign debris may sometimes block egress of the pus from the pocket. Almost invariably, a significant foreign body will have been retained in the pocket but has now been expelled. A classic example is the patient who experiences acute symptoms within a day of eating popcorn, with an entrapped popcorn hull as the culprit. A particularly large calculus deposit is another common source of irritation. Usually, bleeding and/or suppuration will occur on probing of the pocket where the periodontal abscess resides.

Necrotizing ulcerative gingivitis is readily apparent to the patient because of significantly sore gums and halitosis. "Trench mouth," as it used to be called, typically occurs in the patient with poor oral hygiene who is also experiencing several of these conditions: stress, poor diet, sleep deprivation, being a smoker. Distinctive clinical features include significant gingival inflammation, bleeding, and "punched-out" papillae with a pseudomembrane (Figure 9.12). Suppuration may occur and the gingiva is exquisitely tender.

Pain Associated With Tooth Eruption or Pericoronitis

As a normally erupting tooth makes its way into the oral cavity, some discomfort is not unusual. If the tissue over the erupting crown (the **operculum**) becomes traumatized by mastication or contact with the opposing tooth, however, the patient may experience considerable discomfort. Inflammation and swelling may occur, further aggravating the condition and making it even more likely that the operculum will be traumatized. **Pericoronitis** arises when the operculum becomes infected. At this point, the tenderness may extend to surrounding tissues (Figure 9.13). Particularly in the case of a third molar, **trismus** may develop. Suppuration may be present. Inflamed lymph nodes, **lymphadenitis**, on the affected side may be palpated. If left untreated, constitutional symptoms, such as fever and malaise, may develop. Diagnosis is based on history and clinical findings. Presence and position of the erupting or impacted tooth should be confirmed by radiographic imaging.

Pain Associated With Previous Dental Treatment

Patients may experience acute symptoms after dental treatment. Acute sequelae after treatment such as deep caries excavation

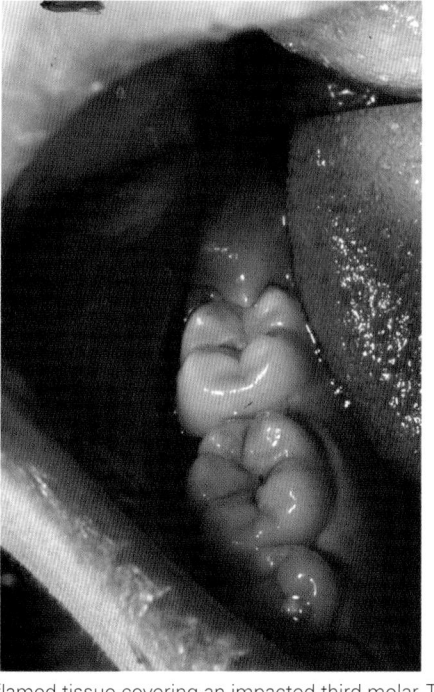

Fig. 9.13 Inflamed tissue covering an impacted third molar. The operculum extends onto the second molar. (Courtesy Ms. Nancy Slach.)

or an extraction or surgical procedure may be expected and are predictable occurrences. In some cases, the discomfort may occur because the treatment was incompletely or improperly done. For example, when an initial and limited debridement is performed on a patient with significant pockets and subgingival deposits, the gingiva may shrink and become firm after the procedure, eliminating the existing pathway for exudate to egress from the periodontal pocket, resulting in a periodontal abscess.

Some acute problems may occur months or years after initial treatment. The demise of the pulp and development of an apical infection years after placement of a deep restoration is a case in point. Another example is the development of a symptomatic lesion (such as a denture sore or ulcer or a denture stomatitis) in response to changes in the tissues under a prosthesis. In most of these situations, a thorough history and careful clinical examination will usually reveal the problem and its source.

When a patient fractures a restoration or prosthesis, they may express concern that the problem *will cause pain in the future*. Immediate treatment is usually not warranted, but the patient deserves an evaluation and a diagnosis that includes a professional opinion regarding the prognosis for the tooth, restoration, or prosthesis, and the likelihood of additional problems. Rendering such an opinion reassures the patient and also has important risk management and practice management benefits.

Other Sources of Oral Pain

A small percentage of patients whose chief complaint is pain have symptoms that are not related to the teeth or periodontium. This diverse group of problems may present diagnostic difficulties, especially if the patient has trouble localizing the pain. In many situations, the dentist develops a list of possibilities, which

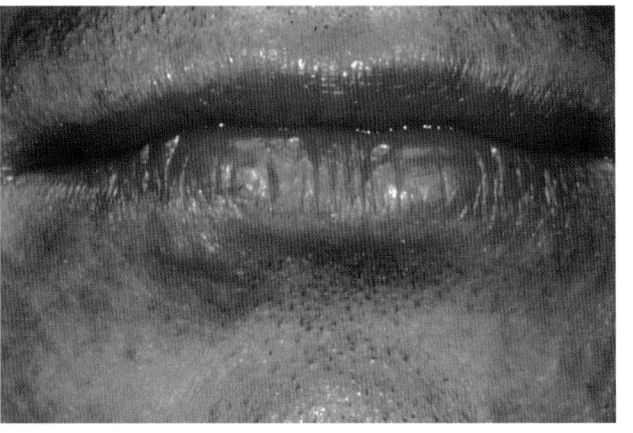

Fig. 9.14 Herpes simplex virus (HSV) lesion of the lower lip. (Courtesy Dr. Michael Finkelstein.)

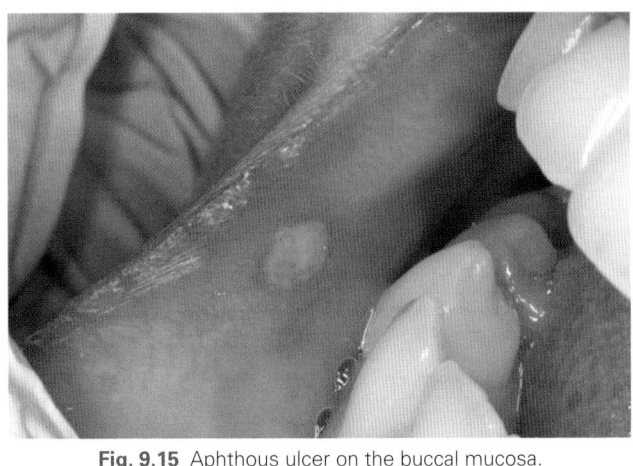

Fig. 9.15 Aphthous ulcer on the buccal mucosa.

by a process of elimination leads to a differential diagnosis. This process can be challenging for the dentist, frustrating for the patient, and time consuming for both. The following paragraphs describe instances of such conditions, along with others that are easier to detect.

Three common types of ulcers may cause problems for patients: **herpetic ulcers, traumatic ulcers**, and **aphthous ulcers**. These are relatively easy to recognize clinically. Herpetic (herpes simplex virus) ulcers are diagnosed using their characteristic history (prodromal symptoms), initiation in vesicular form, and predictable recurrence (Figure 9.14). Patients with **herpes zoster** may experience acute pain and prodromal itching before the outbreak of characteristic vesiculation and ulceration. Zoster is expected to present as a unilateral process distributed in a specific dermatome. Traumatic ulcers are diagnosed by their history and location, usually in proximity to a recognizable source of trauma. **Aphthous ulcers** are usually found on movable tissue in the oral cavity and are typically diagnosed by their characteristic appearance (Figure 9.15). Oral ulcers are often seen in patients with immunocompromised conditions or as a reaction to some medications.

Patients with debilitated health or suffering from an autoimmune disorder may be prone to multiple and recurrent vesicles, bullae, erosions, or ulcers. When these lesions are generalized, they constitute a **stomatitis**. It may be appropriate to refer such patients to an oral medicine specialist, an oral and maxillofacial surgeon, or an internal medicine specialist to confirm the specific cause and recommend treatment.

Acute **temporomandibular disorders** (TMDs) appear in many forms. Acute arthritis usually manifests with pain on opening accompanied by marked crepitation in the temporomandibular joint. A patient may exhibit an acute open lock—be unable to close the jaw and occlude the teeth—or a closed lock, which prevents normal opening of the mouth. Other common manifestations of acute TMD include painful pops or clicks, limited opening, deviation on opening, or painful spasm of one or more of the muscles of mastication.

Neurologic facial pain also can take different forms. **Trigeminal neuralgia** is an exquisitely severe, electric-like, lancinating pain that is related to the distribution of one or more

divisions of the trigeminal nerve. A **neuritis** can be a deep, constant burning pain that runs the course of a nerve trunk. Trauma to a nerve can produce various symptoms ranging from increased sensation (**hyperesthesia**); to altered sensation (**paresthesia**) with burning, itching, or tingling; to complete loss of sensation (**anesthesia**). Patients with this kind of pain usually benefit from referral to a neurologist, an orofacial pain specialist, or an oral and maxillofacial surgeon who has particular expertise in nerve injuries or neurologic disorders.

Acute sinusitis may involve one or both maxillary sinuses. It is characterized by a constant "heavy" debilitating pain that changes intensity with changes in head position and may be accompanied by a foul odor and heavy discharge of mucus or pus from the affected sinus. The maxillary posterior teeth may be painful to chewing and the occlusion may feel high to the patient. Palpation of the sinus wall is positive and the involved sinus cannot be transilluminated. Radiographic imaging may confirm congestion in the sinus.

Complaint of Swelling

Swelling of dental origin is almost always caused by infection (Figure 9.16). The infection may arise in the periapical area as a result of a necrotic pulp tissue, it may be initiated in the periodontal pocket as a result of periodontal disease, or it may develop in the pericoronal tissues concurrent with an erupting or impacted tooth. In some situations, several sites may be involved, as with a periodontal infection that causes swelling and lymphadenitis of a cervical lymph node or a periapical abscess that drains into the maxillary sinus. Any of these situations is likely to bring the patient to the dental office seeking immediate care. A thorough history, clinical examination, pulp vitality testing, and selected imaging usually lead to a definitive diagnosis. Specific diagnoses for acute dental conditions in this group are the same as those listed under *Complaint of Pain.*

Possible sources for oral swelling not associated with the teeth or periodontium are many. These include cysts, benign and malignant tumors, infections, granulomatous diseases, and hyperplastic conditions secondary to medication use. In addition to the health and medication history, clues to diagnosing

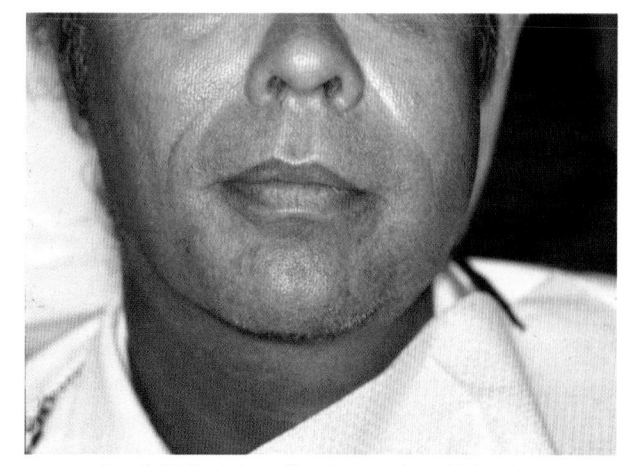

Fig. 9.16 Facial swelling from a dental infection.

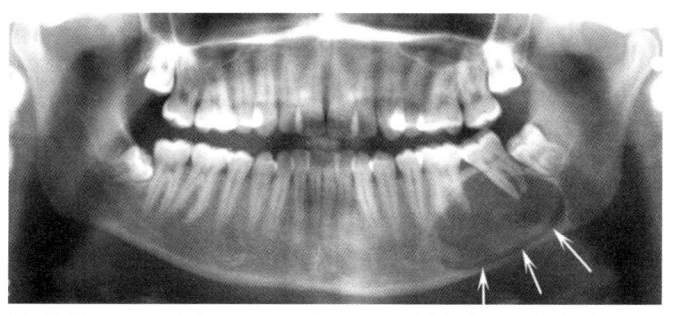

Fig. 9.17 Panoramic image revealing an ameloblastoma within the body of the left mandible that had caused swelling for the patient. (From Mallya S, Lam E. *White and Pharoah's Oral Radiology: Principles and Interpretation.* 8th ed. Elsevier; 2019 [Fig. 18.5].)

these lesions include their duration, the presence or absence of other symptoms, the shape, the texture, the integrity of the surface epithelium, the presence or absence of invasion into surrounding structures, and the presence or absence of lymphadenopathy. With lymphadenopathy, the shape, texture, borders, movability, and sensitivity of the affected lymph nodes can be useful in differentiating preexisting fibrosis or calcification from inflammation, lymphoma, or malignancy. Radiographic images may be helpful in the differential diagnosis of lesions in bone or in close proximity to bone (Figure 9.17). Computed tomography scans, magnetic resonance imaging, and/or a biopsy may be required to make a definitive diagnosis. The major salivary glands may swell from infection or blockage of duct.

Esthetic Complaints

Esthetic complaints are generally simple to diagnose because they are usually apparent to both dentist and patient. Such complaints often arise because of the fracture of a tooth or fracture or loss of a restoration in an esthetic area. Other common causes include fractured porcelain on a crown or fixed partial denture and fracture or loss of a tooth from a removable prosthesis. Although these occurrences would not constitute an emergency (unless accompanied by an abscess or overt infection), they can constitute an urgent need if the patient's appearance or ability to speak is affected adversely.

The underlying cause of esthetic problems not caused by overt trauma may be less apparent than the complaint itself. Was the tooth or restoration in hyperocclusion? Were lateral forces on the tooth excessive? Has there been loss of vertical dimension of occlusion? Was reduction in a crown preparation insufficient? Did the patient abuse the prosthesis in some way? If the underlying cause can be determined and mitigated, the prognosis for a successful repair or replacement will be greatly improved.

Traumatic Injury

When an individual experiences a significant traumatic event, as might be associated with a fall, for example, or playing sports, or a motor vehicle accident involving facial injuries, the dentist is likely to be consulted. Because such an event may simultaneously affect teeth, soft tissues, and bone, all three areas must be assessed.[10] The dentist can also help prevent sport-related orofacial trauma by fabricating mouthguards for patients engaged in contact sports and by sponsoring mouthguard programs in the community.

Tooth injuries may range from the slight loosening of a single tooth (**partial luxation**) to fractures of enamel, dentin, and even into the pulp chamber. One or more teeth may be completely avulsed from the socket. Dental fractures may be **complete (displaced)** or **incomplete (nondisplaced)**. Root fractures can occur independent of coronal fractures and are described in terms of location (apical, middle, or coronal third) and angulation (vertical or horizontal). As a result of the trauma, teeth may have been moved from their normal position—intruded or extruded or displaced facially, lingually, mesially, or distally. Making these descriptive distinctions is valuable as healthcare professionals communicate with each other concerning the nature and severity of the injury.

Classification of a dental injury can be important in the determination of the prognosis for a tooth and in shaping both short- and long-term treatment planning. The assessment of a traumatized tooth includes careful inspection for fractures, mobility testing (for traumatized teeth *and* opposing and surrounding teeth), pulp vitality testing (should be delayed in the case of a displaced or avulsed tooth), and selected radiographic or other imaging. Careful evaluation of the occlusion is critical in helping the dentist identify a displaced or extruded tooth requiring immediate treatment.

Soft tissue injuries typically include lacerations and contusions from lips or cheeks being compressed between the teeth and a foreign object. If the lip or tongue is lacerated, significant bleeding may occur. Edema, induration, and swelling may occur during the healing process. If tissue becomes necrotic, it may slough and ulcerate. The dentist may be called on to diagnose and manage any or all of these conditions. All traumatized tissue must be carefully examined for the presence of foreign bodies or debris. Carefully debriding the site of any foreign material (gravel, glass, or even tooth fragments) is therapeutic and facilitates diagnosis. Selected imaging at a density appropriate for soft tissue can be helpful.

Jaw bones may be crushed or fractured by the impact of a blow. Fractures may be partial or complete, displaced or

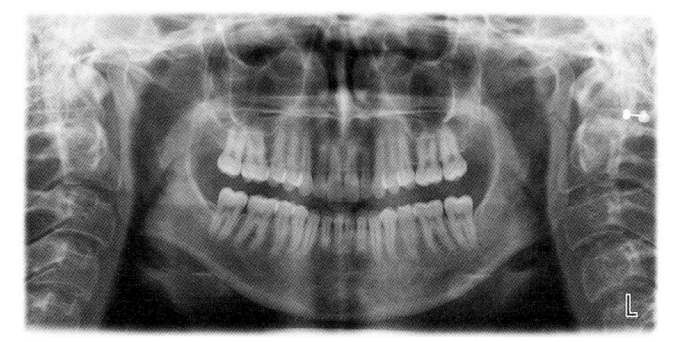

Fig. 9.18 Panoramic radiograph of a fracture of the left condyle.

nondisplaced. The initial diagnosis of a jaw fracture is based on the reported symptoms, findings from the examination, and appropriate imaging (Figure 9.18). A displaced fracture often results in the patient's inability to close the mouth comfortably and altered occlusion of the teeth. Trauma or infection may cause lack of sensation, or paresthesia, to oral and perioral structures. Especially in the compromised host, an infection of the bone, **osteomyelitis**, may occur at the site of fracture. When a jaw fracture is suspected or diagnosed, it is usually appropriate to refer the patient to an oral and maxillofacial surgeon for definitive evaluation, diagnosis, and treatment.

When evaluating a patient with a traumatic injury, dental personnel should screen for signs of domestic violence or child or elder abuse. Such injuries might include fractures of the jaws or other facial bones; fractured, avulsed, or subluxated teeth; lacerations; facial abrasions; or bruising. Careful questioning of the patient in the absence of the domestic partner or caregiver may be necessary and referral to the appropriate agency to prevent further injury may be indicated.

Traumatic injuries may also arise at the time of, or as a result of, dental treatment. Examples include luxation or removal of the wrong tooth, loosening a crown or fracturing a restoration on another tooth during extraction, lacerating the cheek or lip during a restorative or surgical procedure, and injuring a nerve during administration of a nerve block or during surgery. Most of these problems are apparent to the patient and/or clinician at the time, but occasionally necessitate the patient's return to the office on an acute care basis. A careful history, examination of the operative site, and review of the patient record should be sufficient to enable a diagnosis of the problem. In some cases, for example, if paresthesia occurs, referral to an oral and maxillofacial surgeon for consultation, definitive diagnosis, and management may be warranted.

TREATMENT PLANNING FOR ACUTE NEEDS

It would seem logical that treatment planning for a patient's acute needs would be simpler than dealing with the complexities of a comprehensive plan of care. Unfortunately, this is often not the case. Even though the options are usually more limited and the elements in the process are identical, acute phase decision making often must be achieved under adverse circumstances and a much more pressing time constraint.

When confronted with a patient with acute needs, the practitioner must go through several steps before arriving at an appropriate acute phase plan. Typically, these steps are collapsed into a single conversation with the patient in which treatment options are discussed and informed consent is acquired. For the purposes of this discussion and to articulate the elements in this process more clearly, the steps are presented separately.

Defining the Range of Options

For the patient with an acute treatment need, a finite range of options is considered. For purposes of illustration, Table 9.2 includes a list of the more common acute phase diagnoses and the most frequently used short-term therapies associated with each. Also included are possible long-term implications of those treatment options that both dentist and patient should keep in mind.

Factors Influencing Treatment Decisions

Making a treatment planning decision for the acute needs patient is not simply a matter of selecting the best treatment from a standard menu. Numerous influences can affect planning acute phase treatment. Some of these (professional factors) must be determined and assessed by the dentist; some are solely under the control of the patient (patient factors and modifiers); and some are issues that need the perspectives of both patient and practitioner (combination factors).

Professional factors are those that define the limits of what is feasible and possible. At the outset, the dentist must establish parameters for what can be done under current circumstances that will be professionally reasonable and feasible. Important considerations include the patient's general health, the complexity of the dental treatment to be undertaken, the dentist's level of experience in and confidence with a proposed procedure, and the availability of specialists to provide consultation and/or treatment. Occasionally, a patient desperately seeks treatment that is not in his or her best interest—for example, the patient who wants to save "at all cost" a tooth that is not restorable. The dentist must define the limits for treatment and, in this particular situation, has the obligation to refuse the patient's request. It is the dentist's responsibility to identify and present treatment options that are reasonable and professionally appropriate.

Patient factors and modifiers (discussed in Chapter 5) are those patient circumstances or issues that have a direct bearing on the treatment choice selection. These include the patient's interests and priorities, the time and financial resources they are willing and able to expend on the treatment, the quality of oral self-care, and the patient's ability to maintain the dental work. Additional patient factors include whether the patient has available the transportation and home support necessary to engage in the definitive therapy and follow-up under consideration.

It is important to keep in mind that the patient determines this set of issues. Some conversation between patient and dentist is required to delineate which issues are relevant and important for the situation. With the need to expedite treatment, it is easy for the dentist to hasten this conversation and make assumptions

TABLE 9.2 Treatment Options and Recommendations for Selected Acute Phase Problems

Problem	Therapy Options (Short Term)	Treatment Implications (Long Term)
Traumatic Injury		
Avulsed tooth[a]	If <60 min since injury, reinsert and stabilize (short term).	Monitor for changes (resorption) and need for root canal therapy, physiologic splint, extraction
Displaced tooth	Reposition tooth; radiograph and baseline pulp tests; splint as necessary	Monitor for changes (resorption) and possible need for root canal therapy, physiologic splint, extraction
Fractured jaw	If displaced, set fracture and stabilize; if not displaced, pulp test teeth and monitor	Follow carefully for bleeding, infection, root resorption, loss of vitality, malocclusion
Occlusal trauma	If resulting from clenching/bruxism, occlusal adjustment; if resulting from external trauma, radiograph, baseline pulp tests; consider short-term splinting	Consider fabricating occlusal guard or definitive splinting of the teeth
Pain Associated With Individual Teeth		
Cracked tooth syndrome	Adhesive restoration; circumferential banding; provisional full-coverage restoration	Often requires cusp-protective cast restoration; may require endodontic therapy or extraction
Fractured tooth or restoration	Detailed analysis to determine underlying cause, place restoration	Definitive restoration
Irreversible pulpitis/acute apical periodontitis/apical abscess	Analgesics (symptomatic), extraction or root canal therapy (definitive)	Replacement of extracted tooth; definitive restoration of endodontically treated tooth
Pain after restoration placement	Check the occlusion, integrity of restoration; analgesics	May need endodontic therapy
Pain after endodontic therapy	Analgesics; antibiotics; occlusal adjustment; reinstrument if necessary	If tooth is fractured, may require extraction
Postextraction pain	Palliative therapy; antibiotics; antiinflammatory medication; if dry socket, apply dressing	Follow patient, confirm resolution
Reversible pulpitis secondary to caries, fractured restoration, or fractured tooth	Palliative treatment; temporary restoration	Requires definitive restoration
Hypersensitive noncarious cervical lesions	Dentifrice or topical treatment for tooth sensitivity	May require sealant or restoration[b]
Periodontal and Other Soft Tissue Pain		
Pain after periodontal therapy	Analgesic; recheck for residue or debris	Follow patient; confirm resolution; if pain persists, look for other causes
Acute (marginal) periodontitis	Scaling and root planing; irrigate with chlorhexidine	Requires posttreatment evaluation and definitive periodontal therapy; if prognosis is hopeless, extract and discuss long-term treatment options
Acute gingivitis	Scaling, prophylaxis, oral hygiene instruction	Establish regular maintenance program
Periodontal abscess	Scaling and root planing; incision and drainage; irrigate with chlorhexidine	Definitive periodontal therapy or tooth extraction; consider effect of retention vs. extraction on the entire dentition
Periodontal/endodontic lesion	If endodontic in origin, provide root canal therapy and treat periodontal problems secondarily (periodontal treatment may not be necessary); if periodontal in origin, treat periodontal disease and do root canal therapy simultaneously	Definitive restoration after root canal therapy; long-term periodontal maintenance
Soft tissue injury associated with dental treatment	Obtain primary closure; analgesics and antibiotics as needed	Follow patient; communicate and confirm resolution of injury
Third molar pericoronitis	Palliative treatment; antibiotics; local irrigation with saline or chlorhexidine; consider extraction of the opposing third molar	Extraction of the offending tooth; consider extraction of all third molars
Ulcers/stomatitis	Palliative treatment with topical anesthetic and compounds that provide a protective covering of the lesions	Definitive therapy as needed to manage underlying systemic or oral disease; pharmacologic treatment

TABLE 9.2	Treatment Options and Recommendations for Selected Acute Phase Problems—cont'd	
Problem	**Therapy Options (Short Term)**	**Treatment Implications (Long Term)**
Other		
Broken prosthesis	Repair prosthesis	Replace or remake prosthesis if needed
Pain associated with debonded, fractured, or missing provisional restoration	Re-cement, repair, remake provisional restoration	Definitive restoration
Pain associated with orthodontic therapy	Analgesics; cover sharp edges of brackets, bands, or wires	Reevaluation of orthodontic hardware
Swelling without pain (neoplasms, cysts, lymphadenopathy, sialadenopathy, mucocele)	Biopsy, aspiration, or other diagnostic tests as necessary; consult with radiologist, surgeon, or pathologist as needed	Definitive treatment of primary disease may be disfiguring, may require extensive reconstruction
Temporomandibular disorder	Palliative treatment: analgesics, muscle relaxants, splint therapy; applying ice or heat to the painful area, soft diet	Detailed analysis required to determine underlying cause; behavior modification, psychotherapy, pharmacotherapy, physical therapy, or surgical evaluation may be indicated

[a]Fouad AF, Abbott PV, Tsilingaridis G, et al. International Association of Dental Traumatology guidelines for the management of traumatic dental injuries: 2. Avulsion of permanent teeth. *Dent Traumatol.* 2020;36(4):331-342.
[b]Veitz-Keenan A, Barna JA, Strober B, et al. Treatments for hypersensitive noncarious cervical lesions: a Practitioners Engaged in Applied Research and Learning (PEARL) Network randomized clinical effectiveness study. *J Am Dent Assoc* 2013;144(5):495-506.

about the patient's motivation and desire (or lack thereof) for treatment. But these assumptions can be misleading and can lead the dentist to recommend inappropriate treatment options. For instance, a patient with a severely decayed but restorable molar may seem a candidate for extraction, especially if they have other oral problems or appear unable to afford the cost of root canal treatment and a definitive restoration. Removing the tooth may indeed be the most appropriate therapy, but each patient at least should be *offered* the ideal treatment if there is a reasonable prospect of success. If the patient rejects the ideal option, the dentist can then suggest other possible alternatives.

Combination factors are those about which both the dentist and patient have legitimate, although sometimes differing, interests and perspectives. Both perspectives can be critical to making the correct treatment decision. An excellent example can be drawn from the patient whose chief concern is an esthetic issue. A patient may present with a serious esthetic problem involving discolored, crowded, and missing teeth, with the goal of improving their appearance before an imminent job interview. The dentist may mistakenly assume that replacing the missing teeth or masking or straightening the malposed teeth is the top priority, when in fact the patient is far more concerned with just the dark color of the maxillary anterior teeth. This example illustrates the importance of ensuring that the dentist and patient clearly understand all options and goals before any acute or definitive treatment is begun.

Choosing a Plan That Takes Long-Term Implications into Account

Often overlooked when planning treatment for a patient with acute needs are the requirements of long-term follow-up. It is imperative that the patient be made aware of both the consequences of the acute phase treatment and any anticipated future treatment needs. This understanding must be achieved *before* a plan of care for acute treatment is finalized. All too often, the patient presents for an emergency tooth extraction without fully realizing the consequences. The patient must be informed of the risks and hazards to the dentition and overall health that may be associated with the loss of the tooth, including the possibilities of impaired function and movement of the surrounding teeth. The patient must also be made aware of the cost in time and money of future tooth replacement options. Similarly, a patient might insist on saving one tooth at a significant financial cost, when these resources would be better used to preserve other teeth that have a more optimal prognosis.

Acquiring Consent for Acute Care

Informed consent for an acute care treatment plan requires all the same elements as consent for a comprehensive care plan. In both situations, the patient must be fully aware of (1) the diagnosis, (2) all reasonable treatment options (including the option of no treatment), (3) the risks and benefits of each option, (4) the nature of the recommended treatment, and (5) the costs of that treatment, both now and in the future. This is a significant amount of information, and the acute care patient, often in pain and in an anxious state, may have difficulty assimilating the information and making an informed treatment decision. This creates a genuine dilemma for the dentist. Although both the patient and dentist have a strong interest in relieving the patient's pain and satisfying the acute concern quickly, inability to establish fully informed consent may preclude expeditious treatment. It may be necessary to defer irreversible procedures until the patient feels comfortable with the options and can make a definitive decision. Providing short-term palliative care offers one approach to making that transition. The *In Clinical Practice: Decision Making for the Acute Care Patient* box discusses some of the issues associated with this situation.

IN CLINICAL PRACTICE

Decision Making for the Acute Care Patient

"Extraction or a root canal treatment?" In the context of acute care, this simple treatment question is frequently asked by both patient and dentist. Acute pulpal and periapical disease, frequently involving irreversible pulpal pathologic conditions, is the most common problem leading patients to seek urgent dental treatment. In short, only two treatment options effectively eliminate the source of pain: initiation of root canal therapy or extraction.

Initially, the dentist must determine how critical the tooth is to the patient's overall oral health. What is the prognosis for the tooth? Is it restorable? In light of the patient's other dental needs, is it realistic to invest time and resources in trying to maintain the tooth? If so, what endodontic, orthodontic, periodontal, and/or restorative therapy will also be required or recommended?

At the same time, the patient must consider how much time, money, and energy they are willing to invest in saving the tooth. Even in the acute care situation, the dentist has the professional responsibility to be sure the patient fully understands the treatment options and their likely long-term consequences. The patient also needs to know what will be required in the way of follow-up care and be prepared to commit to that. If the patient is not well acquainted with possible dental treatment options, this may require considerable discussion.

In some situations, it is relatively easy to reach consensus and achieve fully informed consent. An example is the patient who has generalized severe periodontal disease, rampant caries, or a tooth with a poor restorative prognosis who wishes to have the affected tooth or teeth extracted. At the other end of the spectrum is the patient who exhibits excellent oral health, values and appreciates optimal treatment (including root canal therapy), and wishes to invest the time and financial resources necessary to save their teeth. In both cases, the treatment objectives are clear and the dentist and patient can readily proceed with treatment.

However, for many patients the decision is not so simple. The dentist may recognize that it is in the patient's best interest to save the tooth, but the patient may insist on having it extracted. Conversely, the patient may wish to save the tooth at all costs, with unrealistic expectations about the extent of treatment required or the prognosis. In many cases, various compelling patient and clinical reasons fall on both sides of the issue, with no clear choice indicated. When this occurs, it is critically important for the dentist to provide the patient with the maximum amount of information on which to base the decision. If the discussion overwhelms the patient so that they become immobilized and cannot make a decision, it may be helpful to include a family member, spouse, partner or friend of the patient in the decision-making process.

In summary, resolving acute problems often results in a difficult decision for the patient and dentist. It is possible, however, to approach the decision-making process in an efficient, sequential, and professional manner, even within the constraints and limitations of the acute care visit. The patient can be provided with sufficient information to make an informed and appropriate treatment decision that meets both short- and long-term needs. To accomplish this thoroughly, professionally, and compassionately, the dentist must develop a pattern for the process that includes various contingency plans that address issues as they arise and a communication technique that conveys unhurried and focused attention on the patient. With practice, this can become a seamless process in which the dentist and the patient are both well served.

Using Medications to Treat Acute Problems

In general, the best treatment alternative is to manage the patient's acute problem with definitive care—for example, an extraction or pulp extirpation, rather than pharmacologically. In some situations, however, it is not only prudent but also preferable to prescribe medications rather than initiate treatment. Examples include the following:

- The problem or offending tooth cannot be identified.
- The patient has a compromising systemic condition that precludes treatment at this time.
- The patient has an active infection, and there is significant risk that surgical intervention or extraction may lead to further pain or spread of the infection.
- The patient is unwilling or unable to provide consent to treatment.

In any of these situations, the dentist's duty does not end with the writing of the prescriptions for antibiotics and/or analgesics. Nonsteroidal analgesics such as acetaminophen and ibuprofen are preferred to opiate containing medications for controlling pain and minimizing adverse events, particularly addiction.[11] Dentists should also carefully instruct patients to not exceed the maximum daily limit of analgesics.[12] To minimize the chance of developing antibiotic resistance, the clinician should prescribe antibiotic medication when there are signs or symptoms of systemic involvement such as fever or malaise.[13] It is the dentist's obligation to provide follow-up to ensure resolution of the problem. Patients should be given an appointment with the dentist or an appropriate specialist for definitive therapy. If the patient fails to keep the subsequent appointment, the responsibility for success or failure of the treatment becomes the patient's and the dentist cannot be faulted.

An after-hours call from a patient with a toothache or other dental complaint to the practitioner at their residence is not an unusual occurrence. If the person is a patient of record and currently under the care of the dentist, it may be appropriate for the dentist to offer to return to the office to provide care or to call in a prescription to treat the symptoms. If the patient is new to the practice or had been in the practice but has since left or been dismissed, the dentist may recommend that the patient be seen in another setting, such as a hospital emergency room. When the patient is treated pharmacologically, especially after hours and over the phone, accurate and comprehensive documentation is essential. This includes many of the items presented in the next section.

DOCUMENTING ACUTE CARE TREATMENT AND FOLLOW-UP

If the acute or potentially acute treatment necessary is recognized during the formulation of an overall plan of care, it is included in the plan in the acute phase of care and is sequenced first. In this situation, a routine progress note in the patient record is sufficient to document the diagnosis and treatment recommendations.

An alternative situation arises when a patient presenting for acute care is either new to the practice or is a patient of record who now has an unanticipated problem. In either of these situations, the practitioner may document the event in a different manner from the usual progress note entry. Adapted from techniques used by our physician colleagues who routinely handle episodic care patients, this format has come to be known as a

SOAP note, an acronym taken from the first initial in each of its four components. The SOAP note is a commonly used method of documenting the visit of an acute care patient in both medicine and dentistry. The components are as follows:

Subjective: This information includes the chief concern or complaint and the history of that complaint (i.e., the history of the present illness) and is recorded in the patient's own words.

Objective: This portion is garnered by the dentist and summarizes the clinical findings gathered during the examination process. Typically, this portion of the note includes visual findings, results of periodontal assessment, clinical tests (palpation, percussion, and vitality tests) and interpretation of radiographs.

Assessment: In a word, this is the diagnosis. If insufficient information is available to arrive at a definitive diagnosis, the dentist records a preliminary or tentative diagnosis.

Plan: This includes the acute care plan for the patient and documentation of informed consent. Any options offered to the patient must be noted here. The patient's wishes and evidence that he or she understands the problem, options, and proposed plan are also included in the writeup.

In a dental practice, the SOAP note is usually preceded by a summary of significant positive or negative findings from the health history and review of systems and a recording of the vital signs on the date of the event, followed by an entry describing the treatment rendered (Figure 9.19).

Whether the patient has been active in the practice for many years, has a newly formulated plan of care, or has recently come to the office seeking only emergency care, they deserve to have the problem handled in a competent, courteous, and professional manner. Additionally, as noted earlier, the dentist's responsibility does not end at the conclusion of the office visit. The dentist may need to manage any complications that may arise from treatment. Specifically, at the conclusion of the visit, the patient should be given:

- Postoperative instructions explaining what has been done and what (if any) oral self-care procedures the patient should carry out to protect and maintain oral health. Similarly, if the patient should avoid certain behaviors or habits (e.g., chewing on hard foods, smoking), these should be explained.
- Prescriptions for antibiotics, analgesics, or other medications as appropriate.
- Guidance on what to do if the original problem persists or worsens. This usually includes a phone number at which the treating dentist can be reached after office hours. If the patient is given a referral to another dentist, that office or clinic should be notified so that any pertinent records and radiographs can be made available.

Irreversible treatment of an acute condition based on a rushed evaluation and performed on an anxious patient who may not be thinking clearly is a volatile combination and has the potential to lead to litigation. The patient who perceives the dentist as unresponsive to problems or concerns arising from the acute or urgent care treatment may accuse the dentist of abandonment (see Chapter 7). Thorough documentation of the patient assessment, diagnosis, treatment plan, consent, treatment rendered, and postoperative conversation can reduce considerably the risk of litigation.

Aside from the risk management benefits, other important reasons for maintaining an open dialogue with the patient throughout the acute care treatment experience are as follows:

- Patients who are better informed tend to be less anxious and generally recover with fewer complications.
- Patients who can share their concerns and questions at the acute care visit are less likely to have questions later and to need to contact the dentist after office hours or to return for unscheduled postoperative visits.
- Patients who know what to expect in the way of possible sequelae and pain are more prepared to tolerate the discomfort and are less concerned if it does arise.

SOAP Note

(Date of Acute Care Visit)
Health status: No allergies, no medications and no contraindications to dental treatment; BP 136/80, Pulse rate: 76. Head, face, and neck examination within normal limits.

S – "Toothache on the upper right for last 2 weeks–getting worse." Patient reports pain to cold and hot, duration 5-10 minutes, loss of sleep and requires ibuprofen 3-4 times per day.

O – Grossly decayed #3, (+) response to percussion; palpation, swelling and periodontal examination is (−); #3 is non-vital to electric pulp testing (EPT), no apical change interpreted on the periapical radiograph.

A – Caries, necrotic pulp, acute apical periodontitis–tooth is restorable.

P – Discussed treatment options including endodontic therapy and crown vs. extraction with pros/cons and risks/benefits of each procedure. Patient prefers root canal therapy and understands that tooth may need a crown lengthening procedure.

Patient given a fee estimate of ____.

(Treatment notes)

Fig. 9.19 SOAP note.

By managing the acute care patient efficiently, compassionately, and professionally, the dentist creates the potential for a sustained referral base of new patients. Many acute care patients, even if they themselves do not return to the office, will recommend the practice and the dentist to their friends. Some, having successfully navigated the initial acute care visit, will become excellent patients in the practice. The acute care visit can be an opportunity to educate the patient about the benefits of contemporary oral healthcare and to demonstrate that dentistry does not have to be an impersonal, agonizing, or painful process. Some of the most appreciative and loyal comprehensive care patients in most any practice are those who began as acute care patients.

CONCLUSION

Incorporating patients with acute needs into an already busy practice is a challenge. To do so with efficiency and compassion represents a genuine achievement. The professional responsibility of carrying out an appropriately detailed evaluation of the patient's general health and dental condition, deriving a diagnosis, developing an acute phase plan of care with complete informed consent, and delivering that care in a timely and professional manner is a necessary part of today's dental practice. When done well, benefits to the patient are inestimable and the dentist receives significant personal and professional rewards.

▋ REVIEW QUESTIONS

- What is the difference between an emergency problem and an urgent problem?
- In what ways does the acute care patient present a unique challenge to the dentist?
- How does the patient evaluation differ between the acute care patient and a comprehensive care patient?
- Describe the common acute problems seen in a dental practice. How is each diagnosed?

- How are acute phase treatment options determined and presented to the patient? How is consensus achieved? How is consent established?
- When is it appropriate to use medications to treat acute problems?
- How should acute care be documented?

REFERENCES

1. Brecher EA, Keels MA, Quiñonez RB, Roberts MW, Bordley WC. A policy review of after-hours emergency dental care responsibilities. *J Public Health Dent*. 2016;76(4):263–268.
2. Fiehn R, Okunev I, Bayham M, Barefoot S, Tranby EP. Emergency and urgent dental visits among Medicaid enrollees from 2013 to 2017. *BMC Oral Health*. 2020;20(1):355.
3. Balenović A, Fazlić A, Mihelčić M, Hoch A, Radujković V. Sociodemographic determinants and common reasons for visiting the emergency dental service in the city of Zagreb. *Acta Stomatol Croat*. 2019;53(3):247–254.
4. American Dental Association. Oral health and well-being in the united states https://www.ada.org/~/media/ADA/Science%20 and%20Research/HPI/OralHealthWell-Being-StateFacts/US-Oral-Health-Well-Being.pdf?la=en.
5. Kim PC, Zhou W, McCoy SJ, et al. Factors associated with preventable emergency department visits for nontraumatic dental conditions in the U.S. *Int J Environ Res Public Health*. 2019;16(19).
6. Sanderson S. Medico-legal considerations in providing emergency dental care in practice. *Prim Dent J*. 2017;6(2):20–25.

7. Aaron S. Key Factors in treating the emergency patient. *Prim Dent J*. 2017;6(2):71–73.
8. Hargreaves KM, Berman LH. *Cohen's Pathways of the Pulp*. 12th ed. Elsevier; 2021.
9. Torabinejad M. *Endodontics - Principals and Practice*. 6th ed. Elsevier; 2021.
10. Chauhan R, Rasaratnam L, Alani A, Djemal S. Adult Dental trauma: what should the dental practitioner know? *Prim Dent J*. 2016;5(2):66–77.
11. Moore PA, Ziegler KM, Lipman RD, Aminoshariae A, Carrasco-Labra A, Mariotti A. Benefits and harms associated with analgesic medications used in the management of acute dental pain: An overview of systematic reviews. *J Am Dent Assoc*. 2018;149(4):256–265.e253.
12. Hommez G, Ongena B, Cauwels R, De Paepe P, Christiaens V, Jacquet W. Analgesia (mis)usage on a dental emergency service: a patient survey. *Clin Oral Investig*. 2018;22(3):1297–1302.
13. U.S. Centers for Disease Control. Checklist for antibiotic prescribing in dentistry. https://www.cdc.gov/antibiotic-use/community/downloads/dental-fact-sheet-FINAL.pdf. Accessed July 6, 2021.

The Disease Control Phase of Treatment

Samuel Nesbit, Carlos Gonzalez-Cabezas, Jonathan Reside, Antonio Moretti,
Peter Tawil, Lee Boushell, Pei-Feng Lim, Gregory Essick, and Kim Sanders

 Visit eBooks.Health.Elsevier.com

OUTLINE

After a thorough examination and diagnostic workup of the patient, both the new and experienced practitioner may be tempted to finalize the treatment plan and move on to actual treatment. Certainly, there is merit in having a single, clear, well-sequenced restorative plan of care. A fundamental question to consider at this point, however, is whether the plan (exclusive of the systemic and acute phase elements discussed in Chapters 8 and 9) should be one continuous successive list, including all periodontal, restorative, orthodontic, endodontic, or surgical treatments required, or will the patient's oral health require a separate **disease control phase** of treatment to establish a stable foundation for future reconstruction?

PURPOSE OF THE DISEASE CONTROL PHASE

Disease control is appropriate when, in the dentist's judgment, the questionable status of the patient's oral health suggests the need for further stabilization before making final decisions on treatment—that is, *treatment uncertainty*. Disease control is also warranted when an intentional reevaluation of the patient is necessary to ensure control of oral disease and infection—that is, *disease status uncertainty*. Finally, in problematic situations that could be characterized as *patient commitment uncertainty*, a disease control phase allows the dentist to preserve, for a time, the maximum number of treatment options while continuing to evaluate the patient's desires, resolve, commitment, compliance

with oral hygiene recommendations, financial status, and comfort in the dental chair.

The purpose of the disease control phase is:
- To eradicate active disease and infection
- To arrest occlusal, functional, and esthetic deterioration
- To address, control, or eliminate causes and risk factors for future disease

The disease control phase allows the practitioner to determine the cause or causes of disease, assess risk factors, and estimate the prognosis for control of disease and various treatment options. The disease control phase also provides both the practitioner and patient with crucial information on which to base treatment recommendations and decisions. In general, when conditions warrant a disease control phase, nonacute and elective orthodontic, endodontic, periodontic, and oral and maxillofacial surgical procedures, as well as any definitive reconstruction, are postponed until the oral disease has been controlled.

A disease control phase is not necessary in a patient whose oral disease is minimal (e.g., patient's only active problem is a slight chronic localized marginal gingivitis) or who does not demonstrate significant risk factors for new disease. It also is not necessary for a patient whose oral disease will be eliminated de facto during definitive treatment. For example, consider the patient with generalized severe alveolar bone loss and clinical attachment loss whose treatment plan includes 14 extractions and the design, fabrication, and placement of complete maxillary and mandibular dentures. Because this treatment generally has a predictable outcome, with disease essentially eliminated by the definitive treatment itself, a disease control phase is usually unnecessary. On the other hand, the patient with five variously sized carious lesions and multiple risk factors for the development of new caries lesions (and who will be retaining the teeth) *will* be likely to benefit from a separate disease control phase of treatment. In this case, it would be inappropriate for the dentist to provide crown restorations before the caries process has been controlled and caries risk factors neutralized or eliminated.

Minimally, the disease control phase should include plans for management of the following:

- Any active oral disease or infection, including but not limited to caries, periodontal disease, and pulpal pathology.
- Teeth requiring stabilization before definitive reconstruction.
- Risk factors that predispose the patient to the development of new or recurrent oral disease, such as smoking or a diet high in refined carbohydrates.

The plan for the disease control phase includes a posttreatment assessment. Although the concept of posttreatment assessment is discussed in detail in Chapter 12, the unique aspects of assessment after a disease control phase merit discussion here because of their importance and timing. Using quantifiable measures whenever possible, such an assessment provides an opportunity for the practitioner to confirm that disease and infection are under control. An example of this is a patient who demonstrates an increased usage of fluoride toothpaste, along with a reduction in frequency of sugar consumption, at the conclusion of the disease control phase. A patient with chronic periodontitis who exhibits a reduction in the percentage of sites with bleeding on probing after scaling and root planing is another.

An assessment at the conclusion of the disease control phase allows both patient and dentist to make a realistic evaluation of feasible and practical treatment options. Previously considered options can be revisited and the prognosis can be determined with more certainty. In addition, the patient will gain a clearer understanding of the level of financial resources, time, and energy they will need to invest in the process. With a track record already established by the patient, the dentist can make individualized treatment recommendations with a clearer sense of expected outcomes.

At the time of the assessment, *new* options for definitive treatment may also become apparent. A patient who, at the outset, only wanted to receive reparative treatment may now be prepared to consider other possibilities. Having successfully completed the disease control phase, the patient may have a new appreciation of self and the improvements that dental treatment can provide. For example, when there is less bleeding during brushing and flossing and anterior teeth have been restored to an esthetically pleasing shape and color, the patient may be prepared to consider orthodontic tooth movement to correct anterior crowding. Before disease control therapy, the patient may not have considered and probably would not have wanted orthodontic therapy. Furthermore, the dentist may have been appropriately reluctant to suggest orthodontic treatment to the patient before a successful outcome to the disease control phase had been assured.

STRUCTURING THE DISEASE CONTROL PHASE

After the dentist has determined the need for a disease control phase, the next step is to formulate and sequence that plan. Many of the principles that apply to the development of the overall plan of care also have application to a plan for disease control. During this phase, however, those principles may take on a unique importance. In addition, other principles are specific to disease control.

As the dentist begins to shape the plan for this phase, there must be a consideration of all reasonable treatment options. In conversation with the patient, a winnowing process that leads to a single mutually agreeable approach to the disease control plan will be necessary. Once a general plan is agreed, the dentist helps the patient to set achievable treatment goals and build realistic expectations for treatment outcomes. The dentist will need to establish clear, specific, and quantifiable standards for success (i.e., outcomes measures), such as setting a target plaque score and bleeding index. The dentist should specify, preferably in writing, the factors that will be evaluated at the posttreatment assessment that closes this phase of care. In addition, the dentist delineates the successive steps to be implemented both when the patient does and does not meet the standards for success. The dentist may also wish to share various definitive phase options that may be appropriate to consider with the patient on completion of the disease control phase. Normally, this discussion should include the options that emerge (1) if the disease control therapy is successful and (2) if disease control therapy is *not* successful. Such a discussion will prepare the patient for either eventuality.

Treatment during the disease control phase is sequenced by priority of patient need rather than by dental discipline. The accompanying *In Clinical Practice* box features keys to a successful disease control phase of treatment.

IN CLINICAL PRACTICE

Keys to Success of Disease Control Phase

Although the disease control phase provides an ideal window of time and opportunity for both patient and practitioner to refine their individual assessments about the best overall course of treatment, that window must be framed and defined clearly. Before engaging in a disease control phase plan of care, it is imperative that the patient understand the purpose, benefits, cost, and time frame of the phase. Specific *goals* must be established and a *definite end point* must be set at which time an evaluation of the outcomes will occur. The dentist must project a clear plan of what the outcome will be—both if the goals are met and if they are not. Despite its numerous advantages, the patient may perceive the disease control phase as a waste of time if it is not carefully developed and properly explained. Without tangible progress or positive reinforcement, the patient may become frustrated and give up. Such a patient may begin arriving late for appointments, delay paying bills, become noncompliant with treatment recommendations, or leave the practice, blaming the dentist for the apparent failure to improve their oral condition. All of these problems can be prevented if a clear understanding of the specific goals for the disease control plan is established between dentist and patient and if honest communication occurs throughout the process. When properly designed and executed, a disease control plan ensures that the patient has achieved and can maintain a healthy oral condition and that definitive care, when provided, will have a high likelihood of success.

In addition to clear goals and ongoing communication with the patient, a key ingredient for the success of the disease control phase is the patient's commitment to the plan. With that commitment, the disease control phase becomes an effective tool with which the dentist can provide the best quality care. Without that commitment, the pace of care slows, dental problems continue to develop, and both patient and practitioner become frustrated. Even when early outcomes seem negative, positive value can be achieved. When handled properly, less than satisfactory outcomes can be seen by both dentist and patient as an opportunity to redirect therapy in a direction more appropriate to the patient's abilities and desires. Sometimes the plan and effort will not succeed as hoped, but if both the patient and dentist share the perspective that the attempt has been made in good faith—and that it has effectively ruled out some treatment options—then the effort will have been worth the effort. The patient who recognizes that effort has been made in their best interests and at their behest will be likely to see the dentist's efforts as ultimately beneficial, even in light of short-term failure. Consequently, if handled effectively, even a negative outcome can strengthen, rather than diminish, the therapeutic relationship between the patient and dental team as they work to define and accomplish the optimal plan of care.

General guidelines for sequencing elements of the treatment plan are discussed in Chapter 5. The following suggestions have particular relevance to the disease control phase.

- *Address the patient's chief concern as early in the plan as possible*, as long as such treatment does not conflict with the primary goals of the disease control phase. Although the psychological value to the patient of addressing the chief concern in a timely fashion is obvious, that approach may sometimes conflict with the demands and goals of disease control treatment. For example, the patient with rampant caries whose primary request is placement of a maxillary anterior fixed partial denture presents the clinician with a dilemma. Although it would not be professionally responsible to place a definitive fixed partial denture before the caries process is controlled, it may be possible to find a provisional solution that meets the patient's needs but does not compromise the standard of care.

- *Sequence by priority—preferably treating the most severe and urgent needs first*. Some notable exceptions will, of course, be necessary. For example, to minimize pain and reduce the need for root canal therapy, it is sometimes preferable to restore a moderately large carious lesion on a vital tooth before initiating root canal therapy with an asymptomatic necrotic pulp or extracting an asymptomatic tooth with a hopeless restorative prognosis (Figure 10.1).

- *Sequence by quadrant/sextant*. Once teeth with gross carious lesions or a questionable restorative prognosis have been extracted or stabilized using provisional (i.e., sedative or protective) restorations, it is most efficient and productive to restore other carious lesions in the same area of the mouth at the same time. Placing direct-fill interim or definitive restorations on multiple teeth in the same quadrant or sextant greatly speeds completion of the disease control phase and may give the patient a much-needed psychological boost as rapid and dramatic progress is experienced.

- *Integrate periodontal therapy into the disease control phase plan*. Many practitioners routinely sequence scaling and root planing or an oral prophylaxis as the first item on the treatment plan. Although it may be easier and more convenient for the general dentist to have a hygienist or periodontist perform the initial periodontal therapy before restorations are attempted, it may not represent the ideal sequence (Figure 10.2). Often, a better approach is to provide both scaling and caries control restorations at the same visit as when that quadrant is anesthetized. In general, treatment of deep caries lesions in vital teeth, symptomatic pulpal problems, and acute oral infections takes precedence over treatment for nonacute periodontitis.

- *Keep definitive phase options open with minimalist treatment in the disease control phase*. It is desirable, during the disease control phase, to look forward to what can be expected to be reasonable treatment options in the definitive phase treatment plan. Toward this end, a priority should be preservation of key teeth and other teeth that are salvageable, but about which there is uncertainty as to whether it will be feasible or desirable for the patient to expend the necessary resources

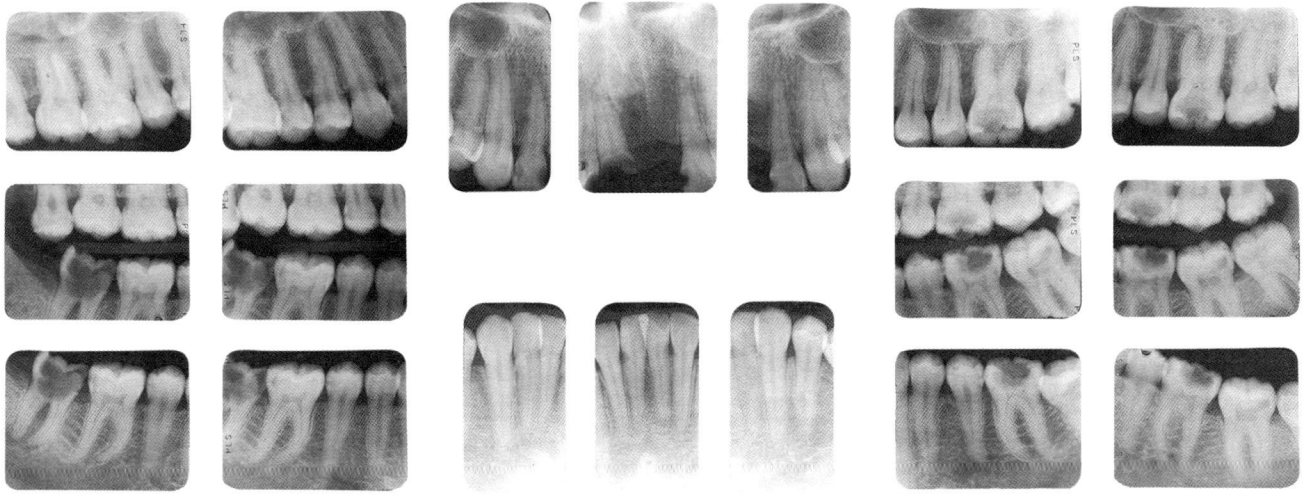

Fig. 10.1 Patient with numerous carious lesions of varying size. The asymptomatic and unrestorable lower right second molar and the asymptomatic and necrotic lower left first molar are not urgent needs. The management of the patient's esthetic problems, initiation of a caries control protocol, and restoration of the numerous moderately sized carious lesions should take precedence over the treatment of these two teeth. (Courtesy Dr. Chai-U-Dom, Chapel Hill, NC.)

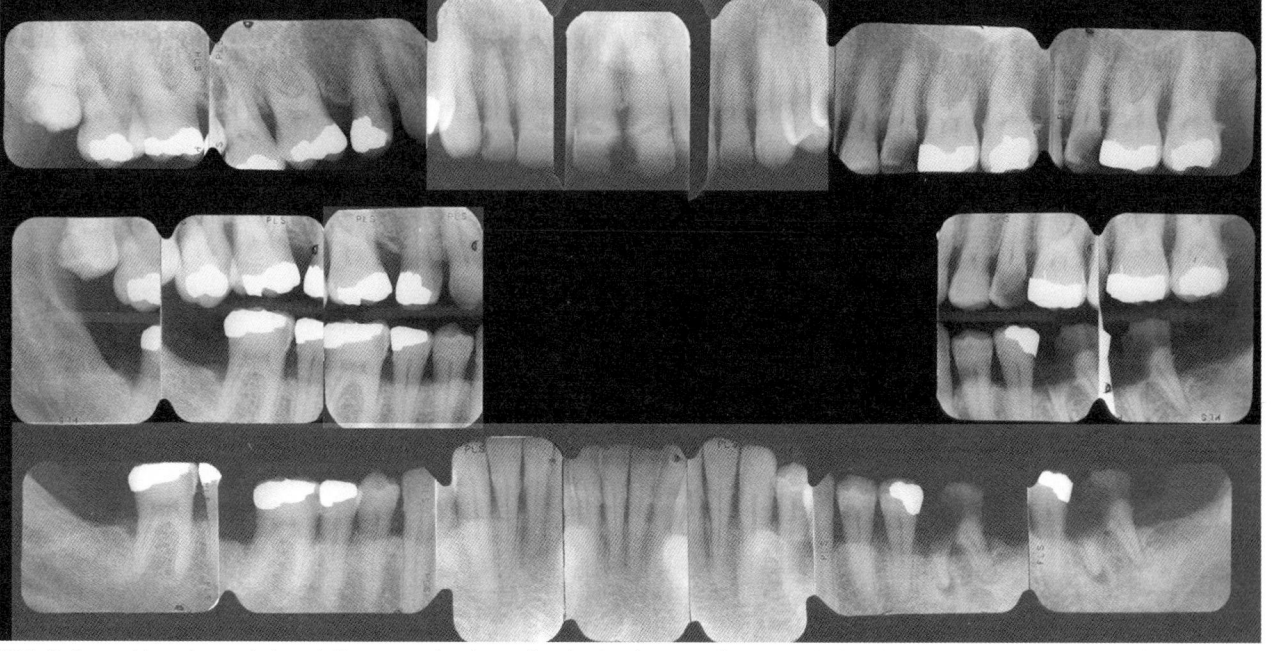

Fig. 10.2 Patient with active periodontal disease and active caries. In the absence of acute periodontal symptoms, management of the deep carious lesions should precede initial periodontal therapy. (Courtesy Dr. I Aukhil, Chapel Hill, NC.)

to restore them definitively. Generally, however, only those procedures necessary to arrest the deterioration and prevent further infection should be undertaken in the disease control phase. In this context, moderate to long-term provisional restorations are preferred to definitive crowns. Pulp capping procedures (when clinically appropriate) are preferred to the initiation of endodontic therapy and pulpotomy and pulpectomy procedures are preferred over definitive root canal treatment. Placement of a protective (sedative or temporary) restoration is commonly done in the disease control phase as an efficient and cost-effective means of restoring multiple large caries lesions in a patient who has an active caries problem. Even in the disease control phase, however, placement of a definitive direct fill restoration is often appropriate and has the benefits of greater longevity for the restoration and avoidance of the need for a definitive restoration at a later date.

Specific circumstances and sound clinical judgment will create many exceptions to each of these general guidelines. Nevertheless, the overarching priority should be to retain key teeth, as well as other teeth that may have an uncertain prognosis, until completion of the disease control phase plan of treatment—at which time the salvageability of the teeth, and the patient's willingness to invest in more extensive and expensive procedures, can be accurately assessed. In other words, it is illogical and inefficient to invest extensive time and resources in an attempt to save teeth that are likely to eventually be lost. Importantly, this approach preserves the option, if the patient later chooses, of retaining the teeth and avoids the scenario of removing all questionable teeth and having the patient later regret that decision. An even worse outcome to be avoided is having the patient blame the dentist for "(needlessly) talking me into taking all my teeth out."

The sequencing of the disease control plan is driven by many factors, including patient desires, symptoms, presence (or absence) of infection, and the other issues previously described in this section.

COMMON DISEASE CONTROL PROBLEMS AND ISSUES

Dental Caries

Worldwide, dental caries continues to be the single most prevalent oral health problem.[1] In countries with developed economies, where caries incidence has declined in recent decades, there are still many individuals who are highly caries active and who are at elevated risk of new caries lesions. For those individuals, restorative procedures alone will not eliminate the disease and they will need to be managed in a strategic, comprehensive, and personalized way.

A functional framework for the overall management of the patient with dental caries activity includes the following elements:
- Comprehensive caries diagnosis, including an evaluation of number of teeth involved, lesion location by surface, and lesion activity (see Chapters 1 and 2).
- An assessment of caries risk level (see Chapter 3).
- A basic caries control protocol for all patients with active lesions or those who are at risk of developing new lesions.
- A supplemental intervention protocol or menu designed to address the specific needs of the patient who, at the outset, is recognized as needing additional measures beyond those in the basic caries control protocol, or those of the patient who, after the initial caries management efforts, remains caries active.
- Maintenance and reevaluation at appropriate intervals to identify new lesions, reinforce caries control protocols, and reevaluate the risk for future caries activity.

Caries Management: Working Definition

The term **caries management** (or **caries control**) is sometimes applied to placement of restoration in teeth that have active cavitated caries lesions. It also is sometimes used to characterize the use of sealants intended to prevent, arrest, and, in some cases, reverse noncavitated (i.e., incipient) lesions. The term has been applied to dietary and/or behavioral approaches, such as reducing frequency of consumption of fermentable carbohydrates between meals or increasing fluoride exposure, intended to prevent new caries lesions or the progression of existing ones. In this text, caries management means any and all efforts to prevent, arrest, remineralize, or restore caries lesions. A caries management protocol is a comprehensive organized plan designed to arrest or remineralize early caries lesions, eradicate overt caries lesions, and prevent the formation of new lesions in an individual who has a moderate or high rate of caries activity or is at increased risk of developing new caries lesions in the future.

Objectives and Scope of the Caries Management Protocol

The primary objective of the caries management protocol is to arrest carious lesions and prevent new lesions from forming. To achieve this objective, it is essential to eliminate or to manage effectively the causes of the disease process. A key aspect of this effort is restoration of the balance between the individual etiologic disease-driving agents—primarily dental plaque or oral biofilm—and the host and protective factors that the patient and dental team can bring to bear. Enamel covered by stagnant dental plaque cycles regularly through periods of demineralization and remineralization, and remains healthy as long as there is not a net loss in mineral content at the site over time (eFigure 10.1). When the amount of mineral content is sufficiently depleted over an extended period of time, a caries lesion begins to develop (eFigure 10.2). Factors affecting this balance are:

- the quality and quantity of plaque;
- the frequency of carbohydrate intake: refined carbohydrates provide nutrients to the plaque bacteria and resulting in acid and extra-cellular polysaccharide (glucans) production that increases the "stickiness" of dental plaque;
- the volume and quality of saliva: saliva provides buffering action, antimicrobial action, the essential minerals to replenish the demineralized enamel, and helps with clearance of food residues;
- any fluoride exposure: fluorides dramatically affect the demineralization and remineralization events in favor of the host.

Modifying these factors and increasing the resistance of the host are goals that require, in most cases, a coordinated effort between the patient and dental team. The patient's caries management plan should use the best evidence available, taking into account the patient-specific causes (risk factors), as well as the readiness of the patient to accept various forms of treatment and behavioral modification. Traditional caries management strategies, including fluorides, sealants, and restorative treatment, have demonstrated efficacy and constitute important components of the caries management program for most patients.

An important tenet of the caries management plan is the implementation of the minimum surgical or restorative intervention that is sometimes necessary to achieve the objective.

Caries excavation can effectively remove the macroscopic caries defect and conventional dental restorative procedures are required to replace destroyed tooth structure. These procedures alone are not enough to arrest caries activity in many caries-active patients, however, and in the absence of other (nonsurgical) therapy, new or recurrent caries lesions might continue to develop.

In most cases, behavioral changes, including diet, oral self-care, and fluoride use, are needed to achieve the objectives of the protocol. Such changes are often difficult to establish and maintain, however, and the dental team needs to be aware of these challenges and realistic about which interventions can be successful. Unfortunately, many caries management plans fail because they are too burdensome to fit into the patient's lifestyle or because of the dental team's overly ambitious attempt to modify those habits of the patient that are considered to be outside the traditional "ideal" oral health behavior. Typically, an evidence-based and personalized preventive plan will have the greatest likelihood of success. Often, a useful strategy is to introduce changes in manageable, sequential steps—engaging the patient in the goal-setting process and doing so at a pace that the patient determines. It is also helpful to encourage and reward the patient for positive changes as they are achieved at each step in the process. Chapter 19 includes an extensive discussion of how to engage and motivate such patients.

Regular assessments of the effectiveness of the caries management program will be essential. Progress can be tracked using one or more of the caries risk assessment and management forms described in Chapter 3.

Caries Management Strategies

Today, many strategies are available to prevent and manage dental caries in individual patients. Most patients will require a multifaceted approach that includes behavioral, chemotherapeutic, and both surgical and nonsurgical restorative therapy. Selection of the appropriate management regimen for each patient must be based on many factors, including the evidence supporting each methodology. Fluorides and pit and fissure sealants are two preventive approaches that have been used for decades to prevent dental caries and have been shown to be effective in multiple randomized clinical trials. These approaches are considered caries management strategies with the highest level of supporting evidence.

An appropriate caries management plan takes into account the patient's risk level (and the reasons for increased risk), the causes of the caries lesions, the patient's willingness to change deleterious behaviors, and their willingness to accept the different modes of therapy. The following sections delineate common caries management strategies and the rationale for each.

Provide fluoride exposure. The benefits of fluoride use in reducing caries incidence and prevalence have been established conclusively over an extended period of time. Multiple reputable professional organizations have publicly supported the use of fluorides in a variety of forms. For example, the American Dental Association and the US Centers for Disease Control have strongly endorsed the addition of a limited amount of fluoride to community-based water supplies as a public health measure. They have also endorsed individual patient use of fluoridated dentifrices and other forms of topical fluoride as caries prevention strategies.

Although there may be some systemic and antibacterial effects, most of the evidence suggests that fluoride works primarily at the topical level, affecting the demineralization and remineralization events occurring between the tooth structure and biofilm fluid. The presence of small amounts of fluoride in the enamel crystals and surrounding fluid decreases the critical pH necessary for enamel dissolution, thereby effectively decreasing demineralization. In addition, the amount and speed of remineralization is enhanced.

Fluoride dentifrices, gels, varnishes, and rinses have all been shown to reduce caries incidence. Brushing teeth with a fluoride-containing dentifrice is the most common oral hygiene practice around the world. Regular use of a (nonprescription) dentifrice with fluoride concentrations between 1000 and 1500 ppm has been shown to be highly effective in reducing caries levels. Dentifrices with higher fluoride levels, 5000 ppm, have also been shown to provide additional benefits, particularly reducing caries at the root surfaces. Fluoride rinses (0.05% NaF), used after brushing or between meals, have also been demonstrated to be effective in reducing caries in patients who are at increased risk. If the patient is using a prescription fluoride dentifrice and/or a fluoride gel as part of the daily regimen, using a fluoride rinse after brushing provides no additional benefit.

An increase in fluoride exposure can also be attained by the regular application of high-concentration fluoride products at the dental office. Professionally applied fluoride products include varnishes, gels, foams, and rinses. Fluoride varnish (typically 5% NaF) is becoming the standard for topical fluoride applications in the dental office because of its ease of use and short time required for application, safety, patient acceptance, and significant level of supporting evidence.

Chemotherapy, in the form of fluoride application, should be selected first over restorative or surgical treatment in the management of reversible noncavitated ("white spot") lesions. When fluoride ions contact the exposed demineralized enamel surface, they are incorporated into the crystalline structure, forming fluorohydroxyapatite. A significant amount of the fluoride is also retained in teeth, soft tissue, plaque, and saliva as a reservoir to be released back later, when the saturation levels in plaque drop (e.g., after the consumption of sugars). In this process, fluoride serves to reduce demineralization and enhance remineralization. This reservoir can be replenished each time a fluoride exposure occurs, making it advantageous for the caries-active patient to have multiple exposures each day. This is most easily accomplished by asking the patient to rinse with a fluoride mouth rinse between meals, in addition to a twice-daily regimen of brushing with a fluoride dentifrice. It is logical to recommend the fluoride dentifrice application after breakfast and at bedtime, when there can be a maximum uptake of the fluoride and extended clearance time. Because fluoride retention and anticaries efficacy have been shown to be affected by the volume of water used to rinse after brushing,[2,3] the patient at increased caries risk should brush with a fluoridated dentifrice,

expectorate the excess, and not rinse with water (or other beverage or fluoride-free rinses) for 30 minutes afterward.

Use of a two-part system of a fluoride dentifrice, along with the daily use of fluoride gel in a custom tray, has been shown to be effective in reducing caries in patients with severe dry mouth (e.g., radiation-induced xerostomia). The advantage of prescription level (5000 ppm) and some over-the-counter (1100 ppm) fluoride gels is that, unlike toothpastes, they include no detergents and abrasives. Gels, therefore, have the potential to increase fluoride bioavailability, as well as decrease irritation of the dry intraoral soft tissues in patients with dry mouth. The daily concurrent use of both toothpaste and gel can become burdensome for the patient (or personal care provider), however, and, as a result, many patients tend to become noncompliant over time. Some investigators have therefore recommended the use of a twice-daily, 2-minute brushing with a prescription dentifrice (5000 ppm) without rinsing after brushing (just expectoration) as an alternative to the two-part regimen, citing similar benefits in caries reduction and better patient compliance.[4]

For young patients at increased caries risk who are not regularly exposed to fluoridated water, prescription of fluoride supplements can be considered. Although the use of fluoride supplements has been associated with a reduction in caries incidence in permanent teeth, there is lack of strong evidence for its efficacy in deciduous teeth.[4,5] In general, the more frequent the fluoride exposures and the greater the concentration, the greater the benefit.[6,7] Providers and patients always need to be aware of the potential for toxicity, however, especially in children, if high-concentration fluorides are ingested indiscriminately.

For frail elderly patients or patients for whom surgical restorative treatment is contraindicated, **silver diamine fluoride (SDF)** is a conservative means of arresting some active primary or secondary caries lesions. Its use in esthetic areas may be limited by the fact that some caries lesions will turn dark following SDF application and be unsightly to the patient.[8]

Plaque management. Before the 1970s, the prevailing theory on caries formation was the nonspecific plaque hypothesis. Consistent with this philosophy was the assumption that all dental plaque is deleterious for oral health and that, to halt caries development, it is essential regularly to remove mechanically all plaque from all exposed tooth surfaces at least daily. Regrettably, traditional mechanical removal methods alone, such as brushing and flossing *without fluoride*, do not seem to be efficacious in controlling active dental caries. A few decades ago, the specific plaque hypothesis was preeminent, positing that only a few pathogenic bacteria were the culprits in the oral diseases (e.g., *Streptococcus mutans* for dental caries). Active and passive vaccines to protect against *S. mutans* were developed and tested, demonstrating some efficacy, but in light of their cost, limited efficacy, and potential side effects, the evidence was not sufficiently persuasive for regulators to approve their use.

Now that there is a clear understanding that dental caries development requires the presence of a stagnant acid-producing oral biofilm that functions to demineralize the tooth structure, the ecological plaque hypothesis has been developed as an alternative. In this model, the presence of disease (caries) is caused by an "ecological catastrophe" in the local dental plaque.[9] In other words, dental plaque may be nondetrimental, as long as it is in homeostasis with the host. Examples of potential factors that can create these "catastrophic" events are poor oral hygiene combined with an inappropriate diet or use of medications that significantly reduce salivary flow. Under this hypothesis, management of dental plaque is not focused on its complete elimination, but rather on bringing it back into balance with the host. Control of factors including plaque level, diet, and salivary flow is essential to creating this favorable plaque that would be in homeostasis. In many situations, a small amount of plaque does not contribute significantly to demineralization and can enhance fluoride efficacy by serving as a fluoride reservoir.[4] Therefore, based on the evidence available today, the dental team should rely less heavily on mechanical plaque control as a central element in the caries management program; rather, the focus should be on targeted plaque removal, with the goal of bringing the biofilm back to homeostasis, to serve as an adjuvant to fluoride therapy, because fluoride efficacy improves with thinner levels of plaque.[10]

Although this may seem contrary to conventional wisdom and to flaunt the long-held mantra that all plaque is bad for oral health, there are two common circumstances in which whole-mouth mechanical plaque control is to be encouraged: the first is if the patient, in addition to being caries active, also has active *periodontal disease* (see Periodontal Diseases, later in this chapter). In the presence of gingivitis, the daily elimination of plaque remains a high priority. Also, the caries-active patient with heavy plaque deposits throughout the mouth will need traditional instruction in plaque removal and will need to be encouraged to engage in daily effective plaque removal. For these two groups, reduction in total plaque score remains an important treatment objective and can serve as a useful benchmark with which to assess the progress and success of the patient's caries management program.

Limit fermentable carbohydrates. Bacterial fermentation of dietary carbohydrates produces the acids that cause localized tooth destruction (i.e., dental caries). Classic studies, such as the Vipeholm study[11] and the Hopewood House study,[12] have clearly demonstrated that dental caries do not develop easily in a diet with limited fermentable carbohydrate exposure and that the frequency and consistency of the carbohydrates are closely associated to their cariogenicity. More recently, numerous studies have shown that a biofilm ecological shift occurs when dental plaque is exposed regularly to fermentable carbohydrates. The regular production of acids by the biofilm creates an environment highly favorable for the development of aciduric bacteria, such as lactobacilli and mutans streptococci, which are also acidogenic and known to be closely associated with caries lesion development and progression. Because of this, it seems logical always to recommend limiting refined carbohydrate intake by caries active and/or at-risk patients. As with other strategies that are patient dependent, however, compliance can be a significant problem. Dietary modification has generally been shown to be minimally effective in reducing caries prevalence, probably most often owing to the general lack of compliance commonly found in at-risk patients. Fortunately, because of the wide use of fluorides, the close association between consumption of dietary fermentable

carbohydrate and dental caries has shifted and currently, most patients who are exposed to fluorides regularly and have reasonably effective oral hygiene routine can consume a limited amount of fermentable carbohydrates daily and still remain caries inactive. On the other hand, **dietary counseling** is definitely appropriate for patients with obviously deleterious behaviors, such as frequent sipping of sugared drinks or consumption of sugared cough drops. For these patients, dietary habits must be modified if caries activity is to be controlled. Of particular importance are reduction of between-meal exposures to refined carbohydrates and switching to other, noncariogenic sweeteners, such as sugar alcohols. The daily use of xylitol-based chewing gum has been shown to inhibit *S. mutans* and to be anticariogenic.[13] The recommendation is to consume between 5 and 10 grams of xylitol per day, divided into three or more consumption periods per day, ideally chewing after meals for approximately 20 minutes.

Pit and fissure sealants. Pit and fissure sealants are placed in high-risk locations to provide a physical barrier to microorganisms and carbohydrates. A resin composite is the material most commonly used as a dental sealant. Specially designed glass ionomer (GI) cements can also be used as sealants. Sealants have been used in dentistry since the early 1970s to prevent caries formation at those anatomical locations. Because numerous clinical studies and systematic reviews have demonstrated that they are highly effective in preventing dental caries,[14] many reputable groups, including the American Dental Association, the American Academy of Pediatric Dentistry, the International Association of Dental Research, and the US Centers for Disease Control, highly recommend their use. More recently, pit and fissure sealants have been recommended not only to prevent the initiation and formation of caries lesions but also to prevent progression of noncavitated lesions. Recent expert reviews of the literature have documented their effectiveness in accomplishing both processes.[15,16] The effectiveness of sealants depends on their long-term retention and when a sealant has been lost or fractured, it should be replaced or repaired to guarantee its continuing effectiveness.

Restorative treatment. Overt caries lesions are typically restored in the disease control phase with GI resin-modified glass ionomer (RMGI) cement, composite, or amalgam. Lesions that closely approach the pulp are often managed with a **selective caries removal** procedure (see Chapter 3 for the rationale and evidence; and the section *Pulpal Therapy and Management of Lesions and Defects Encroaching on Pulp*, later in this chapter, for procedures). In general, GI or RMGI materials are favored when there are multiple large active caries lesions and it will be advantageous to restore several teeth in relatively few visits. When used in this context, protective (or provisional or temporary) restorations constitute what are frequently described as **caries control restorations**. This type of restoration has the advantage of stabilizing the oral environment by eradicating the locus of infection and changing the localized niche of the lesion sites in a minimal amount of chair time. Such restorations also provide the benefit of stabilizing the plaque:host balance. In cases with less urgency and when the caries lesions are smaller, composite or amalgam restorations will serve well. Composites have the advantage of being more esthetically pleasing but should be restricted to sites where a dry operating field can be ensured. Amalgam is often recommended in sites where the patient and dentist prefer a definitive restoration, esthetics is not an issue, and isolation of the preparation is compromised. GI and RMGI restorations have the advantages of being relatively easy to place, bonding to dentin, maintaining a good marginal seal, and providing a modicum of esthetics. They also have the potential benefit of recharging and releasing fluoride—but their ability to prevent secondary caries has not yet been established (see *In Clinical Practice: Do Glass Ionomer Restorations Prevent Recurrent Caries?* box). Indirect restorations are generally contraindicated in the caries management protocol and in the disease control phase.

IN CLINICAL PRACTICE

Do Glass Ionomer Restorations Prevent Recurrent Caries (i.e., Secondary Caries)?

Prevention of recurrent caries is a critical issue in managing the patient with high caries risk. Most patients will benefit from the advantages offered by a restorative material that, through the release of fluoride, will inhibit recurrent caries. Historically, silicate cements have had a proven track record in caries prevention, but they are no longer available. GI cements have been shown to be effective in inhibiting recurrent caries in vitro, but are they effective in vivo?

After an extensive review of the literature and screening of available reports, Randall and Wilson identified 28 appropriately controlled prospective studies.[17] The results were mixed and no clear conclusion could be drawn regarding whether GI restorative materials inhibit secondary caries. To date, the evidence suggests that, although GIs, in general, perform no worse than other restorative materials, no clinical caries-inhibiting benefit has been consistently demonstrated.[17,18] Prudent judgment suggests that where a GI restoration would otherwise be a satisfactory choice as an interim or definitive restoration, this material will be a good choice in the patient with active caries. The dentist should be cautious, however, in assuming that such a restoration will in fact inhibit caries. When used in a caries-active individual, it will be advisable to also provide the patient with frequent repeated fluoride exposure for potential recharging of the restorative material.

RMGIs are the restorative materials of choice for atraumatic restorative treatment (ART) technique on both primary and permanent teeth. ART involves use of hand instruments only to excavate and remove carious tissue, followed by placement of an RMGI restoration (see the World Health Organization website http://www.paho.org/hq/index.php?option=com_content&view=article&id=7411:atraumatic-restorative-treatment&Itemid=39633&lang=en for a more detailed description of the ART technique). ART is most often performed on schoolchildren aged 6 to 15 years, who live in locations where conventional restorative dentistry is not feasible because of costs or geographic location. Although many reports on ART studies have not specifically tested the capacity of RMGIs to prevent recurrent decay, studies have shown that, in terms of acceptable longevity and retention rates, ART with RMGIs is a satisfactory method.[19–22]

Caries susceptibility tests. Caries susceptibility tests (CST) can be a useful adjunct in the diagnosis of the caries condition, the development of behavioral and pharmacologic management strategies for an active caries patient, and for monitoring the progress of the caries management program. See the *In Clinical Practice: Caries Susceptibility Tests* box.

Comprehensive Caries Management

Basic caries control protocol. The basic caries control protocol, shown in Table 10.1, should be implemented for all patients who are caries active (at least one active lesion at the oral examination). Designed for simplicity and effectiveness, most of the products used in the protocol are readily available over the counter and involve techniques that are no more difficult to master than routine oral self-care procedures. Minimal chair time will be required for dentist and staff to explain the protocol and its use to the patient. A sample office handout for this purpose is shown in Figure 10.4.

IN CLINICAL PRACTICE

Caries Susceptibility Tests

CSTs encompass a cluster of specific laboratory and/or chairside analyses of saliva that can help the dentist rule in or out some specific possible causes of caries activity in a patient. Although not proven to be a reliable predictor of caries risk, these tests represent the tools we have to date for ongoing monitoring of caries activity in the oral environment and are an important *quantitative* method available to the practitioner for evaluating an individual patient's current disease state.

Typical CSTs evaluate the following:
- Salivary flow—whole stimulated and unstimulated saliva calculated in milliliters per minute
- Buffering capacity—recorded in final pH
- Concentration of *S. mutans*
- Concentration of lactobacilli

These four tests, except determination of *unstimulated* salivary flow, can all be carried out with a single sample of stimulated saliva. Typically, the patient chews a piece of paraffin wax and expectorates saliva into a collecting tube over a 5-minute period. A microbiology laboratory, set up to run the four specified tests as a block, can provide consistent, accurate, timely results for a reasonable fee. The clinician sends the sample directly to the laboratory, with results reported usually within a week. Alternatively, CSTs can be performed chairside using a variety of generic and commercially produced kits (Figure 10.3).

Several of the notable benefits that can be derived from use of CSTs:

Diagnosis: CSTs serve as a diagnostic instrument to help identify specific causes of the disease, for example, hyposalivation.

Baseline values: CSTs provide baseline values for the number of cariogenic microbes in the patient's mouth and serve as a basis for comparison to judge whether the caries management program has been successful.

Tracking mechanism: CSTs provide a quantifiable method of assessing disease process progression and the efficacy of intervention methods used to date.

Patient education/goal setting/and motivation: CSTs act as a tool for educating the patient about the causes and management of caries as a disease process, establishing goals for the patient and dental team, and motivating the patient to engage in the recommended behavioral changes.

Optional caries interventions. Likely candidates for additional intervention include patients with unusually active or rampant caries or those who have specific identifiable factors suggesting high risk for caries development. Suggestions or guidelines for possible interventions and their indications are listed in Table 10.2.

Management based on caries activity and caries risk. The appropriate strategy for management of the individual patient's dental caries activity will be driven by the patient's current disease activity and caries risk status. In the following discussion, a patient with dental caries is classified in one of three groups and a management strategy is suggested for each classification.

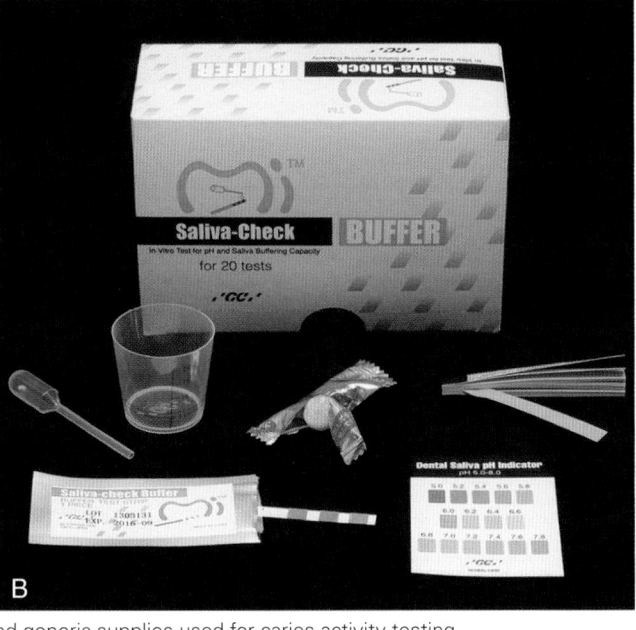
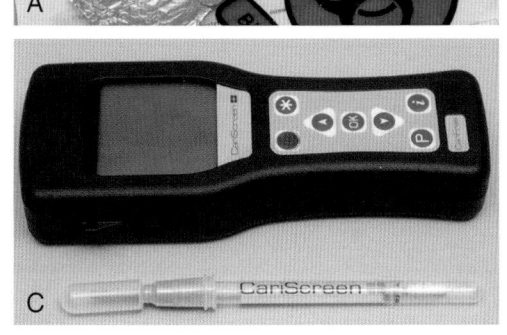

Fig. 10.3 Examples of proprietary and generic supplies used for caries activity testing.

Patient with no active caries lesions and at low risk of future caries. Patients who have cracked or fractured teeth, defective restorations, or other problems associated with previous caries activity do not need and are unlikely to benefit from a basic caries control protocol. Affected teeth should be restored with definitive restorations as appropriate. Selection of restorative materials and techniques for pulpally involved or potentially pulpally involved teeth is discussed later in this chapter. General restorative treatment planning options for individual teeth are discussed in Chapter 11. After restoration and in the continued absence of significant risk for new caries, these patients require only routine maintenance services, as discussed in Chapter 12.

Patient with no clinically visible caries lesions but at moderate or high risk of caries. Patients who fit this criterion may be handled successfully in the following way. The individual should be placed on a basic caries control protocol and reevaluated at specified intervals (usually every 6 months). In some instances, the dentist's clinical judgment may determine that the patient will benefit from additional management. Careful reassessment at the conclusion of the interval is warranted. At that time, if no lesions have developed and the risk potential does not appear to have increased, the patient can be reassured. If caries activity or risk has increased, the patient may need to be managed according to the protocol discussed in the following section.

Patient with multiple active lesions or at high risk of new caries.

Determination of the patient-specific cause. Before proceeding with any nonemergency treatment, every effort must be made to determine the specific causes of the caries problem, beginning with a second-level review of the entire patient history. Does the patient have a systemic disease, such as Sjögren's syndrome that may cause xerostomia? Is the patient taking medications that may cause dry mouth? Has the patient had chemotherapy or radiation therapy for cancer that has affected salivary function? Does the patient have a deleterious dietary habit that promotes rampant caries development? Is the patient's oral environment regularly exposed to fluoride?

The patient's oral home care practices must be reviewed. How effective are the current plaque control measures? The history may suggest and evidence from the initial examination may confirm the effectiveness or ineffectiveness of the patient's oral self-care program. What type of fluoride exposure does the patient have and what is the frequency?

Lifestyle issues must be evaluated. Have there been recent stressful life-changing events that may have caused metabolic changes, altered daily patterns and routines, including oral self-care, or perhaps induced the patient to adopt a diet rich in "comfort foods"? Assessment of the patient's diet at the initial interview may have been cursory, but once the determination of high caries activity or high caries risk has been made, dietary issues require careful scrutiny. The patient should be asked specifically about sources of refined carbohydrates. What form? How much? With what frequency? Sometimes the cariogenic source is obvious (two liters of soda sipped each day), whereas other sources may seem more innocuous (sipping coffee with creamer throughout the day). Other common culprits include sucrose-containing cough drops, breath mints, or lozenges. This aspect of the reevaluation deserves time and attention. If the practitioner suspects a dietary component to the caries problem but is unable to elucidate the source with the questioning process, a 5-day dietary history may be warranted to identify hidden problems.

After a careful review of the patient history and a detailed clinical examination, if doubt lingers concerning the patient-specific cause or causes of the active caries condition, additional testing is warranted to determine whether such factors as diminished salivary output, an abnormally acidic oral environment, or high numbers of specific pathogenic microbes are in evidence.

Implementing the basic caries control protocol. This protocol offers several advantages for the patient with a high level of

TABLE 10.1 **Basic Caries Control Protocol**	
Item	**Rationale**
Caries activity tests	See In Clinical Practice: Caries Activity Tests
Oral prophylaxis (professional)	Removes plaque and plaque-retentive accretions; makes tooth surfaces more receptive to fluoride uptake
Oral hygiene instructions[a]	Removes plaque and reduces potential for developing smooth surface caries
Professional fluoride gel or varnish[b] application at each scaling or preventive (recall/maintenance) visit	Remineralizes tooth structure; potential antimicrobial effect; increases fluoride reservoir short-term; reduces caries incidence; most effective when given at more frequent time intervals (less than 6 months)
Diet recommendations to reduce frequency and duration of acid and sucrose (refined carbohydrate) exposure	Eliminates substrate for cariogenic bacteria; reduces acid-induced dissolution of tooth structure
Over-the-counter fluoride dentifrice and fluoride rinses (use daily)	Remineralizes tooth structure, replenishes intraoral fluoride reservoir, increases caries resistance
Silver diamine fluoride applied to caries lesions	Arrests caries progression; conservative non-surgical treatment (not applicable in esthetic sites)
Sealants on susceptible pits and fissures (e.g., exposed pits and fissures in adolescents or in adults when other pits and fissures have needed restoration)	Eliminates sites of infection and potential for inoculation of other sites; prevention of pit and fissure caries
Restoration of cavitated caries lesions with direct-fill provisional or definitive restorations[c] (Note: definitive indirect restorations are not recommended)	Eliminates nidus of infection; improves cleansability; arrests caries progression

[a]Flossing has not been shown to reduce caries incidence. However, it is logical to encourage its use because of its many other proven benefits, including the reduction of plaque formation and gingivitis.
[b]In general, professionally applied fluoride varnish applications have been shown to be more effective than professionally applied fluoride gel treatments (Bader J, Shugars D, Bonito A. *Community Dent Oral Epidemiol.* 2001;29(6):399–411; and Peterson L, Twetman S, Dahlgren H, et al. *Acta Odontol Scand.* 2004;62(3):170–176).
[c]The merits of GI restorations as a means of inhibiting secondary caries are reviewed in *What's the Evidence? IN CLINICAL PRACTICE: Do Glass-Ionomer Restorations Prevent Recurrent Caries?* (see BOX pp 8–9)

caries activity. In addition to providing an initial treatment to curtail caries activity, the protocol can act as a useful program for increasing the patient's understanding of the nature of dental caries and introducing the concept that caries can be appropriately managed as a disease process. The basic caries control protocol (see Table 10.1), in particular, can be important in refining and confirming the cause of the caries. In addition, the protocol encourages the patient to engage in the management of their own condition and to assume a degree of ownership of the problem.

Selecting from the optional caries interventions. When the cause or causes of the problem have been determined through an examination and a secondary analysis of the patient history, selections that address the patient's particular needs can be made from the optional menu (see Table 10.2). The dentist may develop creative strategies specific to the problem that provide palatable alternatives to the patient. Even the most logical and strategic of therapies is useless if the patient cannot live with the recommendations on a daily basis, however. An example of such a well-intended but misguided approach would be to prescribe and fabricate custom fluoride trays for a patient who has a severe gag reflex or is nauseated by fluoride gels.

Reassessment. During implementation of the caries management plan, multiple reevaluation opportunities arise as strategies are tried and modified, continued, or discarded. At a point clearly established by the dentist at the beginning of treatment, a comprehensive reevaluation of the disease control phase occurs and all aspects of the caries management plan are assessed.

Development of an individualized posttreatment assessment is described later in this chapter and a template for a comprehensive posttreatment assessment is shown in detail in Chapter 12.

This is a critical juncture for both patient and practitioner. If the caries management plan has been successful, definitive treatment can proceed with a high level of confidence in the outcome. If caries management efforts have been unsuccessful, the options are usually limited and less attractive. For a patient who continues to exhibit active caries and/or continues to be at moderate or high risk for new lesions, the two logical options are (1) to recommend extraction of questionable teeth and proceed with interim or transitional (usually removable) prostheses or (2) to enter an extended disease-control phase. For some patients, these two options may merge and the distinction between them becomes blurred. In general, indirect restorations and fixed partial dentures on natural teeth are contraindicated as long as the patient remains at an elevated caries risk.

Although this situation can be frustrating for both the patient and dentist, a positive outcome may still emerge. The patient may be forced to make the hard decision to accept extraction of teeth, a decision that they would have preferred to avoid but that is now inevitable. In other cases, the dentist's refusal to provide definitive treatment may become the impetus to motivate the patient to engage more actively in the caries control practices necessary for halting the disease. If, at this point, the patient decides to terminate the therapeutic relationship, the dentist will at least have the satisfaction of having made a strong effort to manage the caries problem and of having avoided providing

---

Customized Dental Decay Prevention Plan

From: <<Provider>>
UNC School of Dentistry

To: <<patient>>
Date: <<dd/mm/yyy>>

We are committed to helping you eliminate and control your dental cavities (caries). Fillings alone will not stop cavity formation. We need your help to stop the decay process and prevent new cavities from forming.

Based on several factors your caries risk assessment (CRA) is <<level>>

Based on those specific factors we are recommending the following:

☐ Brush and floss using methods discussed in clinic (for all patients, including low CRA)
☐ Brush at least twice a day (morning and bedtime) with a prescription fluoride toothpaste (example: Prevident 5000 Plus) with no or limited rinsing after expectoration (mostly for patients with exposed roots and low salivary flow)
☐ Use proxy brush as instructed (for patients with specific high risk plaque accumulation problems, particularly at margins of restorations and prosthesis; be able to select per patient based on perio architecture)
☐ Purchase and use an electric toothbrush (example: Sonicare or Oral B) (for patients at increased risk having problems removing plaque)
☐ Use gum or lozenges with xylitol (at least 3 times per day between meals, and for a total of 6-15 g per day)(to be considered for all patients as adjuvant therapy)
☐ Rinse for at least one minute with fluoridated 0.05% NaF mouth rinse (example: ACT) at <<specific for the patient>> intervals
☐ Rinse for at least one minute (morning and bedtime) with mouth rinse moisturizer (example: Biotene, Oasis)(for patients with dry mouth symptoms)
☐ Minimize the frequency of tooth contact with acids and sugars between meals (if snacking on cariogenic foods/drinks is frequent)
☐ Substitute non-acidic, high pH foods (e.g., cheeses) for between-meal snacks (if diet is highly cariogenic)
☐ Make appointment to have sealants placed (if P&F are at high risk or present clinical signs of incipient lesions)
☐ Return to recall clinic every 3 months for a cleaning and fluoride varnish application (if high risk)
☐ Return to recall clinic every 6 months for a cleaning and fluoride varnish application (if moderate risk)
☐ Expect updated posterior bitewing radiographs every 6-12 months (if high risk)
☐ Expect updated posterior bitewing radiographs every 12-18 months (if moderate risk)

Fig. 10.4 Sample office handout for a caries-active patient.

TABLE 10.2 Optional Caries Interventions

Problem	Suggested Intervention
Decreased quantity or quality of saliva	Frequent oral hydration, salivary substitutes
Medication-induced zerostomia	After consultation with patient's medical provider, prescribe alternative medication that is less xerostomic
Continued incidence of new caries activity despite previous intervention	Custom fluoride trays for daily home use
Patient at risk for additional root or smooth surface caries	Fluoride varnish application
Patient who would benefit from higher-level fluoride exposure, but is unwilling or unable to accept custom trays	Prescription dentifrice or gel with high-concentration fluoride
Any patient at risk for new caries who likes to chew gum	Ad lib use of xylitol chewing gum (good alternative for persons who crave between-meal high-sucrose snacks or drinks)
Patients with concurrent marginal periodontal disease and/or patients with Streptococcus mutans counts that remain high despite previous intervention	Chlorhexidine mouth rinses

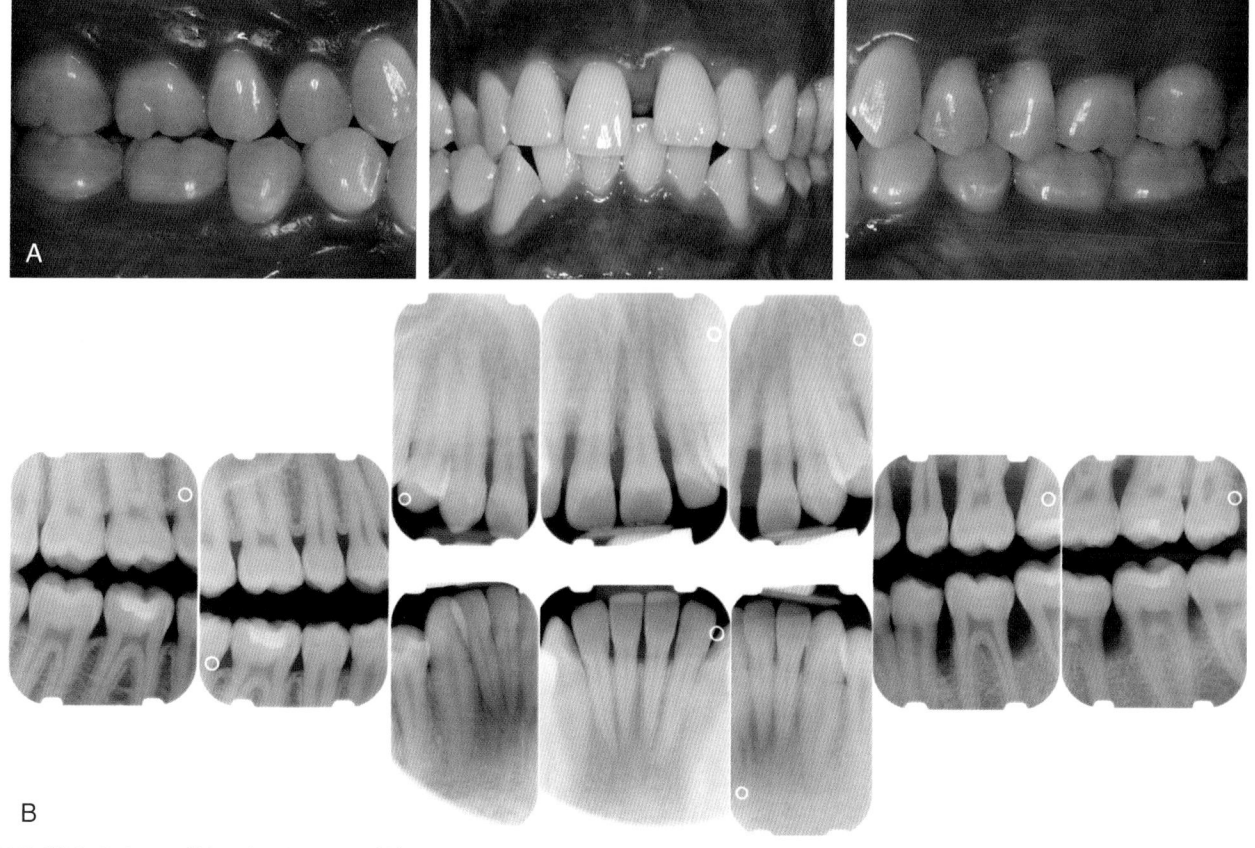

Fig. 10.5 Clinical photos **(A)** and radiographs **(B)** showing a Molar/Incisor Pattern of Periodontitis Stage III Grade C. This is an uncommon form of periodontitis affecting mostly adolescents and young adults. Rapid periodontal destruction is a hallmark feature, with first molars and incisors most frequently involved. These patients are otherwise systemically healthy. Familial aggregation is common; parents, siblings, and children of individuals with this form of periodontitis should be clinically evaluated on a regular basis. In many cases, little plaque or calculus may be detected clinically. The microbial composition of the biofilm may contain elevated proportions of *Aggregatibacter actinomycetemcomitans* and/or Porphyromonas *gingivalis*. Referral to a periodontist is generally necessary for the management of their periodontal needs. (Courtesy Dr. Jonathan Reside and Dr. Antonio Moretti).

therapy that is likely to fail in a short time. This strategy is also wise from a legal risk-reduction perspective.

Periodontal Diseases

Periodontal diseases are not a singular entity, but rather comprise a group of inflammatory conditions affecting the supporting soft tissues around the teeth. Proper diagnosis is critical and, depending on the condition, varying modes of therapy are required, particularly if the patient has a more aggressive or severe form of the disease (Figure 10.5).

In the majority of cases, periodontal disease can be stabilized and controlled through appropriate treatment and maintenance. To minimize the likelihood of disease progression (i.e., clinical attachment loss and bone loss), patients with periodontal disease should expect to require long-term therapy to help retain their teeth. Management of periodontal disease is often a continuous process and may need to be addressed at every stage of the treatment plan.

Before initiating treatment, the practitioner must obtain detailed medical and dental histories (Chapter 1), complete a thorough periodontal examination (Chapter 1), assign appropriate periodontal diagnoses (Chapter 2), consider various etiologic and risk factors (Chapter 3), and assign periodontal prognoses (Chapter 3). With the careful completion of these steps, the clinician will have all of the information needed to develop a control phase treatment plan.

This section focuses on controlling or eliminating modifiable risk factors for, and causes of, periodontal disease, as well as arresting disease progression. Definitive (i.e., surgical) management of periodontal disease and implant therapy are discussed in Chapter 11. Maintenance therapy for periodontitis is discussed in Chapter 12.

Causes of Periodontal Disease

Local factors—pathogenic microbiota, biofilm, and calculus. The presence of **bacterial plaque**, or **biofilm**, is the primary cause of most periodontal diseases (Figure 10.6). Plaque is composed of bacteria organized around the teeth as a biofilm, which is a matrix enclosure providing the bacteria with protection, nutrients, and cooperative niches. Mineralized deposits around the teeth, **calculus**, also contribute to periodontal disease development through two key mechanisms:
1. Calculus provides a rough surface to which biofilm can adhere, making effective mechanical plaque removal more challenging.

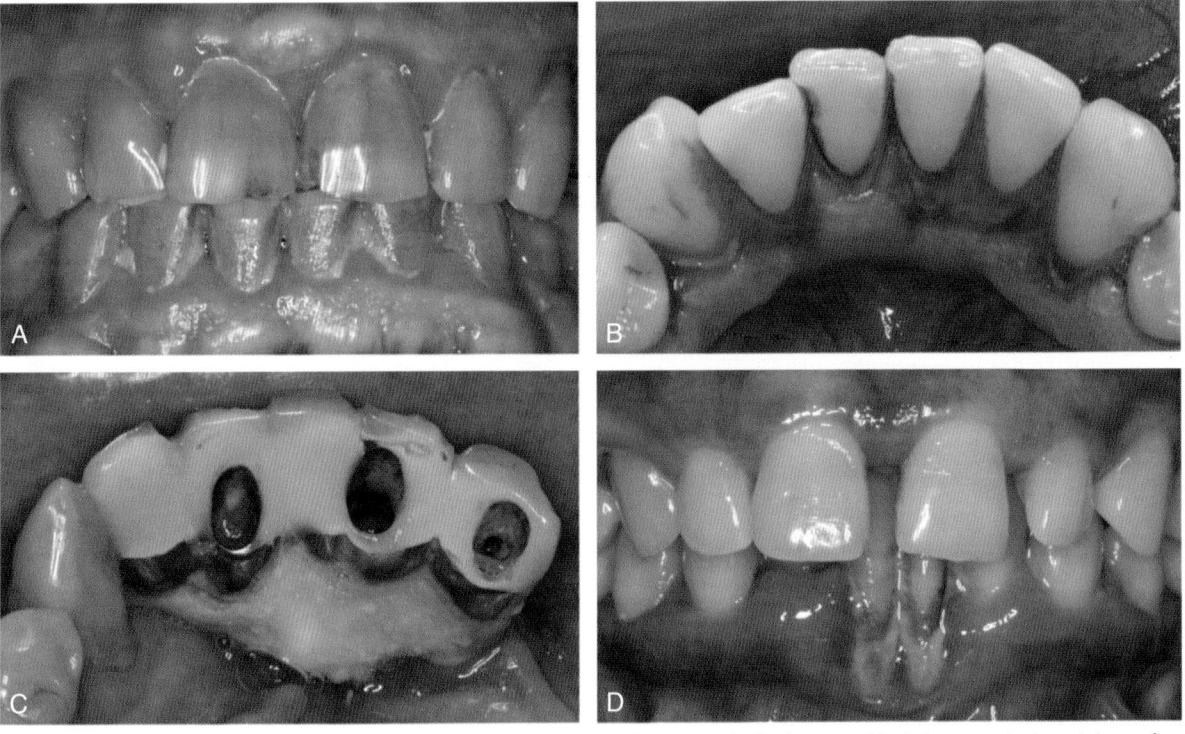

Fig. 10.6 Local factors contributing to the development of periodontal disease. Plaque and calculus are critical elements in the etiology of periodontal diseases. (Courtesy Dr. Jonathan Reside and Dr. Antonio Moretti.)

2. Calculus harbors bacterial toxins and byproducts that contribute to periodontal inflammation and encourage an immune response eventually leading to periodontal tissue destruction.

The initiation and progression of periodontal disease is a complex interaction of a susceptible host and virulent strains of specific pathogens. It is well known that specific pathogens contribute to the development and progression of periodontitis. For instance, *Aggregatibacter actinomycetemcomitans, Porphyromonas gingivalis, Prevotella intermedia, Tannerella forsythia,* and *Treponema denticola* are commonly associated with more severe forms of periodontitis. Mechanical removal of biofilm and local irritants, such as calculus, remains the most effective mode of prevention and treatment for periodontal disease. The importance of removing biofilm and calculus to inhibit or arrest the progression of periodontal disease cannot be overemphasized. Evidence suggests that if the local ecological niche (i.e., the tooth surface adjacent to the ulcerated pocket epithelium) is debrided of toxins and the biofilm is disrupted at regular intervals (by patient and clinician), disease progression can be arrested in the majority of cases.[23,24] An extensive body of literature describes the most effective methods for daily biofilm removal procedures by the patient. Similarly, the creation of smooth tooth surfaces and the removal of biofilm through scaling and root planing and oral prophylaxis procedures are thoroughly described in periodontology textbooks (see Suggested Readings at the conclusion of this chapter).

In some forms of periodontitis, the mechanical removal of biofilm and other local factors may be insufficient to arrest or eradicate the disease, even on a temporary basis. Each patient (and even each site within a patient) presents with a microbial composition and a host response that is unique to them. Consequently, therapeutic interventions must be targeted to address the needs of the patient. *Aggregatibacter actinomycetemcomitans,* for example, may penetrate the periodontal tissues and, as a result, may not be effectively eliminated by scaling and root planing alone. In such cases, antibiotic therapy used adjunctively with scaling and root planing or surgery can be helpful in controlling the disease.

Genetic predisposition. Heredity can be both a risk factor for and a cause of periodontal disease. There is growing evidence that genetics are a factor in periodontitis. Studies have demonstrated that genetic factors may account for approximately 33% of the population variance in common forms of periodontitis, with "higher heritability for more severe [forms of] disease."[25]

Genetics may impact periodontitis in two key ways: (1) a hyper- or hypoactive inflammatory host response and/or (2) the presence of periodontal tissues that are more susceptible to inflammatory breakdown. Studies have also demonstrated that, due to the quality and degree of the inflammatory host response, changes in the subgingival environment may occur which favor the growth of more pathogenic microbiota.[26] Research into the genetic factors associated with periodontitis is ongoing and comprehensive and sophisticated assessments are being made to identify previously unexplored genetic inheritance patterns.[27] Commercial tests are available to assess individual genetic risks for periodontitis and the implications of these data for disease management are currently being studied. Although it is not yet possible to alter genetic inheritance to correct a predisposition for periodontal disease, research on genetic therapy options continues.

The role of epigenetics in the development of periodontal disease must also be considered. Epigenetic changes are reversible genetic modifications resulting in an alteration of gene expression patterns and may lead to gene upregulation or silencing.[28] These changes may be induced by environmental stressors and may ultimately result in an altered inflammatory response. Several factors that may lead to epigenetic modifications (such as tobacco exposure and diabetes) may also contribute to periodontal disease in other ways.

It is important for the patient to understand that presence of the genetic or epigenetic factors described does not make the occurrence or progression of periodontal disease unavoidable. The dental team must ensure that the patient understands that we now have safe and effective methods of treating periodontal disease. Patients who have seen their grandparents, parents, and siblings lose their teeth as a result of periodontitis need the reassurance that—*in most cases*—the disease *is* treatable and the eventual loss of teeth is *not* inevitable. Understanding these issues can have an important influence on the patient's acceptance of recommended therapy. Furthermore, the dentist's understanding of the patient's genetic predisposition for development of periodontal disease may help the practitioner to tailor management strategies and provide more effective treatment.

Systemic factors and immunoinflammatory response. Systemic disease and, in particular, diabetes mellitus, can contribute to the development and progression of periodontal diseases. In the poorly controlled diabetic, microvascular changes, altered circulation and leukocyte chemotaxis, impaired white cell function, and other ill effects of an impaired immune response all contribute to periodontal disease and may negate efforts by the dental team and the patient to control the disease.[29]

Although, in general, the immunoinflammatory response plays a protective role for the host, it may also play a central role in the initiation and progression of periodontal disease. The patient's immune function may foster periodontal disease in two distinct ways:

1. Any condition that diminishes function of the immune system has the potential to increase the severity, complexity, and seriousness of periodontal disease. Common causes for reduced immune system function include human immunodeficiency virus infection, cancer chemotherapy, rheumatoid arthritis, systemic lupus erythematosus, and some blood dyscrasias, such as leukemia.
2. Impaired immune function may predispose patients to periodontal disease or modify the presentation of the disease, for example, as in patients with cyclic neutropenia.[30–32]

Although the immunocompromising condition often cannot be eliminated, effective treatment of the periodontal disease can still be implemented. In such cases, current treatment approaches involve holding the periodontal disease in check until the immunocompromising condition is mitigated or controlled, at which time more aggressive periodontal therapy can be initiated. If the underlying cause cannot otherwise be controlled, it may be possible to augment the patient's immune function with pharmacologic agents.[33]

Paradoxically, although the immune system is essential for control of disease and infection, an overexuberant response to the pathogens at a local site may also cause severe destruction to periodontal tissues. Certain patients appear to exhibit a hyperinflammatory response to periodontal infections. Compared with normal controls, the inflammatory response of such patients release increased amounts of catabolic cytokines and arachidonic acid metabolites in response to bacterial endotoxins.[34] These cytokines and prostaglandins in turn lead to increased tissue destruction and bone loss.

Tobacco use. Tobacco use has serious deleterious effects on periodontal health and individuals who smoke tend to have a higher risk for developing periodontal and peri-implant diseases.[35] Tobacco facilitates the establishment of periodontitis, the progression of disease, and treatment outcomes. In particular, tobacco products have the potential to affect negatively the periodontal microbiota, collagen metabolism, immune system function, wound healing, and other treatment outcomes. On clinical examination, the appearance of the gingival tissue may not be consistent with the extent of disease. Patients who smoke typically have a more hyperkeratotic and fibrotic gingiva, which may mask an underlying inflammatory presence. Tissues typically do not appear erythematic, and bleeding on probing may be less compared with the responses of a nonsmoking patient with a similar periodontal disease presentation.[36,37] Smokeless tobacco can also affect the periodontium, causing a variety of lesions, including gingival recession.

Although the beneficial effects of smoking cessation on the periodontium have been firmly established, the risk for periodontal disease lingers for an extended period of time for former smokers, and reduced treatment outcomes may also be expected compared with nonsmokers.[38] Every effort should be made to provide education about the hazards of tobacco use and encourage cessation.

Other deleterious habits. Some individuals engage in self-destructive activities or behaviors that damage the periodontal tissues at local sites (i.e., factitial injuries) or that may affect the entire periodontium.[39] In some instances, the patient may be unaware of the activity/habit or its effect. For example, a well-intentioned patient may inadvertently contribute to gingival recession through aggressive toothbrushing or be unaware of the potential impact of intraoral piercings on their oral tissues. The dentist should call these findings to the patient's attention, identifying the consequences and encouraging changes to minimize the risk of tissue damage. Additional examples of such habits are listed in Table 10.3.

TABLE 10.3   Habits That May Injure Periodontium

Source	Effect
Trauma from tools, instruments, needles held in the mouth	Localized stripping of the tissue
Placement of caustic medicaments	Tissue burn, slough, ulceration (e.g., aspirin)
Holding acidic foods (e.g., lemons) against the teeth for extended periods of time	Tissue irritation, dental erosion, dentinal sensitivity
Aggressive or obsessive tooth brushing	Gingival recession, cervical notching

Failure to identify and eliminate or modify these habits may result in continued progression of periodontal destruction, despite appropriate care.

Defective restorations. Poorly contoured restorations or crowns, ill-fitting prostheses, or plaque-retentive orthodontic appliances may contribute to food and biofilm entrapment, tissue irritation, and gingival inflammation.[40,41] If unaddressed, the result may be the development of bony defects, periodontal abscesses, or other forms of periodontal disease. When the periodontal problem stems from restorative treatment that is less than ideal, the dentist has an obligation to bring these issues to the patient's attention and must do so in an honest but nonjudgmental manner. The dentist needs to avoid casting blame on the previous provider and the discussion needs to focus on the current condition, its relative importance, and the options in moving forward with treatment (see Chapter 7 for a more extensive discussion of this ethical issue).

Management of the defective or **iatrogenic restoration** is paramount to ensure improvement in the health of the adjacent periodontal tissues. In appropriate cases, recontouring of the restoration may be completed to establish ideal anatomic contours. However, in cases in which recontouring is not possible, replacement of the restoration may become necessary.

Occlusal trauma. Although occlusal trauma does not cause periodontal disease, it can result in increased tooth mobility and may accelerate localized alveolar bone loss, potentially leading to the progression of periodontal disease and hastening the loss of periodontally-involved teeth.[42-44] Management of acute occlusal trauma is discussed in Chapter 9 and management of other forms of occlusal trauma is presented later in this chapter.

Treatment of Periodontal Disease—Initial Therapy

The management of periodontal diseases in the control phase of treatment is often referred to as **initial periodontal therapy**. The key components of this process are described in the following sections.

Systemic considerations. The management of systemic issues is discussed in detail in Chapter 8. Issues of specific concern in the patient with active periodontal disease include the following:

- Identification of, and if possible, mitigation of any diseases, treatments, or medication regimens that may affect periodontal disease pathogenesis, delay healing, or otherwise interfere with recommended periodontal therapy.
- Identification of individuals requiring antibiotic prophylaxis to minimize the risk of infective endocarditis (see Chapter 8) and/or infection associated with prosthetic joint replacements (see Chapter 18).
- Obtaining clearance, as appropriate, from the patient's physician for invasive dental treatment (i.e., confirming as necessary that the patient will be able to tolerate scaling and root planing without detriment to their health).

Oral self-care instructions. Any patients at risk for periodontal disease and/or dental caries should be educated about the etiology of disease and provided with oral self-care instructions tailored to the particular condition. **Oral hygiene instructions** should emphasize the importance of mechanical plaque control. Tooth-brushing techniques should highlight proper positioning and movements of the toothbrush head relative to the teeth and gingiva. Instruction in techniques that emphasize plaque removal without damaging the hard or soft tissues should be provided. Powered toothbrushes have been shown to be slightly more effective in plaque removal and in generating patient compliance compared with manual toothbrushes.[45] Interdental cleaning is paramount in achieving ideal plaque removal. A wide range of products are available to aid patients in effective plaque removal, including dental floss and floss holders, interproximal brushes, wooden toothpicks, wooden and plastic picks, and rubber tip stimulators. Flossing instructions should emphasize careful C-shaped flossing techniques, and additional devices, such as interproximal brushes, may be useful in individuals with wider interdental spaces. Additionally, irrigation devices are available to assist patients with oral hygiene.[46] Tongue debridement should be considered as part of routine oral hygiene to reduce tongue coating (bacterial colonization), while potentially reducing oral malodors.[47]

Patients with limited manual dexterity may require even greater assistance in tailoring specific oral hygiene regimens because of inherent challenges in holding and manipulating hygiene devices. For these patients, the use of manual and/or powered toothbrushes with larger handles, dental floss holders, and irrigation devices may be necessary. Visually impaired patients may benefit from guided hands-on and auditory hygiene instructions to ensure that they are effective in their oral self-care technique.

An important benefit of brushing the teeth twice daily will be the result of the actions of the chemical properties of the dentifrice in preventing caries and/or periodontal disease. Dentifrices that include stannous fluoride or chlorhexidine have been shown to reduce plaque accumulation and gingival inflammation effectively.[48] Mouth rinses that include essential oils, cetylpyridinium chloride, and chlorhexidine have also been demonstrated to be effective in removing plaque and reducing gingivitis.[48]

Regardless of the technique used, it is critical that the patient be able to implement it effectively. Teaching and learning good oral self-care is a complex process and should not be taken lightly by the dental team or patient. The patient must not only be able to hear and understand the instruction, but also must be able to demonstrate the technique in the office and then repeat it at home. The learning process may be slow and laborious and can be frustrating to all parties but is definitely worth the effort, because the rewards are significant and, if the effort fails, the outcome can be devastating to the patient. Once the techniques are learned, the use of each prescribed oral home care aid should be reviewed and reinforced at subsequent visits. (See Video 10.1 Demonstration of Oral Hygiene Instruction on ebooks+.)

Extraction of hopeless teeth. In some instances, it will already have been determined that selected teeth are to be removed because of advanced periodontal disease, nonrestorability as a result of severe caries or fracture, or in preparation for placing prosthodontic appliances. Such extractions should be completed as part of initial therapy. Delay of inevitable extractions may give false hope and leave the patient deflated and discouraged when the teeth are finally lost. Exceptions to this approach may be advisable or necessary in some instances. It may be appropriate to maintain hopeless teeth temporarily until a replacement prosthesis has been prepared, to preserve appearance, if their retention prevents the imminent tipping or extrusion of other teeth, or if their removal would compromise the vertical dimension of occlusion. In these cases, excellent home care and compliance with recall recommendations is paramount to minimize damage to adjacent tissues and reduce the systemic inflammatory burden.

Elimination of iatrogenic restorations and open caries lesions contributing to periodontal disease. Management of carious lesions or defective restorations that interfere with effective plaque removal should be completed either before or in conjunction with scaling and root planing. In general, caries control should be carried out early in the sequence of treatment and the placement of restorations, or the correction of overhanging restorations, should precede scaling and root planing for the following reasons:

- Scaling and root planing procedures are more effective after gross irregularities are removed and the open smooth surface carious lesions are sealed.
- The patient's oral self-care efforts will be more effective and the patient can witness the improvement in tissue health.
- Periodontal tissue healing may be enhanced.
- Caries or leaking restorations can be ruled in or out as the cause of pulpal symptoms or dentinal sensitivity.

Managing other dental problems that contribute to periodontal disease. Conditions relating to tooth anatomy, position, and occlusion may also contribute to periodontal disease. Anatomic defects, such as root fluting, root concavities, or exposed furcations are typically managed in the definitive phase of care. Similarly, orthodontic correction of a root proximity problem normally is delayed until completion of the disease control phase. Marginal ridge discrepancies, open proximal contacts, and plunger cusps may be repairable with odontoplasty in the disease control phase or, if more severe, may need to be corrected with complex restorations during definitive treatment. Although comprehensive occlusal adjustment should not be performed before scaling and root planing, significant occlusal interferences causing acute occlusal trauma or trauma-related mobility should be eliminated through limited occlusal adjustment as part of the disease control phase.

Scaling and root planing. Scaling and root planing constitute central elements in the periodontal aspect of the disease control phase. These procedures provide effective antimicrobial therapy by mechanically removing bacteria and disrupting their organized biofilm structures. Scaling removes plaque, calculus, and stains from affected tooth structures (to include enamel, dentin, and cementum) and root planing is used to eliminate rough or irregular root surfaces and establish smooth root contours. Coupled with careful personal and professional oral hygiene procedures, such measures will help to prevent subsequent biofilm accumulation and maintain periodontal health. These improvements manifest clinically as reduced probing depths and decreased gingival inflammation (i.e., gingival redness and bleeding on probing).

Educating the patient about the value of the procedure represents an important component of this stage of care. When faced with the prospect of worsening periodontal health, the potential need for periodontal surgery, and/or the need for dental extractions, patients may be more inclined to accept this important treatment phase.

Scaling and root planing can be a technically challenging procedure. Tenacious calculus, deep pockets, irregular root anatomy, and the inability of the operator to visualize the tip of the instrument during the procedure make this one of the most demanding tasks for the general dentist, hygienist, or periodontist. To achieve ideal outcomes, this requires patience, persistence, appropriate instruments, and skilled instrumentation. A few clinical practicalities in support of these procedures serve the patient and practitioner well (see *In Clinical Practice: Improving the Efficacy of Scaling and Root Planing Procedures* box).

IN CLINICAL PRACTICE

Improving The Efficacy Of Scaling And Root Planing Procedures

- The use of local anesthetic may help the clinician to perform their best work. In the absence of pain or discomfort, the patient is better able to tolerate the procedure and less likely to become stressed or fatigued. Similarly, if the patient is more comfortable, the procedure will be less fatiguing or frustrating for the clinician and the outcome will be improved. Use of a vasoconstrictor can also establish a cleaner and drier visual field for the clinician and more favorable access to the deposits. Judicious use of a local anesthetic therefore helps the dental team to deliver this treatment in the most safe, efficient, and effective means possible.
- It is better to perform complete scaling and root planing on a smaller area than to scale a larger area superficially, with the result that further scaling and root planing will be required at a later date. The second option may appeal to both patient and provider because it appears that more is accomplished in less time, but the appearance can be both deceiving and counterproductive. Superficial scaling may allow the gingiva to heal and to return to a normal contour and texture, giving both patient and clinician the false sense that the periodontal disease is under control and no additional periodontal therapy is required. In reality, the disease continues unabated at the depth of the pocket and in some cases the healing of the superficial tissues allows the formation of a periodontal abscess.
- If calculus, because of its location, mass, or tenacity, cannot be readily removed using standard means of non-surgical instrumentation, including ultrasonic or sonic scalers, it will be advisable to discontinue the effort, delaying completion of removal until a flap can be reflected surgically. With the calculus exposed, debridement can be more efficient, effective, and thorough.

Pharmacotherapy. In very specific cases, prescribing topical antimicrobial rinses as an adjunct to disease control phase periodontal therapy may be appropriate. Chlorhexidine gluconate (CHX), a commonly used topical antiseptic, can be effective in reducing plaque, gingival inflammation, and bleeding. Side effects may include increased extrinsic stain and calculus accumulation and temporary taste alterations.

The following clinical indications for the use of CHX rinses in initial phase periodontal therapy have been identified:

- Acute conditions, such as necrotizing ulcerative gingivitis.
- Disabled patients who cannot manipulate handheld oral hygiene devices.

- Patients with immunocompromising conditions.
- Patients with severely debilitating systemic disease.
- Overt residual gingival inflammation and bleeding, which persists despite the dental team's and patient's best efforts at initial therapy.

Careful case selection is important when prescribing CHX rinses to patients during initial therapy. The excellent antiplaque and antimicrobial properties of CHX may mask deficiencies in patient's home care techniques, providing a false sense of security about mechanical plaque removal abilities and delaying necessary instructions to remedy these deficiencies. As long-term use is rarely indicated, the discontinuation of CHX in these cases will probably result in a recurrence of plaque accumulation and gingival inflammation. For these reasons, the routine use of CHX with nonsurgical periodontal therapy is not helpful.

Although systemic antibiotic therapy is rarely needed in the management of most forms of periodontal diseases, it is often used as an adjunct to initial scaling and root planing in the management of more severe cases (i.e., Grade C) or cases refractory to treatment.[49] Antibiotic treatment helps eradicate invasive bacteria and also provides improved antimicrobial function for the patient with a compromised immune response. Its administration should be timed so that it coincides with mechanical plaque disruption through scaling and root planing to permit better penetration and action within the plaque biofilm. The distinct disadvantage of this therapy, however, is that it also removes the normal populations of protective bacteria, which may allow repopulation with even more aggressive bacterial pathogens. The clinician must remember that not all bacteria are pathogenic.

If systemic antibiotics are to be used, it can be advantageous to culture plaque from the affected sites and perform antibiotic sensitivity tests to select the most effective antibiotic and the one with the least likelihood of impacting desirable microbiota. Even with appropriate cultures, sensitivity testing, and optimal antibiotic selection, this therapy has potentially serious drawbacks, including the development of drug-resistant organisms, superinfection, and sensitivity to the medication. Although decisions largely remain empirical, the best documented outcomes point toward the combination of amoxicillin and metronidazole.[50] Decisions on integrating systemic antibiotics into a patient's periodontal care and the specific selection of antibiotics used should be based on patient diagnosis, clinical presentation, clinical experience, and knowledge of antibiotic mechanisms of action and pharmacokinetics.

An additional indication for systemic antibiotic use is in the management of acute periodontal conditions, such as necrotizing periodontal diseases and periodontal abscesses (see Chapter 9).

Periodontal Reevaluation

Often overlooked, **periodontal reevaluation** represents a critically important component of the disease control phase of periodontal therapy. (See Box 10.1 for the elements of the periodontal reevaluation.) Reevaluation is necessary to assess the effectiveness of periodontal therapy to date and to provide guidance for future treatment. With a thorough evaluation, the

dentist can assess the efficacy of all aspects of the initial nonsurgical therapy, determine which elements have served their purpose and should be continued, and which have been ineffective and should be discontinued. If the situation calls for additional intervention, strategies can be selected with the advantage of seeing the outcomes of earlier approaches. This is also the ideal time to assess the patient's need for and willingness to accept periodontal surgery.

The periodontal reevaluation should be performed 4 to 8 weeks after the final scaling and root planing visit.[51] This time frame gives the patient ample opportunity to develop an effective oral hygiene routine and, if the therapy has been effective, allows sufficient time for resolution of inflammation. Furthermore, the time interval is brief enough that most patients will not yet have developed significant new calculus deposits.

The practitioner should keep in mind several practical considerations that may facilitate planning the periodontal reevaluation visit. First, if the patient needs both an evaluation of initial non-surgical periodontal therapy and an overall disease control phase post-treatment assessment (i.e., to include assessing control of other pathologic conditions), it is advantageous to do both simultaneously. Many features are common to both evaluations and it is more efficient to combine them when possible. Second, any additional scaling and root planing or amended oral hygiene instructions often can be accomplished at this visit. Third, if the reevaluation suggests that periodontal surgery should be recommended, related issues can be discussed and informed consent for the surgery obtained before the patient leaves the office. If the patient agrees to surgery, the surgery appointment can be made before the patient is dismissed. Combining these efforts not only saves time, but also guides the patient more smoothly into the next phase of therapy. In short, consolidating activities at the periodontal reevaluation appointment benefits both patient care and practice management.

If the initial therapy has been successful, the patient's periodontal needs can now be managed through maintenance therapy (sometimes characterized as supportive periodontal therapy) as described in Chapter 12. If initial therapy has been

---

BOX 10.1 Periodontal Reevaluation Elements

Reevaluation of patient's health status, recognition of any changes or significant continuing systemic conditions

Reevaluation of patient's gingival condition, including description of tissue color, texture, contour, and form

Probing depth and clinical attachment level measurements

Notation of any sites where bleeding on probing occurs and calculation of bleeding index

Calculation of plaque index

Evaluation of teeth for mobility

- Assessment of mucogingival status
- Identification of occlusal factors that may affect periodontal condition

An overall summary of patient's response to initial therapy

Assessment of additional periodontal treatment needs, to include periodontal surgery

Determination of interval for subsequent periodontal maintenance visits

unsuccessful, or if other periodontal needs remain, therapy can be provided during the definitive phase of care.

Pulpal Therapy and Management of Lesions and Defects Encroaching on the Pulp

The following section focuses on assessing and managing chronic pulpal or periapical pathology or those conditions that may cause pulpal pathology. (The diagnosis and management of acute pulpal and periapical conditions are discussed in Chapter 9.) The disease control phase of treatment is an ideal setting in which to provide initial restorative treatment for overt caries lesions, lost or defective restorations, displaced or nondisplaced fractures of teeth, or other tooth abnormalities that, if untreated, may result in loss of pulp vitality (Box 10.2). The disease control phase provides the opportunity for conservative procedures, such as **selective caries removal** (SCR) that, if successful, will result in the formation of tertiary dentin and maintain the vitality of the tooth. The pulpal and periapical response to such therapy can be followed after 3 to 6 months and through the disease control phase. A definitive diagnosis should be confirmed before initiating the definitive phase therapy. If the pulp is already irreversibly compromised, and the expectation is that the tooth will be retained, then it is usually advantageous to do the root canal treatment in the disease control phase plan of care. The disease control phase is also the appropriate time to restore such teeth provisionally, often with foundation restorations (Figure 10.7), in anticipation of the definitive restoration that will follow.

If any of the conditions listed in Box 10.2 exist or if the dentist has concerns about the pulpal or periapical health of a tooth

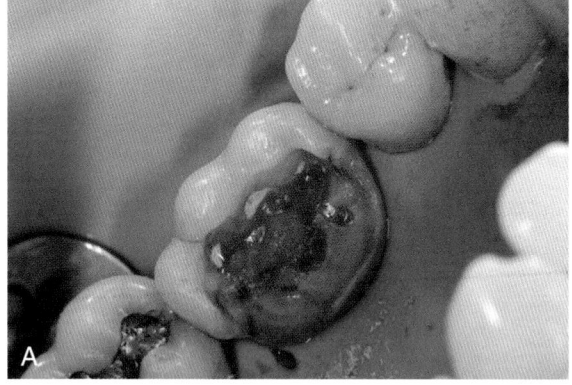

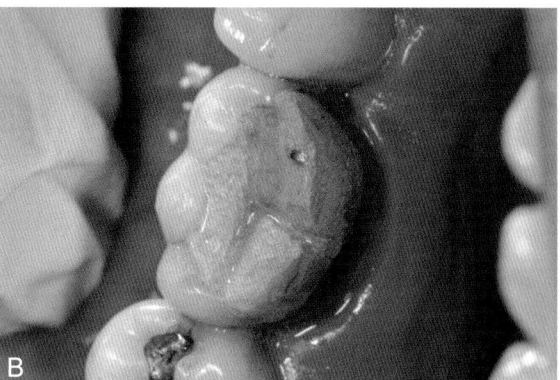

Fig. 10.7 (A, B) Amalgam foundation. (Courtesy Dr. Glenn Garland, Chapel Hill, NC.)

before restoration, an endodontic evaluation is in order. A specific tooth history and pulp vitality testing provide information for evaluating the health of the pulp. Appropriate evaluation of the periapical area includes visual inspection, palpation and percussion testing, and interpretation of a recent periapical radiograph. It is important to have a diagnosis of both the pulpal and periapical condition of such teeth *before* initiating restorative treatment.

The following sections address several approaches to managing and restoring teeth in various conditions of pulpal health during the disease control phase of treatment.

Reversible Pulpitis or a Healthy Pulp when the Caries, Fracture, or Defect Is of Moderate Depth and Pulp Is Not Exposed

The typical approach to this situation is to use a desensitizer (5% glutaraldehyde + 35% HEMA) followed by placement with a direct-fill restoration.[52] The purpose of the desensitizer is to limit the flow of tubular fluid during the restorative procedure.

A traditional base or liner under the restoration is usually not warranted unless less than 2 mm of dentin remains between the depth of the preparation and the pulp. If time does not permit placement of a conventional restoration, an adhesive material (GI cement or resin hybrid) can be placed as a "bandage" over the site. This expedient and atraumatic technique may provide an esthetic solution and, by covering the exposed dentin, eliminate further insult to the tooth. In addition, this approach gives the practitioner time to confirm pulp health and the patient time to consider restoration alternatives before making an irreversible commitment. The obvious disadvantage to this approach is that it necessitates one or more additional visits for definitive restoration of the tooth.

Reversible Pulpitis or a Healthy Pulp, and Healthy Periapical Area when the Caries, Fracture, or Defect Is in Close Proximity to the Pulp

The de facto clinical approach for this situation has become SCR (see Chapter 3 for the evidence-based rationale). In the application of SCR deep caries removal should cease when caries excavation has reached approximately 1 mm from the pulp. It is essential to remove all carious dentin from the *periphery* of the deep lesion (circumscribing the caries in close proximity to the pulp). The remaining affected dentin is commonly covered

---

BOX 10.2   Common Causes of Loss of Pulp Vitality

- Deep caries lesions (Figure 10.8)
- Fractured or leaking restorations
- Displaced fractures in close proximity to pulp
- Nondisplaced tooth cracks or fractures (Figure 10.9)
- Large restorations in close proximity to pulp (Figure 10.10)
- Tooth wear or notching via abfraction, abrasion, attrition, or erosion (Figure 10.11)
- Acute occlusal trauma or extreme chronic occlusal trauma
- Inadvertent exposure of pulp during tooth preparation

with a GI-based liner or base material in the deep recesses of the preparation, sealing the carious tissue. If deep transparent dentin allows the pinkish/red color ("blush") of the pulp to be visualized, calcium hydroxide or mineral trioxide aggregate (MTA) liner material is placed directly on that area of the pulpal/axial wall as an indirect pulp cap (IPC). It is recommended that the IPC and adjacent deep peripheral dentin be covered with a resin-modified GI base. The preparation is then restored with a direct-fill restorative material consistent with the overall approach of the current treatment plan.

Uncertain Pulpal Health, and Healthy Periapical Area When the Caries, Fracture, or Defect Is in Close Proximity to the Pulp

Following a careful history, clinical and radiographic examination, and pulp vitality testing of a symptomatic tooth, there may be uncertainty as to whether the pulpitis is reversible or irreversible. Such a dilemma may arise when the tooth pain is not spontaneous but lasts for more than a minute on stimulation; or a tooth that responds to vitality testing but with a delayed response. Two common treatment alternatives have been developed for this clinical situation. The first, more traditional, approach argues that total caries removal and the final form of the preparation should be undertaken. If the pulp is encountered in the process, endodontic therapy or extraction is recommended. This approach argues that, with a compromised pulp and a higher-than-normal likelihood of developing necrosis, the appropriate course of action is to force the issue and either initiate root canal treatment or extract the tooth. This rationale

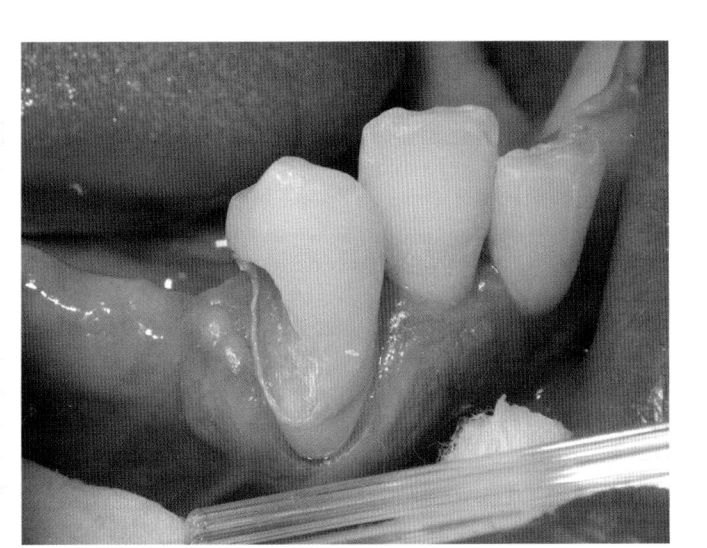

Fig. 10.8 Deep caries lesions. (Courtesy Dr. Carlos H. Barrero.)

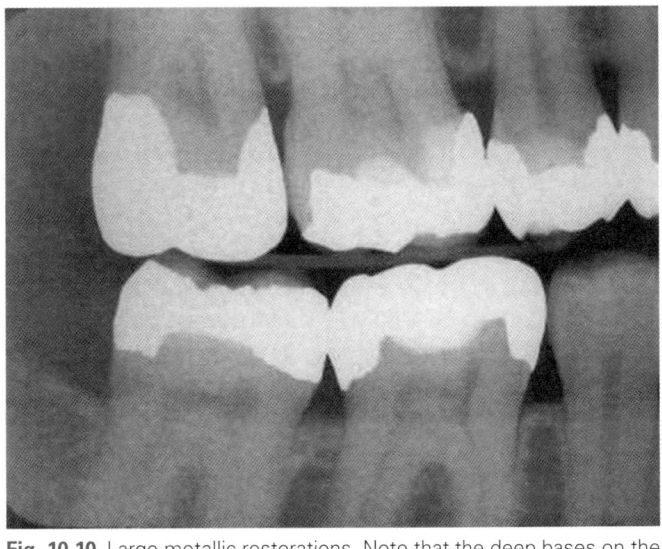

Fig. 10.10 Large metallic restorations. Note that the deep bases on the maxillary second premolar and first molar appear to be in close proximity to the pulp. (Courtesy Dr. J. Ludlow, Chapel Hill, NC.)

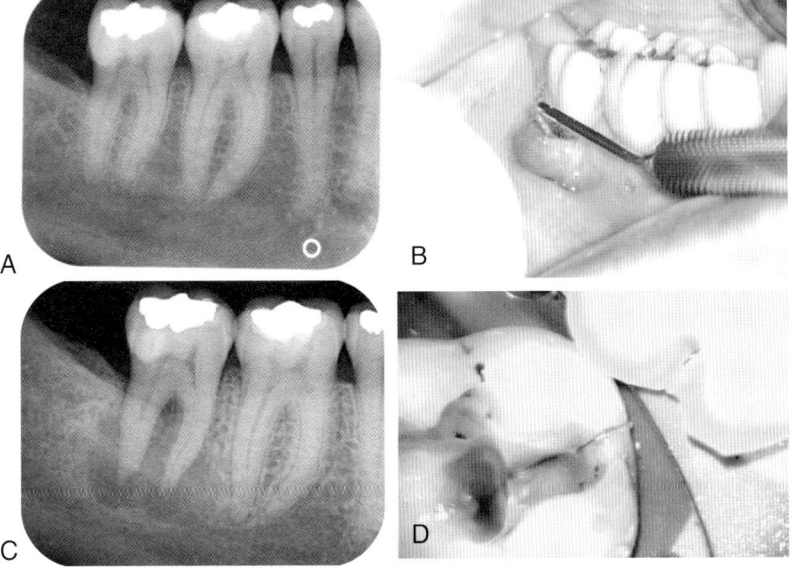

Fig. 10.9 Tooth crack. **(A)** Mandibular second molar at initial visit. **(B)** Second visit (11 months later), chronic apical abscess. **(C)** Second visit, apical rarefying osteitis. **(D)** Second visit, restoration removed and tooth crack exposed. (Courtesy Dr. Peter Tawil, Chapel Hill, NC.)

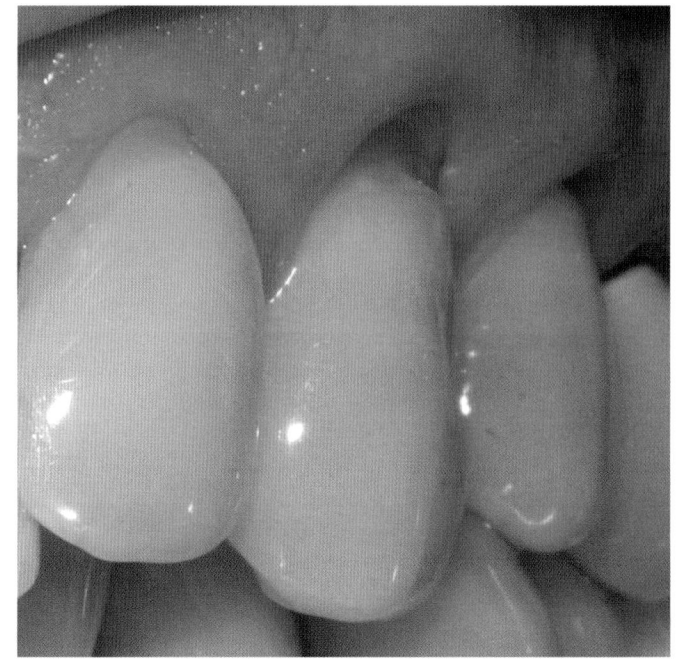

Fig. 10.11 Cervical notching. (Courtesy Dr. Lee Boushell.)

holds that definitive intervention (root canal treatment [RCT] or extraction) will reduce the possibility of future negative sequelae. Furthermore, if RCT should become necessary, it is better to do it preemptively because the root canals are less likely to become calcified and the treatment outcome is more predictable. Classic research has shown that RCT on a tooth with a vital pulp has a long-term success of more than 95%.[53,54]

The second approach, held by many advocates of an SCR procedure, promotes the idea that because an indirect pulp cap has a generally favorable prognosis and as long as the pulp will have a reasonable likelihood of survival, it should be attempted. If successful, root canal treatment (or extraction) and a considerable expense to the patient can be avoided. If unsuccessful, RCT can still be done, although with a somewhat diminished chance of success. Classic research has shown that RCT on a necrotic infected pulp has a long-term success rate of around 85%.[53,54]

The discerning practitioner will recognize that, in certain circumstances, one or other of the two approaches clearly represents a better choice, whereas in other circumstances *either* approach could be selected and that the decision is best made in conversation with the patient. Certain situations call for aggressive treatment, as for example when a "key tooth" is involved and the prognosis for the entire reconstruction depends on its successful retention. If it is important to avoid the necessity of RCT *after* the tooth has been definitively restored, or if root canal treatment would improve the retention and longevity of the final restoration, it would be wise to treat aggressively and not attempt a SCR. If, on the other hand, the patient is unwilling or unable to accept root canal treatment should that become necessary and if the tooth would otherwise be lost, a more conservative approach, the SCR, should be attempted. In intermediate cases, in which there is a realistic choice between the two options, the patient should be engaged in the discussion and involved in the decision-making process.

The practical reality is that because this decision is being made in the context of the disease control phase, there is often uncertainty about the long-term retention of the tooth, as well as the lengths to which the patient is prepared to go to save it. In that state of uncertainty, the conservative treatment (SCR/indirect pulp cap) is usually preferable to root canal treatment on a tooth that may be extracted in the future.

Treatment Options when the Pulp Is Exposed

The tooth pulp may be exposed as a result of tooth fracture, abfraction, attrition, during a caries removal procedure, or inadvertently during tooth preparation for a restoration. What is the best practice for managing a tooth when there has been a pulp exposure? Traditionally many practitioners have held that whenever the pulp is exposed the death of the pulp is almost always inevitable and that a root canal treatment or extraction is the only logical course of action. An alternative treatment, the **Direct Pulp** Cap (DPC) has been espoused for decades but remains controversial. The endodontic community has generally opposed the procedure based on some reports of high failure rate and the hazard of developing calcification within the root canal system that could jeopardize the success of (future) root canal treatment. However, credible practitioners continue to support the technique in selected circumstances.[55] The efficacy of the direct pulp cap has been reviewed extensively with reported 4-5 year success using calcium hydroxide of 56% and 81% using mineral trioxide aggregate (MTA).[56] Several factors are known to be associated with higher success rates[57] absence of spontaneous pain preoperatively, a small exposure, a mechanical exposure, careful isolation and restorative technique, and an effective restorative seal over the pulp. Teeth with a preoperative diagnosis of irreversible pulpitis or pulpal necrosis are not candidates for a DPC. When encountering the pulp, the presence of excessive bleeding (a "hyperemic" pulp) suggests that the pulp tissue has developed a substantial inflammatory response to the previous insult; whereas the presence of a vacant pulp chamber or purulent exudate indicates that the pulp has necrosed. In both instances, pulp capping is contraindicated. Calcium hydroxide or MTA have been the materials of choice for the DPC. MTA has shown slightly better success rates but is also more expensive and is less commonly available in most general dentistry practices. When pulpal necrosis or uncontrollable hemorrhage is encountered at the site of the pulp exposure a partial pulpotomy or a coronal pulpotomy may be attempted. The reported 2 year success rates with a partial pulpotomy are 55% with calcium hydroxide and 85% with MTA.[58] The 1-2 year clinical success rate for a pulpotomy ranged from 92.2 to 99.4%.[59]

A DPC, partial pulpotomy, coronal pulpotomy and a pulpal debridement have particular applicability in the Disease Control Phase of treatment. For the patient with limited financial resources, forcing a decision between doing a root canal treatment or an extraction may be problematic in multiple ways. Expending limited resources for the root canal treatment on that one tooth may restrict the options for other (perhaps many) teeth that have a better prognosis and that are more worthy of the investment. Pending the results of the disease control phase of treatment the patient may come to regret the decision to do the root canal treatment, and in hindsite would have elected extraction. Alternatively, extracting the tooth at this juncture may disrupt the flow of the control phase plan and lead to additional patient visits, especially if the patient is to be referred to another practitioner for the extraction. Premature loss of the tooth may compromise the patient's function and allow shifting of adjacent or opposing teeth. Also, upon successful conclusion of the Control Phase the patient may regret having extracted the tooth. In general it is preferred that the decision whether to extract or do complete root canal treatment on a pulpally involved tooth be deferred until the completion of the disease control phase plan when such decisions can be made in the context of the patient's overall oral condition and in light of the definitive phase plan of care. A DPC, partial pulpotomy, coronal pulpotomy, or pulpal debridement effectively facilitates that process.

At the time the pulp is encountered but before a direct pulp cap is placed, all treatment options, and the possible consequences of each, must be described to the patient, including the fact that the direct pulp cap or other vital pulp therapy may eventually lead to loss of pulp vitality and the future need for root canal treatment or extraction. Some patients will reject this staged approach on the grounds that they are uneasy with the uncertain outcome and the prospect of delaying definitive treatment. Some will be uncomfortable with the knowledge that this is an interim measure and that additional treatment and financial outlay will be require later to save the tooth. In either case the patient may elect to proceed immediately with the root canal treatment or extraction.

Initially, the direct pulp cap, partial pulpectomy or coronal polpotomy should be considered as an interim solution by both patient and practitioner. If, on reevaluation (after 3 to 6 months), the tooth remains asymptomatic, with vital pulp tests and no clinical or radiographic evidence of apical pathology, the expectation of long-term service can be given qualified endorsement. The dentist should continue to monitor the tooth at regular intervals (see Chapter 12). If during the disease control phase a pulpal debridement was performed, or if the tooth develops an irreversible pulpitis, pulpal necrosis, or pulpally induced apical pathology, root canal treatment or extraction will usually be indicated.

Definitive Diagnosis of Irreversible Pulp or Periapical Infection

In this situation, definitive pulpal therapy with root canal treatment or extraction is required. Pulp capping is contraindicated. If the tooth is to be retained, the initial treatment would be to do caries removal and perform a complete pulpectomy (pulpal debridement). A partial pulpectomy or pulpotomy should be considered only if the practitioner is unable to execute a complete pulpectomy (or extract the tooth) at that visit. The patient must understand that a pulpectomy is not a definitive form of treatment and that root canal treatment or extraction will be necessary.

Patient Declines Treatment for an Asymptomatic Apical Periodontitis, Cyst, or Granuloma

When definitive pulp therapy is indicated but the patient is asymptomatic and exhibits no signs of active infection or progressive disease and declines endodontic treatment, the clinician is presented with a dilemma. If the patient is immunocompromised, allowing chronic apical infection to persist would, in most cases, be inappropriate and unacceptable. For a patient with a normal host response, the dentist may elect to reevaluate the condition at specified periods, as discussed in Chapter 12. If the lesion increases in size or is associated with signs of active infection, then intervention will be necessary. Some clinicians never allow chronic apical lesions to go untreated and certainly this approach has merit. Even in cases in which RCT might otherwise be deferred, commonsense dictates that when a restoration is planned for the tooth, the root canal treatment should be performed first.

Single Tooth Restoration in the Disease Control Phase of Care

A tooth that is to be restored as part of the disease control phase normally receives a direct-fill definitive restoration, as discussed earlier in this Chapter. If the tooth is expected to require a crown in the definitive phase of care, a **core** or **foundation** is commonly placed during the disease control phase using a direct-fill restorative material. This treatment acts as both an interim restoration and the base on which the definitive restoration is to be placed. In some situations, usually associated with a compelling esthetic concern for which a composite restoration will not suffice, it may be appropriate to recommend a long-term provisional, or less commonly a definitive, indirect full-coverage restoration.

Teeth receiving RCT need special management. While root canal treatment is in progress, the tooth must have some form of provisional restoration (usually IRM, Cavit, or a GI) that isolates the canal from salivary contamination. Once the root canal treatment is complete, it is critical to maintain an effective seal between the oral cavity and the root canal filling material; it will be very important to place a restoration that will protect the tooth from fracture. A **protective cusp amalgam or composite** or a long-term provisional indirect restoration can serve both of those purposes. In the definitive phase a cusp-reinforcing (covering) indirect restoration is usually recommended. In the disease control phase, when an anterior tooth has had root canal treatment, but insufficient tooth structure remains to support a composite restoration, a provisional post and crown are typically constructed. Another interim solution is to fabricate the definitive post and core and follow up with a long-term provisional full-coverage restoration.

Stabilization of Dental Malalignment, Malocclusion, or Occlusal Disharmony

Problems related to the malposition or malocclusion of teeth are addressed in the definitive phase of the treatment plan and are discussed in Chapter 11. It is usually inadvisable to provide orthodontic treatment before disease control therapy has been successfully completed. In some instances, however, occlusal or limited orthodontic therapy can or should be accomplished as part of a comprehensive disease control program. Examples are discussed in the following section.

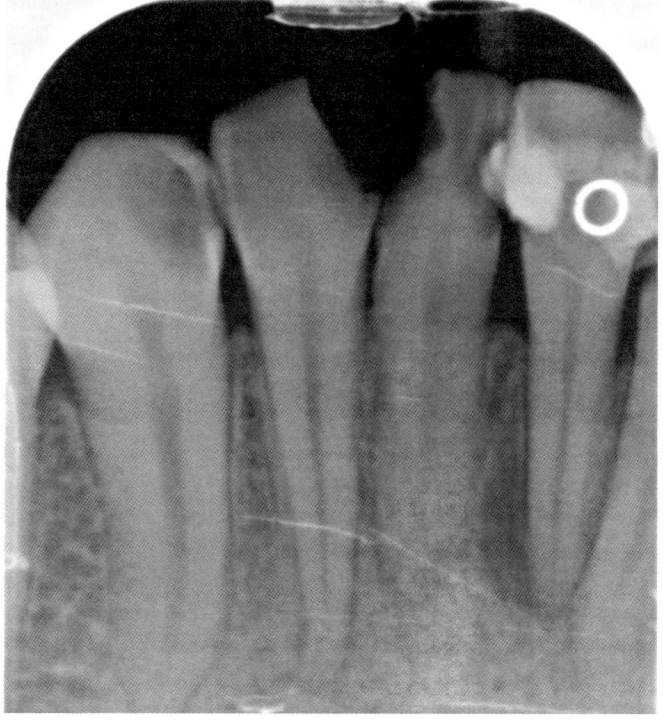

Fig. 10.12 Root proximity problem induced by caries-related space collapse. (Courtesy Dr. R Quinonez, Chapel Hill, NC.)

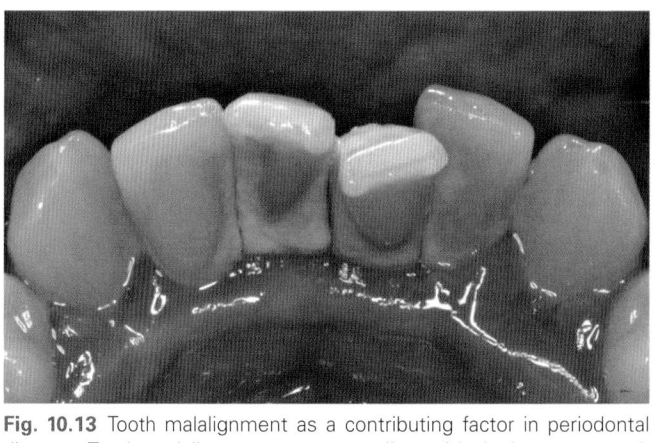

Fig. 10.13 Tooth malalignment as a contributing factor in periodontal disease. Tooth malalignment may complicate ideal plaque removal, encouraging the formation of calculus and potentially leading to periodontitis. Careful oral hygiene instructions must be provided to the patient so they can achieve adequate plaque control. Orthodontic treatment (i.e., tooth alignment) may be completed to help facilitate oral hygiene; however, patients must be cautioned about the risk of accelerated periodontal destruction if their oral hygiene is not adequate during orthodontic movement. (Courtesy Dr. Jonathan Reside and Dr. Antonio Moretti.)

Root Proximity Problem that Precludes Restoration of a Carious Lesion or Fracture

In the presence of a large proximal carious lesion, adjacent teeth may drift together (Figure 10.12). To gain access for caries removal and place a matrix band and restoration with a physiologic contour, it may be necessary to separate the teeth orthodontically.

Plunger Cusp, Open Contact, and/or Marginal Ridge Discrepancy Contributing to Food Impaction and Periodontal Disease

Presence of a "plunger cusp" (a sharp, very prominent cusp that extends deep into the opposing tooth anatomy or proximal embrasure areas) may encourage interproximal food impaction. This chronic condition may cause the soft tissue in the area to become red, bulbous, swollen, and tender. Significant bleeding on probing and deeper periodontal pockets may result. In this situation, a judicious recontouring (enameloplasty) of the offending cusp may be in order. If the problem is caused by an open contact that cannot be remedied by adjusting the opposing occlusion, consideration should be given to altering the proximal surface on one or both of the adjacent teeth through placement of a restoration or restorations. An orthodontic solution may also be considered. Small marginal ridge discrepancies can be corrected by recontouring the "high" tooth or restoration. Larger discrepancies may require orthodontic correction or placement of a restoration.

Severe Crowding

In some patients, severe crowding or malposed teeth may preclude effective plaque removal and can become a cofactor in periodontal disease. When tooth malalignment is an unmitigated factor in persisting gingivitis or periodontitis (Figure 10.13), limited or comprehensive orthodontic therapy may be recommended or necessary. In the case of malposed lower anterior teeth, if one incisor is significantly displaced, it may be possible to solve the problem by removing that tooth. Optional limited orthodontics after the extraction can enhance the patient's ability to remove plaque and further improve tooth alignment and esthetics.

Occlusal Trauma Affecting the Entire Dentition

Occlusal trauma can be classified as primary or secondary (see Chapter 2). A dentition afflicted by primary occlusal trauma may exhibit isolated wear facets or more generalized severe attrition, in some cases exposing dentin. Abfraction lesions often accompany the development of wear facets and/or attrition. Erosion may accelerate tooth loss initiated by attrition or abfraction. More severe occlusal trauma may lead to increased tooth mobility with clinically detectable fremitus. The patient may report sensitivity associated with affected tooth surfaces. In the absence of symptoms, treatment may or may not be indicated (see discussion of bruxism in Chapter 3). If comprehensive occlusal adjustment is indicated, it should generally be implemented at the conclusion of, rather than during, the disease control phase of treatment.

The most common clinical feature of secondary occlusal trauma is significant tooth mobility. Other common findings (in addition to those noted with primary occlusal trauma) include drifting and tipping of the teeth. The maxillary anterior teeth are particularly susceptible to labial flaring and often exhibit obvious fremitus when the teeth are occluded. In some cases, the symptoms may be relieved by a comprehensive occlusal adjustment, which should follow rather than precede initial periodontal therapy. However, isolated secondary occlusal trauma that is associated with a very limited number of teeth should be corrected as soon the resultant fremitus has been detected. In severe cases where the teeth have drifted or exhibit moderate to severe mobility, provisional splinting may be required. Less commonly, orthodontic therapy may be needed, but should be undertaken with great caution and only with a full discussion with the patient regarding the prognosis for treatment.

Occlusal Trauma Affecting Isolated Teeth

The diagnosis and management of acute occlusal trauma is discussed in Chapter 9. Individual teeth with occlusal trauma may exhibit pulpal sensitivity, be clinically mobile (with palpable fremitus), and (because of coexisting occlusal interferences) cause aberrant excursive patterns in eccentric jaw movements. Secondary occlusal trauma may contribute to additional loss of clinical attachment. Gross discrepancies that interfere with smooth function in excursive jaw movements or that cause occlusal trauma normally should be eliminated as part of the disease control phase of therapy. Usually, this can be accomplished with selective occlusal adjustment to eliminate premature contacts or interferences to excursive and/or protrusive mandibular movements. In rare instances, orthodontic or restorative correction is required.

Supraeruption

Supraeruption or **hypereruption** of a tooth or teeth can be problematic, because it may preclude future reconstruction with a normal occlusal plane and, depending on the tooth position and location, there is an increased likelihood of symptomatic interference in excursive movement and function (Figure 10.14). This problem is usually addressed in the definitive phase, after evaluating mounted study casts. It is mentioned here because if the clinician considers a conservative approach such as occlusal reduction without RCT or an indirect restoration, it is often advantageous to begin the process during the disease control phase. Thus, the reduction can be achieved sequentially, with the goal of allowing for the gradual deposition of secondary dentin and maintenance of a healthy pulp. If RCT or an indirect restoration becomes necessary, that therapy can be undertaken immediately. It should be noted that this conservative approach requires consideration also be given to the stabilization of the tooth to prevent further supraeruption.

Impacted Tooth Other Than a Third Molar

Impacted teeth (usually maxillary canines or mandibular premolars) should usually be addressed in the disease control phase of care. If extraction is warranted because insufficient space exists for forced eruption, the procedure should be carried out earlier rather than later to avoid delaying definitive therapy. If forced eruption is a possibility but the outcome is uncertain, the attempt should be made as early as possible, so that by the time the definitive phase is initiated, the outcome will be clear and subsequent therapy, if needed, can be delineated. Potential psychological and health benefits accrue to the patient when impactions are managed in the disease control phase. Delay simply prolongs the inevitable and may give the patient the false sense that treatment can be postponed indefinitely. Delay also

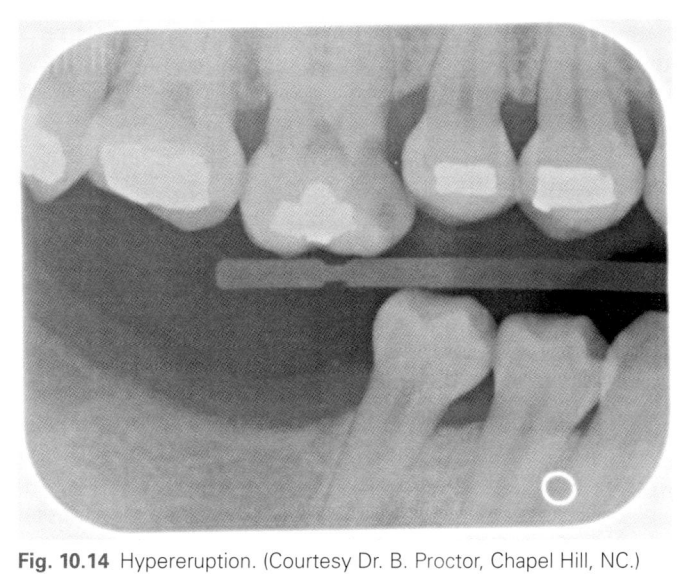

Fig. 10.14 Hypereruption. (Courtesy Dr. B. Proctor, Chapel Hill, NC.)

increases the risk of resorption, periodontal disease, or carious invasion of adjacent teeth.

Decreased Vertical Dimension of Occlusion

Management of **decreased vertical dimension of occlusion** can be complex and challenging. Certainly it is easier for the dentist to defer the decision whether it is necessary or desirable to open the bite until the disease control phase is complete. By delaying the decision, however, the dentist risks being placed in the awkward position of having to recommend extraction of teeth already restored, or re-restoration with definitive (often indirect) restorations at the new vertical dimension. For these reasons, it is important to consider the fundamental question of whether to open the bite and, if so, how that should be accomplished as part of the disease control phase.

If it is determined that reconstruction can be accomplished successfully at the existing vertical dimension, every attempt to save teeth may be justified. If the vertical dimension needs to be opened and the patient cannot afford the required complete mouth reconstruction, a denture or overdenture may be the only alternative. If the vertical dimension needs to be opened and the patient can afford comprehensive reconstruction, it may be prudent to refer the patient to a prosthodontist for the entire reconstruction.

Disorders Associated With the Temporomandibular Joints and/or Muscles of Mastication

Pain or dysfunction of the temporomandibular joint(s) (TMJ) and/or muscles of mastication is commonly referred to as **temporomandibular disorders (TMD)**.[60–63] Symptoms of TMD may have a significant impact on jaw functions and, as a result, should be included in the acute phase (Chapter 9) or disease control phase of treatment. Four of the more common types of TMD are discussed here, with information on diagnosis, relevance to the patient's care, and treatment. In the absence of specific training on the diagnosis and management of orofacial pain (OFP), practitioners are advised to consult with, or refer the patient to, an OFP Specialist.

Disc Displacement With Reduction

Disc displacement (DD) refers to the displacement (usually anteriorly) of the articular disc of the TMJ in the closed month position. During mouth opening, the disc is reduced into its proper location on the superior portion of the condyle. This is known as **disc displacement with reduction (DDR)**. Both opening and closing movements may produce distinct, audible, and/or palpable clicking or popping (also known as reciprocal clicking). Mandibular range of motion is within normal limits. The clicking or popping is usually painless and does not result in mandibular dysfunction. However, patients may seek treatment when the joint clicking is painful or when the click is so loud that it causes social embarrassment. Treatment consists of education and reassurance, self-care measures (such as applying ice or heat to the painful area, massaging the jaw, restricting jaw functions to a painless range, soft diet, oral parafunction awareness, jaw exercises, and jaw muscle relaxation training), nonsteroidal anti-inflammatory drugs (NSAIDs) as needed for pain control, and occlusal splint therapy.

Disc Displacement Without Reduction

Disc Displacement without Reduction, or closed lock, refers to the complete displacement or dislocation (again, usually anteriorly) of the articular disc of the TMJ in both the closed and open mouth positions. Owing to the lack of reduction of the articular disc, TMJ popping or clicking is absent. Both active and passive mouth opening is restricted with a hard end-feel and ipsilateral deflection. Patients typically complain of severely restricted mouth opening accompanied by moderate to severe pain in the acute stage. The TMJ pain is often localized to the joint and may be perceived as an earache because of its proximity to the ear canal. Associated inflammation of the retrodiscal tissue (known as retrodiscitis) results in tenderness of the ear canal to palpation. Treatment consists of self-care measures (as described earlier), NSAIDs, and occlusal splint therapy. Orthodontic treatment and occlusal adjustments are contraindicated. Over time, although the articular disc remains displaced or dislocated, the retrodiscal tissue assumes a "pseudo-disc" formation, resulting in increased mouth opening. On resolution of the acute inflammation, physical therapy can assist with rehabilitation of the TMJ, especially in improving the mandibular range of motion.

TMJ Osteoarthritis

Osteoarthritis of the TMJ is the result of destruction of the articular surfaces of the condyle and/or glenoid fossa secondary to joint inflammation. The etiology of osteoarthritis is complex and can result from micro- or macro-trauma, aging, prior TMJ surgery, or underlying systemic disease (such as polyarthritis or rheumatoid arthritis). Patients may complain of TMJ pain, preauricular swelling, restriction in mouth opening, and joint crepitus (a crunching or grating sound on movement of the TMJ). The pain is usually spontaneous and may worsen with jaw movement. Capsulitis/synovitis of the TMJ may result in a

transient acute malocclusion (disclusion of the ipsilateral posterior teeth and heavy occlusion of the contralateral anterior teeth), which self-corrects after resolution of the joint inflammation. Bony condylar changes, such as erosions and osteophytes, is notable in the CT scan. Treatment consists of self-care measures (as described above), oral NSAIDs or steroids, and occlusal splint therapy. In severe cases, intra-articular steroids and TMJ surgery (such as arthrocentesis, arthroscopy, and total joint replacement) may be indicated.

Masticatory Myalgia

Masticatory myalgia is pain originating from the muscles of mastication. Acute myalgia frequently occurs as a result of trauma (such as prolonged wide mouth opening during dental treatment) or bruxism secondary to stressful events. It differs from TMJ pain in several ways. Myogenous pain is often diffuse and cyclical (waxes and wanes over time) compared with TMJ pain, which is often very well localized with a distinct onset. When asked to indicate the location of pain, patients with TMJ pain typically point to the preauricular area in front of the tragus of the ear, whereas patients with muscle pain will place their hands over the entire side of the face. On clinical examination, myogenous pain can be provoked or aggravated by digital palpation of the masseter and temporalis muscles, with an acknowledgment that the pain is familiar. Active mandibular range of motion is usually restricted because of pain, but passive mandibular range of motion is within normal limits and associated with a soft end-feel. In myofascial pain, taut muscle bands with exquisitely painful areas (known as trigger points) radiate pain in a characteristic pattern. The management of acute masticatory myalgia include self-care measures (as described earlier), NSAIDs and/or muscle relaxants, and occlusal splint therapy.

Acute TMD pain often resolves quickly and uneventfully with conservative self-care measures. In some, TMD pain may become chronic and persistent or recurrent. The etiopathophysiology of chronic TMD is complex and involves pain amplification, elevated psychological distress, environmental factors, and genetic predisposition.[64] Chronic TMD is comorbid with other bodily pain conditions such as fibromyalgia, chronic headaches, irritable bowel syndrome, and low back pain. Patients with chronic TMD are best managed in a multi-disciplinary OFP clinic.

Sleep Disorders

In 2017 the American Dental Association recommended that going forward dentists screen all patients for **obstructive sleep apnea (OSA)**.[65] Those at increased risk should be referred to a medical provider for follow-up evaluation and diagnosis. Risk is determined by the presence of symptoms and signs of OSA, pertinent findings in the medical history (e.g., a history of hypertension, arrhythmia or stroke), and risk indicators identified during the intraoral and extraoral examination of the patient (see Chapter 2). Screening should occur in the disease control phase of dental treatment to avoid subsequent ill-informed treatment decisions. For example, a maxillary occlusal splint for sleep bruxism can exacerbate snoring and increase the severity of OSA.[66] As such, it is recommended that the splint only be treatment planned for OSA-managed patients.[67] Alternatively, a **mandibular advancement device (MAD)** that can both manage the patient's OSA and protect the teeth from bruxism could be a treatment option.

The gold standard treatment for OSA is **continuous positive airway pressure (CPAP)**. Air is forced into the nose or nose and mouth through a mask on the face or tubes inserted into the nares. The pressure required to keep the airway from collapsing is determined during in-laboratory polysomnography (CPAP titration) or directly by some CPAP machines (auto-CPAP). A nasal mask can apply pressure to the maxillary teeth resulting in undesirable dental side effects that can impact dental treatment planning. These side effects include retrusion of the anterior maxilla and palatal tipping of the maxillary anterior teeth.[68] Labial tipping of both the maxillary and mandibular anterior teeth has also been reported from CPAP use.[69] The inferior border of a nasal mask can apply a constant undesirable pressure to the periodontium of the maxillary anterior teeth impacting the health of these tissues.

Although CPAP is often very efficacious in reducing the severity or eliminating OSA, a high percentage of patients cannot tolerate it.[70] For these patients, a mandibular advancement device (MAD) may be indicated. A MAD stabilizes the mandible in an adjustable forward position, thereby decreasing upper airway collapsibility. MADs are recognized as a first-line therapy for patients diagnosed with mild or moderate OSA and for patients diagnosed with severe OSA who cannot tolerate CPAP or who prefer alternative therapy.[71] The devices can also be used to eliminate or reduce primary snoring. The MADs are considered durable medical equipment, not dental devices. For the management of OSA, a referral (prescription or standard written order) from the patient's medical provider is required. The dentist is expected to collaborate with the medical provider throughout the patient's OSA treatment.[72] Once the MAD is fabricated and adjusted by the dentist to achieve symptomatic improvement and to optimize its efficacy, the medical provider orders a sleep apnea test to determine whether the MAD adequately reduces the severity of the patient's OSA. At least annual follow-up of the patient is expected as long as the MAD is used. Dentists should complete specialized training in dental sleep medicine prior to treating patients with MADs. Certification by a non-profit organization such as the American Board of Dental Sleep Medicine is recommended.

Like CPAP, MADs can have dental side effects that vary from patient to patient in their severity. These side effects include the following: decreased overbite and overjet, palatal tipping of the maxillary anterior teeth, labial tipping of the mandibular anterior teeth, anterior cross-bite, widening of the mandibular dental arch, loss of occlusal contacts on posterior teeth, posterior open bite and anterior open bite.[73,74] For patients who use or anticipate using a MAD for OSA, the potential side effects should be taken into consideration during dental treatment planning. For example, restorations planned for the incisal edges of the anterior teeth must be able to withstand the increased occlusal force that results from a posterior open bite, should this occur.

Unwanted tooth movement may prevent full seating of a removable partial denture. A pre-existing MAD may no longer fit the teeth after occlusal restorations are placed. Occlusion on a new restoration may not be indicated if the adjacent teeth are not in occlusion.

Use of Tobacco Products

In the United States, tobacco use, although declining, is still pervasive, resulting in significant morbidity and mortality to both users and nonusers.[75] Worldwide, tobacco use continues to increase. Cigarette smoking is a major risk factor for heart disease, various forms of cancer, stroke, and chronic obstructive pulmonary disease. It is estimated that one in five deaths is related to smoking and that one in four smokers will die prematurely of a tobacco-related disease, losing on average 15 years of life.[76] Women who smoke are at risk of the same adverse effects as men and, in addition, a pregnant woman who smokes puts her unborn child at risk of complications, such as premature birth and low birth weight. Tobacco smoking causes 30% of all cancer deaths in the United States.[75] Tobacco smoking has been cited as the leading preventable cause of mortality and morbidity worldwide.[77] The morbidity and mortality from cigarette smoking are related to the total years of smoking, the number of cigarettes per day, and the depth of inhalation. The use of nonfiltered cigarettes and mentholated cigarettes is also related to increased morbidity.[78] See Chapter 14 for more information on the ill effects and addictive potential of nicotine and tobacco products.

Cigar and pipe smoking are associated with the same health concerns as cigarette smoking, including cardiac and pulmonary diseases, the risk of nicotine addiction, and the creation of indoor air pollution.[79] Cigar and pipe smoking are considered at least as great a risk factor for the development of oral cancer as cigarette smoking.[79,80] The pipe stem (smoke delivery end) delivers smoke that has both thermal effects and hot gasses produced during combustion. These act synergistically with the toxic components in tobacco smoke to enhance the risk of carcinogenesis in chronically exposed tissues, such as lips and soft palate. The habit of holding the lighted end of the cigarette inside the mouth, called "reverse smoking," is also associated with a significantly higher risk of oral cancer.[80,81] Oral effects of pipe smoking are shown in Figure 10.15.

Currently, there are as many as 46 million smokers in the United States[75] and millions of other individuals who are exposed to passive or secondhand smoke indirectly. Secondhand smoke from cigarettes, cigars, and pipes is known to pose health risks to nonsmokers.[82] The oral use of smokeless tobacco (commonly called spit, chew, or snuff) is not a safe alternative to smoking.[82-84] Compelling scientific evidence documents the fact that smokeless tobacco is also dangerous and can lead to nicotine addiction and a number of noncancerous oral pathologic conditions demonstrated in Figure 10.16. Types of smokeless tobacco to be chewed are shredded loose-leaf, pressed brick or plug, or twist, made of dried ropelike strands. Snuff is a powdered or finely cut cured tobacco, which is available as a wet or dry product to be used topically in the mouth or nose. All forms contain nitrosamines and other potentially carcinogenic substances. The risk of

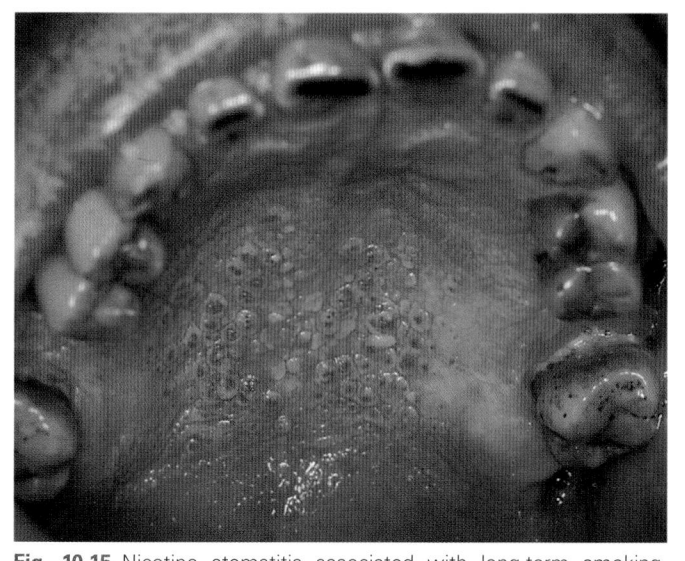

Fig. 10.15 Nicotine stomatitis associated with long-term smoking. From Ibsen OAC, Phelan JA. Oral Pathology for the Dental Hygienist. 6th ed. St. Louis: Saunders; 2014.

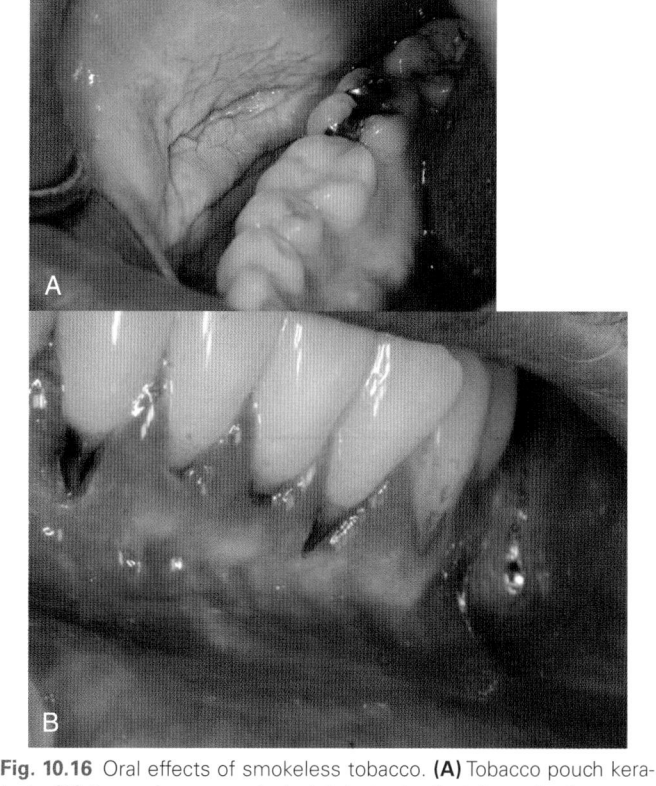

Fig. 10.16 Oral effects of smokeless tobacco. **(A)** Tobacco pouch keratosis. **(B)** Recession, mucogingival defects, tooth stain, and submucous fibrosis. (Courtesy Dr. Ricardo J. Padilla.)

developing oral cancer increases with long-term use of smokeless tobacco.

Vaporizing or vaping of substances (primarily tobacco, cannabis, hashish or opium) began centuries ago. The e-cigarette is the most recent popularized product for vaping. In 2018, 14.9%

of adults reported having used an electronic cigarette and 3.2% were current e-cigarette users.[85] Nine per cent of US adults said they "regularly or occasionally" vape.[86] The National Youth Tobacco Survey in 2021 revealed that more than 2 million middle school and high school students used e-cigarettes and one in four vaped daily in that year (85% used flavored e-cigarettes).[87]

E-cigarettes were introduced as a safer alternative to smoking tobacco products and a means to assist current smokers in their cessation efforts. However, both of these contentions are now being called into question.

A WebMD Connect to Care circulation to the public asserted that e-cigarette use has been linked to lung cancer and lung issues, brain damage, heart issues, and mouth/gum disease.[88] In 2019, the CDC alerted the public and medical community to the existence of EVALI (E-cigarette or Vaping use-Associated Lung Injury) and reported 52 deaths associated with the use of vaping products.[89]

Johns Hopkins in their WWW circular [] *5 Vaping Facts You Need to Know* asserted that[90]:

1. Vaping is less harmful than smoking, but it's still not safe
2. Research suggests vaping is bad for your heart and lungs
3. Electronic cigarettes are just as addictive as traditional ones
4. Electronic cigarettes aren't the best smoking cessation tool
5. A new generation is getting hooked on nicotine

Oral health problems associated with vaping include demineralized enamel and dental erosion, xerostomia, caries, and periodontal disease.[91]

The US Office of the Surgeon General has posted a circular highlighting the particular vulnerability of the teenage population to both the hazards of vaping and the potential for addiction to e-cigarettes.[92]

Smoking Cessation

In light of the current knowledge about the health effects of tobacco use, oral health providers (dentists and dental hygienists) have a professional and ethical obligation to engage in tobacco prevention and promote cessation with patients who use tobacco products. Tobacco intervention is consistent with the goals of oral and dental health promotion and preventive dentistry. When appropriate, tobacco use cessation should be an integral part of the dental treatment plan.[93]

For many patients with limited access to health care, the episodic visit to the dentist may be the primary point of contact with a health care provider. For these patients and for those patients who are regularly seen for periodic dental visits, the dental office can be an ideal setting and opportunity to initiate, manage, and reinforce a patient's smoking cessation program. By seeing the patient at periodic maintenance visits, dental team members can also help manage a relapse of tobacco use, should it occur. All members of the dental practice team can play a role in promoting smoking cessation. First, they should set a good example by being tobacco-free themselves. When addressing issues of patient tobacco use, dental team members should be discrete, diplomatic, and encouraging, but not condescending. All office members should be educated in the harmful oral and systemic effects of tobacco use and aware of current approaches and acceptable strategies for tobacco control.

Information for patients about effects of tobacco. Dental patients who use tobacco should be advised about the adverse effects that tobacco products may have on both systemic and oral health. Patients who smoke tobacco products should be aware of their increased risk for developing lung cancer and the potentially life-threatening pulmonary and cardiac effects of smoking but they may not be cognizant of the direct and indirect effects of smoking on the oral cavity and the effect of smoking or vaping on oral health.[82] Tobacco-induced illnesses affecting the cardiovascular and respiratory systems may contraindicate some elective oral surgical treatment or general anesthesia. For the medically compromised patient who smokes, the detrimental effects can be synergistic and may further limit dental treatment options. Cellular, tissue, and immune system changes caused by smoking can have a negative effect on the outcome of oral surgical procedures.[76,94] This is a particular concern with respect to implants. Because early long-term studies had shown that patients who smoke are more likely to develop peri-implantitis,[95] some practitioners have declined to place implants requiring osseointegration in individuals who continue to smoke and many will require that patients receiving implants refrain from smoking during the postinsertion healing period.

By altering the humoral and cellular immune system response, tobacco use increases the probability that periodontal disease will occur and that it will occur sooner than it would have otherwise. Tobacco smokers are 2.5 to 3.0 times more likely to develop periodontal disease than are nonsmokers.[82,96] Smoking increases the risk of necrotizing gingivitis. A strong association has been found between smoking and tooth loss, as well as alveolar bone loss. There is also a direct relationship between periodontal disease severity and the number of cigarettes consumed daily, number of years of use, and age at initiation of smoking.[96] The smoker's susceptibility to other smoking-related diseases may be correlated with the severity of that smoker's periodontal disease.[96] Smoking can have a significant negative effect on any efforts to treat or prevent the recurrence of inflammatory periodontal diseases. Some evidence suggests that with cessation of smoking, periodontal tissues are more likely to regenerate and rehabilitate.[97-99]

Tobacco use has been associated with other oral conditions as diverse as oral mucosal leukoplakia, localized alveolar osteitis (dry socket),[94] and halitosis. The combustion products of smoked tobacco can stain the oral soft tissue, especially the tongue; tooth structure; dental prostheses; and composite resins. Use of smokeless tobacco is associated with buccal tooth abrasion and gingival recession in the areas of the mouth where the tobacco is held.[67] Some smokeless tobacco products contain sugar, which can significantly increase the risk of developing cervical caries.

Patients who use tobacco products over an extended period have increased risk of developing oral cancer (see discussion in Chapter 3). Tobacco cessation studies have shown that there is a greatly increased risk for a second primary oral cancer in patients who continue smoking after cancer treatment and that the 5-year survival rate is approximately twice as high for nonsmokers than for smokers.[81] Oral cancer can seriously affect ability to eat, chew, talk, and function, as well as significantly altering the individual's appearance and self-image.

Conversely, the benefit of discontinuing to use tobacco products is that the patient can expect reduced risk of encountering the afore mentioned oral health problems.

Box 10.3, to be shared with patients by the dental team, summarizes the major effects of tobacco products in the mouth. Open-source publications on the effects of tobacco and tobacco cessation techniques and programs are available from the National Cancer Institute.[100-102]. These are excellent resources for educating patients and are suitable for use in the dental office.

Smoking and vaping cessation strategies. Smoking cessation can be accomplished through health care providers and health care systems; medications, including **nicotine replacement therapy (NRT)**; individual and group counseling; and computer-based or hard copy self-instructional programs. The most successful programs involve a combination of different strategies, and personal efforts, such as counseling and medications, have proven to be effective with many smokers.[103]

Smoking cessation programs show a predictable success rate of 40% with NRT or 20% without NRT.[78] Established tobacco intervention protocols, such as the one advocated by the US National Cancer Institute, can be easily implemented in the clinical setting, including the dental office. The **5 As of Tobacco Intervention** (Box 10.4)[96] is an evidence-based model that all healthcare providers have been urged to adopt.

BOX 10.3 Patient Pointers on Possible Oral Effects of Tobacco Products

- Discoloration and coating of tongue
- Smoker's palate
- Bad breath
- Staining and wear of teeth and fillings
- Tooth decay
- Irritation and staining of gums
- Receding gums
- Bone loss around teeth
- Gum disease and pyorrhea
- Implant infection
- White or red premalignant lesions
- Oral cancer

BOX 10.4 Five As of Tobacco Intervention

- ASK—Systematically identify all tobacco users at every visit.
- ADVISE—All tobacco users should be encouraged to quit. Advice should be clear, direct, and individualized for each patient.
- ASSESS—Determine the patient's willingness to initiate cessation.
- ASSIST—Aid the patient in quitting. Patients should be advised to remove tobacco products from their environments and to avoid situations that may compromise their efforts to stop using tobacco, such as socializing with active smokers or consumption of alcohol.
- ARRANGE—Schedule follow-up contact. Follow-up contact should occur soon after the quit date, preferably during the first week. A second follow-up contact is recommended within the first month. Schedule further follow-up contacts as needed. Acknowledge success.

Adapted from the National Cancer Institute's tobacco intervention program [www.prevent.org/.../leg-community_health_report_inside_final_web_10...]. Source: http://www.ahrq.gov>slide43

The first step in smoking cessation therapy is recognition that the patient is a user of tobacco products. This information can be gathered routinely, as part of the patient history. If a patient is identified as a tobacco user, they can then be asked about readiness to quit. A discussion with the dentist or dental hygienist focusing on the oral health risks and personal advantages of quitting tobacco use can be a useful method for motivating an individual to make the decision to quit.[104–106] An analysis of the tobacco history becomes the basis for smoking cessation counseling.[107] Tobacco cessation not only involves a behavioral change in breaking a habit, but also recognition of the need to overcome the physical dependence on nicotine. Successful change in behavior is usually predicated on the patient's understanding of the disadvantages associated with the habit and the advantages of cessation.[105,106]

Once a patient's habit is confirmed and their readiness to consider cessation affirmed, it is usually appropriate to engage the patient in a brief (3–5 minutes) intervention.[107] Following the brief intervention, many oral health providers will then elect to refer the patient to a social worker, psychologist or other health care provider trained in addictionology to engage the patient in a cessation program. Alternatively, the patient may be given a recommendation to pursue some of the excellent resources available from the Communicable Disease Center (CDC), US Food & Drug Administration (FDA), National Cancer Institute, or other State programs (e.g. NCQuitline). Box 10.5, lists online resources and Quit Lines to assist patients with their cessation. Some of these sites, including the NC Quitline, have an online portal for referrals, and many providers are therefore finding this to be an easy, streamlined way to screen for tobacco use, provide education to the patient, and refer out for (sometimes no charge to the patient) individual counseling and assistance with accessing NRT.

NRTs have been developed to reduce or eliminate withdrawal symptoms and have been found significantly to increase success in efforts to stop smoking and tobacco use.[78]

These over-the-counter and prescription agents provide individuals with help for the physiological, psychological, and behavioral aspects of their nicotine use once the decision has been made to stop tobacco use. Physical symptoms, such as headache, digestion complaints, sleep disturbances, irritability, anxiety, and increased appetite, are common during nicotine withdrawal and, in addition, the intense craving for nicotine may cause the patient to resume tobacco use.

BOX 10.5   Patient Resources for Smoking and Tobacco Cessation

Online Resources
https://www.cdc.gov/quit
https://www.aafp.org

Quit Links
American Cancer Society 866-784-8454
American Lung Association 800-586-4872
US Department of Health & Human Services 800-784-8669

Source: https://quitlinenc.dph.ncdhhs.gov

There are two types of agents, prescription tobacco cessation drugs and nicotine replacement products. Prescription tobacco cessation drugs, such as bupropion (Zyban) and varenicline (Chantix), do not contain nicotine and work within the central nervous system. Nicotine replacement products supply a specific measured dose of nicotine without exposing the patient to any associated tobacco carcinogens and toxins. Nonprescription NRT agents include nicotine chewing gum, lozenges, sprays, and inhalers that come in generic and brand names Nicorette and Habitrol as well as topical patches that come in generic and brand name NicoDerm CQ. The different products, doses, and expected duration of therapy are listed in Table 10.4. Evidence from a systematic review suggests that antidepressants such as bupropion and nortriptyline help in long-term smoking cessation and that adverse events with either drug are not likely to require stopping use of the medication.[108] The products can be used in combination and, although no one of the delivery systems has been demonstrated to be superior, individual who use tobacco may find that one product or combination of products is more effective than another. The choice of nicotine replacement product should be based on the patient's tobacco use pattern and level of dependence.[104,109] See Table 10.4 for a comparison chart of nicotine replacement products.

Following successful cessation intervention, the dental team should take the opportunity to congratulate the ex-smoker/vaper on their success. If a patient is found to have resumed smoking or vaping, ask if they are ready to try again. Relapses are common and smokers often need four or more attempts to achieve long-term success. Oral health care providers should ask patients who have been on cessation programs about their tobacco use status at every periodic visit. Patients may hold shame and guilt about re-starting tobacco use and therefore they may not offer this information to their provider unless prompted.

Other Forms of Oral Pathology

The disease control phase of the treatment plan is a logical place to deal with oral pathology in its many forms. Lesions that require a biopsy, consultation, or active therapy are usually addressed in the disease control phase. Benign lesions that should be monitored (e.g., fibromas or condensing osteitis) are best addressed in the maintenance phase of care. Soft tissue pathology may appear at any time during the course of the patient's treatment. For that reason and because it may appear in myriad forms and need to be treated in widely divergent ways, the management of oral pathology has application to all phases of the treatment plan and is found in many chapters of this book. Oral manifestations of systemic disease, such as anemia-induced glossitis, are most often managed as a systemic element throughout all phases of care. Acute conditions, such as stomatitis, may be most appropriately handled as an acute phase of care. New lesions that may arise during the course of definitive therapy, such as abrasions caused by dentures or hyperkeratosis, are addressed as they occur.

Any comprehensive attempt to control oral disease should certainly include the management or eradication of any and

TABLE 10.4 Nicotine Replacement Therapy Products[a,b]

Product	Advantage/Uses	Precautions/Adverse Effects
Nicotine Gum Available: 2- and 4-mg strengths. Maximum: 24 pieces per day. Use 4-mg strength only for patients who take their first cigarette within 30 min of waking or smoke > 25 cigarettes/day. Dose: 2 or 4-mg gum piece every 1–2 hours for 6 weeks, then 1 piece every 2–4 hours for 3 weeks, and then 1 piece every 4–8 hours for 3 weeks. If cravings are strong and frequent, may use second piece within an hour.	Available over the counter. Use: Chew gum slowly until it tingles, then park between cheek and gum. When tingle is gone, begin chewing again until tingle returns. Repeat process until most of the sensation is gone (30 min). Using at least 9 pieces/day the first 6 weeks is associated with higher chances of quitting. Short acting makes dosing more flexible.	Adverse effects: Continuous use may cause nausea, dizziness, hiccups or heartburn. Other effects: gastrointestinal disturbances, jaw pain, orodental problems. May worsen TMJ disorder. No food/drink except water 15 min before and while chewing. May use with cigarettes. Duration of use: 6 weeks to 6 months.
Nicotine Lozenges Available: 2- and 4-mg strengths. Maximum: 20 lozenges per day. Use 4-mg strength based on timing of first cigarette similar to gum Dose (as with gum): 2- or 4-mg lozenge every 1–2 hours for 6 weeks, then 1 lozenge every 2–4 hours for 3 weeks, and then 1 lozenge every 4–8 hours for 3 weeks.	Available over the counter. Use: Allow lozenge to slowly dissolve in mouth over 20–30 min. Minimize swallowing. Do not chew or swallow lozenge. Using at least 9 lozenges/day the first 6 weeks is associated with higher chances of quitting. Occasionally rotate to different areas of the mouth.	Cautions similar to gum. Do not use more than 1 lozenge at a time or more than 5 lozenges in 6 hours. Duration of use: 3 months.
Nicotine Nasal Spray Available: 0.5 mg per metered spray. Maximum of 40 mg (80 sprays) per day. Initial dose range 8–40 mg/day depending on level of addiction. Dose: 1–2 sprays in each nostril every hour, taper over 4–6 weeks.	Prescription only. Use: To minimize side effects, do not sniff, swallow, or inhale through nose while using product. Tilt head back slightly when administering. During initial 6–8 weeks of treatment, use at least 8 doses/day Fastest form of nicotine delivery, short acting allows for dosing flexibility.	Adverse effects: nasal irritation and congestion, runny nose, changes in taste or smell (most adverse effects improve after 3 days). Caution in those with underlying chronic nasal disorders or severe reactive airway disease Need for frequent dosing can compromise adherence May be more likely to induce dependence owing to fast onset, poor compliance. Duration of use: 3–6 months.
Nicotine Transdermal Patch: 24 hours Available: 7, 14, 21 mg per 24 hours. Maximum of 21 mg/day transdermally. Start with highest dose if patient smokes >10 cigarettes/day. Dose: Use daily for 6 weeks, then taper by 7 mg/day every 2 weeks.	Available over the counter. Use: Apply new patch to nonhairy, clean, dry skin on upper body or upper outer arm and wear for 16–24 hours. If cravings occur on awakening, wear for 24 hours. If vivid dreams or sleep disturbances occur, remove patch at bedtime. Rotate patch application site daily Can be used in combination with other agents and delivers consistent nicotine levels over 24 hours	Adverse effects: Skin sensitivity and irritation may affect up to 54% of users; also dizziness, headache, nausea, unusual dreams, racing heartbeat. Wash hands after applying or removing patch. Disadvantage: does not treat acute cravings. Duration of use: 8–10 weeks.
Nicotine Oral Inhaler Available: 4 mg/metered vapor in 10-mg cartridge. Maximum of 64 mg/day (16 cartridges). Dose: 6–16 cartridges/day for up to 12 weeks. Initially use 1 cartridge every 1–2 hours, then taper dose over 6–12 weeks.	Prescription only. Use: Inhale into back of throat or puff in short breaths. Do not inhale into lungs like a cigarette but "puff" as if lighting a pipe. Best effects with continuous puffing for 20 minutes. Most successful patients in clinical trials used between 6 and 16 cartridges/day. Recommend at least 6 cartridges/day for the first 6 wks. Mimics hand-to-mouth action of smoking, moderate compliance.	Adverse effects: local irritation of mouth and throat, coughing, rhinitis. Avoid in severe reactive airway disease. Cartridges might be less effective in cold environments (<60oF) Duration of use: 3–6 months.

[a]A 2013 Cochrane review of pharmacologic interventions for smoking cessation ranked various nicotine replacement therapies as being equivalent and second only to varenicline in treatment efficacy.

[b]Precautions for all products: Recent (<14 days) myocardial infarction, underlying cardiac arrhythmias, serious or worsening angina pectoris, adolescents (<18 years), pregnancy, breastfeeding. Taper slowly off all products.

From Nicotine. Drug Facts and Comparisons. Facts & Comparisons eAnswers. Wolters Kluwer Health, Inc. Riverwoods, IL. http://online.factsandcomparisons.com; Cahill K, Stevens S, Perera R, Lancaster T. Pharmacological interventions for smoking cessation: an overview and network meta-analysis. *Cochrane Database Syst Rev.*2013(5); Hartmann-Boyce J, Chepkin SC, Ye W, Bullen C, Lancaster T. Nicotine replacement therapy versus control for smoking cessation. *Cochrane Database Syst Rev.* 2018;5(5):CD0;00146; Palmer KJ, Buckley MM, Faulds D. Transdermal nicotine. A review of its pharmacodynamic and pharmacokinetic properties, and therapeutic efficacy as an aid to smoking cessation. *Drugs.* 1992;44:498-529; Nicotrol (nicotine) inhalation system [prescribing information]. New York, NY; Pfizer; December 2008.; Nicotrol NS (nicotine) nasal spray [prescribing information]. New York, NY: Pfizer; June 2010; Nicorette (nicotine) lozenge [prescribing information]. Moon Township, PA: GlaxoSmithKline Consumer Healthcare; 2014; Nicorelief gum [prescribing information]. Livonia, MI: Major Pharmaceuticals; October 2012; NicoDerm CQ (nicotine) transdermal system [prescribing information]. Moon Township, PA: GlaxoSmithKline; 2014; Nides M. Update on pharmacologic options for smoking cessation treatment. *Am J Med.* 2008;121(4 Suppl 1):S20-S31; Fiore MC, Jaen CR, Baker TB, et al. Treating tobacco use and dependence: 2008 update - clinical practice guideline, U.S. Department of Health and Human Services. May 2008. http://www.ahrq.gov/professionals/clinicians-providers/guidelines-recommendations/tobacco/index.html.

all pathologic diseases and conditions. From a timing perspective, this also makes sense because overt oral pathology requiring treatment should receive priority in scheduling and should therefore precede the definitive phase of care.

Chapter 6 discusses in detail the recognition, diagnosis, and management of oral cancer. For more specific information on the diagnosis and management of the numerous oral pathologic conditions, the reader should consult one of the many currently available texts in oral pathology. Suggested Readings are listed at the end of this chapter.

Replacement of a Missing Tooth or Teeth During the Disease Control Phase

Many patients do not wish to delay tooth replacements until the conclusion of the disease control phase of care. Although tooth replacement usually occurs during definitive phase therapy, it may be necessary and appropriate to place a provisional restoration or prostheses during the disease control phase to satisfy the patient's short-term esthetic or functional needs and maintain arch integrity (Figure 10.17).

Replacement of a missing single tooth in the anterior region is most typically accomplished by bonding in a denture tooth or the crown of the extracted tooth (Figure 10.18) or with a temporary removable partial denture or provisional fixed partial denture. Replacement of multiple missing teeth in the disease control phase is usually implemented with a provisional removable partial denture.

REASSESSMENT

The plan of care for the disease control phase includes a comprehensive reevaluation of the patient. This assessment provides the dentist with the opportunity to evaluate the patient's response to treatment, ascertain the patient's current condition, and determine the risk for future disease. As noted in the introduction to this chapter, this reassessment is sometimes designated as a posttreatment assessment. The disease control phase posttreatment assessment can follow the same general format as the posttreatment assessment described in Chapter 12, but with emphasis on the components in the patient's disease control phase plan of care.

Components of the disease control phase posttreatment assessment and sample questions include the following:

- Systemic status: Includes an update of the health history and vital signs. Have current conditions improved or worsened? Is the patient complying with recommended therapy? Have any new problems developed?
- Chief concern: Have the patient's major concerns been addressed? Are there any new concerns?
- Caries status: Are there new lesions? Has the patient complied with all recommended therapy? What are the results of repeated caries susceptibility tests? What is the current caries risk status?
- Condition of the marginal periodontium (see the section "Periodontal Reevaluation" earlier in this chapter): Is the patient at future risk of periodontal disease?
- Condition of the pulp and periapical tissue of any previously symptomatic teeth or teeth that have had a SCR or direct pulp cap procedure: Are there any residual signs or symptoms? What are the findings on a 6-month postoperative image of the tooth? Current pulp and apical diagnosis?
- Status of the occlusion and tooth alignment: Is there evidence of occlusal trauma? Does the patient have any esthetic concerns or functional limitations? What is the risk for tooth fracture?
- Condition and function of the TMJ complex: Are there signs or symptoms of TMD? Is the patient at risk of TMD?
- If there have been interventions for tobacco use or sleep disorders, have they been successful?
- Health of other oral tissues: Has all previously diagnosed oral pathology been managed or treated? Are there any new lesions? Is the patient at risk of new or recurrent pathologic lesions or conditions?

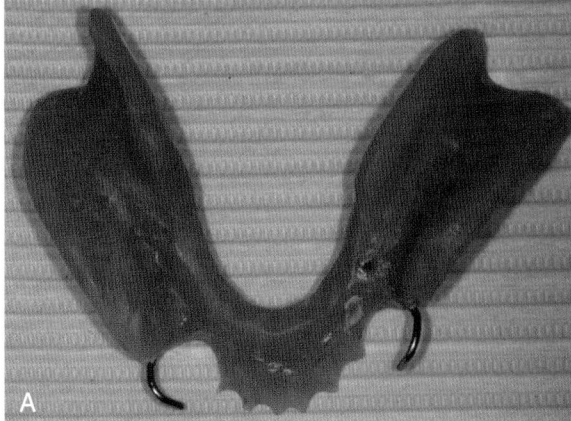
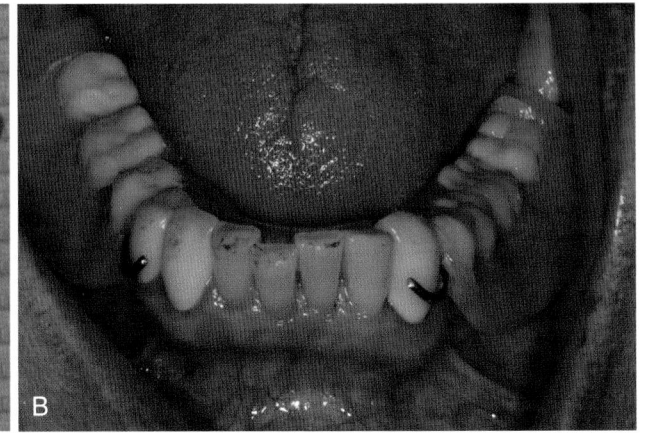

Fig. 10.17 (A, B) Provisional removable partial denture. (Courtesy Dr. Carlos H. Barrero.)

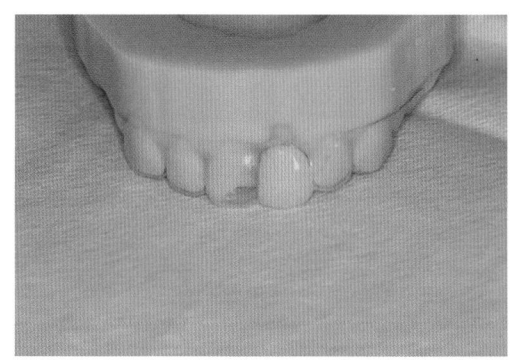
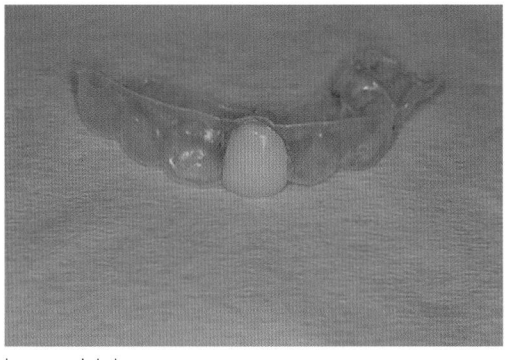

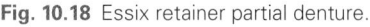

Fig. 10.18 Essix retainer partial denture.

MAKING THE TRANSITION TO THE DEFINITIVE PHASE OF CARE

After the comprehensive reevaluation or disease control phase posttreatment assessment, the dentist determines whether to continue disease control therapy or progress to the definitive phase. Both patient and practitioner will have been working toward definitive care and at this point are hoping to move to the next stage. A setback can be frustrating to both parties and can cause the patient to doubt their own resolve or to question whether confidence in the dentist has been misplaced. Nonetheless, it is also in the interest of both parties that aggressive reconstruction *not* be undertaken until the disease control phase has been completed successfully. To do otherwise is to invite failure of the treatment and an even greater level of frustration for the patient. Failure at that stage also carries greater legal risk for the dentist.

If the dentist deems it appropriate to move to the definitive phase, discussion can begin for the planning of care. If the plan includes fixed or removable prosthodontics, it is recommended that photographs and study casts be generated at this juncture. From these diagnostic records, the dentist can often more easily and accurately determine which treatment options are feasible and should be presented to the patient. This is also an ideal time for options to be redefined in light of the patient's response to treatment. Previous options may be discarded and new ones considered. As the patient engages in the conversation and comes to understand each option with its associated risks, benefits, costs, and demands, the best plan of care for the patient can be selected and informed consent acquired. In this way, the patient will move seamlessly into the definitive phase of care.

▮ REVIEW QUESTIONS

- When is a disease control phase indicated?
- Which elements should be included in a disease control phase?
- How should treatment be sequenced within the disease control phase?
- What is included in the basic caries control package? What is the rationale for each component?
- Which caries control measures may be needed beyond the basic caries control package? What are the indications for each?
- What are the common causes of periodontal diseases?
- Which treatment modalities are included in initial periodontal therapy?
- What are the indications for doing a selective caries removal procedure?
- What are the indications for amalgam, composite, and resin modified GI restorations?
- What single tooth restorative options are available in the disease control phase? What are the indications and contraindications for each?

- Identify common temporomandibular disorders. How do you manage each condition?
- What are causes of sleep disorders and what problems might sleep disorders induce?
- How would you advise and educate a patient who wishes to stop using tobacco products?
- What multiple tooth restorative options are available in the disease control Phase? What are the indications and contraindications for each?
- Which activities should be included in a disease control phase posttreatment assessment?

Practice Enhancements

- Design a management strategy for high caries risk patients in your practice.
- Design a management plan for patients with active periodontal disease.

REFERENCES

1. Marcenes W, Kassebaum NJ, Bernabe E, et al. Global burden of oral conditions in 1990-2010: a systematic analysis. *J Dent Res.* 2013;92(7):592–597.
2. Mellberg JR. The mechanism of fluoride protection. *Compendium Continuing Educ Dent.* 1997;18(2):37–43.
3. Ashley PF, Attrill DC, Ellwood RP, Worthington HV, Davies RM. Toothbrushing habits and caries experience. *Caries Res.* 1999;33(5):401–402.
4. Tavss E, Bontá CY, Joziak MT, Fisher SW, Campbell SK. High-potency sodium fluoride: a literature review. *Compendium Continuing Educ Dent.* 1997;18(2):313–316.
5. Bader JD, Shugars DA, Bonito AJ. A systematic review of selected caries prevention and management methods. *Community Dent Oral Epidemiol.* 2001;29(6):399–411.
6. Walsh T., Worthington H.V., Glenny A.M., Marinho V.C., Jeronic A. Fluoride toothpastes of different concentrations for preventing dental caries. Cochrane Database Syst Rev. 20194;3(3):CD007868.
7. Marinho VC, Higgins JP, Sheiham A, Logan S. Fluoride toothpastes for preventing dental caries in children and adolescents. *Cochrane Database Syst Rev.* 2003;1:CD002278.
8. Slayton RL, Urquhart O, Araujo MWB, et al. Evidence-based clinical practice guideline on nonrestorative treatments for carious lesions: A report from the American Dental Association. *J Am Dent Assoc.* 2018;149(10):837–849. e19.
9. Marsh PD. Are dental diseases examples of ecological catastrophes? *Microbiol.* 2003;149(2):279–294.
10. Pearce EI, Dibdin GH. The effect of pH, temperature and plaque thickness on the hydrolysis of monofluorophosphate in experimental dental plaque. *Caries Res May-Jun.* 2003;37(3):178–184.
11. Gustafsson BE, Quensel CE, Lanke LS, et al. The Vipeholm dental caries study; the effect of different levels of carbohydrate intake on caries activity in 436 individuals observed for five years. *Acta Odontol Scand.* 1954;11(3-4):232–264.
12. Harris R. Biology of the children of Hopewood House, Bowral, Australia. 4. Observations on dental-caries experience extending over five years [1957-61]. *J Dent Res.* 1963;42:1387–1399.
13. Fontana M, Gonzalez-Cabezas C. Are we ready for definitive clinical guidelines on xylitol/polyol use? *Adv Dent Res.* 2012;24(2):123–128.
14. Ahovuo-Saloranta A, Forss H, Walsh T, et al. Sealants for preventing dental decay in the permanent teeth. *Cochrane Database Syst Rev Mar.* 2013;28(3):CD001830.
15. Beauchamp J, Caufield PW, Crall JJ, et al. American Dental Association Council on Scientific Affairs. Evidence-based clinical recommendations for the use of pit-and-fissure sealants: a report of the American Dental Association Council on Scientific Affairs. *J Am Dent Assoc Mar.* 2008;139(3):257–268.
16. Simonsen RJ. From prevention to therapy: minimal intervention with sealants and resin restorative materials. *J Dent Dec.* 2011;39(Suppl 2):S27–S33.
17. Randall RC, Wilson NHF. Glass-ionomer restoratives: a systematic review of a secondary caries treatment effect. *J Dent Res.* 1999;78(2):628–637.
18. Donly KJ, Segura A, Wefel JS, Hogan MM. Evaluating the effects of fluoride releasing dental materials on adjacent interproximal caries. *J Am Dent Assoc.* 1999;130(6):817–825.
19. Raggio DP1, Hesse D, Lenzi TL, A B Guglielmi C, Braga MM. Is atraumatic restorative treatment an option for restoring occlusoproximal caries lesions in primary teeth? A systematic review and meta-analysis. *Int J Paediatr Dent Nov.* 2013;23(6):435–443.
20. de Amorim RG, Leal SC, Frencken JE. Survival of atraumatic restorative treatment (ART) sealants and restorations: a meta-analysis. *Clin Oral Investig Apr.* 2012;16(2):429–441.
21. Mickenautsch S, Yengopal V. Failure rate of atraumatic restorative treatment using high-viscosity glass-ionomer cement compared to that of conventional amalgam restorative treatment in primary and permanent teeth: a systematic review update. *J Minimum Intervent Dent.* 2012;5:63–124.
22. JE1 Frencken, Peters MC, Manton DJ, Leal SC, Gordan VV, Eden E: Minimal intervention dentistry for managing dental caries - a review: report of a FDI task group. *Int Dent J Oct.* 2012;62(5):223–243.
23. Ramfjord SP, Morrison EC, Burgett FG, et al. Oral hygiene and maintenance of periodontal support. *J Periodontol.* 1982;53(1):26–30.
24. Mousques T, Listgarten MA, Phillips RW. Effects of scaling and root planing on the composition of the human subgingival microbial flora. *J Periodontal Res.* 1980;15(2):144–151.
25. Nibali L, Bayliss-Chapman J, Almofareh SA, Zhou Y, Divaris K, Vieira AR. What is the heritability of periodontitis? a systematic review. *J Dent Res.* 2019;98(6):632–641.
26. Loos B.G., Van Dyke T.E. The role of inflammation and genetics in periodontal disease. Periodontology 2000;83(1):26-39.
27. Divaris K, Monda KL, North KE, et al. Exploring the genetic basis of chronic periodontitis: a genome-wide association study. *Hum Mol Genet.* 2013;22(11):2312–2324.
28. Barros SP, Offenbacher S. Epigenetics: connective environment and genotype to phenotype and disease. *J Dent Res.* 2009;88(5):400–408.
29. Grossi SG, Genco RJ. Periodontal disease and diabetes mellitus: a two-way relationship. *Ann Periodontol.* 1998;3(1):51–61.
30. Hart TC, Atkinson JC. Mendelian forms of periodontitis. *Periodontol 2000.* 2007;45:95–112.
31. Kinane DF. Periodontitis modified by systemic factors. *Ann Periodontol.* 1999;4(1):54–64.
32. Kinane DF, Peterson M, Stathopoulou PG. Environmental and other modifying factors of periodontal diseases. *Periodontol 2000.* 2006;40:107–119.
33. Robinson PG. Treatment of HIV-associated periodontal diseases, Oral Dis 3. *S238-S240.* 1997
34. Offenbacher S. Periodontal diseases: pathogenesis. *Ann Periodontol.* 1996;1(1):821–878.
35. Nociti FH, Casati MZ, Duarte PM. Current perspective of the impact of smoking on the progression and treatment of periodontitis. *Periodontology 2000.* 2015;67:187–210.
36. Dietrich T, Bernimoulin JP, Glynn RJ. The effect of cigarette smoking on gingival bleeding. *J Periodontol.* 2004;75(1):16–22.
37. Preber H, Bergström J. Occurrence of gingival bleeding in smoker and non-smoker patients. *Acta Odontol Scand.* 1985;43:315–320.
38. Tomar SL, Asma S. Smoking-attributable periodontitis in the United States: findings from NHANES III. National Health and Nutrition Examination Survey. *J Periodontol.* 2000;71(5):743–751.
39. Blanton PL, Hurt WC, Largent MD. Oral factitious injuries. *J Periodontol.* 1977;48(1):33–37.
40. Lang NP, Kiel RA, Anderhalden K. Clinical and microbiological effects of subgingival restorations with overhanging or clinically perfect margins. *J Clin Periodontol.* 1983;10(6):563–578.

41. Brunsvold MA, Lane JJ. The prevalence of overhanging dental restorations and their relationship to periodontal disease. *J Clin Periodontol*. 1990;17(2):67–72.

42. Deas DE, Mealey BL. Is there an association between occlusion and periodontal destruction? Only in limited circumstances does occlusal force contribute to periodontal disease progression. *J Am Dent Assoc*. 2006;137(10):1381 1383, 1385.

43. Harrel SK, Nunn Me, Hallmon WW:. Is there an association between occlusion and periodontal destruction? Yes – occlusal forces can contribute to periodontal destruction. *J Am Dent Assoc*. 2006;137(10):1380 1382, 1384.

44. Greenstein G, Polson A. Understanding tooth mobility. *Compendium*. 1998;9(6):470–471. 473-6, 478-9.

45. Claydon NC. Current concepts in toothbrushing and interdental cleaning. *Periodontol 2000*. 2008;48:10–22.

46. Ciancio SG. The dental water jet: a product ahead of its time. *Compend Contin Educ Dent*. 2009;30(Spec No 1):7–13.

47. Van der Sleen MI, Slot DE, Van Trijffel E, Winkel EG, Van der Weijden GA. Effectiveness of mechanical tongue cleaning on breath odour and tongue coating: a systematic review. *Int J Dent Hyg*. 2010;8(4):258–268.

48. Gunsolley JC. A meta-analysis of six-month studies of antiplaque and antigingivitis agents. *J Am Dent Assoc*. 2006;137(12):1649–1657.

49. American Academy of Periodontology Systemic antibiotics in periodontics. *J Periodontol*. 2004;75(11):1553–1565.

50. Teughels W, Feres M, Oud V, Martin C, Matesanz P, Herrera D. Adjunctive effect of systemic antimicrobials in periodontitis therapy. A systematic review and meta-analysis. *Journal of Clinical Periodontology*. 2020

51. Segelnick SL, Weinberg MA. Reevaluation of initial therapy: when is the appropriate time? *J Periodontol*. 2006;77(9):1598–1601.

52. Larson TD. Clinical uses of glutaraldehyde/2-hydroxyethlmethacrylate (GLUMA). *Northwest Dent*. 2013;92(2):27–30.

53. Sjogren U, Hagglund B, Sundqvist G, Wing K. Factors affecting the long-term results of endodontic treatment. *J Endod*. 1990;16(10):498–504.

54. Strindberg LZ. The dependence of the results of pulp therapy on certain factors. *Acta Odontol Scand 14*. 1956;Suppl 21:1–175.

55. Christensen GJ. Pulp capping 1998. *J Am Dent Assoc*. 1998;129(9):1297–1299.

56. Cushley S, Duncan H, Cappin M, et al. Efficacy of direct pulp capping for management of cariously exposed pulps in permanent teeth: a systematic review and meta-analysis. *Int Endod J*. 2021;54(4):556–571.

57. Hilton TJ Keys to clinical success with pulp capping: a review of the literature. *Oper Dent*. 2009;34(5):615–625.

58. Taha NA, Khazali MA. Partial pulpotomy in mature permanent teeth with clinical signs indicative of irreversible pulpitis: a randomized clinical trial. *J Endod*. 2017;43(9):1417–1421.

59. Lin GSS, Hisham ARB, Ch Er CIY, Cheah KK, Ghani NRNA, Noorani TY. Success rates of coronal and partial pulpotomies in mature permanent molars: a systematic review and single-arm meta-analysis. *Quintessence Int*. 2021. https://doi.org/10.3290/j.qi.b912685.

60. Orofacial Pain: Guidelines for Assessment,De Leeuw R, KG, ed. *Diagnosis, and Management* 6th ed · Quintessence Publishing; 2018.

61. Peck CC, Goulet J-P, Lobbezoo F, et al. Expanding the taxonomy of the diagnostic criteria for temporomandibular disorders. *J Oral Rehabil*. 2014;41(1):2–23.

62. Schiffman E, Ohrbach R, Truelove E, et al. Diagnostic criteria for temporomandibular disorders (DC/TMD) for clinical and research applications: recommendations of the International RDC/TMD Consortium Network and Orofacial Pain Special Interest Groupdagger. *J Oral Facial Pain Headache*. 2014;28(1):6–27.

63. International Classification of Orofacial Pain, 1st ed (ICOP). Cephalalgia, 2020. 40(2): p. 129-221.

64. Maixner W, Diatchenko L, Dubner R, et al. Orofacial pain prospective evaluation and risk assessment study—the OPPERA study. *J Pain*. 2011;12(11 Suppl):T4–T11. e1-2.

65. https://dentalsleeppractice.com/ada-policy-statement-and-the-role-of-dentistry-in-the-treatment-of-sleep-related-breathing-disorders/

66. Gagnon Y, Mayer P, Morisson F, Rompré PH, Lavigne GJ. Aggravation of respiratory disturbances by the use of an occlusal splint in apneic patients: a pilot study. *Int J Prosthodont*. 2004 Jul-Aug;17(4):447–453.

67. https://www.prosthodontics.org/assets/1/7/16.Role_of_Oral_Devices_in_Managing_Sleep-disordered_Breathing_Patients.pdf .

68. Tsuda H, Almeida FR, Tsuda T, Moritsuchi Y, Lowe AA. Craniofacial changes after 2 years of nasal continuous positive airway pressure use in patients with obstructive sleep apnea. *Chest*. 2010 Oct;138(4):870–874.

69. Pliska BT, Almeida FR. Tooth movement associated with CPAP therapy. *J Clin Sleep Med*. 2018 Apr 15;14(4):701–702.

70. Rotenberg BW, Murariu D, Pang KP. Trends in CPAP adherence over twenty years of data collection: a flattened curve. *J Otolaryngol Head Neck Surg*. 2016;45(1):43.

71. Ramar K, Dort LC, Katz SG, et al. Clinical Practice Guideline for the Treatment of Obstructive Sleep Apnea and Snoring with Oral Appliance Therapy: An Update for 2015. *J Clin Sleep Med*. 2015;11(7):773–827.

72. Levine M, Bennett K, Cantwell M, Postol K, Schwartz D. *Dental sleep medicine standards for screening, treating, and managing adults with sleep-related breathing disorders. J. Dent Sleep Med*. 2018;5(3):61–68.

73. Bartolucci ML, Bortolotti F, Martina S, Corazza G, Michelotti A, Alessandri-Bonetti G. Dental and skeletal long-term side effects of mandibular advancement devices in obstructive sleep apnea patients: a systematic review with meta-regression analysis. *Eur J Orthod*. 2019;41(1):89–100.

74. Sheats RD, Schell TG, Blanton AO, et al. Management of side effects of oral appliance therapy for sleep-disordered breathing. *Journal of Dental Sleep Medicine*. 2017;4(4):111–125.

75. National Cancer Institute. *Tobacco research implementation plan: priorities for tobacco research beyond the year 2000. National Cancer Institute and National Institutes of Health*. Bethesda Md: NIH Publication; 1998.

76. Somerman M, Mecklenburg RE. Cessation of tobacco use. In: Ciancio SG, ed. *ADA Guide to Dental Therapeutics*. Chicago: American Dental Association; 1998.

77. Gelskey SC. Impact of a dental/dental hygiene tobacco-use cessation curriculum on practice. *J Dent Educ*. 2002;66(9):1074–1078.

78. Hartmann-Boyce J, Chepkin SC, Ye W, Bullen C, Lancaster T. Nicotine replacement therapy versus control for smoking cessation. *Cochrane Database Syst Rev*. 2018;5(5):CD000146.

79. U.S. Department of Health and Human Services. *Cigars: health effects and trends. smoking and tobacco control program, monograph 9. National Cancer Institute and National Institutes of Health*. Bethesda Md: USDHHS Publication; 1998:98–4302.

80. Regezi JA, Sciubba JJ, Jordan RC. *Oral pathology: clinical pathologic correlations.* ed 4 Philadelphia: Saunders; 2003.

81. Silverman S. *American Cancer Society atlas of clinical oncology: oral cancer.* ed 5 Hamilton, Ontario: BC Decker; 2003.

82. Mecklenburg RE, Greenspan D, Kleinman DV, et al. *Tobacco effects in the mouth. A National Cancer Institute and National Institute of Dental Research guide for health professionals. National Cancer Institute and National Institutes of Health.* Bethesda Md: NIH Publication; 2000. No. 00-3330.

83. DeWitt KD, Lee N. Benign and malignant lesions of the oral cavity, oropharynx, and nasopharynx. In: Lalwani AK, ed. *Current Diagnosis and Treatment in Otolaryngology—Head and Neck Surgery.* New York: Lange Medical Books/McGraw-Hill; 2004.

84. U.S. Department of Health and Human Services. *Smokeless tobacco or health, monograph 2. National Cancer Institute and National Institutes of Health.* Bethesda Md: USDHHS Publication; 1993.

85. National Health Interview Survey – NCHS Data Brief No 365, April 2020. https://www.cdc.gov>nchs>National Health Interview Survey>Data Briefs>Electronic Cigarette Use Among U.S. Adults, 2018.

86. Gallup 2018. https://news.gallup.com>poll>percentage-americans-vape.

87. National Youth Tobacco Survey. https://www.fda.gov>tobacco-products>Results from the Annual National Youth Tobacco Survey. Accessed October 9, 2021.

88. https://www.WebMD.com>Connect to Care>Vaping>4 Major Health Risks Linked to E-cigarette Use. Accessed October 7, 2021.

89. Centers for Disease Control and Prevention. Outbreak of lung injury associated with the use of e-cigarettes, or vaping, products. CDC Bull12/12/2019. https://www.cdc.gov/tobacco/basic_information/e-cigarettes/severe-lung-disease.htm.

90. https://www.hopkinsmedicine.org>Health>Search>Vaping>5 Vaping Facts You Need to Know. Accessed October 7, 2021.

91. Irusa KF, Vence B, Donovan T. Potential oral health effects of e-cigarettes and vaping: A review and case reports. *J Esthetic Rest Dent.* 2020;32:260–264.

92. US Office of the Surgeon General. e-cigarettes.surgeongeneral. gov>Know the Risks> E-Cigarettes & Young People. Accessed October 7, 2021.

93. American Dental Association Summary of Policy and Recommendations Regarding Tobacco (1964 – Present). https://www.ada.org/ ADA Positions, Policies and Statements/Tobacco and Nicotine. Accessed October 7, 2021.

94. Houston JP, McCollum J, Pietz D, et al. Alveolar osteitis: a review of its etiology, prevention, and treatment modalities. *Gen Dent.* 2002;50(5):457–463.

95. Karoussis IK, Muller S, Salvi GE, et al. Association between periodontal and peri-implant conditions: a 10-year prospective study. *Clin Oral Implants Res.* 2004;15(1):1–7.

96. Tomar SL. Dentistry's role in tobacco control. *J Am Dent Assoc.* 2001;132(Supplement):30s–35s.

97. Bergstrom J. Tobacco smoking and chronic destructive periodontal disease. *Odontology.* 2004;92:1–8.

98. Warnakulasuriya S, Sutherland G, Scully C. Tobacco, oral cancer, and treatment of dependence. *Oral Oncol.* 2005;41:244–260.

99. Dietrich T, Hoffmann K. A comprehensive index for the modeling of smoking history in periodontal research. *J Dent Res.* 2004;83:859–863.

100. https://www.cancer.gov/news-events/cancer-currents-blog/2015/smoking-burden

101. https://www.cancer.gov/about-cancer/causes-prevention/risk/tobacco/cessation-fact-sheet

102. https://www.cancer.gov/about-cancer/causes-prevention/risk/tobacco/help-quitting-fact-sheet

103. Chapman S, MacKenzie R. The global research neglect of unassisted smoking cessation: causes and consequences. *PLoS Medicine.* 2010;7(2):e1000216.

104. Ramseier C. Smoking prevention and cessation. *Oral Health Prev Dent.* 2003:427–439. Supplement 1.

105. Miller WR, Rollnick S. *Motivational interviewing.* New York: Guilford Press; 2002.

106. Prochaska JO, DiClemente CC. Stages and processes of self-change of smoking: toward an integrative model of change. *J Consult Clin Psychol.* 1983;51:390–395.

107. https:www.cdc.gov>materials> The Brief Tobacco Intervention – Quick Reference for Health Care Providers

108. Hughes JR, Stead LF, Hartmann-Boyce J, Cahill K, Lancaster T. Antidepressants for smoking cessation. *Cochrane Database Syst Rev.* 2014;1:CD000031.

109. Fagerstrom KO. Measuring degree of physical dependence to tobacco smoking with reference to individualization of treatment. *Addict Behav.* 1978;3:235–241.

SUGGESTED READINGS

CARIES

Cochrane Collaboration www.cochrane.org/reviews/clibintro.htm/ (see Dentistry and oral health/ Dental caries).

Doméjean S, White JM, Featherstone JD. Caries management by risk assessment (CAMBRA) group validation of the CDA CAMBRA caries risk assessment—a six-year retrospective study. *J Calif Dent Assoc.* 2011

Fejerskov O, Kidd E. *Dental Caries: the Disease and Its Clinical Management.* ed 3 Oxford, UK: Blackwell; 2015.

Ritter AV, Boushell L, Walter R. *Sturdevant's the Art and Science of Operative Dentistry, ed 7.* St Louis. : Mosby; 2018.

Young DA, Fontana M, Wolff MS. Current concepts in cariology. *Dent Clin N Am.* 2010;54(53):v-viii.

PERIODONTAL DISEASE

Berglundh T, Giannobile W, Sanz M, Lang N. *Linde's Clinical Periodontology and Implant Dentistry.* ed 7 Oxford: Wiley-Blackwell; 2021.

Caton JG, Armitage G, Berglundh T, Al. A new classification scheme for periodontal and per-implant diseases and conditions – introduction and key changes from the 1999 classification. *Journal of Periodontology.* 2018;89(suppl 1):S1–S8.

Newman MG, Takei H, Klokkevoid PR, Carranza FA. *Newman & Carranza's Clinical Periodontology.* ed 13 St Louis: Saunders; 2019.

TEMPOROMANDIBULAR JOINT DISORDERS

De Leeuw R, ed. American Academy of Orofacial Pain. *Orofacial Pain—Guidelines for Assessment, Diagnosis and Management*. ed 6 Chicago: Quintessence; 2018.

Okeson JP. *Management of Temporomandibular Disorders and Occlusion*. ed 8 St Louis: Mosby; 2020.

American Academy of Orofacial Pain. https://aaop.org.

ENDODONTICS

Berman LH, Hargreaves KM. Cohen's pathways of the pulp. ed 12 St Louis: Mosby; 2021.

Torabinejab M, Fouad A, Shabahang S. *Endodontics: Principles and Practice*. ed 6 St Louis: Saunders; 2020.

ORAL PATHOLOGIC CONDITIONS

Neville BW, Damm DD, Allen CM, Chi A. *Oral and Maxillofacial Pathology*. ed 4 St Louis: Elsevier; 2015.

Regezi JA, Sciubba J, Jordan RC. *Oral Pathology: Clinical-Pathological Correlations*. ed 7 St Louis: Elsevier; 2016.

11

The Definitive Phase of Treatment

Samuel Nesbit, Jonathan Reside, Antonio Moretti, Tate Jackson, Lee Boushell, Gustavo Oliveira, Peter Tawil, Ibrahim Duqum, Wendy Clark, and Carlos Barrero

Visit eBooks.Health.Elsevier.com

OUTLINE

A **definitive phase of care** is indicated when the patient needs surgical, functional, esthetic and/or restorative therapy or treatment to establish a condition of optimal comprehensive oral health within the scope of their health status, social determinants of health, and autonomous choices. The purpose of the definitive phase is to assist the patient in achieving the best possible state of oral health within the context of the patient's desires, abilities and resources. This phase forms the core of virtually every patient's plan of care. An exceptions is when the patient is currently in a disease control plan (see Chapter 10) and for whom a definitive phase plan cannot yet be determined. Patients who need preventive services (e.g. oral prophylaxis and oral hygiene instruction) but who do not need a disease control plan will have those services completed in the Definitive phase. Commonly the definitive phase will include elective surgical procedures; orthodontic therapy; single tooth restorations, implants; and any definitive tooth replacements.

Before engaging in definitive phase treatment, the practitioner should affirm that the following requisites have been met:
- For patients who required a disease control treatment plan, all such therapy must have been completed and all active disease and infection eliminated, arrested, or otherwise addressed. After a posttreatment assessment, the

success or failure of the control phase should be discussed with the patient. If the objectives of the disease control phase have not been met, it is imperative that appropriate additional control phase treatment be instituted or that the definitive phase plan be adjusted to accommodate this new reality.
- All reasonable definitive phase treatment options must have been thoroughly evaluated and discussed with the patient. If this process occurred at an earlier point (possibly at the time that the disease control plan was formulated), the plan should now be reviewed and reconsidered.
- Finally, the dentist must reach an informed consent agreement with the patient. This will involve a clear understanding of the diagnoses, the advantages and disadvantages of the various treatment options, and the details of the proposed plan including associated risks and hazards, contingencies, prognosis, time required for completion, and costs.

In general, the discussion of these topics in the following pages reflects the spectrum of today's practice of general dentistry. The aim of this chapter is to suggest the range of clinical options available for representative situations. For each topic, professional considerations and patient considerations that influence and shape the decision-making process are discussed. For more in-depth coverage of specific areas, several excellent texts are available for each of the clinical disciplines of dentistry covering diagnosis, treatment planning, and therapy (see Suggested Readings at the end of this chapter).

DEFINITIVE PHASE TREATMENT OPTIONS

PERIODONTAL THERAPY

After initial therapy, additional treatment may be indicated for diseased sites where periodontal pockets and bleeding persist after scaling and root planing. In some cases antibiotic therapy delivered locally or systemically may be a useful adjunct. When nonsurgical reinstrumentation is planned, reflecting gingival flaps to improve access and increase visibility of root deposits may be necessary. Surgical interventions to noninflammatory periodontal conditions may also be considered for esthetic problems such as excessive gingival display or black triangles. Surgery is necessary to correct ridge deficiencies or gingival recession with tooth root exposure and can be an invaluable adjunct to restorative correction of tooth defects caused by external resorption. Candidates for implant-supported prostheses with inadequate alveolar bone dimensions may require bone and/or sinus augmentation in preparation for implant placement. Concurrent occlusal therapy (discussed later in this chapter) may be indicated to reduce **secondary occlusal trauma**.

Periodontal Disease and Related Conditions

The following clinical situations related to the periodontal tissues and structures are commonly addressed in the definitive phase of treatment.

Periodontitis not Responsive to Initial Therapy

As discussed in Chapter 10, initial therapy for periodontitis usually consists of meticulous scaling and root planing (often performed under local anesthesia); specific instruction in oral hygiene; and, after a 4- to 8-week period, a detailed reevaluation including new periodontal charting.[1] Although most patients respond favorably to this regimen, some do not. Others may respond well at some sites and not so well at others. The causes of failure may include the presence of periodontally pathogenic bacteria, poor oral hygiene, site-specific impediments to plaque/biofilm control, or inadequate host response as a result of systemic factors, such as cigarette smoking and/or poorly-controlled diabetes.

Bone Loss

Alveolar bone loss contributes to the formation of deeper periodontal pockets and frequently impairs access for biofilm removal. The loss of alveolar support also exposes underlying root concavities and other anatomic niches to the oral environment, favoring biofilm accumulation that is difficult to access and predisposing the tooth to caries or periodontal disease. Although the ultimate impact of bone loss will vary based on tooth type, root length, and various anatomic factors,

teeth with untreated, progressive bone loss generally have a poorer prognosis.

Bone loss occurs either horizontally or vertically. The type of bone loss is initially determined radiographically, using an imaginary line connecting the interproximal cementoenamel junctions of the adjacent teeth and comparing it with the underlying crestal bone contours/angulation. Vertical, or angular, bone loss is further classified according to the number of remaining bony walls (i.e., one-, two-, or three-walled defects), which are typically identified during the course of periodontal surgery. Vertical bone loss poses an additional challenge to the management of periodontal disease because of the difficulties in accessing the depth of the defect during treatment. It is important to rule out root fractures or periodontal-endodontic lesions when a vertical bone defect is identified.

Anatomic Issues

Furcation Involvement. When progressive alveolar bone loss advances to the furcation area of a multirooted tooth, the condition is described as **furcation involvement**. The furcation defect may be further classified depending on the pattern and extent of bone loss in the furcation area. Several furcation classification systems have been developed, such as the Hamp Classification System[2] and the Glickman Classification System.[3]

Patients have an increased likelihood of developing furcation involvement when they have a short root trunk. Cervical enamel projections and enamel pearls also predispose a patient to more readily developing a furcation defect. Given the difficulty accessing the furcation by the patient for daily home care and the oral health care profession at maintenance visits, plaque/biofilm control in furcation defects is often very challenging. Consequently, the presence of furcation involvement almost without exception worsens the prognosis of the tooth.

Root Proximity. The close proximity of roots, as a result of natural occurrence or orthodontic treatment, presents an additional obstacle to the management of periodontitis. In the presence of inflammation, the narrow interradicular bone is more vulnerable to rapid and dramatic destruction, affecting two or more teeth concomitantly.

Third Molars. Malposed third molars may lead to bone loss, periodontal pocketing, and dental caries on the distal aspect of the adjacent teeth. In these cases, timely management is indicated to minimize the risk of attachment loss around or irreversible damage to the second molars.

Grooves. Palatogingival, or distolingual, grooves may be seen on maxillary incisors caused by aberrant tooth development. These grooves cross the cingulum and extend to various levels on the root, making adequate biofilm control in these areas extremely difficult. It is not uncommon to see localized deep probing depths and bone loss adjacent to these grooves.

Open Proximal Contacts. Open contacts are susceptible to food impaction and, potentially, discomfort for the patient. Although their impact in predisposing a site to gingival inflammation, increased probing depths, and bone loss is contended, careful oral hygiene is recommended nonetheless to ensure periodontal health.

Cleft lip or palate. In the presence of a cleft lip, the patient may be self-conscious about the defect and experience social embarrassment and low self-esteem. A cleft palate may result in airway problems, aspiration of food or fluids, respiratory infections, difficulty swallowing, or altered speech.

Congenital or Medication-Associated Gingival Enlargement

Gingival enlargement can occur as a result of a genetic predisposition or in response to certain medications, including anticonvulsants such as phenytoin (Dilantin), calcium-channel blockers (e.g., Nifedipine), or the immunosuppressant drug cyclosporine.[4] Gingival enlargement may compromise esthetics and often inhibits effective oral hygiene (Figure 11.1). In extreme instances, if it extends past the coronal surfaces of the teeth, overgrowth can interfere with mastication.

Mucogingival Deformities and Conditions

Mucogingival conditions are defined as altered relationships between the gingival margin and mucogingival junction that either do not allow control of inflammation or are associated with progressive gingival recession. Common clinical findings include singular or multiple areas of gingival recession, minimal or absent keratinized gingiva, and probing depths that extend beyond the mucogingival junction. Mucogingival defects can result from local factors or from mechanical trauma to the tissue, such as toothbrush trauma (Figure 11.2). Patients with a **thin gingival phenotype** are more susceptible to gingival recession than those with a thick gingival phenotype. Special attention should be given to sites with thin and narrow bands of keratinized tissue, especially when subgingival margin placement or orthodontic tooth movement is planned.

High Frenal Attachment

If the maxillary labial frenum is coronally inserted, it may contribute to the presence of a diastema that the patient may regard as unesthetic. High buccal or facial frenula may complicate denture construction (Figure 11.3).

Other Esthetic and Architectural Defects or Problems

Some patients present with periodontal conditions that they perceive to be unesthetic. Examples include a high lip line, short clinical crowns, excessive gingival display, gingival pigmentation, and loss of interproximal papilla. Tissue piercing and oral jewelry often contribute to the development of periodontal tissue loss. Traumatic injuries and surgical removal of lesions in the oral cavity can cause defects in the jaws and oral soft tissue.

Keys to Decision Making
Professional Considerations

Before considering retreatment, new surgical periodontal therapy, or other adjunctive periodontal procedures, the dentist should evaluate the importance of any relevant systemic factors, tooth-related problems, and localized periodontal conditions. Systemic factors of note could include diabetes or a history of tobacco use. If the patient is a smoker, has smoking cessation been recommended? (See Chapter 10 for discussion of smoking cessation.) If medication-induced problems are present (e.g., medication-induced gingival enlargement), can the drug regimen be altered with concomitant approval by the patient's medical provider? If periodontal surgery is considered, will the patient's general health be a limiting factor?

Tooth-related issues include an assessment of whether the teeth in question have a good restorative prognosis independent of the periodontal findings. Is there a tooth-related cause for the

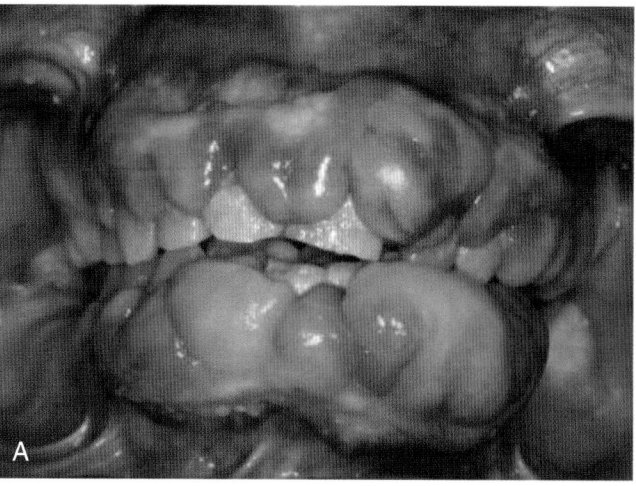
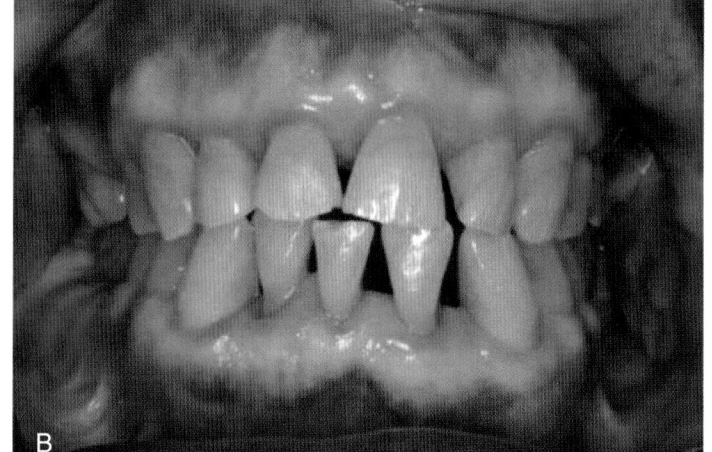

Fig. 11.1 Drug-Influenced Gingival Enlargement. (A) 54 year-old female with amlodipine-induced gingival overgrowth. **(B)** 7 months after full mouth gingivectomy and modification of her anti-hypertensive drug regimen. (Courtesy: Dr. Alex Gillone, Greenville, N.C.)

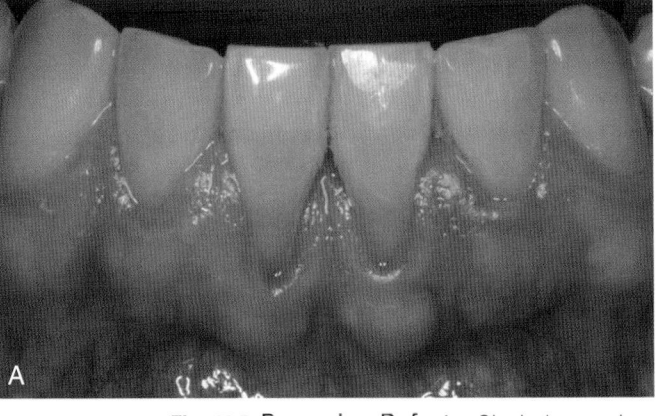
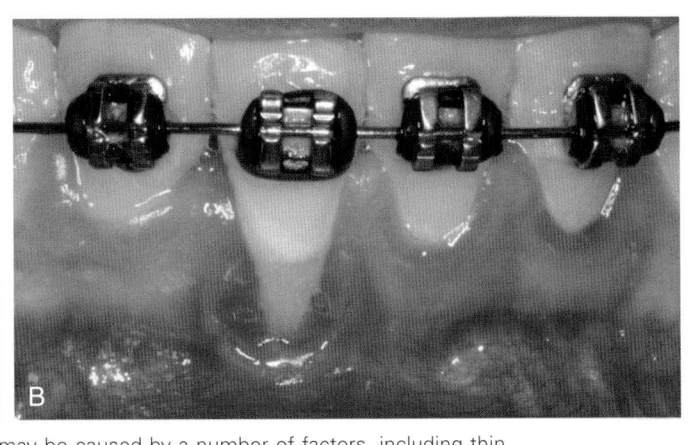

Fig. 11.2 Recession Defects. Gingival recession may be caused by a number of factors, including thin gingival biotype, periodontal disease, improper tooth position (i.e., facial tooth positioning), and trauma (i.e., heavy toothbrushing). Gingival recession may be confined to the keratinized tissue or extend to the mucogingival junction leading to a loss of attached gingiva. Various soft tissue augmentation procedures have been developed to help address recession defects. (Courtesy Dr. Jonathan Reside and Dr. Antonio Moretti.)

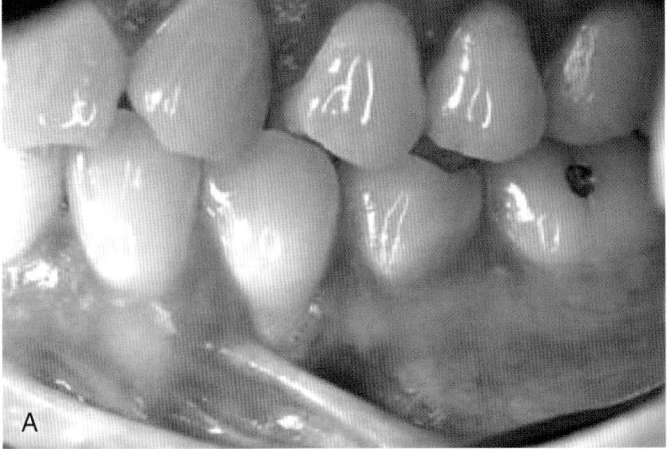
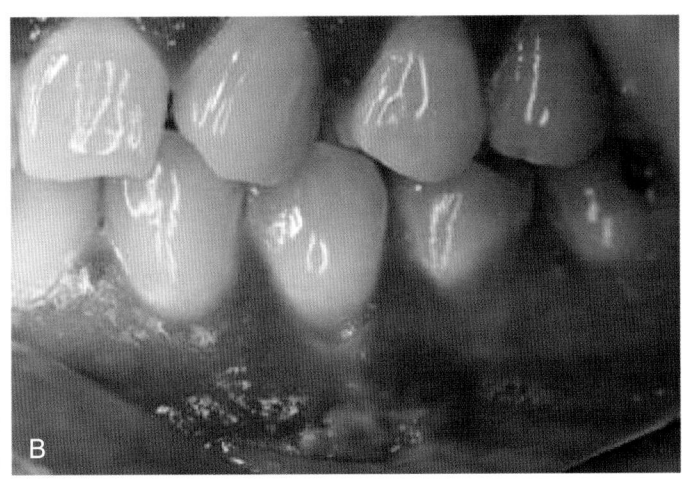

Fig. 11.3 Frenum pull **(A)** before surgery and **(B)** 2 weeks after surgery. (Courtesy Dr Antonio Moretti.)

current periodontal problem, such as an open proximal contact, calculus, or a poorly contoured restoration? How important is retention of the tooth (or teeth) to the patient's overall oral condition?

Localized periodontal factors that should be assessed include plaque accumulation, bleeding on probing, soft tissue and bone topography, probing depths, clinical attachment levels, furcation invasions, mucogingival relationships, tooth mobility, and occlusal factors (Figure 11.3). In addition to conventional methods of evaluation, the patient's periodontal status may warrant use of additional diagnostic procedures, such as microbial testing or medical laboratory tests. Other factors that the dentist will assess include the level of overall patient compliance and response to previous therapy and oral self-care instructions. In addition, the prognosis for any treatment

options under consideration, including the option of no treatment, should be weighed.

Patient Considerations

Some behavioral issues can be pivotal to the treatment decisions for the periodontal tissue–related conditions described earlier. Does the patient engage in a healthy lifestyle and maintain good control of any systemic conditions? Does the patient use any tobacco products? Does the patient understand and value the importance of the proposed treatment? Is the patient motivated to preserve the teeth in question? If not, can they be motivated to accept and appreciate the treatment?

Patient-specific issues may affect the planning, timing, and sequencing of definitive periodontal therapy. Is the patient in discomfort or experiencing any symptoms related to the condition? Are there personal reasons motivating the patient to have the treatment (e.g., esthetics, halitosis)? If so, the dental team will need to be sure that these concerns are addressed in the course of therapy. Does the patient have a preference for a particular form of therapy? Are they willing to undergo the removal of hopeless teeth? Are they willing to accept treatment for teeth with a guarded prognosis? Are they willing to undergo the postoperative discomfort of a surgical procedure?

Other important questions to ask before proceeding with definitive care include: Does the patient have the necessary time and financial resources for the treatment? Is the patient willing to follow through with long-term maintenance therapy?

Procedures for Treating Periodontal Disease

Local Delivery Antimicrobials

Local delivery antimicrobials have been an important addition to the periodontal disease treatment armamentarium. The site-specific use of antimicrobials is recommended when a few localized and persistently inflamed pockets have been unresponsive to conventional therapies, including initial scaling and root planing and/or periodontal surgery.[5] The use of these agents in most periodontitis patients is not a substitute for periodontal surgery and should be considered only after conventional periodontal therapies have been completed. Other indications would be the presence of isolated deep probing depths in an immunocompromised host, severe forms of periodontitis, and select peri-implant defects (Box 11.1).

Three commercially available local antibiotic-antimicrobial delivery systems are currently approved for use in the United States: (1) Atridox (doxycycline in a polylactic acid polymer), (2) Perio-Chip (CHX chlorhexidine in a gelatin chip), and (3) Arestin (minocycline in a polyglycolide-co-DL-lactide carrier). These agents are resorbable and, in many jurisdictions, may be placed by a dental hygienist. A meta-analysis of more than 50 studies has confirmed that the subgingival application of local delivery antimicrobials results in statistically significant improvements in probing pocket depth and clinical attachment levels.[6] Although evidence supports the use of these products as an adjunct to debridement in deep periodontal pockets or sites with persistent gingival inflammation, the magnitude of clinical benefits is typically modest. Some patients, however, may achieve high therapeutic benefits, as demonstrated in multiple number-needed-to-treat studies.[7] Careful clinical judgment and proper patient and/or site selection is advised.

Host Modulation

The clinician should consider **host modulation** as part of periodontal management to enhance treatment outcomes for select cases or in the treatment of cases that are poorly responsive to traditional treatment modalities. While most periodontal therapies target the bacterial etiology, host modulation is based on the principle of modifying or influencing the host's immune response to bacterial challenge.[8] Currently, there is only one Food and Drug Administration (FDA)-approved agent for

BOX 11.1   ADVANTAGES AND DISADVANTAGES OF LOCAL DELIVERY SYSTEMS

Advantages of Local Delivery Systems
- Patient compliance is not an issue.
- High doses of the medication are established at the disease site without altering the ecology of the remainder of the oral cavity.
- Side effects and adverse reactions are minimized.

Disadvantages of Local Delivery Systems
- Cannot inhibit or kill all pathogenic organisms.
- May depopulate normal oral flora.
- Will only affect adjacent tissues.
- The patient remains susceptible to reinfection.

systemically administered periodontal host modulation: a sub-antimicrobial dose of doxycycline. At low doses, doxycycline acts as an anti-collagenolytic agent and minimizes connective tissue turnover and alveolar bone resorption associated with inflammation. Other pharmacologic agents may indirectly interfere with inflammatory-driven periodontal tissue metabolism, such as NSAIDs, bisphosphonates, and statins. Due to the potential for adverse effects, prescription for dental use is not recommended but patients may receive benefits when taking them for other medical purposes.

Periodontal Surgery

Periodontal surgery performed in the management of periodontitis typically involves flap reflection to gain visual access to the root surfaces and alveolar bone. After reflection, the dentist removes granulation tissue and performs scaling and root planing (Figure 11.4). Gingival and osseous tissue heights and contours may be altered to idealize the bony architecture and reduce probing depths. Because of challenges with home care and professional access, periodontal surgery is recommended for residual probing depths of 6 mm or greater following conventional non-surgical therapies. Recurrent periodontal inflammation associated with probing depths of 4–5 mm and/or furcation-involved teeth may also benefit from surgical intervention. Periodontal surgery is also strategically used for the correction of gingival overgrowth, mucogingival defects (Figure 11.5), high frenal attachments, and other esthetic and/or architectural problems.

Periodontal surgery has a relatively high success rate, especially in healthy patients who do not use tobacco, who have good oral self-care, and who have high compliance with maintenance therapy recommendations. Postoperative complications of surgical therapy, although uncommon, can include bleeding, pain, and infection. Long-term negative outcomes may include dentinal hypersensitivity, gingival recession, and loss of periodontal attachment.

Periodontal Regeneration Therapy

Periodontal regenerative therapy draws on multiple techniques and biomaterials, including placement of bone grafts,

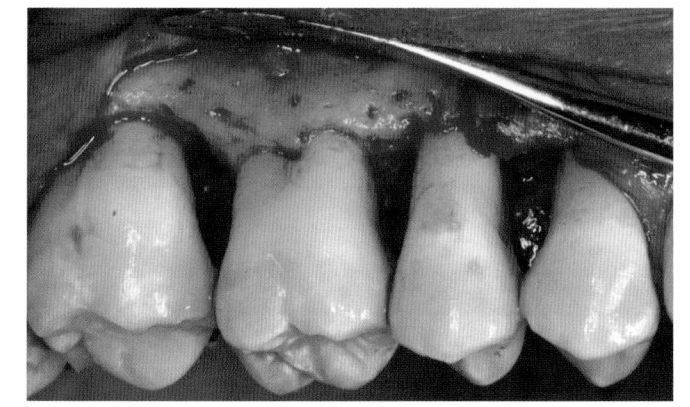

Fig. 11.4 Periodontal Flap Surgery. The careful elevation of a full-thickness mucoperiosteal flap permits improved access to the tooth root to facilitate complete debridement (i.e., scaling and root planing). It also provides access to the underlying alveolar bone for further considerations regarding possible periodontal regeneration and/or bone recontouring. (Courtesy Dr. Jonathan Reside and Dr. Antonio Moretti.)

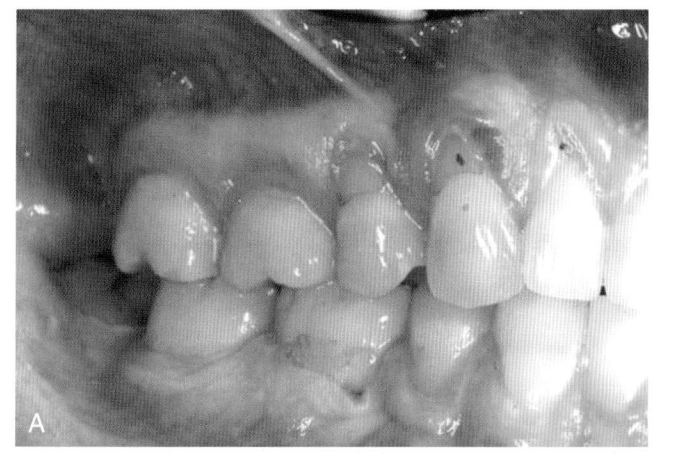

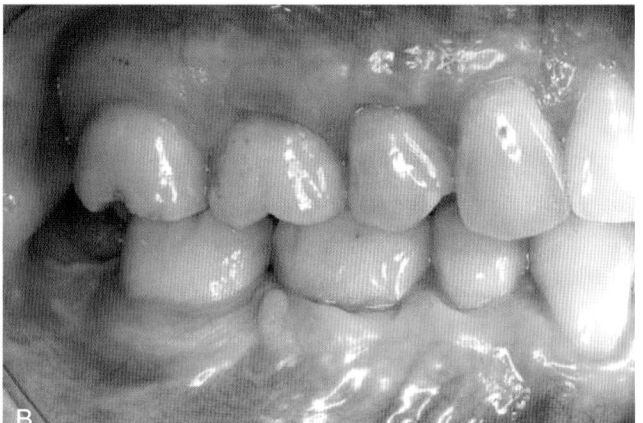

Fig. 11.5 Gingival Recession. Maxillary and mandibular teeth with recession **(A)** before and **(B)** after surgery. (Courtesy Dr Antonio Moretti.)

infrabony periodontal defects. Regeneration is also possible in select furcation and recession defects. Complications occurring after placement of these biomaterials are similar to those associated with periodontal flap surgery. In addition, biomaterial placement increases the cost and the time required for treatment. The use of commercially available growth factors (such as enamel matrix derivative, recombinant BMP-2, and recombinant PDGF-BB) may be considered to enhance treatment outcomes.

Summary

Not all patients or disease sites respond acceptably or equally to periodontal therapy. When trying to manage periodontitis that

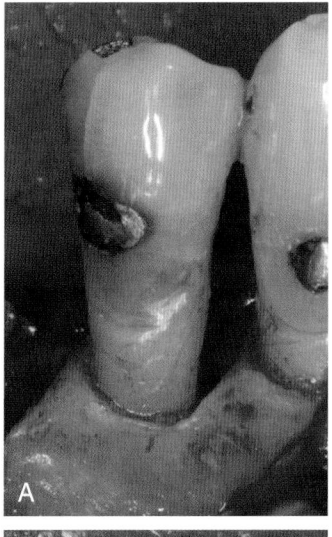
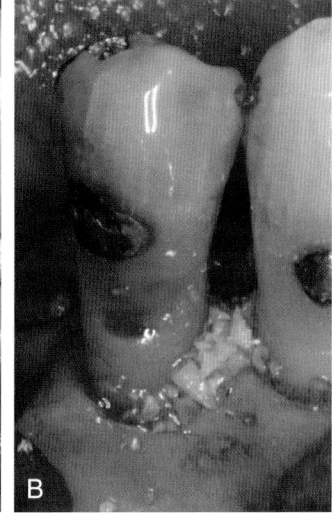
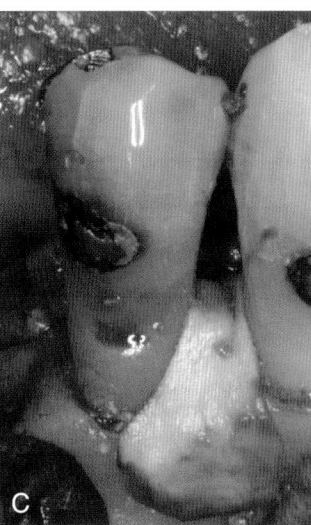

Fig. 11.6 Placement of Materials for Periodontal Regeneration. In some cases it may be possible to regenerate the periodontal attachment apparatus previously lost because of severe disease. Vertical osseous defects and some furcation defects are the most favorable for successful regeneration. After complete degranulation of the osseous defect and scaling and root planing **(A)**, bone graft particles are placed within the defect and covered with a barrier membrane **(B and C)**. In addition, today's practitioner has a variety of biologic material choices available to consider in treatment, such as enamel matrix derivative or recombinant platelet-derived growth factor. (Courtesy Dr. Jonathan Reside and Dr. Antonio Moretti.)

barrier membranes, and biologic agents to induce bone formation and/or provide a substrate for the regeneration of previously lost alveolar bone, periodontal ligament, and cementum (Figure 11.6). Case selection for these procedures is important; the success rate is best for deep three walled

has not responded to initial therapy, any of the professional or patient modifiers discussed earlier may significantly affect the outcome. Successful periodontal therapy requires a sound plan, good execution, and a motivated patient. Long-term success depends on an appropriate maintenance program. Patient noncompliance with maintenance therapy can lead to disease recurrence or progression. A subset of patients may experience recurrent or progressive disease despite adequate maintenance therapy. For these patients, additional treatment may be indicated.

eTable 11.1 summarizes guidelines for the selection of common treatment options for each of the seven periodontal tissue related conditions discussed.

ORTHODONTIC TREATMENT

Indications for orthodontic care are frequently esthetic, with a benefit in dentofacial appearance and psychosocial health as primary outcomes. For patients of all ages, however, it is also important to recognize functional or other health-related indications for care. For example, in growing patients, interceptive care may help avoid the adverse effects of impacted teeth, particularly impacted cuspids, and deliver a full complement of teeth to the arch. Similarly, in younger patient growth, modification or maxillary expansion may allow for more optimal skeletal and occlusal relationships that help to limit functional issues ((Figure 11.4) think of a crossbite with a functional shift). For adults, the vertical dimension of occlusion may need to be increased to limit excessive incisal wear, and an orthodontic approach may be the least invasive and most efficient way to accomplish this goal. Restorative or periodontal therapies may be enhanced by uprighting tipped teeth before the fabrication of a fixed partial denture (FPD) or placement of implants in an edentulous space. No matter what the reason, the patient deserves to be informed when orthodontics is a reasonable treatment option and what the potential benefits of orthodontic treatment may be. Malocclusion and tooth position problems may be treated with orthodontics alone or with orthodontics in combination with restorative and/or surgical procedures.

Malocclusions and Related Conditions

In Chapter 2, the sections *Occlusal Abnormalities* and *Esthetic Problems* identify common oral health problems that are treated orthodontically. This section highlights examples of tooth or jaw malalignment that the general dentist will encounter and will need to be knowledgeable about, so that they can be conversant with their patients and make appropriate recommendations for consultation, referral, and/or treatment.

Angle Class I Malocclusion

This diagnosis typically involves tooth-arch discrepancies in which the cumulative anteroposterior dimension of the teeth is greater than the length of the available alveolar bone (Figure 11.7). Often the opposing first molars and canines are in normal relationship relative to each other. This type of malocclusion is most often characterized by crowded or malposed

teeth, but also may be associated with rotated or tipped teeth, impactions, or isolated cross-bites. It is important to note that a patient may have a Class I relationship of the molars and cuspids, but a nonideal overbite and/or overjet relationship. Often improving overbite and overjet and, therefore, the functional occlusal relationship of their anterior teeth can be a key goal for a patient who is Class I.

Impacted Maxillary Canines

The occurrence of this condition presents the dentist with a unique treatment planning challenge. Because of their arrival in the eruption sequence after the incisors and premolars, the maxillary canines are more likely to be impacted or blocked out of the normal dental arch configuration. Maintaining these teeth in a proper alignment has unique and important advantages given their long root length and their pivotal functional and esthetic role.

Anterior Open Bite

This condition occurs when the posterior teeth are in maximum intercuspation and there is vertical space between one or more pairs of maxillary and mandibular anterior teeth. Depending on the size of the open bite, this occurrence may represent a significant esthetic, phonetic, or functional problem for the patient (Figure 11.8).

Skeletal Abnormalities

Several abnormalities of maxillary or mandibular size, form, or relationship can be recognized and diagnosed by the general

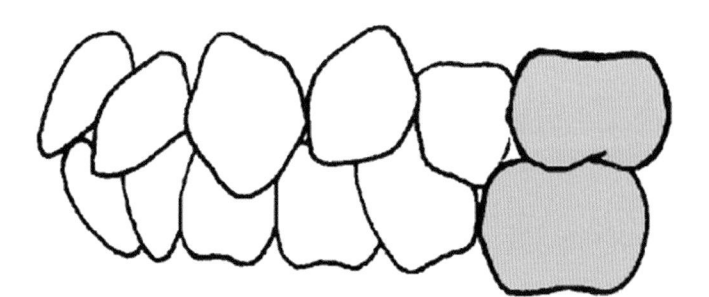

Fig. 11.7 Angle Class I Malocclusion. (From Proffit WR, Fields HW, Sarver DM. *Contemporary Orthodontics.* 5th ed. St Louis: Mosby; 2013.)

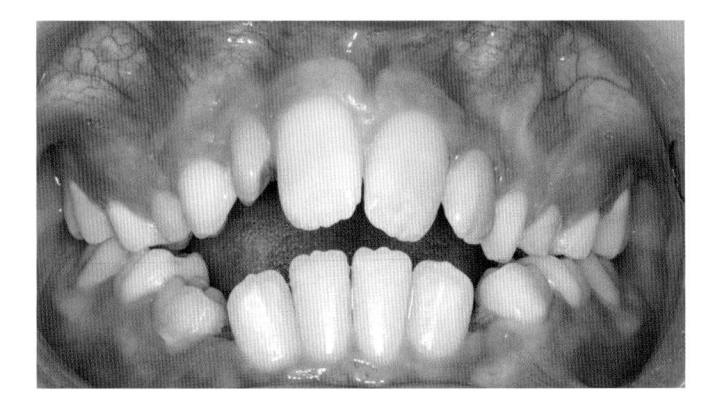

Fig. 11.8 Anterior open bite in an adolescent. (Courtesy Dr. Emile Rossouw.)

dentist. These include Angle class II or III malocclusions, micrognathia, macrognathia, transverse cross-bite relationships, and complex open bite.

Keys to Decision Making
Professional Considerations

Before a decision can be made to engage in orthodontic treatment, the dentist must carefully assess the patient's condition and any potential modifiers to the treatment. Individually or collectively, these items may have a bearing on deciding whether to treat, how to treat, and when treatment should take place. For each situation previously discussed, a definitive orthodontic case analysis is in order, such as the "Facial Form Analysis," developed by Proffit and Fields (see Chapter 17). Commonly, panoramic radiographs, a complete full mouth series of radiographs, and digital models of the complete dental arches are required. In those cases in which a skeletal component to the malocclusion exists, cephalometric radiographs and a cephalometric analysis are also necessary.

Unless the general dentist has had considerable additional training in orthodontic assessment and treatment, it is usually prudent to enlist the services of an orthodontist during this treatment planning process. Key questions include determining the scope of care (limited vs. comprehensive), whether extractions are necessary or desirable, and whether the option of orthognathic surgery should be pursued. For some adult patients, it may be best to displace teeth relative to the supporting bone to compensate for an underlying jaw discrepancy. This repositioning of teeth primarily for improving facial esthetics is referred to as **camouflaging** and is often a viable alternative to orthognathic surgery.

Before considering orthodontic treatment, the dentist must be certain that the patient does not have active caries or periodontal disease and is not at significant risk of future development of these conditions. The teeth and restorations must be in a stable state and capable of supporting the retention of orthodontic appliances for the duration of treatment. It is also the dentist's responsibility to identify any apical pathology or root abnormality, such as resorption, before orthodontic treatment is initiated. In addition, the dentist should assess the scope and magnitude of the problem for which orthodontic treatment is considered. If the problem goes untreated, will any significant negative sequelae arise? Is the problem causing, or is it likely to cause, a functional or esthetic problem? In some cases, identifying the specific cause of the problem is critical to the outcome of treatment. For example, if the dentist or orthodontist attempts correction of an anterior open bite without recognizing and addressing the underlying cause, such as degenerative joint disease, it is likely that relapse will occur and the treatment will ultimately fail.

Other issues to be considered include the generalist's training, expertise, and level of confidence in providing orthodontic treatment. Every general dentist should be able to recognize the clinical problems described in this section and converse with the patient about them. Some general dentists prefer to refer all orthodontic treatment to specialists. Others will manage limited tooth movement cases. A few generalists who have had extensive additional training can handle more complex malocclusions. In any case, it is wise for the general dentist to define carefully the limits of their knowledge and ability and treat only those cases that offer a high likelihood of success. It is also advisable for the general dentist to cultivate a close working relationship with an orthodontist and an oral and maxillofacial surgeon so that cases can be discussed and referrals made when appropriate.

Patient Considerations

A fundamental determinant in orthodontic treatment planning is the patient's own perceived need for that treatment. For most patients, the willingness to accept orthodontic treatment is motivated by a desire to improve appearance; a direct correlation can be made between the strength of that desire and the motivation to receive orthodontic treatment. Changes in the patient's personal life or career can be extremely powerful and effective motivators for initiating orthodontic treatment. Some influences, such as the desire to please a spouse or family member, can be short-lived and if the patient lacks a strong internal motivation to continue, the outcome of treatment may be in jeopardy. The wise practitioner carefully investigates these issues before engaging the patient in orthodontic treatment.

It is important to gain a sense of the patient's expectations about the treatment. Are those expectations realistic? Is the patient interested in limited treatment or comprehensive care? If limited care is preferred, is it technically possible to achieve the patient's goals? If comprehensive orthodontic care is favored, does the patient have any misperceptions that the treatment can be accomplished in a matter of weeks or by putting braces on a few selected teeth? Does the individual have an aversion to either fixed or removable orthodontic appliances or retainers? If so, will this compromise the treatment?

It is also important to ensure that the patient has a full appreciation of the costs of treatment in terms of both financial resources and the time and inconvenience that may be required. Is the individual aware of the number of visits that may be required and the number of months over which the treatment will extend? Do they recognize that there may be some discomfort to the teeth and soft tissue? Most importantly, can the patient maintain the health of the oral cavity with effective daily oral self-care despite the impediments to plaque removal that orthodontic appliances may raise? If orthognathic surgery is recommended or required, is the patient fully aware of the costs, hazards, inconvenience, and discomfort that the procedure may entail?

Procedures for Treating Malocclusion
Comprehensive Orthodontics

Comprehensive orthodontics involves the movement of multiple teeth, usually in multiple sextants and in both arches, to improve tooth alignment, function, and esthetics. Usually the practitioner bonds brackets to the teeth, coupled with arch wires and elastic bands. A newer form of treatment that has gained considerable popularity with patients and within the profession involves the use of Invisalign clear aligners. These appliances are more esthetic than some other types and are tolerated well by most patients.

Extraction of some teeth may be necessary in conjunction with comprehensive orthodontic treatment. The treatment time varies and can range from 1 to more than 3 years depending on the individual characteristics of the case. Orthodontic treatment has predictable success rates and outcomes when done by a skilled provider using sound treatment principles and evidence-based techniques. Potential negative sequelae include root blunting and resorption, gingival recession, increased caries activity, and discomfort to the teeth, periodontium, and other soft tissue during treatment.

Limited Orthodontic Tooth Movement

Limited orthodontic tooth movement involves tipping, rotation, or bodily movement of a limited number of teeth (usually no more than six), usually in just one arch. Several techniques are available to the dentist and include both fixed and removable appliances. Treatment is usually accomplished in less than a year. Counterintuitively, some limited orthodontic care can have a higher chance of unwanted side-effects, such as unwanted movement of anchor teeth. A specific example of limited tooth movement is forced eruption of an anterior tooth in which caries or fracture of the crown (and root) has compromised the biologic width. Another frequently implemented minor tooth movement involves uprighting tipped posterior teeth in preparation for use as prosthodontic abutments or to facilitate implant placement (see In Clinical Practice box).

IN CLINICAL PRACTICE

Uprighting a Tipped Molar Tooth

When a posterior tooth has been removed and is not replaced, over time the potential exists for any remaining distally positioned posterior teeth to move or tip mesially into the edentulous space (Figure 11.9). If, at a later date, the patient wishes to replace the missing tooth or teeth, a significantly tipped molar may not be optimally positioned to serve as an abutment for a fixed or removable partial denture, or to provide adequate space for implant placement in the bounded edentulous site. Two options are available: (1) attempt placement of a prosthesis or implant despite the presence of the tipped adjacent tooth or (2) upright the tooth orthodontically before prosthesis fabrication.

Professional Considerations

What is the periodontal prognosis with and without molar uprighting?

Would gingival contours, risk of food impaction, or the patient's ability to remove plaque from the adjacent tooth be favorably or unfavorably altered with molar uprighting?

Can occlusal function be improved with uprighting? If so, will the effect be significant?

With molar uprighting, will the tooth be retained for a longer or shorter length of time? Or will there be no difference either way in expected time for retention?

If the molar is not uprighted, what restorative compromises must be made (such as alteration in size, shape, or contour of the replacement tooth or adjacent teeth)?

Are there other compelling professional issues that favor or contraindicate molar uprighting?

Commonly Asked Questions by Patients

- What are the reasons for doing this?
- Must I do this?
- What will happen if I don't do this?
- Are there other alternatives?
- Will I have to wear braces? How visible will they be? What will they look like?
- Will they be uncomfortable?
- How much will it cost?
- How long will I have to wear them?

Reaching a Decision

If the dentist determines that significant periodontal, functional, or restorative advantages can be gained through molar uprighting and if the patient concurs, uprighting is the ideal and best course of action. Often, however, the patient is not enthusiastic even though orthodontic uprighting is the best and the recommended treatment from a professional perspective. The patient may think the appearance or feel of orthodontic appliances will be unpleasant. They may be apprehensive about the expected discomfort and commitment of time to undergo orthodontic care. The patient may not see the procedure as worth the required expenditure of financial resources. Whether the patient accepts or declines the recommendation to implement the uprighting, the consent discussion must be documented in the patient's record. If the patient declines orthodontic treatment, the dentist must clearly explain to the patient the consequences of that decision and document the conversation. At that point, the dentist must make the final decision whether to proceed with restorative treatment despite the possibility of a compromised result or decline to attempt to replace the missing tooth on professional grounds.

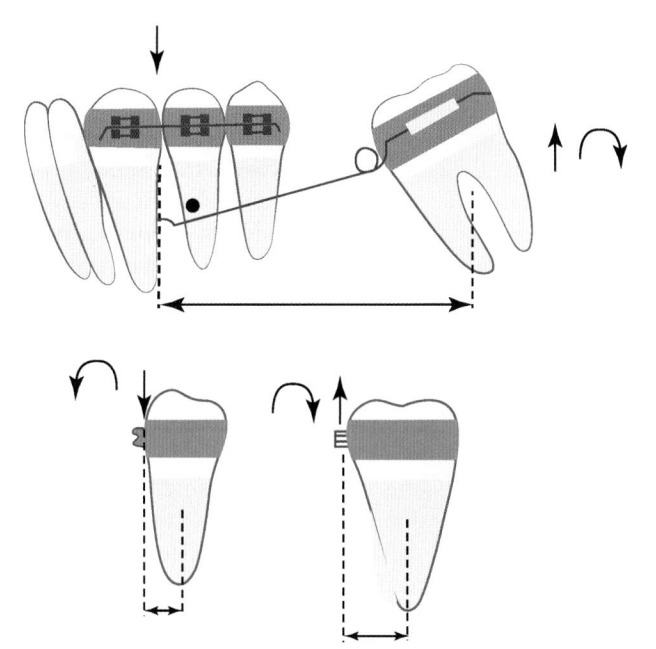

Fig. 11.9 Schematic diagram of a typical appliance for molar uprighting. (Courtesy Dr. L. Bailey.)

Orthognathic Surgery

Orthognathic surgery may be indicated when the patient has significant skeletal abnormalities in addition to a dental malocclusion. These procedures, usually performed by an oral and maxillofacial surgeon in a hospital setting, involve surgical realignment of the jaws or repositioning of dentoalveolar segments. Surgical treatment is usually preceded by, and carried out simultaneously with, comprehensive orthodontic treatment.

Orthognathic surgery may be the only satisfactory option for correcting a severe skeletal defect, especially in adult patients. Significant swelling and pain can be associated with the procedure and 1 to 2 days of hospitalization will usually be required. Nerve damage during surgery may result in areas of paresthesia involving the teeth, lips, tongue, and other surrounding tissues. This usually resolves in weeks or months but in some cases may be permanent.

Typical treatment options for four common problems that can be treated with orthodontics are summarized in eTable 11.2 with guidelines for selecting the most appropriate option.

For more in-depth discussion of the diagnosis and treatment of orthodontic problems the reader is encouraged to look at the Suggested Resources at the end of this chapter.

OTHER OCCLUSAL THERAPIES

Occlusal therapy incorporates those treatment modalities available to the dentist to manage occlusal abnormalities that can cause damage to the teeth and periodontium. Common clinical problems in this group include acute or chronic occlusal trauma, occlusal plane discrepancies, and **parafunctional habits**, such as bruxism, clenching, or nail biting. Some patients with occlusal abnormalities may experience increased inflammation in the muscles of mastication and/or temporomandibular joint(s) with resultant acute or chronic pain in the associated structures. When careful occlusal analysis confirms the presence of occlusal disharmony, strategic modification of maxillary/mandibular occlusal relationships of individual teeth (occlusal adjustment) may help resolve the problem.

Occlusal treatment is often indicated in preparation for prosthodontic rehabilitation. In some cases it may be provided in conjunction with adjunctive or comprehensive orthodontic treatment. Individuals who engage in contact sports or other physical activities that place the teeth at risk for blunt trauma are good candidates for protective occlusal (athletic) guards.

Procedures for Treating Occlusal Problems
Athletic Guard

A soft, plastic, removable appliance, the athletic guard is designed to protect teeth from blunt injury trauma (Figure 11.10). Most frequently prescribed for younger patients who engage in contact sports such as football and wrestling, the athletic guard can benefit adults too, particularly those who play basketball and racquet sports. If used consistently, the athletic guard effectively protects teeth from damage.

Patients can make their own guards using kits available in sporting goods stores or the dentist can fabricate a custom-fitted appliance by vacuum-forming the guard material onto a cast of the patient's maxillary arch. To maintain an adequate fit for children, the guard may need to be remade periodically as deciduous teeth are lost and new teeth erupt. The most significant limiting factor is the failure of some patients to always use the athletic guard when engaged in contact sports.

Occlusal Guard

An **occlusal guard** (also referred to as a **bite guard** or **night guard**) is a custom-fitted device commonly used to prevent additional occlusal tooth wear in patients who have marked bruxism or attrition. The dentist may use also such a device to assess the patient's tolerance for an increased vertical dimension of occlusion before prosthodontic rehabilitation. It is usually fabricated from a hard or slightly flexible acrylic material and fits over the maxillary occlusal and lingual tooth surfaces. Commonly the occlusion is flat plane and developed from a simple maximum intercuspation bite. Fitting is usually uncomplicated and follow-up adjustments and reevaluation are rarely necessary.

Occlusal Splint

An **occlusal splint**, also referred to as a **bite splint**, is a custom-fabricated acrylic device that fits over the occlusal and incisal surfaces of the maxillary or mandibular teeth (Figure 11.11). Occlusal splints have several uses. For patients with symptoms of temporomandibular dysfunction (TMD), the use of a splint promotes a more orthopedically stable temporomandibular

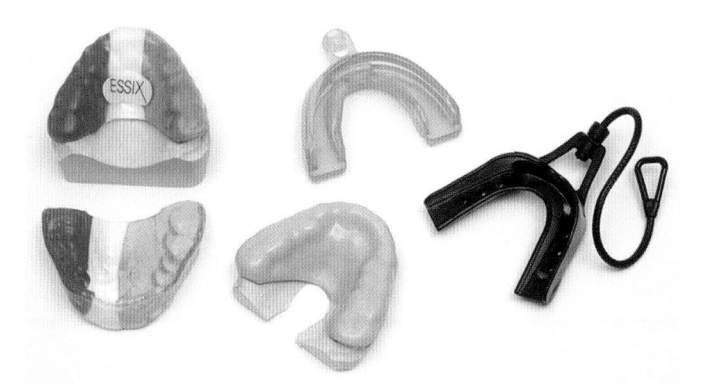

Fig. 11.10 Examples of different types of athletic guards. (Courtesy Dr Ralph Leonard.)

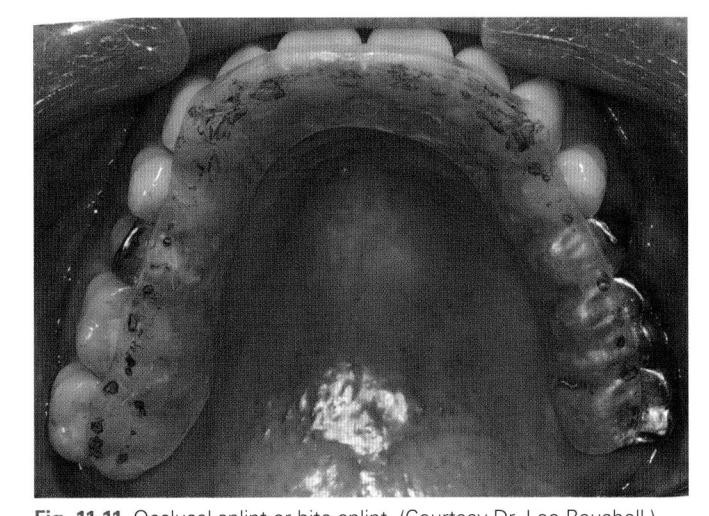

Fig. 11.11 Occlusal splint or bite splint. (Courtesy Dr. Lee Boushell.)

joint (TMJ) position and fosters reorganization and reduction of neuromuscular reflex activity. Decreased hyperactivity of the masticatory muscles allows resolution of associated inflammation-mediated pain. Along with providing some measure of relief from pain symptoms for the patient, use of the splint may also confirm the diagnosis of an occlusal component contributing to the patient's TMD.

To gain maximum benefit from the occlusal splint therapy, the dentist must carefully adjust the splint at the time it is delivered and periodically thereafter. Adjustment of the device should allow even centric occlusal contacts for anterior and posterior teeth. Furthermore, the design must utilize anterior and condylar guidance to ensure disclusion of all posterior teeth during protrusive, excursive, and any parafunctional mandibular movements. Initial adjustment of the functioning surface of the splint may require multiple visits to allow modification as masticatory muscle tonus and TMJ inflammation/effusion begin to resolve.

A major advantage to an occlusal guard and an occlusal splint is that the treatment is reversible and noninvasive. Both require patient cooperation, however, because the device is only effective when the patient is wearing it.

Occlusal Adjustment

Occlusal adjustment, also referred to as **occlusal equilibration**, involves selective grinding of tooth surfaces with the goal of improving tooth contact patterns and the associated masticatory muscle response. The treatment can be an adjunctive therapy used to alleviate symptoms of temporomandibular dysfunction or, more commonly, to complement comprehensive prosthodontic reconstruction. Treatment goals for selective grinding include establishment of an acceptable centric relation contact position for the patient, providing atraumatic lateral and protrusive guidance, and establishing an acceptable plane of occlusion with adequate interarch space for any prosthesis replacing missing teeth.

Occlusal adjustment is an irreversible procedure and the dentist must conscientiously study the patient's existing occlusion before removing any tooth structure for this purpose. This often includes analyzing articulated diagnostic casts, intraoral confirmation of occlusal/incisal wear facets, and use of articulating paper or occlusal indicating wax to verify occlusal patterns. Before performing the procedure, the dentist should inform the patient that grinding the teeth may cause tooth sensitivity in some individuals. Areas of adjustment are strategically planned so that the vertical dimension of occlusion is not modified and interferences to normal mandibular movement are removed from offending cusp inclines. The patient also needs to be aware that when gross occlusal reduction is used to correct an occlusal plane discrepancy—such as that caused by a hypererupted or extruded tooth—root canal treatment, surgical crown lengthening, and/or a crown restoration may also be required.

RESTORING INDIVIDUAL TEETH

Single tooth restorations replace tooth structure lost because of caries, tooth fracture, abrasion, attrition, abfraction, erosion, or a combination of these conditions. These restorative techniques may also be used to improve the appearance of teeth, establish more normal contours, or close proximal contacts. Some restorative materials are designed to desensitize tooth surfaces, or to seal areas that have the potential to decay. Commonly, new restorations are necessary to replace older restorations that have failed because of secondary caries, fracture, material loss, marginal leakage, or stain. Because amalgam, composite resin, or ceramic inlay restorations are usually placed in preparations that are *within the confines of* teeth, they are, therefore, considered to be **intracoronal restorations. Extracoronal restorations**, such as the gold or ceramic onlay, or full cast, porcelain fused to metal (PFM), or all-ceramic crown, encompass most or all of the coronal surface of the tooth.

Keys to Decision Making

Throughout this text, an overriding perspective has been that the patient should be involved in the decision making for their dental treatment. As discussed in Chapter 5, it is the role of the dentist to determine the reasonable and feasible treatment options for any given situation and to present those options to the patient. When dentist and patient are faced with the single tooth restorative options described in this section, a well-informed and knowledgeable patient can and should be able to make the final treatment decision. In some cases, however, compelling professional issues such as the structural integrity of the tooth and the forces of occlusion will be paramount. In such situations, it will be appropriate for the dentist to limit the choices offered to the patient or to make a stronger recommendation for one of the available options.

Professional Considerations

When recommending single tooth restorative options to the patient, the dentist will need to consider several issues. The following are frequently encountered clinical questions that the dentist may need to address to be able to inform the patient properly about the treatment options and thereby assist the patient in making the best treatment choice:

- What is the diagnosis? Is the caries lesion active or arrested? Is it incipient or overt? These issues are discussed in Chapters 1 and 2.
- Is a restoration needed? Can the condition (such as an incipient caries lesion) be managed nonsurgically with chemotherapeutic or other noninvasive treatment? Which negative outcomes might arise if restorative intervention is not undertaken? Frequently, the dentist will recognize that an existing restoration is not ideal, but the patient is asymptomatic and is not currently suffering any deleterious effects from the defect. The concept of minimalist dentistry holds that the dentist should not intervene surgically unless necessary. In any case, the patient needs to be informed in an unbiased way about the risk and benefits of the surgical and nonsurgical options and of no treatment.
- What is the patient's caries risk? The concept of caries management by risk assessment (CAMBRA) is described in Chapter 3. If the patient is at relatively low risk of caries, more conservative and less invasive measures are preferred.

See Chapter 10 for more information on managing the active caries patient.

- Does the patient need a disease control phase plan of care? In the disease control phase, if restorations are indicated, interim restorations or direct-fill definitive restorations are preferred; definitive indirect restorations are almost always contraindicated.
- What is the fracture potential for the proposed restoration and for the tooth? Some restorations, depending on the restorative material, the patient's occlusion, and the tooth's position in the mouth, are inherently more prone to fracturing. Also, some restorations (e.g., full coverage crowns) will usually reduce the risk for tooth fracture though others (e.g., large amalgam in a tooth with compromised cusp integrity) may actually increase the risk for fracture.
- Is the restoration likely to cause significant attrition to or abrade the opposing tooth or restoration? Over time, glass ceramic materials (e.g., porcelain, lucite-reinforced porcelain, lithium disilicate) will abrade natural teeth. From a wear perspective, gold and highly polished zirconia are most compatible with tooth enamel. It is desirable to have restorations that oppose each other fabricated out of the same material (i.e., metal occluding with metal; ceramic occluding with ceramic).
- What are the esthetic benefits or deficits of the various restorative options? Esthetic (i.e., tooth colored) restorative materials vary in translucence, surface texture, polishability, and effectiveness at concealing intrinsic stains. Some can be characterized to match other teeth or restorations, but others cannot. The dentist must make a determination as to what type of material and what particular brand and formula will be best suited to the situation.
- What is the expected longevity of the restoration? See Chapter 3, *What's the Evidence? How Long Do Restorations and Prostheses Last?* box for a detailed evidence-based summary of restoration longevity.
- What will the cost be to the patient for the restoration and the alternatives?

Patient Considerations

If the patient has teeth that are sensitive or that display visible dark areas, they will probably request treatment. In either of these situations, however, the patient is unlikely to have a full understanding of the available treatment options or the inherent limits and risks of each. Although the patient will be the final decision maker, considerable education may need to take place before an informed decision about the treatment can be made.

Unlike problems involving the periodontal tissues, malocclusion, or missing teeth, single tooth restorative needs may not be self-evident to the patient. This presents the dentist with a twofold challenge: first, to explain to the patient that there is an existing or potential problem, and second, to describe the available surgical and nonsurgical options in an unbiased manner.

Some patient issues are indispensable to single tooth treatment decision making. If restorative treatment is not mandatory,

as would be the case with a stained but sound composite resin restoration, the decision to treat or not treat is left to the patient. Certainly, the patient's willingness to invest time and financial resources will have a significant bearing on the decision. What benefits does the patient perceive? How highly are those benefits valued? How committed is the patient to improving esthetics or warding off future problems? Are they willing to accept the risks and hazards if treatment is not provided?

When restorative intervention is necessary and the patient accepts this, the patient may contribute significant input to the selection of restorative material. Is the patient averse to amalgam? Do they prefer, or insist on, a tooth-colored restoration? Will a metal margin on a crown present an esthetic problem? What are the individual's priorities: longevity of the tooth and restoration or the cost in time and financial resources required for the immediate work? Is optimal treatment preferred now in the hope of preventing future problems? Or does the individual prefer to wait and see, accepting the fact that the tooth may break or even be lost prematurely?

Single Tooth Restorative Procedures
Pit and Fissure Sealant

Sealants are low-viscosity unfilled or filled resin materials designed primarily to be used to prevent caries development in susceptible pits and fissures of posterior teeth in children and adolescents. With time, however, sealants have gained wider application and are commonly used for patients of all ages, not only to prevent the formation of new carious lesions but also to interrupt caries progression in areas with shallow incipient carious lesions.[9] Frequently, the dentist will be faced with the diagnostic challenge of differentiating between deep fissures with stains, and incipient caries. Placement of a sealant in this circumstance is an inexpensive, noninvasive approach with a proven benefit provided the sealant is placed under well-controlled conditions. Consistent with the concept of minimally invasive dentistry, sealants will be preferred to a composite or amalgam restoration—both of which require tooth preparation and removal of some tooth structure. Sealants are even more likely to be recommended rather than a more invasive restorative procedure if the patient is at low caries risk and will be able to return for regular maintenance visits.

When placing sealants, some have advocated the use of mechanical instrumentation (enameloplasty or prophylactic odontotomy) if there is a high degree of probability that demineralization has occurred in the depth of the fissure. However, research has suggested that this is not recommended for a noncavitated pit or fissure.[9] Sealant resins have many other uses, including sealing slight voids or surface imperfections and defects in enamel or composite materials, resurfacing a new or existing composite, and sealing dentin tubules as a desensitizing treatment.

Composite Resin Restoration

Composite resin is a direct-fill, tooth-colored restorative material (Figure 11.12). Composites were first used to restore anterior teeth but are now routinely used in conservative occlusal

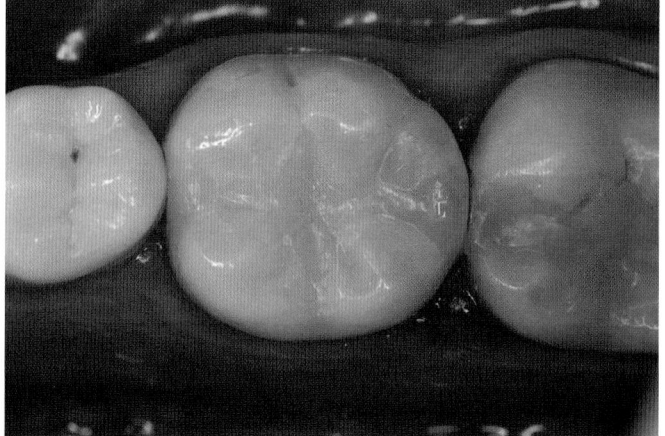

Fig. 11.12 Composite restorations. (Courtesy Dr. Lee Boushell.)

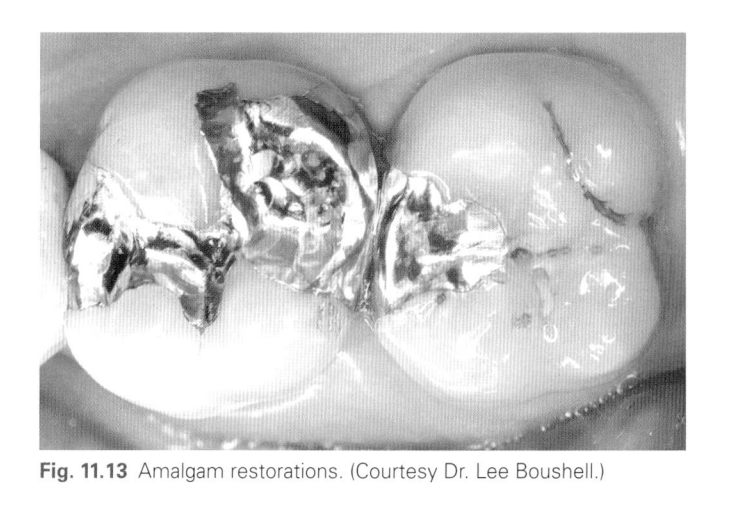

Fig. 11.13 Amalgam restorations. (Courtesy Dr. Lee Boushell.)

and proximal preparations on posterior teeth. Composite resin restorations exhibit excellent color-matching characteristics and the material is versatile and relatively easy to manipulate. Light-cure composite material has almost unlimited working time. Disadvantages include the possibility of microleakage, staining, and wear, especially when used in large posterior preparations. Recent nano-filled composite restorations do not suffer from the same level of wear as previous resin formulations. Composite resin restorations in posterior teeth have increased risk of development of secondary caries, as compared with amalgam, in patients who are at high risk of caries.[10]

Composite restorations can fail because of secondary caries, fracture of the restoration, or fracture of adjacent tooth structure. It is frequently possible to repair previously placed composite restorations with new composite material and, thus, extend the life of the initial restoration. Composite resin restorations are more technique-sensitive than amalgam restorations. Isolation of the operative field from contamination (e.g., saliva, gingival sulcular fluid, hemorrhage, handpiece lubricants, water) is necessary for good bonding and long-term success of the restoration.[11]

From a treatment planning perspective, posterior composites are usually advocated: (1) for relatively small preparations, (2) when all margins of the preparation can be isolated and dried, (3) when esthetics is an overriding concern for the patient, and (4) when the patient has a documented allergy/sensitivity to metallic alternatives. Special consideration should be given to the reduction of caries risk as prerequisite to posterior composite resin restorations. Outside the United States, composite is often the preferred material for all direct-fill posterior restorations.

Glass Ionomer Restoration

Glass ionomer restorations can be used in various applications when a tooth-colored material is preferred. This material is commonly used to restore carious and noncarious cervical lesions (that have a multifactorial etiology that includes erosion, abrasion and abfractive forces from occlusal function). It has often been recommended for use as an interim or definitive restoration in

caries-active patients and in the atraumatic restorative treatment technique (see Chapter 10). Because a glass ionomer restoration will bond to dentin and enamel, cavity preparation may not be necessary in areas of cervical notching or erosion although restoration adhesion is improved with removal of any smear layer with a mild polyacrylic acid prior to restoration placement. Glass ionomers set quickly in bulk and are ideal as a temporary or provisional direct-fill restoration for large carious lesions, endodontic access openings, and cusp fractures. Glass ionomer restorations are more prone to fracture and wear than composites. Compared with composites, esthetics are generally regarded as inferior because shade ranges are more limited, and the materials have a more opaque appearance. Compomers and resin-modified glass ionomer materials have properties that blend the qualities of glass ionomer and composite in various combinations.

From a treatment planning perspective, glass ionomer restorations should be considered for the high-risk caries patient when esthetics is a consideration and composite resins may not be the best choice. For many practitioners, glass ionomer cements are the material of choice for xerostomic patients and for patients with root caries.[12,13]

Glass ionomer cements are also widely used as temporary restorations in the acute care setting.

Amalgam Restoration

Amalgam is a direct-fill material used primarily for restoring lesions or defects on the mesial, distal, occlusal, and lingual surfaces of posterior teeth (Figure 11.13). Amalgam can be used to replace missing cusps, especially nonfunctional cusps, and as a build-up material for a core (foundation) before placing a crown.

Dental amalgam is inexpensive, easy to handle, strong, durable, resistant to fracture and marginal leakage, and can be expected to have a relatively long service life in the patient's mouth. It is also expected to perform better in the posterior teeth of patients at high risk of caries than composite resin.[10] It is the preferred restorative material for posterior teeth where operator visibility is compromised or where isolation of the preparation from contamination is a problem. Disadvantages include the fact that its color does not match tooth structure, and additional sound tooth structure may have to be removed to provide adequate retention for the restoration. Amalgam

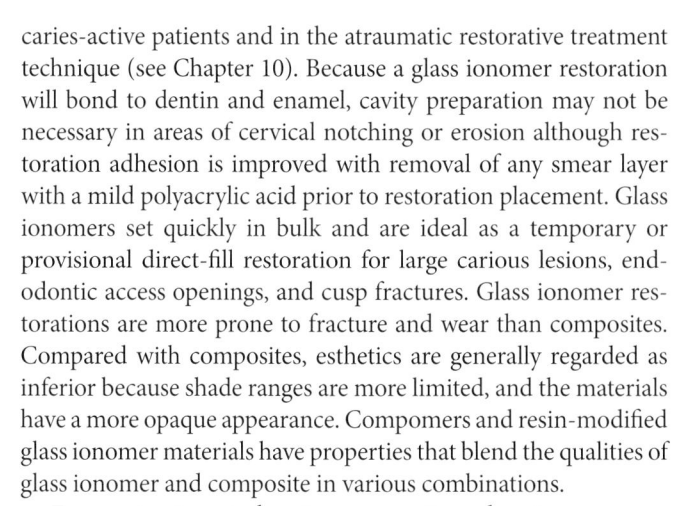

restorations may fail because of secondary caries, fracture of the restoration, or fracture of adjacent tooth structure. Although numerous studies support the safety of amalgam, some patients and dentists choose to avoid using it citing health and safety reasons (see In Clinical Practice: Responding to the Patient Who Wants No "Silver Fillings" box). In some European nations, the use of amalgam has been severely limited because of environmental concerns, which focus on the handling and disposal of the mercury in dental amalgam.

IN CLINICAL PRACTICE

Responding to the Patient Who Wants No "Silver Fillings"

For various reasons, patients may be opposed to having amalgam restorations in their mouths. These reasons may include esthetic concerns, allergy to metal fillings, or concerns for the toxic effects of mercury (or other metals) on their body. A few healthcare providers have advocated the elimination of amalgam restorations as a means of promoting optimal oral health and as an approach to eliminating various systemic diseases, including chronic depression, multiple sclerosis, and cancer. The American Dental Association (ADA) has issued a clear statement on this issue affirming that, except in the presence of a confirmed allergy, no scientific evidence justifies the removal of otherwise sound amalgam restorations for the sole purpose of promoting the health of the patient.[1] Despite the evidence-based position of the ADA, some healthcare providers and some patients still insist on the removal of all amalgam or other metallic restorations. To complicate the issue further, some dentists do not themselves use amalgam and others have eliminated all metallic restorations (dental amalgam, gold alloys) from their practice.

Before making any judgments or decisions, the dentist needs to listen carefully to the patient's concerns, responding to any questions. If the patient has a legitimate health concern, such as an allergy to amalgam, an alternative treatment should be provided. Reasonable *dental* indications may also justify replacing amalgam restorations, such as a defective restoration or the patient's desire for a more esthetic restoration.

If a patient wants to replace restorations, ostensibly for health reasons, and the likelihood of a health benefit is in doubt, the dentist must carefully consider the options. If the existing restorations are intact and serviceable and no obvious dental benefit to replacing them can be cited, the dentist is justified in refusing to provide the treatment. This is particularly true when the replacement restoration, a composite for example, may be less durable than amalgam.

Unfortunately, many cases are not so clear-cut. Often the ostensible health benefits are not obvious to the dentist but cannot be totally discounted and the replacement restorations would not be expected to provide significant improvement in function or longevity than their predecessors. Recognizing the potential for the patient to incur substantial cost, particularly if gold or ceramic restorations are the only alternative, is it ethical or professionally responsible for the dentist to proceed with removing the amalgam? One approach is to respectfully decline the patient's request. Another approach is to proceed with the requested replacement but only after ensuring that *full informed consent has been achieved* and the patient fully understands that the *dentist is not promising or expecting that the patient's health will be improved* as a result of the restoration replacement.

In an effort to find acceptable middle ground, the dentist may offer to replace only those restorations that would improve the patient's dental condition. Indeed, environmental issues and the development of a more ideal and esthetic posterior restorative material may eventually eliminate the use of dental amalgam, but until that occurs, the dental practitioner will have to face this treatment planning challenge.

Reference

1. ADA principles of ethics and code of professional conduct, April 2012. http://www.ada.org/~/media/ADA/About%20the%20ADA/Files/code_of_ethics_2012.ashx (Section 5, paragraph 5.A. 1–Dental Amalgam).

Inlays and Onlays

An **inlay** is an indirect intracoronal restoration that can be made of gold, composite resin, or ceramic material (Figure 11.12). Newer alternatives are the ceramic optimized polymers, also known as ceramers or polyglass, which are highly filled bondable materials that combine the esthetics of ceramics with the flexural strength and shade control of a resin. Generally, the ceramic optimized polymers have not performed well over time. Current lithium disilicate materials are demonstrating superior clinical performance when tooth colored inlay/onlay materials are indicated. Traditionally, a laboratory indirectly fabricates the restoration on a cast of the prepared tooth. The prepared tooth is **temporized** during this interval. The final restoration is tried in the mouth and, after occlusion and proximal contacts have been adjusted, is cemented in place.

Composite and ceramic inlays have the advantages of excellent esthetics with increased resistance to abrasion and occlusal wear compared with direct-fill composites. It is currently unknown whether long-term strengthening of tooth structure is achieved by adhesively bonding to conditioned tooth surfaces. As with other indirectly fabricated restorations, more precise control of contours and proximal contacts can be achieved. Disadvantages (compared with direct-fill restorations) include increased chair time, increased cost, and the technical demands of preparation and cementation. Chairside computer-assisted milling of ceramic inlays, onlays, and crowns (CAD/CAM) is currently available, making same-day delivery possible. With time, more dentists are likely to have this technology and to offer this service in their offices. The initial cost for such systems is considerable and, after an initial fairly steep learning curve, incorporation into dental practice has the potential to add efficiencies to the delivery of dental care.[14]

An **onlay** is an indirect restoration covering one or more cusps of a posterior tooth (Figure 11.14). It is designed to strengthen a tooth that has been weakened by caries, tooth fracture, or a previously placed large restoration. Resin, cast gold, or glass-ceramic may be used. An onlay is defined as an extracoronal restoration covering most of the occlusal surface and up to five-eighths of the surface tooth structure. An onlay that covers or "shoes" all of the cusps provides excellent protection against fracture, but tooth preparation is technically challenging. A digital or elastomeric impression must be taken and, absent CAD-CAM technology, a temporary restoration placed while the onlay is indirectly fabricated. Glass-ceramic onlays, which are available through conventional and CAD/CAM technology, provide excellent esthetics and have durability that has continued to improve over time when used as indicated. Glass-ceramic materials fail by fracture development secondary to heavy cyclic occlusal loading. Patients who are prone to parafunctional habits such as clenching or clenching/grinding (bruxism) may have more clinical success with cast metal onlay restorations.

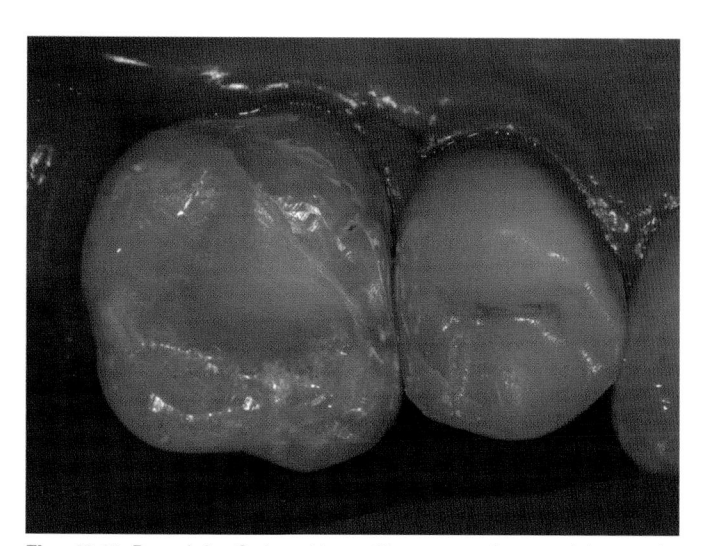

Fig. 11.14 Porcelain Onlay. Note: Glass ceramic materials require resin cement luting as well as post-insertion attention to detail such as excess cement removal and careful polishing after refinement of occlusion. (Courtesy Dr. Hanan Elgendy.)

Full Coverage Indirect Restoration (Definitive Crown)

A **crown** covers five-eighths or more of the external tooth surface and is made of gold (Figure 11.15), ceramic (Figure 11.16), or PFM. Like the onlay, a crown provides protection for a tooth that has been severely compromised by caries or fracture. Because a crown is fabricated indirectly, improved proximal contacts and occlusion can be obtained. PFM and all-ceramic crowns are good esthetic replacements for lost tooth structure. As with an onlay, a digital image or elastomeric impression of the preparation is required. With CAD/CAM technology chairside fabrication and same-day delivery is possible.

In the case of severe caries or breakdown of the tooth, it may be necessary to replace missing structure by performing root canal therapy and placing a foundation or a prefabricated or cast **post and core** (Figure 11.17). This cost, when added to that of the crown and the root canal therapy, may make restoration of the tooth cost-prohibitive for the patient.

Common restorative problems, treatment options, and keys to decision making are presented in eTable 11.3.

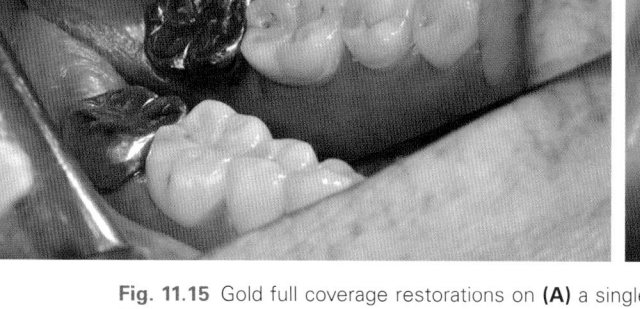

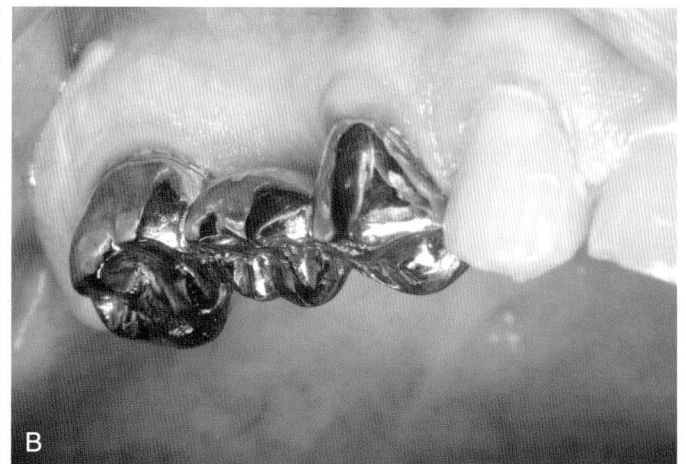

Fig. 11.15 Gold full coverage restorations on **(A)** a single tooth and **(B)** multiple teeth. (Courtesy Dr. Carlos H. Barrero.)

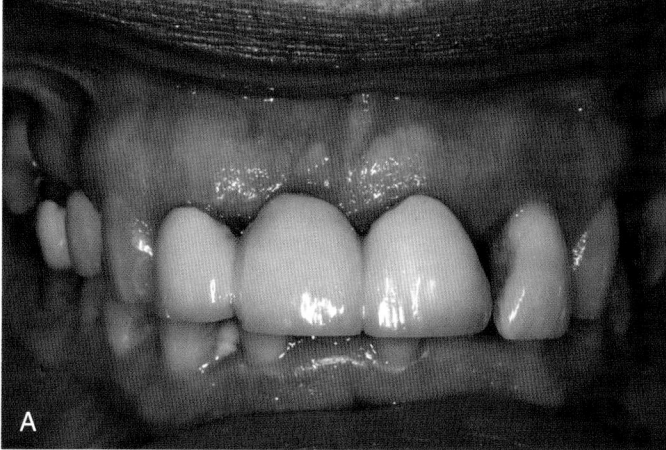

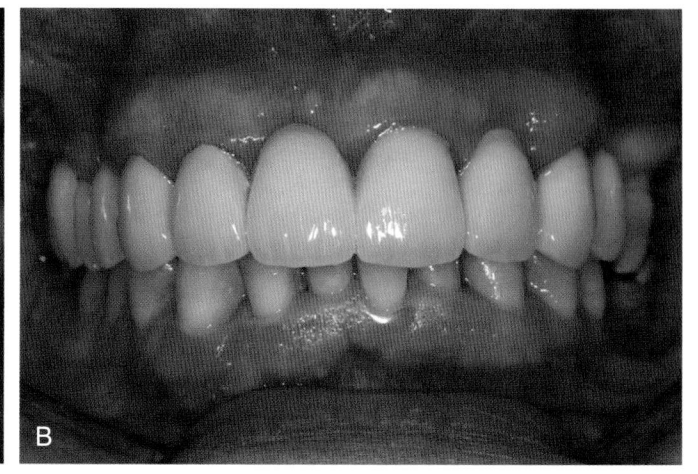

Fig. 11.16 Example of how **(A)** poor esthetics can be remedied with **(B)** a full coverage porcelain restoration. (Courtesy Dr. Ed Kanoy.)

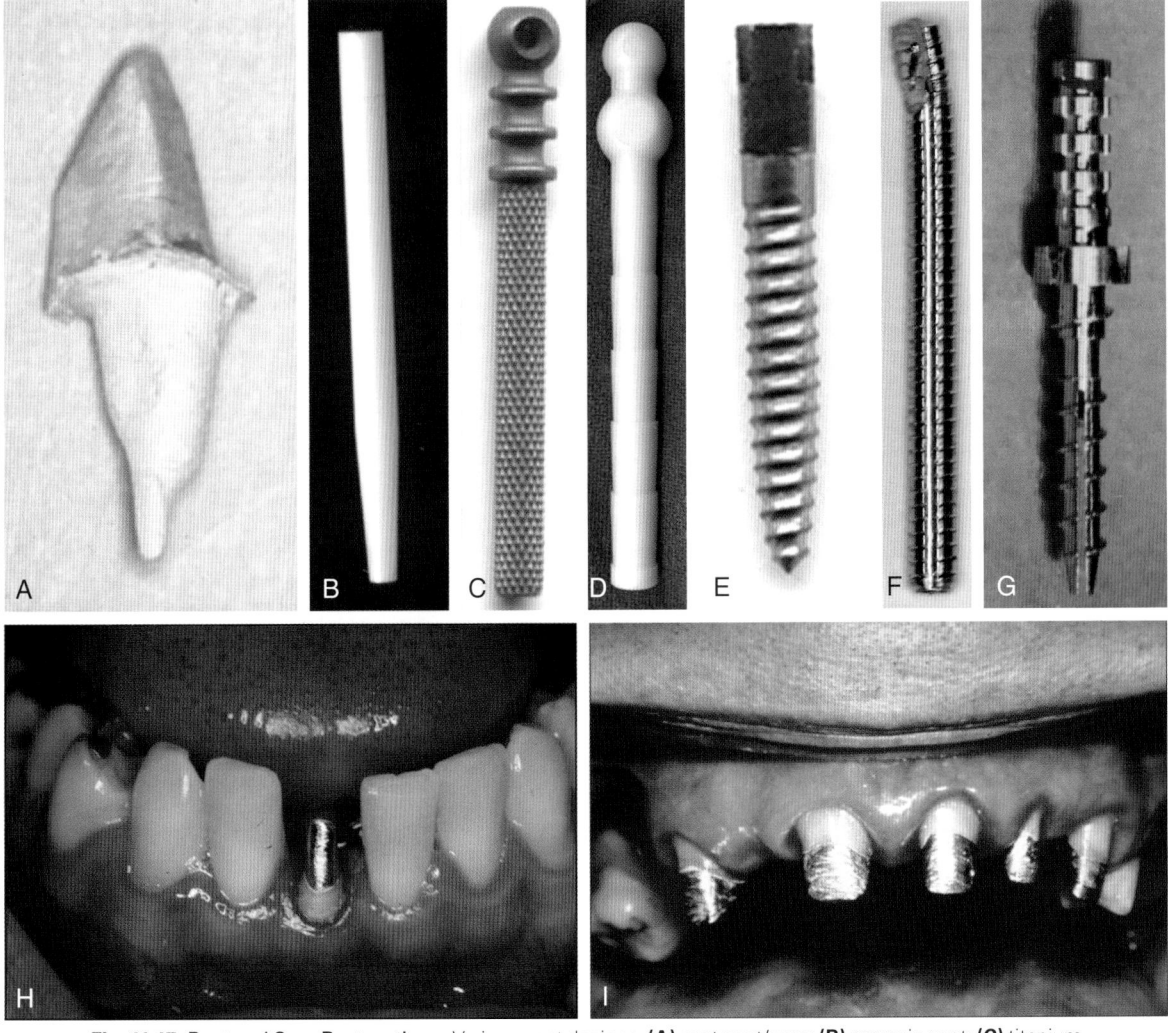

Fig. 11.17 Post and Core Restorations. Various post designs: **(A)** cast post/core; **(B)** ceramic post; **(C)** titanium post; **(D)** fiber post; **(E)** old style threaded post; **(F)** original parallel sided prefab, parapost (stainless steel); **(G)** more recent style threaded post. **(H and I)** full crown restoration preparations on post and core build-ups. **(A–E,H,I)**courtesy Dr. Thomas Ziemiecki; **(F)** courtesy Dr Stephen Stefanac; **(G)** TV Padmanabhan, V Rangarajan, Textbook of Prosthodontics, second edition, 2017, Hackensack, NJ.

ESTHETIC DENTISTRY

Since the middle of the 20th century providing patients with a pleasing smile has been an integral part of general dental practice. The population awareness of esthetic dental procedures, and the development of techniques for changing the color and shape of teeth have driven this cultural and professional shift. This section focuses on esthetic treatment options for individual teeth. Esthetic treatments for skeletal abnormalities, malocclusion, and gingival architectural defects are addressed in other sections of this chapter.

Esthetic treatments for individual teeth vary in terms of their degree of invasiveness (eTable 11.4). At one end of the spectrum are over the counter whitening toothpastes that affect tooth color only minimally, primarily by removing extrinsic stains. At the opposite end is the full coverage indirect restoration, which usually requires significant reduction of enamel and dentin to allow space for the restoration. Procedures discussed in this section include resin infiltration, micro and macro abrasion, tooth reshaping, bleaching of vital and nonvital teeth, veneers, and full coverage indirect restorations.

Keys to Decision Making
Professional and Patient Considerations

Before the start of any esthetic dental treatment, the dentist must carefully assess the patient's concerns and diagnose the perceived problem correctly. Not uncommonly, the patient's concern may be different from our initial professional presumption of the patient's need. Misreading the patient at this stage can lead the patient to believe that we are wanting to "overtreat" and incorrectly identifying what we assume is the "problem" may be interpreted as insensitivity on our part. Misunderstanding at this stage may be detrimental to the doctor–patient relationship, and in some cases may lead to litigation. Several questions need to be asked and explored, such as: What are the patient's expectations for treatment? Are those expectations realistic? Can the expectations be met within the context of the patient's general health, oral health, social determinants of health, and financial resources? The dentist has the responsibility to explain the diagnosis(es) and delineate the relevant treatment options to resolve the patient's concern. The informed consent discussion will need to include the risks, benefits, and costs of each option as well as the expected outcomes and the expected longevity of each of the interventions. If the patient is reluctant to engage in extensive elective treatment at this time or if limited financial resources preclude ideal but more extensive intervention, it may be advantageous to recommend a sequential treatment approach that starts with the most conservative treatment options (such as composite restorations). In time, in accordance with the patient's desires and as circumstances and finances permit, more extensive treatment (e.g., onlays and crowns) may be undertaken.

At the initial examination visit, the dentist must appropriately document the patient's condition. For single tooth treatments, this may simply be an entry in the patient's record describing the present appearance and proposed treatment objectives. In the presence of a discolored tooth or restoration, the dentist should determine and record the original shade of the tooth, and adjacent teeth, using a physical shade guide or color matching instrument. Documentation for patients with more extensive treatment plans commonly includes study casts (with or without face bow and mounting), intraoral scanning, and digital or conventional diagnostic wax-up. Intraoral photographs should be part of the documentation process for most esthetic cases and are now becoming standard of care for single or multiple tooth restorations in the esthetic zone. Computer software designed to aid the analysis of facial and dental esthetics may be helpful when discussing the case with the patient (see Chapter 4). It can help to clarify and document the patient's expectations and the mutual objectives of the treatment.

Representative Esthetic Problems and Treatment Procedures

Resin Infiltration, Microabrasion, and Macroabrasion

Resin infiltration, (Figure 11.18) **microabrasion** (Figure 11.19) and **macroabrasion** (Figure 11.20) are considered safe and conservative methods of removing superficial stains and defects of the enamel surface. They are used to treat conditions such as mild to moderate fluorosis, postorthodontic demineralization, and superficial enamel hypoplasia.[15] The indications for these treatments are similar and the esthetic outcomes of resin infiltration and microabrasion appear to be comparable after 12 months.[16] A transilluminator may help to determine the depth of the lesion and thereby help select the most appropriate treatment option. Of the three techniques, resin infiltration is considered to be least invasive and macroabrasion the most.

The resin infiltration technique uses a combination of erosion of the most superficial and less porous layer of the enamel,

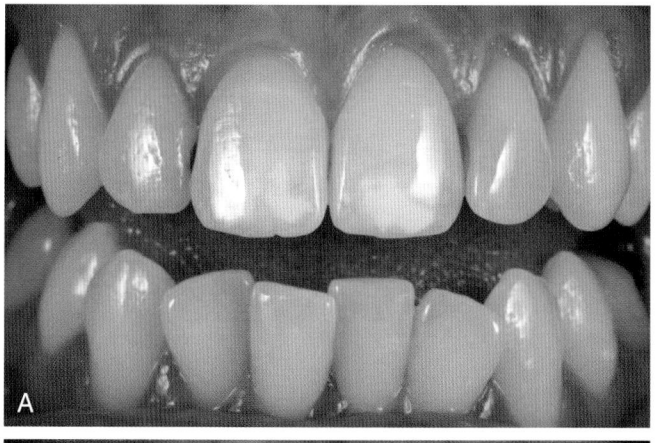
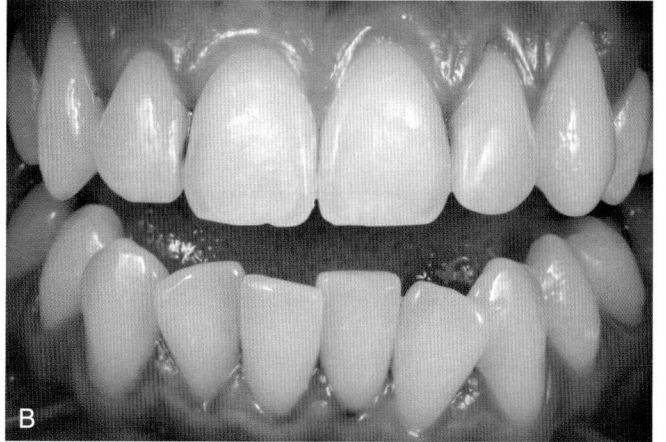

Fig. 11.18 Resin infiltration. (Courtesy Dr. Ali Altak.)

with the infiltration of a low-viscosity resin through the internal porosities of the enamel. This is achieved by capillary action. This technique can be used to treat incipient caries lesions, or white spot lesions, on labial surfaces of anterior teeth, and to mask noncarious enamel discolorations. The procedure is initiated by the application of a solution of hydrochloric acid on the surface of the enamel with an applicator tip. Following removal of the acid solution, the enamel is dried and ethanol solvent is applied on the etched surface as an aid to predict the color change. Additional rounds of acid application may be needed until desired color change is observed. When that objective is achieved, the low-viscosity resin is infiltrated into the porous areas of the enamel. The appearance of the enamel is improved as a result of a change in the light scatter within the newly infiltrated enamel.[17]

When microabrasion is the treatment of choice, the defective surface layer of enamel is removed using a combination of abrasion and erosion. This is usually achieved by using an acid, such as hydrochloric acid, along with an abrasive powder, such as silicon carbide particles. A paste formed from mixing hydrochloric acid with the abrasive powder is commonly applied with a low-speed handpiece and rubber cup or hand application device to gently remove the outermost layer of enamel. Clinically, the microabraded surface looks smooth and esthetically pleasing because the procedure causes a prismless layer of enamel to form. Care should be taken to

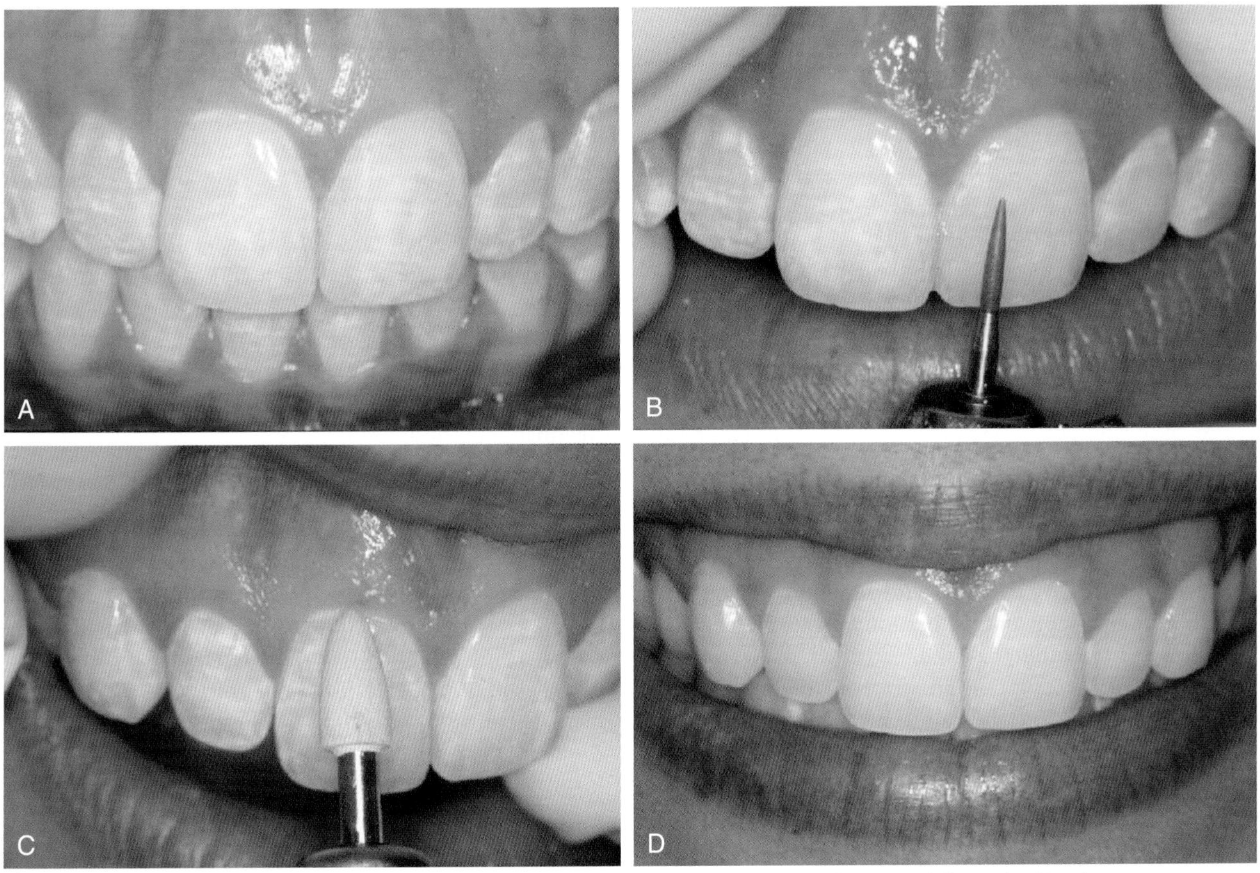

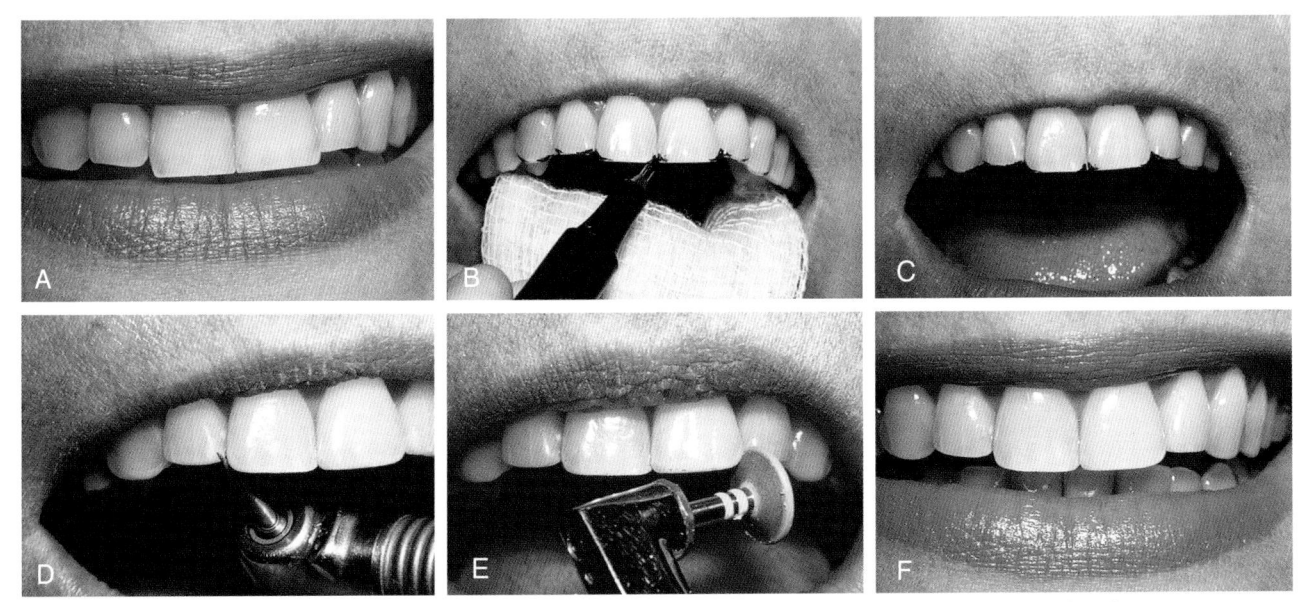

Fig. 11.19 Microabrasion. (From Ritter AV, Boushell LW, Walter R. *Art and Science of Operative Dentistry.* Elsevier; 2019.)

Fig. 11.20 Macroabrasion. (From Ritter AV, Boushell LW, Walter R. *Art and Science of Operative Dentistry.* Elsevier; 2019.)

protect the soft tissues from spatter by using a rubber dam during the procedure.[18]

Macroabrasion is another treatment option for removing localized, superficial stains and defects that cannot be remineralized. The procedure involves the utilization of a fine (12-fluted)

carbide or a fine-grit finishing diamond bur in a high-speed handpiece to reduce or remove the defect. An ultra-fine finishing bur (30-fluted) is used following removal of defects to refine the surface and remove facets and striations created by previous instrumentation. Occasionally, on shallow stains, the ultra-fine finishing bur may be used alone. It is important to maintain a light pressure to control the removal of enamel and avoid unnecessary tooth damage. If an electric handpiece is utilized, lowering the speed (rpm) may provide additional help to control the amount of enamel reduction. The procedure should be done under air–water spray to dissipate heat and to avoid tooth dehydration. When teeth are dehydrated white spots may become more visible and the dentist will need to use caution to avoid unnecessary reduction of tooth structure. Once the procedure is completed, an abrasive rubber point is used to provide the final polishing of the tooth structure.

Although these procedures can usually provide significant improvement, some patients may require more invasive procedures, such as composite resin restorations, veneers, or full coverage restorations.

Esthetic Reshaping of Teeth

Esthetic reshaping or recontouring of natural teeth is a method to conservatively improve esthetics and function without the need for tooth preparation and restoration. It is useful to refine the appearance of fractured, chipped, extruded, or overlapped teeth, or prevent further chipping and fractures of incisal edges. The procedure may include rounding incisal angles, altering facial line angles, opening incisal embrasures, or smoothing rough incisal edges to improve symmetry. It may be beneficial to use a smile design software to illustrate the possible clinical outcome before initiating treatment. Teeth are typically recontoured using rotary instrumentation. The sequence of steps may begin with finishing burs or diamonds and abrasive discs and points, followed by fine-abrasive impregnated rubber points, cups, or discs. Finishing strips are sometimes useful for polishing proximal surfaces of the dentition. Contraindications to contouring include hypersensitive teeth, thin enamel, and situations in which contouring would expose dark or discolored dentin in the esthetic zone.

Vital Bleaching

Bleaching vital teeth involves application of a bleaching agent to change tooth color (Figure 11.21). Typically, the bleaching agent consists of hydrogen peroxide or carbamide peroxide, and it can be used in a variety of different concentrations and application techniques. For many patients, use of over-the-counter trayless strip delivery system (Figure 11.22) can be an inexpensive and generally innocuous means of achieving the desired effect. Lack of proper fitting of the strips and low concentration of peroxide are some of the shortcomings of this option. For patients who desire to have the treatment directed by the dentist, other modalities are available. Bleaching treatment can be provided in-office and out-of-office.

The in-office modality is referred to as power bleaching and the out-of-office is referred to as at-home bleaching. Both options are done under the dentist's supervision. The in-office treatment may be appealing to some patients as it is more expeditious than other techniques. In-office bleaching utilizes a high concentration of hydrogen peroxide and different methods to speed up the process, such as incorporating metal ion into the agent formulation, increasing the pH of the agent, or applying a heat source. Some of the initial results from in-office bleaching can be attributed to teeth dehydration. The dehydration process usually occurs in a few minutes under relative or rubber dam isolation.[19,20] Within 24 hours of the in-office bleach, the teeth will rehydrate and there will be an expected rebound from the immediate office bleach shade.[21] A combined approach of in-office and at-home bleaching is often prescribed to complement the initial results of the in-office treatment. Light sources are widely utilized during the in-office bleaching procedure, because it is commercially claimed that light sources can improve and speed up the process. However, the validity of this claim has not been proven scientifically regardless of the concentration of hydrogen peroxide utilized in the process.[22]

The nightguard vital bleaching, or at-home bleaching technique, consists of a bleaching gel applied to the teeth via custom-fitted plastic trays fabricated by the dental team (Figure 11.23). Usually, the bleaching gel used in this modality is less concentrated than the gels used for in-office bleaching. Most common concentrations vary between 10% and 20% carbamide peroxide. Treatment time for this method is usually 1 to 2 weeks.

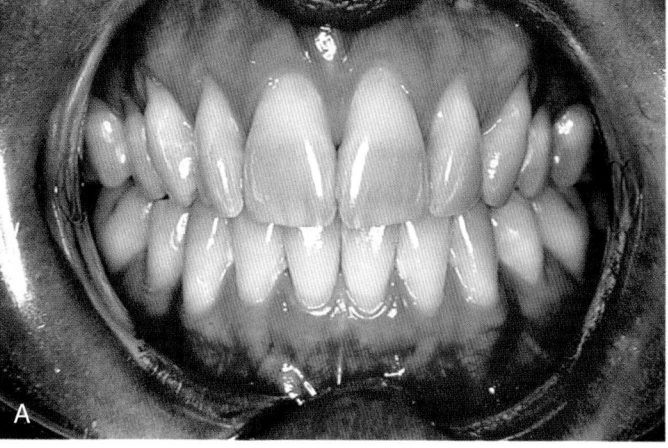
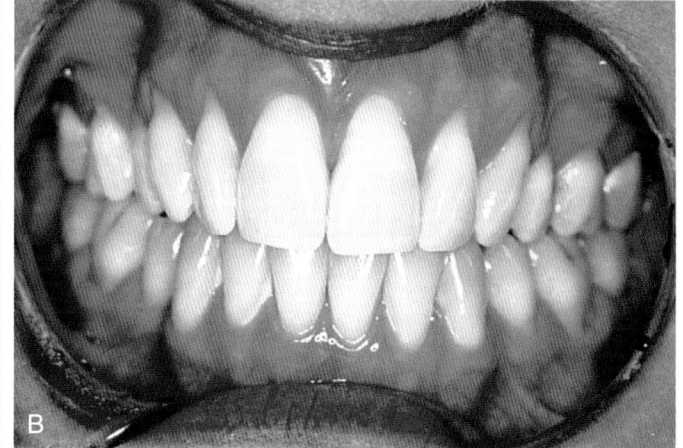

Fig. 11.21 Vital bleaching before/after. (From Ritter AV, Boushell LW, Walter R. *Art and Science of Operative Dentistry.* Elsevier; 2019.)

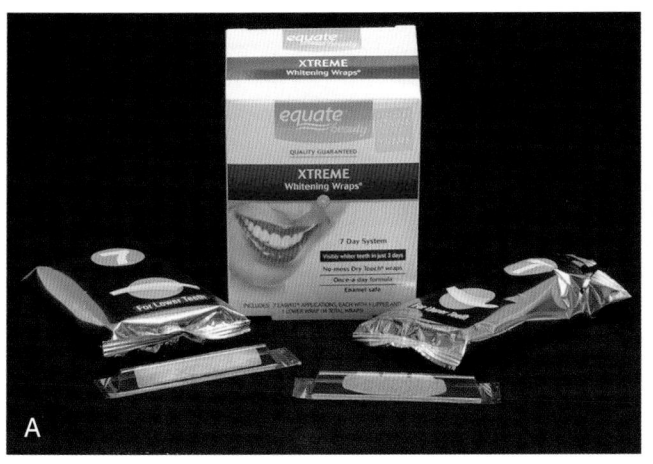
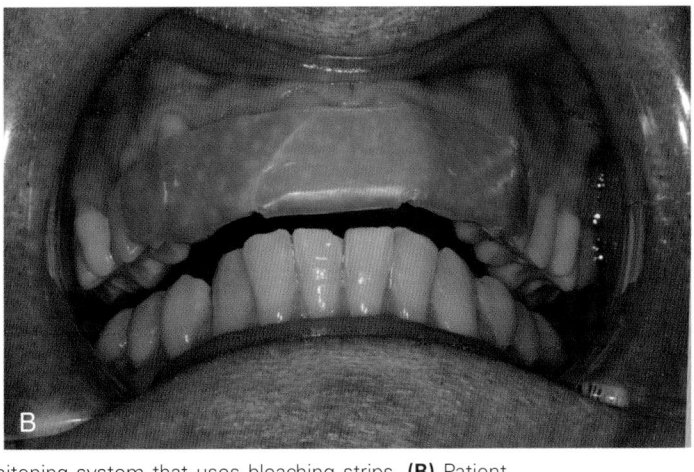

Fig. 11.22 **(A)** Example of over-the-counter tooth whitening system that uses bleaching strips. **(B)** Patient wearing plastic strip that contains bleaching material. (Courtesy Dr. Sam Nesbit.)

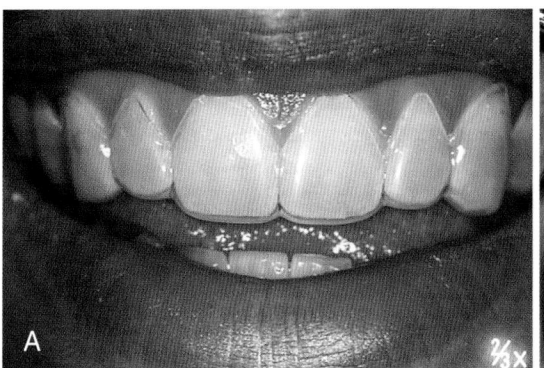
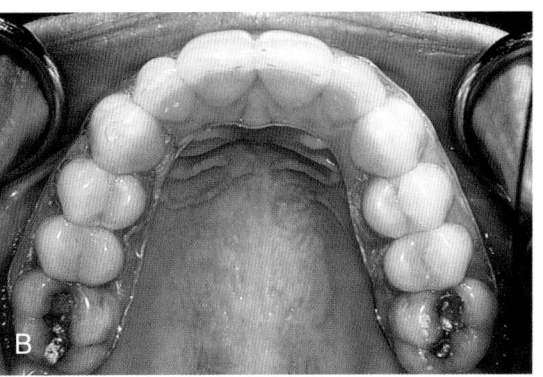

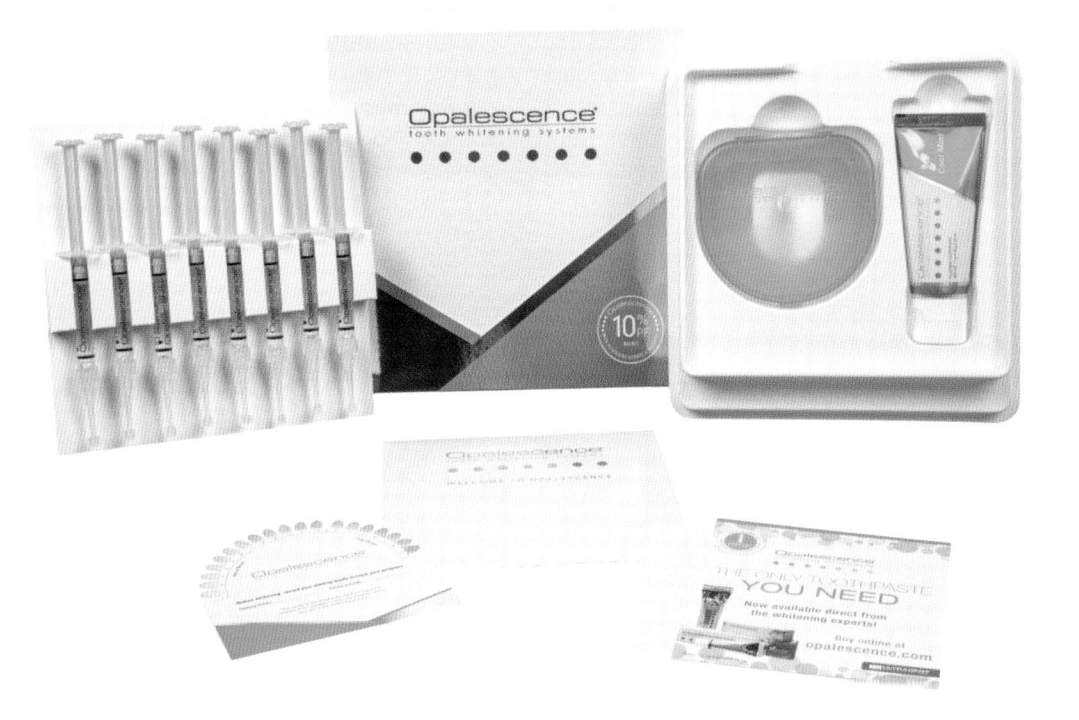

Fig. 11.23 Example of proprietary vital bleaching materials: Opalescence Tooth Whitening System (Ultradent Products, Inc.) (Courtesy Dr. Ralph Leonard.) **(A and B)** Bleaching trays inserted in patient's mouth.

The primary disadvantage associated with bleaching vital teeth is the risk of pulpal sensitivity, usually manifested as sensitivity to heat and cold. Sensitivity occurs more frequently with the in-office technique because of the use of bleaching agents with high concentration of peroxide. In contrast, the sensitivity to heat and cold that some patients experience as a result of home bleaching relates to frequency of use of the bleaching agent.[23] With either technique, most side-effects are transient. Home bleaching has been shown to be effective and safe for patients when implemented as directed.[23] Careful consideration must be given where there are visible existing composite restorations on anterior teeth. Patients need to be informed that facial restorations may need to be replaced after the bleaching procedure because of a mismatch of the existing restoration and the newly bleached tooth shade. For this reason it is usually recommended that where new restorations are planned bleaching is done prior to, rather than after, the re-restoration. Patients with hypersensitive teeth may not be good candidates for vital bleaching. If the treatment is prescribed for patients with tooth sensitivity, bleaching agents with low concentration of peroxide in combination with desensitizing agents should be considered. Some types of tooth discoloration, such as moderate to severe tetracycline stain, do not respond to vital bleach treatment.[23]

Bleaching Nonvital Teeth

For discolored teeth that have undergone endodontic therapy, **nonvital bleaching** treatment can help lighten the hue of the tooth structure (Figure 11.24). The treatment can be accomplished in the dental office (in-office nonvital bleaching or power bleaching technique) or it can be initiated in the professional setting and passively completed outside the dental office. With the in-office nonvital bleach technique, the tooth is isolated, the pulp chamber cleansed and etched, and a highly concentrated bleaching agent (38% hydrogen peroxide) applied in repeated applications until a satisfactory result is achieved. Alternatively, the out-of-office technique ("walking bleach"), is achieved by sealing a bleaching agent such as a sodium perborate paste into the pulp chamber for several weeks.[24]

Bleaching nonvital teeth is an effective technique that can produce excellent esthetic results with minimal trauma or discomfort. However, there is a risk of the dessvelopment of external cervical resorption. If the coronal portion of the root canal is not sealed effectively during the bleaching process with a sealing cement such as resin-modified glass ionomer (RMGI), nonvital bleaching may induce external resorption. To avoid this complication, the dentist should remove gutta-percha 1–2 mm apical to the clinical crown and place an RMGI liner to seal the root canal filling and isolate the bleaching agent within the coronal portion of the pulp chamber.[24] Some teeth do not respond to nonvital bleaching therapy and relapse can occur; in either case, an external bleaching technique may be attempted as an alternative treatment option.

Veneers

Veneers are restorations that can be applied to the facial surface of a tooth to improve esthetics by changing the color, contour, or size of the tooth. The materials commonly used as veneers are composite, feldspathic porcelain, (Figure 11. 25) or lithium disilicate (Figure 11.26). Veneer restorations can be fabricated using a direct (chairside) or indirect (laboratory fabricated) technique. The direct technique using composite resin generally provides a more conservative and less costly alternative to indirect veneers, but it does not afford the same resistant to staining, wear, and abrasion as indirect veneers (see the discussion of composite resin restorations in the section *Restoring Individual Teeth* for more information.)

With indirect veneers, the teeth are typically prepared by removing 0.3 to 0.6 mm of enamel on the facial and 1 to 1.5 mm from the incisal surfaces. In some cases, preparations can be minimal due to existing conditions such as significant erosion or abrasion of the facial surface of the tooth (sometimes termed a "no-prep veneer"). The traditional workflow for indirect veneers involves the following steps: the preparation is completed, conventional impressions are taken, a temporary restoration is fabricated, the veneer is manufactured by a laboratory, and then bonded in place. The workflow can also be done digitally using an intraoral scanner and the veneers can be milled and stained chairside with a computer-aided manufacturing system and ceramic oven.

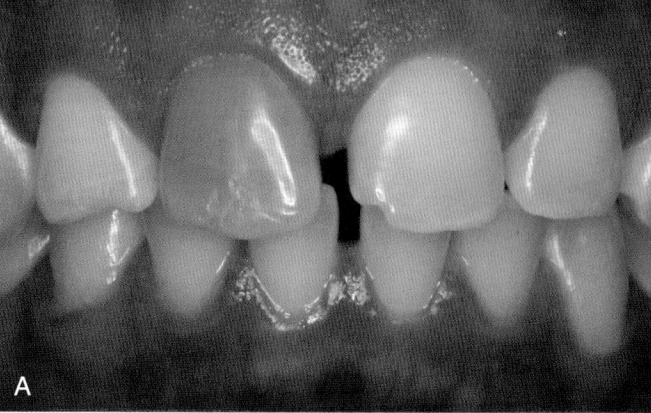 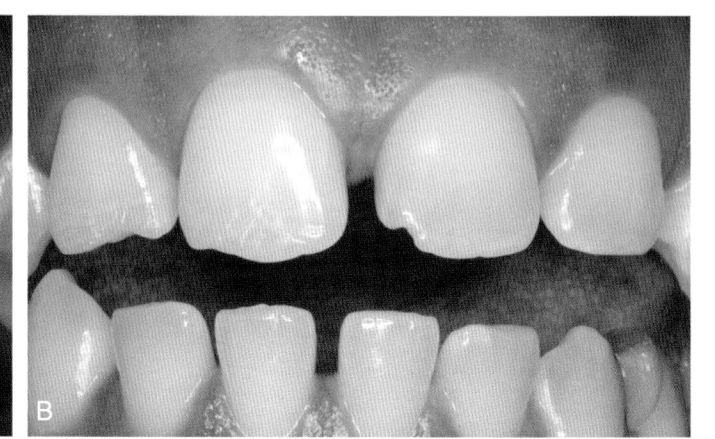

Fig. 11.24 Bleaching nonvital teeth before/after. (Courtesy Dr. Glen Ajith Karunanayake.)

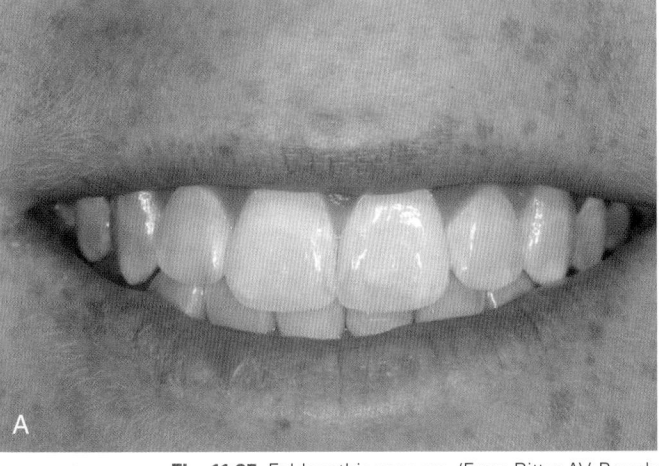
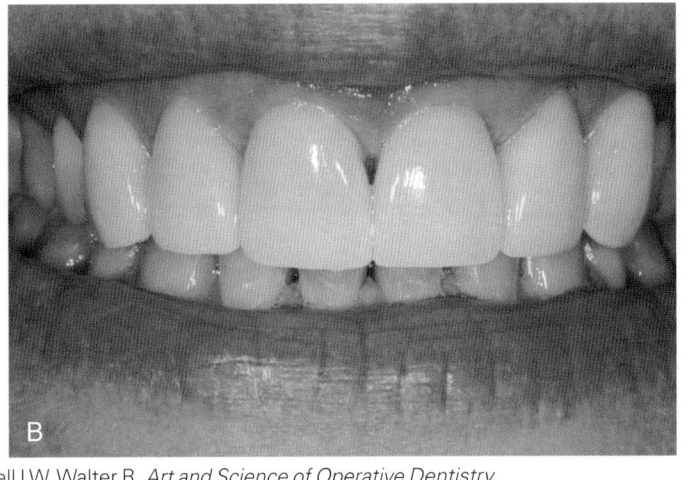

Fig. 11.25 Feldspathic veneers. (From Ritter AV, Boushell LW, Walter R. *Art and Science of Operative Dentistry.* Elsevier; 2019.)

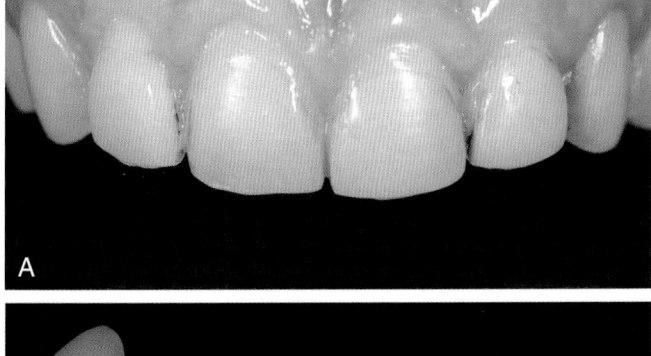
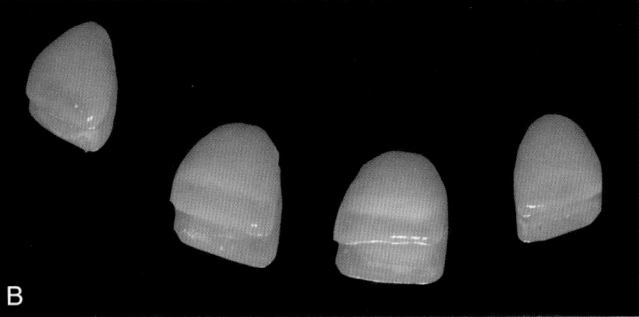
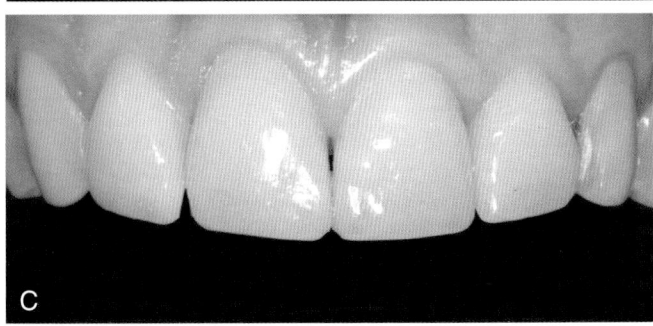

Fig. 11.26 CEREC milled lithium disilicate veneers (e.max) **(A)** before preparation, **(B)** ready for cementation, **(C)** after placement. (Courtesy Dr. Zaid Badr.)

Veneers may be indicated in cases involving extreme enamel discoloration, such as is seen with tetracycline staining or fluorosis. If an attempt is going to be made to bleach the affected teeth, bleaching should precede the veneering procedure and veneering should be delayed 7 to 10 days after the completion of any

bleaching phase of treatment because peroxide residue will negatively affect the bond strength of the veneer. Veneers can also be used to close diastemas, lengthen short teeth, or to replace small amounts of missing tooth structure (Figure 11.19). Feldspathic porcelain has historically been the material of choice for indirect veneers because it has been able to provide ideal esthetics, and durability. In recent years, medium-strength glass-ceramic materials such as lithium disilicate have been used increasingly for indirect veneers. This material can be pressed or milled and combines excellent esthetics with favorable physical and mechanical properties. Regardless of the material selection, every attempt should be made to avoid extending the veneer preparations into dentin as most failures associated with bonded porcelain veneers occur when the veneer is bonded largely or entirely to dentin substrate.[25]

Indirect veneers are contraindicated for patients who have habits such as bruxism or pencil chewing[25] because of the fracture potential when heavy persistent loading force is placed on the restoration. Similarly, patients with Class III and end-to-end bite relationships may not be suitable candidates for veneering. Teeth with existing direct restorations on the proximal surface may need full coverage rather than an indirect veneer. Considerable technical skills are required to prepare teeth for indirect veneers and successfully cement them in place.

Full Coverage Indirect Restorations

If a partial veneer restoration is warranted but insufficient tooth structure remains to support it, a full coverage restoration is appropriate. Throughout the 20th century, the most common and esthetic full coverage restoration for a maxillary anterior tooth was the feldspathic porcelain crown and its successor, the aluminous porcelain with layered feldspathic **porcelain jacket crown** (PJC). The PJC has translucence similar to that of natural tooth structure and therefore has a lifelike appearance. However, it has two significant limitations. It requires a significant reduction in the tooth structure for the crown to have sufficient strength and the PJC fractures easily making it unsuitable for patients presenting oral parafunctional habits. Through the late 20th century and into the 21st century, the PFM crown has been the mainstay when an indirect full coverage esthetic restoration is warranted. The PFM crown is fabricated with an internal metal coping, an opaque layer to block the metal color, and a porcelain layer surrounding the metal coping. It has significantly improved fracture resistance over that of the PJC and can provide excellent esthetic results, especially in the hands of an expert laboratory technician/ceramicist. Drawbacks have been the need for significant tooth reduction, sometimes blue grey shadowing at the gingival margin where the metal coping substructure may show through, or excessive opacity ("headlighting") in areas of insufficient facial tooth reduction. A collarless design where the metal substructure is cut back to allow a porcelain butt margin can effectively provide excellent esthetics and mitigate or eliminate possible color issues. Although PFM crowns continue to be a viable restorative option, the use of sintered, pressed, cast or milled ceramic crowns is rapidly increasing. Contemporary ceramic systems such as lithium disilicate (Figure 11.27) and zirconia (Figure 11. 28) can provide optimal esthetics, have improved fracture resistance, may require less

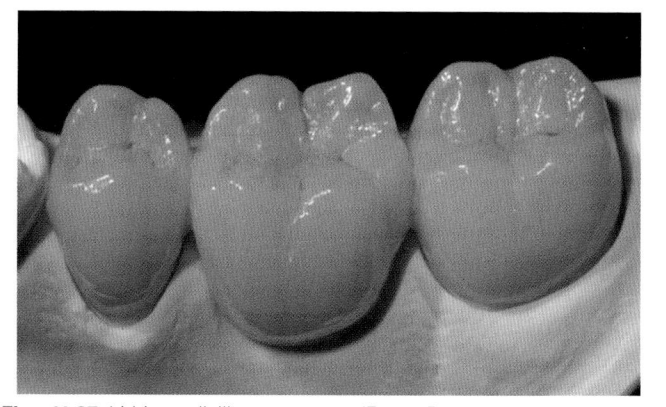

Fig. 11.27 Lithium disilicate crown. (From Ritter AV, Boushell LW, Walter R. *Art and Science of Operative Dentistry.* Elsevier; 2019.)

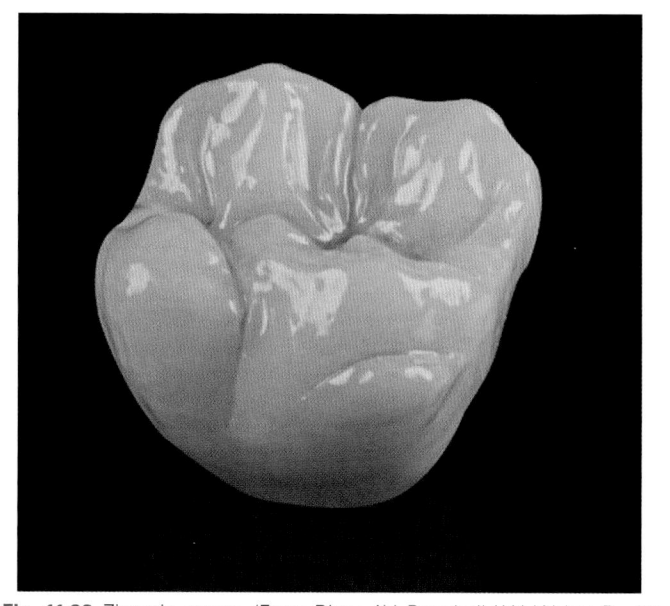

Fig. 11.28 Zirconia crown. (From Ritter AV, Boushell LW, Walter R. *Art and Science of Operative Dentistry.* Elsevier; 2019.)

tooth reduction, are less costly to produce, and can be fabricated chairside in some cases. Lithium disilicate, a glass-based ceramic, is usually favored in esthetic-demanding situations. Zirconia is favored in situations of significant occlusal load due to its high flexural strength and fracture resistance.[26]

ELECTIVE (NONACUTE) ENDODONTIC TREATMENT

Endodontic procedures (pulpal debridement or root canal treatment) are often provided for teeth with pulpal or periapical disease during the acute phase of care (Chapter 9) because the patient is experiencing pain or swelling; or in the disease control phase (Chapter 10) to halt the progression of pulpal or periapical disease, or to prevent acute problems from developing. Endodontic procedures performed in the definitive phase include conventional root canal therapy, endodontic retreatment, and apical microsurgery.

Endodontic therapy is indicated when there is a diagnosis of irreversible pulpitis, pulpal necrosis, or apical pathology (see Chapter 2, *Pulpal and Periapical Diagnoses*). During the disease control phase, the patient may have experienced signs of chronic infection (chronic apical periodontitis) but treatment was deferred in light of uncertainty about the patient's willingness, or need to, retain the tooth. At the outset of the definitive phase the patient's condition will need to be reassessed and the current treatment options discussed with the patient.

During the definitive phase, endodontic therapy may also be appropriate in the following situations:

- Apical pathology associated with a necrotic pulp represents a prime indication for root canal therapy. The patient and the dentist may not detect such a problem until the tooth darkens in appearance or distinctive signs are visible on periapical radiographs.
- Teeth with a large portion of the crown missing (usually caused by caries or fracture), teeth with deep or large direct-fill restorations, and teeth treatment planned for an indirect restoration, may benefit from elective root canal treatment. If the dentist determines that there is a high probability that the tooth will eventually need root canal treatment, the patient should be presented with the option of root canal treatment prior to fabrication of the indirect restoration. An even more compelling rationale for root canal treatment is if the retention and integrity of the indirect restoration would be improved by doing the root canal treatment and either anchoring the foundation into the pulp chamber or placing a post and core.
- Elective endodontics should be considered for teeth that will be devitalized in the process of overdenture construction or for those hypererupted teeth in which the pulp is likely to be devitalized in the process of altering the occlusal plane.

Retreatment (Figure 11.29) of a previously endodontically-treated tooth or **apical microsurgery** (Figures 11.30 and 11.31) may be necessary when signs of reinfection (i.e., contamination of the root canal system) appear. This may become apparent clinically in the form of a parulis or

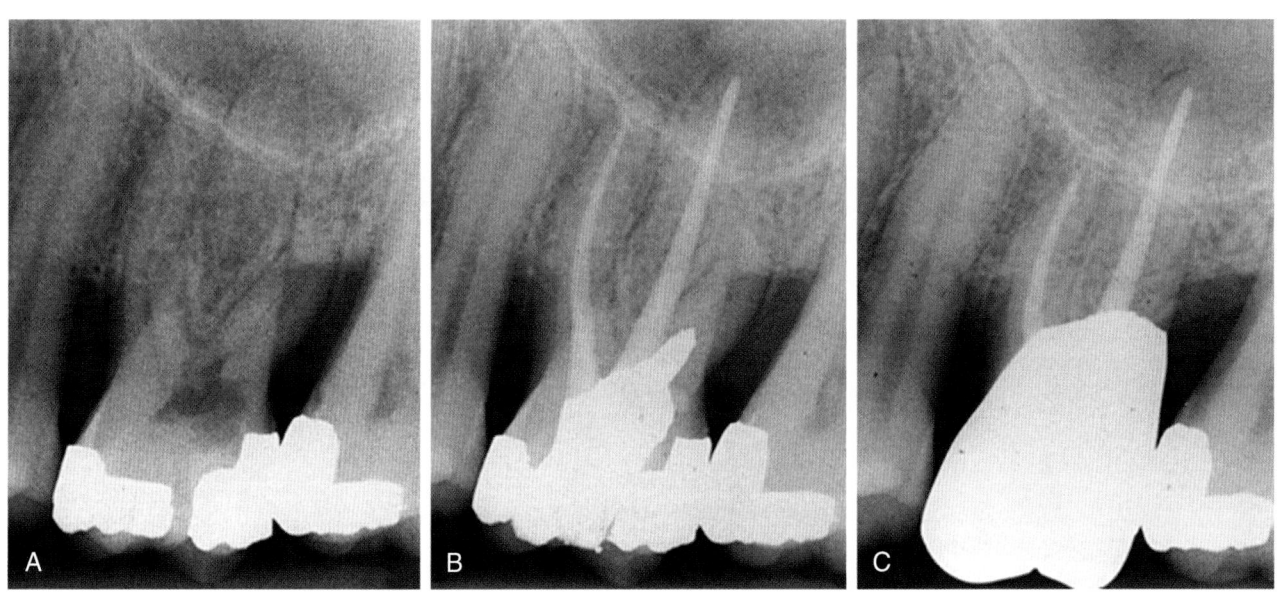

Fig. 11.29 Successful root canal treatment. (From Mahmoud Torabinejad, Ashraf F. Fouad, Shahrokh Shabahang; Endodontics: Principles and Practice, Sixth Edition © 2021)

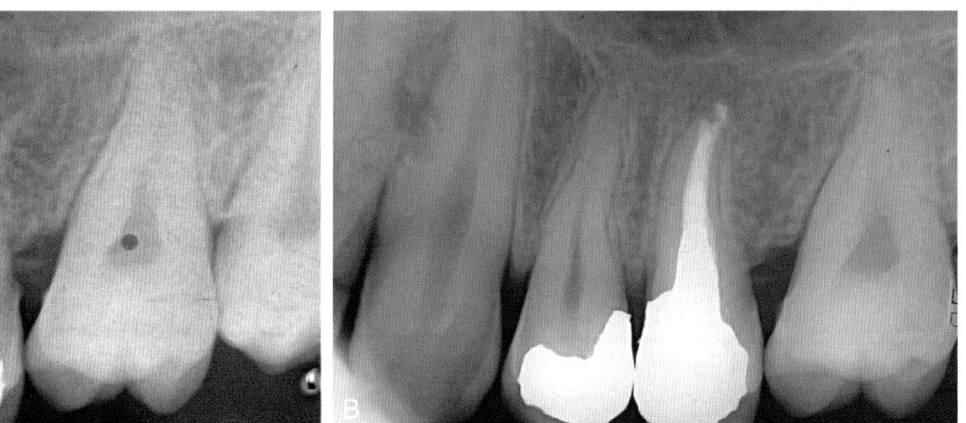

Fig. 11.30 Successful root canal retreatment. (From Robert A. Convissar; Principles and Practice of Laser Dentistry, Third Edition, Copyright 2023.)

fistula, or radiographically as an unresolved, new, or enlarged apical rarefying osteitis (see Chapter 3 for evidence-based discussion of this topic).

Keys to Decision Making
Professional Considerations

Before proceeding with endodontic therapy, the dentist must first assess the clinical significance of the involved tooth in relation to the other teeth and to the overall treatment plan. Although an important goal of dentistry is to help patients retain teeth, it may not be in the patient's best interest to invest the time and financial resources on endodontic therapy for a particular tooth. An example is a patient whose third molar would require root canal therapy if it were to be retained. The tooth's position in the arch and its often complex canal anatomy make it difficult to treat with root canal therapy. Even more compellingly, the lack of functional benefit to retaining the wisdom tooth and

the potential for caries or pericoronal or periodontal infection, often make extraction the best alternative.

After establishing the value of retaining a tooth, the dentist assesses whether the tooth can be restored and which procedures will be required to retain it. The question of restorability commonly hinges on how much tooth structure remains coronal to the alveolar crest. Often a bite-wing radiograph can help facilitate that analysis (Figure 11.32). In questionable cases, to reliably assess restorability, it may be necessary first to remove the caries. If there is infringement of the biologic width or if there is insufficient ferrule to retain a crown, a crown lengthening procedure (CLP) may be appropriate. If the tooth already has significant clinical attachment loss the CLP may be contraindicated because such a procedure could contribute to an unfavorable crown-to-root ratio and a poor periodontal prognosis. Endodontically treated teeth are often inherently fragile as a result of the loss of tooth structure to caries, large restorations, cuspal fractures, and even the root canal therapy itself. A full

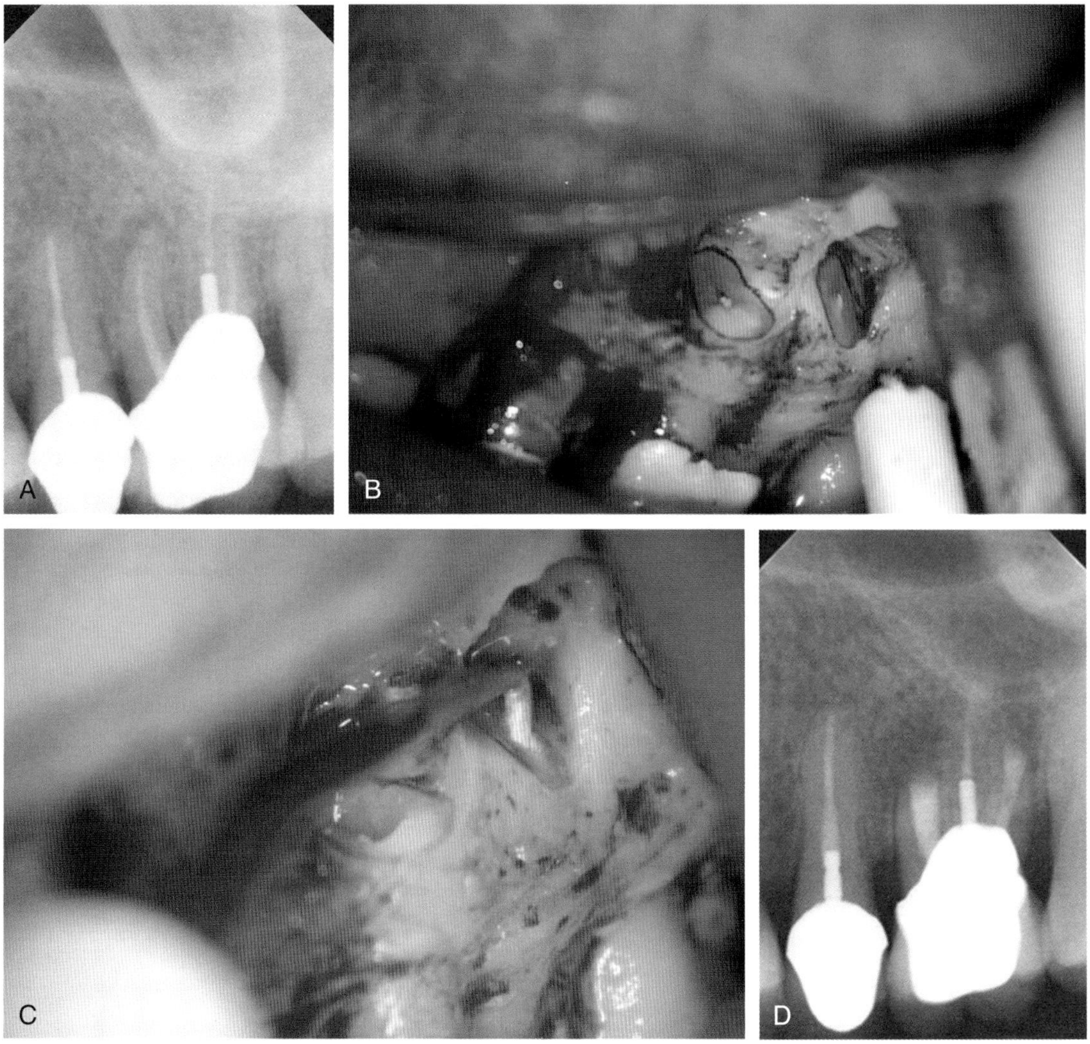

Fig. 11.31 Apical surgery. **(A)** Preoperative radiograph. **(B)** Root apices exposed. **(C)** One root apex resected and another root apex restored. **(D)** 3-month postoperative radiograph. (Courtesy Dr. Peter Tawil.)

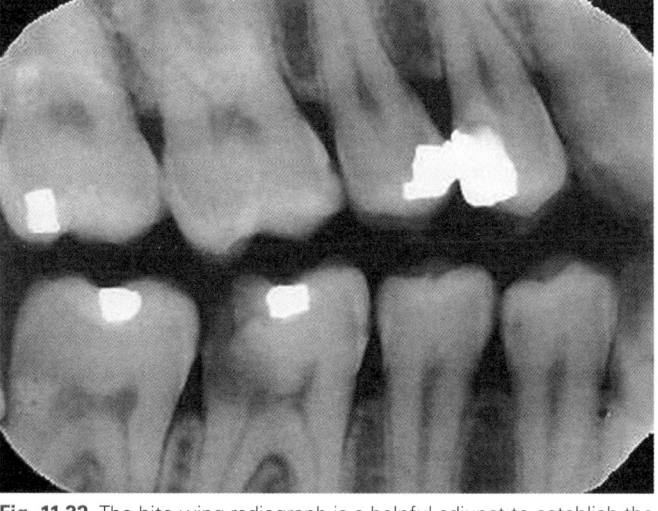

Fig. 11.32 The bite-wing radiograph is a helpful adjunct to establish the relationship of a proximal carious lesion to the bone crest, as with this lower first molar, because it helps in the assessment of the need for a crown lengthening procedure and helps to determine the restorative prognosis for the tooth. (Courtesy Dr. J. Ludlow.)

coverage restoration, such as a crown, is often needed to restore the tooth to function. A related issue that must be addressed is the prognosis for such a heavily restored tooth. Having determined that a tooth can be restored, how does the long-term prognosis for the tooth compare with what it would be after the usual treatment alternative of an extraction and an implant-retained crown? (See Chapter 3, *In Clinical Practice: A Common Dilemma–Deciding Between Extraction and Placement of an Implant Retained Crown Versus Restoration With a Root Canal Treatment, Foundation, and Crown* for an evidence-based discussion of this issue.)

The dentist must also assess whether there are anatomic or other treatment issues that may affect the outcome of root canal treatment. **Root dilacerations**, calcified canals, or poor access (e.g., limited opening) can make treatment more challenging and the prognosis less favorable. A related issue is for the dentist to determine, and discuss with the patient, when it is appropriate to refer the patient to a specialist for the endodontic treatment (see In Clinical Practice: When a Dentist May Consider Referral to an Endodontist box.)

When a Dentist May Consider Referral to an Endodontist

- Difficult patient management
- Complex medical history necessitating short appointments or other significant modifications to treatment
- Significant calcification of the pulp cavity
- Root dilaceration
- Maxillary premolars with three canals
- Mandibular premolars with split (fast break) canal
- Access through a crown
- Molars
- Retreatment
- Apical microsurgery
- Congenital anomalies
- Difficult isolation with rubber dam
- Root resorption (cervical, inflammatory, replacement, or internal)
- Caries with significant marginal periodontitis and questionable prognosis
- Immature teeth: open apex

Adapted courtesy Dr Lisiane Susin, Chapel Hill, NC

The American Academy of Endodontics AAE Endodontic Case Difficulty Assessment Form and Guidelines [https://www.aae.org/specialty/wp-content/uploads/] is a helpful tool in this regard.

Upon completion of root canal treatment, it is imperative that a definitive seal be placed to prevent recontamination of the root canal system. This seal may be in the form of a definitive direct-fill restoration (amalgam or composite) or a foundation. If a definitive indirect restoration is planned for the tooth, it is recommended that this be implemented as soon as practicable. If, however, the patient still has disease control treatment requirements (see Chapter 10) or if there are other more pressing definitive phase needs at this time and placement of an indirect restoration needs to be deferred, it is important to protect the tooth by:

- placing a cusp protective provisional or foundation restoration on the tooth; or at a minimum, reducing the occlusion and placing a durable interim direct-fill provisional restoration, such as glass ionomer;
- advising the patient to be cautious when chewing and to avoid applying heavy force on the tooth;
- informing the patient about the possibility of tooth fracture and the negative outcomes that may result, and documenting that conversation;
- examining the tooth at regular intervals for signs that the restoration is deteriorating or that the seal may be compromised.

Patient Considerations

The plan for definitive restoration, the prognosis for endodontic and restorative treatment, and the anticipated fees for all associated treatment, must be presented to the patient before beginning endodontic treatment. For some patients, the added cost of the procedures required to restore the tooth to function, such as crown lengthening, a post and core, and a crown, may make

the expense of the root canal treatment prohibitive. The patient may instead choose to have the tooth extracted. For medicolegal reasons, the dentist should document in the patient's record that all treatment options, including endodontic therapy, have been discussed before moving to extraction.

If endodontic treatment is not done in the practice or if the patient presents with challenges that would warrant treatment by an endodontic specialist, the consent conversation would need to include a discussion of the referral process, what each provider will be doing, and the charges for each entity. The lack of easy access to, or the cost for treatment by, a specialist may be a deterrent to the patient. Some patients may prefer to have endodontic treatment done in the general dentistry office for reasons of cost, convenience, or because they trust their dentist and are reluctant to see an unfamiliar specialist provider in spite of the additional training, experience, and equipment (microscope). This can be an ethical challenge for the general dentist who would like to see the patient retain the tooth, but who will be held to the standard of care for an endodontist.

Some patients may choose to have root canal therapy to retain a tooth but then delay definitive restorative treatment on the tooth because of cost or other considerations. Such a delay will leave the tooth at risk of a catastrophic fracture and endodontic treatment failure. Patients must be informed of this risk and the conversation needs to be documented in the patient record.

EXTRACTIONS AND PREPROSTHODONTIC SURGERY

Tooth Extraction

An extraction may be warranted when the patient has acute pain or infections (see Chapter 9) or in conjunction with disease control phase treatment (see Chapter 10). In the definitive phase of treatment there are also many circumstances where tooth extraction should be considered. When a tooth is hopelessly compromised from a restorative or periodontal standpoint, extraction may be necessary. Examples include teeth that have extensive caries, are split or have an irreparably fracture, or that have pulp and periapical involvement and conventional root canal treatment or apical surgery is not feasible or desired by the patient. Extractions can be used to facilitate succedaneous tooth eruption; and to prevent, mitigate or better manage malocclusion during and following the mixed dentition stage of patient development (see Chapter 17). Extractions are sometimes indicated for optimal management of tooth arch discrepancies and in conjunction with comprehensive orthodontic treatment and/or orthognathic surgery. Extraction is often the treatment of choice for impacted teeth, most commonly, third molars (see the In Clinical Practice: *Should Asymptomatic Third Molars Be Removed?* box). Teeth must sometimes be removed in conjunction with excision or block removal of a cyst, tumor, or carcinoma. Teeth with a guarded prognosis that would be in the portal of radiation therapy for oral cancer are generally extracted prior to cancer treatment. Teeth may need

IN CLINICAL PRACTICE

Should Asymptomatic Third Molars Be Removed?

The Issues

Third molars, also known as wisdom teeth, are sometimes viewed as unnecessary and potentially problematic and are often seen as candidates for extraction. Some practitioners have recommended their universal removal as a means of preventing infection, cysts, tumors, caries, periodontal disease, or destruction to adjacent teeth. Extraction of third molars has been the definitive treatment of choice for the prevention or elimination of pericoronitis. Patients may request their removal to preclude crowding of the anterior teeth, a projected outcome that has now been discredited. Research has cast doubt on the value and the necessity of routinely removing asymptomatic and clinically sound, but impacted, third molars.[1] Public health studies assessing the cost/benefit ratio of third molar removal continue to be divided.[2,3]

There is evidence that when pockets with bleeding on probing are found adjacent to third molars, the microbes in those sites are the same as those found in chronic periodontal disease. There is also evidence to suggest that the two disease processes are the same and that both have a similar association with markers for systemic inflammation.[4,5] Although this evidence is not compelling enough to suggest the necessity of removing all periodontally involved third molars, it does suggest the need to assess carefully the periodontal health of third molars especially for individuals with immunocompromising conditions, including the inflammatory arthropathies. Patients with chronic debilitating conditions and the inability to achieve effective daily plaque control will be at greater risk of periodontal disease and comorbid systemic diseases. In light of sometimes conflicting evidence, the dentist must consider carefully whether or not to recommend extraction.[6]

The requirements of informed consent make it necessary that the patient be an active partner in the decision-making process.

Reaching a Decision

A healthy 19- to 25-year-old patient whose impacted third molars have caused repeated episodes of pain from pericoronitis is a good candidate for extraction. When there is no reasonable prospect for the wisdom teeth to become properly aligned and fully functional and the patient has a strong desire to stave off future potential problems, consideration should be given to removal. Third molars that have a poor periodontal or restorative prognosis are usually best removed. Aside from these fairly clear-cut situations, the decision whether or not to extract becomes the purview of the patient after the dentist has presented the arguments for and against extraction in detail. Although there are no absolutes, the following general guidelines may help form the basis of the consent conversation with the patient.

- Younger and healthier patients (ASA I or II) generally have an easier time with the surgery, heal faster with fewer complications, and can be expected to exhibit more normal architecture in the edentulous ridge after healing. It is usually recommended that impacted third molars be removed by the time a patient reaches their mid-30s.[7]
- When the risk of future complications or problems associated with the third molars is high (e.g., caries, periodontal disease, pericoronitis), more weight should be given to extraction.
- When the possibility of surgical complications (e.g., paresthesia, fracture, dry socket, infection, or injury to the maxillary sinus) is high, more weight should be given to avoiding extraction.
- If there is a reasonable probability that the wisdom tooth may be needed in the future as an abutment for a prosthesis, as an anchor for orthodontic treatment, or to maintain the occlusal plane, more weight should be given to retention of the tooth or teeth.
- If loss of the third molars will compromise the patient's occlusion, function, or mastication, more weight should be given to retention.

In addition to these issues, the patient will want to weigh other personal considerations, such as the financial cost, potential loss of time at work, pain and anxiety control, and the timing of the procedure in relation to other life events. Two often unspoken but relevant considerations are the patient's prior experience with elective surgical procedures and personal philosophy in dealing with risk or uncertainty. Some patients have had unfortunate past experiences with surgical procedures and, as a result, are extremely apprehensive about such procedures. These patients are convinced that they are more likely to have complications or postoperative problems and will therefore often decline extraction unless it becomes imperative. These patients are resigned to dealing with the consequences if and when they arise. In contrast, other patients have a proactive orientation and seek to avoid preventable problems. Such patients typically elect to have the extractions if they have confidence the procedure will help them avoid pain, infection, or other clinical problems in the future. The wise practitioner is attentive to these varying perspectives and helps the patient factor them into the decision-making process.

References

1. Tulloch JF, Antczak-Bouckoms AA. Decision analysis in the evaluation of clinical strategies for the management of mandibular third molars. *J Dent Educ.* 1987;51(11):652–660.
2. Tulloch JF, Antczak-Bouckoms AA, Ung N. Evaluation of the costs and relative effectiveness of alternative strategies for the removal of mandibular third molars. *Int Technol Assess Health Care.* 1990;6(4):505–515.
3. Hounsome J, Pilkington J, Mahon J, et al. Prophylactic removal of impacted mandibular third molars: a systematic review and economic evaluation. *Health Technol Assess.* 2020;24(30):1–116.
4. White RP. Third molar oral inflammation and systemic inflammation. *J Oral Maxillofac Surg 63(8).* 2005;Supp 1:5–6.
5. Ruvo AT, Moss KL, Mauriello SM, et al. The systemic impact of third molar periodontal pathology. *J Oral Maxillofac Surg.* 2005;63(8). Suppl 1:69.
6. https://www.aaoms.org/docs/govt_affairs/advocacy_white_papers/white_paper_third_molar_data.pdf
7. Rofetto LK. Managing Impacted Third Molars. *Oral Maxillofac Surg Clin North Am Aug.* 2015;27(3):363–371.

to be removed in conjunction with as the treatment of a gunshot wound or blunt force trauma. **Autotransplantation** must include tooth extraction.

Simple dental extraction typically involves the removal of a tooth or root fragments with elevation and forceps delivery. A surgical extraction is often indicated for severely broken down or impacted teeth. This entails elevating a gingival flap for access and removing bone around the tooth and/or dissecting a multirooted or impacted tooth to facilitate its removal. The most common complications associated with extraction include bleeding, postoperative pain, dry socket (localized alveolar osteitis), infection, injury to an adjacent tooth or restoration, fracture of alveolar process, and injury/abrasion/tearing of soft tissues.

Professional Factors

From a professional perspective there are several important questions for the dentist to ponder before offering or recommending an extraction to a patient:

- Are there general health implications associated with doing the extraction? In some cases there are significant benefits to a patient when an extraction resolves an active infection or prevents future infection. Conversely, elective extractions may be contraindicated when a patient is severely debilitated, immune compromised, has a severe coagulation problem, or is at high risk of medication-related osteonecrosis of the jaw. If there are significant health risks associated with the extraction procedure, are they outweighed by the benefits? Can they be mitigated or managed safely and effectively?

- What are the dental indications for the extraction? Are they compelling? Do the benefits outweigh the risks? What are the consequences if the tooth is not extracted?
- Does the tooth have a favorable periodontal prognosis? If not, can the periodontal prognosis be improved with surgical or nonsurgical treatment? Is the patient capable of undergoing the necessary periodontal therapy and of maintaining the tooth in a healthy state?
- Is the tooth restorable? If so, what procedures are needed to restore and maintain the tooth (e.g., crown lengthening, root canal treatment, foundation, crown)? Sometimes the recommendation to extract is made because, if retained, the teeth would not act as satisfactory abutment for a prostheses or it might jeopardize the prognosis for the surrounding teeth.
- Has the patient been given sufficient information to make an informed decision, i.e., a balanced and fair presentation of the treatment options, including the risks, benefits, costs, prognosis, and expected outcomes both with and without treatment?
- Who will be doing the extraction? Are some extractions done in the general dental office? If so, is this an extraction that can be done safely and predictably in the same office or does it present with issues that make it better suited for a specialist or other provider who has more skill, training or experience?

Patient Factors

The patient may have an implicit bias either for or against extractions. Someone who had a difficult experience with a previous extraction may be unduly hesitant to have another tooth removed even under serious and compelling circumstances. Conversely, a patient with a family and personal dental experience thought to be "hopeless" may be overly fatalistic and unwilling to invest even modest resources in saving teeth that could have a favorable prognosis. Both of these scenarios will require the dental team to invest time and energy in developing a trusting relationship with the patient and to attempt to instill in the patient a realistic perspective regarding the diagnoses, disease risk, and treatment alternatives. In some cases, teeth may be salvageable, but the patient believes that they do not have the time, financial resources, or the interest in undergoing the necessary treatment required to save them. Such patients may be inclined to make a hasty decision to extract in order to "solve the problem quickly" or to "save money." That decision may be regretted later when the patient realizes the negative consequences of the extraction (impaired esthetics, function) and the eventual cost of tooth replacement.

Most definitive phase dental procedures are elective and extractions are irreversible. In light of these realities it is imperative that the patient understand the diagnoses and be given the opportunity to make a treatment decision with a clear understanding of the options with the attendant risks, benefits, and costs of each. Taking the time to have an open and impartial dialogue with the patient, listening and responding to their questions and concerns, and sharing honestly and compassionately regarding both the short-term and long-term consequences of the treatment decision is essential when establishing informed consent and is the essence of person-centered care.

Preprosthetic Surgery

Surgical procedures may be necessary or beneficial before fabrication of dental prostheses. Common preprosthetic surgical procedures include removing soft tissue or bone that will interfere with fabrication, insertion, or function of a denture; maintenance of bone following extraction, known as **site preservation** or **ridge preservation;** and implant placement. In some situations, preprosthetic surgery is mandatory to achieve a successful prosthetic outcome. In others, the surgery is optional. When faced with the cost, time, and inconvenience of undergoing preprosthetic surgery, some patients may decline, but all patients who could potentially benefit from the surgery should be presented with the option.

Patients scheduled to receive fixed or removable partial or complete dentures should have healthy and supportive soft and hard tissues underlying the prosthesis. Four clinical conditions that often require surgical intervention are discussed in this section and summarized in eTable 11.5 on the ebooks+.

Exophytic Soft Tissue Lesions

Many different conditions or pathologies can be included under this heading. Some of the more common diagnoses are hypertrophic or hyperplastic (flabby) ridges, epuli, and denture (palatal) papillomatosis. If minor, these lesions may be inconsequential, but in an advanced state they may make successful denture wearing impossible. Regardless of the severity of these conditions, diagnosing and managing them properly is paramount for a successful prosthodontic therapy outcome.

Bulbous Tuberosities

Enlarged tuberosities may consist of excess soft tissue, bony tissue, or both. Overextended "drooping" tuberosities can alter the occlusal plane, limit the space for teeth or denture base material, interfere with retention, and in extreme cases, render the denture unusable. In these cases, surgical intervention is needed to facilitate the prosthetic rehabilitation and create enough restorative space.

Exostoses and Tori

Like enlarged tuberosities, large exostoses may impair the seating of prostheses and their presence may impede the retention, fit, strength, and function of a denture. Bony exostoses often result in undercuts in the denture base. They are notorious for causing denture sores because the overlying soft tissue tends to be thin, friable, and easily abraded or traumatized during denture function, and placement and removal of the prosthesis.

Deficient Edentulous Ridges

Some patients have extensive bone loss and ridge resorption in the edentulous areas and this pattern may be progressive over the patient's lifetime.[27] The severity and pattern of bone loss varies by individual and site but can progress to become unsatisfactory as denture-bearing areas, lacking a long-term stable foundation for a conventional removable partial or complete denture. One common example, also known as **combination syndrome**, occurs when the maxillary anterior teeth have been missing for an extended period during which the mandibular anterior teeth have been present and in occlusal function, leading to severe resorption of the maxillary anterior ridge.

If a conventional denture is the chosen course of treatment in the presence of ridge atrophy, then modifying the alveolar ridge to improve the ridge shape and increase the size of the denture-bearing area may be the only recourse. **Vestibuloplasty** or repositioning of the vestibular fold more apically—often with concurrent placement of grafts from skin or oral mucosa—can effectively increase the usable ridge height and area. Some cases may require osseous surgical procedures, such as a total or segmental bone graft, a palatal osteotomy, or a maxillary sinus floor graft. **Distraction osteogenesis** is an alternative to conventional augmentation procedures.[28] With this procedure, the edentulous ridge is enhanced by incrementally separating the buccal and lingual plates horizontally, or the alveolar bone from the basal bone vertically, and encouraging new bone deposition to develop between the bony segments.

A deficient ridge in a bounded edentulous space can compromise the pontic site in fixed prosthodontic therapy. Absent tissue augmentation procedures, the pontic site may be unusually large, esthetically unappealing, difficult for the patient to clean and may be a site for frequent food entrapment.

Surgical Procedures Associated With Implant Placement

Depending on the volume (height and width) of alveolar bone available in the planned dental implant site(s), bone augmentation and/or sinus floor elevation procedures may be necessary. Ridge preservation or site preservation refers to the placement of bone graft material within an extraction site immediately after tooth removal with the purpose of preserving bone height and width. Following tooth extraction, the alveolar ridge undergoes dimensional changes resulting in a reduction in both the height and width of the site.[29] Site preservation helps to minimize the extent of these changes,[30] theoretically helping to facilitate dental implant placement by reducing the need and/or likelihood for later bone augmentation. In edentulous sites with insufficient bone volume for dental implant placement, **guided bone regeneration (GBR)** may be necessary. In cases where the ridge volume is deficient such that implant placement is precluded, GBR is performed to increase the ridge dimension using a variety of materials, including bone grafts, barrier membranes, biologic agents, and/or space maintaining devices (tenting screws, titanium mesh, etc.). In this staged approach, GBR typically precedes dental implant placement by 3 to 6 months. In select cases, however, GBR may be completed in conjunction with dental implant placement, assuming that primary[31] implant

stability is obtained. Current technologies such as 3D imaging and digital implant planning allow very accurate assessment of the pretreatment condition and to preview the plan for not only the implant placement but for any necessary bone augmentation procedure. Generally, when bone augmentation procedures are included, the treatment duration will be longer to accommodate healing.

Because of individual patient anatomy and/or sinus pneumatization, the floor of the maxillary sinus may limit the availability of vertical bone in the posterior maxilla for dental implant placement. In these cases, subantral sinus floor elevation may be necessary. The two most commonly used techniques for sinus floor elevation include a **lateral approach** via a Caldwell-Luc procedure and a **transalveolar approach**. When the lateral approach is used, bone is removed from the lateral aspect of the alveolus overlying the planned implant site, permitting access to the underlying Schneiderian membrane lining the sinus cavity. The membrane is gently elevated by the clinician and bone graft materials are placed to elevate the sinus floor. Using this procedure, simultaneous or delayed implant placement may be completed, depending on the clinician's ability to achieve primary implant stability. The transalveolar approach is most commonly recommended when at least 5 mm of vertical bone height is present.[32] When this technique is used, osteotomes are introduced into the dental implant preparation site and are used to elevate the sinus floor locally. Particulate bone graft materials are commonly placed to retain the new contour of the sinus floor. If the implant fixture is stable in the prepared site, it is also placed during that same visit.

Short dental implants have been introduced to provide anchorage and stability in situations where there is inadequate bone height in the posterior maxilla or the posterior mandible. These implants usually have a wide body (diameter) and, according to multiple recent systematic reviews, have survival rates and marginal bone loss comparable to that of regular sized implants. Advantages of utilizing short implants include avoiding invasion of vital structures such as the maxillary sinus and the inferior alveolar nerve, reducing treatment time and morbidity, and reducing the need for bone augmentation and therefore treatment cost.[33,34]

REPLACING MISSING TEETH

The replacement of missing teeth has long been one of the fundamental services provided by dentists. Teeth are commonly missing or lost due to congenital reasons, extensive caries, advanced periodontal disease, or catastrophic fracture. When a tooth is lost in the **esthetic zone** or if loss contributes to speech or functional problems, the patient is usually highly motivated to replace the tooth or teeth.

Traditional modalities of tooth replacement include complete dentures, removable partial dentures, and FPDs. These continue to be viable modes of treatment and are now supplemented and enhanced by an additional wide array of fixed and removable implant-retained and supported dental prosthetic options. The following section discusses commonly utilized tooth replacement therapies and their attributes.

Keys to Decision Making
Professional Considerations

A fundamental question that the dentist must first answer is whether the missing tooth or teeth *need(s)* to be replaced and how compelling that need is. Significant issues in this regard include whether the absence of teeth has caused limitation of function, speech, or esthetics. Has the patient experienced a loss of self-esteem because of the tooth loss? Another important concern is occlusal stability. Has there been any tipping, drifting, or extrusion of the teeth, or collapse of arch form or loss of vertical dimension of occlusion; and what is the potential for any of these to occur in the future? These issues are critical to making a treatment versus no treatment recommendation to the patient. And if a treatment recommendation is made, how strong should it be?

When it has been determined that the patient will benefit from tooth replacement and is interested in having the procedure, the dentist must determine whether any systemic problems limit or contraindicate prosthodontic treatment.

Oral health (disease control) needs to be established before definitive prosthodontic therapy can begin. Active oral disease, including dental caries and periodontal and periapical disease, must be eliminated. If teeth are to be retained, the patient's oral disease risk must be assessed and mutable risk factors addressed with the patient and mitigated or eliminated. A related factor is the dentist's assessment of the effectiveness of the patient's oral self-care, which can have a significant impact on the optimal selection of treatment by dentist and patient and on the prognosis for the definitive plan of care.

Given the stability, functionality, longevity, and esthetics of implant-retained prostheses, they have become the desired and recommended solution for replacing missing teeth in many situations. If an implant-retained prosthesis is not feasible or if implant options are ruled out by the patient, other nonimplant retained prosthetic options are available; and each of those will have attendant professional considerations to be weighed. For tooth-borne prostheses, any potential abutment tooth must be carefully evaluated for its suitability in the appropriate restoration design. Overall occlusion should be evaluated for irregularities in the occlusal plane, loss of vertical dimension of occlusion, malalignment or malpositioning of the abutment teeth, and guidance patterns in excursive movements. Each of these considerations may affect which type of prosthesis, occlusal scheme, and material selection will have the best prognosis. When managing bounded edentulous spaces, additional matters of interest include a detailed analysis of tooth vitality and pulpal status, bone support, periodontal status, and crown-to-root ratio of the abutment teeth. The length of the edentulous span can have a bearing on the number of abutments required and on the long-term prognosis for an FPD. Specific areas of concern when dealing with an unbounded edentulous space include the viability and suitability of the potential abutments; the height, width, and form of the edentulous ridge; available interocclusal space for restorative material; the location and size of tooth and bony undercuts; and any other factors that may be associated with the various prosthetic designs under consideration.

One of the greatest challenges and responsibilities for the dentist is to be able to provide the patient with an honest assessment of the prognosis for each of the reasonable treatment options. Given the many variables that may influence the prognosis determination (see Chapter 3), the level of certainty about the prognosis for one or more of the considered options may be low. Regardless, the patient needs to be provided with the best available information before a fully informed consent decision can be reached.

Attendant with the consent discussion is consideration of who will be providing the prosthetic treatment for the patient. Patients who need prosthodontic services and have complex medical problems, or who are deemed to be particularly challenging from a management or legal risk perspective, may be good candidates for referral to a prosthodontist. Similarly, patients should be given the option of referral to a prosthodontist when it is apparent that the additional, training, knowledge, or expertise of the specialist would be of benefit to the patient. Most general dentists will be comfortable and capable of handling what Dr Frank Celenza termed "conformative dentistry," i.e., any restorative procedures done within the confines of existing tooth form and occlusal relationships.[35] When the reconstruction involves multiple teeth where there will be a change in the contour of the teeth (e.g., full mouth rehabilitation) or when opening the vertical dimension is needed (other than with a full denture), it is normally prudent and wise to discuss with the patient the option of referral to a prosthodontist or another dentist who has had advanced training and has demonstrated skill in performing the procedure.

Patient Considerations

As with other treatment options discussed in this chapter, key patient considerations drive the decision making. In this treatment category, modifiers can be briefly summarized in three questions: What does the patient want? How strongly do they want it? How much is the patient willing to invest in the process? If the patient declines treatment, there may or may not be significant adverse consequences. Replacement of teeth may offer a significant benefit in the overall quality of life and in the patient's sense of self-esteem, but those benefits can only be achieved if the patient desires the treatment and is willing to invest the required time, energy, and resources required to achieve it.

The first question then is "**Does the patient want the missing tooth or teeth replaced**?" If the patient is not interested in tooth replacement, the dentist should be sure that the patient is aware of the possible consequences of not doing so. If the patient does seek replacement, the dentist should review with the patient why this option is perceived as worthwhile. Is it for esthetic, functional, preventive, or other reasons? Are the patient's anticipated outcomes realistic? Follow-up questions should determine whether the patient is fully informed as to the replacement options. Do they have a preference for a fixed or removable treatment option? Have implants been considered? Will visible metal clasps or other aspects of the prosthesis be esthetically acceptable? Is the patient willing to undergo adjunctive orthodontic treatment or preprosthetic surgery if it is deemed necessary?

It is essential for the dentist to provide the patient with information regarding the relative importance of replacing missing teeth in their unique situation. There are notable clinical situations where the need for tooth replacement is more compelling. For example, when the patient has a lack of occlusal stability, loss of periodontal attachment, or a history of shifting and drifting of teeth, there is evidence to suggest that tooth replacement is needed to prevent more adverse consequences. For younger patients, the need is usually even more pressing.[36]

The second major question, "**How strongly does the patient want the treatment?**" offers a means of assessing the extent to which the patient is motivated to receive the treatment in light of the challenges that they will be expected to face. Patients who have a strong desire for the treatment and are well informed about the risks, hazards, and possible negative consequences can be expected to be better able to adapt, more accepting of problems should they arise, and more likely to attach a high value to the outcome. Engaging the patient in the decision-making process and encouraging the patient to take ownership in their oral health condition are powerful motivators and are associated with patient perceived positive outcomes of treatment.[37] Conversely, the patient who has a low tolerance for pain and who does not trust oral health professionals will usually not be a good candidate for a full-mouth reconstruction involving extensive fixed prosthodontics.

The third major question, "**How much is the patient willing to invest?**" relates to the individual's commitment to the process. Do they have the time and the energy to engage in the treatment and see it to completion? Are they willing to endure the discomfort and inconvenience that may occur during the course of treatment? Can they comply with oral self-care recommendations and maintain the prosthesis and their oral health during the treatment and for years to come? Do they have the necessary financial resources to cover the cost of the treatment? For example, the individual on a subsistence level fixed income may not be a candidate for an implant-retained prosthesis or extensive rehabilitation. On the other hand, a patient with the necessary financial resources may not be willing to spend the time or undergo the inconvenience of having implants placed in order to have an implant-retained prosthesis.

If the patient lacks the motivation, commitment, or resources to engage in ideal treatment, we still have an ethical and professional responsibility to provide appropriate care for the patient to alleviate pain and help the patient achieve the best possible level of oral health in light of their general health and life circumstances. Chapter 13 frames the discussion of how to care for patients with special needs, and Chapter 19 specifically addresses care provision for patients who are motivationally or financially challenged.

Procedures for Replacing Missing Teeth
Fixed Partial Dentures

For decades, **FPDs** have provided a stable, reliable, and functional means of restoring bounded edentulous spaces (Figure 11.33). If done well and maintained properly, an FPD can provide a long-lasting restorable solution that can be esthetic,

functional, and satisfactory for both the patient and the dentist. But if this treatment modality is not done based on solid fundamentals, the results can be disappointing and result in further tooth loss and morbidity. An FPD usually consists of at least two tooth-borne **retainers** attached to one or more artificial teeth or **pontics**. The retainers with pontics are then permanently cemented to abutment teeth. FPDs may be fabricated of cast metal, porcelain-fused-to-metal, ceramics, and reinforced resin. The retainers for most FPDs are full-coverage restorations but may be partial coverage (an inlay or onlay). Another notable exception is the resin-bonded FPD, for which the retainers are etched ceramic or metal wings that are bonded directly to the abutment teeth taking advantage of advances in adhesive dentistry (Figure 11.34).

The major advantage of an FPD is that the replacement teeth are fixed in place and provide a stable and natural-appearing alternative to a removable prosthesis. An FPD generally provides good esthetics, function, and preservation of arch form. Patients must keep the FPD plaque free because the abutment teeth remain susceptible to recurrent caries and periodontal disease. The presence of the pontic is often an impediment to oral self-care and can be responsible for increased plaque retention. An FPD may compromise the abutment teeth, making them susceptible to future treatment needs, such as root canal therapy or even extraction (necessitated because of a tooth or root fracture). An FPD is not indicated if the restorative and periodontal condition of the abutment teeth cannot support it.

With the increased use of an implant-retained crown as a replacement for a single missing tooth, the conventional FPD is now used more sparingly. There are still some notable indications for the FPD, however. Patients who have a bounded edentulous space and who for medical, financial, or other reasons are not good candidates for implants, may be good candidates for an FPD. For patients who have an aversion to oral surgical procedures of any kind, an FPD may be a good alternative to an implant-retained prosthesis. The prime dental indication for placing an FPD is the patient whose abutment teeth are heavily restored and who is otherwise a good candidate for full coverage restorations on those teeth.

Removable Partial Dentures

A conventional **removable partial denture (RPD)** consists of a metal framework (can be cast, milled, or printed) with an acrylic base and replacement teeth (Figure 11.35). The forces on the partial denture are transferred to the abutment teeth via the framework and clasps and to the edentulous ridge from the acrylic bases. Relatively inexpensive and stable, this prosthesis can provide a measured level of esthetics and function. Some patients may find a partial denture unappealing because it must be removed for cleansing and maintenance of tooth and tissue health and because it may have visible metal clasps. The abutment teeth are at a statistically higher risk for caries and increased mobility. As with complete dentures, particularly in the absence of adequate oral self-care, the RPD may cause traumatic ulcers, stomatitis, or epuli formation and may accelerate bone atrophy in the edentulous areas. The prosthesis itself is prone to occlusal wear,

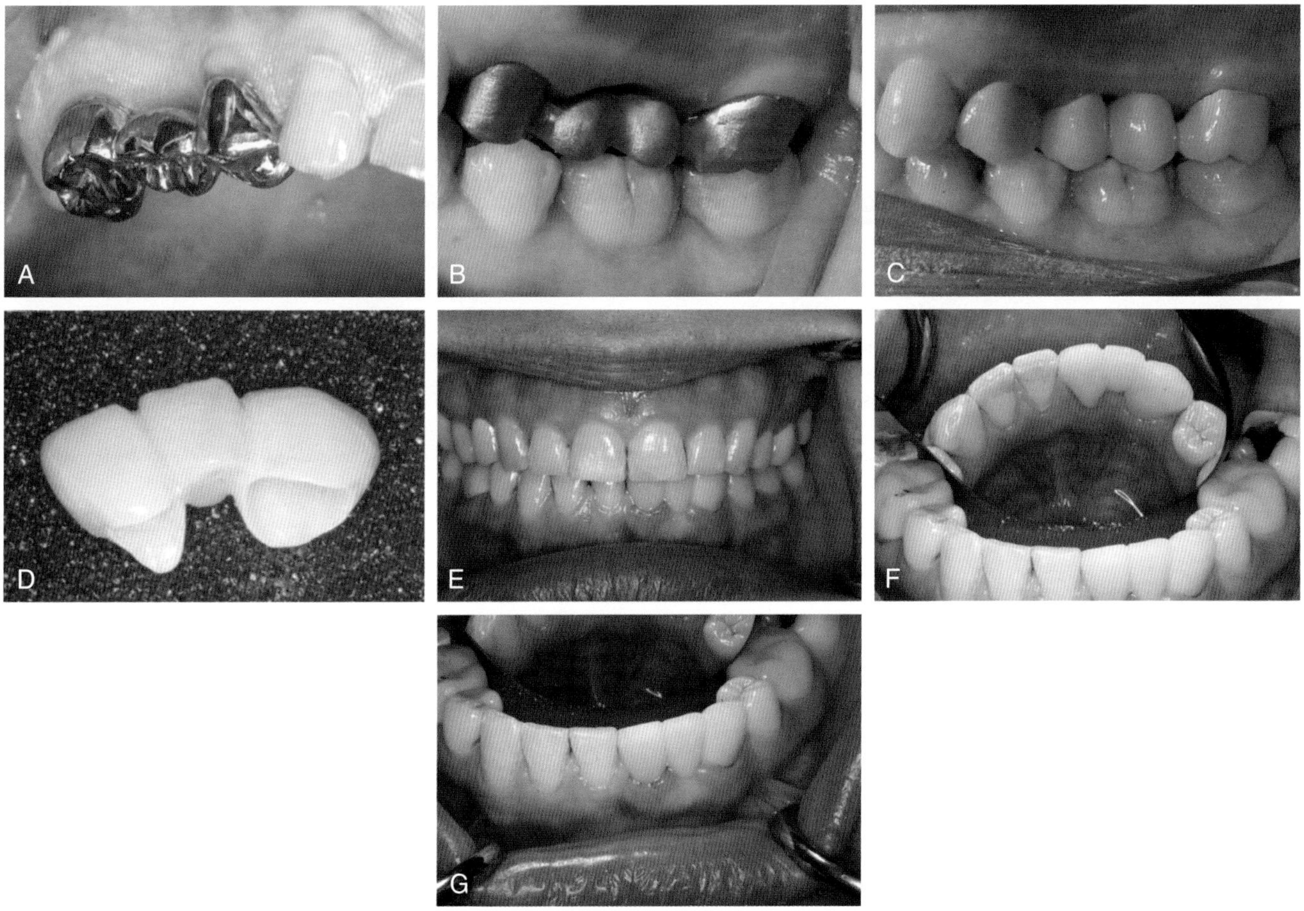

Fig. 11.33 Fixed partial dentures (FPD). **(A)** All-gold FPD; **(B and C)** PFM FPD framework try-in and after cementation; **(D–G)** All-ceramic FPD. (Courtesy Dr. Carlos H. Barrero.)

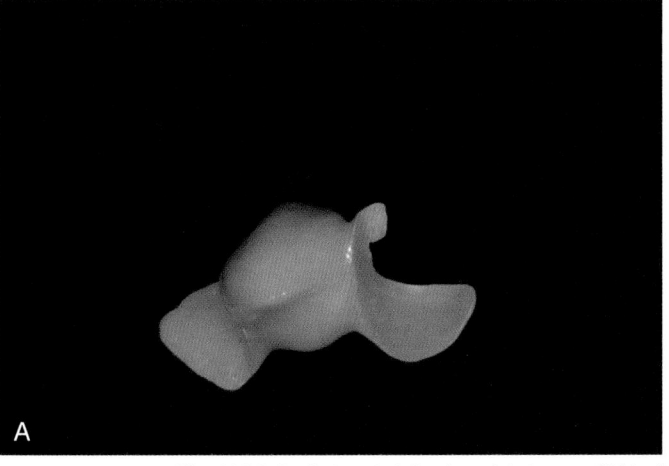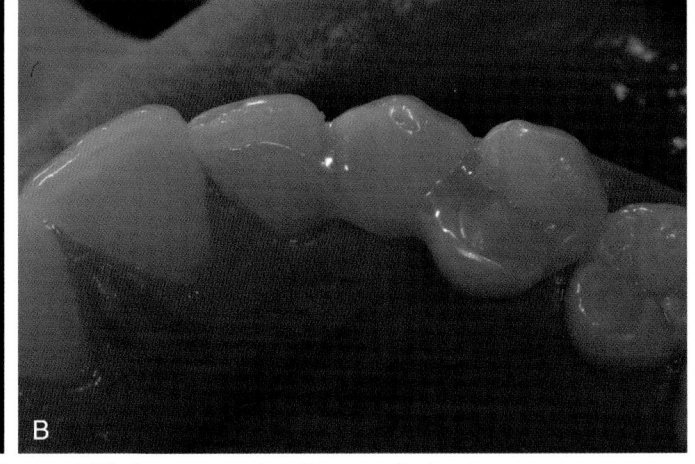

Fig. 11.34 Resin-bonded fixed partial denture **(A)** before, and **(B)** after cementation. (Courtesy Dr. Ingeborg De Kok.)

fatigue of the clasps, fracture of the cast metal components or acrylic saddles, or loss of denture teeth. The most notable disadvantage, however, is the significantly reduced function when compared with natural teeth, FPDs, or implant-retained prostheses. If the patient will accept a removable partial denture but does not want to have visible metal clasps, tooth color clasps made of clear, white, and pink resin can be used to retain these prostheses.

If the patient has an allergy or aversion to the metal components in removable partial dentures, an RPD can be fabricated in acrylic. There are three main categories of acrylic RPD materials: (1) all-acrylic (PMMA) resin, with or without wrought wire clasps (2) flexible resin, (3) a more durable resin framework such as acetyl resin. The first category, all acrylic PMMA resin, is often used as a temporary or interim RPD (sometimes colloquially called a "flipper.") These are the most quickly and

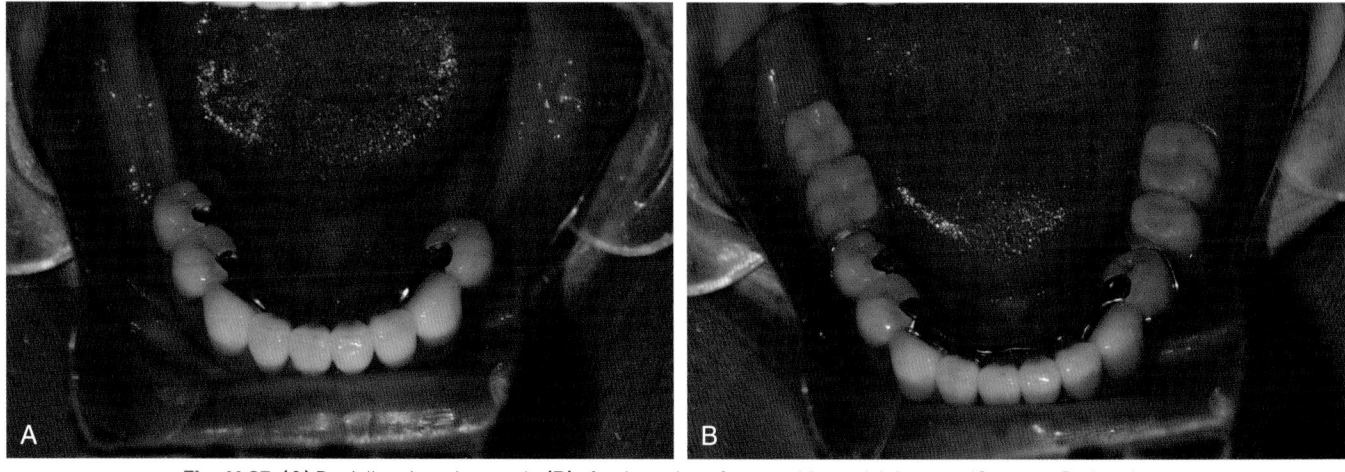

Fig. 11.35 **(A)** Partially edentulous arch; **(B)** after insertion of removable partial denture. (Courtesy Dr. Ingeborg De Kok.)

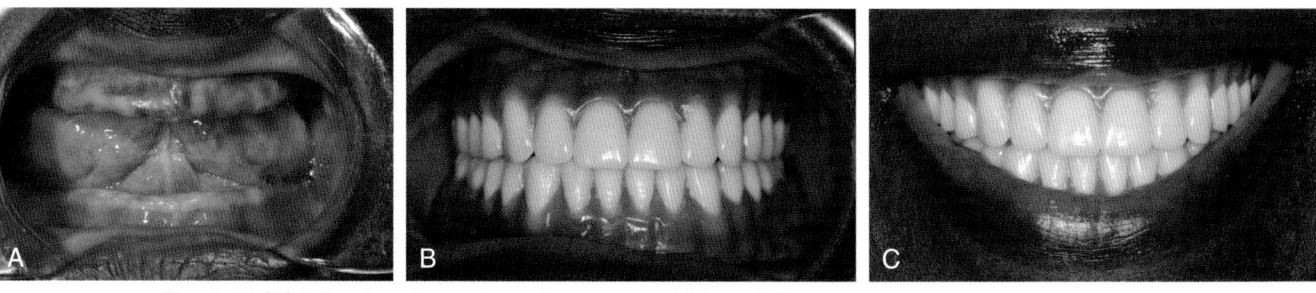

Fig. 11.36 **(A)** Fully edentulous arches; after insertion of **(B)** and **(C)** maxillary and mandibular complete dentures. (Courtesy Dr. Wendy A Clark.)

easily fabricated and have the lowest cost. The second category, flexible RPDs (i.e., Valplast, Duraflex) are fabricated from flexible acrylic resin with nylon fibers. Both all-acrylic and flexible RPDs have a shorter lifespan than a conventional RPD with a framework. In general, they are less retentive, less durable, more prone to fracture and more likely to entrap plaque and allow caries development. Consequently, their primary use is as an interim prosthesis for patients who have multiple undercuts caused by recession and loss of clinical attachment. A more recent alternative is the third category, an RPD that contains a framework made with a non-metal material such as polymer-based Acental Resi.[51] These prostheses resemble a conventional RPD with a cast frame in their stability and retention and tend to have a longer lifespan than other non-metal RPDs. With the advent of digital dentistry and the revolution of digital manufacturing through milling and 3D printing, polymer-based RPD options are expanding and providing more choices for esthetic, light-weight, and functional prostheses.

Complete Dentures

A **complete denture** is a removable acrylic replacement for teeth, soft tissue, and bone in a completely edentulous arch (Figure 11.36). Complete dentures are relatively economical, easy to fabricate and repair, and provide a level of esthetics and function acceptable to many patients. Common complaints by patients with complete dentures include lack of retention and reduced ability to taste and chew compared with natural teeth. It may be possible to reduce these problems by retaining a few selected teeth in an arch to serve as overdenture abutments. These are commonly endodontically treated roots with a capping restoration (direct-fill restoration or gold coping), that may also include a retentive, e.g., Locator or ERA, attachment on which the denture rests and attaches. Such abutments provide increased stability to the denture as compared with the traditional full denture and also help to preserve the residual ridge. Some patients report retaining a proprioceptive "feel" on chewing with a natural tooth overdenture. A disadvantage of this type of overdenture is that the retained natural teeth remain vulnerable to caries and/or periodontal disease. For patients who are fully edentulous and who want a more retentive and stable alternative to a conventional complete denture, the implant-retained overdenture is usually the best solution.

Typical treatment options for the conditions relating to missing teeth are summarized in eTable 11.6 on the ebooks+.

Implant-retained Prostheses

Dental implants are biologically compatible materials surgically placed within the bone to replace the roots of missing teeth. Currently in clinical practice dental implants are most commonly made of titanium and its alloys. Zirconia and tantalum implants are also available and are being used with increasing frequency. When the titanium surface is exposed to oxygen, it forms a biocompatible coating of titanium dioxide that enables the bone cells to attach to the implant in a process called osseointegration. This process begins at the time of implant placement and continues over the life of the implant. Currently, several implant systems are available to dentists. Typical components of an implant system include implant fixtures (body), healing abutments/cover screws, abutments, protective caps, impression copings/scan abutments, and laboratory replicas (analogues) and copings (Figure 11.37). Each major manufacturer has its own custom design for the various components and their interlocking mechanisms (Figure 11.38).

There are different approaches for implant healing and loading protocols. In a **one-stage technique**, the implant fixture is surgically placed in the bone and a healing abutment is secured into place. The healing abutment will occupy the soft tissue transition zone and the top of it is exposed to the oral environment. After an adequate healing time for osseointegration to occur (typically 3 to 6 months), the healing abutment is removed and an impression of the fixture and the surrounding tissue (fixture level impression) is made. An alternative approach is to place a prefabricated abutment and then take an impression of the abutment following an abutment-level impression protocol. Subsequently, a crown, FPD, or other prosthesis is fabricated and retained on the implant and abutment. When an implant fixture is placed in the tooth socket at the time of its extraction, it is described as an **immediate implant placement**. If an abutment and provisional prosthesis are placed at the time of the fixture placement, the process is described as **immediate provisionalization** and often referred to as **immediate loading**.

In a **two-stage technique**, the fixture is placed and covered (submerged) with oral soft tissue at the first surgical appointment. The patient returns for another surgical visit, usually 3 to 6 six months later, to uncover the fixture and place either a healing abutment or a definitive abutment. If it is a healing abutment, additional time is allowed for soft tissue healing and maturation before taking an impression. A fixture or abutment level impression can then be made using an impression post. A restoration is fabricated in similar manner as with the one-stage technique.

For many patients and dentists, implants have become the preferred treatment option for the reconstruction of bounded and unbounded edentulous spaces, and for fully edentulous arches. Notable advantages include improved patient satisfaction, preservation of remaining tooth structure, maintenance of bone, increased stability of removable prostheses, and a realistic and esthetically pleasing appearance. The primary disadvantages are cost, the length of the healing period during which the patient wears a temporary prosthesis, and the fact that the patient must undergo one or more surgical procedures. Usually, an 8 to 12 week waiting period is recommended between tooth extraction and implant placement in a delayed (nonimmediate) implant placement situation. A minimum healing time of 3 months is usually recommended following fixture placement (nonimmediate loading) to allow osseointegration of the implant fixture. With immediate placement and immediate loading these waiting periods are eliminated but can carry a higher risk of surgical or prosthetic complication.

Keys to Implant Decision Making
Professional Considerations

A multidisciplinary approach to the treatment planning of implants has some distinct advantages but is not mandatory. Depending on the local access to specialty care and the comfort level, training, and expertise of the dental professionals involved, implant treatment planning can be a team approach (at a minimum, a surgeon, a restorative dentist, dental laboratory technician, and a staff team coordinator), may be the sole responsibility of a single practitioner, or may be referred by the primary provider, usually a general dentist, for selected components of the treatment. Regardless of who orchestrates the

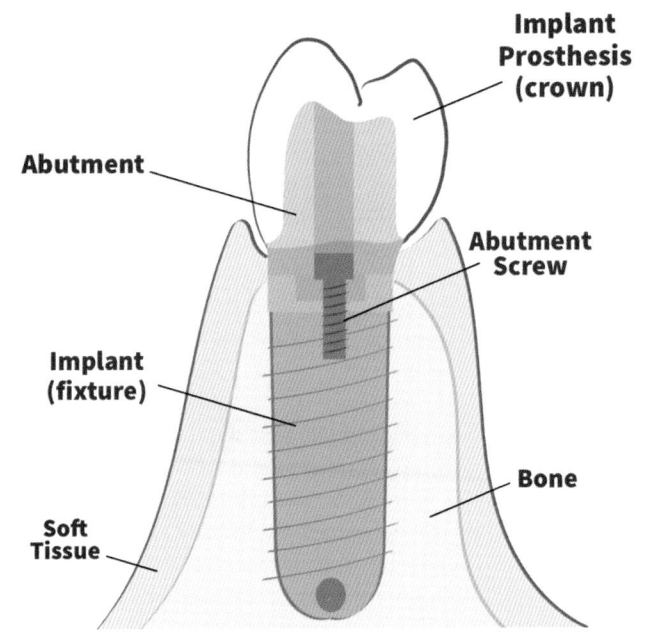

Fig. 11.37 Implant schematic. (Courtesy Dr. Wendy A Clark.)

Implant Prosthesis (crown)

Abutment

Abutment Screw

Implant (fixture)

Bone

Soft Tissue

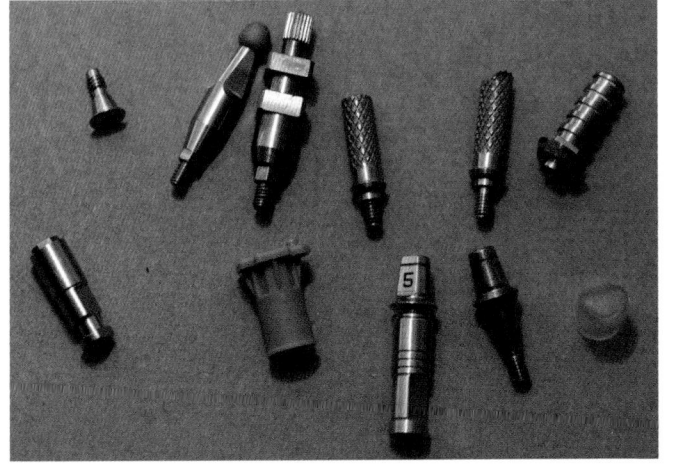

Fig. 11.38 Various components from multiple implant systems. (Courtesy Dr. Wendy A Clark.)

implant treatment, with certain types of patients or situations, the expertise of an oral and maxillofacial radiologist, an oral and maxillofacial surgeon, a periodontist, and/or a prosthodontist can be valuable. The following listing briefly describes the professional tasks and responsibilities required in the process of evaluating, diagnosing, treatment planning, and providing implant treatment and maintenance.

- *Initial patient contact.* The patient or the dentist may find it appropriate to raise the prospect of implant therapy at the initial examination appointment; or the issue may come up much later in the therapeutic relationship when the patient's dental condition has changed, perhaps with the loss of a fractured tooth. In either scenario, the general dentist can play two important roles that can prepare the way for the provision of implant services: (1) assessing the need for disease control treatment and implementing it if warranted (see Chapter 10) and (2) initiating a discussion with the patient about the various treatment options. If the general dentist is not directly involved with implant treatment, a referral to another practitioner for an implant consultation would be in order.

- *General health assessment.* Systemic conditions, such as poorly controlled diabetes, osteoporosis, radiation therapy to the head and neck, and immunocompromising conditions can sometimes be a contraindication to implant placement. Because cigarette smoking impairs healing and osseointegration, many practitioners will decline to place implants until the patient has stopped smoking. If the patient is a current cigarette smoker, this would be an appropriate time to provide smoking cessation resources to the patient (see Chapter 10) or suggest referral to a healthcare provider who provides tobacco use cessation therapy.

- *Assessment of the intraoral condition.* A thorough evaluation of the patient's oral condition in preparation for implant therapy is required. Site evaluation for a single tooth implant must include an assessment of bone height, width, contour, and density; mesial-distal interdental space; amount and quality of attached gingiva, and interarch space. Articulated casts and photographs are always a helpful adjunct and are often essential to this process. In the esthetic zone, particular attention must be paid to esthetic parameters including the lip line and support; incisal edge position; prospective restoration gingival zenith position; the shade, form and alignment of the surrounding teeth; the facial gingival and bone architecture; and the height, density, and translucency of the facial gingiva. The dentist must also carefully consider the specific esthetic desires and expectations of the patient. It is helpful in these cases to generate a diagnostic wax-up, a diagram or rendering of the expected result, or a corrected digital photographic (2D) image to help the patient better understand what can be expected. A powerful tool that is being used increasingly is digital smile design (DSD). There are many software programs and apps available to complete either a 2D image to share with the patient or to design a 3D rendering that can be tried in the patient's mouth. The 2D or 3D[38–40] design can be completed by the clinician or the dental laboratory technician. Be aware that an exacting patient may have

unrealistic expectations; with these patients an individualized consent form explaining details, limitations, and possible complications of treatment is mandatory.

- Intraoral assessment in preparation for patients who may need implant-retained FPDs, fixed complete dentures, or overdentures must include all of the preceding items plus evaluation of the TMJ, maxillomandibular relationship, vertical dimension of occlusion, occlusal plane, arch form and size, occlusal relationships, and guidance patterns in excursive movements. For complex cases, the standard of care in contemporary dental implant practices requires mounted diagnostic casts; and DSD and 3D mock-ups are particularly beneficial in these situations. When anterior esthetics are involved, the dentist must evaluate the lip support and position, midline, smile line, and gingival display. The location and size of the edentulous areas must be considered because they will have a significant impact on the placement of the implants and the prosthesis design. Any natural teeth and/or existing prostheses remaining in the arch must be assessed for integrity, stability, and prognosis. Decisions about any implant prostheses must be made in the context of the patient's overall comprehensive restorative plan and should never be made in isolation.

- *Psychosocial assessment.* Patients may have significant psychosocial issues that limit or contraindicate implant therapy. On the other hand, a patient with a severely compromised oral condition, who has tried diligently but unsuccessfully to wear a removable prosthesis in the past, may be an extremely motivated and ideal candidate for an implant prosthesis. Related issues are discussed in the Patient Considerations section.

- *Radiographic imaging.* Single tooth implants will necessitate, at a minimum, periapical and/or panoramic radiographs. Patients to receive multiple implants—especially if implants are to be placed in unbounded edentulous spaces—are usually be best served by use of advanced imaging techniques, most commonly cone beam computed tomography (CBCT). Radiographic images are required to establish the relationship of the considered implant site or sites to various anatomic structures, including the maxillary sinus, nasal cavity, mental foramen, and mandibular canal. The angulation and position of the roots of adjacent teeth must also be considered. Radiographic templates are useful in identifying the relationship of these anatomic structures to the prospective restoration, particularly in multitooth edentulous sites and fully edentulous arches. These utilize radiopaque tooth replicas or markers that appear white on the digital image, allowing the dental team to analyze thoroughly the space available and plan the surgical and prosthetic treatment better. Advances in computer technology have allowed the practitioner to integrate radiographic and surgical templates into one.[41–43] There is a growing number of software programs that allow clinicians to treatment plan implant placement, specify the location, angulation and depth for the implants, and create a laboratory fabricated surgical guide to be used by the dentist when placing the dental implants (e.g., Simplant, coDiagnostiX, Blue Sky

Bio). Additionally, a conventional or digital wax-up can be merged in the software, allowing for a prosthetically driven implant plan.

- *Finalize the plan with informed consent.* Following a detailed analysis of the issues described and having obtained a clear perspective of the patient's wishes, the dentist will need to define the range of treatment options, with or without implants. The consent discussion follows. Consultation should be implemented between the surgeon, restorative dentist, and other team members as to the number and position of implants, prosthesis design, the need for grafting or other adjunctive procedures, and the need for provisional restorative care. The final design of the prosthesis will depend on many factors, including the location and physiologic characteristics of the edentulous sites; the experience of the general dentist, the specialists, and the laboratory technician involved in the case; and the accessibility of surgical, restorative, and supportive treatment for the patient. When the treatment plan has been established and approved by the patient, it will be beneficial to present the patient with a copy of the treatment plan, which includes all procedures in appropriate sequence, costs for each component, and identification of all dental care providers to be involved in the process.

- *Monitor and coordinate the treatment.* Because multiple steps, and in some cases several providers, will be involved in the process of planning and executing implant therapy, someone will need to coordinate that activity. This role can be filled by the dentist but is often most efficiently and effectively implemented by a staff person—a treatment plan or care coordinator. This is especially true when several dental care providers are involved. Appointments may need to be made with several providers and, if so, these must be timed and sequenced appropriately. Surgical kits and necessary implant parts must be ordered to be available as needed. The patient may have questions or concerns that arise during the course of treatment and these will need to be addressed by the dental team.

- *Provide supportive care during and after implant treatment.* Implant surgical complications are usually managed by the dentist that provided the patient's surgical treatment and restorative complications are usually attended to by the clinician that provided the prosthetic care. Provisional restorations or prostheses may need to be fabricated, adjusted, or repaired during any phase of implant therapy, including planning, presurgical, surgical, or postoperative care, or during prosthodontic reconstruction. The implant surgeon will usually take responsibility for any issues or problems relating to the implant fixture and the restorative dentist can usually address any needs related to the abutment, crowns, or prostheses, but these roles can be interchangeable. Following placement of the definitive prosthesis, the restorative dentist will usually accept primary responsibility for maintaining the reconstruction and providing any indicated supportive care. If questions arise about the stability of the fixture or the hard and soft tissue response to the implant, referral back to the implant surgeon is indicated. The patient will need to be

seen at regular intervals by a hygienist, restorative dentist, and/or periodontist for maintenance therapy. Ideally, probing around the implant should be done with a plastic probe to minimize the potential for scratching the fixture or abutment. When practicable, plastic scalers should be used to remove accretions from the implant surfaces. Also, it is prudent to check occlusal contacts with a thin articulator paper to assess and evaluate intensity of occlusal contacts. Heavy occlusal or eccentric contacts can be detrimental to the stability of dental implants. As patients with parafunctional habits (clenching and bruxing) are at a statistically higher risk for complications, an occlusal guard is often fabricated. If so, this should be checked for fit, function, and stability at future care appointments.[44]

Patient Considerations

The consent discussion is an essential part of the process of formulating any treatment plan. When implants are a viable treatment option, there are typically many restorative options to choose from and because the treatment is more complex, and often being carried out by a team of clinicians, the consent discussion must be both extensive and detailed. Usually, the dentist will begin the process by gaining an understanding of the patient's treatment desires, objectives, expectations, and concerns. The patient should be offered all reasonable treatment options, with and without dental implants. The patient must be informed about the risks and benefits associated with each of the options and the expected outcomes of the proposed treatment. This may be difficult for the patient to conceptualize and appreciate. If the patient has had previous experience with a conventional removable partial or complete denture, they are more likely to appreciate the benefits of an implant-retained prosthesis because they are familiar with the limitations conventional removable prosthodontics therapy presents. Information must be provided about how the treatment will be staged, what each care provider will be doing at each stage of the treatment, how long each stage will take, and what the sequence of the treatment visits will be. The patient should also understand that they may need to wear a provisional prosthesis and that adjustments and relines may be necessary during transitional periods while extraction sites or bone grafts are healing and as osseointegration is occurring subsequent to implant placement.

A discussion of treatment fees is an important part of the implant planning. The patient must be given realistic estimates, if not a firm commitment, relating to the fees to be billed by the various providers. These fees will often include implant diagnostic evaluation, imaging, fixture placement, placement and provisionalization of abutments, and the final prosthesis. If adjunctive surgical procedures are indicated, the patient will also need to know what those treatment fees may be. Initially, it may appear that placement of a single tooth implant-retained crown is more expensive than a conventional FPD in the same location. However, if a core build-up, root canal treatment, and/or crown lengthening procedure are required on one or both of the abutment teeth for the FPD, that difference may be negated. Furthermore, given the longer expected usefulness of the implant crown, the implant may be a better option for the patient in the long run. (See Chapter 3 for a more extensive discussion of this topic.)

Some important questions and issues that must be addressed with the patient include: Is the individual committed and motivated to receive implant therapy? If not, what are the perceived barriers? Can they be overcome? Is the patient averse to receiving a surgical procedure? Are they willing to wait for the period of time required to heal before placement of the final restoration? Will the patient be able to tolerate and function with the provisional prosthesis? Are they capable of making the financial commitment? Will they be willing and able to maintain the prosthesis, carry out daily oral self-care instructions, and return to the dental office for regular periodic visits and supportive therapy?

In short, this can be a difficult and confusing process for the patient. The dental team will need to be supportive, understanding, and forthright in answering all of the patient's questions and concerns. More than one visit may be necessary for the patient to weigh and discuss all the options and to select the plan that is most appropriate. The beneficial outcome of this process will be a committed, informed patient who is confident and enthusiastic about the treatment plan, eager to receive treatment and appreciative of its benefits; and is taking ownership of their oral health.

A variety of implant-retained prosthodontic options are available, both fixed and removable. Five clinical conditions are presented here and the implant options for each are described.

Implant-Retained Single Crown

The implant-retained single crown is a prosthetic replacement for a missing tooth held in place by a single dental implant (Figure 11.39A–E). In most cases, an implant should be the primary option when replacing a single missing tooth, especially in cases where there is sufficient bone density and volume to retain the implant and where the adjacent teeth are either unrestored or minimally restored and healthy. Advantages of an implant-supported crown compared with a FPD include longevity and the fact that it is easier for the patient to clean and maintain. Perhaps most important is the fact that healthy tooth structure on the adjacent teeth need not be sacrificed in the preparation of the abutment, as would be the case for a tooth-borne FPD. This calls to mind the classic quote of M.M DeVan on this topic:[45] "Our goal should be the perpetual preservation of what remains rather than the meticulous restoration of what is missing".

Placement of a single tooth implant in the esthetic zone can be a challenge and requires special attention, including careful evaluation of the patient's midline, smile line, position, and angulation of adjacent teeth relative to each other and to the bone base, gingival display, existing tissue contours, and the thickness of the free gingiva. Orthodontic treatment is usually the best means of correcting an undesirable midline deviation. When the angulation or position of the roots of the adjacent teeth do not allow space for a dental implant to be placed, this problem can sometimes be resolved with limited orthodontic treatment (using brackets or clear aligners). If there is appropriate space between the roots to place the implants,

but restorative space is lacking, recontouring of the proximal surface of adjacent teeth to increase mesial-distal space may be sufficient. But if the space is too large, or asymmetric, adjunctive treatment may be needed to meet the patient's esthetic expectations, including orthodontics, cosmetic crown lengthening, or composite or veneer restorations. To achieve an emergence profile that resembles that of a natural tooth, implant fixtures are generally placed more apically in the anterior region (approximately 3–4 mm apical to the gingival zenith of the prospective restoration or below the cementoenamel junction of the adjacent teeth). Periodontal surgery may be needed to establish adequate ridge form and density or to correct excessive gingival display (see earlier sections in this chapter on periodontal surgery and preprosthodontic surgery). It can also be a challenge to match the soft tissue contours of the adjacent natural teeth to those around the implant. If the soft tissue contours are deficient before implant placement, the patient must be advised that the final soft tissue contours will probably not look natural and additional procedures may be necessary. Esthetic periodontal surgery before implant placement, at the time of implant placement, or with a separate surgical procedure later, can often help create a more pleasing gingival architecture. Also, advances in dental ceramics now allow the use of gingival shade ceramic to mimic soft tissue in restorations, creating the illusion of the presence of gingiva and masking the appearance of increased crown height.

Implant-Retained Fixed Partial Denture

An implant-retained FPD is, as the name suggests, an FPD that is retained by implants rather than natural teeth (Figure 11.39F–H). The FPD is either attached directly to the implant fixtures or cemented or screw-retained onto prefabricated multiunit abutments. Some general principles apply to the use of implant-retained FPDs:

- More implants should be placed where heavier occlusal forces are expected or where bone is less dense.
- Fewer implants are generally needed in the anterior region or when the implants oppose a removable prosthesis.
- Implant-retained FPDs in the esthetic zone will need the same precise and detailed consideration as noted for single implant-retained crowns.[46]
- Significant advantages of an implant-retained versus a tooth-borne FPD include:
  - A tooth-borne FPD is susceptible to caries; an implant retained FPD is not.
  - An implant-retained FPD can be placed in an unbound or long-span edentulous space, whereas in most situations a tooth-borne prosthesis cannot.
  - An implant-retained FPD can usually be repaired or replaced more easily than a tooth-borne FPD.

In individuals with a long edentulous span, it may be necessary to replace not only the missing teeth, but missing soft and bony tissue as well. In this situation, a hybrid-type restoration may be indicated. These hybrid restorations typically include pink restorative material, combining the features of both fixed and removable prosthodontics. They typically use a more advanced type of implant prosthetic design

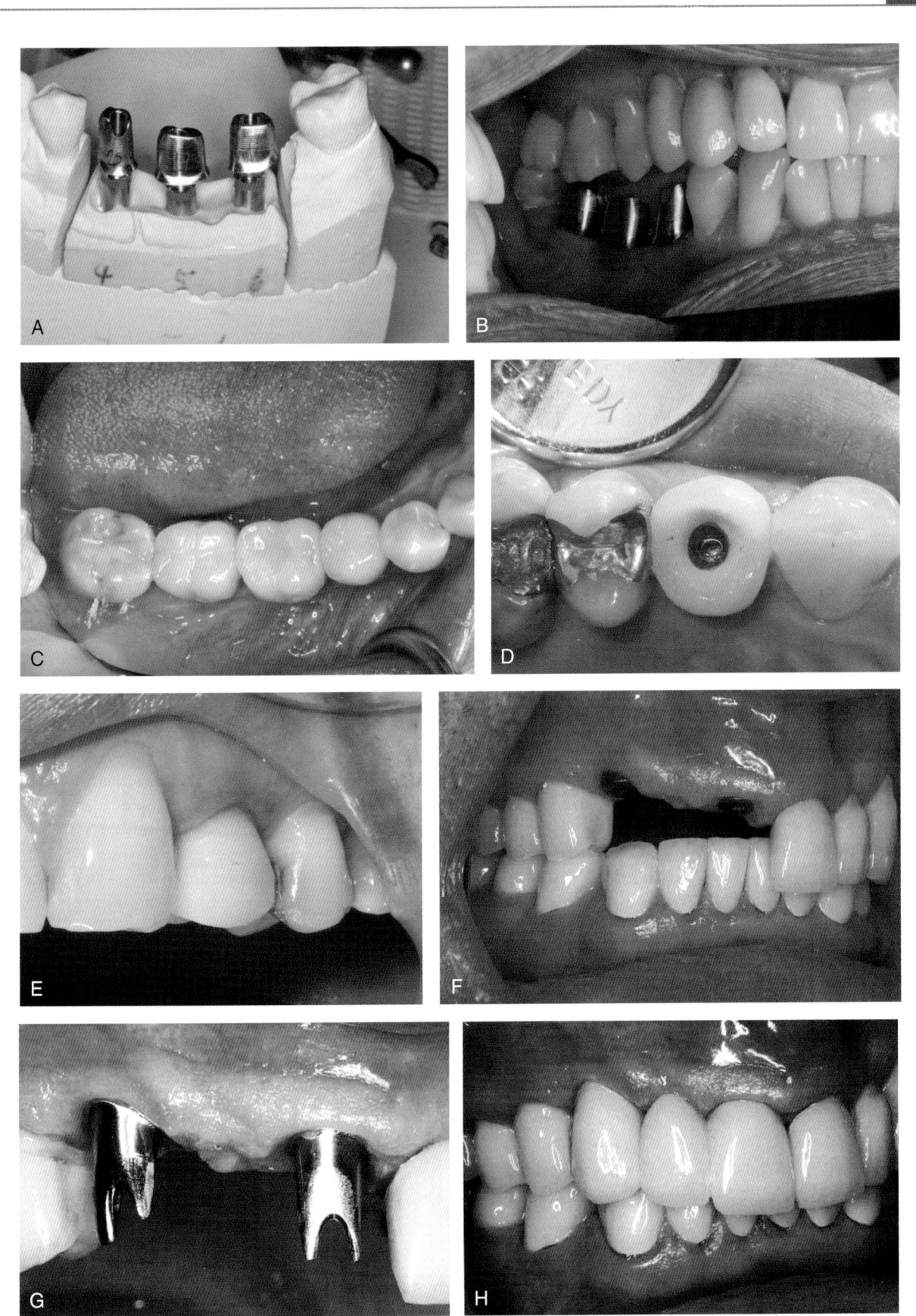

Fig. 11.39 Implant retained prostheses. **(A–C)**, Cement-retained implant crowns; **(D and E)**, screw retained implant crown; **(F–H)**, implant retained fixed partial denture. (**A**–**E**, Courtesy Dr, Carlos Barrero; **F–H**, courtesy Dr. Ibrahim Duqum, Chapel Hill, N.C.)

including components such as bars, attachments, or multi-unit abutments. These restorations can be fabricated with a range of design options and the treatment should be planned with a clinician who has extensive restorative experience or training.

Implant-Retained Removable Partial Denture

Tooth-borne removable partial dentures may not be an option if the proposed abutment teeth have an unfavorable crown:root ratio, have significant loss of clinical attachment, or need extensive restorative work with a less than ideal restorative prognosis. In this situation, the placement of dental implants can act as retention to a removable partial denture with the primary advantage that this removable appliance will not induce additional loading force on what may be an already compromised abutment tooth. Additionally, these prostheses can be utilized to improve esthetics by strategically placing them to avoid clasp assemblies on anterior abutment teeth. In many situations a combination of tooth and implant supported overdentures can be utilized to improve retention, support and esthetics. These prostheses can also be fabricated with a wide variety of materials and designs.

Implant-Supported Fixed Complete Denture

An implant-supported fixed complete denture is a non-removable solution for the completely edentulous patient. They are often described by the materials of which they are composed: metal acrylic (or hybrid prosthesis) (Figure 11.39I–K), metal-ceramic (or porcelain-fused-to-metal), and zirconia (monolithic or layered).The **hybrid prosthesis** is composed of a milled or cast alloy framework layered with polymethyl methacrylate (PMMA) denture base resin and denture teeth. Because the pink PMMA can be easily customized, this restoration readily compensates for moderate bone loss and missing soft tissue contours. When there is minimal loss of bone, **the metal ceramic restoration** can be an esthetically pleasing, but often more complex and costly, alternative. A more contemporary option is the **zirconia prosthesis**. With fewer components and materials, this solution is often easier to fabricate for both clinicians and laboratory technicians. Stains and layering allow the zirconia to be colored to match gingival or tooth structure. Therefore, the zirconia implant-supported fixed complete denture may provide acceptable esthetics even in the presence of excessive bone loss. Regardless of material, the prosthesis is fixed (screw-retained or cemented) so that the patient cannot remove it for cleaning or other purposes. This type of prosthesis is substantially more stable and retentive than conventional complete dentures. Other advantages of this treatment option compared with conventional complete dentures include less food entrapment and no need for denture relines, rebases, and/or denture adjustments. From a psychological perspective, many patients prefer a fixed prosthesis as the function more closely resembles that of natural teeth and it avoids the instability and inconvenience that is often associated with conventional complete dentures.

It should be noted that there are a few important contraindications to fixed implant-supported complete dentures. Patients who require extensive lip and soft tissue support (as with a denture flange) usually cannot achieve support from fixed implant restorative. Any attempt to do so would create a restoration that is not cleansable and would put the implants at risk. Additionally, this solution is not ideal for patients with poor home care or who lack the dexterity to clean between the prosthesis and tissue. This restoration is one of the most challenging to clean and maintenance is critical for its longevity. For patients who cannot reliably clean this prosthesis, a removable option is generally preferred. As with other forms of implant reconstruction, the biggest disadvantages are the time required for office visits, the time required for osseointegration, and the cost, which increases with each additional implant. The factors that are most influential in ensuring the success of the treatment are case selection and the experience and training of the restorative dentist and surgeon.

Complete Implant Overdenture

A complete implant overdenture is a complete denture retained in an edentulous arch by implants. It is a removable solution for a fully edentulous arch that can provide improved function and quality of life when compared with a conventional complete denture. Although maxillary or mandibular overdentures can be fabricated, mandibular overdentures are more common and are discussed first. Mandibular complete dentures prove to be more challenging to wear because of edentulous anatomy. Consequently, most patients have a greater functional benefit from a mandibular implant overdenture versus a maxillary. Most commonly, it is designed as a complete denture that is supported by, but not definitively attached to, two dental implants placed in the anterior mandible (Figure 11.40). Currently, the most common approach to connecting the denture to the implants is by utilizing a Locator abutment connected to the implant and a replaceable attachment embedded inside the denture base. Because fewer implants are needed, the overdenture is a less expensive option for the edentulous patient than an implant-retained fixed complete denture. Because of the dense type one bone, and lack of anatomic structures in the anterior mandible, the surgery is usually simple and relatively risk free.[47] Given the modest cost, positive risk:benefit ratio and the expected significant improvement in quality of life for the patient, this solution has become the generally accepted and preferred treatment for the completely edentulous mandible. In selected cases, implants may be connected by a metal bar and the bar or connected individual attachments retain(s) the denture. As with the individual Locator attachments, this type of overdenture can be removed and reinserted by the patient. The implant-supported overdenture with a bar attachment provides an additional measure of retention, which is particularly beneficial in cases of severe ridge atrophy. This prosthesis requires more vertical height (and corresponding interarch space) than an individual attachment complete denture. It also necessitates more

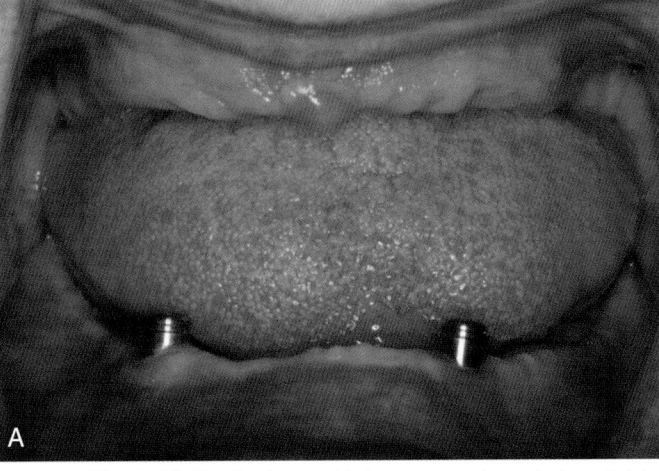 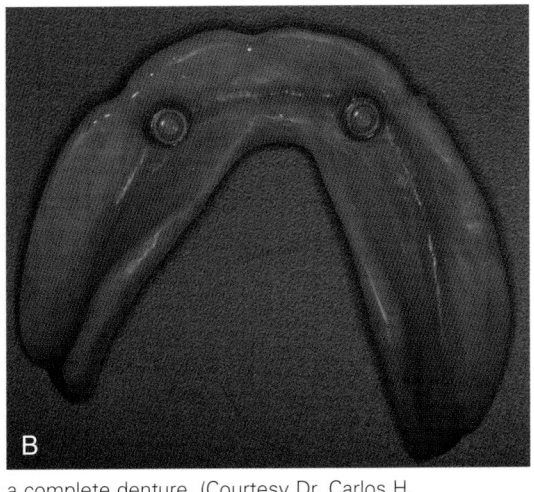

Fig. 11.40 Two implants with Locator attachments for retaining a complete denture. (Courtesy Dr. Carlos H. Barrero.)

sophisticated laboratory technique and support and, consequently, is also more expensive for the patient.

When considering the maxillary arch, the bone tends to be less dense than the mandibular arch. Consequently, more implants are needed to support a maxillary overdenture. Although there are different philosophies, most practitioners and outcomes studies recommend placement of a minimum of two implants on the mandible and four on the maxilla.[48] It is also recommended that there be cross-arch support on the maxilla to best distribute the forces to the implants.[49] This could be in the form of a connecting bar rigidly splinting the implants together, a metal framework embedded in the overdenture, or maintaining full palatal coverage.

There are several factors to consider when determining whether or not to choose an implant overdenture. Compared with a conventional complete denture, overdentures tend to have higher patient satisfaction, fewer sore spots, and improved stability and retention.[50] When compared with fixed complete dentures, facial esthetics are often enhanced by support of the lip with labial flanges. Additionally, the ability to remove the prosthesis at night also carries significant benefits.

With daily cleaning, plaque can be effectively removed. This helps prevent malodor, candidiasis, denture stomatitis, and peri-implant mucositis. Nighttime removal also ensures that the patient can avoid any destructive forces resulting from nocturnal parafunctional habits. Another advantage of this design is that the retentive inserts/attachments are easy to replace when fatigued.

CONCLUSION

This chapter sets forth the range of definitive surgical, functional, esthetic, and/or restorative therapeutic options that are available. Indications and contraindications for each procedure have been identified. along with a review of important dentist- and patient-based considerations that will have an impact on formulation of the patient's plan of care. The ultimate goal of the definitive phase is to help the patient achieve the best possible state of oral health within the context of the patient's desires, abilities, and resources. At the conclusion of the definitive phase, the patient's care moves to the maintenance phase, that is discussed in Chapter 12.

▊ REVIEW QUESTIONS

- In what situations is definitive periodontal care indicated?
- What treatment options are available for the adult patient with malposed teeth?
- When is orthognathic surgery indicated?
- What is the difference between an occlusal guard and an occlusal splint? What are the indications for each?
- In what situations would the material of choice for restoring a posterior tooth be amalgam? Composite resin? A gold or ceramic crown?
- List treatment options for changing tooth color and sort them by order of invasiveness. When might you be cautious about providing these services for a patient?
- What are some reasons, other than pain, for providing endodontic therapy?

- When would you recommend to a patient *not* to have third molars removed?
- When would you recommend preprosthodontic surgery?
- With regard to implant placement, when might you consider immediate placement? Immediate loading?
- What are the challenges in placing a single tooth implant in the esthetic zone?
- Which *professional considerations* have a bearing on whether and how to replace a missing tooth or teeth? Which *patient considerations* have a bearing on these questions? How is the final decision made?

PRACTICE ENHANCEMENT

Design a "treatment options list" as a guide for patients in your practice setting. Include a complete array of procedures provided by your practice. Descriptors should include (but need not be limited to) approximate charges, number of visits, expected length of service, and advantages and disadvantages to the patient.

REFERENCES

1. Segelnick SL, Weinberg MA. Reevaluation of initial therapy: when is the appropriate time? *J Periodontol.* 2006;77(9):1598–1601.
2. Hamp SE, Nyman S, Lindhe J. Periodontal treatment of multi rooted teeth. Results after 5 years. *Journal of Clinical Periodontology.* 1975;2:126–135.
3. Glickman I. *Clinical Periodontology.* 2nd ed. Philadelphia: W. B. Saunders; 1958:694–696.
4. American Academy of Periodontology. Drug-associated gingival enlargement. *J Periodontol.* 2004;75(10):1424–1431.
5. American Academy of Periodontology. Systemic antibiotics in periodontics. *J Periodontol.* 2004;75(11):1553–1565.
6. Herrera D, Matesanz P, Martin C, Oud V, Feres M, Teughels W. Adjunctive effect of locally delivered antimicrobials in periodontitis therapy. A systematic review and meta-analysis. *Journal of Clinical Periodontology.* 2020;47(Suppl 22):239–256.
7. Greenstein G. Local drug delivery in the treatment of periodontal disease: assessing the clinical significance of the results. *Journal of Periodontology.* 2006;77:565–578.
8. Caton J, Ryan ME. Clinical studies on the management of periodontal diseases utilizing subantimicrobial dose doxycycline (SDD). *Pharmacol Res.* 2011;63(2):114–120.
9. Wright JT, Crall JJ, Fontana M, et al. Evidence-based clinical practice guideline for the use of pit-and-fissure sealants. *J Amer Dent Assoc.* 2016;147(8):672–682.
10. Rasines Alcaraz MG, Veitz-Keenan A, Sahrmann P, Schmidlin PR, Davis D, Iheozor-Ejiofor Z. Direct composite resin fillings versus amalgam fillings for permanent or adult posterior teeth. *Cochrane Database Syst Rev.* 2014;3:CD005620.
11. Ritter AV. Posterior composites revisited. *J Esthet Rest Dent.* 2008;20(1):57–67.
12. Haveman CW, Summitt JB, Burgess JO, et al. Three restorative materials and topical fluoride gel used in xerostomic patients: a clinical comparison. *J Am Dent Assoc.* 2003;134(2):177–184.
13. McComb D, Erickson RL, Maxymiw WG, et al. A clinical comparison of glass ionomer, resin-modified glass ionomer and resin composite restorations in the treatment of cervical caries in xerostomic head and neck radiation patients. *Oper Dent.* 2001;27(5):430–437.
14. Boushell LW, Ritter AV. Ceramic inlays: a case presentation and lessons learned from the literature. *J Esthet Restor Dent.* 2009;21:77–88.
15. Croll TP. Enamel microabrasion: Observations after 10 years. *J Am Dent Assoc.* 1997;128:45S–50S.
16. https://pubmed.ncbi.nlm.nih.gov/30719932/
17. https://pubmed.ncbi.nlm.nih.gov/23374407/
18. https://pubmed.ncbi.nlm.nih.gov/9120146/
19. https://pubmed.ncbi.nlm.nih.gov/33352224/
20. https://pubmed.ncbi.nlm.nih.gov/30801926/
21. https://pubmed.ncbi.nlm.nih.gov/32573090/
22. https://pubmed.ncbi.nlm.nih.gov/29289725/
23. Boushell LW, Ritter AV, Garland GE, et al. Nightguard vital bleaching: side effects and patient satisfaction 10 to 17 years post-treatment. *J Esthet Rest Dent.* 2012;24(3):211–219.
24. Plotino G, Buono L, Grande NM, Pameijer CH, Somma F. Nonvital tooth bleaching: a review of the literature and clinical procedures. *J Endod.* 2008;34(4):394–407.
25. Swift H, Friedman EJ. MJ: Porcelain Veneer Outcomes. *Part 1 J Esthet Rest Dent.* 2006;18(1):54–57.
26. https://pubmed.ncbi.nlm.nih.gov/18768903/
27. Burger EH, Klein-Nulen J. Responses of bone cells to biomechanical forces in vitro. *Adv Dent Res.* 1999;13:93–98.
28. Boyne PJ, Hersford AS. Distraction osteogenesis of the nasal and antral osseous floor to enhance alveolar height. *J Oral Maxillofac Surg Suppl.* 2004;62(9):123–130.
29. Araújo MG, Lindhe J. Dimensional ridge alterations following tooth extraction: an experimental study in the dog. *J Clin Periodontol.* 2005;32(2):212–218.
30. Ten Heggeler JM, Slot DE, Van der Weijden GA. Effect of socket preservation therapies following tooth extraction in non-molar regions in humans: a systematic review. *Clin Oral Implants Res.* 2011;22(8):79–88.
31. Bazrafshan N, Darby I. Retrospective success and survival rates of dental implants placed with simultaneous bone augmentation in partially edentulous patients. *Clin Oral Implants Res.* 2014;25(7):768–773.
32. Rosen PS, Summer R, Mellado JR, et al. The bone-added osteotome sinus floor elevation technique: multicenter retrospective report of consecutively treated patients. *Int J Oral Maxillofac Implants.* 1999;14(6):853–858.
33. Telleman G, Raghoebar GM, Vissink A, den Hartog L, Huddleston Slater JJ, Meijer HJ. A systematic review of the prognosis of short (<10 mm) dental implants placed in the partially edentulous patient. *J Clin Periodontol.* 2011;38(7):667–676.
34. Anitua E, Alkhraisat MH. 15-year follow-up of short dental implants placed in the partially edentulous patient: Mandible Vs maxilla. *Ann Anat.* 2019;222:88–93.
35. Celenza FV, Litvak H. Occlusal management in conformative dentistry. *J Prosthet Dent.* 1976;36:164–170.
36. Faggion CM Jr, Giannakopoulos NN, Listl S. How strong is the evidence for the need to restore posterior bounded edentulous spaces in adults? Grading the quality of evidence and the strength of recommendations. *J Dent.* 2011;39(2):108–116.
37. Reissmann DR, Bellows JC, Kasper J. Patient Preferred and Perceived Control in Dental Care Decision Making. *JDR Clin Trans Res.* 2019 Apr;4(2):151–159.
38. Coachman C, Georg R, Bohner L, Rigo LC, Sesma N. Chairside 3D digital design and trial restoration workflow. *J Prosthet Dent.* 2020;124(5):514–520.
39. Jafri Z, Ahmad N, Sawai M, Sultan N, Bhardwaj A. Digital Smile Design-An innovative tool in aesthetic dentistry. *J Oral Biol Craniofac Res.* 2020;10(2):194–198.
40. Coachman C, Calamita M. Digital smile design: a tool for treatment planning and communication in aesthetic dentistry. *Quintessence Dent Technol.* 2012;35:103–111.
41. Chen P, Nikoyan L. Guided Implant Surgery: A Technique Whose Time Has Come. *Dent Clin North Am.* 2021;65(1):67–80.

42. Kernen F, Kramer J, Wanner L, Wismeijer D, Nelson K, Flügge T. A review of virtual planning software for guided implant surgery - data import and visualization, drill guide design and manufacturing. *BMC Oral Health*. 2020;20(1):251.

43. Bornstein MM, Horner K, Jacobs R. Use of cone beam computed tomography in implant dentistry: current concepts, indications and limitations for clinical practice and research. *Periodontol 2000*. 2017;73(1):51–72.

44. Goodacre BJ, Goodacre SE, Goodacre CJ. Prosthetic complications with implant prostheses (2001-2017). *Eur J Oral Implantol*. 2018;11(Suppl 1):S27–S36.

45. DeVan MM. The nature of the partial denture foundation: suggestions for its preservation. *J Prosthet Dent*. 1952;2:210.

46. Misch CE. Rationale for Dental Implants. In: Misch CE, ed. *Contemporary Implant Dentistry*. 3rd ed. St. Louis: Mosby; 2008:3–21.

47. Zarb GA, Schmitt A. The longitudinal clinical effectiveness of osseointegrated dental implants in anterior partially edentulous patients. *International Journal of Prosthodontics*. 1993;6(2):180–188.

48. Sadowsky SJ, Zitzmann NU. Protocols for the maxillary implant overdenture: A systematic review. *Int J Oral Maxillofac Implants*. 2016;31(Suppl):s182–s191.

49. Raghoebar GM, Meijer HJ, Slot W, Slater JJ, Vissink A. A systematic review of implant-supported overdentures in the edentulous maxilla, compared to the mandible: how many implants? *Eur J Oral Implantol*. 2014;7(Suppl 2):S191–S201.

50. Sivaramakrishnan G, Sridharan K. Comparison of implant supported mandibular overdentures and conventional dentures on quality of life: a systematic review and meta-analysis of randomized controlled studies. *Aust Dent J*. 2016;61(4):482–488.

51. Duqum I, Barker S, Marshall E, Wang R, Preisser JS, Khan A. The effect of single tooth implant restorations on the survival, morbidity, pulpal, and periapical health of adjacent teeth: a chart review. *Clin Implant Dent Relat Res*. 2018;20(4):479–482.

SUGGESTED READINGS

PERIODONTICS AND PERIODONTOLOGY

Berglundh T, Giannobile W, Sanz M, Lang N. *Linde's Clinical Periodontology and Implant Dentistry*. 7th ed. Oxford: Wiley-Blackwell; 2021.

Caton JG, Armitage G, Berglundh T, et al. A new classification scheme for periodontal and per-implant diseases and conditions – introduction and key changes from the 1999 classification. *Journal of Periodontology*. 2018;89(suppl 1):S1–S8.

Newman MG, Takei H, Klokkevoid PR, Carranza FA. *Newman and Carranza's Clinical Periodontology*. 13th ed. St Louis: Saunders; 2019.

ORTHODONTICS

Graber NVR, Vig K, Huang G. *Orthodontics, Current Principles and Techniques*. 6th ed. 2017.

Proffit W, Fields H, Larson B, Sarver D. *Contemporary Orthodontics*. 6th ed. St Louis: Mosby; 2018.

OCCLUSION

Dawson P. *Functional Occlusion: from TMJ to Smile Design*. St Louis: Mosby; 2006.

Nelson J. *Wheeler's Dental Anatomy, Physiology and Occlusion*. 11th ed. St Louis: Elsevier; 2020.

Okeson J. *Management of Temporomandibular Disorders and Occlusion*. 8th ed. St Louis: Mosby; 2019.

SINGLE TOOTH RESTORATIONS AND DENTAL MATERIALS

Shen C, Rawls H, Esquivel-Upshaw J. *Phillips' Science of Dental Materials*. 13th ed. St Louis: Elsevier; 2022.

Ritter AV, Boushell L, Walter R. *Sturdevant's the Art and Science of Operative Dentistry*. 7th ed. St Louis: Mosby; 2018.

Sakaguchi R, Ferracane J, Powers J. *Craig's Restorative Dental Materials*. 14th ed. St Louis: Mosby; 2019.

ESTHETIC DENTISTRY

American Academy of Cosmetic Dentistry.

Aschheim KW. *Esthetic Dentistry: a Clinical Approach to Techniques and Materials*. 3rd ed. St Louis: Elsevier; 2014.

Freedman GA. *Contemporary Esthetic Dentistry*. St Louis: Elsevier; 2012.

Geissberger M. *Esthetic Dentistry in Clinical Practice*. Oxford: Blackwell; 2010.

Goldstein R, Chu S, Lee E, Stappert F. *Esthetics in Dentistry*. (2 vols). 3rd ed. Oxford: Wiley; 2018.

Magne P. *Biomimetic Restorative Dentistry*. Chicago: Quintessence; 2022.

Mistry S. Principles of smile demystified. *J Cosmetic Dentistry*. 2012;28(2):116–124.

ENDODONTICS

AAE Endodontic Case Difficulty Assessment Form and Guidelines https://www.aae.org/specialty/wp-content/uploads/

Berman L, Hargreaves K. *Cohen's Pathways of the Pulp*. 12th ed. St Louis: Mosby; 2021.

Torabinejab M, Fouad A, Shabahang S. *Endodontics: Principles and Practice*. 6th ed. St Louis: Saunders; 2020.

ORAL AND MAXILLOFACIAL SURGERY

Fonseca R. *Oral and Maxillofacial Surgery*. 3rd ed. St Louis: Elsevier; 2017.

Hupp J, Tucker M, Ellis E. *Contemporary Oral and Maxillofacial Surgery*. 7th ed. St Louis: Elsevier; 2018.

Miloro M, Ghali G, Larsen P, Waite P. *Peterson's Principles of Oral and Maxillofacial Surgery*. 4th ed. New York: Springer Verlag; 2022.

PROSTHODONTICS AND IMPLANTS

Carr AB, Brown DT. *McCracken's Removable Partial Prosthodontics*. 12th ed. St Louis: Mosby; 2010.

Shillingburg H, et al. *Fundamentals of Fixed Prosthodontics*. 4th ed. Chicago: Quintessence;; 2012.

Rosenstiel S, Land M, Fujimoto J. *Contemporary Fixed Prosthodontics*. 5th ed. St Louis: Mosby; 2015.

Sarmet DP, Peshman B. *Lexi-Comp's Manual of Dental Implants*. 2nd ed. Ohio: Lexi-comp;; 2009.

Misch CE. *Dental Implant Prosthetics*. 2nd ed. St Louis: Mosby; 2014.

Misch CE. *Contemporary Implant Dentistry*. 3rd ed. St Louis: Mosby; 2007.

Palmer RM, Howe LC, Palmer PJ. *Implants in Clinical Dentistry*. 2nd ed. London: Informa;; 2011.

Sandowsky SJ, Bedrossian E. Evidence-based criteria for differential treatment planning of implant restorations for the partially edentulous patient. *J Prosthodont*. 2013;22(4):319–329.

The Maintenance Phase of Care

Jeff Wang, Jennifer Harmon, Jennifer Brame, and Samuel Nesbit

 Visit eBooks.Health.Elsevier.com

OUTLINE

After completion of definitive phase therapy, there will often be issues that remain to be addressed, and previously rendered treatment that must be reevaluated. Some of these concerns will need attention for as long as the dentist–patient relationship exists. In addition to their importance to patient care, good **maintenance phase** plans provide the patient-specific elements essential to the development of an organized, practice-wide system of periodic care that serves as the backbone of a successful and productive dental practice.

Although this aspect of the treatment plan may seem less important at the outset, the maintenance phase represents a critical component of any complex treatment plan. In many cases, the long-term success or failure of the treatment depends on it. As this chapter unfolds, it will become clear why the dentist should discuss with patients how long-term periodic care is essential to maintaining an optimal state of oral health. Furthermore, the rationale for initiating this discussion at the time that the original treatment plan is presented will also become apparent.

Prevention of future problems is, of course, the guiding principle of the maintenance phase. The astute practitioner works throughout all phases of treatment to educate the patient in strategies for maintaining a healthy oral condition and

preventing future oral disease. Certain aspects of a systemic phase may include activities that are preventive in nature. The acute phase may also include treatment that has the effect of preventing disease progression. The disease control phase, by its nature, is preventive in orientation, and numerous references to preventive therapies are made in Chapter 10. Because restorations are delivered in the definitive phase there will be an opportunity and necessity to discuss with the patient their role in maintaining the restorations and prostheses and in the prevention of recurrent disease.

But several components of patient education may occur primarily during the maintenance phase, including modification of oral and systemic health-related behaviors and the reinforcement of oral homecare practices. For that reason and because this chapter provides a convenient location to consolidate the broad range of preventive and maintenance strategies that are available to both patient and the dental team, preventive concepts and preventive therapy are emphasized here.

The maintenance phase must be flexible and individualized, with timing and content specifically tailored to each patient's needs. Although formulated at the treatment planning stage, it will have been modified during the disease control and definitive treatment phases, and will take its final form at the posttreatment assessment, which is discussed in the following section. The dentist implements maintenance phase care through the periodic visit as discussed in detail later in this chapter. The American Dental Association (ADA) sanctioned procedure coding system uses the designation "Periodic Oral Evaluation." Consistent with that perspective, the terms "periodic examination" and **periodic visit** are used in this text. Because of common usage, the terms **recall visit** and **recare visit** are also included here.

POSTTREATMENT ASSESSMENT

The posttreatment assessment is a dedicated, structured appointment scheduled at the conclusion of the disease control phase of treatment, if the original plan includes disease control, and at the conclusion of the definitive phase. The purposes of the assessment are to evaluate the patient's response to treatment, comprehensively to assess current oral health status, to determine any new treatment needs, and to develop a specific plan for future dental and oral health care. If accomplished during the first periodic evaluation and visit, the posttreatment assessment will commonly include oral homecare instructions, selected scaling as needed, and oral prophylaxis.

Most colleges of dentistry have developed a formalized process for the clinical examination that will be made when the patient is about to exit the patient care program. The following discussion utilizes one such system as an example. Because each practice or institution will have unique needs, the decision regarding development of a **posttreatment assessment protocol** will be made on an individual basis. Whatever mechanism the dentist decides on, the emphasis will be on the importance of engaging the patient in a comprehensive reevaluation and reassessment at the conclusion of the disease control phase of treatment and/or at the conclusion of the entire plan of care. For instance, comprehensive periodontal reevaluation should be performed at a designated interval following nonsurgical or surgical periodontal treatment. Any remaining local or systemic factors that are not fully controlled should be documented. The dentist needs to communicate to the patient any recommendations for further treatment or oversight management. Many practitioners prefer *not* to formalize this process, declining to take the time to develop a specific protocol or form for recording findings. The current **standard of care** in practice does not dictate a mandatory posttreatment assessment protocol. The standard of care does require, however, that patients be provided maintenance services and *continuity* of care. In that context, the concepts described here should have application to any practice. Each practitioner is encouraged to incorporate some type of patient maintenance program into the office policy manual and to implement use of that program with each patient. The information included here can be used as a guide for that purpose.

Objectives for the Posttreatment Assessment

The purpose and intent of the posttreatment assessment is to enable the practitioner to evaluate the following:

- The patient's current oral and medical condition
- Outcomes of treatment rendered by the dental team

- The patient's satisfaction with the care that has been provided
- Present and future treatment needs of the patient

The posttreatment assessment provides a foundation for planning any additional treatment and **maintenance therapy** that the patient will need.

Elements of the Posttreatment Assessment

Items to be included in the posttreatment assessment and recorded in the patient record will vary with the nature and scope of the dental practice, the individual patient profile, and the patient's need. Typical elements in a posttreatment assessment include the following:

- Update of the general health history and review of systems
- Recording vital signs
- A head/face/neck examination to reassess any previously diagnosed conditions and to determine whether any new oral pathology is present
- Updating radiographs according to the practice or institutional protocol and the patient's individual need
- Comprehensive caries diagnosis and caries risk assessment
- Evaluation of the alignment of the teeth and jaws; the occlusion; the temporomandibular joint; and the patient's ability to speak, chew, and function
- Assessment of all periapical areas, with particular focus on teeth that have received root canal therapy
- Comprehensive periodontal assessment and periodontal risk assessment
- Assessment of dental implant health
- Evaluate adherence to homecare advisories, reinforce oral homecare instructions
- Evaluation of all existing restorations and prostheses
- Statement describing the patient's satisfaction (or dissatisfaction) with the treatment rendered; were all the patient's expectations met?
- Summary of the patient's response to treatment; was the patient adherent with attendance and professional recommendations?
- Description of any remaining restorative needs and how those needs will be addressed
- Specific plan to address any other ongoing or emerging issues that will need future attention
- Provide preventive and therapeutic product recommendations
- Establish an appropriate recare interval

Reassessment and Perpetual Planning

Although there may be common elements to the maintenance phase with different patients, rarely will a standardized "cookie cutter" approach be appropriate. Each patient will present with unique circumstances that will require specificity and personalization of the plan. Depending on the risk profile of the patient, individual elements in the maintenance plan will need to be evaluated with a more (or less) critical eye, and at a more (or less) frequent interval. The caries active patient is one such example. If the patient is at high risk of caries, more frequent examination intervals, more frequent radiographic intervals, more careful attention to dietary and preventive regimes would be in order. More critical evaluation of previously identified incipient caries lesions is also warranted. Interdental cleaning should be reinforced and the daily application of prescription high-fluoride tooth paste to the site may also be recommended. If there is evidence of lesion progression, caries removal and restoration should normally be performed sooner rather than later.

The maintenance needs of a patient will also change as the general health and oral health condition of the patient continues to evolve. A patient may have deep periodontal pockets that are stable and healthy for many years, but in the presence of new autoimmune disease the periodontitis morphs into an active and aggressive state. The treatment and management of a patient in a long-term stable condition will be significantly different from that of a patient with a newly developed Stage 3 Grade C periodontitis. It is also noteworthy that a patient with a history of periodontal disease may undergo rapid disease progression in the absence of periodontal maintenance or when there is compromised periodontal maintenance.

As the patient ages and life circumstances change so too may the patient's desires for and expectations of treatment. Many of the concerns and remaining issues will also change. An elderly patient in declining health will sometimes require creative and less invasive strategies as treatment goals and the expectations of the patient (and family) narrow in focus. Elective treatment that at an earlier stage of life carried the promise of better health and higher quality of life, may now be judged to be of minimal benefit and limited utility to a patient whose "things worth living for" are defined in the most simplistic of terms. At the other end of the spectrum, a patient who is a cancer survivor and is now invigorated and has a new vision and fuller expectation of what life has to offer, may be an excellent candidate to engage in comprehensive preventive services and elective dental treatment that holds the promise of improved oral health, function and self-image.

Changing oral and general health conditions and changing patient expectations, wishes, and desires will require periodic reassessment of the maintenance plan. These conversations need to be carried out with the patient openly, honestly, and compassionately with the decision making left to the patient. It is important to record these discussions in the patient record because these will become the foundation for the next stage of maintenance phase as it continues to evolve.

Documenting the Posttreatment Assessment

The posttreatment assessment may be documented in the progress notes in a narrative or bullet format, with or without a predetermined outline to guide the process. If the practice has multiple providers, a common outline or format should be developed for consistency and efficiency. In an institutional setting, it is usually advantageous to develop a form specifically for that purpose (Figure 12.1).

RATIONALE FOR INCLUDING A MAINTENANCE PHASE IN THE TREATMENT PLAN

The primary purpose of the maintenance phase is to ensure long-term oral health, optimum function, and favorable esthetics for the patient. In the maintenance phase, continuing systemic issues can be managed; disease control measures can be reevaluated and strengthened; and restorations and prostheses can be repaired, cleaned, polished, recontoured, or relined as needed.

Posttreatment Assessment	
Patient concerns/expectations met?	
Patient response to treatment	
Medical history current (date of most recent update)	
Radiographic examination (date & type of most recent images)	
Head & neck, extraoral/intraoral examination (date of most recent exam) and notation of (+) findings	
Periodontal condition (date of last recall appointment)	
Pulp and periapical health	
Occlusal/orthodontic/functional status	
Caries/restorative condition of the teeth	
Caries risk assessment	
Risk for occlusal/functional problems or tooth fracture	
Risk for periodontal disease	
Preventive recommendations for patient	
Disposition (remaining or new Tx needs and how they will be addressed)	
Established recall interval	
Type of recall:	☐ D1110 Adult prophylaxis ☐ D4910 Periodontal recall

Fig. 12.1 Example of posttreatment assessment form.

Success or failure of previous treatment must be reassessed and any necessary additional treatment planned. Multiple benefits derive from a comprehensive and strategically crafted plan for the maintenance phase. These benefits can be clustered into three categories: (1) issues that remain unresolved at the close of the definitive phase of treatment, (2) patient-based issues, and (3) practice management issues.

Address Ongoing Patient Needs

Follow-Up of Untreated Diagnoses

At the conclusion of the definitive treatment phase, previously diagnosed but untreated conditions may require reevaluation. These might include reactive soft tissue lesions, asymptomatic chronic bone lesions, defective but not problematic restorations, or teeth with incipient carious lesions. The maintenance phase provides an ideal time to reassess these issues, discuss them with the patient, and develop consensus on how to manage them going forward.

Monitoring Chronic Conditions That Can Affect Oral Health

Patients may have systemic diseases that influence plans for or the delivery of dental treatment (e.g., diabetes [Figure 12.2]), systemic diseases with significant oral manifestations (e.g., **Sjögren's syndrome**), or chronic oral diseases (e.g., periodontal disease). The maintenance phase provides an opportunity to reassess such chronic conditions, to determine whether new intervention or retreatment is warranted, and address any new sequelae or related conditions that may have arisen since the last appointment.

Revisiting Elective Treatment Issues

Earlier in the course of treatment, patients may have raised dental concerns or aspirations that for various reasons (e.g., time, finances, anxiety) they chose to defer. Similarly, the patient may have earlier declined certain elective treatments that the dentist recommended, such as removal of asymptomatic third molars or replacement of missing teeth. The maintenance phase provides an ideal opportunity to revisit these issues.

Perpetual Care

Patients who remain at elevated risk of oral diseases including oral cancer, caries, and periodontal disease, will benefit from long-term regular maintenance.[1,2] Dentate patients with a history of periodontitis are expected to have better oral health outcomes (see Chapter 3) and may have better general health[3,4] outcomes when they receive **perpetual oral health care**.[5]

Person-Centered Care

Rapport Building

Patients return to their dentists for periodic care for many reasons beyond the obvious recommended scaling and oral prophylaxis. The importance of the professional trust that patients place in their dentists and the personal security obtained from the relationship should not be underestimated or taken for granted. Consciously or unconsciously, most patients have a strong expectation that their dentist is diligently looking out

for their best interests and will do what is best to promote and ensure their oral health. Periodic visits do much to cement the relationship and fulfill the patient's expectations.

Patient Education

The maintenance phase serves as an effective platform to educate and motivate the patient, with the primary goal of long-term successful management of oral health. As the dentist plans the maintenance phase with the patient, discussion should include the rationale and long-term goals for maintenance.

Discussing the maintenance phase helps to educate the patient about the details of care provided during the periodic visits and the patient's own contribution to maintaining a healthy oral condition. This is the ideal opportunity to inform the patient about oral homecare practices that will help maintain the periodontal tissues, preserve restorations and prostheses, and ensure an acceptable range of disease presence. Continuous an ongoing communication should include optimal oral healthcare suggestions.

Inclusion of the maintenance phase in the overall treatment plan is necessary to engage the patient. It reiterates that the patient is also involved in efforts to maintain disease control. A synergistic relationship between the dentist and the patient promotes the value of maintaining a long-term therapeutic relationship.

Emphasis on Individualized Care

Individualized patient care focuses on tailored treatment, targeting specific needs by utilizing risk assessments, social, medical and dental history, and other data that impact oral health. Creation of individualized care shows investment in the patient's oral and overall health. The benefits to the patient include more meaningful homecare routines and treatment recommendations that provide a foundation for a more successful outcome. By tailoring treatment and preventive recommendations to the needs of each individual, rather than relying on a single lock-step approach, patients gain a sense of ownership and responsibility for their own care.

Health Promotion and Disease Prevention

The well-constructed maintenance phase places the emphasis on promoting and sustaining optimal oral health and function, rather than on restoration and reconstruction resulting from past disease. Routine visits for maintenance care promotes prevention rather than focusing on problem-based care.

Anticipating Additional Treatment Needs

A thoughtful, comprehensive maintenance phase plan includes any issues that can realistically be expected to require reevaluation, reconsideration, or re-treatment in the future. Specific notes, such as "reevaluate tooth no. 29 with poor periodontal prognosis" or "reassess patient need and/or desire for crown on tooth no. 19 with compromised cusp integrity" confirm that the patient has been alerted to potential risks and hazards. These types of documentation examples place the responsibility for accepting the consequences of deferring treatment on the patient rather than the dentist. A casual review of the original treatment plan (or progress note if recorded there) quickly brings the issue to the patient's attention again.

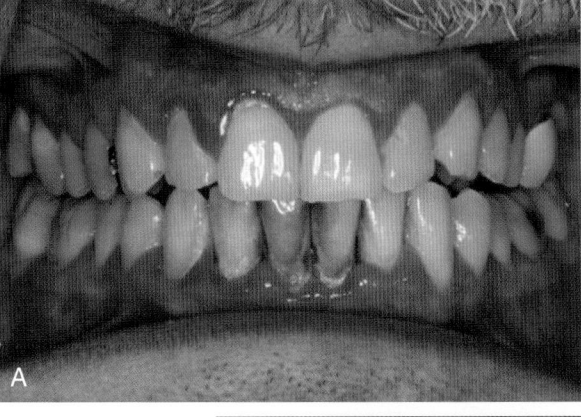
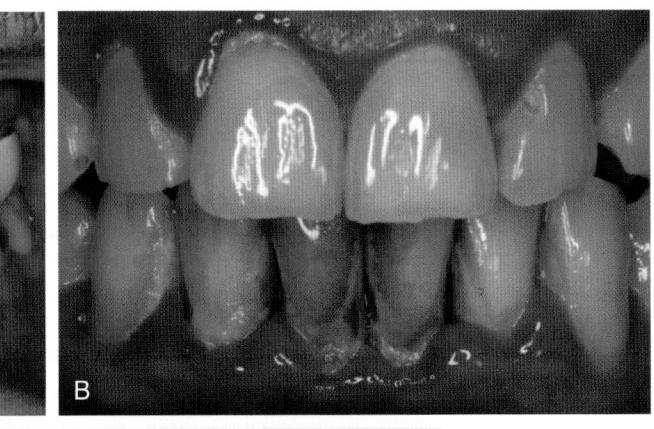
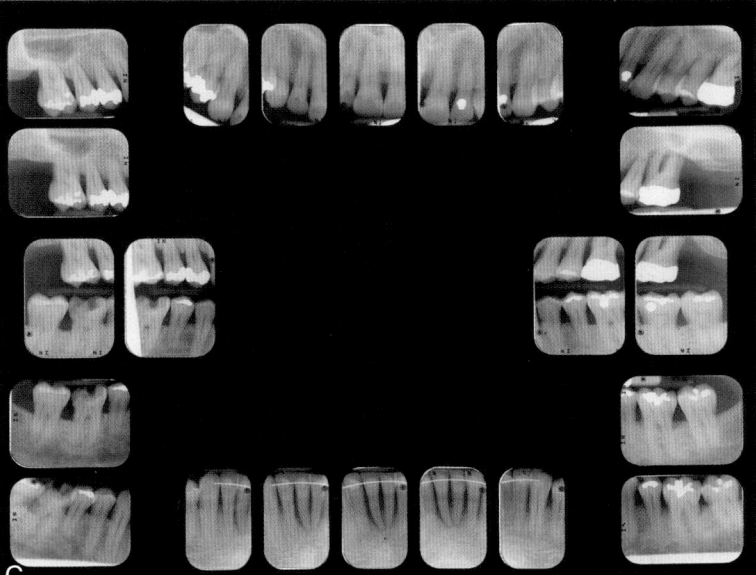
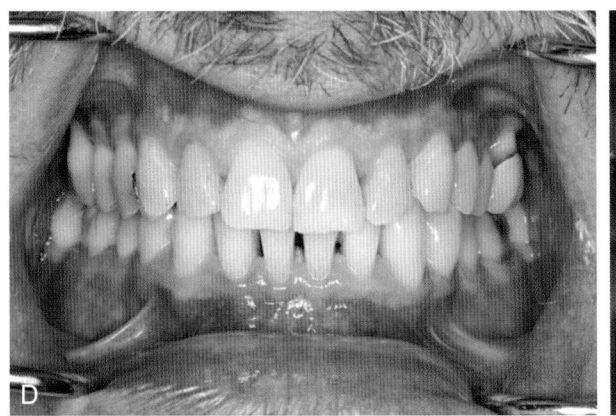
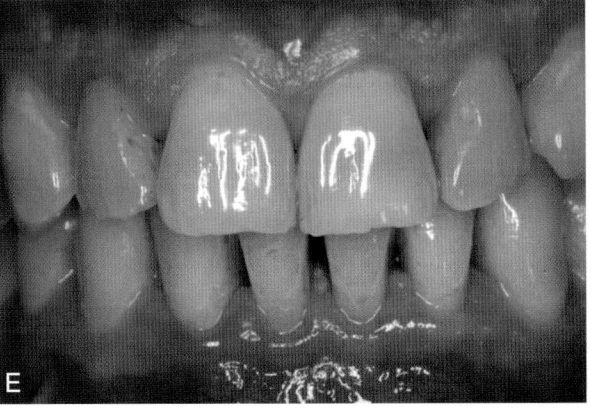

Fig. 12.2 Diabetic patient with periodontal disease. **(A-C)**, Demonstrates advanced periodontal disease and a very poor periodontal prognosis; **(D)** and **(E)**, show the patient after periodontal therapy and successful management of the diabetes. Remarkably, the patient has been able to retain the teeth and the periodontal prognosis is greatly improved. (Courtesy Dr. Thiago Morelli, Chapel Hill, N.C.)

Without a clearly articulated maintenance phase, the patient may assume that any new problems that arise are, at least in part, the responsibility of the dentist. The tooth with longstanding severe periodontitis that must now be extracted or the tooth with a large amalgam restoration that now fractures are examples. Recording these potential problems in the treatment plan and calling them to the patient's attention at the outset of the maintenance phase avoids any potential for future misunderstanding, mistrust, or conflict.

Implementation of a comprehensive and individualized maintenance phase ensures quality patient care, and benefits to the dentist, staff, and practice.

Practice Management Benefits

Professional Competence

Informing patients about the need for maintenance therapy and procedures is an important part of our ethical and professional responsibility.

Collectively, the entire patient record-—if it includes a comprehensive, accurate, and complete database, diagnosis, plan of care, and consent-—provides excellent evidence of professional competence. A thorough, well-written maintenance phase is part of that continuum. Faced with a patient record that documents your comprehensive efforts to provide professionally appropriate person centered care will often discourage a disgruntled patient (and their attorney)from pursuing litigation.

Efficient Delivery of Care

Thorough documentation is used as an effective tool to alert the dental team to oral and overall health issues that should be addressed during periodic visits. Awareness of such issues and concerns will make the visit more focused, organized, and personalized. With a recorded plan, the entire staff approaches the periodic visit proactively and efficiently.

Reducing Patient Emergencies

An informed patient who understands that oral health problems can arise may be more likely to take preventive action before a crisis develops. Patients who follow a routine maintenance program will enable the dental team to identify and anticipate early oral health problems, thus reducing the need for urgent care visits.

Partnering With Patients

The maintenance plan encourages the patient to become a partner in the long-term management of his or her oral health, rather than simply a client. The maintenance phase provides an effective way to engage the patient in co-therapy with the dental team. With informed and collaborative decision making, the patient has greater perceived value of, and is willing to accept more responsibility for, their long-term oral health.

ISSUES TO CONSIDER IN THE MAINTENANCE PHASE OF CARE

To list all the items that could be included in the maintenance phase would be an overwhelming undertaking. To give the reader a realistic perspective on this issue, the authors suggest the following list of categories that are common to many maintenance phase plans (see Box 12.1).

This list can also act as a template from which you can develop a menu to use in your own practice. Although no individual patient would be expected to require attention to all of the areas listed here, it can be anticipated that most patients will need several.

General Health Condition and Medical Risk

Specify all items from the systemic phase that will require follow-up, reevaluation, or intervention as part of the patient's

---

> **BOX 12.1   Issues Commonly Included in the Maintenance Phase**
>
> General health considerations
> Oral home care instructions
> Oral prophylaxis
> Periodontal maintenance
> Caries control
> Restorations and prostheses
> Implant assessment and maintenance
> Endodontic reevaluation
> Management of chronic oral soft tissue disease
> Management of radiographically-evident abnormalities and pathologies
> Orthodontic assessment
> Radiographic images
> Elective treatment
> Continued care interval

perpetual care. Examples include physician consultation in the presence of chronic life-threatening disease, such as liver cancer, premedication for anxiety or infective endocarditis, reevaluation of previously diagnosed hypertension or other chronic conditions, and treatment modification because of an immuno-compromising condition, such as rheumatoid arthritis.

Oral Health Condition and Risk Assessment

Any perioral or intraoral abnormalities that were identified at the initial examination, but will not be actively managed in the patient's plan of care, should be flagged for reevaluation in the maintenance phase plan. Oral health problems that were recognized at the outset to need long-term maintenance should also be included. Patients who have been at elevated risk of oral cancer, caries, periodontal disease, or occlusal trauma or other occlusal abnormalities will need careful assessment of their risk status and determination whether intervention is warranted.

Patient Concerns

When a patient presents for an initial exam and treatment plan, they may have some requests or concerns that cannot be definitively addressed in the initial plan of care. Commonly, when the patient needs a disease control phase plan of care it would not be possible to determine the definitive phase plan of care. In such cases, it is essential that the maintenance phase plan include a reevaluation of the patient's original and current concerns, desires, and treatment objectives. Doing so reaffirms to the patient in a tangible way that the original concerns are not being "forgotten" and that the dental team places a high priority on addressing those concerns, albeit at the appropriate time.

Malocclusion, Parafunctional Habits and the Patient's Ability to Function

If at the initial diagnosis and treatment planning visit the patient expressed concern about their ability to chew or if the dentist identified that the patient had malocclusion, parafunctional habits or TMD, the need to reevaluate any of these problems should be included in the patient's maintenance phase plan.

Oral Self-Care and Preventive Trajectory

It is expected that patients will need a reassessment of their plaque control, oral self-care practices, and their **preventive trajectory** as part of their maintenance phase plan. Optimal oral health is achieved through a partnership of professional maintenance and oral self-care. An essential element in establishing and maintaining gingival, periodontal, and dental health is biofilm control. There are a multitude of home preventive and therapeutic aids to assist the patient in that effort such as toothbrushes, interdental cleaners, floss holders and chemotherapeutic agents. Product recommendations and instructions should be specific to the patient's needs, preferences, and circumstances.

Whenever the patient has been given specific instructions regarding prescriptions, devices, or techniques, those instructions need to be documented in the patient's record and the maintenance phase plan is often a convenient and efficient place to record such recommendations.

Caries Control

This aspect of the maintenance phase plan is a continuation of the caries control plan described at length in Chapter 10. For patients who are at elevated risk of caries, the maintenance phase should include a reassessment of the patient's risk; careful examination of incipient, white spot, or "suspicious" lesions that were identified at the comprehensive exam visit; detailed review of the interventions and treatments in the caries management plan; and examination for new caries lesions.

Periodontal Condition and Stability

For a patient with gingivitis, the maintenance phase will commonly include an oral prophylaxis at intervals of 6–12 months. For a patient with periodontitis, this would include periodontal maintenance appointments at specified intervals usually no greater than 3 months depending on the individual risk for disease progression. The maintenance phase plan should identify specific problems, such as isolated deeper pockets, areas of furcation involvement, or mucogingival defects that need to be examined and may require additional therapeutic treatment, e.g., localized scaling and root planing or placement of local chemotherapeutic agents. Depending on the outcome of the disease control phase and definitive phase therapy, antibiotics may be administered locally or systemically. Antimicrobial rinses may also be prescribed. In the presence of aggressive or refractory periodontitis, the patient must be comprehensively reassessed for additional interventions.

Condition of Restorations, Prostheses, and Implants

Often during the course of the initial comprehensive examination, restoration defects are identified and treatment options discussed with the patient Examples include ditched amalgams; composites that are stained, poorly contoured or have defective margins; or crowns that have chipped porcelain, bulky contours, or open margins. In the case of absent caries or a compelling esthetic concern on the part of the patient, the dentist may judge the restoration to be "not ideal" but still "clinically acceptable" because there would be no imminent harm to the patient if left untreated. In some cases it may be possible to polish or recontour the restoration. The ideal treatment in most of these situations would be to veneer or to replace the restoration with a similar or more extensive restoration, but the patient may choose to defer treatment because of cost, time, or other considerations. When a patient elects to defer treatment, the issue needs to be included in the maintenance phase and revisited at future visits.

The maintenance phase should also include the reevaluation of any suspect direct or indirect restorations, or any existing fixed or removable dental prostheses. Implants will need to be reevaluated for stability and the presence of peri-mucositis or peri-implantitis.

Radiographic Images

The maintenance phase should include specific recommendations concerning when to consider the need for follow-up radiographs. General guidelines for radiographic examination are presented in Chapter 1 (Table e1.1). If a third molar assessment will be needed, a panoramic radiograph is usually recommended. At the completion of the definitive phase or in the maintenance phase, new periapical radiographs are recommended of teeth that have received extra-coronal or large direct-fill restorations (Figure 12.3). Teeth that have received restorations in close proximity to the pulp (selective caries

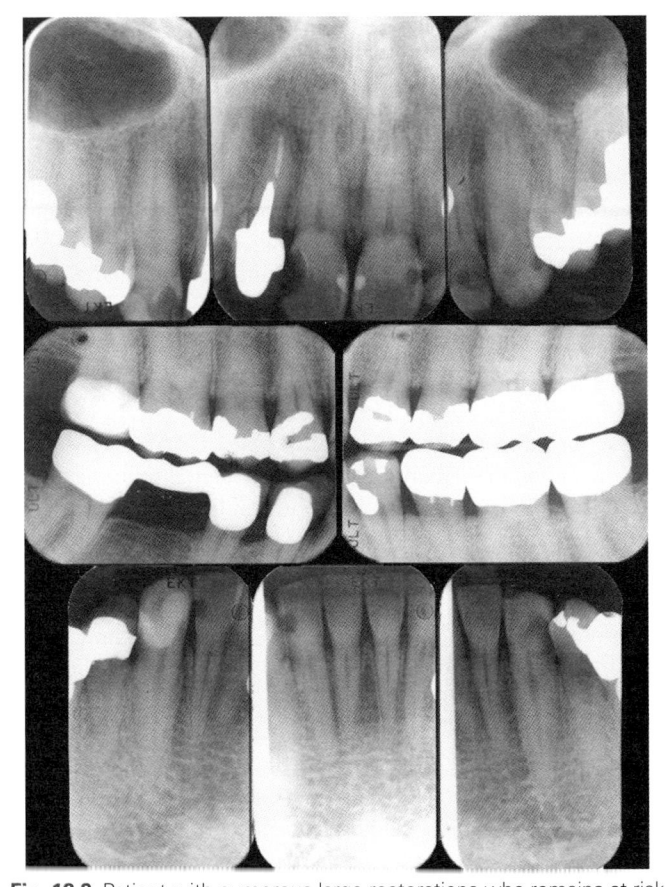

Fig. 12.3 Patient with numerous large restorations who remains at risk of caries—a prime indication for taking radiographs more frequently. (Courtesy Dr. J. Ludlow, Chapel Hill, NC.)

removal) should be slated for reevaluation and updated radiographs in the maintenance phase. Asymptomatic radiographic lesions for which the initial treatment decision was to observe should also be identified for radiographic follow-up in the maintenance phase.

In general, patients with a history of periodontal disease should be evaluated for a complete mouth radiographic series at 2- to 3-year intervals, depending on disease activity. Vertical bite-wing radiographs are recommended for patients with Stage III or IV Periodontitis. Similarly, patients with a history of active caries should be evaluated with bite-wing radiographs at 2-year intervals and more frequently in the presence of increased caries activity. In the absence of caries, periodontal disease, or other issues, such as those previously mentioned, it is often appropriate to delay taking bite-wing radiographs for up to 3 years and a complete mouth or panoramic radiographic survey for up to 6 years. These suggestions will vary with specific patients, practices, and patient populations.

Elective Treatment

At the time that the original treatment plan was formulated, treatments may have been proposed that the patient was unwilling or unprepared to commit to. Examples include fixed or removable partial dentures, implants and implant retained prostheses, and orthodontic treatment. The maintenance phase is the ideal time to discuss these options again with the patient.

Recare Interval

In the generation of the maintenance phase plan of care it is common to indicate an estimation of how frequently the recare visit should occur for the patient. For a patient with active caries (moderate or high caries risk) or active periodontal disease, that interval may be 2–4 months. For patients with no active disease and for whom there is no specific indication necessitating a return to the office (e.g., to reevaluate a soft tissue lesion), a **recall interval** of 6–12 months will often be appropriate (see the next section).

COMMON PROCEDURES DONE AT THE RECARE/PERIODIC VISIT

Implementation of the maintenance phase occurs at the periodic visit, i.e., the patient's return to the dental office at designated intervals, usually several months in length. The purposes of the periodic visit are to review the patient's oral health status, attend to any new problems that have emerged, and discuss any additional treatment needs. The periodic visit includes several components: evaluation, therapy, plan for ongoing and future treatment, and documentation in the progress note. Each of these components is discussed in sequence.

Evaluation

The periodic examination of the dentate patient normally includes the following components. Some elements will be omitted for the edentulous patient. Additional items should be added to this list as appropriate to meet the specific needs of individual patients.

WHAT'S THE EVIDENCE?

What's the Evidence that Maintenance Visits Should Occur at Particular Intervals and that They Are Beneficial to Oral Health? (Why 6-Month Recall Intervals?)

There is little evidence to support the frequently cited standard that "You should visit the dentist every 6 months," yet insurance companies will often cover two, but no more than two, recall visits per year.[6,7] Additionally, systematic reviews have found that there is insufficient evidence to support one specific interval for all individuals.[8,9] Some suggest that the origin of the 6-month interval came from the 1950s Bristol-Myers Co. toothpaste commercials with the character Bucky Beaver whose slogan advised listeners to use Ipana toothpaste and see the dentist twice a year.[6]

Research has shown that, in patients with gingivitis, a 6-month periodic visit including an oral prophylaxis is insufficient to control the problem.[10] Uncontrolled gingivitis will commonly lead to periodontitis. It must be recognized that each individual has different susceptibility to periodontal disease.

Some patients will experience rapid progression whereas a smaller (~10%) group will remain resistant to inflammation-induced alveolar bone loss.[11] Therefore, risk stratification to determine a personalized recare interval is essential. Many studies have shown that routine prophylactic recall visits are important in treating periodontal disease.[12–18] Maintenance visit intervals for individuals with periodontitis range from a few weeks to 6 months, but 2- to 3-month intervals are the most common.[19,20] Patients with continuously high plaque scores are more likely to exhibit recurrent gingivitis or periodontitis and should be appointed at shorter intervals. Advanced cases of periodontitis can be adequately maintained with properly spaced maintenance visits and good oral.[21,22] However, if adequate plaque control cannot be achieved, an interval of 2–3 months is still advised.[17]

As implant therapy has become more commonplace, it has become apparent that quality implant maintenance plays an important role in assuring that the implants will be retained and have a favorable outcome. Clinical trials and studies investigating the incidence of peri-mucositis and peri-implantitis in relationship with the frequency and interval of the maintenance visits have been illuminating. Less frequent recall intervals have been associated with higher incidence of peri-implantitis both at implant and patient-level.[23] It has been suggested that the recall interval be a minimal 5–6 months in low risk individuals and that the recall interval be 2–3 months for higher risk patients (e.g., patients with a history of periodontal disease).[24]

Another important consideration in determining the appropriate recall interval for a patient is their caries activity and their caries risk. Important markers for caries activity include the development of new lesions and the progression of previously diagnosed incipient, primary, or secondary lesions. Other findings that would suggest significant risk of caries include lack of patient compliance with previous behavioral recommendations, elevated plaque score, dry mouth, a diet that is aciduric or with high levels of fermentable carbohydrates, immune compromise, or debilitated general health. Patients who are at elevated risk of caries will need more frequent recalls and shorter recall intervals.[25–27]

Update of the Health History Questionnaire

At the periodic visit, the patient history must be updated. Particular attention must be paid to any new medical conditions or allergies. Are preexisting conditions being effectively controlled? Review the current medications to identify any changes and confirm compliance. Any limitations or contraindications to dental treatment on this date must be documented. The record must reflect that the medical history has been reviewed and updated.

Vital Signs

The vital signs routinely taken at the periodic visit include the blood pressure and pulse; in selected circumstances it may also be appropriate to evaluate respiration and temperature. Vital signs are helpful in identifying undiagnosed or poorly controlled hypertension or cardiovascular disease, medical contraindications to certain modes of treatment, and establishing an essential baseline of information should a medical emergency arise in the course of the dental visit.

Head and Neck Exam/Extraoral/Intraoral Examination

The head and neck, extraoral and intraoral exam is an essential component of the periodic visit. Careful screening for oral cancer is a professional responsibility and, in most jurisdictions, a legal obligation. It also provides the patient with peace of mind when they are assured that no pathology is present. Early detection of oral cancer (Figure 12.4) is important because it may improve the prognosis for the disease and the patient's quality of life and life expectancy.

Evaluation of Patient Concerns

The dental team should inquire about the chief concern, and other concerns, at each periodic oral health visit. Understanding

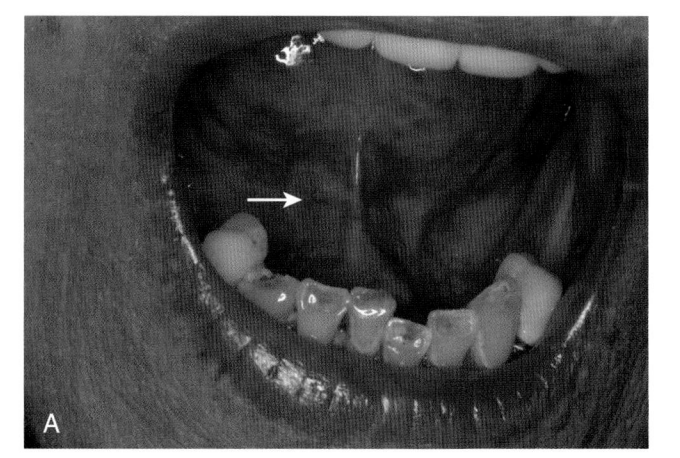

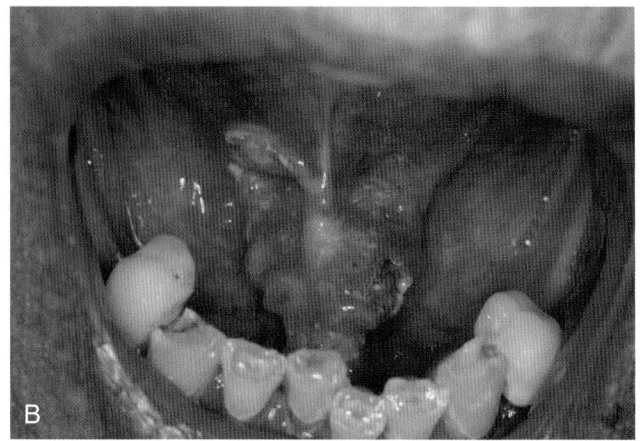

Fig. 12.4 (A) A suspicious lesion at initial presentation. The patient initially declined a biopsy and did not come in for their first follow-up appointment. **(D)** The same patient returned many weeks later – note the dramatic change in the size and appearance of the lesion. The biopsy definitively confirmed the lesion to be a squamous cell carcinoma. (Courtesy Dr. Ricardo Padilla, Chapel Hill, N.C.)

and responding to the patient's chief concern, or chief complaint, is important in developing and maintaining rapport with the patient. Oral health care professionals may inquire about the chief concern by simply asking, "What brings you in today?" Patients may not necessarily have a symptomatic chief concern at the periodic visit, but giving the patient an opportunity to raise questions or concerns can lead to early intervention and help to alleviate problems before they become more significant or acute. If the patient does have an acute concern, the normal procedures at the periodic visit may need to be modified as the dental team focuses on resolving the patient's urgent need.

Procuring and Interpreting Radiographic Images

Using selection criteria discussed earlier in this chapter, radiographic images are obtained at the recare visit. A symptomatic chief concern, evidence of new or recurring caries activity, progression of periodontal disease, or the appearance of a dental problem that may warrant complex restorative work, are common findings to indicate the need for new radiographs.

Occasionally, as described in the accompanying *In Clinical Practice: The Patient Who Refuses to Update Radiographs* box, the dentist may encounter patients who do not want to update radiographs. Most opposition can be overcome if the dentist and staff are prepared to respond to the patient's concerns.

After radiographs have been taken, special attention should be given to interpreting the images and recording the findings. Having ordered the images, the dentist is obligated to view all of them comprehensively. Regardless of the type of image, any and all structures evident on the radiograph must be assessed and the findings recorded. The practitioner must develop a disciplined and systematic approach to radiographic interpretation. Typically, the pattern is similar to that of the clinical examination: beginning with the more general and the more peripheral structures followed by the periapical areas, then the

---

IN CLINICAL PRACTICE

The Patient Who Refuses to Update Radiographs

At the periodic visit, patients may question the need for obtaining updated radiographic images. The following stepwise formulaic is helpful in addressing these concerns.

- Discern the patient's reasons for not wanting to have radiographic images taken:

  Many patients have a deep underlying concern and want to avoid any exposure to ionizing radiation. This concern may have evolved from information in blogs, the popular media and/or social media, which have highlighted a one-sided perspective on the hazards of x-rays in any form. Others may have had therapeutic radiation therapy for cancer and seek to avoid any additional exposure. Others may be pregnant (or are hoping to become pregnant) and wish to avoid anything that may be harmful to the fetus.

  Some patients want to avoid having radiographs because they consider them to be "unnecessary." These patients may have given credence to the urban legend that "dentists take too many x-rays." They may not be convinced that there is any real benefit and they are willing to take the risk of not having the radiographs. Patients who are missing many or all of their teeth may think that radiographs are irrelevant.

  There are also some patients who argue that "I can't afford it." This is often a relative issue as the patient has the financial means but believes that the radiographs are not as important as other needs and wants. These patients may also use finances as a stated rationale for one or more of the other underlying concerns noted previously. For those patients with a true financial hardship and who do not have the required financial resources, the dentist may elect to reduce or waive the fees (see Chapter 19 for more discussion of options).

- Explain the use of selection criteria as a guide (2012 Food and Drug Administration and ADA Recommendations[28]), which takes into account the patient's dental history, current symptoms, past and current disease activity, current restorative condition, and future treatment needs.
- Discuss the specific *benefits* to the patient of obtaining radiographic images in the context of the patient's past dental history and current dental condition.[28,29]
  - If the patient has symptoms or signs of new or reactivated oral infection or disease and new images will aid in making a correct diagnosis, the benefit of obtaining new images is obvious.
  - If the patient is considered to be at an elevated risk of caries, periodontal disease, or periapical pathology, radiographic images are an important element in verifying whether the risk is static, has become elevated, or is diminished.
  - In the presence of implants, root canal treatments, or large existing restorations, images may facilitate the early discovery of new or recurrent disease.
  - With early detection and accurate diagnosis of new disease or recognition of newly elevated disease risk, preventive strategies may be more effective, interventions more successful and less costly, and more serious outcomes, such as loss of teeth, may be avoided.[28]
  - New radiographic images can, when no pathology is evident, give patients the peace of mind of knowing that they are disease-free at this juncture. This may be especially meaningful to patients who have had oral cancer or who have other forms of cancer and want to be sure there is no metastasis to their jaw.
- Discuss the *risks* of obtaining the images and processes for limiting ionizing radiation exposure.
  - All dental practices should routinely practice the ALARA (As Low As Reasonably Achievable) principles. Informing a patient of efforts your office has made in this regard is appropriate and is usually appreciated by the patient.
  - Significant advances have been made in recent years to minimize the ionizing radiation exposure from dental radiographs.[28–30] The benefits of changing from D Speed to F Speed (Insight) and from round to rectangular collimation are illustrated in Table 12.1.
- The Consent Discussion

  The consent discussion should be carried out in a thoughtful, dispassionate, professional manner, with the dentist listening carefully to the patient's questions and responding to their concerns. If the patient has specific concerns not already addressed in the risk/benefit discussion, those concerns should be addressed at this time. A pregnant patient is a good example. A fundamental question for pregnant patients may be which images are absolutely necessary at this juncture and which can be deferred until after the birth. The American Dental Association Council on Scientific Affairs states that no justified diagnostic examination should be deferred because of pregnancy.[28,29] The health physics society has confirmed that there is no known association between in utero birth defects and dental imaging.[31] If the history and clinical exam suggest the serious possibility of new active disease (caries, periodontal disease, pulpal or apical disease) and new images will assist with the diagnosis and treatment, new images should be taken. If the patient is asymptomatic, however, and has no clinical evidence of caries, periodontal disease, or other oral pathology, it may be prudent to defer routine images until after the birth. However, if the dentist has determined that the patient is at high risk of

developing an oral infection during the pregnancy, the images should be taken without delay. A factor that might weigh against taking elective radiographs during pregnancy would be the patient's high level of anxiety about radiation exposure (which could in itself increase the risk of an untoward event).

If the patient continues to decline recommended radiographs, some practices have developed a consent form: ***Informed Refusal to Take Radiographs***. In some settings, this has become the pro forma response to any patient resistance to the suggestion that new radiographs be taken. Although accepting the patient's position without discussion and asking the patient to sign the Refusal form might save time and avoid what can sometimes be a lengthy and challenging conversation, this approach violates professional ethical principles. Furthermore, it is not clear that a patient can legally consent to nontreatment that can be considered negligent and does not meet the standard of care. Nor is it clear in case law that the dentist is not responsible for failure to diagnose and treat clinical problems that would have been evident on radiographs had they been taken (see Chapter 7).

If, after comprehensive discussion with the patient, the patient still refuses to allow indicated images to be taken, the dentist may be faced with no other alternative but to dismiss the patient from the practice. This may be the only recourse if the dentist is confident that they cannot in good conscience continue to treat the patient without violating their own ethical standards and the professional standard of care. If dismissal is decided on, the patient must be given due process as discussed in Chapter 7. In many cases, however, the prospect of having to leave the practice and find another dental home may cause the patient to reconsider the issues and consent to have radiographs taken. Regardless of the outcome, the consent discussion must be thoroughly documented in the patient record.

marginal periodontium, and concluding with abnormalities of the teeth and restorations. A panoramic image will also require an evaluation of the temporomandibular joints and the maxillary sinuses. Findings from this analysis must then be recorded in detail, usually in the progress notes.

Periodontal Evaluation

For all patients, the periodontal portion of the recall exam should include:

1. Careful evaluation of the color, shape, contour, and texture of the gingiva, including notation of recession, clefting, and any mucogingival defects (Figure 12.5).
2. Plaque score and assessment of the patient's effectiveness with oral homecare and identification of the worse area of plaque accumulation for a customized oral hygiene instruction.
3. Full mouth periodontal probing and a recorded Bleeding Index.

For patients with significant gingival recessions, clinical attachment loss and width of the keratinized tissue (location of mucogingival junction) should also be recorded (see periodontal re-evaluation in Chapter 10 for details).

Caries/Restorative Evaluation

In general, examination of the teeth and restorations should follow the other more universal parts of the examination. Otherwise, the focus tends to be primarily on the teeth and, if notable restorative items arise, they are sometimes discussed immediately with the patient, thereby delaying, abbreviating, or bypassing other aspects of the examination. This can easily be prevented simply by doing the caries/restorative examination *last*.

TABLE 12.1 Effective Dose and Risk from Dental Radiographic Examinations

Examination Type	Collimation	Average Effective Dose (μSv)	Background Equivalent Days (μSv)[a]	Probability of x in a Million Fatal Cancer[b]
Bite-wings (BW) (Adult) Four Images				
D-speed film[c]	Circular	80	9	4.4
D-speed film	Rectangular	25	3	1.4
PSP	Circular	32	4	1.8
PSP	Rectangular	10	1	0.6
DD	Circular	16	2	0.9
DD	Rectangular	5	<1	0.3

69% = Average dose reduction from collimation.
94% = Potential dose reduction switching from D-film to DD with collimation.

Full Mouth Series (Adult) 18 Images				
D-speed Film	Circular	215	25	11.8
D-speed Film	Rectangular	135	16	7.4
PSP	Circular	86	10	4.7
PSP	Rectangular	54	6	3.0
DD	Circular	43	5	2.4
DD	Rectangular	27	3	1.5

37% = Average dose reduction from collimation.
87% = Potential dose reduction switching from D-film to DD with collimation.

Panoramic (Adult)[d]				
DD		19	2	1.0
Panoramic + BW (Adult)				
DD	Circular	35	4	1.9
DD	Rectangular	24	3	1.3

[a]Values are rounded to nearest whole day. Based on 3.1 mSv annual per capita natural background dose in United States. NCRP Report No.177.
[b]Dose in μSv x 0.055. 6-cm circular collimator. Optimized rectangular collimator.
[c]The value provided is the average dose from dedicated panoramic array detector. A large range may be encountered because of detector type.
[d]D-speed film dose determined by a factor of 2.5 respective PSP dose. PSP dose values result from exposure parameters optimized for both PSP and F-speed film.
DD, Direct digital; PSP, photostimulable phosphor.
Table information sourced from Brandon Johnson et al. (2021), Chapel Hill, NC
Effective dose calculations are based on the revised guidelines of the International Commission on Radiological Protection.

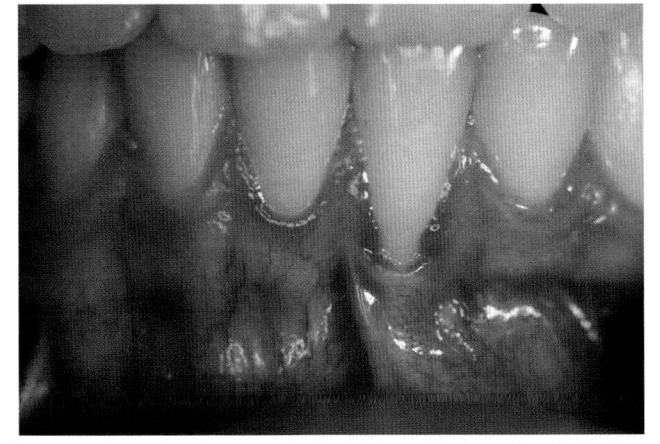

Fig. 12.5 Example of a mucogingival defect. (Courtesy Dr. J. Moriarty, Chapel Hill, NC.)

The teeth must be examined carefully for new or recurrent caries lesions. Here the detailed notes in the maintenance phase of the plan of care (or in the patient record from previous periodic visits) are particularly helpful because they direct the dentist and staff to specific sites where incipient lesions are present or other areas that need reevaluation for signs of caries.

Existing restorations should be evaluated for occlusal and proximal contacts, contour, and esthetics. In addition, restorations should be examined for fractures, marginal defects, improper contours, or missing restorative material. Again, it is helpful to the staff and the dentist if previously noted defects and problems that were to be watched or observed have been specified on the maintenance phase plan or on a periodic visit progress note.

If the patient had previously been judged to be at risk of future caries and a caries control plan has been developed, any remaining aspects of the plan should be attended to. If new intervention is necessary or if previous caries control measures need to be reinstituted, they should be implemented at this visit. If the patient has not previously been caries active or determined to be at elevated risk for caries, but present evaluation confirms that the patient is now caries active or at increased risk, a caries management protocol should be instituted.

Endodontic Treatment Revaluation

Many endodontists evaluate the response to root canal therapy at regular intervals to confirm that all symptoms have resolved, that signs of infection have disappeared, and that bone has filled in the periapical area. Initially, these visits may occur at set intervals and continue until complete healing has occurred. If the root canal therapy has been done in the general dentist's practice or if the endodontist is not completing a reevaluation, it is in the patient's best interest that these reevaluation procedures be followed as part of the patient's regularly scheduled periodic examination. If signs or symptoms consistent with tooth fracture or clinical infection are found, the site of the root canal therapy must be carefully scrutinized. Referral to an endodontist may be warranted. Following conversation with the patient, a decision must be made as to whether to extract the tooth, to provide endodontic retreatment, to intervene surgically, or to reevaluate the situation in the future. The final decision and evidence of patient consent must, of course, be documented in the patient's record. In the absence of signs or symptoms, it is usually prudent to take a follow-up radiograph 6 to 12 months after root canal therapy. If apical periodontitis or an apical rarefying osteitis remains visible on the radiograph, the patient must be informed about treatment options, risks and benefits, the likelihood of success for each, and the potential consequences if no additional intervention is implemented.

Special Considerations for Implants

Common patient concerns related to implants include the presence of food impaction, unsightly black triangles, gingival irritation, loosening of implants or implant retained abutment or crown. When any of these concerns arise at the periodic visit, they, or any other concern, will need to be carefully investigated and diagnosed and options for resolution discussed with the patient. At the recare visit each implant must be examined carefully for mobility, pocketing, swelling, exudate, bleeding on probing and any signs of inflammation in the peri-implant tissues. To avoid scratching the implant, it is generally recommended that probing be implemented with a plastic probe. In the presence of increased recession, advancing probing depths (attachment loss), suppuration, extensive bleeding on probing, or implant mobility, a new radiograph (or radiographs) is indicated. Deeper probing depths are common around dental implants and, when present, may be associated with a healthy periodontium or a peri-implantitis. Monitoring the bone levels on sequential radiographs can be helpful in making that distinction. For the first 3 years, annual radiographs to assess bone level are recommended.[2]

The patient's effectiveness in removing plaque must be carefully evaluated. Retention of biofilm is the most common cause

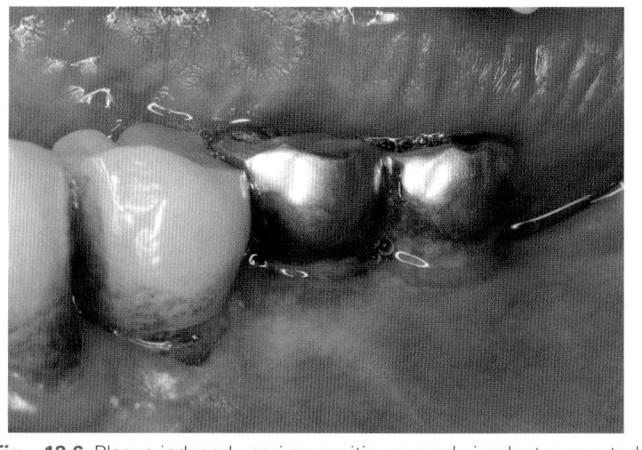

Fig. 12.6 Plaque-induced peri-mucositis around implant-supported crowns. (Courtesy Dr J Wang, Ann Arbor, MI.)

of peri-implant mucositis. Early detection of peri-implant mucositis (Figure 12.6) and preventing it from developing into peri-implantitis is an important goal of the periodic visit. In addition to biofilm retention, other common causes for peri-implantitis are the presence of calculus or adherent excess cement at the crown margin.

It is also important to look for the presence of parafunctional occlusal contacts on implant-retained restorations. Implant prosthetic complications such as crown loosening are more common in the presence of traumatic occlusal forces or if the patient is a bruxer.

Special Considerations for Fixed Partial Dentures

Fixed partial dentures are susceptible to several common problems. These include debonding; recurrent caries; gingivitis; periodontal disease; pulpal necrosis and associated periapical disease; occlusal trauma; fracture of the prosthesis (usually the porcelain); unesthetic margins, shade or contour (Figure 12.7). Acid-etch retained prostheses have a particularly high rate of debonding. Resin-bonded bridges present a particular concern if one retainer loosens and another remains stable, in which case the abutment with the loose retainer is vulnerable to rapidly advancing caries. With these concerns in mind, it is mandatory that the fixed partial denture be thoroughly evaluated for mobility, fracture, occlusal trauma, pulpal health, soft tissue and periodontal response, presence of plaque, food impaction, caries, marginal integrity, function, and esthetic problems.

Special Considerations for Removable Prostheses

Abutment teeth for a removable partial denture or a toothborne overdenture are subject to the same problems as abutments with fixed partial dentures. Natural tooth overdenture abutments are particularly susceptible to caries. Removable partial dentures may become loose or exhibit fracture of a clasp, the framework component, or the acrylic. Denture teeth are prone to occlusal wear, fracture, and detachment. Complete dentures are subject to midline fractures, flange fractures, and loss of retention (Figure 12.8). Any removable prosthesis may become stained or accumulate calculus. Implant-retained removable prostheses are susceptible to wear or dislodgment of the attachments.

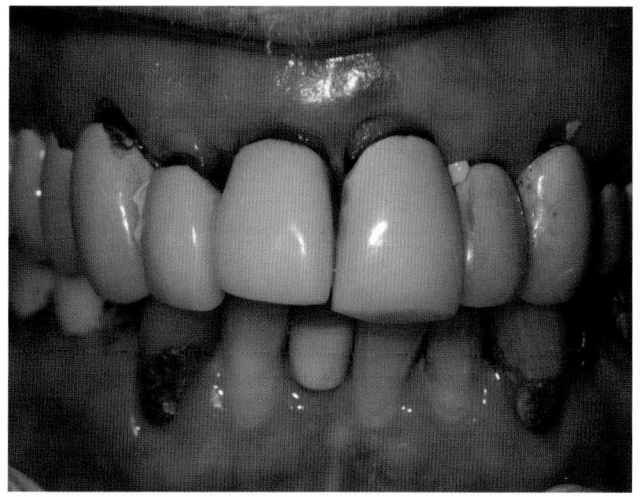

Fig. 12.7 Example of failed fixed partial denture. (Courtesy Dr. B.E. Kanoy, Chapel Hill, NC.)

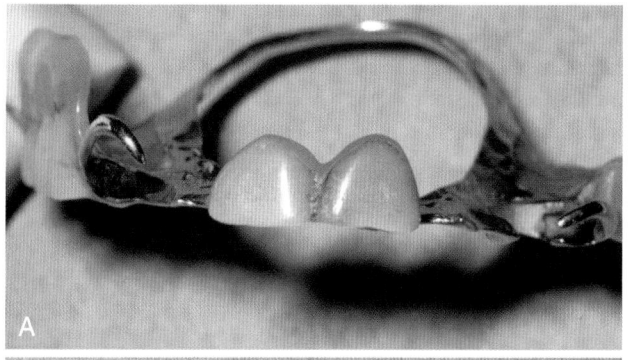

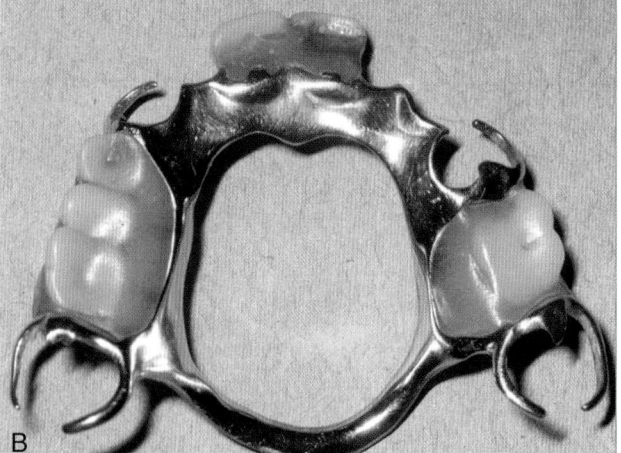

Fig. 12.8 Worn removable partial denture. (Courtesy Dr. A. Guckes, Chapel Hill, N.C.)

With any removable prosthesis, the dentist may find it helpful to segment the evaluation into three components: (1) information derived by the dentist from the clinical exam, (2) information obtained from the patient, and (3) issues to be assessed by both patient and dentist.

1. Dentist-derived issues include: an evaluation of the occlusion, stability, adaptation, integrity, and retention of the prosthesis; tissue response; and the effectiveness of the patient's oral homecare.

2. Patient-derived issues include any patient reports of symptoms or problems with the fit or function of the prosthesis.

3. A third category includes those concerns that are important to both patient and practitioner, and for which each may have a different perspective. Esthetics provides a useful example. When opinions differ concerning an esthetic issue, the patient's perspective should usually prevail. However, the dentist must provide appropriate information so that the patient is able to make an informed decision. For example, if the patient thinks the teeth in the partial denture are "too short," the dentist's role is to explain why the teeth were selected, positioned, and shaped as they are (e.g., consistency with the form of adjacent teeth, available interarch space, occlusal wear, etc.), describe available alternatives including how such alternatives may affect esthetics and function, and at what cost. In this situation, assuming the request is reasonable and the patient has realistic expectations for the outcome, the ultimate decision to modify or remake the prosthesis is left to the patient.

Orthodontic/Occlusal/Temporomandibular Joint Examination

Unless the patient raises concerns, this area rarely needs extended discussion. In most cases, a simple inquiry as to whether any problems with chewing, the bite, or the jaw joint have arisen is sufficient to elicit any concerns that may require evaluation or treatment. If the patient is a candidate for elective orthodontic, occlusal, or prosthodontic therapy, but has declined such treatment in the past, the periodic visit is a good time to raise those issues again. The In Clinical Practice Discussing Elective Procedures With Patients box offers an approach to this.

IN CLINICAL PRACTICE

Discussing Elective Procedures With Patients

Patients with significant bruxism or severe occlusal attrition should be reminded periodically that an occlusal guard can be fabricated to protect the teeth from continued wear, sensitivity, pulpal pathology, or loss of vertical dimension. Similarly, patients who have previously declined the option of correcting malpositioned, maloccluded, or missing teeth deserve to have these issues revisited. Often with a change of life circumstance, the patient's receptivity and desire for elective treatment will also change. The subject should be raised in a relaxed, nonthreatening manner so that the patient can listen carefully to all aspects of the issue and make an informed decision without feeling pressured. Printed material may be useful to the patient so that the options can be discussed with family members or friends.

The practitioner must be sensitive, however, not only to the patient's need to be informed about the dental problem and its attendant treatment options, but also to the patient's level of trust in healthcare providers and willingness to tolerate repeated discussions of the same issue. Some patients need and appreciate repeated discussion of comprehensive restorative and orthodontic options and are only able to make a decision after several lengthy conversations. In contrast, others are decisive at the first opportunity and view follow-up discussions as intrusive selling of unnecessary services. Both types of patient deserve to have the benefit of the dentist's professional expertise, but the nature, complexity, timing, and frequency of those discussions should be tailored to the individual patient. In any case, it is essential to document these conversations and the patient's response in the patient record.

Management and Maintenance Care

A therapeutic component is almost always appropriate during the periodic visit after completion of a thorough evaluation. If the patient's plan of care includes a disease control phase, the periodic visit procedures will include a continuation of the disease control phase therapy. In any case, a well-written maintenance phase plan or a disease control or definitive phase posttreatment assessment will guide and shape what occurs at the initial periodic visit. Subsequent visits are shaped in turn by the findings at the previous visit and the corresponding recommendations made and recorded in the progress notes.

Typical therapies provided at a periodic visit may include (but are not limited to):

- Responding to any general health/systemic phase issues (e.g., appropriate premedication)
- Oral prophylaxis
- Oral homecare instructions (with particular emphasis on problem areas, orthodontic retainers, and any prostheses)
- Scaling and root planing
- Any necessary disease control measures required for the elimination or prevention of caries or periodontal disease. This may include caries activity tests, dietary counseling, fluoride treatment and/or varnish, prescription of fluoride dentifrice, fluoride gel, trays or rinses, xylitol-based chewing gum, salivary substitutes, or antibiotics (locally applied, topical, or systemic).
- Recontouring, polishing, or providing simple adjustment to chipped teeth, stained composites, or ditched amalgams. This may include such procedures as elimination of easily accessible restoration overhangs or plunger cusps that contribute to food impaction.
- New or replacement restorations. The patient will typically need to return on a separate day with a designated appointment for restoration repair, placement, or replacement.
- Fixed partial denture maintenance may require recementation, repair, or removal to investigate possible caries or pulpal disease. Root canal therapy, periodontal surgery, or replacement is prescribed as necessary.
- Denture maintenance typically includes ultrasonic cleaning. Adjustments to tighten the clasps, replace worn implant attachments, or for relief of denture sores can usually be made on the day of the periodic visit. Repairs can be made on the same day or rescheduled if the complexity of the problem requires more time or laboratory support.
- Implant maintenance. Implants should be scaled with plastic instruments to prevent scarring or scratching the implant surface. If an implant-retained crown or retainer is loose, it may be possible to replace the retention screw and re-torque and replace the access restoration (if screw-retained); or re-cement the crown (if cement-retained). The broken component of a fractured retention screw or abutment can be removed and replaced with a healing cap. Extensive repair, or replacement of an abutment or crown will usually necessitate another visit.
- Occlusal guard maintenance. Patients who wear an occlusal guard may need an occlusal adjustment or, less commonly, a reline of the appliance. These procedures can normally be accommodated at the periodic visit if the patient brings the guard to the appointment. If an occlusal guard is completely fractured, it may be best to remake it rather than to try to repair it.

Manage General Health Considerations

If the patient presents at the recare visit with a new general health problem that has not been diagnosed or a preexisting problem that is not well controlled, a consultation with the patient's primary care provider may be in order. It is essential to confirm that it is safe to proceed with dental treatment on this date. If the patient needs premedication (for example for anxiety or because of risk of endocarditis), it will need to be prescribed and taken by the patient prior to the visit. The periodic visit is an opportune time to resume previous efforts to advance the patient's general health goals such as smoking cessation efforts, diet counseling, and encouragement of healthier lifestyle and behaviors. This can also be a good time to inform the patient how their oral health goals intersect with their general health goals and to affirm the patient's relationship with other healthcare providers. During the maintenance phase the patient's long-term health trajectory will become apparent. The periodic visits will reinforce the patient's understanding and experience that oral healthcare providers are an important link in their interprofessional and interdisciplinary healthcare system (see Chapter 6).

Management of New Soft Tissue Lesions and/or Chronic Oral Pathology

Any chronic oral pathologic conditions not eliminated in the earlier stages of the plan of care should be revisited as a part of maintenance care. The need for periodic reevaluation and the scheduling to reevaluate the lesion or condition must be discussed with the patient and documented. Examples include unresolved mucous extravasation phenomenon, dysplasias, erosive lichen planus, or chronic candidiasis (Figure 12.9).

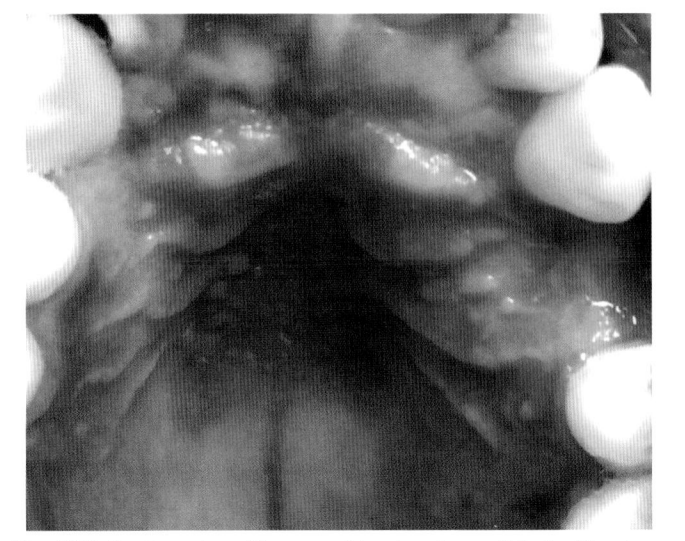

Fig. 12.9 Denture stomatitis caused by chronic candidiasis. (Courtesy Dr. V. Murrah, Chapel Hill, NC.)

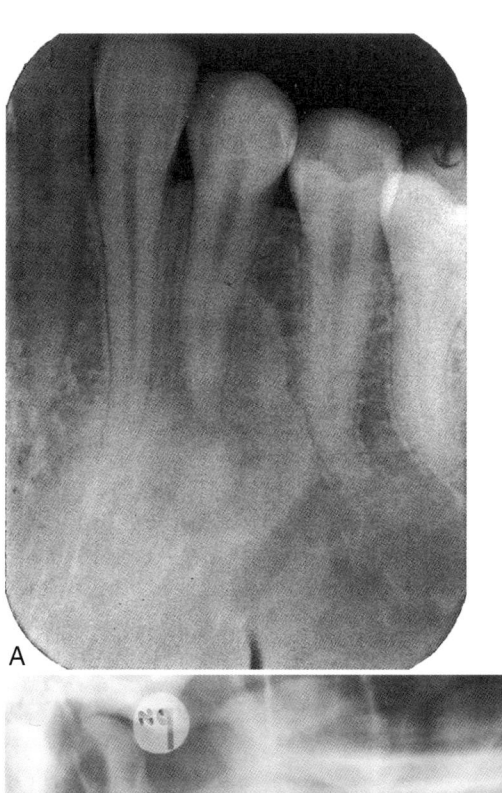

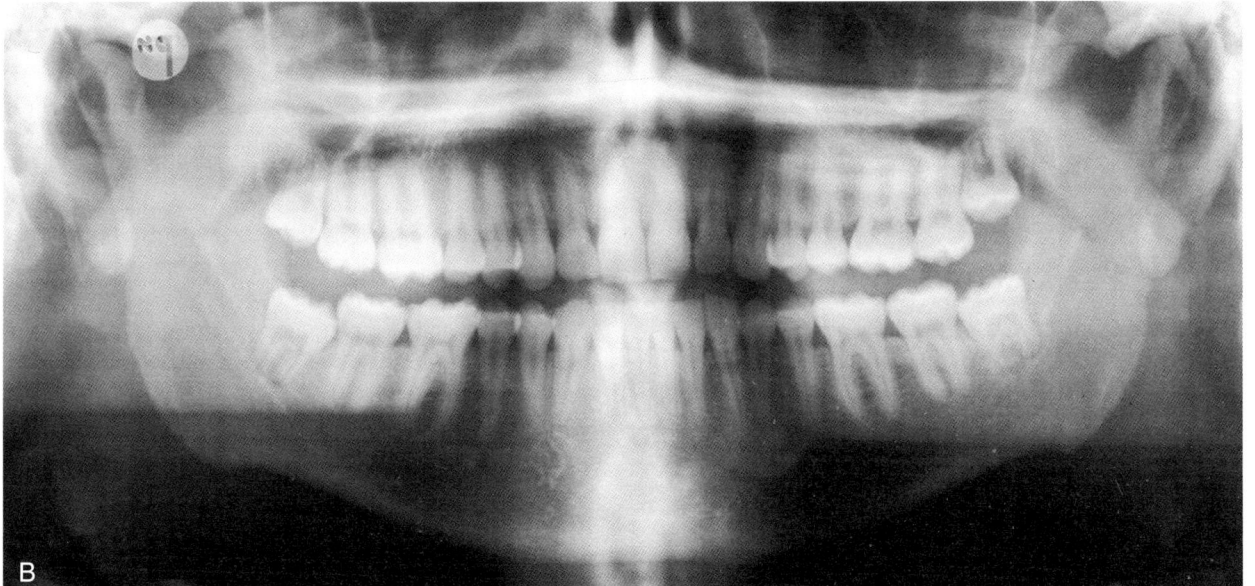

Fig. 12.10 An 18-year-old patient with cemento-ossifying fibroma—an example of a condition that needs to be reevaluated at periodic visits. **(A)** Periapical radiograph. **(B)** Panoramic radiograph. (Courtesy S. Addison, Chapel Hill, NC.)

Management of Radiographically Evident Abnormalities and Pathologies

Asymptomatic radiographic lesions of bone (Figure 12.10), such as cysts, periapical cemental dysplasia, florid osseous dysplasia, or impacted teeth for which treatment has been deferred should be reevaluated periodically with radiographs and other examination techniques.

Oral Hygiene Instructions and Homecare Therapy

Oral hygiene instructions play a vital role in the long-term maintenance of a patient's oral health and the overall success of the maintenance phase. As an integral aspect of the individualized patient care plan, homecare instructions should be thoughtfully developed and based on the status of the dentition, the history of restorations, any periodontal or caries risk, and the anticipated level of patient adherence. The dental team will need to attend to, and to teach the patient how to manage, areas that may be susceptible to trapping biofilm such as open contacts, extensive restorative work, and periodontal defects. Oral physiotherapy aids need to be recommended based on specific patient needs such as an end-tuft brush for a third molar area or a floss threader for bridgework (Figure 12.11 and Table 12.2). Additional preventive and therapeutic agents such as prescription-level dentifrices and antibacterial mouth rinses

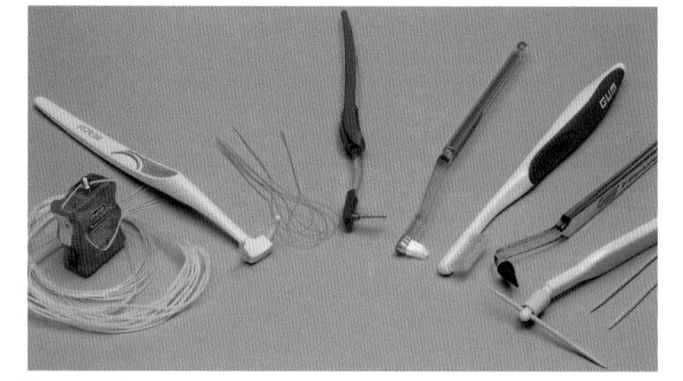

Fig. 12.11 Supplementary oral physiotherapy aids.

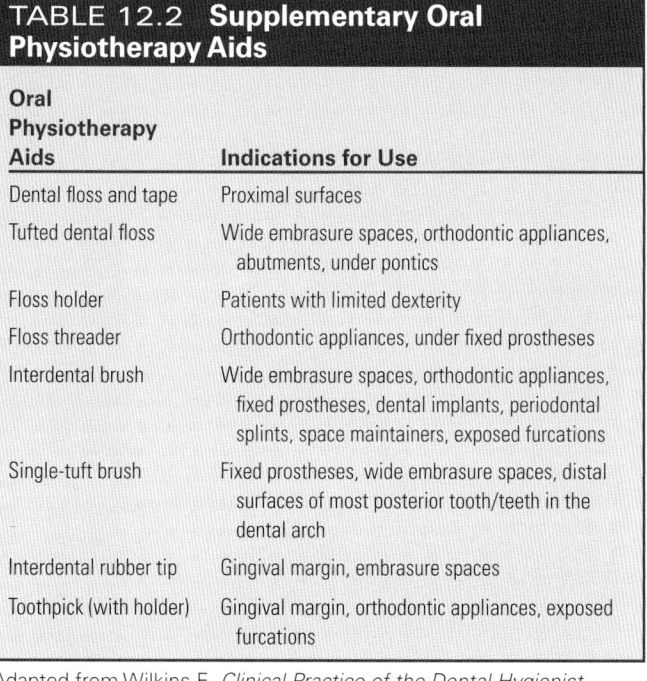

TABLE 12.2	**Supplementary Oral Physiotherapy Aids**
Oral Physiotherapy Aids	**Indications for Use**
Dental floss and tape	Proximal surfaces
Tufted dental floss	Wide embrasure spaces, orthodontic appliances, abutments, under pontics
Floss holder	Patients with limited dexterity
Floss threader	Orthodontic appliances, under fixed prostheses
Interdental brush	Wide embrasure spaces, orthodontic appliances, fixed prostheses, dental implants, periodontal splints, space maintainers, exposed furcations
Single-tuft brush	Fixed prostheses, wide embrasure spaces, distal surfaces of most posterior tooth/teeth in the dental arch
Interdental rubber tip	Gingival margin, embrasure spaces
Toothpick (with holder)	Gingival margin, orthodontic appliances, exposed furcations

Adapted from Wilkins E. *Clinical Practice of the Dental Hygienist.* 11th ed. Philadelphia: Lippincott, Williams & Wilkins; 2013

should be considered and recommended as needed. Document all recommendations and instructions made to the patient including any prescribed oral physiotherapy aids, materials, and techniques; and the advisable frequency of future maintenance visits.

Oral Prophylaxis

In the United States, a licensed dental hygienist or dentist is qualified to determine the need for an oral prophylaxis (https://www.adha.org>American Dental Hygienists' Association Position Paper on the Oral Prophylaxis). An adult prophylaxis is a preventive procedure where deposits are removed to control irritational factors (https://www.ada.org>ICD and CDT Codes/ Americal Dental Association). A patient who presents with gingivitis, calculus deposits, and localized or generalized bleeding on probing would warrant an oral prophylaxis. Patients who do not have periodontitis but who exhibit localized gingival

recession and gingival inflammation would also benefit from this procedure.

An oral prophylaxis is a routine treatment where calculus, stain, and biofilm are removed from the teeth and restorations using an ultrasonic scaler and hand-scaling instruments; and polishing of the teeth with prophylaxis paste applied with a cup or brush on a rotary instrument. For patients with elevated risk of caries, the oral prophylaxis is frequently followed up with application of fluoride varnish to all exposed tooth surfaces.

The interval for care is based on the specific needs of the individual patient.

Periodontal Maintenance

A patient who has been diagnosed with periodontitis and who has completed active periodontal therapy will need periodontal maintenance as long as they remain dentate. These patients commonly present with reduced periodontium, residual deep periodontal pockets, and furcation involvement. The periodontal maintenance visit normally includes a detailed periodontal examination, diagnosis of the current condition and risk status, determination of the prognosis, oral hygiene instructions, and select sites of manual subgingival scaling and root planing. Special attention is required to debride an exposed furcation thoroughly.

When, at the periodic visit, periodontitis is newly disgnosed, or reemergent because of a lapse in periodontal maintenance visits, nonsurgical periodontal therapy (scaling and root planing) is indicated and an appointment for a periodontal reevaluation should be scheduled – usually 4–8 weeks after completion of the scaling and root planing (see *Periodontal Reevaluation* in Chapter 10 for further discussion).

Caries Control Procedures and Recommendations

See Chapter 10 *The Disease Control Phase of Treatment* for extensive discussion of the reevaluation and maintenance procedures and processes for the patient with active caries and/or elevated caries risk.

Adjust or Refurbish Restorations and Prostheses

Common procedures in this category include: removing restoration overhangs; recontouring, polishing or veneering existing restorations; repairing or relining dentures, adjusting clasps on partial dentures; adjusting or relining occlusal guards or occlusal splints.

Implant Maintenance

Maintaining a healthy periodontium adjacent to an implant is essential for the long-term stability and retention of the implant. In the absence of a clear evidence-based protocol for implant maintenance, several guiding principles have emerged. Effective daily is recognized to be the most important strategy for ensuring long-term implant survival. Recognizing where there are areas of plaque retention and educating the patient how to remove the biofilm is an essential part of the periodic visit. Removal of any calculus or excess luting agent is also important. Currently, there is no standardized protocol for cleaning around dental implants.

When using manual or powered scaling instruments, providers need to be careful to avoid damaging porcelain surfaces or scratching implant surfaces. When calculus is detected, it may be prudent to remove it with plastic scaling instruments (rather than metal).[32] However, plastic scalers might not be effective at removing calculus or cement on hindered platform or supracrestal abutment surfaces (Figure 12.12); therefore in those situations a titanium instrument may be needed. In addition, use of subgingival irrigation or an airflow polishing device (Figure 12.13) may be a safe effective alternative when cleaning narrow deep spaces and rough surfaces. Antibacterial agents may also be beneficial in reducing biofilm and controlling gingivitis; but lower pH citric acid should be avoided because research has shown it may erode the implant surface and elute titanium particles.[33]

Another facet to implant maintenance to the need to assess the occlusion. Articulating paper should be used to check for excessively heavy MI (maximum intercuspation) contacts, or excursion interferences. Although a dental implant does not move after osseointegration, its relationship with the adjacent and opposing teeth is still dynamic and may change overtime. Judicious limited occlusal adjustment to relieve excessive MI contacts or excursive interferences is encouraged at the periodic visit.

Management of Orthodontic-Related Problems

At least three possible situations can be described in which the general dentist may be involved with maintenance during and after orthodontic treatment.

Ongoing Orthodontic Treatment by an Orthodontist

In this situation, the general dentist and the orthodontist each has a responsibility to reevaluate the patient periodically. The orthodontist is responsible for the progress of the orthodontics and any urgent or ongoing problems that arise directly from orthodontic brackets, bands, arch wires, fixed or removable orthodontic appliances, or retainers. The general dentist is usually responsible for the management of any oral diseases or conditions not directly caused by the orthodontic therapy, such as tooth fracture, restoration failure, newly emerging periodontal disease, or oral medicine problems. In areas of overlap, however, both practitioners bear responsibility. Both the general dentist and the orthodontist must be vigilant in watching for signs and symptoms of recurrent caries (Figure 12.14), root resorption, periapical pathology, occlusal trauma, reactivation of preexisting periodontal disease, or soft tissue lesions induced by the orthodontic appliances. Although

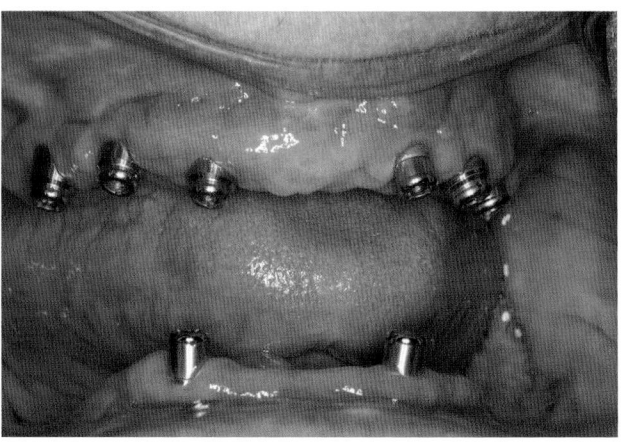

Fig. 12.12 Implant-supported hybrid prosthesis poses a challenge for maintenance care. (Courtesy Dr J Wang, Ann Arbor, MI.)

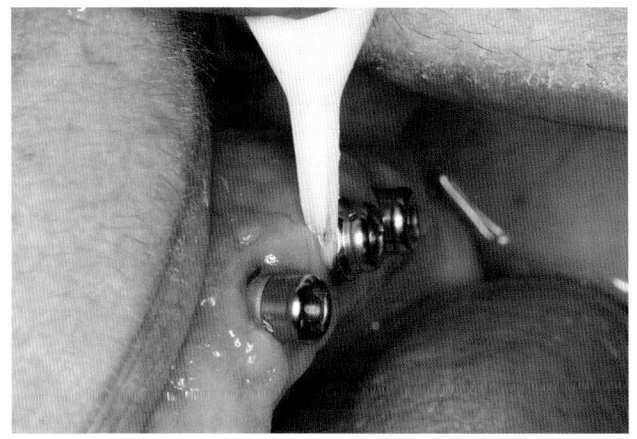

Fig. 12.13 The use of airflow for implant maintenance. (Courtesy Dr J Wang, Ann Arbor, MI.)

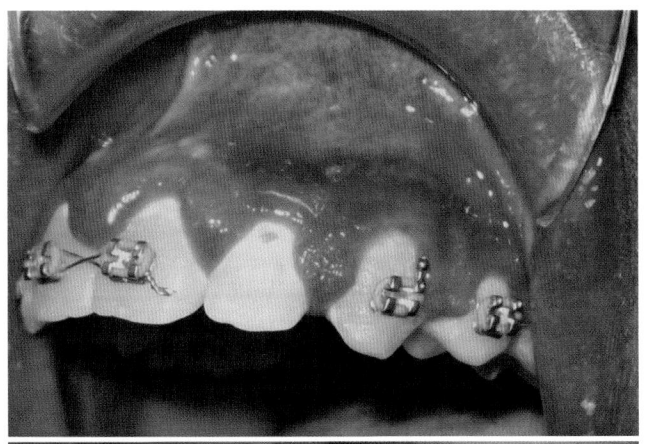

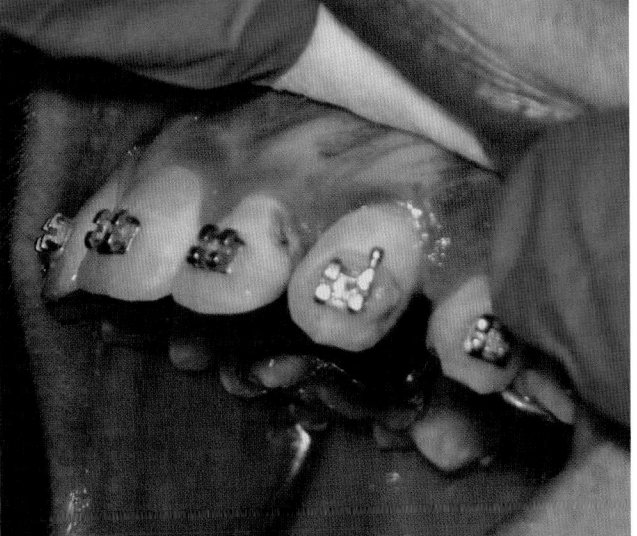

Fig. 12.14 (A) Orthodontic patient with active caries. **(B)** Patient with demineralization apparent on removal of elastics and arch wire. (Courtesy Drs. R. Beane and L. Bailey, Chapel Hill, NC.)

recognition of these problems is the responsibility of the practitioner who sees the patient first, both general dentist and orthodontist need to examine regularly for new caries activity. Management of the problem depends on the issue, its complexity, and the expertise of each of the practitioners involved.

In general, if the first practitioner to recognize the problem can address the issue successfully, they should do so. In any case, the two practitioners must communicate and clearly document in both patient records the diagnosis, the management plan, and who is responsible for each aspect of the plan. *It remains the responsibility of both practitioners to ensure that the problem is managed and resolved.*

Ongoing Orthodontic Treatment by the Patient's Regular General Dentist

In this situation, the general dentist is responsible for all of the issues discussed in the previous section. Although the problems with referral of the patient and communication between the providers are eliminated, the general dentist takes on a significantly higher level of responsibility and the importance of comprehensive record keeping and documentation becomes even more important.

Orthodontic Treatment Has Been Completed

If caries develop after the orthodontic treatment has been completed, the patient can be managed in much the same manner as the patient without orthodontic treatment. If the patient wears a removable retainer, it must be removed periodically (usually during waking hours) and both retainer and teeth must be kept meticulously clean. If the patient has a fixed orthodontic retainer that collects plaque and inhibits effective oral home care, it may be desirable or necessary to replace it with a removable retainer. If so, this procedure would be carried out by the orthodontic treatment provider. If the patient continues to be caries active even in the presence of the basic caries control protocol, it may be helpful to replace the existing retainer with a mouth guard designed to serve as both an orthodontic retainer and a reservoir for fluoride gel during sleep.

Reconsider Previously Declined Elective Treatment

At the original comprehensive examination, diagnosis and treatment planning visit or series the patient may have been offered one or more treatment options that for financial reasons, time constraints, competing life priorities, or other reasons, the patient declined. At the periodic visit those options can be revisited and reconsidered. This is an ideal time to allow the patient to ask questions and to explain in as much detail as the patient would like to hear, the options and their attendant risk/benefits/costs/contingencies/prognosis and expected outcomes.

Establish Continuing Care Interval and Plan

At the conclusion of the recall visit, the dental team will need to develop a plan for the next treatment and/or recall visit. Based on comprehensive knowledge of the patient's oral and general health, current state of disease activity, assessed risk of future disease, and the patient's particular expectations and concerns,

plans for the next visit are formulated via a consent discussion with the patient. The patient needs to be informed of the plan and any expectations that the dental team may have for the next visit(s). The patient must be given the opportunity to ask questions and confirm that they understand and agree with the proposed plan. The consent discussion and any expectations that the dental team may have for that visit are recorded in the patient record. An immediate restorative need will normally be addressed at an appointment in the near future. If there are no immediate treatment needs, specific items to be reassessed or addressed at the next recall visit are recorded.

Progress Note

Documentation of the periodic visit should be recorded in the progress notes in the patient record. The note should include the following information:

- General health status summary and record of the vital signs (confirm that patient has taken premedication if indicated).
- Summary of all positive, and significant negative, findings from the periodic examination.
- Diagnosis of all conditions that require recognition, management, or treatment.
- Description of all treatment rendered including local anesthetic, materials used, medicaments applied, prescriptions written, and oral homecare instructions given to the patient.
- Notation of the patient's response to treatment.
- A written plan for the next visit. If the next visit is for a restorative procedure, the note should include the tooth numbers, surfaces, the material and procedure planned, and evidence of patient consent. The time interval for the next maintenance visit should be specified. (See e-Fig12.1 for sample periodic visit progress note.)

Electronic patient records may include templates used for development of the progress notes. Various systems may have a skeleton outline, with narrative entries to be added. A template for such a system is illustrated in Box 12.2. An alternative approach is to have a rather complete and detailed narrative already included, with the provider filling in critical blanks with options from appropriate dropdown menus and editing the prepared text as appropriate.

DOCUMENTING THE MAINTENANCE PHASE PLAN

The maintenance phase can be recorded in the patient record in several different ways. The simplest and easiest way is to place it directly on the original treatment plan (see Box 12.3 for a Sample Maintenance Phase Plan of Care). Alternatively, maintenance phase needs can be listed in the progress notes. Although the latter method ensures that the information is included in the patient record, it may be difficult to locate since it will be superseded by new progress notes as they are continually added.

Another alternative is to generate an office-specific form for recording maintenance plans and treatment. This form can be designed to indicate what treatment is to be provided with the time interval for each activity. It can be made operator specific

BOX 12.2 Sample Template for Recall Visit Progress Note

- Patient concerns (and history):
- Health history update and considerations:
- Vital signs:
- Radiographic images (type of images and date):
- Extraoral exam findings:
- Intraoral exam findings:
- Findings from exam of teeth/ restorations/ prosthesis/ occlusion:
- Gingival and periodontal findings:
- Plaque index:
- Bleeding index:
- Oral homecare and prevention recommendations:
- Treatment rendered:
- Posttreatment instructions:
- Return to clinic (immediate treatment needs):
- Recare plan (recall interval; goals and expectations for next recall visit):

BOX 12.3 Sample Maintenance Phase Plan of Care

- Monitor Type 1 diabetes
- Reevaluate denture stomatitis associated with maxillary removable partial denture; confirm proper oral home care practice; prescribe antifungals as necessary
- Reassess tissue response to a bulky crown on the maxillary left second premolar; discuss patient need and/or desire for new crown
- Periodontal maintenance therapy at 3-month intervals; vertical bite-wings at 24 months; remove chlorhexidine stain
- Reevaluate caries activity:
- Repeat caries activity tests
- Confirm that patient has eliminated sugar-containing beverage habit
- In presence of new lesions or elevated *Streptococcus mutans* or *Lactobacillus* counts, fabricate custom fluoride trays and dispense fluoride gel for home use

(hygienist, dental assistant, or patient education specialist), with a means for recording completion dates, outcomes, and patient performance. Although somewhat more labor intensive because the entire staff participates, this method, if used regularly, becomes an excellent tool for educating the patient, setting goals for the maintenance phase, organizing preventive activities, and ensuring that the patient receives the highest quality continuous long-term care.

CONCLUSION

The maintenance phase of treatment establishes the platform for a mutually beneficial long-term relationship between the patient and the dental team. Benefits to the patient include the satisfaction of recognizing a partnership with the dentist and practice that is invested in the improvement of the patient's oral health for the long term; and the sense of confidence and trust that ongoing and future dental needs will be provided in a timely and efficient manner for as long as the patient remains in the practice. The maintenance phase is an essential part of the comprehensive care provided to each patient to support long-term stable and sustainable oral health.

IN CLINICAL PRACTICE

Tips for Developing an Effective Maintenance Care Program in Your Practice

- Create a mission statement for your practice maintenance program.
- Specify the component parts of the program and services to be performed.
- Develop standard documentation for each periodic visit and a plan for each subsequent visit, including the details of *what* will be done and when.
- Develop list of responsibilities and delegate responsibilites to specific team members.
- Formalize the program in an office manual.
- Periodically reevaluate the effectiveness of your system.

REVIEW QUESTIONS

- What are the benefits of a maintenance phase of care?
- What issues are typically addressed in the maintenance phase of care?
- What is a posttreatment assessment? What is its purpose? What are its elements?
- Which services are commonly provided to the patient at the periodic visit?

- How will you respond to a patient who declines having recommended radiographs?
- At the periodic visit what assessments are recommended, and what services are provided, for a patient who wears a removable complete or partial denture?

PRACTICE BUILDER

Develop a practice policy that covers all aspects of a periodic visit:

- What is to be done?
- What is the sequence of events?
- Who is responsible for each of the steps in the process?

- What information is communicated to the patient, and how?
- What arrangements will be made for follow-up or future care?
- How is the information to be recorded?
- Create a simple form that will be used in your practice to document each periodic visit. Include all items that should be evaluated, treated, and/or reassessed at future visits.

SUGGESTED RESOURCES

Bowen DM, Pieren JA. *Darby and Walsh Dental Hygiene Theory and Practice*. 5th ed. St Louis: Elsevier; 2019.

Wilkins EM. *Clinical Practice of the Dental Hygienist*. 12th ed. St Louis: Mosby; 2017.

REFERENCES

1. Ghaffari M, Rakhshanderou S, Ramezankhani A, Noroozi M, Armoon B. Oral health education and promotion programmes: meta-analysis of 17-year intervention. *Int J Dent Hyg*. 2018;16(1): 59–67.

2. Gambhir RS, Brar P, Singh G, Sofat A, Kakar H. Utilization of dental care: An Indian outlook. *J Nat Sci Biol Med*. 2013;4(2):292–297.

3. Sen S, Giamberardino LD, Moss K, et al. Periodontal disease, regular dental care use, and incident ischemic stroke. *Stroke*. 2018; 49(2):355–362.

4. Sharma P, Cockwell P, Dietrich T, Ferro C, Ives N, Chapple ILC. INfluence of Successful Periodontal Intervention in REnal Disease (INSPIRED): study protocol for a randomised controlled. *Trials*. 2017;18(1):535.

5. Vargas CM, Arevalo O. How dental care can preserve and improve oral health. *Dent Clin North Am*. 2009;53(3):399–420.

6. O'Hehir TE. Is the six-month recall a realistic interval of care? *RDH*. 1993;13(10):18.

7. Tomar SL. There is weak evidence that a single, universal dental recall interval schedule reduces caries incidence. *J Evid Base Dent Pract*. 2011;11:89–91.

8. Patel S, Bay RC, Glick M. A systematic review of dental recall intervals and incidence of dental caries. *JADA*. 2010;141(5): 527–539.

9. Riley P1, Worthington HV, Clarkson JE, Beirne PV. Recall intervals for oral health in primary care patients. *Cochrane Database Syst Rev*. 2013;12 CD004346.

10. Listgarten MA, Schifter CC, Laster L. 3-year longitudinal study of the periodontal status of an adult population with gingivitis. *J Clin Periodontol*. 1985;12(3):225–238.

11. Löe H, Anerud A, Boysen H, Morrison E. Natural history of periodontal disease in man. Rapid, moderate and no loss of attachment in Sri Lankan laborers 14 to 46 years of age. *J Clin Periodontol*. 1986;13(5):431–445.

12. Axelsson P, Lindhe J. Effect of controlled oral hygiene procedures on caries and periodontal disease in adults. *J Clin Periodontol*. 1978;5(2):133–151.

13. Axelsson P, Lindhe J. The significance of maintenance care in the treatment of periodontal disease. *J Clin Periodontol*. 1981;8(4):281–294.

14. Axelsson P, Lindhe J. Effect of controlled oral hygiene procedures on caries and periodontal disease in adults. Results after 6 years. *J Clin Periodontol*. 1981;8(3):239–248.

15. Axelsson P, Nystrom B, Lindhe J. The long-term effect of a plaque control program on tooth mortality, caries and periodontal disease in adults. Results after 30 years of maintenance. *J Clin Periodontol*. 2004;31(9):749–757.

16. Knowles JW, Burgett FG, Nissle RR, et al. Results of periodontal treatment related to pocket depth and attachment level. Eight years. *J Periodontol*. 1979;50(5):225–233.

17. Ramfjord SP, Morrison EC, Burgett FG, et al. Oral hygiene and maintenance of periodontal support. *J Periodontol*. 1982;53(1): 26–30.

18. Suomi JD, Greene JC, Vermillion JR, et al. The effect of controlled oral hygiene procedures on the progression of periodontal disease in adults: results after third and final year. *J Periodontol*. 1971;42(3):152–160.

19. Shick RA. Maintenance phase of periodontal therapy. *J Periodontol*. 1981;52(9):576–583.

20. Wilson Jr TG, Glover ME, Schoen J. Compliance with maintenance therapy in a private periodontal practice. *J Periodontol*. 1984;55(8):468–473.

21. Lindhe J, Nyman S. The effect of plaque control and surgical pocket elimination on the establishment and maintenance of periodontal health. A longitudinal study of periodontal therapy in cases of advanced disease. *J Clin Periodontol*. 1975;2(2):67–79.

22. Lindhe J, Nyman S. Long-term maintenance of patients treated for advanced periodontal disease. *J Clin Periodontol*. 1984;11(8):504–514.

23. Monje A, Aranda L, Diaz KT, et al. Impact of Maintenance Therapy for the Prevention of Peri-implant Diseases: A Systematic Review and Meta-analysis. *J Dent Res*. 2016;95(4):372–379.

24. Beirne PV, Clarkson JE, Worthington HV. Recall intervals for oral health in primary care patients. *Cochrane Database Syst Rev*. 2007;17(4). CD004346.

25. Clarkson JE, Amaechi BT, Ngo H, Bonetti D. Recall, reassessment and monitoring. In Pitts N. Detection, Assessment, Diagnosis and Monitoring of Caries. *Monogr Oral Sci*. 2009;21:188–198.

26. Jenson L, Budenz AW, Featherstone JD, Ramos-Gomez FJ, Spolsky VW, Young DA. Clinical protocols for caries management by risk assessment. *J Calif Dent Assoc*. 2007;35(10):714–723.

27. National Health Service, National Institute for Clinical Excellence Guideline *Dental recall: Recall interval between routine dental examinations*. London: NICE; 2004.

28. American Dental Association, Council on Scientific Affairs; US Department of Health and Human Services, Public Health Service, Food and Drug Administration. Dental radiographic examinations: recommendations for patient selection and limiting radiation exposure. http://www.ada.org/sections/professionalResources/pdfs/Dental_Radiographic_Examinations_2012.pdf.

29. American Dental Association Council on Scientific Affairs The use of dental radiographs: Update and recommendations. *JADA*. 2006;137:1304–1312.

30. Johnson KB, Ludlow JB. Intraoral radiographs: A comparison of dose and risk reduction with collimation and thyroid shielding. *JADA*. 2020;151:726–734.

31. Brent R. Pregnancy and radiation exposure. https://hps.org/hpspublications/articles/pregnancyandradiationexposureinfosheet.html.

32. Louropoulou A, Slot DE, Van der Weijden FA. Titanium surface alterations following use of different mechanical instruments: a systematic review. *Clin Oral Implants Res*. 2012;23(6):643–658.

33. Wheelis SE, Gindri IM, Valderrama P, Wilson Jr TG, Huang J, Rodrigues DC. Effects of decontamination solutions on the surface of titanium: investigation of surface morphology, composition, and roughness. *Clin Oral Implants Res*. 2016;27(3):329–340.

Planning Treatment for Unique Populations

13

Patients With Special Needs

Allen Samuelson and Christine Downey

 Visit eBooks.Health.Elsevier.com

OUTLINE

This chapter introduces Section IV of *Diagnosis and Treatment Planning in Dentistry*. The scope of this chapter is intentionally broad and will address the diagnosis, treatment planning, and management of a wide range of patient conditions that can be considered to reflect special needs.

The management of several important selected clinical needs is discussed in greater detail later in this text. Treatment planning for the substance-abusing individual, the anxious or phobic patient, patients with psychological problems, adolescents, older adults and patients who are motivationally compromised or financially limited is addressed in the other chapters of this section. This chapter serves as an overview and introduction to those chapters and, in addition, discusses a variety of special needs conditions not specifically addressed elsewhere in the book.

The U.S. government defines persons with disabilities as individuals with a physical or mental impairment that substantially limits one or more major activities of daily living (ADL). Census 2010 identified 85.3 million individuals in the United States with some type of long-lasting condition or disability. In developed countries, the elderly who are commonly included within the population of special needs patients, constitute an increasingly large component of the population. It is now estimated that almost 21% of the US population will be older than 60 years by 2030.[1,2]

This group is prone to health problems in general and to oral health problems in particular. Patients with disabilities, especially frail elderly patients frequently reside in assisted living facilities. In 2019 the Communicable Disease Center (CDC) reported that the United States had approximately 15,600 nursing homes with 1.7 million licensed beds and 1.4 million patients.[3] Moreover, with the growing numbers of older adults worldwide, nursing homes will be expected to provide residence and care for a significant portion of this population.

A strong relationship between disability status and oral health status has been identified.[4-10] Individuals with special needs are more likely to exhibit gingivitis or periodontitis and to have poor oral hygiene. Improvement of oral health in individuals with special needs can lead to improved quality of life. Unfortunately, however, many of these individuals have limited access to oral healthcare, and their oral health needs remain unmet.[11-15]

Patients with special needs may provide the dental team with unusual and interesting challenges in both planning and delivering dental treatment. Treatment modifications may range from slight (e.g., giving the patient more time to communicate or providing physical support in the dental chair) to complex (providing treatment for a patient who is bedridden and requires full-time skilled nursing care). The range of oral health services runs the gamut from simple pain relief to complete oral rehabilitation. All patients seek high-quality treatment delivered with compassion, integrity, and safety, and the patient with special needs is no different. These patients will often be unusually appreciative of the time and effort that the dental team invests in their care.

The stated goal of special care dentistry is "to improve the oral health of individuals and groups in society who have a physical, sensory, intellectual, mental, medical, emotional, social impairment or disability, or, more often, a combination of a number of these factors."[16] The process of achieving that goal can be challenging, but it also presents unique opportunities and inestimable rewards for all the members of the dental team. The mission of the authors of this chapter is to help the reader develop both the skill set and comfort level to diagnose the problems of such a patient, devise a treatment plan that promotes oral and general health within the limits of the patient's circumstances and temperament, and deliver treatment in a manner that is safe, effective, compassionate, and affirming of the patient's sense of self (Box 13.1).

> ### BOX 13.2 Factors that Promote Optimal Oral Health
>
> 1. Limited or adapted medical burden
> 2. In-tact or adapted physical capacity
> 3. In-tact or adapted* cognitive capacity (*adaptation can be achieved through a caregiver)
> 4. In-tact or adapted psychological capacity
> 5. In-tact social support system/SES/Access to Care
> 6. The will to comply/learn/grow and fit oral health into daily health routine
> 7. In-tact or mitigated salivary integrity
> 8. Patient engagement in an oral health-promoting diet – carbohydrate discipline
> 9. Exposure to fluoride/recaldent/etc.
> 10. Engages in effective oral hygiene - awareness, ability and technique
> 11. Habit Cessation – tobacco, illicit drugs, alcohol etc
> 12. Minimally restored dentition
> 13. Attends to periodic dental evaluations.

Most of these patients can be managed very successfully within the context of a general dentistry practice. Armed with this knowledge and with a willingness to try, providing care can be a rewarding opportunity for the dentist, and in some instances, a life-changing experience for the patient.

There are various ways that oral health and the function of the stomatognathic complex is protected and preserved in a given patient. The oral health practitioner and the health care team should be cognizant of these issues and how the presence or absence of each may impact on the oral health status and functioning of the patient (Box 13.2).

A patient with special care needs will commonly have challenges in many of these areas. Some of the issues listed above may be mitigated or naturally improve over time; others will not. In any case, is incumbent on the oral health care team to identify and fully explain these challenges to the patient and/or caregivers. Failure to do so may allow the patient, family or caregivers to harbor unrealistic expectations about the outcomes of treatment or the difficulties that will be encountered in the treatment process, and to lose confidence in the oral health care team. These conversations need to be clearly documented in the patient record and periodically recapitulated.

IDENTIFYING THE PATIENT WITH SPECIAL NEEDS

The distinction between the patient designated as "special care" or "special needs" and the more typical dental patient who may need small accommodations to be comfortable or to facilitate efficient treatment may sometimes seem indistinct. Indeed, all patients deserve individualized compassionate and, in a manner of speaking, "special care." Every patient has the right to be treated as a unique individual by the dental team. This may be manifested in small but significant ways, such as addressing the patient in a preferred manner, or using a mouth prop to reduce strain on a sensitive temporomandibular joint (TMJ).

> ### BOX 13.1 Treatment Planning Principles for the Special Needs Patient
>
> Dignity – All patients regardless of any background or disability deserve the Hippocratic ideal of dignity
>
> Safety – Patients rightfully expect and deserve a safe, clean, cordial environment that considers their health in all things.
>
> Comfort – Is the patient in pain? All oral health professionals should work toward having the patient as pain free from oral disease as possible.
>
> Function – What is their level of function? This is critical to ascertain as a baseline and this helps shape and define the nature and scope of the treatment.
>
> Health – What are their habits? Can we get the patient engaged in health? What is their preventive trajectory and prognosis for improvement (when improvement is called for)?
>
> Esthetics – Are their goals and desires realistic given their preventive trajectory?

The patient with special needs, although typically seeking the same types of services and therapy, will require an even more intentional, strategic, and individualized approach to care. *Broadly speaking, patients with special clinical needs are those patients who live with significant mental, physical, psychological, or medical challenges and who, as a result, require significant modifications to treatment planning and delivery of oral healthcare.* The following list of physical or mental conditions can be categorized as "special care" or "special needs":

- Autism
- Mentally Handicapped (e.g. Down syndrome)
- Traumatic brain injury
- Cerebral palsy
- Mental illnesses (psychoses or neuroses of various diagnoses)
- Medically compromised conditions (e.g., congestive heart failure, unstable angina, cancer, transplant, human immunodeficiency virus [HIV]-acquired immunodeficiency syndrome [AIDS])
- Severe dental anxiety or phobia
- Craniofacial abnormalities (craniofacial syndromes, Cleft lip and palate)
- Certain congenital illnesses (e.g., hemophilia, sickle cell anemia)
- Various dementias (Alzheimer, Parkinson diseases, multi-infarct dementia)
- Severe depression or pseudodementia
- Physical disability, such as severe rheumatoid arthritis or developmental diagnoses

Patients with special needs may require modifications in both the kind and scope of dental treatment. Certainly, specific physical, medical, psychological, or psychosocial problems will have a bearing on the kinds of modifications to the dental treatment plan that will be necessary. Equally important, the *severity* of the disorder will have an effect on what the necessary modifications will be. For example, an individual with mild autism who can cooperate during restorative procedures and is responsive to preventive therapy may be treated with minimal or no modification to treatment. At the other extreme, a patient in the late stages of Alzheimer's disease is a poor candidate for anything beyond basic preventive and acute care services.

ROLE OF THE GENERAL DENTIST IN MANAGEMENT OF THE PATIENT WITH SPECIAL NEEDS

Recognizing, managing, and treating all oral healthcare problems presented by individuals with special needs is within the scope of general dentistry. The general dentist has several roles to play in the management of the patient with special needs:

- Recognize that a patient *has* special needs.
- Perform an initial oral examination, making adjustments to the process as appropriate. as well as documenting why these adjustments were made.
- Consult with other oral healthcare providers as needed regarding the patient's condition and treatment.

- Referral to a hospital dentistry unit or an academic health center when indicated.
- Generate a plan of care for the patient, the complexity of which will depend on multiple factors, including (1) patient's dental needs, (2) anticipated level of cooperation, (3) patient's ability to carry out effective oral self-care, (4) availability and extent of support from a caregiver, and (5) the patient's preventive trajectory.
- Engage the patient, and surrogates as indicated, to achieve informed consent.
- Educate the patient and caregivers in the importance of oral health and its relationship to systemic health; work with them to establish a daily oral care program.
- Educate the patient and caregivers about realistic expectations and prognosis based upon the patient's level of cooperation and preventive trajectory.
- Execute the plan of care in a compassionate and professional manner.
- Provide long-term maintenance care.
- Engage and encourage the participation and support of caregivers during all steps of the therapeutic process: examination, treatment plan formulation, active treatment, and maintenance therapy.
- Document your assessment of the patients preventive trajectory, level of cooperation and coordination; and how those considerations will impact on the prognosis and scope of care.
- Respond to physician's requests regarding the following:
  - Oral health assessment
  - Clearance before medical surgery
  - Management or treatment of oral infections or other oral health problems

The dental team has the responsibility to help the patient with special needs maintain a functional, healthy oral condition. For such patients, this can necessitate considerable time, effort, and creativity. The ultimate goal is to help the patient achieve an optimal state of oral health consistent with what his or her mental and physical condition will permit.

ACCESS TO CARE

Access to care is an important issue in the management of the patient with special needs. If the patient is homebound, can dental services be brought to that location? If the patient is living independently, does he or she have transportation to the dental office? Once brought to the dental office, are environmental modifications in place to accommodate his or her needs? If the patient lives in a residential facility, can dental services be provided on site, or should the patient be brought to the dental office? Four components of the access to care issue are considered in this section.

Transportation

Many modes of transportation can be used to bring a patient to a dental appointment, including personal conveyance, public transportation (bus or taxi), ambulance, or van (sponsored by social services, government, transit authority, or private enterprise). Often a personal friend or relative will offer to bring the patient in the patient's or the friend's or relative's own vehicle. The mode of transportation may have an effect on the appointment scheduling for a patient. For instance, the dentist may try to provide more treatment or an extended appointment time for an individual conveyed by ambulance.

Residency

Many patients with special needs live in facilities other than a private home, apartment, or condominium. Such facilities include rest homes, nursing homes, and continuing care retirement centers. Several approaches to delivering dental care to these individuals are available.

- **In-house dental unit**. The facility may have a fully equipped dedicated dental operatory permanently on site or may share a room equipped for dental care that is also used at other times by a hair stylist or podiatrist.
- **Comprehensive mobile dental operatory**. This can be a complete dental operatory with all the amenities, including a full-sized dental unit with wheels built into the chair base. All equipment, materials, and supplies are packaged and transported by truck. Typically, the mobile operatory is delivered to the facility and set up to be fully operational on the same day. This format allows the dentist to provide a complete range of oral healthcare services on site.
- **Portable units**. Portable dental units are easily transportable "fold-up" units stored in cases/containers and assembled on site by the dental team. These self-contained units typically include their own sources of water, suction, and compressed air. If electricity is not available, a portable generator can provide power. Designed primarily to serve in the mission field or at temporary military installations, this type of setup is adaptable to a wide variety of settings. Although in theory, a full range of services can be provided, the limited suction and air capacity, less ergonomic chair, and lack of many of the comforts and amenities of a fixed base setting make it difficult for the dentist and staff to carry out extended or complex procedures day after day.
- **Vans or buses with dental facilities on board**. In this type of installation, a complete dental operatory with dental chair, x-ray head, sources for compressed air and suction, and a complete array of dental equipment, instruments, and supplies is housed and ready for use in a fully functioning van or bus. Using this mode of operation, the dental team drives to a convenient parking area, hooks up to an existing electrical and water supply, if available, and is prepared to see patients who need only to be brought to the van to receive dental treatment.
- **Delivery to the dental office**. In some cases, patients living in nursing homes or continuing care facilities are transported to a dental care facility. Often it is a caregiver, family member, or friend who brings the patient in, or it may also be someone on the dental team.

Additional information on alternative modes of care delivery is provided in Chapter 18.

BOX 13.3 Suggested Environmental Features to Accommodate Patients With Special Needs

- Handicapped parking clearly marked
- Ramps for wheelchair access
- Automatic doors (wide enough for wheelchair or gurney)
- Reception window accessible from a wheelchair
- Handicapped-accessible restrooms (automatic doors)
- Operatory door wide enough for wheelchairs or gurney*
- Operatory size large enough to accommodate wheelchair, gurney,* staff, and dental equipment
- Extended tubing length on the dental unit
- Control of noise

*Higher-level accommodations that may not be practical or possible to retrofit in an existing office.

Some of the options described previously (portable units, dental van or bus, delivery to the dental office) can be implemented for the home-bound patient. In addition, the dental team may provide in-home rudimentary dental services, as described in Chapter 18.

Office Accommodations

If the dental team elects to treat special needs patients in the dental office, the facility must be properly designed and equipped to deliver care in a manner that is comfortable and safe for the patient, and efficient for the dental team (Box 13.3). (See Video 13.1, Tour of an Operatory for Special Needs Patients on ebooks+.)

American dental offices must comply with standards established in the Americans with Disabilities Act. Some state and local jurisdictions may also have laws or ordinances that are relevant. The dentist who anticipates seeing patients with disabilities should consult the document "Americans with Disability Act Standards for Accessible Design".[17]

Funding Sources

As with all other patients, the dental team must establish with the patient and/or caregiver how dental treatment will be paid for. Several potential funding sources can be considered.

Private Pay

Many special care patients have their own or family financial resources with which to pay for oral health services. If a designated power of attorney or legal guardian has taken over financial responsibilities, costs of treatment and financial resources will be discussed with this individual.

Medicare[18,19]

In the United States, Medicare is a health insurance program for persons 65 years or older, some individuals with disabilities who are younger than age 65, and individuals with end-stage renal disease requiring dialysis or renal transplant. There are strict limitations as to the types of dental treatment covered by Medicare, however. For example, Medicare does not cover routine dental treatment, such as cleanings, restorative treatment, dentures, or extractions. However, Medicare Part A (hospital insurance) will pay for certain dental procedures performed while a patient is in the hospital. As of 2020, Medicare will pay for the following:

1. Comprehensive examination in a hospital inpatient setting preceding kidney transplantation or heart valve replacement.
2. Extractions in preparation for radiation treatment for oral cancer. (The patient is responsible for the cost of any prosthetics, however.)
3. Dental services that are an integral part of a medical procedure, such as reconstruction of the jaw after an accident or facial tumor removal.

It is important to note that, according to cms.gov, coverage of dental care is not determined by the necessity of the dental care but by the type of service provided and the anatomic structure involved in the procedure. Therefore it is important to verify with Medicare which dental procedures are covered before initiation of treatment.

Medicaid

In the United States, Medicaid is the federally sponsored, state and/or county-administered insurance program for blind, disabled, and indigent individuals. Medicaid dental coverage for both adults and children varies from state to state. For the patient to benefit from this form of assistance, the dental team must be knowledgeable about and comply with all the rules and restrictions, as well as with the fee schedule for the Medicaid plan in the patient's jurisdiction.

Other Sources

Other possible sources of financial support for the special care patient in the United States include Supplemental Security Income (SSI), pensions, and religious or other nonprofit groups. Social workers and case managers are well trained in optimizing federal, state, and community-based resources for clients under their care.

Throughout the world, there is great variability in the level of governmental support for oral healthcare. Western European countries have traditionally placed a high priority on the provision of basic dental services both to their general population and to special needs populations, such as the elderly, infirmed, and impaired. Programs and benefits are determined for the most part by national policy.

PLANNING FOR SPECIFIC CONDITIONS

As noted earlier in this chapter, many conditions can be appropriately designated as "special needs." The following paragraphs discuss briefly six relatively common special needs conditions that are not addressed in depth elsewhere in this text.

Patients With Developmental Delay or Cognitive Disorders

At the outset, the patient's level of cooperation must be diagnosed to help the dental team determine which treatments can

be performed and in what setting. Prevention is of paramount importance. Oral home care coaching and dietary analysis and counseling are extremely important. The caregiver must be heavily involved in providing the patient's oral home care and maintenance of the patient's oral health. If the patient is fully cooperative, routine dental care can be provided in the office setting. If the patient is combative or uncooperative, however, the decision needs to be made as to the setting where care will be provided. Alteration or modification of the treatment goals from the ideal is often necessary. If a complete examination, radiographs, and treatment are necessary, then general anesthesia is usually indicated. When the patient is partially cooperative, the decision becomes more difficult. If the patient is not both clinically and legally competent, then treatment goals, risks, benefits, and limitations of each mode of treatment must be explained fully to the caregiver. Often times, an initial attempt to accomplish care in the office setting will provide a sound basis for determining whether treatment in a hospital or other setting is appropriate or necessary.

Traumatic Brain Injury

Patients with a history of traumatic brain injury may be treated similarly to individuals with cognitive disorders. The level of potential cooperation must be assessed as noted previously. Similar decisions regarding setting and extent of treatment will be made for patients with head injuries. It must be recognized, however, that the functionality of the patient with traumatic brain injury can change dramatically over time. The patient may progress from an uncooperative, combative individual to one who is fully cooperative. The dental treatment plan can be changed, sometimes drastically, with changes in the patient's physical ability and cognitive function. Although initially, dental treatment may be limited to palliative and acute care, with full recovery, the patient may become an ideal candidate for comprehensive definitive treatment. From the time of the injury and throughout the recovery phase, the caregivers often must be intensely involved in providing for the general and oral healthcare needs of these patients.

Severe Coagulopathies

Hemophilia A and B and von Willebrand's disease are three well-known congenital coagulopathies requiring specific management plans. If invasive therapy is anticipated (including mandibular blocks), then factor replacement is generally necessary. Postoperatively, an antifibrinolytic agent (e.g. tranexamic acid) may be prescribed to assist in stabilizing the initial clot. There are instances of hemophiliacs with inhibitor to the very factor they require for coagulation. For example, the hemophilia A patient with inhibitor will exhibit an immune response to the administered factor and will thus require a continuous infusion to clot properly. Discussion with the patient's hematologist, describing the nature of planned dental procedures, should take place before dental treatment. These patients often require infusion of coagulation factor or by-pass agents (e.g. factor VIIa for Classic Hemophilia with inhibitor) before and after dental procedures.

Additionally, several anticoagulant medications that are frequently prescribed to prevent thrombi, strokes, coronary artery occlusions, and/or myocardial infarctions may have implications for the provision of some dental procedures. For patients on Coumadin, a current international normalized ratio (INR) value (preferable to a prothrombin time) is an important preoperative measure. The INR provides a standard measure of coagulability. However, the patient who requires oral surgery or any dental treatment likely to cause bleeding (including uncomplicated tooth extractions) typically does not require alteration of Coumadin dosage unless the individual's INR is greater than 3.0-3.5, provided that local hemostatic measures such as Gel foam® and suture closure are used.

Other oral anticoagulants, such as antiplatelet medications (e.g., dipyridamole, ticlopidine, aspirin, ibuprofen), direct thrombin inhibitors (dabigatran etexilate), or factor Xa inhibitors (rivaroxaban, apixaban, edoxaban, betrixaban, darexaban, eribaxaban, and idrabiotaparinux) may need to be discontinued or dosages decreased before surgery depending on anticipated blood loss and extent of the planned surgery. Discussion with the patient's physician, including a thorough explanation of the planned dental procedure, should take place before invasive dental treatment. Furthermore, risks and benefits of discontinuing or decreasing the dosage of these medications should be discussed. Often, discontinuance is not necessary if appointments are planned conservatively and staged in a safe manner.

Acquired Immunodeficiency Syndrome

The dental team must be vigilant in recognition of the occurrence or progression of the oral manifestations of HIV/AIDS, including Kaposi's sarcoma, candidiasis, oral hairy leukoplakia, HIV-associated periodontal diseases, or other opportunistic infections. Good oral health and hygiene instruction and oral home care are critical to managing the oral health of the patient with AIDS. If invasive treatment is planned, a complete blood count (CBC) must be evaluated. The platelet count should be at least 50,000, and the absolute neutrophil count should be higher than 1000. If the absolute neutrophil count is lower than 1000, antibiotic premedication should be considered. Physician consultation is advisable when invasive treatment is planned. Viral load and CD4 counts are indicators as to the level of control of the illness.

Patients Under Hospice Care

By definition, the patient in hospice care has an anticipated life expectancy of 6 months or less. Frequently, it is much less than 6 months, because hospice care is often called late in the disease process. Palliative care and pain control are of great importance. If invasive treatment is planned, depending on the diagnosis, a thorough review of the medical record is necessary. Any patient-requested dental treatment that is not life threatening should be provided if feasible. For example, if the patient desires a reconstruction, and the dental team is capable of providing this care, then it is justifiable to proceed. Informed consent must be obtained, listing diagnoses, alternatives, and costs. Code status should be designated (e.g., Do Not Resuscitate/Do Not Intubate/Full Code). [see the *In Clinical Practice: Physician*

Orders Related to Resuscitation box later in this chapter]). Occasionally, the dental team may be called on to evaluate a patient who is losing weight because of a refusal to eat. In this situation, it is appropriate for the dentist to do a limited evaluation to discern whether the refusal to eat results from oral pain or, for example, an ill-fitting denture. Here, a comprehensive assessment may not be necessary, and the dental treatment can be limited to strategic efforts to alleviate the pain or improve the functionality of the denture. An oral health care consultation also provides the dentist an opportunity to rule out oral diagnoses as the cause for systemic concerns such as fever or weight loss.

PATIENT EVALUATION

Ideally, the patient with special needs will be identified at the time of the initial appointment through a matter-of-fact query by office staff: "Do you have any physical or other limitations that we can assist you with on your arrival?" If the patient answers affirmatively, he or she should first of all be assured of a welcome to the practice and that any necessary effort to provide accommodation will be made. The patient should be asked to bring any available medical records and names and contact information for other healthcare providers; a list of all medications; and any available dental images or records. An effort should be made to determine whether the patient has a guardian or caregiver. If such a person has been designated, that person should be invited to attend at least the initial visit. Some dental offices find it useful to develop a specific form or questionnaire for such patients that will characterize any special needs and individual expectations. On arrival, the patient should be greeted warmly and given an explanation of what to expect at this first visit. If the patient has brought any documentation, forms, questionnaires, or images, these should be received, recorded, and copied, and returned to the patient or caregiver as appropriate. If a caregiver or family member accompanies the patient, he or she should be recognized and thanked for assistance in providing care for the patient.

After introductions, the patient is escorted to the operatory, and the examination process begins. The patient may be more comfortable if the caregiver or family member is also present during the examination, and that should be encouraged. A patient with special care requirements is evaluated with the same basic approach as described in Chapter 1 of this text. Although an initial attempt should be made to complete a typical examination, depending on the level of the patient's ability to cooperate, parts of the examination may not be completed effectively. Strategies for managing such a situation will be described later in section, *Physical and Oral Examination*.

Initially, the patient may have difficulty becoming acclimated to the new and strange surroundings. The dental team must be flexible and accepting of the patient's behavior and limitations. As the team converses and interacts with the patient in a kind, gentle, and caring manner, the patient will often lower defenses and anxiety will abate. The patient may become sufficiently comfortable to allow at least a brief look, a moderately complete examination or, in a best-case scenario, a complete oral examination. If the examination is not completed at the initial visit, the dentist (in consultation with the caregiver) may reappoint the patient, with the goal of completing the examination at a future date when the patient is less stressed and more comfortable with the dental office setting. If the patient is physically unable or mentally incapable of cooperating for a comprehensive evaluation, some form of anxiolysis, sedation or general anesthesia may be necessary.

Chief Concern and History of the Chief Concern

To properly address specific needs that the patient or the caregiver perceives to be important, it is critical to evaluate the patient's chief complaints or concerns. Characterization of the chief concern often gives the dentist a sense of the patient's or caregiver's oral health philosophy and knowledge. If the patient is unable to articulate his or her wishes and concerns, the chief complaint can be derived from a variety of other sources, including family members, physician, caregiver, social worker, or case manager. If the dentist believes that addressing the chief concern is unrealistic or unreasonable, then the issues involved must be explained to the patient and caregivers or other individuals who may be involved in the decision making. For example, if the family of an individual with dementia desires complex restorative treatment, but the patient appears uncooperative and lacking in the capacity for preventive care, then the family must be informed as to why this option cannot be implemented. Addressing the chief concern is often the starting place for identification of issues central to the ultimate management of the patient and will provide a touchstone from which to begin the education of the patient and caregivers.

General Health History and Review of Systems

Although important as a baseline of information for all patients, obtaining a thorough and complete health history for the special care patient can be of life-preserving significance. Answers to questions regarding hospitalizations, major illnesses, surgical procedures and complications, medications, and allergies are essential if the patient is to be treated safely and effectively. Because of the complex physical status of many of these patients, an exclusive use of only a standard health history form with close-ended questions will generally be inadequate.[20] Instead, an open-format mode of questioning, or a questionnaire supplemented with follow-up questions, is frequently necessary to provide a complete history. In addition to the patient interview, the history can be taken from a variety of other sources, including family members, caregivers, nurses, physicians, case managers, and the patient's medical records.

The phrasing of questions must be consistent with the patient's level of understanding and education. Layperson's terms and colloquialisms can appropriately be used to take a good history. Even with this open format, however, it is imperative that the dentist use a standardized and consistent "branching-tree" series of questions (Box 13.4).

The **review of systems (ROS)**, an integral part of the health history, consists of a sequential series of questions about each organ system. Inherent in this process are checks and balances that prompt the patient to remember aspects of his or her history

> ### BOX 13.4 Example of a "Branching-Tree" Questioning Process
>
> The branching-tree questioning process refers to a method in which, after an affirmative response to a general question, more-specific questions are asked to ascertain the dimensions of a particular condition, problem, or concern. For example, if the patient gives an affirmative answer to the question, "Do you suffer from angina pectoris?" the following questions are commonly asked:
> - What is the frequency of the pain?
> - When does the pain typically occur? (after meals, related to exertion, specific time of day)
> - What is the duration of the pain?
> - What is the character of the pain (sharp/dull/crushing)
> - What is the severity of the pain? (mild/moderate/severe/intolerable)
> - What exacerbates the pain? (exercise, position, or posture)
> - What alleviates the pain? (rest, nitroglycerin)
> - Does the pain radiate? If yes, where?
> - Do you take antianginal mediation? (frequency, amount)
> - Have you visited an emergency room for this condition? (frequency, treatment received)

> ### BOX 13.5 Common Issues Included in a Review of Systems
>
> Head, Eyes, Ears, Nose, Throat—hearing, vision, glaucoma, sinus/allergies, mouth ulcers, oral cancer
> Neurologic—strokes, seizures, trauma, lightheadedness, Parkinson's disease
> Neck—arthritis (spondylitis), trauma, subluxation, mobility, masses
> Cardiovascular—myocardial infarction, angina pectoris, valvular disorders/murmurs (nature of, how diagnosed), atherosclerosis, hypertension, peripheral vascular disease
> Pulmonary—tuberculosis exposure, asthma, smoking, emphysema, bronchitis
> Gastrointestinal—polyps, ulcers, reflux, indigestion, liver/gallbladder disorders
> Genitourinary—kidney/bladder disorders, incontinence, renal failure (dialysis and type)
> Endocrine—adrenal gland, diabetes, thyroid disorders, pituitary
> Hematologic—bleeding disorders, clotting problems, anemia (type)
> Musculoskeletal—weaknesses, prosthetic joints, arthritis
> Other—cancer, chemotherapy, radiation, metabolic disorders (for head and neck cancer, need dosages and portals of radiation, history of hyperbaric oxygen)

that may have been missed in the questionnaire or in previously discussed sections of the history. Key topics to be listed in a typical review of systems are included in Box 13.5.

Oral Health History

Many questions on the oral health history are the same as for all patients (for example, frequency of check-ups and oral prophylaxis), but there are additional questions that have particular relevance and importance for the patient with special care requirements. It will be helpful to learn the setting for past dental care (i.e., general dental office, hospital-based clinic, operating room [OR], or other). Did the patient receive sedation or general anesthesia? It is also important to learn what type of specialty care the individual has received and the nature of the treatment. The dentist should inquire about each of the dental specialties in an effort to gain a comprehensive understanding of the patient's dental experience. The patient's specific daily oral care regimen should be ascertained. It may be necessary to ask caregivers to describe their routines for cleaning the patient's mouth. In fact, it is important to determine whether the patient's mouth *can* be cleaned, and whether he or she is cooperative with such care. Important questions to be asked of the patient or caregiver include the following:

- How often do you brush your teeth? What times during the day? How much time do you spend brushing? Do you use a mechanical or a manual toothbrush? What type of toothpaste do you use?
- Do you clean in between your teeth? How often and when? What, specifically do you use?
- Do you use other cleaning devices?
- Do you use mouth rinses? Gels? Other forms of fluoride?
- Do you have plaque or tartar buildup?

Caregivers should be asked whether a mouth prop is needed when assisting the patient with oral home care.

Also included in this section of the patient history is a dietary analysis. The patient or caregiver should be questioned about the following:

- How much table sugar do you use?
- Do you consume soft drinks, sweetened beverages (e.g.tea) or sodas? If so, how often? With meals? How quickly consumed (sip or gulp)?
- Do you consume two or more fruit drinks or juice per day?
- Do you eat hard candy or other sweets including cough drops? If so, what type? How often?
- Do you ingest acidic foods or beverages (such as citrus fruits, artificially sweetened soft drink or soda, sports drinks, energy drinks, hot sauce or other vinegar based condiments) on a regular basis (especially between meals)?
- How often do you consume snacks or baked goods?

An understanding of the nutritional intake and dietary history is important for any patient but can be critical for the patient with special needs. Sugary "comfort foods" may be readily available and more appealing than healthier foods. Caregivers may use such foods to pacify their patients and reduce the required caregiving time or lessen caregiver stress. Especially when coupled with poor oral home care, such patients will often be afflicted with many active carious lesions and be at high risk for new caries development.

It is critically important to educate patients and caregivers about the hazards of a cariogenic diet (carbohydrate discipline) and suboptimal oral home care.

Patients who are deemed to be at high risk for caries are good candidates for the use of a diet diary. Patients with active caries, for whom the cause of the dental caries is not clearly evident, can definitely benefit from the compilation of a comprehensive diet history. The diet diary can be used to identify hidden and overt sugar and acid sources and can serve as the basis for counseling relating to dietary habits and those food items detrimental to dental and oral health. The patient is usually instructed to keep a diet diary for 5 to 7 days, writing down *all* food items and beverages consumed (Box 13.6).

When the patient returns to the office, a member of the team reviews the diary in detail with the patient and caregiver when appropriate. It is often helpful to circle those food items harmful to the patient's teeth. Dietary recommendations are then made

> ### BOX 13.6   Example of a Single Day From a Patient's Diet Diary
>
> **Breakfast**
> Sugared cereal
> Toast and grape jam
> 2 glasses of OJ
> Cup of coffee with tablespoon of sugar and milk
>
> **Lunch**
> Meatloaf
> Black beans
> Fruit cup
> Bread and butter
> Candy bar
> 1 regular soda
>
> **Dinner**
> Hunan chicken and vegetables
> Fried rice
> Pecan pie
> Fruit Loops and milk (during evening)

> ### BOX 13.7   Dietary Tips for Special Needs Patients and Their Caregivers
>
> - Limit consumption of refined sugars, especially between meals. Drinks such as pure fruit juice and fruit drinks, milk, and dietary supplements often contain large amounts of fermentable carbohydrates and can cause cavities— particularly in the absence of good plaque control.
> - Limit consumption of acidic substances and beverages—especially between meals. Acidic substances, including carbonated beverages, can dissolve tooth structure and contribute to cavities. Diet sodas are particularly damaging.
> - After consuming acidic or sugary between-meal snacks, rinse the mouth with water to flush away sugars and dilute acids in the mouth and o not brush for at least 30 minutes after acid exposures.
> - Fresh fruits, vegetables, meat products, whole grains, cheeses, and water are generally good foods for oral health.
> - Fluoride use should be encouraged—fluoridated toothpaste, mouth rinse, gels, and varnish have all been shown to be helpful for patients who are at risk for cavities.

to the patient and/or caregiver (Box 13.7). After this review, it is often helpful to compose a follow-up letter for the patient and caregiver reviewing relevant dietary and oral home care issues and formalizing the dental team's recommendations and goals for the patient (Box 13.8). Such a letter can be an important part of the process of educating, encouraging, and empowering the patient and/or caregiver.

Psychosocial History

A psychosocial history, useful for any comprehensive care dental patient, often has particular relevance and importance for the patient with special care needs. Information about basic issues, such as the patient's ability to ambulate and get to the dental office, is essential to the effective provision of dental care. Does the patient need an accompanying person? Who will that be? Does the patient need transportation? If so, how will that

---

BOX 13.8   Example of a Follow-Up Letter to a Patient Regarding His or Her Oral Health and Recommendations for Oral Disease Prevention

May 1, 20___

Dear Mr. Smith,

My staff and I have appreciated the opportunity to work with you to improve your oral health during the past two appointments. I believe that we have made real progress in oral health promotion in preparation for restoring your dentition and getting you on the road to keeping your teeth for your entire lifetime! I hope that all your questions about brushing/flossing techniques and diet have been answered. If not, please do not hesitate to contact me or to bring them up at our next appointment.

As we discussed, several areas in your diet raise concerns relating to good oral health:

1. Fruit Loops and other sweet cereals are particularly devastating if oral hygiene procedures are not carried out soon after eating.
2. Sugar in coffee is acceptable, but again I recommend a quick brushing afterward.
3. Sodas are EXTREMELY detrimental to your dentition. It would be best to limit or discontinue their use. When you do consume them, be sure to rinse your mouth out with water and brush afterward.
4. Any consumption of sweets should be followed with oral hygiene procedures as soon after as feasible.
5. Considering your past caries activity, I recommend a thorough brushing and flossing two to three times a day. I also recommend use of an electric toothbrush.
6. Remember, preserving your teeth is primarily up to you with support from our dental team! I am very encouraged by your positive attitude and feel confident that you will follow through with our recommendations!

Thanks and please contact me if you have any questions or concerns. I know some of these changes may be difficult, but with you as a co-therapist, I think we can accomplish much.

Professionally,

Allen D. Samuelson, DDS
Clinical Associate Professor

BOX 13.9   Activities of Daily Living

A range of common activities whose performance is required for personal self-maintenance and independent community residence.

Physical ADLs (basic self-care activities)
1. Dressing
2. Toileting/continence
3. Transferring
4. Eating
5. Mobility
6. Bathing

Instrumental ADLs (complex abilities needed for independent living)
1. Shopping
2. Traveling/transportation
3. Using the telephone
4. Preparing meals
5. Housework/laundry
6. Taking medicine
7. Managing money

Depending on the level of function that the patient exhibits, treatment planning may need to be altered. An analysis of the patient's ability to perform ADLs is predictive of how well he or she may be able to perform oral hygiene. For instance, if the patient has limited mobility (e.g., severe arthritis), he or she may not be able to get to a lavatory to perform basic oral hygiene, and modifications, such as basins and towels brought to the bed, may be necessary to facilitate daily oral care.

---

biting; "doodling" with needles, nails, and other objects; obsessive use of oral health aids; bruxism; and mouth breathing.

One might inquire as to whether the patient is currently employed or volunteers, and in what capacity. It may also be helpful to know the patient's level of education and areas of study; as well as any hobbies or outside interests.

Functional History

The **functional history** reviews the patient's past and present ability to live independently and function in society. Typically, this includes an analysis of the patient's capacity for the **ADLs**. Review of the ADLs is important because it allows the practitioner to evaluate the patient's physical and cognitive ability to follow through with a preventive, restorative, and maintenance plan of care. The patient's ability to perform ADLs is predictive of how effectively he or she will perform oral self-care. Furthermore, depending on the level of function exhibited by the patient, treatment planning may need to be altered. For example, if the patient has limited mobility (e.g., severe arthritis), getting to the bathroom to perform oral hygiene may be difficult. Modifications such as basins and towels brought to the bedside may be necessary to facilitate daily oral care.

Importantly, a query regarding as to whether the patient has a functional occlusion and how well they can masticate their food is critical in planning care. A fully functional occlusion coupled with a disease-compromised dentition is cause for great caution in planning and will require a thorough informed consent and counseling with regards to alterations to the occlusion such as multi-tooth removal, complete dentures, or removable partial dentures.

ADLs are divided into two major groups: basic and instrumental (Box 13.9).

be arranged? It should not be assumed that because a patient is elderly or handicapped, they are not employed. An understanding of the patient's past and present career and employment can have a bearing on the nature and extent of dental treatment that may be desired or appropriate, the timing of dental visits (to accommodate the patient's work schedule), and financial resources. An understanding of the patient's support system, schooling, and domiciliary arrangements can give the dentist an idea of how well the patient may be able to follow through with a preventive and restorative plan.

Taking a good psychosocial history also affirms the patient's humanity and integration into the family unit and society. Trust is gained from the patient and family by this affirmation. A thorough personal history will disclose relevant habits, including the use of alcohol, tobacco, and illicit drugs (discussed in in Chapters 1 and 14). Oral habits can be commonplace in patients with special needs and may impede the success of preventive therapy and negatively affect the outcome of dental treatment. Some common deleterious habits include fingernail or object

Obtaining Additional Information From Other Healthcare Providers

For the typical dental patient, the dentist completes all parts of the patient evaluation and, if warranted, obtains a physician consultation. In the case of patients with complex health concerns and multiple medications, however, this sequence may need to be modified. If the individual comes to the office unattended, he or she may have some difficulty communicating all the necessary health and drug information to the dental team. If the individual comes with an attendant or family member who is not the primary caregiver, the attendant may not have the necessary information either. If the patient lives in a residential care facility, the medical record (or a general health problem list and summary of current medications) can be requested and brought with the patient on the initial visit. It still may be necessary to consult with the patient's primary care physician, pharmacist, primary caregiver, close family member, or other responsible party who is knowledgeable about the details of the patient's general health. In many cases, it may be prudent to do this before initiating the invasive portions of the clinical examination. This is usually accomplished most effectively by making an immediate telephone contact. Where this is not possible, follow-up contact via phone, fax, or e-mail can be made (with the patient's permission) before the next visit. Otherwise, arrangements can be made to have other medical records or documentation brought to the next visit. Examples of useful documentation include: a copy of a recent medical history and physical examination; a hospital discharge summary from within the last 12 months; and laboratory reports such as an electrocardiogram (ECG), chest x-ray (CXR), echocardiogram, and CBC with differential.

Although in many cases a consultation with the patient's primary care health provider is warranted, it is usually not necessary that it occur before the clinical examination. Often, the dental team can complete those portions of the intraoral and extraoral examination and the noninvasive portions of the clinical examination that the patient is able to cooperate with, make a general determination of what dental treatments may be recommended to the patient, and *then* obtain a medical or other consultation. The procedure and documentation for a referral to a medical provider follow guidelines discussed in Chapters 1, 6, and 8. Specific cases in which a referral letter is warranted include the following:

1. A patient with special needs presents for dental treatment and has no established or current relationship with a physician.
2. The dental team believes that a complete or accurate health history has not been obtained.
3. The patient exhibits signs of an emerging health problem or signs that a preexisting condition is not under adequate control.

Generally, referral should be to a primary care physician or a specialist in internal medicine or geriatrics. The referral letter should include a brief explanation of planned treatment, anticipated blood loss and time in the chair, and medications to be used. The physician should be queried about the diagnosis and management of any health problems that are relevant to dental treatment. The physician can be expected to respond with recommendations and suggestions regarding how any health problems should be managed in the dental setting. The ultimate rationale behind a physician consultation is to gain a complete and accurate understanding of the patient's general health problems, conditions, and treatments so that dental care can be delivered as safely as possible. This should be explained to the patient or care provider before the referral.

Physical and Oral Examination in the Dental Office

The objectives of the physical examination are no different for these patients, but the methodology and scope may need to be altered to accommodate the patient's limitations. The dental team must be prepared to receive patients who present to the appointment in a wheelchair, gurney, or geri-chairs. (Information on conveyance methods and transport techniques is presented later in this chapter.)

The physical examination should occur after the history has been obtained. Good lighting, magnification, positioning, and, in some cases, gentle restraint are important for an effective examination. The same instruments can be used as with the standard patient, but care must be taken to prevent the patient from biting down on metal instruments and damaging teeth or intraoral soft tissue. A mouth prop may be useful to allow for better access. The "tell, show, do" approach is helpful for many patients because it promotes understanding and trust and can be effective in reducing the patient's anxiety. It may also help the dentist carry out the examination with greater ease and efficiency.

Important preliminary components of the physical examination include assessing general appearance, body build, facial appearance, and ability to ambulate and transfer. This process begins as the patient is escorted to the operatory. Such observations provide the dental team with a rapid assessment of the general disposition and behavior of the patient and suggest what accommodations may be necessary during the examination and at future visits.

The same structures and tissues are examined as with the more typical dental patient. Patients with special needs are more likely, however, to exhibit certain oral problems. For example, they may have limited opening and decreased range of motion, and often have difficulty following instructions regarding jaw movements. They may exhibit oral injuries, including oral ulcers and evidence of soft tissue trauma. They may present with substantial plaque and calculus deposits, gingivitis, periodontitis, gingival hyperplasia, gingival abscesses, severe tooth mobility, rampant caries, and attrition. Signs of general attrition and aberrant tooth wear caused by habits such as nail or object biting need to be diagnosed, because they have a potential impact on the restorative plan. For example, successful retention of a seemingly simple Class IV restoration on an anterior tooth may be significantly compromised if the patient has a severe nail biting or other parafunctional habit. The dental team should anticipate that the findings from the examination will vary substantially depending on the nature and scope of the patient's problem and the patient's individual circumstances.

Behavior exhibited at the initial examination is usually an indication of how cooperative the patient can be expected to be for other procedures. If it becomes apparent during the initial examination that the patient's level of cooperation will limit the nature and scope of dental treatment, then it is prudent to inform the patient and caregiver at that time. It is important to be aware, however, that the patient's level of cooperation may improve over time. With trust established, anxiety relieved, and comfort with the office setting and personnel achieved, the patient may become more engaged and cooperative. The following section describes management strategies related to the level of the patient's cooperation that can be developed at the initial examination visit.

Actively Cooperative Patients

The actively cooperative patient is able to undergo all typical examination procedures. For those patients, the examination can be carried out in the same manner as for the typical adult patient (see Chapter 1).

Passively Cooperative Patients

The passively cooperative patient is not resistive, but is unable to understand or respond appropriately to some or all directives (for example, a patient who opens his or her mouth, but doesn't cooperate with specific requests to move the lower jaw or close the mouth). Dental team members need to be calm, patient, and sensitive to the patient's needs. The examination will typically require extra time.

Actively Uncooperative or Combative Patients

Patients with dementia, autism, severe phobias, or significant mental illness may be actively uncooperative for the examination and, in a small proportion of cases, combative. If the patient is uncooperative or unwilling to allow a detailed visual examination, it may be possible to perform a digital examination, palpating for gingival abscesses, broken teeth, or other gross pathology. In these situations, the caregiver must be informed that a complete examination is not possible at the present time and an accurate diagnosis cannot be obtained. A modified examination may be acceptable if it is evident from a brief look that reasonably good oral hygiene appears to be practiced and that there are no visible caries. The caregivers must be informed, however, that latent dental disease may be present, and the conversation must be documented. If, in the dentist's judgment, a more thorough examination is imperative, then some form of sedation or general anesthesia is warranted. The risks of the sedation/anesthesia must be weighed against the relative benefits of an improved diagnostic process. If broken teeth, abscesses, or gross visible caries are present, then an OR procedure under general anesthesia is indicated. General anesthesia is certainly a means through which an ideal radiographic series can be taken and a comprehensive examination and comprehensive treatments can be performed.

Passively Uncooperative Patients

The passively uncooperative patient, although not actively avoiding examination or treatment, exhibits facial or body movements that make both examination and treatment delivery extremely difficult. An initial attempt should be made to examine and treat these patients on an outpatient basis. If successful, a variety of control phase procedures can be planned and executed. If not, treatment under general anesthesia may be required.

Imaging

Imaging should occur after the physical and oral examination. Selection criteria for images are the same as those for normal dental patients (see Chapter 1). During the examination, the dentist can usually discern whether the patient can be expected to be cooperative for imaging. Guidelines for obtaining images for the patient with special care needs can be categorized based on the patient's level of cooperation:

- Cooperative and coordinated patients (actively cooperative)—standard techniques can be used.
- Cooperative but uncoordinated patients (passively cooperative; e.g., mild to moderate mental handicap)—a lead apron and glove can be worn by the dentist or assistant and the film held manually with a hemostat as the images are exposed. This is similar to the technique often used when generating intraoral images in the OR and clinically acceptable images are generally possible.
- Uncooperative or combative patients—it may not be possible to obtain images with an uncooperative patient in an outpatient setting. In such cases, the caregiver or family member must be informed, and a candid discussion of relevant options conducted. Generally, if the caregiver or family member is interested in having treatment performed, then he or she will agree to generating appropriate intraoral images in the OR while the patient is under general anesthesia.

Special Diagnostic Tests and Procedures

The criteria for performing pulp vitality tests, laboratory tests, and other diagnostic studies for the special needs patient are no different from those for other patients. Caution must be exercised, however, so as not to alarm the patient by initiating procedures unexpectedly. The "tell, show, do" approach is helpful in allaying anxiety by giving the patient a realistic sense of what to expect. This is especially important when attempting any tests or procedures, such as electric pulp testing, that can be expected to cause discomfort. Because of cognitive changes in many patients, the findings from those tests that require patient interpretation and communication, such as pulp vitality tests, may be unclear or unreliable. In lieu of accurate clinical tests, a diagnosis can often be made after a careful interview of the caregiver. A caregiver who is aware of and monitors the patient's behavior on a regular basis is in an excellent position to provide an accurate and meaningful review of new or ongoing patient symptoms. Changed eating habits, grabbing at the face or mouth, or crying out may be indicative of infection or other forms of an acute oral problem. If testing is performed (cold pulpal testing, palpation, percussion), careful examination of the reaction of the eyes and/or wincing, grimacing, and withdrawal may be helpful in making a diagnosis.

As with other aspects of the patient evaluation, when compromises or departures from the regular diagnostic process must be made to accommodate the patient, it is essential to document the rationale for any deviations from the normal protocol. In all cases, the dental record must clearly document the rationale for using diagnostic procedures and treatments that do not fit norms for the typical dental patient. Failure to make such documentation may allow the later suspicion that the dentist did not use good clinical judgment or meet the standard of care.

Occlusal Records

As with any patient, study casts are generally indicated if removable or extensive fixed prosthodontic care is planned. Other indications for obtaining study casts or digital occlusal records include the presence of occlusal symptoms, decreased vertical dimension of occlusion (VDO), the need for forensic records, and the fabrication of shims or other dental devices, such as orthotics. Gagging is a frequent problem with these patients. Most often, this is a gagging response, not a true gag reflex. In other words, the patient can place and hold food, cigarettes, lozenges, or other items in the mouth without difficulty, but dental treatment elicits a gagging response. Suggesting that the patient avoid food before the procedure and the use of a topical anesthetic may facilitate impression taking on a patient with a history of gagging. Sedatives may also diminish this response. For the patient who is uncooperative or who has severe coordination problems, it may not be possible to obtain study casts on an outpatient basis.

ARRIVING AT A DIAGNOSIS

The dentist has the obligation to identify and document diagnoses for all comprehensive care patients, including those with special needs. Not surprisingly, patients with special needs tend to have more general health problems and more oral health problems. All diagnoses should be listed, including the following:

- Medical Risk issues
- Behavioral diagnoses (level of cooperation and coordination)
- Oral self-care/dietary/habit diagnoses as well as a general statement regarding preventive trajectory and prognosis for improvement
- Musculoskeletal diagnoses (including ambulation, ADL's, speech, swallowing, mastication)
- Oral/cutaneous pathology diagnoses
- Periodontal diagnoses
- Dental diagnoses
- Occlusal/functional diagnoses
- Other relevant information (e.g., financial, scheduling challenges, transportation)

This list becomes the foundation for the patient-specific plan of care and provides the justification for every item on the treatment plan. Patients must be informed of the diagnoses. This discussion is an integral part of the process of developing informed consent for the plan of care. Patients should be included in this process to the maximum of their abilities.

> ### BOX 13.10 Examples of Common Diagnoses for Patients With Special Needs
>
> Minimal cognitive function or physical coordination, limiting ability to follow through on a preventive plan
>
> Minimal psychological motivation for a preventive plan (e.g., a mentally impaired patient)
>
> Combative patient not allowing examination or treatment in the clinical environment (as with a severely demented patient)
>
> Minimal neuromuscular coordination, limiting possibility of engineering a dental prosthesis (e.g., a mildly uncooperative but uncoordinated autistic patient)
>
> Absent/poor/fair/good/excellent oral home care—assessment dependent on level of plaque control and effectiveness of home care
>
> Dietary risk factors not under control—this may be surmised from either a written or verbal diet diary
>
> Head and neck finding—includes abnormalities of TMJ and neuromuscular complex, and various forms of orocutaneous pathology
>
> Missing teeth with edentulous spaces, signifying lack of arch integrity and the possible need for replacement
>
> Dysfunctional occlusion (subjectively and/or objectively), signifying the need for occlusal treatment and/or restorative dentistry
>
> Dentofacial/craniofacial deformity, signifying the need for multidisciplinary and interdisciplinary treatment
>
> Caries and caries risk, signifying the need for disease control and prevention before definitive restorative dentistry
>
> Recurrent caries (may indicate heightened caries risk or confirm that caries infection has never been under control)
>
> Defective restorations with clinical indications for replacement
>
> Esthetic concerns
>
> Periodontitis
>
> Gingivitis
>
> Aberrant tooth wear (attrition, abrasion, erosion)
>
> Mouth breathing
>
> Habits (continuing tobacco use—30 pack/year history)

When the patient with significant cognitive disorders cannot participate in clinical decision making, the dentist must discuss dental and behavioral diagnoses with family members and/or a legal representative. It is critical that the proxy decision maker understand the diagnoses of the individual under his or her care so that informed consent can be given and an informed decision for treatment can be made by the caregivers.

Diagnoses commonly found in patients with special needs are listed in Box 13.10.

TREATMENT PLANNING FOR THE PATIENT WITH SPECIAL NEEDS

Unique Aspects of Treatment Planning for the Special Care Patient

Throughout this text, the importance of the proper sequencing of events in the treatment planning and treatment delivery process is a consistent theme. Like successive rows of blocks in the foundation for a building, each layer or step in the sequence must be complete and solid to support the next-higher row. In simple terms, the sequence is as follows: comprehensive oral examination → diagnosis → framing of treatment objectives and options → consent discussion and plan selection → development and approval of a sequenced plan of care → execution of the plan → maintenance therapy. Although this process is valid for the patient with special care needs, some distinct differences in emphasis can be noted. Sometimes subtle, these differences can be significant and can drastically alter treatment planning and management of therapy. Six focal differences are highlighted here: the importance of general health issues, the importance of functional and behavioral issues, considering the need for sedation, scope of care, sequencing of the plan and timing of treatment, and preventive and maintenance services.

Importance of General Health Issues

Although recognition of general health issues is relevant to the dental treatment of any patient, for most, these issues are generally isolated and can be easily integrated into the systemic phase of care, which is discussed in Chapter 8. For the patient with special needs, however, physical health and psychological issues are not simply adjuncts to the dental plan of care, but frequently represent major life-altering conditions that must shape the dental treatment planning and may drastically limit the type of treatment that can be provided. For the dentist, in attempting to construct a treatment plan for a patient with special care needs, a fundamental and complete understanding of the patient's physical and psychological condition and the relationship of that condition to dental care delivery is critical. The following key questions will aid in this discovery process:

- What are the patient's general health problems? Psychological problems? Developmental problems?
- What medications is the patient taking? Do any of these medications have significant oral side effects or interact with local anesthetics or other agents used in dentistry?
- Is more information needed from other healthcare professionals?
- What effect will these issues have on the delivery of dental treatment?
- Can dental care be provided safely on an outpatient basis, or should the patient receive dental care in another setting?
- Are there limitations or contraindications to dental treatment? If so, what are they?

As these questions are explored, the dentist can begin to define the range of reasonable dental options that can be offered to the patient. This winnowing process is a sometimes challenging but critical task, with the goal of offering all reasonable options to the patient, caregiver, and family, while excluding those that are not feasible given the patient's physical or psychological impairment. One unheralded benefit to this process is that patients (and their caregivers) are often more willing to accept limitations to the treatment plan offerings if those limitations are based on their general health, rather than on behavioral grounds or criteria relating specifically to the delivery of dental treatment.

The following Box 13.11 delineates particular issues that need to be addressed if surgical procedures are planned for the patient.

BOX 13.11 Surgical Treatment Concerns for the Special Needs Patient

Many patients with special care needs (including frail elderly) have challenging medical problems, polypharmacy and psychosocial impediments to predictable and safe care. It behooves the oral health practitioner to gain access to the medical record to evaluate progress notes, laboratory studies, test results (EKG/ECHO/Cardia Cath/Pacemaker-Defibrillator status and readouts etc). The general list below should be considered in advance of treatment -especially, invasive therapies.

1. Disease/Constitutional stability (ASA Class)
2. Immune integrity – verifying medications list and CBC w/diff
3. Hemostatic integrity (vascular /platelets / clotting pathways / plasminogen) – Platelet count and integrity (if applicable in pts with inherited disorders or renal disease); INR for VKA; Informed consent for DOACs etc.
4. Wound healing – bisphosphonates; antiangiogenics; corticosteroids; chemotherapeutics; radiation hx.
5. Medical emergencies – anticipatory preparation for emergencies given health history
6. Hydration – can the patient maintain hydration in light of their condition and treatment undergone?
7. Nutrition/Weight maintenance – can they maintain weight in light of their condition and treatment undergone?
8. Management of co-morbidities in light of tx.

Importance of Functional and Behavioral Issues

Behavioral issues may be relevant in planning dental treatment for any patient. Patients who are not diligent with their oral self-care are more likely to experience the ravages of caries, periodontal disease, and other oral health problems. Patients who are motivationally compromised may require a wide array of special management techniques, as discussed in Chapter 19. For the patient with special needs, however, behavioral problems often go far beyond the challenge of finding a means to motivate the patient to be more diligent with oral home care. The patient with special needs may be unable to open his or her mouth, or respond to simple commands, or be oriented to person, place, and time. Behavioral issues, like issues related to general health, can have a major effect on the patient's ability to communicate, function in society, and perform ADLs. Some important functional and behavioral questions that must be addressed in the process of developing the treatment plan include the following:

- Was the patient able to adequately cooperate for radiographic and clinical examinations?
- Will the patient allow caregivers to provide oral care?
- Can the patient physically tolerate the time in the chair necessary to complete treatment limited or complex restorative or surgical treatment?
- Will the patient follow through with a preventive regimen?
- Has a relationship been established with the patient and the caregiver? How knowledgeable is the caregiver about oral disease and its prevention? How interested is the caregiver in improving the oral health condition of the patient? How much support can the caregiver be expected to provide to the patient?

The patient with special needs functional and behavioral limitations, along with his or her general health issues, provide the basis for narrowing the range of treatment options. Behavioral issues can severely limit both the scope and nature of the treatment that can be provided on an outpatient basis. For example, engineering indirect restorations, such as crowns, bridges, or implant-supported prostheses, may not be feasible because of lack of neuromuscular coordination. Therefore it is important to take the time to explain such limitations to both the patient and the caregiver. These limitations should never be seen as a failure on the part of the patient, the caregiver, or the dentist. If the patient, either unassisted or with the help of a caregiver, is able to establish an effective level of oral home care, then the long-term prognosis for his or her oral condition is favorable.

The passively cooperative patient may be able to accept and engage in some treatments but not others. In most cases, however, simple extractions, nonsurgical periodontal therapy, and direct-fill restorative procedures can be completed with minimum difficulty, and the dental team can expect to bring a passively cooperative patient to a disease-free and functional state. Some procedures, such as complex fixed prosthodontics, may not be feasible or practical for the actively uncooperative or combative patient. The decision as to whether to use general anesthesia must be made with the informed consent of the patient, legal guardian, or responsible family member.

An important consideration when planning treatment for the special needs patient is whether the individual can respond to necessary requests. For example, if a single unit crown is placed, can the centric and functional aspects of the occlusion be evaluated? If such an evaluation cannot be achieved, then indirect restorations may not be feasible.

Furthermore, the patient whose exceptionally strong or active orofacial musculature makes examination of oral structures difficult or impossible may be otherwise generally cooperative (i.e., does not raise his or her hands or attempt to get out of the chair). Use of light sedation may be sufficient to allow completion of the examination, but if this option is not realistic and a comprehensive baseline is necessary, then general anesthesia may be warranted.

Consider the Need for Sedation

An essential question when planning treatment for the special needs patient is whether the patient will be cooperative at dental visits and for the duration of the dental treatment. Specifically, can comprehensive dental care be achieved in a dental office either with or without sedation? If the patient is uncooperative and cannot be managed in an outpatient setting, will general anesthesia be required? For example, if a patient is resistive and actively uncooperative, then it would be expected that only minimally invasive dental treatment and simple restorative procedures can be performed without sedation. If the patient is *passively* uncooperative, then it may be possible to provide a full range of treatment with only minimal oral sedation. Furthermore, if the patient is actively uncooperative and the treatment objectives include definitive restorative procedures that necessitate generating diagnostic casts and complete mouth radiographic images, then general anesthesia is usually warranted.

The patient's and caregiver's wishes and the dentist's comfort with various sedation techniques will also be the determinants of what, if any, technique will be used. Each technique has notable benefits and limitations. The following section briefly summarizes the indications for the various forms of sedation (see also Chapter 15 for more detail).

Iatrosedation. The term **iatrosedation** has been applied to all nonpharmacologic modes of anxiety control and sedation. Although it may include behavioral therapies, such as desensitization therapy, relaxation therapy, or hypnosis, its essence is the "sedative" effect that is provided by the patient's trust and confidence in the dental team.[21] Often, this is all the "sedation" that is necessary to treat the patient effectively. However, if the patient remains uncooperative, other approaches can be tried. The efficiency of most forms of sedation is dependent on the level of iatrosedation experienced by the patient. If the patient trusts the dental team and feels emotionally supported and listened to, other forms of sedation will work more efficiently.

Nitrous oxide and oxygen analgesia. Nitrous oxide and oxygen is an efficient form of analgesia, but to be used successfully the patient must be able to breathe normally through the nose piece. If the patient is unable or unwilling to be cooperative, allowing nitrous oxide to escape around the mask, or if he or she persists in mouth breathing or talking, then the staff and dentist will be inhaling the nitrous oxide and the effectiveness on the patient will be greatly reduced. There are documented environmental risks for the dental team with this medication, most notably obstetric and reproductive complications.[22-24]

Oral sedation/anxiolysis. Oral sedation can be an effective and relatively inexpensive approach. Several protocols are available for the oral conscious sedation technique. These range from simple anxiolysis (for which, in most jurisdictions no permit is needed) to incrementally administered oral sedatives to achieve a desired effect. Airway protection and management are of paramount importance with the use of any pharmacologic sedation. The patient's level of cooperation and the dentist's experience will determine when and how the oral sedative agents are to be used. In extremely fearful or agitated patients, the dosage required to provide effective sedation may be so high that anesthetic risks (unconsciousness or fatal overdose) become unacceptable. It is important to note that in many jurisdictions throughout the world a permit is required to administer enteral sedation. Please reference your local dental board or other authority for applicable laws, rules and regulations.

Intravenous sedation. Intravenous (IV) sedation is an efficient method of sedation but will necessitate additional cost to the patient. In many jurisdictions, use of IV sedation requires additional training and incurs additional malpractice liability and expense to the dental practice. The drugs can be easily titrated to effect and are very predictable. If general dentistry is planned, however, great caution must be observed to protect the airway from particulate matter. Also, completing all treatment in a timely and safe manner can be quite challenging with this modality if many teeth are to be restored, extracted, or treated endodontically.

General anesthesia. The decision to place the patient under general anesthesia for general dental care takes into account the behavioral diagnosis as well as the projected treatment needs. If a comprehensive examination (particularly a baseline exam) and dental treatment are planned for an uncooperative patient, then general anesthesia is warranted (Figure 13.1). If a brief office examination of an uncooperative patient reveals no evidence of acute or active infection, or suspicion of oral cancer, the risks vs benefits of deferring a comprehensive examination under general anesthesia can be made a matter of consideration with the patient's care provider, HCPOA or responsible family member A recent physical examination, consent (also called an *operative permit* in the hospital setting), and anesthesia consultation must occur preoperatively. The following procedures can typically be performed while the patient is under general anesthesia:

- Complete series of dental radiographs.
- Comprehensive examination.
- Deep scaling and root planing.
- Operative dentistry procedures.
- Oral surgery, including biopsy.
- Periodontal surgery.
- Fixed prosthodontic procedures. This is more challenging, because more time is typically required than for the other procedures for preparation, impression taking, and fabrication of a provisional restoration. If the patient must also be sedated to *deliver* the prosthesis, then an additional trip to the OR for general anesthesia will be required. In general, if hygiene, diet, and physical coordination are inadequate, definitive indirect fixed prosthodontic restorations tare not indicated.
- Concurrent treatment procedures by other medical services in the hospital (e.g., gynecologic, ear-nose-throat [ENT], or ophthalmology examinations).

Many options are available for the provision of sedation by the general practitioner. The dentist may administer the sedation, in which case the practitioner must be aware of and comply with all applicable rules and restrictions relating to the use of sedation in an outpatient dental setting. The dentist may also have the patient admitted to the hospital and perform the treatment in an OR environment, in which an anesthesiologist or certified nurse anesthetist (CNA) performs the sedation. Occasionally, the dentist may hire an anesthesiologist or CNA to come into the dental office and perform sedation on site.

Scope and Levels of Care

The range of feasible treatment options appropriate for the patient with special needs may be more diverse than for the typical dental patient. General health and behavioral issues may necessitate creative and unusual approaches to dental care

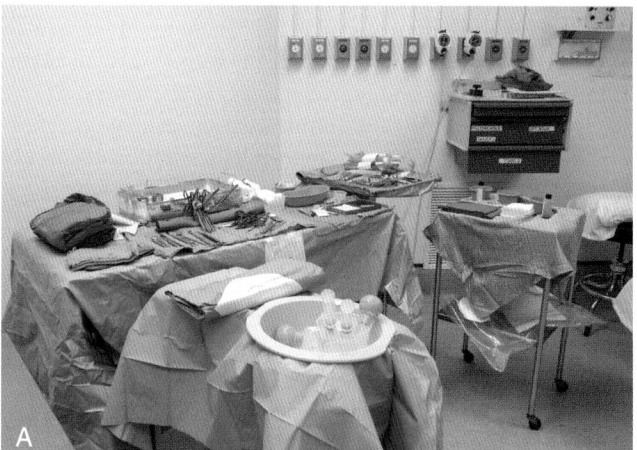
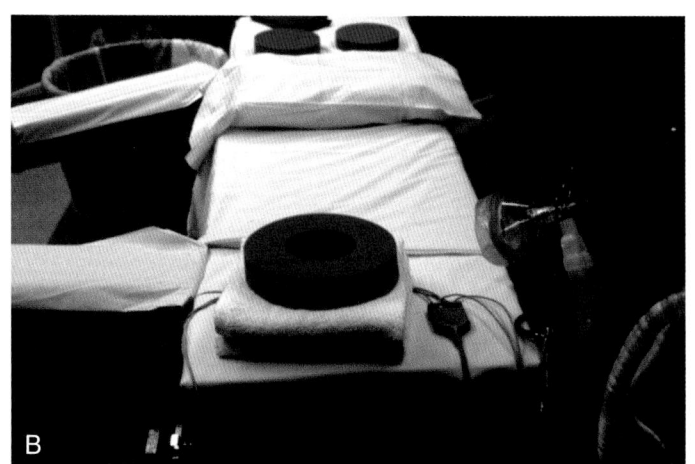
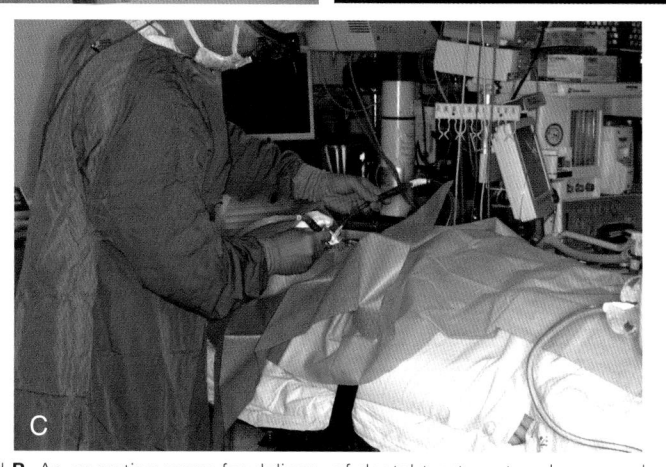

FIG. 13.1 A and **B**, An operating room for delivery of dental treatment under general anesthesia **C**, Dental treatment being preformed in a hospital operating room. (**C**, Courtesy Dr. Allen Samuelson, Chapel Hill, N.C.)

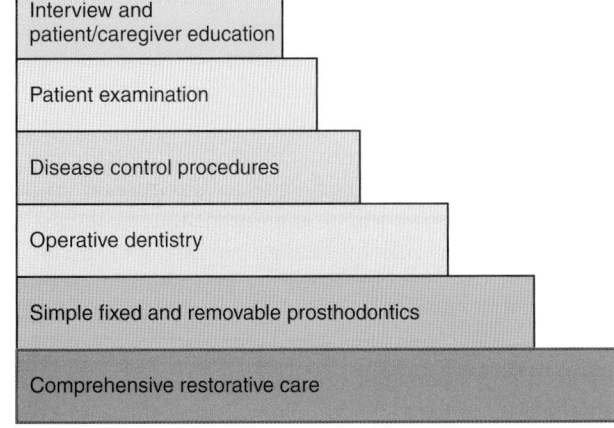

FIG. 13.2 Levels of care.

Interview and patient/caregiver education

Patient examination

Disease control procedures

Operative dentistry

Simple fixed and removable prosthodontics

Comprehensive restorative care

delivery. Differing levels of care can be offered depending on the patient's intellectual capacity, physical status, level of cooperation and interest, and ability to tolerate the rigors of dental treatment. Because of significant health problems or limitations with the patient's cognition, compliance, cooperation, or function, it is often necessary to limit both the scope and complexity of the dental plan of care.

The range of treatment options for the patient with special needs is described here and summarized in the schematic diagram in Figure 13.2.

Interview and patient education. If the patient is actively or passively uncooperative, an interview with the caregivers may be all that is feasible. A discussion of proper diet and oral home care is always beneficial. Encouragement and empowerment of the caregiver will benefit the patient and help to promote trusting relationships among the three principals: dentist, patient, and caregiver. Affirmation of the humanity of the patient is also extremely important. Eliciting a brief life history is particularly apropos for a patient with dementia. Understanding the patient's past and present life circumstances can provide the dental team with valuable insights into goals and expectations that the patient, family, and/or caregiver may have for the patient's oral condition. This conversation also demonstrates to the caregiver that the dentist sees the patient as an individual, not simply as a source of income for the practice.

Patient examination. Although many patients are able to comfortably undergo a complete examination, some can tolerate only a limited (digital only) or modified examination. The dentist should complete as many normal procedures in the initial oral examination as the patient can cooperate with and accept. Oral self-care instructions and dietary recommendations should be shared with caregivers. The focus at this point is to identify acute needs. It may be appropriate to prescribe antibiotics and/or analgesics, especially if the patient is uncooperative. Establishing an ongoing relationship with the caregiver is important to ensure that the dental team will be apprised of changes with the patient. Initially, the patient may not be cooperative or receptive to any restorative treatment, but if the patient's condition improves, even briefly, there may be a window of opportunity for intervention and provision of some restorative or other needed services.

Disease control procedures. The next level of intervention would include an oral prophylaxis, caries control procedures (including direct-fill sedative or provisional restorations as the patient will allow), scaling and root planing, supportive periodontal care, and elimination of sources of oral infection and disease (see Chapter 10).

Operative dentistry. Operative dentistry in this context includes any definitive direct-fill restorations, such as amalgams, composite resins, or glass ionomers. Completion of the operative dentistry plan is predicated on the patient's ability to tolerate and cooperate with the treatment and his or her level of adherence to recommended preventive therapy.

Limited fixed and removable prosthodontics. Some patients may be candidates for select indirect fixed prosthetic restorations and/ or uncomplicated removable partial or complete dentures. These treatments must be reserved for those patients who are sufficiently coordinated to allow the dentist to engineer the prosthesis, and for whom there is a demonstrated ability to maintain the prostheses. Before such treatment is initiated, it is essential to establish that the preventive regimen recommended by the dental team is being adhered to. Patients who are unable to duplicate functional movements or cannot cooperate with taking occlusal records are not good candidates for prosthodontics.

Comprehensive restorative care. Comprehensive occlusal and restorative reconstruction should be undertaken only if the patient is fully cooperative, appropriately coordinated, motivated, and fully able (with the assistance of a caregiver if necessary) to maintain a healthy oral condition. Treatment involving reconstruction in multiple quadrants, alteration of occlusal planes, or the establishment of anterior guidance should be reserved for only the highest-functioning patients with excellent preventive trajectories, excellent cooperation and coordination.

Sequencing the Plan and the Timing of Treatment

As discussed throughout this text, sequencing for most dental patients is driven by patient priorities and the relative urgency of and need for each procedure in the plan of care. Sequencing of the plan for a patient with special care needs often must be based on entirely different criteria. The following are some issues that may affect the sequence of the plan of care and the timing of treatment for this patient.

Transportation and availability. For patients with special needs, access to the dental office may depend on the availability of transportation and the schedules of caregivers. These factors may affect the timing, frequency, and length of appointments.

Planning care to be performed under general anesthesia. If the patient needs general anesthesia for some but not all of the dental treatment, sequencing will be ordered according to which treatments must be performed in the OR. Given the costs, health risks, and logistical challenges of scheduling the patient for dental care in the OR under general anesthesia, it certainly makes sense to cluster all services that are to be delivered under general anesthesia, and to try to minimize the number of such visits.

Support from caregivers. It may be necessary for caregivers to provide assistance to the patient in many ways, including transfer to and from the dental chair, facilitating communication between patient and dentist, provision of oral home care, dispensing medications, implementing postoperative instructions, and providing education and encouragement. If it is necessary for the caregiver to be present before, during, and/or after the visit, timing and sequencing of procedures will necessarily need to be made in conformity with the caregiver's schedule.

Patient cooperation. As the treatment plan is developed, if there is uncertainty as to the level of the patient's cooperation, simple preventive and restorative procedures should be performed before more-demanding treatments, with time-consuming treatments deferred until an appropriate level of cooperation has been confirmed. If acute symptoms develop before patient cooperation has been established, it may be advisable to treat the problem with medication, with more definitive therapy to be provided after behavioral issues have been addressed.

Patient endurance. Although sequencing by quadrant is normally the most efficient and productive way to manage restorative treatment, this may not be the best approach for the patient with special needs. Anxiety, difficulty in comprehending what is happening, and reduced energy levels all may limit the patient's endurance and preclude performance of multiple restorations at a single visit. For such a patient, it may be most expedient to use the limited available working time to treat those teeth and situations in which the ability of the patient to maintain good oral hygiene is high and for which the long-term prognosis is most favorable. Extraction of teeth that cannot be maintained for the long term at a future dedicated appointment, and under general anesthesia if necessary, may be a better option.

Preventive and Maintenance Services

The treatment plan for a typical dental patient may include a maintenance phase [see Chapter 12], with a brief reference to anticipated periodic visits. For most dental patients, maintenance needs and procedures will be determined at the completion of the definitive (restorative) therapy. This simply is not sufficient for patients with special care needs. Many will present initially in a precarious state of oral health and in a condition of serious disrepair with active disease. For many, the inability to understand the need for healthy lifestyle practices and the benefits of good oral health will be a significant problem. Others may understand these issues but will be physically unable to perform basic oral self-care. In the absence of a competent, engaged caregiver, the outlook will indeed be bleak.

For these patients, preventive services become their lifeline—often the only thing that keeps at bay oral infection, pain, the inability to chew, and impaired oral function. Preventive and maintenance therapy for these patients must be the frontline of services provided, and it must be melded into each appointment and each stage of the treatment.

Various physical or emotional issues may interfere for extended periods or indefinitely with the patient's ability or willingness to return to the dental office. During times when active treatment is suspended, the ability of the patient and caregiver

to carry on with basic oral self-care will have a significant bearing on whether the patient will be able to retain his or her teeth.

Referral Options

In some situations, it is appropriate and necessary to refer the patient to a dental specialist or another dental practitioner. In some cases, the referral will be for a selected portion of the plan of care, and in others, it will be appropriate to refer the patient to another dental provider for total patient care. If the treatment plan includes specialty care that is not provided in the general dentist's practice (e.g., periodontal surgery or molar endodontics), then referral to an appropriate specialist is warranted. (See Chapter 6 for an example of a referral letter.)

The referral process should follow the guidelines described in Chapter 6. Additional time may be needed to ensure that the patient and caregiver clearly understand the reasons for the referral, the details of the appointment time and place, the kind of treatment that will be provided at that visit, and when the patient will be returning to the referring practice. Caution should be exercised, however, when the patient appears to need multiple specialty referrals. Bouncing from specialist to specialist, some of whom may make conflicting treatment suggestions and plans, can confuse, frustrate, and overwhelm the patient and often tends to fragment care. Given the choice between performance of a procedure, such as a root canal treatment, in the general dentist's office, with known surroundings and familiar staff, and referral to an endodontic practice, the patient may prefer the former, despite the greater experience and qualifications of the endodontist.

If the dentist determines that the patient's needs are too complex to be handled in a safe, professional manner in his or her practice, then it will be appropriate to refer the individual to another dentist for comprehensive care. Professionalism and common courtesy to the patient and caregiver require an examination and a proper referral with an accompanying letter. Hospitals, academic health centers, and dental offices specializing in the treatment of patients with complex needs are common referral sites.

Before dismissing a patient and making a referral to another dentist for total patient care, appropriate discussion with patient and caregiver about alternative treatment settings must occur. Patients with complex special needs and their caregivers may often feel ostracized and helpless. Isolated and handicapped by their physical and psychological problems, they sometimes have difficulty finding help and may have previously encountered rebuffs by unsympathetic healthcare providers. Referral to another dental practice may be perceived as just another rejection by a busy and detached dental team.

For these reasons, the dentist should carefully weigh the options before making such a referral. If the referral is truly warranted and in the best interests of the patient, then the dentist should personally explain the situation to the patient and caregiver, taking the time necessary to dispel any misunderstandings. An offer to provide additional assistance if the referral does not work out will ease the transition and help reaffirm the dentist's genuine concern to the patient and caregiver. If, after self-examination, the dentist determines that the referral is being made not because of patient safety or the dentist's level of expertise, but rather because of his or her own convenience or comfort, then the issue should be reconsidered.

Because most patients with special needs have rather basic dental treatment needs, their dental care is usually well within the scope of what the general dentist can provide. These patients and their caregivers, when informed, are usually understanding of the limitations of dental treatment and recognize the challenges that they present to the dental team. Most are not unusually demanding beyond the accommodations required by their disabilities. In many instances, they can be treated very effectively in a general dental practice setting, and this often will be their preference.

Phasing Treatment

As described in Chapter 5, comprehensive care involves several phases of treatment that are important to the care of each dental patient. The following section highlights the importance and relevance of each phase of care for the patient with special needs.

Systemic Phase

It can be anticipated that all special needs patients will require systemic phase management. For these patients, the focus will be to prevent medical emergencies in the dental office, provide dental care in a safe and efficient manner, and make appropriate accommodation for the patient's physical, mental, and/or behavioral limitations in the planning and delivery of dental care. Typical systemic phase issues include the following:

1. *Antibiotic prophylaxis* may be necessary for a variety of reasons, including patient risk of infective endocarditis; the presence of renal, ventriculoperitoneal, or ventriculoatrial shunts; or if the patient is severely immune compromised
2. *Anxiolytic premedication* may be needed for anxiety or behavioral control.
3. *Bleeding disorders:* Coagulation problems may be medication induced, as with Coumadin therapy, or disease related, as occurs with hemophilia A or von Willebrand's disease. At a minimum, these conditions will require presurgical coagulation consultation and management. (See section *Severe Coagulopathies*, earlier in this chapter.)
4. *Hemodynamic instability* may be associated with hypertension, congestive heart failure, atherosclerosis, coronary artery disease, or other conditions. Vasoconstrictors should be used with caution and vital signs recorded preoperatively and at appropriate intervals during treatment. Significant hemodynamic instability may necessitate performing extensive or invasive procedures in a hospital setting.
5. *Endocrine disorders*, such as diabetes, hypoglycemia, hyperthyroidism, and (medication-induced) cushingoid condition, may require modification to the dental plan of care.

Guidelines for managing these and other systemic conditions are discussed in Chapters 8 and 18.

Acute Phase

Patients with special needs may have acute oral healthcare needs. The diagnostic process for these problems is similar to that for routine dental patients, but as discussed earlier in this chapter, accommodation may be needed to manage the patient's specific physical or cognitive limitations. The timing and setting for delivering urgent dental care may also vary. For example, if a patient who is severely demented and uncooperative presents with a facial swelling and must be treated expeditiously then treatment under general anesthesia in the operating room may be warranted.

Disease Control Phase

Many patients with special needs have active oral infection or disease and will benefit from disease control therapies. Such patients may be appropriate candidates for comprehensive disease control phase therapy (discussed in detail in Chapter 10). As with acute phase therapy, treatment may need to be delivered in varying settings, depending on the patient's condition and ability to cooperate.

Holding Period [see also Chapter 5 Developing the Treatment Plan]

The concept of a holding period or "holding phase" may have particular application and relevance in the management of the patient with special care needs. The purpose of the holding period is to maintain a patient with recognized ongoing oral disease in a stable state, preventing further deterioration, until his or her overall physical condition allows further dental treatment to be provided. The holding period involves recognition of the fact that although the patient's oral condition is not ideal, because of physical, behavioral, or health-related constraints, it will be impractical or impossible to correct all of the problems. The emphasis is on *managing* oral disease in a way that preserves function to the extent possible and prevents further deterioration and maintains longevity of oral function despite ongoing and sometimes ever present oral disease. Urgent care needs are addressed as they arise. Preventive and maintenance therapies are integral to the holding phase. This phase may have a duration of many months, or even several years or for the life of the patient.

Such a patient is advanced to the definitive phase only after the dental team is satisfied that physical, behavioral, or health-related constraints have been alleviated, and the patient is able to undergo needed comprehensive restorative procedures. After recovery from a stroke or traumatic brain injury, for instance, the patient may become a good candidate for definitive phase care. The dental team must recognize, however, that relapse may occur. The general health or psychological issues that originally defined the special needs condition may recur, and the patient may once again need to be managed in a holding phase—in some cases, for the duration of life. Again, the patient's preventive trajectory is of key importance in the decision-making process.

Definitive Phase

This phase of care is reserved for those patients who have excellent oral home care, who have balanced and optimal dietary patterns, and who are sufficiently cooperative for the delivery of comprehensive dental procedures. In exceptional instances, at the request of interested family members or caregivers, definitive phase treatment may be provided to patients who do not fit these criteria. An example might be the passively uncooperative patient who has been unable to maintain an acceptable level of oral home care. Before definitive therapy is undertaken for this patient, a diagnosis must be made and explained to the caregivers, and a documented informed consent discussion should occur. During this discussion, the problematic prognosis must be made clear to the guardian and/or caregivers, along with the potential negative outcomes of implementing treatment under the current adverse circumstances.

Maintenance Phase

Preventive and oral health maintenance therapies are central components in the plan of care of any patient with special needs. The objectives of the maintenance phase of treatment for the special care patient are comparable to those for the able patient. Disease control and prevention of the occurrence of new disease are of paramount importance. The goal is to help the patient establish and maintain a pain-free, well-functioning, clean, and healthy oral condition in accordance with his or her wishes, circumstances, and abilities. In addition to providing preventive services, the dental team has the responsibility to inform and educate the patient and caregiver, providing realistic diagnostic and prognostic information.

Especially for the patient with special needs, this will be a dynamic process. Changes must be anticipated in the patient's physical or psychological condition, oral health, and level of cooperation and ability to perform oral home care procedures. As these changes occur—whether for better or worse—the dental team will need to adjust the approach and modify the preventive program accordingly.

Diligent and impeccable home oral healthcare can sometimes mitigate the ill effects of a cariogenic diet, but this is often difficult for the special needs patient to achieve. In many cases, the patient does not have the ability to carry out effective oral self-care procedures and is resistant to efforts by caregivers to assist. When a patient needs assistance with oral home care and is not responsible for his or her own dietary choices, it will be particularly important for the caregiver to modify a cariogenic diet Box 13.5 details dietary tips for patients and their caregivers. Serious efforts should be made daily to both reduce plaque and provide a non-cariogenic diet. But of the two, diet may actually be the more important variable in the long run.

It is worth noting that all education relative to diet, oral healthcare, and habits should be given with the realization that the caregiver may have already attempted multiple strategies relating to these issues. It will be important for dental team members to listen carefully to patient and caregiver stories and creatively design preventive strategies that take that information into account.

Maintenance intervals are established on the basis of the patient's oral health status, disease activity, and level of assistance from family and caregivers. Two- to three-month recall intervals are often appropriate for this type of patient. Guidelines on what should be addressed at the periodic visit are detailed in

Chapter 12. Specific health or systemic problems, vulnerabilities to oral health problems, and susceptibility to specific oral diseases and problems will need the attention of the dental team at each periodic visit. Patients requiring special care are more likely to require reevaluation, management, or treatment of many different oral problems.

Specific maintenance phase procedures and processes are detailed in Chapter 12 of this text. Some techniques and methods of particular application to the special needs population are noted here. Electric toothbrushes, prescription-strength fluoride toothpaste, chlorhexidine rinses, stannous fluoride gels, and fluoride varnishes can be useful and effective adjuncts to the preventive plan. Finger brushes, interproximal (proxy) brushes, interdental stimulators, sulcular brushes, and floss aids should be prescribed when needed to assist with plaque control. Mints and gum with xylitol to replace cariogenic candies and sweets can be helpful in managing the patient with active caries.

As discussed earlier in this chapter, providing patient and caregiver education is also an important role for the dental team. A daily oral care plan should be developed by the dental team and communicated to caregivers to ensure optimization of the patient's oral health. Proper diet and oral home care are issues that must be reinforced at each periodic visit. In addition to verbal directions, it is helpful to provide written instructions regarding oral home care procedures, diet modification, and habit cessation to the patient and caregiver.

Caregivers are typically familiar with the physical limitations of the patient but may be less aware of how those limitations affect the patient's oral condition. It is important for the dental team to provide the caregivers with specific oral healthcare strategies and techniques that compensate for or overcome the patient's limitations. Mouth props, good lighting, and, sometimes, portable suctioning devices can be prescribed to assist caregivers in the daily oral care of the patient. The caregiver should be informed as to the limits of the dental treatment that can be provided to the patient. At times, the patient may become frustrated that the dental team cannot do more to help. In those circumstances, the informed caregiver can be an effective ombudsman and educator on behalf of the dental team. Periodically, caregivers change. When this occurs, the new caregiver will need to be engaged and educated by the dental team.

Encouragement and emotional support provided to the patient and caregiver are crucial and often mean the difference between the success or failure of the maintenance program.

Informed Consent

Acquiring informed consent is often challenging with patients who have special care needs. In the process of developing and establishing informed consent, the dental team must be prepared to interface with a variety of individuals, including family members, caregivers, legal representatives, physicians, and social workers. As with all patients, persons with special needs must have a complete understanding of the diagnoses and treatment alternatives, and their risks and benefits, as well as the costs in time, effort, and money for the proposed treatment. In some instances, however, the patient is legally competent but clinically unable to participate in a dental treatment decision—for example, the patient who is in an early stage of dementia. In such a circumstance, the primary caregiver, responsible family member, and/or legal representative must be brought into the discussion. All parties to the decision making should be informed of treatment risks, benefits, and alternatives and involved in the consent discussion. This may become problematic if different family members have varying ideas as to what dental treatment, if any, should be provided. The dentist may need to become both the patient's advocate and the mediator in this discussion.

In some situations, the caregiver or patient declines the recommended treatment. In other circumstances, the patient's physical or mental limitations may preclude provision of the treatment that the patient or caregiver requests. In either of these scenarios, the patient and caregiver must be informed of the potential risks of possible negative outcomes *in the absence* of treatment.

If a portion of the proposed treatment would involve referral to another dental professional, this information must be included in the consent discussion. Similarly, if the necessity for sedation or general anesthesia is anticipated, or if procedures must be performed in a hospital setting, a specific consent for these eventualities must be provided.

The consent process is dependent on the decision-making capacities and legal status of the patient. The decision-making capabilities of patients can be categorized under one of four descriptions. The dental team can expect to work with persons in each of these groups:
1. Legally competent with decision-making capacity
2. Legally competent with impaired decision-making capacity
3. Legally incompetent with decision-making capacity
4. Legally incompetent with impaired or no decision-making capacity

The individuals in categories 3 and 4 will usually have had a legal representative appointed (see *Ethical and Legal Issues*, later in this chapter), and the dental team must work with this individual to obtain informed consent.

A patient in category 2 may pose a particular challenge if he or she has not named a durable power of attorney for healthcare (HCPOA). The patient may have difficulty understanding treatment alternatives, and it may be unclear who should make treatment decisions on his or her behalf. Most often, clinicians turn to immediate family members to participate in decision making. Lack of agreement between family members can complicate the process of decision making. Often, an effective strategy will be to encourage the surrogate decision makers to focus on what they believe the patient would want, rather than what they would want for themselves. This process of substituted judgment may help to reduce conflicts between family members and help all parties to arrive at a mutually agreeable plan of care that is ultimately in the patient's best interest.

If the dental team is concerned that the patient is unable to render a decision about treatment, and family members continue to be in conflict about the decision making, then pursuing guardianship is a logical step. The process of obtaining guardianship, particularly by a family member, can be time consuming, costly, and stressful. Related legal issues are discussed in more detail in the section *Ethical and Legal Issues*, later in this chapter.

DELIVERY OF CARE

Appointment Scheduling

When scheduling appointments for the patient, the dental team should be as sensitive to the caregiver's schedule as is feasible, recognizing that times when it is convenient for the caregiver to bring the patient to the dental office may be limited. On the other hand, the caregiver should be advised as to the effect that any scheduling limitations may have on care. For example, if the caregiver for a severely developmentally disabled adult with many carious lesions requiring immediate attention can only bring the patient at sporadic intervals, it must be made clear that treatment outcome may not be as predictable or effective, and that the patient is at greater risk for acute oral problems and infection than if he or she could be seen in a more expeditious manner.

Many other factors may affect the scheduling, timing, and duration of the patient's appointments, including transportation availability, coordination with other healthcare providers, predictable times during the day when the patient is more cooperative, and the patient's stamina and endurance. Inevitably, appointments with special needs patients require more time.

Patient Positioning and Transfer
Precautions With Transfers

To prevent injury, each patient must be assessed individually before attempting a transfer. Some physical considerations may make a transfer challenging. Urinary catheters must be handled gently and transferred before the patient or along with the patient, or else the catheter may be displaced from its location. Sore joints and bandaged limbs, must be handled with great care so as not to further injure the patient during transfer.

If the dental team is performing or anticipates performing transfers, it may be beneficial to bring in a physical therapist to provide instruction in doing transfers safely, including ways of preventing and caring for back strains or injury should they arise.

Patients Who Are Gurney-Bound

If possible, it is preferable to move the patient from the gurney to the dental chair. This can be accomplished with a self-transfer (and sliding board), one-person transfer, two-person transfer, or lift. Techniques are comparable with those described under *Patients Using Wheelchairs*. If necessary, most procedures can be provided with the patient on the gurney. The dental unit hoses must be long enough to accommodate over-the-gurney delivery. Ergonomics are not ideal, as the dentist and assistant will usually need to bend over to access the patient's oral cavity.

Patients Using Wheelchairs

Many patients with special needs arrive in wheelchairs. (See Video 13.2 Anatomy of a Standard Wheelchair on ebooks+.) The most convenient wheelchairs for dental treatment are those that are fully mechanized and tilt back into an ergonomically stable treatment position similar to the position of an inclined dental chair. Some wheelchairs can be tilted back manually, or a wheelchair tilt device can be used. (See Video 13.3 Use of a Wheelchair Tilt Device on ebooks+.) If the wheelchair does not have a headrest, the dentist may use a portable headrest to facilitate comfort and positioning. If the dental chair cannot be moved, then the hoses on the unit typically need to be lengthened to accommodate chair positioning (Figure 13.3).

Transfers from a wheelchair to a dental chair. Some patients can self-transfer from the wheelchair to the dental chair independently or with assistance. If the patient is unable to self-transfer, several other options are available.

One-person transfer. A single individual can transfer most patients. To use this technique, the patient must be able to support his or her own weight on at least one leg. The key to this technique is weight distribution and transfer. The wheelchair is parked at approximately a 45-degree angle to the dental chair, and the brakes are engaged. The patient is asked to move as far forward in the chair as possible. A transfer belt is placed around the patient, and the dentist braces the patient's knees against his or her own. On the count of three, the patient stands as the dentist pulls, using leg strength, and pivots the patient onto the dental chair. It is critically important for the dentist to use his or her weight to relocate the patient's weight in a controlled manner into the chair. Lightweight individuals can transfer very heavy patients using mechanical advantage and proper form. (See Video 13.4 Transferring a Patient Using the Single-Person Technique on ebooks+.)

Two-person transfer. If the patient is unable to support any weight on his or her legs, a lift is ideally used, but, in the absence of a lift, a two-person transfer can be attempted. It is important to recognize that there are inherent risks in the two-person transfer. The possibility of back injury in susceptible individuals should be considered before attempting this transfer. With this technique, the dental chair and wheelchair are positioned so that both face the same direction, with the wheelchair parallel with and positioned as close to the dental chair as possible. The dental chair should be positioned slightly lower than the wheelchair to allow gravity to assist as the patient is transferred. The arm rails, footrests, and headrest of the dental chair should be removed to provide a clear path for transfer. The brakes on the wheelchair need to be engaged. The individual standing behind the patient locks his or her arms under the arms of the patient, and the second individual cradles the knees. At the count of three, the patient is lifted and transferred to the dental chair. *(Please note that the patient's arthritis or other musculoskeletal disease may preclude being grasped as described, making this type of transfer infeasible.)* (See Video 13.5 Transferring a Patient Using the Two-Person Technique on ebooks+.)

At the conclusion of the visit, the process is reversed, with the dental chair seat positioned slightly higher than the level of the wheelchair seat.

Sliding board. A sliding board may allow an individual to self-transfer to the dental chair. The dental chair is positioned and prepared similarly to preparations for a two-person transfer. A smooth wooden board is slid under the patient, and the patient then grasps a fixed object on the dental chair and pulls himself or herself onto the dental chair. (See Video 13.6 Transferring a Patient Using a Sliding Board on ebooks+.)

Lifts. A lift is the best way to transfer the individual who cannot transfer with a one-person assist and is too heavy for a two-person transfer. A lift is also safer if the dental team members are not sure that they are physically strong enough to transfer a particular patient. A lift is a mechanically or electrically powered hoist that raises the patient completely out of the wheelchair (or gurney) to be reseated in the dental chair.

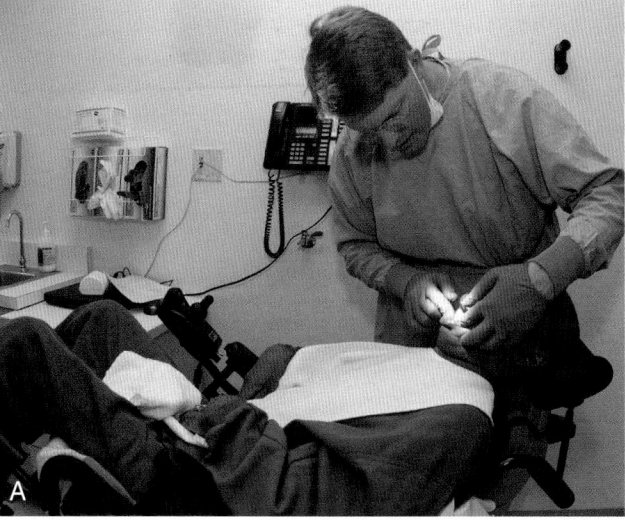 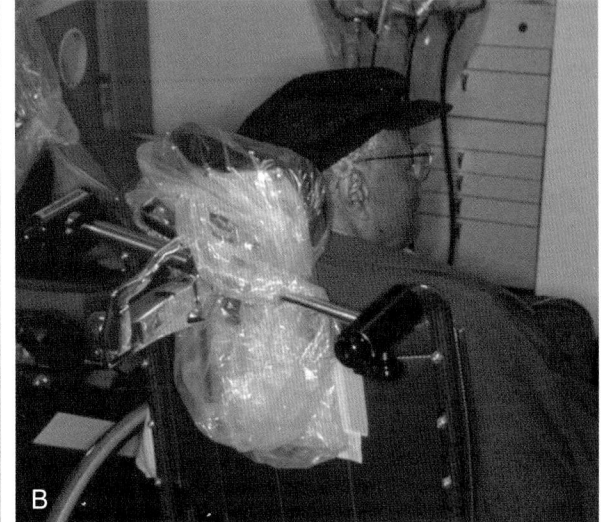

FIG. 13.3 A, The patient receiving treatment is seated in a fully mechanized wheelchair. Note: the doctor has pulled down his mask to facilitate communication with the patient to reduce his anxiety. **B,** A portable headrest can be attached to a wheelchair to facilitate treatment.

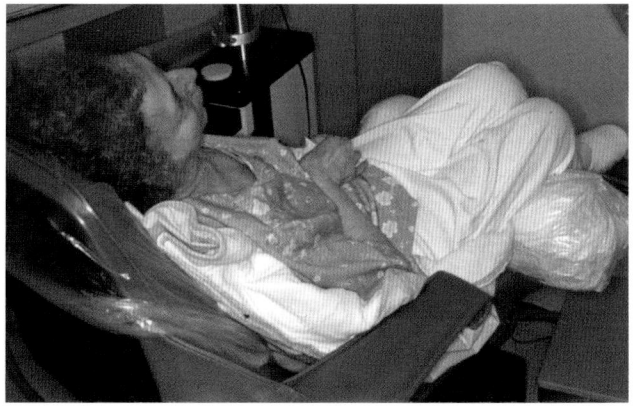

FIG. 13.4 Cushions may be used to support the patient in a comfortable and safe position while treatment is performed.

Supports

Once the patient has been transferred, he or she may require supports under certain limbs or all limbs because of contractures or awkward postures caused by disease (e.g., kyphosis). Pillows or other supports can be placed under the knees, feet, arms, lower back, and neck, enabling the patient to remain comfortable for the lengthy periods of time required (Figure 13.4).

Posture

A patient may be treated either seated or prone, depending on physical condition. Severe congestive heart failure or pulmonary disease often precludes a patient's lying flat, which places the lungs in a dependent position. Severe spinal arthritic disease (i.e., ankylosing spondylitis) may preclude a supine treatment position as well. An individual with lower back pain may need to be treated in a supine position.

Restraints

If the patient is not cooperative, he or she may require restraint. Chemical or physical restraint may be used. Please note that it is extremely difficult to restrain some patients depending on strength, size, and general demeanor. Chemical restraints typically involve benzodiazepines or other sedative/hypnotics. Physical restraint ranges from manually restraining a patient to papoose boards. It is essential to inform family members or the legal guardian as to the kinds of restraint that are planned. Informed consent must be obtained.

Communication With Special Care Patients

Some patients with special care needs may have difficulty communicating normally. The underlying problem may be a lack of comprehension, difficulty with sentence formulation, or impairment of the ability to articulate speech. Depending on the nature of the problem, signing, writing tablets, a computer, or communication boards can be used to converse with the patient. Maintaining eye contact with the patient is essential. Nonverbal communication can be a very effective tool in making the patient aware of your concern and attention. Moreover, a family member or caregiver can occasionally "translate" the

patient's signs, voice inflections, or utterances. The caregiver can be of invaluable assistance in facilitating the communication process by helping the dental team understand the patient's concerns and questions and conveying or reinforcing information from the dental team to the patient. Patients with hearing or visual impairment can be challenging to communicate with effectively. According to the American with Disabilities Act, hospitals and other medical facilities must provide effective means of communication for those individuals who are hearing or visually impaired. Sign language interpreters, oral interpreters, cued speech interpreters, and computer-assisted real time transcription can be utilized for those who are deaf. Qualified readers, Braille, or large print might be used for the visually impaired.[25]

Role of the Family

Family members may be either a great asset or a great liability to the dentist-patient therapeutic relationship. Often, a family member is the primary caregiver for the patient, taking care of most, if not all, of the patient's physical and emotional needs. This dedication and perseverance in providing care to a loved one can monumentally improve the patient's health and quality of life, but can also be an emotionally draining and frustrating duty. It can be difficult, having known the family member intimately for many years and remembering what a productive and engaging person he or she may have been, and now having to watch and be intimately involved in the slow, continuing decline of a once-vibrant person. Fatigued, emotionally charged, and in some cases depressed, the family member may have difficulty participating in the decision making in a positive way and may not have the physical stamina to provide the needed oral home care for the patient. Despite these limitations, and often sustained by latent guilt or a passionate sense of duty, the family member may be unwilling to relinquish any part of the caregiver role.

Faced with this situation, the dental team may be able to fill a valuable role in helping the "burned out" family member to find some relief. Working with a social worker or other family members or encouraging the family member and caregiver to temporarily hire a professional caregiver, may provide some much-needed recovery time. If the family member can be reenergized and reinvigorated in the caregiver role, then the benefit to the patient in improved oral and general health can be significant.

Role of the Patient's Caregiver

As a result of their mental or physical disabilities, many patients with special needs cannot fully take care of themselves. Unable to perform the ADLs, a decision is made by the patient, family, or social service agency to obtain assistance. A caregiver—who may be a parent, child, other family member, friend, nurse's aide, or other healthcare professional—is appointed, hired, or volunteers to fill this role. It is imperative that the dental team enlist the help of the patient's daily caregiver or caregivers. In many instances, the patient may become more cooperative if the caregiver is in the room or close by. The caregiver's voice alone may calm an apprehensive patient. A caregiver can assist with gentle restraint if necessary. As emphasized throughout this chapter, the dental team must educate the caregiver about the condition of the patient's mouth and how best to take care of the teeth, oral structures, and dental appliances. Caregivers play an essential role in implementing the daily oral care plan of those they care for.

Several points are worth considering when giving the caregiver instructions on how to provide oral home care for the patient. The dental team should not assume that the caregiver has a good grasp of oral home care techniques. Appropriate time should be taken to explain all the nuances and details. The caregiver should be encouraged in return to demonstrate each of the techniques to confirm that he or she understands and can successfully carry out the necessary procedures. The team should also make themselves available to the caregiver by phone or via a HIPAA compliant electronic communication platform, in case there are questions. With such an opportunity for follow-up, the caregiver is more likely to pursue rather than abort home oral care efforts when challenges arise. Follow-up telephone conversations (or return office visits) can fill in knowledge gaps, such as when the caregiver nodded in agreement during the instructional session, but when at home "cannot quite remember how to do it." Telephone contact can also be beneficial when the caregiver, for whatever reason, has been reluctant to ask questions of the dental team in the patient's presence.

Involving the patient's caregiver in the treatment planning and decision making is also helpful. The caregiver may have insight into the practical aspects of how the treatment can be carried out and maintained. The caregiver is more likely to accept responsibility for the delivery of oral preventive care if he or she is involved at the initial decision-making stage and understands the negative outcomes that may result from the treatment or the decision to not treat. The caregiver must be apprised of limitations, risks, and alternatives for dental care. It is helpful for the caregiver to be alerted to any oral conditions that may need urgent treatment.

Included here is a simple classification system for assessing need for assistance that can be useful for caregivers and any healthcare providers who work with special needs patients. The dentist or hygienist classifies the patient based on the individual's cognitive and functional level. Note that this classification may change over time—for example, the patient with traumatic brain injury whose condition improves over time in rehabilitation.

The classes are as follows:
1. Requires no assistance with daily oral care, is cognitively and physically able to carry out a plan for daily oral care
2. Requires assistance, needs help with daily oral care, but can complete some care independently
3. Requires full assistance; is unable to carry out any oral self-care

The usefulness of this classification is in the specific delineation of the kinds of oral home care procedures that can be carried out by the patient or caregiver, or that will be shared. Once a designation of responsibilities is established, the dental team

---

BOX 13.12   Signs of Elder Abuse

- **Physical Abuse** occurs when an elder is injured, assaulted or threatened with a weapon, or inappropriately restrained.
- **Sexual Abuse or Abusive Sexual Contact** is any sexual contact against an elder's will. This includes acts in which the elder is unable to understand the act or is unable to communicate.
- **Psychological or Emotional Abuse** occurs when an elder experiences trauma after exposure to threatening acts or coercive tactics. Examples include humiliation or embarrassment; controlling behavior ; social isolation; disregarding or trivializing needs; or damaging or destroying property.
- **Neglect** is the failure or refusal of a caregiver or other responsible person to provide for an elder's basic physical, emotional, or social needs, or failure to protect them from harm.
- **Self-neglect** occurs when vulnerable elders fail or refuse to address their own basic physical, emotional, or social needs.
- **Abandonment** is the willful desertion of an elderly person by caregiver or other responsible person.
- **Financial Abuse or Exploitation** is the unauthorized or improper use of the resources of an elder for monetary or personal benefit, profit, or gain.

From Centers for Disease Control and Prevention, National Center for Injury Prevention and Control, Division of Violence Prevention. http://www.cdc.gov/violenceprevention/elderabuse/definitions.html. Accessed November 17, 2015.

---

must be prepared to revisit the issue at subsequent appointments. As the patient's condition improves or deteriorates, the roles of patient and caregiver will need to change as well.

It is important to note that the stress of daily caregiving is generally high, and caregivers may develop health problems of their own. It is imperative that the dental team be aware of this potential problem and sensitive to the caregiver's attitudes and demeanor. The caregiver's role is critical to the oral health and well-being of the patient, so supporting and encouraging the caregiver becomes just as important as providing care directly to the patient.

The dental team also must be aware that, because of the high level of stress in the caregiver's role, elder abuse may occur. The dentist, hygienist, and all staff need to be cognizant of the indicators of elder abuse (Box 13.12). When the dental team becomes aware of signs or symptoms of elder abuse, the primary focus must be on the well-being of the patient. It is incumbent on the team to report such findings to a local social services agency or law enforcement authorities.

Other Professional Resources

Management of the patient with a high degree of impairment will often require a complex, multidimensional approach to oral and general healthcare. At times, the dental team will interface with allied health, social services, and pharmacy professionals. Professionals and paraprofessionals with whom the dental team may need to interact, and their respective roles, are described here and discussed in detail in Chapter 6.

Social Workers

Sometimes referred to as a *case manager*, a social worker can often provide essential support to the patient/client, caregiver, and family. When the patient, the patient's family or friends, or the community at large becomes aware that an individual is no longer able to effectively provide for his or her own daily needs, a social worker is often called to assist. The social worker's role typically includes locating, activating, and facilitating the provision of medical care, social services, transportation, home care, and assisted living or nursing home care as needed for the patient. Such individuals are skilled in identifying funding sources, such as private insurance, public assistance, religious groups, nonprofit charitable organizations. In so doing, they help patients meet basic needs, improve quality of life, and identify resources to pay for oral and general healthcare. Social workers can also provide valuable medical, social, and financial information about the patient to the dental team.

Physician Assistants

Physician assistants (PAs) are healthcare professionals licensed to practice medicine under the supervision of a physician. PAs (usually medical, not surgical, PAs) frequently provide direct patient care in facilities such as nursing homes or group homes. They can provide detailed medical information and may write medical orders for their patients.

Registered Nurses

Registered nurses (RNs) work closely with physicians and can provide valuable medical information. The director of nursing (DON) and the assistant director of nursing (ADON) are often the primary medical contacts for physicians and dentists providing care in nursing home facilities.

Licensed Practical Nurses

A licensed practical nurse (LPN) is a nurse who has been trained to provide home health or nursing care under the supervision of a nurse with a higher level certification (RN) or a medical doctor. These individuals, along with nurse's aides, provide direct patient care, such as oral cleansing.

Nurse's Aides/Assistants

Nursing assistants work directly with patients, providing assistance with activities of daily living, including oral home care.

Pharmacists

Pharmacists can provide valuable information on drug interactions and contraindications. The dental team can contact the patient's pharmacist to obtain a listing of the individual's medications. Pharmacists can also be an excellent resource, suggesting strategies for improving the patient's compliance in taking the medications and improving the drug efficacy. Some pharmacists can also compound drugs as prescribed by the dentist when commercial drugs are not available or when custom formulations will better suit the patient's needs.

Audiologists/Speech and Language Pathologists

Patients with a suspected hearing deficit can often benefit from the services of an audiologist. Patients who have had a stroke or suffered head trauma may commonly have speech and swallowing difficulties that may be improved, mitigated, or corrected by working with a speech pathologist. An improved ability to communicate with the patient can have multiple benefits for the dental team and will make the provision of oral healthcare services both more efficient and more effective. Swallowing safely will allow the patient a higher quality of life, improve affect nutritional intake, and facilitate safe dental procedures while minimizing aspiration risks.

ETHICAL AND LEGAL ISSUES

Several important legal issues are associated with the delivery of care to special needs patients. In most instances, informed consent can be obtained only from an individual who is at least 18 years of age, has the capacity for decision making, and is informed about the proposed treatment. The consent to treatment must be voluntary. As discussed previously, a variety of conditions may result in an individual's being unable to make rational decisions on his or her own behalf. In an ideal situation, the person will have previously contemplated the possibility of becoming incapacitated and formalized his or her wishes for future healthcare in one or more documents known as **advance directives**. Advance directives are legally recognized documents containing instructions as to how an individual wishes his or her medical and health decisions to be handled in the event that he or she becomes incapacitated. In the United States, advance directives can be generated by any individual older than 18 years with the mental capacity to do so. It is certainly preferable to have such intentions documented before admission to a hospital. If the patient becomes mentally incapacitated, as in a motor vehicle accident, and is hospitalized without having written advance directives, the patient's wishes may not be discernable—or family members may have varying perceptions about those wishes—leaving caregivers, family, and medical personnel in a moral or ethical quandary. Patients with degenerative or chronic illnesses are strongly encouraged to implement advance directives.

The **living will** is one form of an advance directive. A typical living will describes the specific types of care the person wishes to receive in the event that he or she becomes permanently or irreversibly unconscious or is considered terminally or irreversibly ill. Often, the living will specifies what type of life support (oxygen, respirator, feeding tube), resuscitative efforts, or pain control is desired or not desired. Although most advance directives do not contemplate dental care, the patient's preferences for treatment or nontreatment can become relevant to the delivery of dental care if a patient suffers a stroke, cardiac arrest, or other life-threatening event while undergoing dental treatment in a hospital setting. If such a medical emergency arises during the course of dental treatment in a general dental practice setting, the patient is typically transported to the hospital, and the advance directives would not become relevant until the patient transfer is complete.

After discussion with the patient and/or family, doctor's orders can be written for the patient that govern how the medical and dental staff will handle certain prespecified health-related conditions and circumstances. Examples of such doctors' orders are as follows:

- **Do not intubate (DNI)** directs that the patient will not have any breathing apparatus inserted into the trachea to control breathing should respiratory arrest occur.
- **Do not resuscitate (DNR)** means that no advanced cardiac life support or basic cardiopulmonary resuscitation (CPR) will be rendered in the event of cardiopulmonary arrest.
- **Full code** means that the patient desires advanced life support in addition to basic life support in the event of cardiopulmonary arrest.

A DNR order could become relevant during a medical emergency in a dental office. (See the related *In Clinical Practice: Physician Orders Related to Resuscitation* box.)

IN CLINICAL PRACTICE

Physician Orders Related to Resuscitation

Nursing home residents and other patients may have a physician's order stating DNR/DNI or Do Not Resuscitate and Do Not Intubate. This order needs to be respected, and a copy of the DNR/DNI sheet needs to be in the dental chart. A DNR/DNI order signifies that CPR should not be instituted in case of cardiac arrest. This decision is generally made by the patient or the patient's legal representatives (e.g., HCPOA, legal guardian).

Consent forms for dental and medical treatment, particularly in the hospital setting, may ask the patient or legal representative to mark whether to suspend or continue the DNR/DNI, depending on the setting in which the care is provided and the particular treatment the patient is receiving.

A discussion with the patient, the patient's physician, and the patient's family, where appropriate, should occur before treatment to make certain all involved are clear about what to do in case of an emergency in the treatment setting that might require CPR. Also, the DNR/DNI order sheet MUST be present at any appointment. A simple order in a chart is NOT the same as a DNR/DNI order sheet (Figure 13.5).

As described in Chapter 7, once a patient has named a designated guardian or a sanctioned and active durable HCPOA, then that person (or agency) named in that document must approve the dental plan of care and provide consent for future dental treatment.

There are two special circumstances in which the dental team (with the caregiver) can make independent decisions on behalf of a patient who is legally incompetent. These relate to a situation in which the patient requires urgent dental treatment for a potentially life-threatening problem (such as an acute dental abscess or infection of a facial space) and either (1) the patient does not have a surrogate decision maker or (2) the surrogate decision maker cannot be contacted. In either case, the *best-interest standard* or *substituted-judgment standard* can be

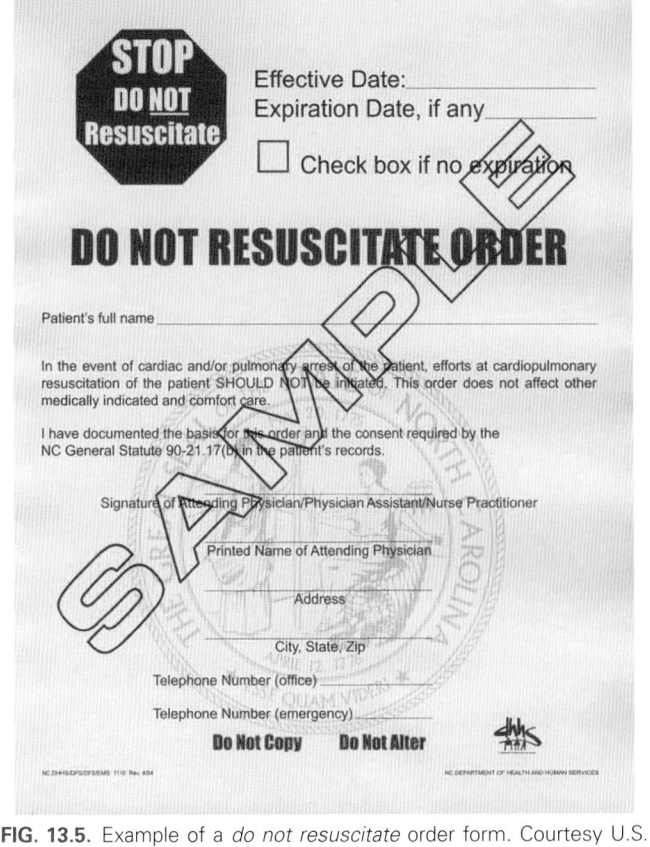

FIG. 13.5. Example of a *do not resuscitate* order form. Courtesy U.S. Department of Health & Human Services.

used to make a treatment decision. The decision must also be made in terms of any advance directives the patient may have in place (see Chapters 7 and 18 for further discussion).

CONCLUSION

When treating patients with special needs, it is important to develop a caring, strategic, and professional approach that is both realistic and flexible. This population has a diverse set of oral and general health needs. The assessment, diagnosis, treatment planning, and delivery of dental treatment for these patients will necessitate the use of special resources, techniques, and strategies on the part of the dental team. Although the team may be challenged to identify creative and individual solutions for the patient's unique needs and problems, the provision of oral healthcare in a compassionate and professional manner will have inestimable benefit to the patient, the patient's family, and caregivers. It can also be rewarding for dental team members. The benefits of such care go far beyond the dental team's primary goal of improving the patient's oral condition. High-quality oral healthcare delivered in a compassionate manner affirms the patient's humanity and can provide some peace of mind to those who care for the patient day by day.

REVIEW QUESTIONS

- Who are dental patients with special needs?
- What is the role of the general dentist in the diagnosis, management, and treatment of the patient with special needs?
- How does patient evaluation differ between the patient with special needs and the "typical" dental patient?
- What are some unique aspects to treatment planning for dental patients with special needs?
- Describe management strategies when treating patients with:
  Developmental delay
  Traumatic brain injury
  Terminal cancer (hospice)

  AIDS
  Severe coagulopathies
- What is the role of the patient's family in the management of a dental patient with special needs?
- What is the role of the caregiver in the delivery of dental care to a patient with special needs?
- Demonstrate a one-person and a two-person wheelchair-to-dental-chair transfer.
- What ethical and legal issues must be considered when treating a dental patient with special needs?

PRACTICE ASSESSMENT

Does your practice have a plan for managing patients with special needs?

Is there a policy regarding how patients with specific disabilities will be managed (include criteria for whom you will treat, and when and where to refer)?

Does the policy include staff roles and functions when treating patients with disabilities?

Does the office have appropriate (ADA Compliant) physical accommodations?

Do all members of the dental team espouse, believe and exercise person centered care in all of their patient related activities?

REFERENCES

1. Older Americans 2020 Federal Interagency Forum on Aging Related Statistics https://agingstats.gov/docs/LatestReport/OA20_508_10142020.pdf. Accessed February 9, 2021.
2. Katz PR. An international perspective on long term care: focus on nursing homes. *J Am Med Dir Assoc.* 2011;12:487–492.
3. Jaber MA. Dental caries experience, oral health status and treatment needs of dental patients with autism. *J Applied Oral Sci.* 2011;19(3):212–217.
4. Rojas CF, Wichowska-Rymarek K, Pavlic A, Vinereanu A, Fabjanska K, Kaschke I, Marks L. Oral health needs of athletes with intellectual disability in Eastern Europe: Poland, Romania and Slovenia. *Int Dent J.* 2016;66(2):113–119.
5. Makkar A, Indushekar KR, Saraf BG, Sardana D, Sheoran N. A cross sectional study to evaluate the oral health status of children with intellectual disabilities in the National Capital Region of India (Delhi-NCR). *J Intellect Disabil Res.* 2019;63(1):31–39.
7. Anders PL, Davis EL. Oral health of patients with intellectual disabilities: a systematic review. *Spec Care Dentist.* 2010;30:110–117.
8. Kumar M, Chandu GN, Shafiulla MD. Oral health status and treatment needs in institutionalized psychiatric patients: One year descriptive cross sectional study. *Indian J Dent Res.* 2006;17(4):171–177.
9. Seidel-Bittke D. Oral healthcare for patients with disabilities. *Dent Today.* 2005;24(3):56–59.
10. Mitsea AG, Karidis AG, Donta-Bakoyianni C, Spyropoulos ND. Oral health status in Greek children and teenagers, with disabilities. *J Ped Dent.* 2001;26(1):111–118.
11. Horner-Johnson W, Dobbertin K. Dental insurance and dental care among working age adults; differences by type and complexity of disability. *J Public Health Dent.* 2016;76(4):330–339.
12. Mahmoudi E, Meade MA. Disparities in access to health care among adults with physical disabilities:analysis of representative national sample for a ten-year period. *Disabil Health J.* 2015;8(2):182–190.
13. Gordon SM, Dionne RA, Snyder J. Dental fear and anxiety as a barrier to accessing oral health care among patients with special health care needs. *Spec Care Dent.* 1998;18:88–92.
14. Stiefel DJ. Dental care considerations for disabled adults. *Spec Care Dent.* 2002;22(3 Suppl):S26–S39.
15. Dolan T, Atchison K, et al. Access to dental care among older adults in the United States. *J Dent Educ.* 2005;69(9):961–975.
16. Specialist Advisory Committee for Special Care Dentistry: *Faculty of Dental Surgery. The Royal College of Surgeons of England. Specialty Training Curriculum, 2012.* http://www.gdc-uk.org/Dentalprofessionals/Specialistlist/Documents/SpecialCareDentistryCurriculum2012.pdf/. Accessed February 24, 2015.
17. Guidance on the 2010 Standards for Accessible Design. https://www.ada.gov/regs2010/2010ADAStandards/Guidance2010ADAstandards.htm Accessed December 17, 2020.
18. Center for Medicaid and Medicare Services: *Medicare dental coverage.* http://www.cms.gov/Medicare/Coverage/MedicareDentalCoverage/index.html?redirect/MedicareDentalCoverage/. Accessed December 17, 2020.
19. Official U.S. Government Site for Medicare: *Your medical coverage: dental services.* https://www.medicare.gov/coverage/dental-servicesAccessed December 17, 2020.
20. Klasser G, Leeuw R. Self-report health questionnaire: a necessary and reliable tool in dentistry. *Gen Dent.* 2005;53(5):348–354.
21. Malamed S. *Sedation: a guide to patient management.* ed 6 St Louis: Mosby; 2017.
22. Howard WR. Nitrous oxide in the dental environment: assessing the risk, reducing the exposure. *J Am Dent Assoc.* 1997;128(3):356–360.
23. Rowland AS, Baird DD, et al. Nitrous oxide and spontaneous abortion in female dental assistants. *Am J Epidemiol.* 1995;141(6):531–538.
24. Szymanska J. Environmental health risk of chronic exposure to nitrous oxide in dental practice. *Ann Agric Environ Med.* 2001;8:119–122.
25. US Department of Justice, Civil Rights Division, Disability Rights Section; Effective Communication, ADA Requirements Bulletin 2014.

SUGGESTED READINGS

Americans with Disabilities Act Standards for Accessible Design. https://www.ada.gov/2010ADAstandards_index.htm Accessed September 9, 2021.

Centers for Medicare and Medicaid services. http://www.cms.hhs.gov/. Accessed September 9, 2021.

UNC Carolina Institute for Developmental Disabilities http://www.cidd.unc.edu/ (accessed 9/21/2021)

Hooyman NR, et al. *Social gerontology: a multidisciplinary perspective.* ed 10 NY, New York: Pearson; 2021.

Little JW, Miller C, Rhodus NL, Falace D:. *Dental management of the medically compromised patient.* ed 9 St Louis: Elsevier; 2018.

Odom SL, Horner RH, Snell ME, Blacher J, eds. *Handbook of developmental disabilities.* New York, NY: Guilford Press; 2007.

Patton LL, Glick M. *The ADA Practical Guide to Patients with Medical Conditions.* ed 2 Hoboken: John Wiley and Sons, Inc.; 2016.

Orient J. *Sapira's Art and Science of Bedside Diagnosis.* ed. 5 Philadelphia: Wolter; 2018.

Saunders MJ, Martin WE:. *Developing a dental program for the nursing home facility: a manual for dental office staff.* ed 3 Texas: American Society for Geriatric Dentistry and SWAP-C/STGEC at UTHSCSA; 2005.

14

Patients Who Are Substance Dependent

John William Claytor Jr., Romesh P. Nalliah, and Stephen Stefanac

 Visit eBooks.Health.Elsevier.com

OUTLINE

INTRODUCTION

A patient who engages in alcohol abuse or the abuse of other substances presents significant problems to themselves, their healthcare providers, and to society. These problems are prevalent in many countries worldwide.[1] **Substance use disorders** are common and cause significant social, psychological, and health problems among users and those around them. The substance-abusing patient is more likely to suffer from a variety of physical, psychological, and oral problems and presents unique challenges that will call on skills and sensitivities that are not regularly required of the dental team.

The purpose of this chapter is to discuss ways in which the general dentist and care team can recognize alcohol and other substance abuse in patients, how they can contribute to addiction management support in those patients, and how they can plan and safely carry out the treatment needed to rehabilitate and maintain the oral health of the patient who is actively using and those who are in recovery.

CHALLENGES FOR THE DENTIST

The dental practitioner will face many challenges and frustrations in the management of the patient who abuses alcohol or other substances. Both the active and the recovering user typically bring many fears and some measure of guilt to the dental setting.[2] The recovering user may fear uncontrolled pain or exhibit an underlying anxiety of relapse into substance abuse. The individual may be concerned that they will be treated differently and that the dentist and staff will be judgmental about the addiction, the individual's appearance, oral condition, and/or lack of oral self-care. The active substance user may contrive elaborate fabrications to explain their neglected oral health, chronic lateness, or missed dental appointments. Such patients will often deny responsibility for their poor oral health and may exhibit argumentative behavior, have difficulty sitting still, and need frequent bathroom breaks: behaviors that can cover for drug use during the dental appointment.[2]

Recognition of Patient Substance Abuse

Early identification of substance abuse is important to prevent injury to and even death for the patient. Dentists may see these patients before other healthcare professionals and thus have an excellent opportunity to assist the patient in recognizing and confronting a substance abuse problem. In such a situation, the dentist can provide substance abuse prevention information and direct the patient to a substance abuse evaluation and treatment center or a substance abuse professional. The dental team can also screen for potential liver disease, prolonged bleeding, delayed wound healing, or other systemic conditions that can influence dental care and are often seen with substance abusing patients.

The substance-abusing patient, particularly the active user, may not be forthcoming about their medical and drug history. It is not unusual for these patients to be defensive, evasive, and untruthful in communicating health-related information to the dentist. If the individual has a history of substance abuse, they may be reluctant to divulge the information for fear of loss of medical benefits or insurance coverage, loss of social position, employment, or self-esteem. Some individuals may be in denial and may not recognize or be willing to admit to having a problem. Others may be aware of the addiction but will go to great lengths to hide, rationalize, explain away, or minimize the importance of the chemical dependence. Unfortunately, some dentists may also be reluctant to delve into the issue of a patient's substance abuse because it may seem too intrusive or because they view the disorder as a moral shortcoming rather than a valid psychiatric disorder. It is imperative that this reluctance and fear on the part of both the patient and the provider be overcome to be able to safely treat the patient.

Delivery of Dental Care

The patient receiving dental treatment while under the influence of alcohol or drugs creates an unsafe and difficult working environment for the entire dental team and can place themselves at higher risk of a medical emergency while in the dental office. Patients under the influence of some drugs may be difficult to communicate with, uncooperative, and not adhere to prescribed therapeutic regimes. Often, they have poor oral hygiene, lack interest in achieving oral health, and are not motivated to receive regular dental care, seeking only relief of pain or infection. Other patients may exhibit initial overt enthusiasm for high-quality dental care but soon lose that enthusiasm and fail to follow through with the treatment that they have committed to. It is not uncommon for the abusing patient to cancel, be late, or not show for their dental appointments. Similarly, such individuals may be erratic or late in paying for dental services. They may also present to the dental visit while under the influence to relax or prepare for the anxiety associated with the dental visit.

Special precautions must be taken when prescribing medications for substance-abusing patients. Analgesics, sedatives, and antibiotics that are likely to cause adverse reactions with alcohol or psychiatric medications should be avoided. For example, the opportunity for severe respiratory depression can occur when a patient mixes alcohol with other central nervous system (CNS) depressants such as narcotics, sedatives, or benzodiazepines. Taken together, these substances have an additive effect that may have lethal consequences.

Behavioral and Compliance Issues

The behavioral problems exhibited by the abusing patient can include aggressiveness, deep sadness, and/or euphoria and may be a direct effect, side effect, or residual effect of the substances being abused. Some antisocial behaviors may be a manifestation of withdrawal symptoms after stopping an abused substance. Some patients may display defensive, secretive, manipulative, or excusatory behavior that may be part of a conscious or unconscious effort at self-rationalization or self-denial. These patients can become remarkably adept at hiding the addiction and simultaneously maintaining the appearance of a normal lifestyle with the accompanying benefits of social acceptance and the appearance of success.

Behavioral problems in the dental office can be a major disruption. Patients may have unexpected emotional reactions to treatment or become belligerent. Less dramatic, but just as detrimental, is the abusing patient who becomes distant, remote, unemotional, and disengaged. This behavior can be a direct effect of the abused substance, a side effect of therapeutic medications, or an otherwise induced mental depression—a secondary effect of the substance abuse.[3]

Many behavioral changes can be evoked by substance use and these may become apparent at any time during treatment. The dentist should especially be suspicious of behavioral anomalies that occur at the initial examination visit. Patients who regularly abuse alcohol or ingest other mind-altering substances, either alone or in combination, may exhibit the following:

- Denial, avoidance behaviors (cancelling, not showing or being late for appointments)
- Anxiety, fidgeting, excitation, nervousness
- CNS depression, lethargy, altered affect, and loss of motivation
- Lowered pain threshold and increased dental, gingival, and oral sensitivity
- Gagging and inappropriate behaviors in the operatory
- Unrealistic expectations about the nature and extent of treatment
- Noncompliance with oral hygiene measures and other instructions
- Diminished ability to pay for treatment

PATIENT ASSESSMENT FOR SIGNS AND SYMPTOMS OF SUBSTANCE ABUSE

Reviewing the Patient's Health History

Obtaining a thorough medical and dental history is an essential first step before initiating comprehensive dental treatment for any patient. Reviewing the health history for a substance-abusing patient is essential to learning any associated health problems that the patient might have. An evaluation of the health history can help divulge complications of the addiction, which could require modifications to dental treatment including postponing care, providing antibiotic prophylaxis, and avoiding certain medications.

The importance of establishing a trusting relationship with the patient, and doing so as quickly as possible, cannot be overemphasized. The social stigma associated with alcoholism and other forms of substance abuse may cause the patient to avoid disclosing a history of the problem. For the abuser, it is easy to find reasons to deny the abuse patterns and, in the mind of the abuser, there are potential risks associated with divulging such a condition. It is important for the practitioner to reaffirm to the patient the confidentiality of the interview and of the findings. Similarly, it is important to explain to the patient why questions related to substance use and abuse are relevant and necessary to the practice of dentistry.

The methods for obtaining a dental and medical health history are the same as those used with other adult comprehensive care patients (see Chapter 1). The goal is to obtain complete and accurate information so that dental care can be delivered in a safe manner and in a manner that is in the patient's best short- and long-term interests. The patient should be treated with respect and questions should be expressed in an objective, nonjudgmental manner with an awareness of the clinician's unconscious biases. The patient should be sitting upright facing the interviewer. Making eye contact is important to reinforce the idea that the dentist is interested in the patient's oral health and overall well-being. The dentist should be aware of the patient's demeanor and body language throughout the interview process. When asked a difficult question, the patient may exhibit diminished eye contact and/or a defensive posture such as crossing arms, possibly signaling an avoidance response. If the patient's answers are vague or there appears to be an effort made to circumvent answering a question, it may indicate a sign of denial of a substance abuse problem. The practitioner must also be aware that an anxious patient or a patient with psychological problems who feels falsely accused can appear to be similarly defensive and less than forthcoming with historical information.

The patient should be asked about the type, frequency, and amount of alcohol consumption or recreational drugs, and the use of any prescription or nonprescription medications. The dentist cannot assume that the patient is a substance abuser simply because they are using a medication for an atypical reason or taking a higher-than-normal amount of a mind-altering drug. For example, many individuals who suffer from chronic, acutely painful conditions use high doses of morphine or methadone for legitimate and medically appropriate reasons. Any current or past history of tobacco use should also be recorded. For individuals who have smoked cigarettes, a pack-year history is a useful way to capture and record that information (see Chapter 1).

A positive response to any of the initial substance-related queries on the health questionnaire, or during the patient interview, should be pursued with additional open-ended questions to determine whether an abuse problem exists. This may lead the clinician to consult with another healthcare provider and/or to modify the patient's treatment plan. In the United States, **Prescription Drug Monitoring Programs (PDMPs)** are an

excellent resource to view a patient's past prescriptions for controlled substances such as narcotics and benzodiazepines. These databases are maintained by each US state and the information is often shared with other states. If not initially reported, the dentist should clarify the type of drug, the quantity, frequency, most recent time of use, and pattern of use. Follow-up questions relating to a family history of substance abuse and the consequences of that abuse may also be appropriate. With the patient's permission, additional useful information about types of substance abuse, amount of use, and the behavioral effects and level of control of the addiction can often be obtained from family members and friends. This information may reveal a patient with a substance use disorder that has been diagnosed by a healthcare professional in addiction medicine. The diagnosis is determined by using the **Diagnostic and Statistical Manual-5 (DSM-5)** that describes the criteria for substance use disorder with sub-classifications of mild, moderate, or severe (see Figure 14.1).[4]

A careful review of the patient's health history may reveal risk indicators or conditions associated with the development of alcoholism or other forms of substance abuse. There are also

Criteria for Substance Use Disorder

1. Substances often taken in larger amounts or over a longer period than was intended.
2. Persistent desire or unsuccessful efforts to cut down or control substance abuse.
3. Great deal of time spent in activities necessary to obtain substances, use substances, or recover from its effects.
4. Craving, or a strong desire or urge to use substances.
5. Recurrent substance use resulting in a failure to fulfill major role obligations at work, school, or home.
6. Continued substance use despite having persistent or recurrent social or interpersonal problems caused or exacerbated by the effects of substances.
7. Important social, occupational, or recreational activities are given up or reduced because of substance abuse.
8. Recurrent substance use in situations in which it is physically hazardous.
9. Substance use is continued despite knowledge of having a persistent or recurrent physical or psychological problem that is likely to have been caused or exacerbated by substances.
10. Tolerance, as defined by increased substance use to achieve intoxication and/or a diminished effect with continued use of the same amount of the substance.
11. Withdrawal, as manifested by taking the substance that relieves the withdrawal symptoms.

Number of Criteria	Diagnosis
0–1	No Diagnosis
2–3	Mild Substance Use Disorder
4–5	Moderate Substance Use Disorder
6 or More	Severe Substance Use Disorder

Fig. 14.1 Criteria for having a diagnosis of substance use disorder.

several medical conditions which, if reported on the patient's health history, may suggest substance abuse, particularly alcoholism. These include a history of cardiac problems, liver and kidney disease, and diabetes. Although these conditions are not pathognomonic, taken collectively they should raise questions as to a significant substance abuse problem. There are also many physical and behavioral signs associated with a patient's drug use that may affect dental treatment planning and treatment (see Box 14.1).[5]

Intraoral/Extraoral Examination

The process of performing an extraoral and intraoral soft tissue examination for the patient with known, suspected, or potential substance abuse is the same as for any other patient. This portion of the examination often provides valuable clues for the dental team as to whether or not there is an abuse problem and the nature and severity of the problem, as well as the specific oral problems that will need to be addressed during dental treatment (see Table 14.1). Some of these findings may be evident when the patient first enters the operatory or they may emerge (or reemerge) at subsequent visits. Does the individual exhibit a staggering or halting gait or slurred speech? Does the individual make eye contact? Does the patient have a wasted appearance? Are they lethargic or do they have memory issues? Some patients may have unclean clothing and hair and exhibit body and breath odors. During the extraoral examination, the dentist should look for dermatologic conditions such as palmar or facial erythema, spider angiomas, or peripheral edema of the extremities. Does the patient's skin, mucosa, or the sclera of the eyes appear jaundiced, suggestive of liver damage? Are there any inflammatory nasal mucosal changes, such as chronic rhinitis, nasal septal defects (from powdered cocaine), facial or lip burns (due to crack cocaine use), dilated or constricted pupils, red eyes, venipuncture sites or needle tracks, stained fingers (marijuana and tobacco), excessive thirst, or unusual decay patterns? Other important findings include hypertension, tachycardia, or other cardiovascular disorders. Relevant extraoral findings may include hand tremor, bloated appearance, baggy eyes or puffy facial features, excessive perspiration, bilateral swelling of the parotid glands (Figure 14.2), red or ruddy complexion, and telangiectasias.

Common intraoral findings seen with substance-abusing patients include dry lips, angular cheilitis, persistent oral ulceration or infection, dry mouth, and candidiasis. The mucosa may exhibit an anemic pallor. Intraoral signs of an associated coagulopathy often include petechiae, purpura, and bruising. Mucosal erosion and ulceration are not uncommon. The patient may exhibit a swollen or inflamed tongue or gingival bleeding. Many substance-abusing patients exhibit signs of poor oral hygiene with accompanying gingivitis, periodontitis, and root caries. The teeth may show evidence of erosion, cracks, fractured cusps, bruxism, cervical notching, and attrition.[6]

Substance users often also use tobacco. With tobacco use, the clinician may notice the patient is using nicotine patches or snuff pouches instead of smoking. For smokers, lesions such as smoker's keratosis or nicotine stomatitis may be seen. Alcohol and tobacco are major contributing factors in the pathogenesis

---

BOX 14.1   Clinical Signs of Potential Drug Use

Physical Signs

- Frequent uncontrolled movement of the jaw, back and forth.
- Inability to sleep, awake at unusual times, unusual laziness.
- Loss of or increase in appetite, changes in eating habits.
- Cold, sweaty palms; shaking hands.
- Extreme hyperactivity; excessive talkativeness.
- Slowed or staggering walk; poor physical coordination.
- Puffy face, blushing, or paleness.
- Runny nose; hacking cough.
- Irregular heartbeat.
- Needle marks on lower arm, leg, or bottom of feet.
- Frequent rubbing of the nose.
- Deterioration of hygiene or physical health.
- Red, watery eyes; pupils larger or smaller than usual.
- Unusual smells on breath, body, or clothes.
- Nausea, vomiting or excessive sweating.
- Tremors or shakes of hands, feet or head.
- Bruising
- Anemia
- Altered immune response
- Hypertension
- Seizures
- Insomnia
- Anxiety
- Irritability
- Stomach problems
- Recurring episodes of ill-diagnosed oral pain
- Chronic headaches
- History of recurrent decay due to lack of proper brushing and flossing

Behavioral Signs

- Silliness or giddiness.
- Paranoia, moodiness, irritability, or nervousness.
- Possession of a false ID card.
- Change in personal grooming habits.
- Sudden oversensitivity, temper tantrums, or resentful behavior.
- Difficulty in paying attention and forgetfulness.
- Changes in friends; new friends are known drug users.
- Unexplained need for money, stealing money or items.
- Complaints of a sore jaw (from teeth grinding during an ecstasy high).
- Change in activities or hobbies.
- Change in overall attitude/personality with no other identifiable cause.
- Drop in grades and tardiness at school.
- Possession of drug paraphernalia.
- Chronic dishonesty and secretive behaviors.
- General lack of motivation, energy, self-esteem. An 'I don't care' attitude.
- Missing, lost, or destroyed prescription pills.
- Excessive need for privacy; unreachable by phone.
- Change in habits at home, loss of interest in family and family activities.
- Decrease in work performance.
- Dissatisfaction and poor experience with other care providers.
- Requesting sedation before the dentist has even examined the patient
- Asking for specific (narcotic) analgesics by name, "street name", or local slang
- Noncompliance with prescribed therapy
- Tardiness or failure to show for appointments
- Emotional fluctuations
- Constant excessive movement or inability to sit still, crying without reason, or other behavior that cannot be explained by other causes (such as psychological disorders, as discussed in Chapter 16)
- Repeated car accidents or unexplained injuries or visits to a hospital emergency department

TABLE 14.1   Potential Findings in Patients Who Abuse Alcohol and Other Mind-Altering Substances

Clinical Finding	Associated Substance
Jaundice of skin, mucosa, sclera	Alcohol
Chronic rhinitis	Powder cocaine
Nasal septal defects	Powder cocaine
Facial/lip burns	Crack cocaine/methamphetamine
Dilated pupils	Stimulants/hallucinogens/inhalants
Constricted pupils	Narcotics/opiates
Venipuncture sites/needle tracks	Heroin
Stained fingers	Cannabis/tobacco
Red, bloodshot eyes	Cannabis
Excessive thirst	Methamphetamine
Unusual dental decay patterns	Methamphetamine

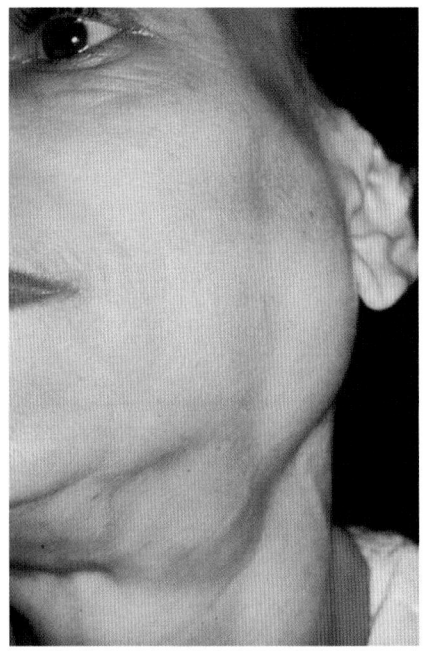

Fig. 14.2 Swelling of the salivary glands in an alcoholic patient. (From Neville BW, Damm DD, Allen CM, et al. *Oral and Maxillofacial Pathology*. 4th ed. St. Louis: Saunders; 2016.)

of oral cancer. Consequently, it is imperative that a thorough intraoral examination be conducted to detect premalignant or malignant lesions. While carrying out the examination, the dentist has an opportunity to inform the patient about the effects of alcohol, tobacco, and other substances on the oral cavity, and discuss oral cancer prevention. If the patient exhibits signs of tobacco use, it is incumbent on the dentist to educate the patient about the health risks of tobacco, including its harmful effects on the oral structures and its relationship to heart disease, hypertension, and lung cancer.[7]

EFFECTS AND IMPLICATIONS OF INAPPROPRIATE DRUG USE

Unpredictable Drug Metabolism

Patients who abuse substances can have unpredictable drug metabolism, therefore an understanding of all medications and their interactions is imperative. For instance, in mild to moderate alcoholic liver disease, heightened enzyme action results in increased tolerance of local anesthetics, sedative and hypnotic drugs, and general anesthesia medications. Larger than normal doses of medications may therefore be required to achieve the desired results. Drug metabolism will be markedly diminished for individuals with significant liver damage. For those patients who are more likely to take larger doses of medication to achieve the desired effect, this can result in the ingestion of a potentially lethal dose of the drug.[8]

Patients will often use combinations of tobacco products, alcohol, prescription drugs, and other mind-altering substances. These may have simultaneously additive, synergistic, or conflicting pharmacologic effects. Unpredictable and variable euphoric, depressive, hallucinogenic, and sedative effects may result. Even more disturbing for the dentist or healthcare worker is the potential for highly unpredictable and extremely variable systemic effects with drugs that depress respiration or speed up the heart rate. Systemic problems from a combination of abused substances with prescription and over the counter drugs can be difficult for medical personnel to treat effectively and may have potentially life-threatening consequences.[9]

If alcoholic hepatitis or cirrhosis is present, the dentist should generally reduce the normal dosages of all drugs that are metabolized in the liver or avoid their use altogether if possible or consult with the patient's healthcare provider. Aspirin should be avoided before any surgical procedures in patients with liver dysfunction or thrombocytopenia because of the potential for excessive bleeding. Acetaminophen should be used with caution in patients with impaired liver function, because granulocytopenia and anemia may be intensified. If acetaminophen is used in conjunction with alcohol, severe hepatocellular disease with potentially fatal consequences may occur.[10] Patients who eat, smoke, or frequently vape high levels of cannabis may experience increased hypertension, tachycardias, and arrhythmias. Table 14.2 provides a summary of some precautionary actions a dentist should consider at the preoperative visit and throughout the treatment process when treating a patient who abuses substances.

Infectious Diseases, Infective Endocarditis, and Nutritional Deficiencies

Patients who have a history of intravenous (IV) drug use are at risk for infectious diseases such as hepatitis B or C, human immunodeficiency virus (HIV), and infective endocarditis. Patients who are known to be IV drug users and who have not had a cardiac evaluation should be referred to a physician for evaluation and possible echocardiogram, with the objective of determining their risk status for endocarditis. If the patient is

TABLE 14.2   Preoperative Considerations for Patients Who Abuse Substances

Condition	Precautionary Action
Alcoholic hepatitis/ Cirrhosis	Avoid or reduce the normal dosages of all drugs metabolized by the liver (e.g., amide local anesthetics such as lidocaine)
Liver dysfunction/ Thrombocytopenia	Avoid aspirin before any surgical procedure Be aware of excess bleeding; obtain laboratory coagulation values prior to treatment
Impaired liver function	Use acetaminophen with caution because granulocytopenia and anemia may be exacerbated If acetaminophen is used with alcohol, severe hepatocellular disease with potentially fatal consequences may occur
Cardiovascular effects	Patients consuming, vaping, or smoking cannabis, cocaine, and methamphetamine can be more prone to tachycardias, arrhythmias and increased hypertension

determined to be at risk of endocarditis, it is appropriate to provide antibiotic prophylaxis before dental treatment if bleeding is anticipated. Substance-abusing patients are also vulnerable to acquiring sexually transmitted diseases because of both their altered immune response and their high-risk behaviors. Patients with alcohol and other substance abuse problems often sacrifice balanced nutritional intake for the sake of maintaining their drug use and to prevent the pain and discomfort of withdrawal. Craving to feed their drug habit, they often have limited discretionary money and may have altered mental judgment, which can both contribute to poor nutrition. Some consequences of poor nutrition may include folic acid and thiamine deficiencies, which can lead to anemia and weight loss. As a result of poor dietary habits, anemia and malnutrition may occur with the attendant problems of a depressed immune response, poor wound healing, and persistent local or systemic infection.

Substance-abusing patients in general, and patients with alcoholism, are more prone to develop serious systemic infections. It has been recognized that bacterial infections are more serious in patients with alcoholic liver disease—sometimes with fatal consequences. The dentist must be cognizant of the fact that oral surgical procedures, sites of oral infection or trauma, and periodontal diseases may all function as a nidus of infection. For high-risk patients—for example, those with confirmed compromised immune systems—systemic antibiotics may be considered. In the absence of ongoing infection, studies have not shown that systemic antibiotic prophylaxis is warranted before invasive dental procedures.[11]

Psychological Issues

Substance-abusing patients may develop psychological disorders, including cognitive impairment, anxiety disorders, antisocial behavior, and affective disorders such as depression and bipolar disorders. In severe cases, permanent neurologic damage may occur and these patients may develop alcohol amnestic

disorder, rendering them unable to recall previously known material or learn new material. Patients may also have alcohol-related blackouts and some individuals may develop dementia and/or severe personality changes. In such cases, professional psychiatric support is required and the dental treatment plan may need to be significantly curtailed.[12]

About 50% of people who experience a mental illness in their life will also experience a substance use disorder and vice versa.[13-15] Research further indicates that adolescents with a substance use disorder have high co-occurring mental illness and over 60% also met diagnostic criteria for another mental illness.[16] High rates of comorbid substance use disorders and anxiety disorders have been reported, including generalized anxiety disorder, panic disorder, and post-traumatic stress disorder.[14,17-19]

Other conditions prevalent in substance abusing patients may include depression and bipolar[20] disorder, attention-deficit hyperactivity disorder (ADHD),[21,22] psychotic illness,[23] borderline personality disorder, and antisocial personality disorder.[24] Patients who exhibit schizophrenia often have higher rates of alcohol, tobacco, and drug use disorders than the general population.[25]

A large US study suggests an increased risk of nonmedical (recreational) use of prescription opioids in people who have mental, personality, and substance use disorders. Forty-three percent of substance abuse disorder patients in treatment for opioid use suffer from anxiety and depression.[26] It is estimated that 40%–60% of an individual's vulnerability to substance use disorder is attributable to genetics.[27] An active area of comorbidity research involves the search for the connection that might predispose individuals to develop a substance use disorder and other mental illnesses or to have a greater risk of a second disorder occurring after the first appears.[28,29]

ALCOHOL ABUSE

Alcohol, when consumed in moderation, is recognized to have cardiovascular and other health benefits. When reviewing the health history of patients, it is important to determine and document how many standard drinks are consumed per day or per week (see Figure 14.3).

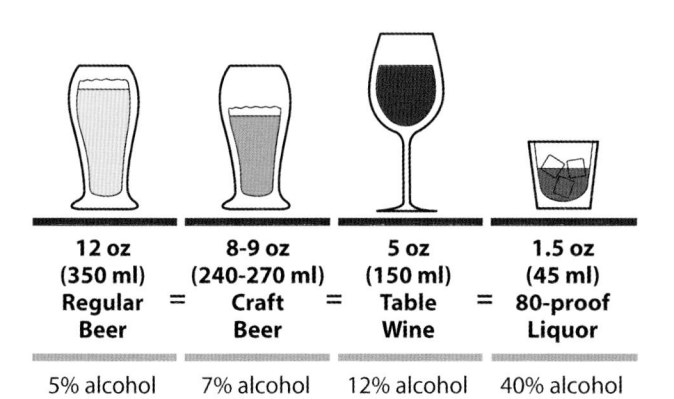

Fig. 14.3 US standard alcohol drink chart. (Adapted from Centers for Disease Control and Prevention. Alcohol use and your health, 2021. https://www.cdc.gov/alcohol/fact-sheets/alcohol-use.htm)

Individuals who drink moderately may be less likely to develop an **alcohol use disorder (AUD)**.[30] The definition of "moderate" differs for men and women. Heavy alcohol consumption for men has been defined as no more than four drinks on any single day and no more than 14 drinks per week. For women, no more than three drinks on any single day and no more than seven drinks per week is considered to be moderate consumption. To stay at low risk for AUDs, individuals must keep within both the single-day and weekly limits[31]. According to the US Department of Health and Human Services and the US Department of Agriculture, adults of legal drinking age can choose not to drink or to drink alcohol in moderation by limiting intake to two drinks or less in a day for men and one drink or less in a day for women.[32]

An individual who has consumed one or two alcoholic drinks often feels more energetic and outgoing. This stimulating effect of alcohol is really a disinhibition of the patient's personality. Instead of functioning as a stimulant, alcohol is actually a CNS depressant. Alcohol consumption slows normal brain function, with the sedating effect becoming stronger with increasing amounts of alcohol. In higher doses, alcohol can even become a general anesthetic.

A healthy dental patient who consumes a limited amount of alcohol typically presents no limitation or contraindications to dental treatment. Patients who use alcohol to excess or patients who often use mind-altering substances, however, may have problems consenting to, receiving, or completing dental treatment. Significant behavioral and medical issues can arise with the substance-abusing patient and may necessitate modification to the dental treatment plan. In some cases, treatment may need to be deferred, limited in complexity, or sequenced differently than for the normal patient.[33]

Prevalence of Alcohol Abuse

Alcohol is the most used addictive substance and its abuse has been identified as the number-one drug problem in the United States.[34,35] It is estimated that 14.1 million adults aged 18 years and older meet the diagnostic criteria for AUD. This includes 8.9 million men (7.3% of all men in this age group) and 5.2 million women (4.0% of all women in this age group).[36] Several million more engage in risky drinking patterns that could lead to alcohol abuse. More than 50% of all US adults have a family history of alcoholism or problem drinking[37] and more than 8 million children live in a household in which at least one parent is dependent or has abused alcohol.[38] AUD can be found in individuals of any race, gender, age, or socioeconomic group. An estimated 95,000 people (approximately 68,000 men and 27,000 women) die from alcohol-related causes annually, making alcohol the third leading preventable cause of death in the United States[39] exceeded only by tobacco use, poor diet, and physical inactivity.[39] Current evidence suggests that excessive alcohol use may reduce an individual's life expectancy by up to 24–28 years.[40]

Alcohol use alone or in combination with other drugs, such as benzodiazepines, is estimated to be responsible for more overdose deaths in the United States than any other agent alone.[41] Approximately one-half of all individuals who are diagnosed with alcohol abuse or dependence have additional psychiatric illnesses. These patients are said to have a "dual diagnosis." Additional illnesses may include anxiety, bipolar disorder, antisocial personality, or major depressive disorders. Although these patients are treated for and receive psychiatric medications for their diagnoses, they are unlikely to abstain from alcohol use and are at greater risk of experiencing alcohol-associated morbidity and mortality. It is common for alcoholics to have multiple addictions, which may include abuse of, or dependence on, other substances such as cocaine and nicotine.[42,43]

AUD is often associated with problems such as those associated with other abused substances (e.g., cannabis, cocaine, heroin, amphetamines, sedatives, hypnotics, or anxiolytics). Alcohol may be used to alleviate the unwanted effects of other abused substances or to substitute for them when they are not available. Symptoms such as behavior problems, depression, anxiety, and insomnia frequently accompany heavy drinking and sometimes precede it.[44–46] Once a pattern of repetitive and intense use develops, individuals with AUD may devote substantial periods of time to obtaining and consuming alcoholic beverages.

Owing to the extremely unpleasant symptoms experienced during withdrawal, individuals may continue to consume alcohol, despite the adverse consequences, simply to avoid or relieve withdrawal symptoms. Some withdrawal symptoms (e.g., sleep problems) can persist at lower intensities for months and may contribute to relapse.[47]

Pathophysiology of High Alcohol Use

Repeated intake of high doses of alcohol can affect nearly every organ system, in particular the gastrointestinal tract, cardiovascular system, and central and peripheral nervous systems. Gastrointestinal effects include gastritis, stomach or duodenal ulcers, and, in approximately 15% of individuals who use alcohol heavily, cirrhosis and/or pancreatitis. Alcohol abusers experience an increased rate of cancer of the esophagus, stomach, and other parts of the gastrointestinal tract.[48,49]

Excessive alcohol ingestion can also damage cardiac muscle tissue, affecting myocardial contractility with resulting cardiomyopathy and congestive heart failure. These factors, along with marked increases in levels of triglycerides and low-density lipoproteins, and cholesterol, contribute to an elevated risk of heart disease. A common problem is the development of low-grade hypertension, which, in combination with increased levels of cholesterol, fosters an elevated risk of cerebrovascular and coronary artery disease.[50]

Peripheral neuropathy may also be seen in individuals who use alcohol heavily as evidenced by muscular weakness, paresthesia, and decreased peripheral sensation. More persistent CNS effects include degenerative changes in the cerebellum, cognitive deficits, and severe memory impairment. These effects are related to the direct effects of alcohol or associated trauma and to vitamin deficiencies, particularly of the B vitamins, including thiamine.[51]

Alcohol abuse frequently results in inadequate nutritional intake. Because alcohol ingestion often accounts for one-half of the daily caloric intake, it displaces dietary proteins, minerals, and important trace elements such as magnesium and zinc. To compound this problem, chronic alcohol ingestion also causes the malabsorption of folic acid, B-complex vitamins; thiamine (B1), riboflavin (B2), pyridoxine (B6), extrinsic factor (B12), and vitamins D, E, and K.[52-54]

Alcohol abuse has a deleterious effect on neural development. Acetylcholine and dopamine receptors are damaged, leading to motor and sensory disturbances. Neuronal cell death and atrophy of several regions of the brain can occur. Clinically, these anatomic changes correlate with deficits in judgment and decision-making ability, reduced attention span, short-term memory loss, reduced emotional stability, and impaired coordination.[55-57] Any alcohol-dependent individual may develop these psychological conditions, along with concomitant cognitive impairment. Alcoholic individuals have a propensity to develop depression as a result of the CNS effects from long-term alcohol abuse and may have alcohol-related blackouts or develop dementia and severe personality changes.

Other adverse effects of long-term alcohol abuse include impairment of the liver's ability to produce coagulation factors and metabolize medications, impairment of white blood cells' chemotactic abilities, and impairment of the bone marrow's production of platelets. The first changes in alcoholic liver disease are the fatty infiltration of hepatocytes. The hepatocytes become engorged with fatty lobules, creating enlargement of the liver. This process is usually reversible.[58]

Alcoholic hepatitis, a more serious form of liver disease, is characterized histologically by a widespread inflammatory infiltrate and cellular destruction. This condition may be irreversible, leading to necrosis, sometimes resulting in death if the damage is widespread. The clinical presentation of alcoholic hepatitis includes nausea, vomiting, anorexia, malaise, weight loss, and fever.[58] The serious form of liver disease is cirrhosis, the tenth-leading cause of death among adults in the United States. This condition is considered irreversible and is characterized by progressive fibrosis of the liver tissue and loss of its excretory and metabolic function, leading to hepatic failure and associated morbidity. In the case of alcoholic cirrhosis, the liver has a diminished ability to detoxify drugs and may develop bleeding problems that are secondary to the inadequate formation of prothrombin and fibrinogen. This may have eventual toxic effects on the bone marrow. Individuals with cirrhosis are prone to anemia, hypoglycemia, hematemesis, blood in the stool, and lung abscesses. In advanced cases, cirrhosis can lead to hepatocellular carcinoma and ultimately death.[59]

As described previously, there are severe systemic and social effects associated with alcohol abuse. Patients may have cardiovascular disease, liver disease, malnutrition, compromised immune systems, and poor self-care. It is important to recognize that these additional conditions, although common among those who abuse alcohol, may not be diagnosed or treated. Dentists must respectfully and consistently screen for alcohol abuse because rates of abuse can vary across the patient's lifespan.[60]

OTHER ABUSED SUBSTANCES

Caffeine

Caffeine is a stimulant and the most widely used behaviorally active drug in the world. It is found in a variety of products, including coffee, tea, soft drinks, weight-loss aids, cold remedies, over-the-counter analgesics, dietary supplements, and chocolate. In the United States, most of the caffeine in a person's diet comes from coffee, tea, and carbonated beverages.[61]

Implications for Dental Treatment Planning and Treatment

Patients should be evaluated preoperatively about their caffeine consumption. While moderate daily consumption of caffeine is considered safe, excessive caffeine consumption can cause problems.[62,63] Excessive caffeine consumption is defined as greater than 400 mg per day, or more than four, 8-oz cups of brewed coffee per day (Table 14.3). High doses of caffeine use may cause patients to exhibit symptoms such as nervousness, flushed face, overexcitement, gastrointestinal disturbance, excessive urination, muscle twitching, tachycardia, or a cardiac arrhythmia.[64] Patients should be questioned about caffeine consumption if their heart rate is high (>100 beats/min). Smoking and other stimulant drugs can also cause tachycardia.

Oral implications of excessive caffeine consumption include halitosis, xerostomia, and stained teeth. Because the half-life of caffeine is 5 hours,[65] dental treatment time may need to be delayed if the patient exhibits signs and symptoms of excessive caffeine consumption.[65,66]

TABLE 14.3 Sources of Caffeine	
Source	Average Amount of Caffeine[a] (mg)
Coffee brewed 8 oz (237 ml)	96
Instant Coffee	62
Decaffeinated	2
Espresso 1 oz (30 ml)	64
Cappuccino 8 oz (240 ml)	75
Latte 8 oz (240 ml)	75
Black tea 8 oz (240 ml)	47
Green tea	28
Iced tea	47
Herbal Tea	0
Soft drink—Cola 12 oz (350 ml)	29
Soft drink—Citrus	54
Energy drink 8 oz (240 ml)	130–300
Energy shot	230
Cocoa beverage 6 oz (175 ml)	5
Chocolate milk beverage 8 oz (240 ml)	5
Solid milk chocolate 1 oz (28 gm)	9
Solid dark chocolate 1 oz (28 gm)	12

[a]Excessive caffeine consumption is greater than 400 mg/day

Nicotine

Nicotine use, especially smoking cigarettes, is a leading cause of preventable disease, disability, and death in the United States. In 2018, about 34 million adults smoked cigarettes, about 10% of the population. Cigarette smoking causes more than 480,000 deaths annually, including 41,000 deaths from secondhand smoke. Over 80% of the world's 1.3 billion tobacco users live in low- and middle-income countries.[67] Nicotine delivery from tobacco carries a significant number of chemical poisons, toxins, and cancer-producing substances and some 600 additives are used in the manufacture of American cigarettes.[68]

Nicotine in small doses acts as a stimulant to the brain. In high concentrations, it is a lethal poison that can affect the heart, blood vessels, and hormones. Nicotine in the bloodstream acts on nicotinic acetylcholine receptors to release neurotransmitters such as dopamine, glutamate, and gamma-aminobutyric acid, which have a calming effect for the smoker. The release of dopamine in the brain may affect the neuroendocrine system in a manner similar to cocaine, heroin, or other addictive drugs. Nicotine acts quickly: once smoke or vapor is inhaled into the lungs, the nicotine reaches the brain in only 6 seconds. The addiction is so powerful that many individuals habituated to the nicotine in cigarettes will continue to smoke despite serious tobacco-related physical symptoms or diseases, such as oral, throat and lung cancer, chronic obstructive pulmonary disease (COPD), and heart disease.

Implications for Dental Treatment Planning and Treatment

It is important for the clinician to document and investigate any history of tobacco or nicotine use by a patient. For a cigarette smoker, this is usually expressed in packs per year. For instance, a person who has smoked a half a pack of cigarettes (20 cigarettes) for 30 years has a 15-pack/year history of smoking. If a patient smoked in the past, the clinician should also record when smoking stopped and the pack/year usage until that time.

Both smoked and smokeless tobacco can affect oral tissues (Figure 14.4). In addition to bad breath and stained teeth, there are strong associations between tobacco smoking and oral cancer and periodontal disease. For instance, if smoking was eliminated in the population, it is estimated that the prevalence of periodontitis would decrease by 14%.[69] There is also an association between smoking tobacco and an increased prevalence of periapical pathology.[70]

The use of e-cigarettes has been increasing in the United States, particularly among teenagers.[71] Although many of the additives and carcinogens in tobacco have been reduced, there are other toxins and ultrafine particles in addition to nicotine in vapor.[72] These chemicals, along with nicotine, may still have an association with increase oral cancer and cardiovascular and pulmonary pathology.[73] The use of e-cigarettes is increasing in the United States and has been approved by the US Food and Drug Administration to decrease the number of individuals using tobacco products, especially among teenagers.[74]

As part of the disease control phase, dentists and dental staff can inform patients about tobacco cessation programs and other preventive measures to help reduce the risk of developing oral cancer. There are multiple resources available to implement tobacco cessation programs and help patients quit using tobacco. Three excellent resources are from the US Centers for Disease Control,[75] the American Dental Association,[76] and the

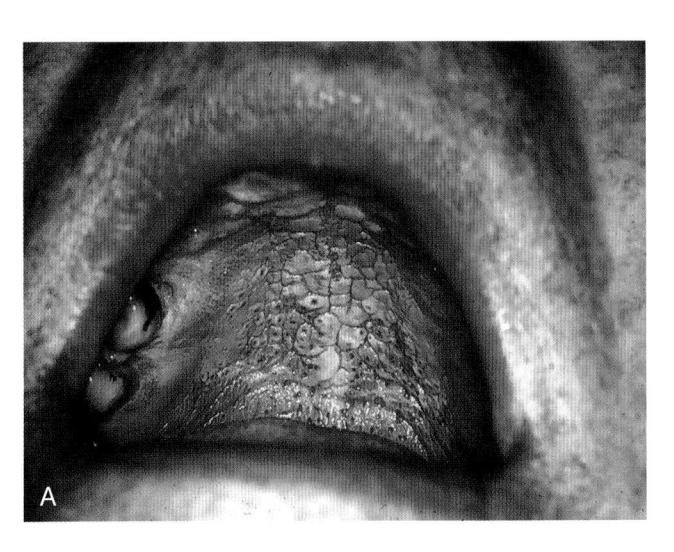

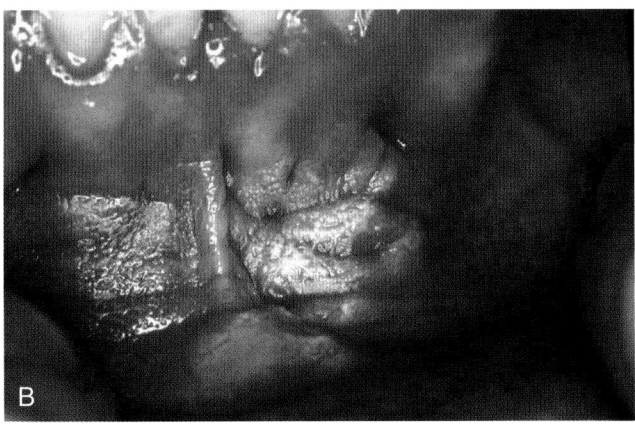

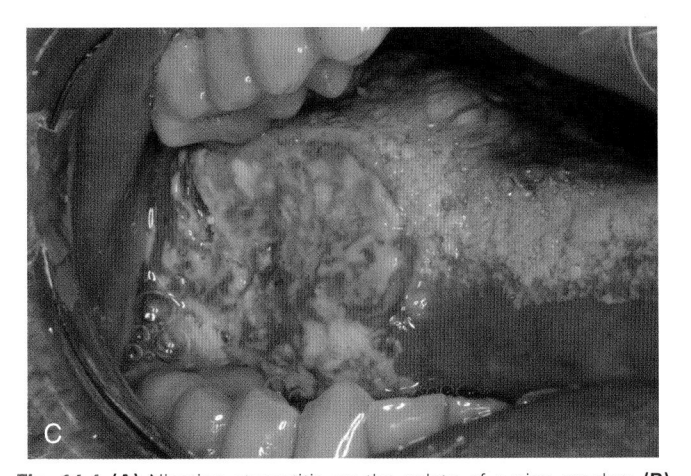

Fig. 14.4 (A) Nicotine stomatitis on the palate of a pipe smoker. **(B)** Snuff dipper's pouch hyperkeratosis. **(C)** Large squamous cell carcinoma on the lateral border of the tongue of a cigarette smoker.

American Cancer Association.[77] Additional information about tobacco cessation can be found in Chapter 10.

Cannabis

Cannabis is the third most used, and potentially abused, substance in the United States after tobacco and alcohol. According to the US Centers for Disease Control and Prevention, cannabis is the most used illegal drug in the United States, with approximately 22.2 million users each month.[78] In 2020, cannabis was the most used illicit drug worldwide with currently 250 million cannabis users.[79] The use of cannabis is expected to rise as more countries and US states decriminalize its sale, possession, and use for either medicinal and/or recreational use. The US National Institute on Drug Abuse (NIDA) reports that repeated cannabis use can lead to dependence, known as **cannabis use disorder**, which takes the form of addiction in severe cases.[80] Recent data suggest that 30% of those who use cannabis may have some degree of cannabis use disorder.[80] People who begin using cannabis before the age of 18 years are four to seven times more likely to develop a cannabis use disorder than adults.[81] In addition, there has been a significant increase in vaping cannabis by adolescents in the United States and Canada.[82]

Tetrahydrocannabinol (THC) is the primary component in cannabis that causes euphoria for the recreational user. Some methods of using cannabis such as vaping and eating may deliver very high levels of THC. THC affects the thought processes, mood, senses, and emotions of the user. Short-term effects include euphoria or a feeling of happiness and excitement as well as heightened senses. There can also be impaired body movement, difficulty with thinking and problem-solving, and impaired memory. Long-term effects include problems with brain development, particularly with young chronic users.[83] Some users may display lower initiative and persistence at performing tasks.[84]

Cannabidiol (CBD) can be found in both marijuana and hemp plants and is the primary component of many medical marijuana products. Unlike THC, CBD does not cause euphoria and may be helpful in the treatment of anxiety, some seizure disorders, insomnia, chronic pain, and addiction to other drugs.[85]

Implications for Dental Treatment Planning and Treatment

With its increasing availability, clinicians should expect to treat more patients who use cannabis recreationally or for medicinal purposes. Adding questions about cannabis/marijuana use to the health questionnaire can be helpful to start a conversation. Determining the frequency and method of use (smoking, eating, vaping) can help the clinician decide whether they can safely treat the patient.

Many of the intraoral effects of smoking cannabis are like those found with tobacco use such as staining of teeth, inflammation of the gingival and other oral tissues, xerostomia and the potential for oral cancer and periodontal disease. Many other effects on the hard and soft tissues are like those seen with other abused substances and may be a result of a diet high in refined carbohydrates, poor oral hygiene, and infrequent dental visits. The major physiologic effects of using cannabis are tachycardia, red bloodshot eyes, and slower respiration. There is also the potential for high blood pressure or orthostatic hypotension

when standing up quickly.[86] The THC in cannabis can also affect cognition and memory.[87]

Because of the euphoria, heightened senses and physiologic and cognitive effects, patients who recreationally use cannabis should be encouraged to abstain from using the substance before a dental visit. The amount of time is variable and most euphoric effects of smoking cannabis subside in 2–3 hours.[88] Heavy cannabis users, particularly those who vape high levels of THC may require up to 27 hours of abstinence before one plasma half-life of THC is reached.[89]

Obtaining informed consent for treatment may be challenging, particularly if the patient is also using alcohol or other substances. The patient should be encouraged not to use any substances of abuse for at least 8–12 hours before the appointment. The clinician should evaluate the patient's ability to understand and retain the details of proposed treatment. In addition to oral instructions the clinician may also wish to provide information in writing, since cannabis use can affect a patient's short-term memory and attention span. Further information on obtaining informed consent can be found in Chapter 7.

Prescription Medication

Some prescription drugs can alter brain activity and lead to dependence when abused. Commonly abused classes of prescription drugs include opioids (prescribed to treat pain), CNS depressants (often prescribed to treat anxiety and sleep disorders), and stimulants (prescribed to treat narcolepsy, ADHD, and obesity). Commonly used opioids include hydrocodone (Vicodin), meperidine (Demerol), oxycodone (OxyContin, Percodan, and Tylox), hydromorphone (Dilaudid), and Tramadol (Table 4.5). Common CNS depressants include barbiturates such as pentobarbital sodium (Nembutal), and benzodiazepines such as diazepam (Valium) and alprazolam (Xanax). Stimulants include dextroamphetamine (Dexedrine) and methylphenidate (Ritalin).[90]

Rates of prescription opioid addiction have soared across the United States and Canada. Eighty percent of the world's opioids are consumed in the United States, even though the population of the United States represents only about 5% of the world's population. In the United States, among high school seniors, hydrocodone is commonly abused, second only to marijuana.

Worldwide, about 500,000 deaths are attributable to drug use, with more than 70% of these deaths related to opioids and more than 30% of those deaths caused by overdose.[91]

On average in 2019, 38 people in the United States died daily from overdoses involving prescription opioids, totaling more than 14,000 deaths.[92] Although prescription opioids were involved in over 28% of all opioid overdose deaths in 2019, there was a decrease of about 7% in prescription opioid-involved mortality from 2018 to 2019.[92] According to the National Institute on Drug Abuse, approximately 16% of opioid overdose deaths include a benzodiazepine.[93]

Deaths from drug overdose, both prescription and non-prescription, have been rising steadily over the past two decades and have become the leading cause of injury and death in the United States.[94-96] In 2019, in the United States, about 130 people died every day because of drug overdose. The COVID-19 epidemic has had a devastating effect on the opioid epidemic. Over 81,000 drug overdose deaths occurred in the United States in the 12 months up to May 2020, the highest number of overdose deaths ever recorded in a 12-month period.[97] An important aspect of the problem is the nonmedical use of prescription painkillers, using drugs without a prescription, or using drugs just for the "high" they cause.

Taking more than the recommended dosage of any prescribed medication can be dangerous. Medical supervision is also necessary to avoid dangerous drug interactions, as well as potentially serious side effects, including accidental overdose. Another issue with prescription medication is the potential for addiction. There has been a dramatic increase in treatment admissions owing to abuse of prescription pain relievers. This increase is seen among all ages and ethnic groups in the United States.[98]

As mentioned earlier in the chapter, most states in the United States have prescription drug monitoring programs (PDMPs) that permit health professionals to see the controlled substance prescription histories for individual patients. PDMPs continue to be among the most promising state-level interventions to improve opioid prescribing, to inform clinical practice, and to protect at-risk patients. Although the findings are mixed, the evaluations of PDMPs have demonstrated changes in prescribing behaviors, less use of multiple providers by patients to obtain controlled substances, and decreased admissions for substance abuse treatment. States have implemented a range of ways to make PDMPs easier to use and access and these changes have significant potential for ensuring that the utility and promise of PDMPs are realized.[99]

Implications for Dental Treatment Planning and Treatment

Prescription medication abuse can affect all age groups and dentists must be vigilant to identify drug-seeking behaviors. Some common signs may include patients seeking pain medication in lieu of dental treatment, frequently switching providers and making specific pharmacological requests prior to being diagnosed by the dentist. The prescription drugs most often abused include opioid painkillers, anti-anxiety medications, sedatives, and stimulants. Signs and symptoms of prescription drug abuse depend on the specific drug.

There are serious consequences when a patient abuses the following drugs.[100]

- Opioids: hypotension, bradypnea, miosis, coma, and overdose death.
- Anti-anxiety and sedatives medications: memory problems, hypotension, bradypnea, withdrawal symptoms associated with suddenly stopping medication resulting in seizures and nervous system hyperactivity, coma, and overdose death.
- Stimulants: Dangerously high body temperature, heart problems, hypertension, seizures or tremors, motor tics, dyskinesias, hallucinations, aggressiveness, and paranoia.

Common oral findings in the opioid and benzodiazepine abuser include xerostomia, advanced caries, occlusal wear, bruxism, red inflamed nostrils, and nasal septal damage. The dentist should consider treating the xerostomia and providing occlusal guards, bite splints, and topical fluoride treatments.

Dental appointments should be scheduled at least 12 hours from last active use if possible. Potential drug interactions may occur with an opioid abuser if fluconazole or rifampin is prescribed. Caution should be taken with patients who are abusing benzodiazepines to prevent cross-addiction with alcohol and opioids.

Heroin and Fentanyl

According to a 2020 report, the global prevalence of opiate (heroin, opium, and pharmaceutical opioids) use in 2018 was estimated at 1.2% of the population, or 57.8 million people.[101] Heroin is an illegal drug produced from morphine, which itself is derived from the opium poppy. The number of heroin users in the United States has increased from 373,000 in 2007 to about 808,000 in 2018.[102] The largest increase in use is for people who are 26 years old. A study in 2020 found that one in three high school seniors who misuse prescription opioids later use heroin.[102] The opioid epidemic is strongly impacting emergency departments in the United States. Data from 2018 indicate that there was a 30% increase in visits for opioid overdose from July 2016 to September 2017.

After smoking, inhaling, or injecting heroin, the user reports a surge of euphoria. This is accompanied by warm flushing of the skin, dry mouth, and heavy-feeling extremities. After this initial euphoria, the user alternates between a drowsy and wakeful state. Mental functioning slows owing to CNS depression. These effects usually last for a few hours. The long-term effects of heroin use appear after repeated use of the drug. Chronic users often develop collapsed veins, abscesses, cellulitis, liver disease, and infections of the heart lining and valves. Because heroin is a CNS depressant, it can affect the user's respiration rate. Heroin abusers frequently have pulmonary complications, including various types of pneumonia. Heroin abuse has been associated with fatal overdose from the drug, spontaneous abortion, and, particularly in users who inject the drug, infectious diseases, including hepatitis B and HIV/AIDS.

As the heroin user develops tolerance with regular use, more of the drug is needed to achieve the same intensity of effect and physical dependence and addiction develop. Withdrawal typically begins a few hours after the last drug administration, with the individual experiencing several side effects including drug craving, restlessness, muscle and bone pain, diarrhea and vomiting, cold flashes with goose bumps, kicking movements and insomnia. Major withdrawal symptoms peak between 48 and 72 hours after the last dose and subside after about a week. In heavily dependent users who are in poor health, sudden withdrawal is occasionally fatal, although heroin withdrawal is considered less dangerous than that associated with alcohol, barbiturate, or benzodiazepine.

Fentanyl is a synthetic opioid invented in 1959 that is 50 to 100 times as powerful as morphine (see Table 14.4). The drug is available legally to control severe and chronic pain. Because fentanyl is not plant-based and can be fabricated from chemicals, its illegal production and distribution has increased. Illegal fentanyl can be added to cocaine and heroin to increase potency and is also available illegally in powder and pill form. The high availability and concentrations of

TABLE 14.4	Approximate Potency of Opioids Compared With Morphine
Drug	**Potency Compared With Morphine**
Codeine	0.1
Hydrocodone	0.67
Morphine	1
Oxycodone	1.5–2
Hydromorphone	4–7.5
Methadone	5–10
Heroin	25–50
Fentanyl	50–100

Adapted from WHO Guidelines for the Pharmacological and Radiotherapeutic Management of Cancer Pain in Adults and Adolescents. Geneva: World Health Organization; 2018. Table A6.2. https://www.ncbi.nlm.nih.gov/books/NBK537482/table/appannex6.tab/

fentanyl have contributed to an epidemic of drug overdose deaths in the United States where over 100,000 individuals died in one year in 2021.[103]

Implications for Dental Treatment Planning and Treatment

Because of the potential for liver and cardiovascular damage, the dentist will need to consult with a physician before removing teeth or providing any other surgical procedures for a patient who uses heroin or fentanyl. The physician can order tests such as a complete blood count, prothrombin time, and partial thromboplastin time. They can also evaluate the patient's cardiovascular status and advise on whether antibiotic prophylaxis is indicated.[104] The patient should also be tested for hepatitis B and HIV, because these infectious diseases are more prevalent in intravenous drug abusers.

Regular dental care is a low priority for most patients who are chronic abusers of heroin and fentanyl. As a result, there is often increased caries and tooth loss because of the dry mouth caused by the drugs, which is often further aggravated by poor oral hygiene and a diet high in refined carbohydrates.[105] Other conditions seen with heroin abuse include periodontal disease, oral candidiasis, mucosal infection, mucosal dysplasia, and bruxism.[106] The use of nitrous oxide inhalation sedation can be helpful to reduce patient anxiety prior to treatment and is preferred to other sedation techniques. Naloxone is a rescue medication that reverses an opioid overdose[107] and the American Medical Association's Opioid taskforce recommends physicians to co-prescribe the rescue drug whenever prescribing opioids.[108] Although there are currently no specific guidelines recommending this practice by dentists, co-prescribing naloxone could save lives and carries relatively limited risk.[109] In addition, the dentist may want to add naloxone to their emergency medicine kit.

Dental treatment should include treatment for xerostomia, fabrication of occlusal guards, and topical fluoride treatment. The recovering patient may be receiving medication used for opioid use disorders such as naltrexone, buprenorphine, or methadone.[110]

Cocaine

Cocaine is a drug refined from the South American coca plant and used medically as a topical anesthetic. Cocaine is one of the only anesthetics with vasoconstrictive properties. When used recreationally it is a highly addictive stimulant that can be taken through the nose or injected intravenously. Cocaine can also be processed into a crystalline state, often referred to as crack, which is smoked.[111] In 2016, there were nearly 1.9 million or 0.8% of the US population aged 18 years or older who used cocaine.[112]

Small amounts of cocaine usually make the user feel euphoric, energetic, talkative, mentally alert, and hypersensitive to sight, sound, and touch. The drug can also temporarily decrease the need for food and sleep. Physiologic effects include constricted blood vessels, dilated pupils, nausea, increased blood pressure, and a fast or irregular heartbeat.[111] Patients who inject cocaine are at greater risk of having HIV or hepatitis B.

Implications for Dental Treatment Planning and Treatment

Common dental conditions seen in cocaine abusers include xerostomia, tooth erosion, occlusal wear, rampant caries, and bruxism.[113] Dental treatment planning and treatment should focus on mitigating dry mouth symptoms, applying topical fluoride, and fabricating occlusal guards. Definitive care should be deferred until the patient stops using the drug.

Chronic cocaine users should not be given local anesthesia containing epinephrine until at least 6 hours after the last use of the substance because the vasoconstrictive effects of epinephrine may lead to an acute hypertensive crisis.[114] Although most cardiovascular effects of cocaine diminish a few hours after use, blood pressure can remain elevated. Even if the patient states that they have stopped using the drug, it is imperative to check their blood pressure before initiating treatment.

Methamphetamine

Methamphetamine is a strongly addictive drug with an extremely high potential for abuse. According to the 2019 National Survey on Drug Use and Health, in the United States approximately two million people (0.7% of the population) reported using methamphetamine in the past year.[115] The average age of new methamphetamine users in 2016 was 23.3 years old.[116] An estimated 964,000 people aged 12 years or older had a methamphetamine use disorder in 2017, meaning that they reported clinically significant impairment because of their drug use. This number is much higher than the 684,000 people who reported the same in 2016.[116]

Although methamphetamine's chemical structure is like that of amphetamine, it has more pronounced neurotoxic effects on the central nervous system. Like amphetamine, it causes increased wakefulness and physical activity, decreased appetite, and a general sense of well-being. After the initial rush of euphoria, there is typically a state of high agitation that for some individuals can lead to violent behavior.[117] The effects may persist for 6–8 hours. Chronic, long-term use may lead to psychotic behavior, hallucinations, and stroke. Another illicit drug, fenethylline, also referred to as Captagon, is a combination of amphetamine and theophylline and is prevalent in the Middle East and other Arab countries and communities.[118]

Methamphetamine can cause a variety of cardiovascular problems, including a rapid and irregular heart rate and increased blood pressure. Methamphetamine abusers may also have episodes of violent behavior, paranoia, anxiety, confusion, and insomnia. Heavy users also exhibit progressive social and occupational deterioration and their physical appearance can degrade, with loss of weight and the appearance of aging in the face and neck areas. Psychotic symptoms can sometimes persist for months or years after methamphetamine use has ceased.[119]

Implications for Dental Treatment Planning and Treatment

Methamphetamine-addicted patients commonly exhibit oral manifestations such as dry mouth, gingivitis, periodontal disease, cracked teeth, and severe dental caries (Figure 14.5). The xerostomia seen in these patients is caused by methamphetamine's inhibitory effect on the salivary glands. Diminished salivary flow contributes to gingivitis, stomatitis, and dental caries. Methamphetamine also affects the microvasculature through vasoconstriction, with resultant impeding of blood supply to the periodontal tissues. Typically, superimposed on these physiologic problems are the ill effects of the unhealthy lifestyle choices made by the methamphetamine user, including poor oral and general healthcare, poor nutritional intake, and episodes of intoxication and loss of consciousness that may lead to antisocial or criminal behavior and/or traumatic injury. Poor oral self-care and frequent or binge consumption of large volumes of highly sweetened carbonated drinks are frequently associated with drug abuse. Generally, caffeinated beverages are preferred by the abuser because they are more likely to sustain the methamphetamine high between ingestion episodes. Collectively, these issues can have devastating consequences for the oral cavity, particularly with the development of rampant caries.[119,120] As with patients who abuse cocaine, dentists should use local anesthetics without a vasoconstrictor for patients who use methamphetamine.[113]

With methamphetamine use, oral changes begin with the yellowing of the user's teeth, gingival inflammation and bleeding, rapidly deteriorating flaking enamel, loosening of the teeth, bleeding gingival tissues with swelling, and sometimes acute periapical or periodontal infection. These changes eventually leave the teeth looking grayish-brown or black-stained, decayed to the gumline, and often unrestorable. Cases can advance so rapidly that some patients in their late teens and early twenties require full-mouth extractions.[113]

The typical decay pattern for methamphetamine users starts at the gum line and eventually spreads over the entire tooth surface, demineralizing large areas of enamel. The rapid destruction of tooth enamel is thought to be a result of the toxic chemicals produced in the associated vapor from smoking methamphetamine. Flaking of the enamel, fracturing of cusps, and whole tooth fractures are also common features. In many cases, these are initiated by caries, but they are also aggravated

by severe clenching and bruxing patterns secondary to the user's intense feelings of anxiety and paranoia while under the influence of the drug. The destruction caused by these processes is usually irreversible.

The quality of life is poor for patients who abuse methamphetamine. Patients may be embarrassed by the appearance of their teeth. They may also have general mouth soreness, a lack of taste, and inability to eat certain foods.[121] The severe caries and bruxism may lead to few treatment options other than extraction. Planning for definitive care must be postponed until the patient is no longer using the drug.

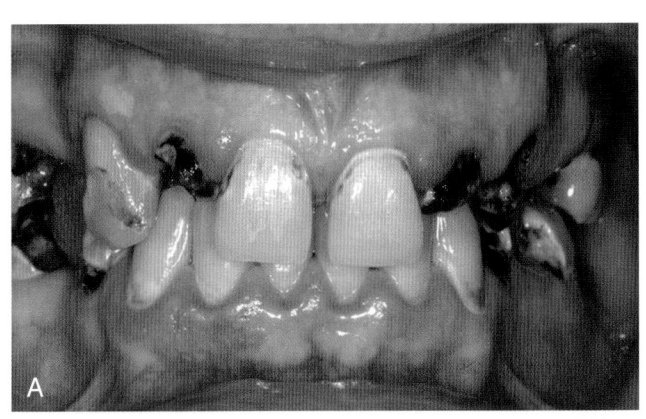
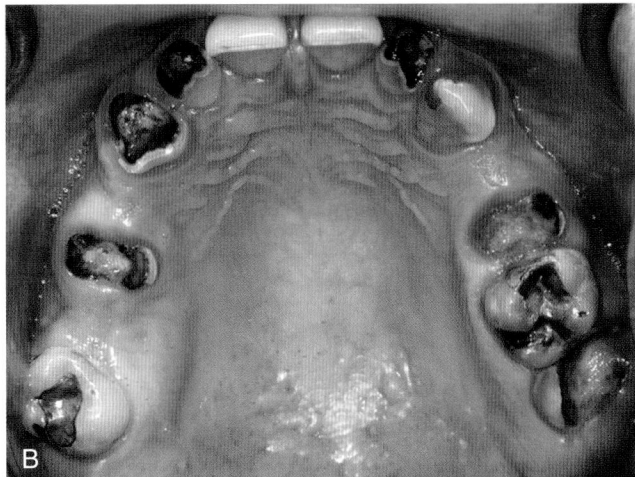
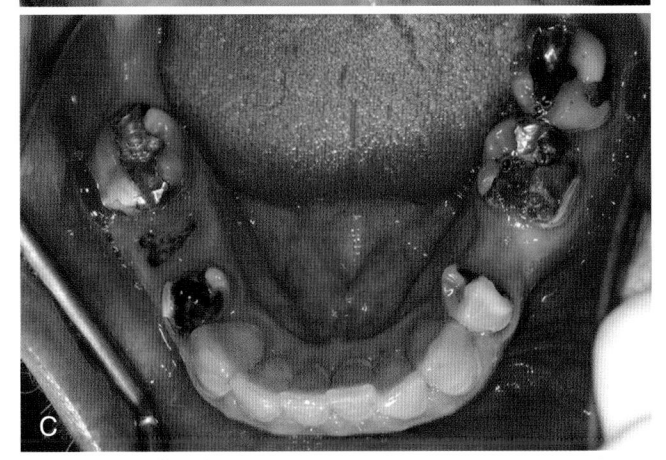

Fig. 14.5 (A–C) Examples of a patient with "meth mouth."

PHYSICIAN CONSULTATION AND LABORATORY TESTING

Consulting with the patient's healthcare provider or medical clinic is warranted when there is suspicion of substance abuse, or the patient is not forthcoming about their abuse history. The patient may acknowledge substance use or abuse or present with signs or symptoms of systemic disease that have not been addressed. The patient may also be unable to supply sufficient information for the dentist to provide treatment safely. The dentist is responsible for providing treatment in a manner that will not jeopardize the health of the patient. Clarification is necessary regarding any associated systemic problems and their effect on the proposed treatment.

The consultation with the healthcare provider should only be implemented with the patient's knowledge and consent. If the patient refuses to allow the dentist to consult with their physician, it may be necessary for the dentist to decline to provide treatment. Before refusing to treat the patient, however, there needs to be an open and honest conversation with the patient and a clear and genuine need on the part of the dentist to obtain the health information. It is unprofessional and unethical for a dentist who may not want to treat a patient with substance abuse to use the patient's refusal to see a physician as a reason to dismiss the patient from the practice.

A request to the patient to consult with their physician must be implemented with tact, compassion, and preservation of the patient's dignity. It is incumbent on the dentist to make it clear to the patient why such a referral is necessary and what specific information will be asked of the physician. Patients must be assured that the conversation and information obtained will be kept confidential. Every effort should be made to explain to the patient that the sole motive in seeking medical consultation is to provide the best oral health care in a manner that is both safe and effective for the patient.

The format of the consultation request is similar for the substance-using patient as for other patients (see Chapter 8). The nature of the medical concerns, however, may be different from those of the typical dental patient. The effects of substance use are more far reaching, raising concerns about addiction management, concurrent psychiatric problems, communication and social interactions, in addition to concern about the patient's general health. The complexity of the issues that can influence the dental treatment plan require the dentist to be thoughtful and organized when composing the referral letter or speaking with the healthcare provider. Vague questions such as, "Does the patient have a drug problem?" and "Should I be concerned?" are likely to elicit a similarly vague and generally unproductive response from the healthcare provider. The dentist needs to be specific about their concerns regarding substance abuse control and any potential for medical complications. The dentist can ask whether any treatment modifications are necessary during the delivery of dental care. These can include identifying which medications should be avoided and whether local anesthetics can be used safely and which analgesics can be used if the patient is in pain. The physician should be asked to list all the patient's medical and psychiatric diagnoses, particularly depression,

schizophrenia, and anxiety. If the dentist has concerns about how well the medical and/or psychiatric conditions are being controlled, those concerns also need to be communicated.

In some cases, the healthcare provider may not be able to answer all the dentist's questions. Questions regarding progress with the addiction management should be deferred to the addiction medicine doctor, psychologist, or counselor who is treating the patient. The dentist should also expect that the consultation will become an ongoing dialogue. The therapeutic relationships between the patient and the dentist, patient and physician, and patient and therapist are, in most cases, ongoing and dynamic. As these three relationships evolve, the nature of the dental treatment, counseling services, and medical care that are provided, will often change—and all three healthcare providers (as well as the patient) will benefit from the professional interaction. If there is ongoing open communication between all the care providers, there is a far greater likelihood that the patient will be treated comprehensively, efficiently, and effectively.

Laboratory testing has relevance for the substance-using/abusing patient. Given the risk of bleeding disorders, malnutrition, anemia, liver dysfunction, infection, and immune compromise in this group of patients, it is often recommended that laboratory testing be done before procedures with significant

---

BOX 14.2   Commonly Used Laboratory Tests for Patients Who Use Alcohol and Other Substances

Platelets

When vessels are damaged, the platelets become sticky and aggregate, forming a mechanical plug. They then release serotonin, which causes vessel constriction, and phospholipids, which are necessary for coagulation. Platelets fail if they are too few or if they do not become sticky. Aspirin destroys the stickiness of platelets.

Normal values: 150,000-450,000/mm³

Bleeding Time

This tests platelet function. Using Ivy's method, the forearm is punctured. The cut is blotted with filter paper every 30 seconds until the bleeding has stopped.

Normal bleeding time: 1–6 minutes

Coagulation (Fibrin Clot Formation) Two Pathways

PT tests the extrinsic pathway, used to test patients on Coumadin.
PTT tests the intrinsic pathway.
Normal values:

PT (extrinsic system Factor VII)	11–15 seconds
PTT (intrinsic)	25–35 seconds

Long PT and normal PTT: defect in extrinsic pathway.
Long PTT and normal PT: defect in intrinsic pathway.

INR

Test for patients on Coumadin therapy, determines effects of oral anticoagulants.
Patients on Coumadin therapy usually have an INR of 2.5–3.0.
For dental therapy to be safe, the INR should be 1.5–2.5.

INR, international normalized ratio; *PT*, prothrombin time; *PTT*, partial thromboplastin time.

bleeding. The physician or the dentist may order the tests. A complete blood count, prothrombin time, partial thromboplastin time, international normalized ratio, and liver function panels are some of the more commonly prescribed tests. Box 14.2 summarizes commonly ordered tests, their purpose and use, normal values, and their relevance in dental practice.

CONFRONTING SUBSTANCE ABUSE WITH THE PATIENT

For the active user who denies a dependency problem, the dentist will have no choice but to confront the patient about the addiction. Admittedly, this is not an easy conversation for either party. One concern is that the patient will take offense at the intrusion into their privacy and leave, become angry, or even hostile. Even if the patient remains calm, however, parting on bad terms is not a pleasant experience for anyone involved. But the alternative of ignoring the problem could have dire consequences for the patient's health.

One method of addressing the problem is using a three-step process: Screening, Brief Intervention, and Referral to Treatment, referred to as **SBIRT**.[122] The screening process involves a review of the patient's health history and identifying any sign or symptoms of substance abuse. Some public health dental clinics use specific questionnaires to learn more about a patient's alcohol and drug using behavior. The brief intervention consists of an objective and empathetic discussion with the patient regarding their substance abuse behavior and supports their autonomy to make decisions on their own. The dentist can use this opportunity to discuss the effect that the substance abuse is having on the patient's medical and dental condition. Last, once the patient agrees, the referral for treatment to a local outpatient program can be made, which is discussed in the next section.

The keys to success in all these endeavors is for the dentist and the rest of the dental team to remain calm, professional, understanding, and rational. There is a chance that the patient may later recall the event in favorable terms and return to the dental office with a respectful, if not apologetic, demeanor. The dentist and staff should keep in mind that the patient's outward behavior reflects the addiction and not the person. When managed successfully, this confrontation may lead to the patient's managing their addiction more effectively and the dental team's being enabled to provide comprehensive dental care safely and efficiently, moving toward establishing and maintaining optimal oral health for the individual.

ASSISTING THE PATIENT IN MANAGING THE ADDICTION

The role of the dentist in the management of a patient's alcohol or substance abuse problem is first and foremost to recognize that there is a problem and to refer the patient for professional therapy. With the patient who refuses to admit to a substance abuse problem or who recognizes that there is a problem but refuses to seek professional help, the dentist is faced with a difficult decision. In the United States and many other countries, the patient cannot be legally forced to engage in therapy unless there is evidence that the person is a danger to themself or others. If a patient demonstrates suicidal ideation or demonstrates hostile or criminal behavior, it is appropriate to notify the relevant mental health or legal authorities.

Before referring a patient for substance abuse counseling, the dentist should be aware of the local resources available. In some communities there are mental health units that can provide alcohol and drug counseling by a social worker or psychologist and also provide excellent referrals. Some communities have private practitioners, such as an addiction psychiatrist or physician or facilities that specialize in substance abuse rehabilitation. Most academic health centers, hospitals, and community-based health clinics provide these services. Having a conversation with the patient about previous therapy experiences, available options, and financial resources can help focus the list on a few of the most appropriate options. In many cases, a letter of introduction or referral from a healthcare professional (dentist or physician) is helpful or even mandatory. The management and treatment of the addiction should be left to a trained professional. It is generally helpful for the dentist to have an ongoing relationship with the substance abuse facility. Not only does this make the initial referral easier, but it also makes ongoing communication more efficient. It is important for the substance abuse specialist and dentist to maintain contact as the behavioral and dental therapies are implemented.

Many forms of therapy for alcohol and substance abuse are available. It is generally recognized that it is difficult for the chemically dependent individual to control their substance use disorder without help. Traditional and long-standing 12-step programs have varying success rates. Alcoholics Anonymous (AA) and Narcotics Anonymous (NA) programs share the goal of total abstinence. Both are based on the premise that the person with a substance use disorder seeks guidance from a higher power and that the individual benefits from joining a community with other people with substance use disorders. In some communities, AA and NA groups hold joint meetings, whereas in other communities, they meet separately and have their own separate identities. Because of the propensity for an abuser of one substance (e.g., alcohol) to be susceptible to other forms of substance abuse (e.g., barbiturates), many substance abuse therapists will insist that the person suffering from substance use disorder refrain from indulging in *any* form of substance abuse.

PRACTICE MANAGEMENT ISSUES

Several overarching principles and challenges are unique when treating a chemically dependent patient. They include preserving the patient's rights, confidentiality, and protecting the patient from harming themselves. Individual staff members in the dental office similarly have the right to safety and security. Furthermore, the dental team has the right to protect the integrity of the clinical practice from security breaches and from being accused of being dishonest. The practice must also endeavor to conduct its business and professional activities in such a way as to reduce legal risk. In general, the axioms of "do no harm" and "do what is in the best interest of the patient" will serve both the dentist and the practice well.

IN CLINICAL PRACTICE

Preventive Therapy for the Chemically Dependent Patient

A patient with a substance use disorder may require substantially more help with preventive services and oral healthcare instruction. Patients who abuse alcohol tend to have more gingival inflammation, plaque, and calculus than other patients. Contributing factors include metabolic and immune deficiencies, as well as neglect of general and oral self-care. Such individuals will often need more frequent periodic visits and will benefit from additional oral self-care instruction, focusing on specific problem areas and issues. These patients may need more treatment time, an increased amount of local anesthesia, and additional anxiolytics. It is often appropriate to delay extensive dental care until the patient can demonstrate the ability to establish and maintain a healthy oral condition.

Patients who smoke tobacco, marijuana, methamphetamine (and, to a lesser extent, crack cocaine), tend to have heavily stained teeth. These patients require substantially more chair time, create more work for the hygienist, and need more frequent oral prophylaxis. These visits do offer excellent opportunities for encouraging patients addicted to tobacco to enroll in a tobacco cessation program.

Methamphetamine users are also likely to have much higher than normal caries activity and to be at increased risk of enamel, cusp, and whole-tooth fractures. Such patients will benefit from dietary counseling, as they commonly consume large volumes of sugar containing carbonated beverages. They, too, are likely to exhibit significant tooth enamel extrinsic stains and calculus deposits. Patients who abuse amphetamine, methamphetamine, or cocaine tend to be more anxious and fearful of dental treatment than other patients. They have difficulty remaining still in the dental chair for extended periods of time, necessitating more frequent and shorter appointments.

The Dental Office as a Source of Drug Procurement

Historically, some patients with substance use disorders have found dental offices to be an easy target for obtaining narcotic analgesics, either to be used or sold on the street. It is relatively easy for a patient to act as if they are experiencing dental pain and enter a busy practice at an inopportune time, requesting specific painkillers, "To get by until I can get to my regular dentist." Typically, a patient will attempt this ploy with multiple dental offices in the same area until the ruse is uncovered, at which point the individual moves on to another area. Similarly, the patient with substance use disorder may call the dentist at home, seeking a telephone prescription for narcotic medications. In general, these ploys can be thwarted by insisting that the source of the pain be evaluated and treated and not simply managed with analgesics. A long-duration local anesthetic such as bupivacaine can be used to provide pain relief for 1–2 days if definitive care needs to be delayed. If an analgesic is determined to be indicated, it is wise to prescribe only nonnarcotic analgesics.

Refusing to call in prescriptions for patients who are not currently active in the practice is professionally prudent and consistent with the expectations of many US state dental practice rules. Networking with pharmacists, physicians, dentists, and other healthcare providers to identify drug seekers is also effective in many cases. As mentioned earlier, one effective method is utilizing the Prescription Drug Monitoring Program, which gives the dentist the ability to check an electronic database that records controlled substance prescriptions in their state.[123]

Dentists should be careful with drug samples kept in the office, making sure the samples are securely locked away where they cannot be taken by staff or after-hours custodial workers. All controlled substances stored in the office must be monitored with a perpetual inventory that documents how much and to whom the substances have been given.

Theft/Burglary

Although the dental office is often regarded by the dentist and office staff as an unlikely target for burglary and vandalism, in fact, cash, cancelled checks, syringes, prescription pads, and medications—anything that can be used as drug paraphernalia or can be used by an abuser or turned into cash on the street—constitutes a prime target. The necessity for keeping the office secure is obvious. It is important to keep supplies of drugs, syringes, and prescription pads out of the view of patients. When treating an individual who is a suspected substance abuser, it is prudent to take inventory of the operatory before and after each patient visit.

Dental offices have been broken into when they are a known source of nitrous oxide. Sometimes this is the focus of an impromptu party on the premises. In other cases, the nitrous tanks are removed for later use or sold on the street. The need for security and monitoring of inventory is self-evident.

Substance Abuse by a Member of the Office Team or Other Dental Healthcare Professional

Unfortunately, substance abuse is a significant problem for the dental profession. Most US state dental licensing boards, in cooperation with local and state dental societies, have developed responsible and humane programs that are effective in helping the abusing professional to recover and continue to practice in the profession.[124]

The American Dental Association is an excellent resource for dentists to find help for themselves or office staff if they suspect substance abuse, mental illness, and **burnout**. Burnout is physical or mental collapse caused by overwork or stress. As a result of the nature of clinical practice and the personality traits, dentists are more prone than the average individual to anxiety disorders, clinical depression, and professional burnout.[125] The signs and symptoms of burnout are increased stress, substance use, and suicidal ideation or attempted suicide. Recognizing the signs and symptoms of burnout in the life of a dentist is paramount. A dentist experiencing burnout may demonstrate personal energy depletion and a lack of interest in people while not feeling very effective at what they do. This can be a concerning combination of factors for a dentist to deal with each day. Burnout is not necessarily age-related. It can occur at any time in one's life. Burnout is the result of three conditions: (1) emotional exhaustion, (2) depersonalization, and (3) reduced personal accomplishment. Six driving factors in the workplace that may contribute to developing burnout are (1) work overload, (2) lack of control, (3) insufficient rewards, (4) breakdown of community, (5) absence of fairness, and (6) conflicting values.[126]

A dentist who is in the throes of burnout may experience an overwhelming decrease in hope and motivation, detachment from work and life demonstrated by sarcasm and cynicism, plus a reduced sense of accomplishment and purpose. It is important to differentiate between stress and burnout as they are not the same. Stress is recognized by overactive emotions, loss of energy, anxiety disorders, and often the individual can self-recognize the condition. In contrast, burnout is associated with disengagement with blunted emotions, a sense of helplessness, and/or hopelessness with a lack of purpose. Burnout is easier to prevent than to treat, but it is treatable. However, burnout can be very difficult for the individual to recognize. A dentist who is not experiencing burnout is engaged in work and life, feels a purpose in life, and recognizes their effectiveness at work.

CONCLUSION

The dental management and treatment of a chemically dependent patient presents both unique challenges and rewards for the dental team. A patient who abuses alcohol or other substances is likely to have significant health and psychosocial problems, which will influence dental treatment and treatment planning. Unlike most health problems, this patient may have a vested interest in not disclosing their addiction and will go to great lengths to mask the signs and symptoms of the addiction. This can be troublesome, because the unwary dentist may initiate dental treatment that will be ineffective or potentially harmful to the patient. In a worst-case scenario, the dentist may precipitate a difficult-to-control hemorrhagic episode or potentially fatal cardiac event. If an addiction is recognized or suspected by the dental team, the necessity to confront the patient is clear, although it may be an unpleasant encounter. The chemically dependent patient is prone to the development of many forms of oral pathology, all of which the dental team must strive to prevent and eradicate. The referral of the patient to specialists for consultation, management of the medical issues, and control of the dependency problem are all important aspects of the dentist's role.

As with any patient, the goal of the dental team is to provide the chemically dependent patient with safe, effective dental care that is compassionately delivered in a way that demonstrates respect for the individuality of the patient. The medical and comorbid psychological problems of such patients, as well as their resistive behavior, often make this a much greater-than-normal challenge. The rewards, however, of assisting dependent patients in their recovery, and helping them achieve an optimal state of oral health in a safe, efficient, and humane manner are extremely gratifying.

REVIEW QUESTIONS

- What are the health consequences of excessive alcohol use? Does alcohol affect women differently from men? If so, how?
- Name some commonly abused substances and describe how their use can affect the general and oral health of patients.
- Describe (or name) some forms of therapy used to treat patients with alcohol or substance abuse problems.
- What types of behavior might a patient exhibit that could suggest alcohol or substance abuse?
- What findings from a patient's medical and oral health histories can be indicative of a substance abuse problem?
- What modifications may be necessary when planning or executing treatment for a patient who is abusing alcohol or other substances? Would any of these modifications apply to the recovering patient?
- How might a dental office become a source of drugs for addicted individuals?
- How might a dentist use SBIRT to help invite a patient into a conversation about their potentially dangerous alcohol or drug use?
- What are the three main signs of a dentist experiencing burnout?
- What are the causes in the workplace that can lead to burnout

REFERENCES

1. Degenhardt L, Dierker L, Chiu WT, et al. Evaluating the drug use "gateway" theory using cross-national data: consistency and associations of the order of initiation of drug use among participants in the WHO World Mental Health Surveys. *Drug Alcohol Depend.* 2010;108(1-2):84–97.
2. Sarkar A., Characteristics of drug-dependent people. National Institute on Drug Abuse, 2004. https://www.drugabuse.gov/international/abstracts/characteristics-drug-dependent-people.
3. Wagner MK. Behavioral characteristics related to substance abuse and risk-taking, sensation-seeking, anxiety sensitivity, and self-reinforcement. *Addict Behav.* 2001;26(1):115–120.
4. National Institute on Alcohol Abuse and Alcoholism, National Institute of Health, Alcohol use disorder: A comparison between DSM-IV and DSM-5, 2021. https://www.niaaa.nih.gov/publications/brochures-and-fact-sheets/alcohol-use-disorder-comparison-between-dsm.
5. College of Dental Hygienists of Ontario. Substance use disorder, 2019. https://www.cdho.org/Advisories/CDHO_Factsheet_Substance_Use_Disorder.pdf.
6. Baghaie H, Kisely S, Forbes M, Sawyer E, Siskind DJ. A systematic review and meta-analysis of the association between poor oral health and substance abuse. *Addiction.* 2017;112(5):765–779.
7. American Cancer Society, Health risks of smoking tobacco, 2020. https://www.cancer.org/healthy/stay-away-from-tobacco/health-risks-of-tobacco/health-risks-of-smoking-tobacco.html.
8. Compton WM, Thomas YF, Stinson FS, Grant BF. Prevalence, correlates, disability, and comorbidity of DSM-IV drug abuse and dependence in the United States: results from the national epidemiologic survey on alcohol and related conditions. *Arch Gen Psychiatry.* 2007;64(5):566–576.
9. American Addiction Centers, Lethal drug combinations. https://drugabuse.com/drugs/lethal-drug-combinations/. Accessed 12/26/21.
10. Seeff LB, Cuccherini BA, Zimmerman HJ, et al. Acetaminophen hepatotoxicity in alcoholics: a therapeutic misadventure. *Ann Intern Med.* 1986;104:399–404.
11. Torrens M, Gilchrist G, Domingo-Salvany A. Psychiatric comorbidity in illicit drug users: substance-induced versus independent disorders psyCoBarcelona Group. *Drug Alcohol Depend.* 2011;113(2-3):147–156.

12. Brady KT, Haynes LF, Hartwell KJ, Killeen TK. Substance use disorders and anxiety: a treatment challenge for social workers. *Soc Work Public Health*. 2013;28(3-4):407–423.

13. Skinner HA. The drug abuse screening test. *Addict Behav*. 1982;7(4):363–371.

14. National Institute on Drug Abuse, National Institute of Health, Common comorbidities with substance use disorders research report, 2020. https://www.drugabuse.gov/download/1155/common-comorbidities-substance-use-disorders-research-report.pdf?v=5d6a5983e0e9353d46d01767fb20354b.

15. Davis L, Uezato A, Newell JM, Frazier E. Major depression and comorbid substance use disorders. *Curr Opin Psychiatry*. 2008;21(1):14–18.

16. Ross S, Peselow E. Co-occurring psychotic and addictive disorders: neurobiology and diagnosis. *Clin Neuropharmacol*. 2012;35(5):235–243.

17. Hser YI, Grella CE, Hubbard RL, et al. An evaluation of drug treatments for adolescents in 4 US cities. *Arch Gen Psychiatry*. 2001;58(7):689–695.

18. Kelly TM, Daley DC. Integrated Treatment of Substance Use and Psychiatric Disorders. *Soc Work Public Health*. 2013;28(0):388–406.

19. Magidson JF, Liu S-M, Lejuez CW, Blanco C. Comparison of the Course of Substance Use Disorders among Individuals With and Without Generalized Anxiety Disorder in a Nationally Representative Sample. *J Psychiatr Res*. 2012;46(5):659–666.

20. Conway KP, Compton W, Stinson FS, Grant BF. Lifetime comorbidity of DSM-IV mood and anxiety disorders and specific drug use disorders: results from the National Epidemiologic Survey on Alcohol and Related Conditions. *J Clin Psychiatry*. 2006;67(2):247–257.

21. De Alwis D, Lynskey MT, Reiersen AM, Agrawal A. Attention-deficit/hyperactivity disorder subtypes and substance use and use disorders in NESARC. *Addict Behav*. 2014;39(8):1278–1285.

22. Harstad E, Levy S, Abuse C on S. Attention-Deficit/Hyperactivity Disorder and Substance Abuse. *Pediatrics*. 2014;134(1):e293–e301.

23. Hartz SM, Pato CN, Medeiros H, et al. Comorbidity of severe psychotic disorders with measures of substance use. *JAMA Psychiatry*. 2014;71(3):248–254.

24. Pennay A, Cameron J, Reichert T, et al. A systematic review of interventions for co-occurring substance use disorder and borderline personality disorder. *J Subst Abuse Treat*. 2011;41(4):363–373.

25. Lubman DI, King JA, Castle DJ. Treating comorbid substance use disorders in schizophrenia. *Int Rev Psychiatry Abingdon Engl*. 2010;22(2):191–201.

26. Goldner EM, Lusted A, Roerecke M, Rehm J, Fischer B. Prevalence of Axis-1 psychiatric (with focus on depression and anxiety) disorder and symptomatology among non-medical prescription opioid users in substance use treatment: systematic review and meta-analyses. *Addict Behav*. 2014;39(3):520–531.

27. Wang J-C, Kapoor M, Goate AM. The genetics of substance dependence. *Annu Rev Genomics Hum Genet*. 2012;13:241–261.

28. Pelayo-Terán JM, Suárez-Pinilla P, Chadi N, Crespo-Facorro B. Gene-environment interactions underlying the effect of cannabis in first episode psychosis. *Curr Pharm Des*. 2012;18(32):5024–5035.

29. Cerdá M, Sagdeo A, Johnson J, Galea S. Genetic and environmental influences on psychiatric comorbidity: a systematic review. *J Affect Disord*. 2010;126(1-2):14–38.

30. National Institute on Alcohol Abuse and Alcoholism. Published April 2021. https://www.niaaa.nih.gov/publications/brochures-and-fact sheets/understanding-alcohol-use-disorder.

31. Centers for Disase Control and Prevention, Alcohol use and your health, 2021. https://www.cdc.gov/alcohol/fact-sheets/alcohol-use.htm

32. United States Department of Agriculture, Dietary guidelines for Americans 2020-2025, https://www.dietaryguidelines.gov/sites/default/files/2020-12/Dietary_Guidelines_for_Americans_2020-2025.pdf. Accessed Dec 27, 2021.

33. Cuberos M, Chatah EM, Baquerizo HZ, Weinstein G. Dental management of patients with substance use disorder. *Clinical Dentistry Reviewed*. 2020;4(1):14.

34. Ericson N. Office of Justice Programs, US Department of Justice (May 2001). Substance Abuse – the nations number 1 helath problem. https://www.ojp.gov/pdffiles1/ojjdp/fs200117.pdf.

35. Flórez-Salamanca L, Secades-Villa R, Budney AJ, García-Rodríguez O, Wang S, Blanco C. Probability and predictors of cannabis use disorders relapse: Results of the National Epidemiologic Survey on Alcohol and Related Conditions (NESARC). *Drug Alcohol Depend*. 2013;132(0):127–133.

36. U.S. Social Security Administration, Drugs used with alcohol or with 2 hours of alcohol use on most recent use of alcohol in past month among past month alcohol users aged 12 or older, by age group and underage and legal drinking age groups. https://www.samhsa.gov/data/sites/default/files/reports/rpt29394/NSDUHDetailedTabs2019/NSDUHDetTabsSect6pe2019.htm#tab6-21b.

37. Miller, S. Alcoholism and alcohol abuse, Recovered, 2021. https://www.ncadd.org/about-addiction/alcohol/facts-about-alcohol#:~:text=More%20than%20half%20of%20all,aspects%20of%20a%20person's%20life.

38. SAMSA, Children living with parents who have a substance use disorder, 2017 https://www.samhsa.gov/data/sites/default/files/report_3223/ShortReport-3223.html

39. National Institute on Alcohol Abuse and Alcoholism, Alcohol facts and statistics, June 2021. https://www.niaaa.nih.gov/publications/brochures-and-fact-sheets/alcohol-facts-and-statistics#:~:text=An%20estimated%2095%2C000%20people%20(approximately,poor%20diet%20and%20physical%20inactivity.

40. Westman J, Wahlbeck K, Laursen TM, et al. Mortality and life expectancy of people with alcohol use disorder in Denmark, Finland and Sweden. *Acta Psychiatr Scand*. 2015;131(4):297–306.

41. Schuckit MA, Daeppen JB, Tipp JE, Hesselbrock M, Bucholz KK. The clinical course of alcohol-related problems in alcohol dependent and non-alcohol dependent drinking women and men. *J Stud Alcohol*. 1998;59(5):581–590.

42. Daeppen JB, Smith TL, Danko GP, et al. Clinical correlates of cigarette smoking and nicotine dependence in alcohol-dependent men and women. *Alcohol Alcohol*. 2000;35:171–175.

43. Kessler RC, Nelson CB, McGonagle KA, et al. The epidemiology of co-occurring addictive and mental disorders: implications for prevention and service utilization. *Am J Orthopsychiatry*. 1996;66:17–3.

44. Schuckit MA. *Drug and Alcohol Abuse: A Clinical Guide To Diagnosis and Treatment*. 6th ed. New York: Springer; 2006.

45. Schuckit MA, Smith TL. Onset and course of alcoholism over 25 years in middle class men. *Drug Alcohol Depend*. 2011;113(1):21–28.

46. Schuckit MA, Smith TL, Heron J, et al. Testing a level of response to alcohol-based model of heavy drinking and alcohol problems in 1,905 17-year-olds. *Alcohol Clin Exp Res*. 2011;35(10):1897–1904.

47. Saitz R. Introduction to alcohol withdrawal. *Alcohol Health Res World*. 1998;22(1):5–12.

48. Choi YJ, Lee DH, Han KD, et al. The relationship between drinking alcohol and esophageal, gastric or colorectal cancer: A nationwide population-based cohort study of South Korea [published correction appears in PLoS One. 2018;13(5): e0197765]. *PLoS One*. 2017;12(10):e0185778.

49. National Institute on Alcohol Abuse and Alcoholism, Alcohol's effects on the body, 2021. https://www.niaaa.nih.gov/alcohols-effects-health/alcohols-effects-body.

50. Nelson RH. Hyperlipidemia as a risk factor for cardiovascular disease. *Prim Care.* 2013;40(1):195–211.

51. Martin PR, Singleton CK, Hiller-Sturmhöfel S. The role of thiamine deficiency in alcoholic brain disease. *Alcohol Res Health.* 2003;27(2):134–142.

52. Nicolás JM, Fernández-Solá J, Fatjó F, et al. Increased circulating leptin levels in chronic alcoholism. *Alcohol Clin Exp Res.* 2001; 25:83–88.

53. Cravo ML, Camilo ME. Hyperhomocysteinemia and chronic alcoholism: relations to folic acid and vitamins B6 and B12 status. *Nutrition.* 2000;16:296–302.

54. Markowitz JS, McRae AL, Sonne SC. Oral nutritional supplementation for the alcoholic patient: a brief overview. *Ann Clin Psychiatry.* 2000;12:153–158.

55. Oscar-Berman M, Valmas MM, Sawyer KS, Ruiz SM, Luhar RB, Gravitz ZR. Profiles of impaired, spared, and recovered neuropsychologic processes in alcoholism. *Handb Clin Neurol.* 2014;125:183–210.

56. Sullivan EV, Deshmukh A, Desmond JE, et al. Cerebellar volume decline in normal aging, alcoholism, and Korsakoff's syndrome: relation to ataxia. *Neuropsychology.* 2000;14:341–352.

57. Little J, Falace D, Miller C, Rhodus N. *Dental Management of the Medically Compromised Patient.* 8th ed. St. Louis: Mosby; 2013.

58. Osna NA, Donohue Jr TM, Kharbanda KK. Alcoholic liver disease: pathogenesis and current management. *Alcohol Res.* 2017;38(2):147–161.

59. Matsushita H, Takaki A. Alcohol and hepatocellular carcinoma. *BMJ Open Gastroenterol.* 2019;6(1):e000260.

60. Barry BL, Blow FC. Drinking across the lifespan: focus on older adults. *Alcohol research: current reviews.* 2016;Vol 38:1. https://arcr.niaaa.nih.gov/alcohol-use-among-special-populations/drinking-across-lifespan-focus-older-adults.

61. National Consumers League, Get smart about caffeine, March, 2016. https://nclnet.org/caffeine_facts/.

62. Bioh G, Gallagher MM, Prasad U. Survival of a highly toxic dose of caffeine. *BMJ Case Rep.* 2013;2013 bcr2012007454.

63. McCarthy DM, Mycyk MB, DesLauriers CA. Hospitalization for caffeine abuse is associated with abuse of other pharmaceutical products. *Am J Emerg Med.* 2008;26(7):799–802.

64. Better Health Channel, Caffeine. https://www.betterhealth.vic.gov.au/health/healthyliving/caffeine. Accessed 12/28/2021.

65. Cherney K. How long does caffeine stay in your system? Healthline, Nov, 2018. https://www.healthline.com/health/how-long-does-caffeine-last#how-long-symptoms-last.

66. Bertazzo-Silveira E, Kruger CM, Porto De Toledo I, et al. Association between sleep bruxism and alcohol, caffeine, tobacco, and drug abuse: a systematic review. *J Am Dent Assoc.* 2016;147(11):859–866.e4.

67. World Health Organization, Tobacco, July 2021. https://www.who.int/news-room/fact-sheets/detail/tobacco.

68. American Lung Association, What's in a cigarette? July 2020. https://www.lung.org/quit-smoking/smoking-facts/whats-in-a-cigarette.

69. Leite FRM, Nascimento GG, Scheutz F, López R. Effect of smoking on periodontitis: a systematic review and meta-regression. *Am J Prev Med.* 2018;54(6):831–841.

70. Aminoshariae A, Kulild J, Gutmann J. The association between smoking and periapical periodontitis: a systematic review. *Clin Oral Investig.* 2020;24(2):533–545.

71. Truth initiative, E-cigarettes: Facts, stats and regulations, June/2021. https://truthinitiative.org/research-resources/emerging-tobacco-products/e-cigarettes-facts-stats-and-regulations.

72. MacDonald A, Middlekauff HR. Electronic cigarettes and cardiovascular health: what do we know so far? *Vasc Health Risk Manag.* 2019;15:159–174.

73. Glantz SA, Bareham DW. E-cigarettes: use, effects on smoking, risks, and policy implications. *Annu Rev Public Health.* 2018;39:215–235.

74. FDA, FDA permits marketing of E-cigarette products, marking first authorization of its kind by the agency, Oct 2021. https://www.fda.gov/news-events/press-announcements/fda-permits-marketing-e-cigarette-products-marking-first-authorization-its-kind-agency.

75. Centers for Disease Control and Prevention, Quit smoking, Sept 2021. https://www.cdc.gov/tobacco/quit_smoking/index.htm.

76. American Dental Association, Tobacco use and cessation, Oct 2021. https://www.ada.org/en/member-center/oral-health-topics/tobacco-use-and-cessation.

77. American Cancer Society, How to quit smoking, Jan 2020. https://www.cancer.org/latest-news/how-to-quit-smoking.html.

78. Centers for Disease Control and Prevention, Marijuana fast facts and fact sheets, May 2017. https://www.cdc.gov/marijuana/fact-sheets.htm#:~:text=Marijuana%20is%20the%20most%20commonly,22.2%20million%20users%20each%20month.&text=Research%20shows%20that%20about%201,rises%20to%201%20in%206.

79. Statistica, Estimated number of cannabis users worldwide from 2011 to 2019, by region. 2021. https://www.statista.com/statistics/264734/number-of-cannabis-users-worldwide-by-region/#statisticContainer.

80. National Institute on Drug Abuse, Is marijuana addictive? https://www.drugabuse.gov/publications/research-reports/marijuana/marijuana-addictive. Accessed 12/29/2021.

81. Winters KC, Lee C-YS. Likelihood of developing an alcohol and cannabis use disorder during youth: Association with recent use and age. *Drug Alcohol Depend.* 2008;92(1- 3):239–247.

82. Lim CCW, Sun T, Leung J, et al. Prevalence of adolescent cannabis vaping: a systematic review and meta-analysis of US and Canadian studies. *JAMA Pediatr.* 2022;176(1):42–51.

83. National Institute on Drug Abuse, What is marijuana, Dec 2019. https://www.drugabuse.gov/publications/drugfacts/marijuana.

84. Lac A, Luk JW. Testing the amotivational syndrome: marijuana use longitudinally predicts lower self-efficacy even after controlling for demographics, personality, and alcohol and cigarette use. *Prev Sci.* 2018;19(2):117–126.

85. Grinspoon P. Cannabidiol (CBD) – what we know and what we don't. Harvard Health Publishing, Sept 2021. https://www.health.harvard.edu/blog/cannabidiol-cbd-what-we-know-and-what-we-dont-2018082414476.

86. Grafton SE, Huang PN, Vieira AR. Dental treatment planning considerations for patients using cannabis: a case report (2016). *J Am Dent Assoc.* 2016;147(5):354–361.

87. Colizzi M, Bhattacharyya S. Does cannabis composition matter? differential effects of delta-9-tetrahydrocannabinol and cannabidiol on human cognition. *Curr Addict Rep.* 2017;4(2):62–74.

88. Joshi S, Ashley M. Cannabis: a joint problem for patients and the dental profession. *Br Dent J.* 2016;220(11):597–601.

89. Schep LJ, Slaughter RJ, Glue P, Gee P. The clinical toxicology of cannabis. *N Z Med J.* 2020;133(1523):96–103.

90. National Institute on Drug Abuse, What are prescription CNS depressants?, Prescription CNS depressants drug facts, March 2018. https://www.drugabuse.gov/publications/drugfacts/prescription-cns-depressants.

91. World Health Organization, Opioid overdose, Aug 2021. https://www.who.int/news-room/fact-sheets/detail/opioid-overdose.

92. Centers for Disease Control and Prevention, Prescription opioid overdose death maps, March 2021. https://www.cdc.gov/drugoverdose/deaths/prescription/maps.html#:~:text=In%20 2019%2C%20an%20average%20of,totaling%20more%20than%20 14%2C000%20deaths.&text=While%20prescription%20opioids%20 were%20involved,rates%20from%202018%20to%202019.

93. National Institute on Drug Abuse, Benzodiazepines and opioids, Feb 2021. https://www.drugabuse.gov/drug-topics/opioids/benzodiazepines-opioids.

94. Centers for Disease Control and Prevention (CDC): *Prescription painkiller overdoses in the U.S.* http://www.cdc.gov/vitalsigns/PainkillerOverdoses/index.html/. Accessed February 19, 2015.

95. Centers for Disease Control and Prevention (CDC): Prescription drug overdose in the United States: fact sheet. http://www.cdc.gov/homeandrecreationalsafety/overdose/facts.html/. Accessed February 19, 2015.

96. Centers for Disease Control and Prevention (CDC): Compressed mortality file: underlying cause-of-death. http://wondcr.cdc.gov/mortsql.html/. Accessed February 19, 2015.

97. Centers for Disease Control and Prevention, Overdose deaths acceleration during COVID-19, Dec 2020. https://www.cdc.gov/media/releases/2020/p1218-overdose-deaths-covid-19.html#:~:text=Over%2081%2C000%20drug%20overdose%20 deaths,Control%20and%20Prevention%20(CDC).

98. Crane E., Emergency department visits involving narcotic pain relievers, Substance Abuse and Mental Health Services Administration, Nov 2015. https://www.samhsa.gov/data/sites/default/files/report_2083/ShortReport-2083.html.

99. Centers for Disease Control and Prevention, Prescription drug monitoring programs (PDMPs), May 2021. https://www.cdc.gov/drugoverdose/pdmp/states.html.

100. Mayo Clinic, Prescription drug abuse, Oct 2018. https://www.mayoclinic.org/diseases-conditions/prescription-drug-abuse/symptoms-causes/syc-20376813.

101. Habal R. What is the global prevalence of heroin use?, Medscape, Dec 31, 2020. https://www.medscape.com/answers/166464-159460/what-is-the-global-prevalence-of-heroin-use.

102. McCabe SE, Boyd CJ, Evans-Polce RJ, McCabe VV, Schulenberg JE, Veliz PT. Pills to powder: a 17-year transition from prescription opioids to heroin among us adolescents followed into adulthood. *J Addict Med*. 2021;15(3):241–244.

103. Caryn Rabin R. Overdose deaths reached record high as the pandemic spread, NY Times, Nov 17, 2021. https://www.nytimes.com/2021/11/17/health/drug-overdoses-fentanyl-deaths.html?algo=combo_als_clicks_decay_96_50_ranks&block=5&campaign_id=142&emc=edit_fory_20211119&fellback=false&imp_id=448469726&instance_id=45754&nl=for-you&nlid=51888241&pool=pool%2Ffa8f6616-7b25-42bd-bdbf-7abdec20107e&rank=1&regi_id=51888241&req_id=380863347&segment_id=74783&surface=for-you-email-rotating-health&user_id=372051d50e7aaaa3549920dbe0c687fe&variant=1_combo_als_clicks_decay_96_50_ranks.

104. Abed H, Hassona Y. Oral healthcare management in heroin and methadone users. *Br Dent J*. 2019;226(8):563–567.

105. Amiri S, Shekarchizadeh H. Oral health-related quality of life among a group of patients with substance use disorders in rehabilitation treatment: a cross-sectional study. *BMC Oral Health*. 2021;21(1):409.

106. Shekarchizadeh H, Khami MR, Mohebbi SZ, Ekhtiari H, Virtanen JI. Oral health status and its determinants among opiate dependents: a cross-sectional study. *BMC Oral Health*. 2019;19(1):5.

107. National Institute on drug abuse. Naloxone drug facts. https://www.drugabuse.gov/publications/drugfacts/naloxone. Accessed 12/15/21.

108. American Medical Association Opioid Taskforce. Help save lives: Co-prescribe naloxone to patients at risk of overdose. https://www.aafp.org/dam/AAFP/documents/patient_care/pain_management/co-branded-naloxone.pdf. Accessed 12/14/21.

109. van Dorp E, Yassen A, Dahan A. Naloxone treatment in opioid addiction: the risks and benefits. *Expert Opin Drug Saf*. 2007;6(2):125–132.

110. O'Neil M. (ed). The ADA Practical Guide to Substance Use Disorders and Safe Prescribing. 2015.

111. NIDA. Cocaine DrugFacts. 2021. https://nida.nih.gov/publications/drugfacts/cocaine. Accessed 10/11/2022.

112. Drug Policy Alliance, How many people use cocaine? https://drugpolicy.org/drug-facts/cocaine/how-many-people-use-cocaine. Accessed 11/15/2021.

113. Nassar P, Ouanounou A. Cocaine and methamphetamine: pharmacology and dental implications. *Can J Dent Hyg*. 2020;54(2):75–82.

114. Little JW, Miller C, Rhodus NL. *Little and Falace's Dental Management of the Medically Compromised Patient*. 9th ed. St. Louis MO: Elsevier; 2018:590.

115. Substance Abuse and Mental Health Services Administration, National survey on drug use and health, Sept 2020. https://www.samhsa.gov/data/sites/default/files/reports/rpt29392/Assistant-Secretary-nsduh2019_presentation/Assistant-Secretary-nsduh2019_presentation.pdf.

116. National Institute on Drug Abuse, What is the scope of methamphetamine use in the United States?, Oct 2021.https://www.drugabuse.gov/publications/research-reports/methamphetamine/what-scope-methamphetamine-misuse-in-united-states.

117. National Institute on Drug Abuse, What are the immediate (short-term) effects of methamphetamine misuse?, Oct 2019. https://www.drugabuse.gov/publications/research-reports/methamphetamine/what-are-immediate-short-term-effects-methamphetamine-misuse.

118. Hubbard B, Saad H, On Syria's ruins, a drug empire flourishes, The New York Times, Dec. 5, 2021. https://www.nytimes.com/2021/12/05/world/middleeast/syria-drugs-captagon-assad.html.

119. Stanciu CN, Glass M, Muzyka BC, Glass OM. "Meth mouth": an interdisciplinary review of a dental and psychiatric condition. *J Addict Med*. 2017;11(4):250–255.

120. Pabst A, Castillo-Duque JC, Mayer A, Klinghuber M, Werkmeister R. Meth mouth—a growing epidemic in dentistry? *Dent J (Basel)*. 2017;5(4):29.

121. Mukherjee A, Dye BA, Clague J, Belin TR, Shetty V. Methamphetamine use and oral health-related quality of life. *Qual Life Res*. 2018;27(12):3179–3190.

122. Viswanath A, Barreveld AM, Fortino M. Assessment and management of the high-risk dental patient with active substance use disorder. *Dent Clin North Am*. 2020;64(3):547–558.

123. Centers for Disease Control and Prevention, Prescription drug monitoring programs (PDMPs), 2021. https://www.cdc.gov/drugoverdose/pdmp/index.html.

124. American Dental Association, State well-being program directory. http://www.dentistwellbeing.com/pdf/ADA_Dentist_WellBeing_Program_Dir.pdf. Accessed 12/29/2021.

125. Rada RE, Johnson-Leong C. Stress, burnout, anxiety and depression among dentists. *J Am Dent Assoc*. 2004;135(6):788–794.

126. Rampton J. The 6 causes of professional burnout and how to avoid them. Forbes magazine. May 13, 2015. https://www.forbes.com/sites/johnrampton/2015/05/13/the-6-causes-of-professional-burnout-and-how-to-avoid-them/?sh=2b6531781dde.

15

Patients With Anxiety, Fear, or a Phobia of Dental Care

Sarah Getch, Erinne Kennedy, and Cindy L. Marek

🛜 Visit eBooks.Health.Elsevier.com

INTRODUCTION

Person-Centered Care

High levels of dental **anxiety** and **fear** are common among individuals in the United States and across the globe.[1-4] Approximately 20% of US adults in private dental practice settings report a moderate level of dental fear and 6% report a high level.[1] Smith and Heaton reviewed 19 published reports involving more than 10,000 adults in the United States and concluded that the rate of dental anxiety and/or fear has remained stable over the past 50 years.[5] Globally, national surveys in Iceland, Taiwan, Finland, and Australia document that at least some dental fear is experienced by between 21% and 50% of adults.[6-8] Studies of children have shown a global variation in the prevalence estimates of dental anxiety ranging between 3% and 43%.[9] Methods used to assess dental fear vary across studies complicating attempts to make direct comparisons both within and between populations, practice settings, and countries. None the less, dental fear impacts the global delivery of dental care.

    Person-centered healthcare is defined by the World Health Organization as the healthcare team and system empowering people to take charge of their own health rather than being passive recipients of services. The benefits of person-centered care are continuing to be explored and some include increased self-care, physical and mental status, patient dignity, systems of care, self-efficacy, and quality of life. Additionally, research shows a decrease in symptom burden, health care costs, and general uncertainty regarding healing.[10] Patients who have anxiety, fear, and/or phobias about receiving dental care benefit from a person-centered approach to oral health care delivery.[11] This chapter is designed to help the practitioner understand patients with anxiety, fear, and/or phobias and provide safe and effective oral health care using a person-centered approach. The following sections will familiarize the reader with (1) the nature and scope of the problem; (2) the characteristics of patients with fear or anxiety; (3) approaches to reducing fear during the phases of patient care; and (4) practical behavioral and pharmacologic interventions to help patients reduce or eliminate their fear. Case examples (Box 15.1) will be given throughout the chapter to provide the practitioner with the knowledge and skills necessary for the assessment, diagnosis, and treatment of anxious patients.

BOX 15.1   Case Examples of the Four Categories of Dental Anxiety

Case 1: Distrust of Medical and Dental Staff

Cheryl, a stay-at-home mother, would not describe herself as an anxious person. She has four children at home, a household to run, and is involved with various community service projects. Despite being high functioning and organized, Cheryl has some difficulty attending her dental appointments. Cheryl has had few positive experiences with dentists throughout her childhood and into adulthood resulting in a mistrust of dentists and dental staff. Dental visits put her on edge, make her tense and even sometimes confrontational.

Treatment Recommendations:
1) Establish trusting relationship
2) Provide information and *explanation*
3) Present the treatment plan in writing and inform of any changes made to it
4) Emphasize patient's autonomy in own treatment
5) Request permission for each stage of treatment

Case 2: Fear of Specific Stimuli

Christian has just graduated from college and started a fulltime job. He considers himself a worrier and often finds himself overwhelmed by his persistent worry about his finances, his health, work performance and relationships. Christian hates letting people down and can be embarrassed by how his anxiety affects his behavior. Often, his anxiety will get the best of him resulting in multiple missed appointments and instances of poor oral health that have led to emergency situations.

Treatment Recommendations:
1) Refocus or redirect as necessary
2) Relaxation
3) Systematic desensitization through early introduction of feared stimuli
4) Coping strategies (deep breathing, mindfulness)

Case 3: Generalized Anxiety

Adam is fidgety, restless, and very nervous about receiving dental care. While he does not experience high levels of anxiety daily, today his heart is racing and his muscles are tense. In fact, he turned around twice on his way to the dentist today resulting in him being 15 minutes late. Adam is a former college athlete and avid runner who has experience with pain but worries about whether his dentist will have to use the drill and the pain it will cause.

Treatment Recommendations:
1) Refocus or redirect as necessary
2) Relaxation techniques and gradual exposure (multiple appointments)
3) Consider pharmacological support
4) Positive reassurance before, during, after
5) Focus on present moment

Case 4: Fear of Medical Catastrophe

Teresa is a software engineer who is genuinely gripped by fear throughout most of medical visits. Each dental visit, she waits in the waiting room clutching her throat and mumbling to herself, which can sometimes put other patients and the dental staff on edge. The night before the dental visit she had trouble sleeping and found herself pacing the room with her heart racing, dizziness, and fear that she was going to die. She worries that she might choke or have an allergic reaction to local anesthesia during the visit.

Treatment Recommendations:
1) Rule out potential allergies/education of allergies and medication
2) Systematic desensitization through early introduction to feared body sensations
3) Relaxation
4) Psychological referral and/or consult

CHARACTERISTICS OF DENTAL ANXIETY, FEAR, AND PHOBIA

Anxiety results in an emotional, behavioral, cognitive, and physical response to an anticipated experience that the individual perceives as threatening. Anxiety can range in severity from mild to severe and can be generalized or a result of specific stimuli. Severe anxiety, as seen with Case 4, Teresa, may significantly limit the individual's ability to function effectively in everyday life. When daily functioning is impaired to the point of negatively impacting work performance or personal relationships, psychological or psychiatric intervention may be necessary. When the dentist observes symptoms of extreme generalized anxiety such as severe, chronic worry about a number of things, the patient should be referred to an appropriate behavioral healthcare provider.

Anxiety and fear are related but distinct emotions. **Fear** is a multifaceted response to an immediate and present danger and is most closely associated with a flight or fight reaction.[12] Anxiety, however, is a response to uncertainty about the future, the unknown, or a future negative event. Research has indicated that fear and anxiety are represented by distinct neural circuitry. Fear-arousal is associated with activity in the amygdala while anxiety is associated with activity in the bed nucleus of the stria terminalis.[13] In its extreme form, persistent, excessive, unrealistic fear of any stimulus can interfere with the ability to perform daily tasks. When the fear of a particular stimulus affects an individual's life to a significant extent and the individual goes to great lengths to avoid the stimulus, it is described as a **phobia**. Sometimes such fears become generalized to multiple stimuli. Dental phobia is a special case of dental fear characterized as a consistent and persistent fear that interferes with a person's social functioning (e.g., relationships) or role functioning (e.g., caregiving) and often leads to avoidance of almost all dental treatment. Medical and mental health professionals draw distinctions between anxiety, fear, and phobias, but a patient may use the terms interchangeably and therefore the dentist will need to provide the appropriate anxiety assessment to determine the nature of the problem/symptoms.

Patients with anxiety, fear, or phobias often report that they are frightened by specific dental stimuli.[14] The feared object or objects may include the needle, office sounds (suction, drilling, or buzzing of machinery), drill, or even smell of products used in the office including cleaners, gloves, or dental materials.[15] Case 3, Adam, is a great example of a patient with fear of specific dental stimuli. Adam is convinced that the drill will cause him pain and as a result engages in avoidant behavior such as turning around on his way to the appointment. Some of the interventions that we will discuss later in the chapter will address his specific fear. Patients may also report distrust of dental personnel or fear of a catastrophe, such as a heart attack or choking during treatment. Other patients may not have fear of specific stimuli, but rather report generalized anxiety about another aspect of life, for example an underlying fear of pain.[16,17] We see examples of generalized anxiety in Case 2 when Christian describes the multiple areas of his life that result in persistent worry from his health to relationships to finances. Patients who catastrophize a situation may be concerned about pain or pain-related procedures, magnify the threat value of the pain, and cope less effectively with pain if it occurs.[18]

Anxiety affects the whole person and symptoms may present on emotional, behavioral, somatic, and cognitive levels. Affective emotional symptoms include the feelings often associated with being anxious. Patients may report feeling on edge, uneasy, nervous, tense, scared, or even terrified. It is also possible that some patients experiencing anxiety present as irritable or impatient. Understanding that there is a wide range of emotion related to anxiety will help the practitioner to identify anxiety early.

Behaviorally, anxiety may present as shaking, freezing, stuttering or stammering, or even impaired coordination. Anxious individuals may also avoid feared situations or stimuli resulting in missed appointments, difficulty driving, impaired relationships, or an inability to move throughout the world as desired. Although avoidance of feared situations allows individuals to feel less anxious in the moment, the long-term effects can be damaging to careers, relationships, and overall quality of life.

Although emotions are often thought of as a purely psychological phenomenon, emotions have a physical component to them. **Somatic symptoms**, or the physical expression of stress or emotions associated with anxiety can range from nausea and vomiting to rapid breathing and weakness. Broadly, the physical responses to anxiety can be cardiovascular (heart palpitations, increased blood pressure, feeling of faintness), respiratory (rapid breathing, shortness of breath, choking sensation/lump in throat), muscular (tremors, wobbly legs, **startle reaction**, rigidity), gastrointestinal (vomiting, nausea or upset stomach, heartburn, abdominal pain, diarrhea), genitourinary (frequent urination or pressure to urinate), and changes in the skin (flushed, pale, sweating, hot or cold spells). Case 3 describes Adam who can identify the physical symptoms that are associated with his moderate anxiety quite well. He reports the physical symptoms of heart palpitations (cardiovascular) and tense muscles (muscular symptoms). The thoughts associated with anxiety may be vague and diffuse fears about the future leading to a state of apprehension and uneasiness while other thoughts may be much more specific. Thoughts that distort a person's reality are often at the core of anxiety and depression. These faulty or unhelpful ways of thinking contribute to negative thinking patterns and often perpetuate symptomology described previously. Examples of faulty thinking include catastrophizing or thinking the very worst will happen, attending to selective information or only paying attention to the negative, making broad rules based upon little evidence, categorizing things to extremes or black and white thinking, or negatively labeling or blaming oneself after an experience. Thoughts provide a window into how the patient manifests their anxiety as well as an opportunity to intervene and reframe ways of thinking.

ETIOLOGY

The cause of dental fear is multifactorial, complex, and cumulative.[19,20] Although dental fear may appear at any age, current data suggest that approximately one-half of adults believe that their fear began during their preteen years.[21] Researchers have identified personal traits and external factors, circumstances, and events that contribute to dental anxiety patients.[22,23]

Early onset dental anxiety has been linked to cumulative lifetime experience of dental caries, patients who seek care only when symptomatic, and patients with concern (anxious, prone to worry, sensitive, or vulnerable).[24] For example, children who received restorative or surgical dental treatment as 9-year-olds are more likely to report dental anxiety as 12-year-olds if they have episodic dental care and do not have regular dental visits between those ages and events.[25] Direct conditioning experiences and modeling play important roles in the development of fear in children who have a family history of dental fear.[26] Research on intergenerational transmission of fear and anxiety has shown that parents' fears/anxieties about dentistry are associated with adolescents' dental fear. This research also suggests that the father's dental fear is more predictive for transmission to adolescent family members.[27] Adult patients whose fears developed during childhood or early adolescence are less trusting toward the dentist than other patients and are more likely to exhibit high levels of generalized anxiety. These fears may lessen with maturity and after positive experiences with the dentist.[25]

For some patients, dental fear persists into adulthood and for others dental fear is categorized as late onset and is developed in adulthood. Late onset dental anxiety has been linked to cumulative lifetime experience of dental caries, losing at least one tooth in early adulthood, symptomatic users of dental services, and lower scores representing an internal locus of control.[24] Approximately one-quarter of fearful patients are believed to first develop their fear as adults.[21] Research suggests that consistent appointments for treatment that include time spent building trust and encouraging good oral self-care behaviors lessen the presence of dental fear. This research suggests that episodic and emergent appointments should be avoided when possible; however, sometimes treatment planning limited care patients is necessary.[28] When possible, a **dental home** should be established to provide regular preventive and comprehensive dental care.[28]

PAIN PERCEPTION AND MEMORY IN PATIENTS WITH DENTAL FEAR AND ANXIETY

The relationship between pain perception and anxiety is a complex experience.[29] The International Association for the Study of Pain defines **pain** as "an unpleasant sensory and emotional experience associated with actual or potential tissue damage or described in terms of such damage."[30] The sensation of pain as it is experienced by a patient is more than a simple reflection of the amount of tissue damage that has occurred. Pain is subjective and includes biological, psychological, and social dimensions that contribute to the patient experience. Sessle proposed that orofacial pain may be more complex than pain in other regions of the body because of the "special emotional, biologic, and psychological meaning" it holds for the person.[31] In addition, sensory nerves are heavily concentrated in the oral cavity, increasing the likelihood that individuals are acutely aware of their mouths.

Evidence suggests that anxiety and fear have different effects on a patient's pain threshold. In a landmark experiment, Rhudy and Meager showed that experimentally induced anxiety led to increased pain reactivity with a lower pain threshold, whereas high levels of fear led to decreased pain.[32,33] Among adults, anxiety may be associated with the patient's current assessment of the dentist's likelihood to inflict pain.[28] Evidence suggests that patients who experience anxiety starting in childhood and persisting into adulthood may overestimate the level of pain they will experience during dental treatment.[34] This overestimation of pain can lead to a high level of anxiety during dental treatment. From a biological perspective, if patients ruminate about a scheduled treatment and experience anticipatory anxiety, it will result in increased autonomic arousal and high levels of anxiety, which produce heightened levels of plasma catecholamines. Laboratory studies have shown that increased levels of plasma catecholamines lower the pain threshold and the patient's pain tolerance.[35] These data offer an explanation for highly anxious patients who show elevated levels of pain reactivity during dental treatment compared with less anxious patients.[36]

In addition to patient experience, dental anxiety also contributes to the level of pain that dental patients remember. One study asked patients to recall their perception of pain during root canal treatment 1 week after treatment and again 18 months later.[37] All patients had an accurate recall of the pain level at the 1-week interval, but, after 18 months, the patients with a higher level of anxiety remembered the pain as being greater than was recorded at the time of the treatment. Experimental pain research has shown that the recall of pain intensity is reasonably accurate immediately after a painful experience and after a short delay of approximately 2 weeks. But after 6 months, the memory of pain delivered within a stressful context becomes exaggerated, with women especially recalling more pain than men.[37] Moreover, exaggerated pain memories can alter brain pathways, further sensitizing the individual to painful stimulation.[38] These findings illustrate the importance of anxiety management at the time of dental treatment to minimize the patient's long-term recollection of the averseness of dental treatment and their anticipation of pain at future visits.

DENTAL ANXIETY AND HISTORY OF ABUSE

Patients who have experienced sexual or physical abuse are likely to have increased dental fear and to catastrophize about receiving dental care. Increasingly, evidence suggests that women with high levels of dental fear are more likely to have a history of sexual/physical abuse than other women.[39] Among children in the United States, 1 in 5 girls and 1 in 20 boys have experienced sexual abuse.[40] The prevalence of patients who have experienced sexual abuse suggest that dentists are probably treating patients who have experienced abuse. A greater understanding of the effect of abuse on anxiety, fear, and phobias of dental care that these patients may experience will help both the patient and dentist to complete care successfully.

For example, a study of sexually abused European women who were categorized by whether they had been exposed to sexual touching, intercourse, or oral penetration showed that women in the oral penetration group scored significantly higher on dental fear than women in the other two groups.[41] Women with a history of childhood sexual abuse and high levels of dental fear consider interpersonal factors related to the dentist as more important than do women with high levels of dental fear but without a history of childhood sexual abuse. These interpersonal factors include not believing that the dentist can be trusted and the absence of a sense of control. Specific symptoms, such as gagging, are also associated with both dental anxiety and a history of sexual abuse and these patients often have a tendency to believe a situation is far worse than it actually is.[42,43]

THE IMPACT OF ANXIETY, FEAR, AND PHOBIAS

Social Determinants of Health

Although much of the initial interview with a patient will and should focus on general health history, medication history, and oral health history, each patient also presents to treatment as an individual operating within the conditions under which they were born, grow, work, live, and age. These conditions and the wider set of forces and systems that continuously shape their lives are referred to as **social determinants of health** (SDOH) (Figure 15.1). SDOH have been shown to have a major impact on physical, mental, and oral health as well as overall well-being, quality of life, and contribute to healthcare disparities inequalities.[44]

Therefore, each patient interaction need not focus solely on the content of their visit, but also on the context of their visit within a much broader social framework in order to provide the most effective care and treatment planning. For example, you may have a patient present reporting moderate anxiety similar to Case 2, Christian. However, during the interview you learn that Christian also drives 3 hours for dental visits because he lives in a small rural community that does not have a dentist. Addressing Christian's anxiety in the context of his commute is important. If you plan too much during the visits initially, Christian may become overwhelmed and not attend his visits. However, if you plan too little, Christian may not be able to make the frequent trips required to address his oral health concerns. Understanding Christian's needs in the context of the SDOH that impact his ability to access oral health care is paramount for treatment plan success.

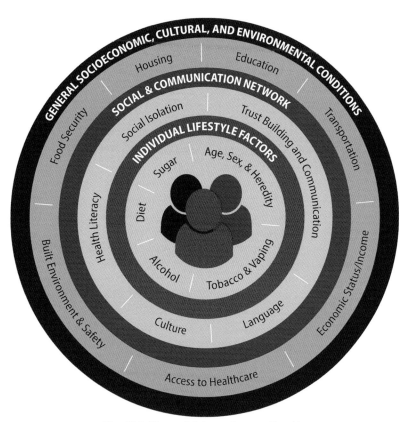

Fig. 15.1 The social determinants of health.

Access to Care[45]

One SDOH that impacts all aspects of health is access to care. Patients may have varied access to care because of where they live, their income or education level, or limitations resulting from their place of work. The **Three Delays Model** is a model that has been used in low- and middle-income countries to understand the barriers for women receiving healthcare in Haiti and explain the high maternal mortality rate.[46] This model has been validated and explored in multiple countries, across various healthcare specialties, and with varying research protocols.[47] The three categories of barriers are known as: Delay 1, Deciding to seek appropriate care; Delay 2, Reaching an appropriate facility; and Delay 3, Receiving appropriate quality care. Dental fear impacts all three areas of delays.[48-50] In some families, several generations of individuals have suffered ill health, oral infection, acute and/or chronic dental pain, loss of oral function, and loss of self-esteem—all because of anxiety or cultural practices about seeking dental care and treatment. In Cases 2 and 3, Christian and Adam, they reported missing appointments and having difficulty reaching the appropriate facility on time because of their dental fear.

Dental fear contributes to access to care barriers when patients enter the cycle of dental fear.[51] Some patients may avoid seeking oral health care and other patients may find the courage to schedule an appointment but will fail to attend appointments regularly or avoid scheduling certain types of appointments (e.g., root canal therapy or surgery). Delayed or nonexistent maintenance and preventive care frequently results in the

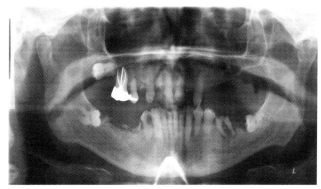

Fig. 15.2 Delaying dental treatment can result in increased cost to treat conditions such as rampant caries and replace missing teeth.

patient experiencing pain and the episodic emergency related care. In addition, the care required by the patient will probably be for more complex care, often at increased cost (Figure 15.2).

RECOGNITION, DIAGNOSIS, AND MANAGEMENT OF DENTAL ANXIETY

Standardized Indices

One of the goals for consistent and comprehensive patient care is to assess anxiety and fear in all patients. Including one of several surveys in a data collection appointment for all new patients is an objective way to collect this patient data. The Modified Dental Anxiety Scale (MDAS) (eFigure 15.1 found in the expanded chapter on ebooks+) has good psychometric properties, can be completed in only a few minutes, and can be quickly scored and interpreted.[4,52] The MDAS consists of five items scored on a Likert-type scale ranging from "not anxious" to "extremely anxious." Total scores are achieved by summing the five items. Total scores range from 5 to 25 with higher scores indicating higher levels of anxiety. Research indicates that a cutoff score of 19 can be used to identify individuals experiencing high dental anxiety.[52] Similarly, the Index of Dental Anxiety and Fear (IDAF-4C) (eFigure 15.2 found in the expanded chapter on ebooks+) contains eight questions and assesses the emotional, behavioral, cognitive, and physiologic components of fear.[53] The IDAF-4C consists of eight items measured on a Likert-type scale ranging from "disagree" to "strongly agree." Total scores are achieved by summing the items with higher scores indicating higher levels of anxiety. These scales are free, provide a standardized way of obtaining information, and afford the patient a nonconfrontational way of revealing fears and concerns about dental treatment. However, these indices are not diagnostic, rather, they provide information about a patient's symptoms, triggers, and level of dental fear/anxiety.

MANAGING A FEARFUL AND ANXIOUS PATIENT

When managing patients with anxiety, fear, or phobias, it is important to recognize that their symptoms will probably impact each appointment and each component of an appointment in different ways. Within a dental visit, various activities or time points may result in increased feelings of anxiety or fear. These time points include making and cancelling appointments, arrival at the office, the visit itself, as well as treatment planning and consent (Figure 15.3). Each time point offers an opportunity for the dentist and their team to identify and intervene on these waves of anxiety, fear, or phobia. The following section details each time point and provides instructions for assessment and intervention.

Accessing Care

According to the American Dental Association Health Policy Institute report, 4.1% of US adults avoid accessing dental care because of dental-related fear or anxiety.[54] Dental assistants and front desk personnel are in the position to observe these indicators and gather information from the patient that can help reduce their barriers to accessing dental care. The role of the dental team members it to understand the reason for a patient canceling appointments so that the appropriate resource can be provided. For patients exhibiting these behaviors, a question such as, "I noticed that sometimes you have trouble getting here for your appointment. What can I do to help you make your dental appointment?" Or, "Does going to the dentist make you nervous?" allows the patient to acknowledge the fear or to identify other barriers about which the dentist should know. For some patients, taking a virtual or in-person tour of the office prior to their first dental visit can help reduce the anxiety during their exam. Becoming familiar with the office surroundings and meeting the team can ease the anxiety the patient might

have for their first dental visit. For Christian, Case 2, he reports multiple missed appointments, and a history of seeking limited care. He may benefit from individual appointments that have a clear goal. For example, he may book separate appointments for a tour and meeting team, treatment appointments, and case presentation appointments. This will help Christian limit his worry or concern to one component of the dental experience.

Arrival and Introduction

Anxiety or fear about dental treatment may be apparent to the administrative and clinical assistants when a patient first enters the office. Research suggests creating a calm waiting room and clinical environment with soft music or white noise sounds, warm lighting, cooler temperatures or inviting posters or pictures. Some offices may encourage the use of essential oils to manage the triggering smells of a dental office and other offices may have fragrance policies barring this technique.[55] Patients may share information with the oral health team about previous dental experiences that will help explain why they feel anxious or fearful. Your team can be trained to identify the signs and symptoms of anxiety as patients often have enlarged pupils and sweaty or cold hands and are extremely fidgety in the waiting room or dental chair. Patients may talk excessively or not want to talk at all. When you notice these signs and symptoms, you can learn more about the patients concerns by saying "You seem a little nervous. Am I right about that?" followed by, "Is there anything I can do to help you be more comfortable?" Welcoming the patient and helping them through each step of the patient care process creates a positive experience and a less-stressful environment. In Case 3 described earlier in the chapter, Adam reported feeling fidgety or restless in the waiting room of the dental office. For Adam, your team will probably notice his anxious movements and will be able to personalize the waiting room experience and clinical environment to help reduce his anxiety.

Interview, Examination, and Diagnosis

Upon introduction to the patient, the oral health care professional will complete a full medical, dental, and social history. Using a specific question on the patient medical-dental health history questionnaire, such as, "Are you anxious about receiving dental treatment?" can be useful for identifying patients with dental fear or anxiety. If the patient responds positively, a series of oral follow-up questions regarding the patient's perception of the cause(s) of the anxiety can lead to fruitful revelations about specific averse issues, materials, and techniques. See Video 15-1, Interview of an Anxious Patient. Additionally, the use of a standard interview protocol whether a written questionnaire with oral follow-up questions, a semi-structured interview, or a complete open-ended format, as discussed in Chapter 1 may facilitate interviewing patients who present with dental fear.[55] The clinician can use open and closed questioning to learn more about the patient's symptoms and experience. For example, if the fearful patient is not talking, the clinician could ask open-ended questions to leave space for the patient to respond. If the patient is talking excessively, closed-ended questions will help the clinician focus the interview on the important information. A mix of open and closed questions produces the most effective

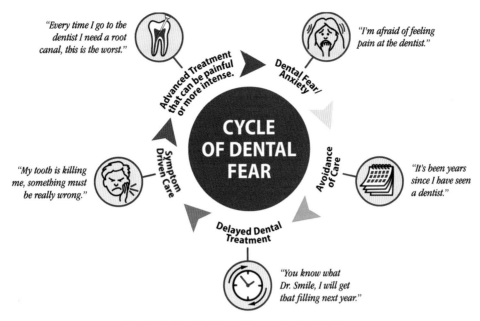

"Every time I go to the dentist I need a root canal, this is the worst."

Advanced Treatment that can be painful or more intense.

"I'm afraid of feeling pain at the dentist."

Dental Fear/ Anxiety

CYCLE OF DENTAL FEAR

Avoidance of Care

"It's been years since I have seen a dentist."

Symptom Driven Care

"My tooth is killing me, something must be really wrong."

Delayed Dental Treatment

"You know what Dr. Smile, I will get that filling next year."

Fig. 15.3 Model of the vicious cycle of dental fear.

interview and facilitates an ongoing dialogue. Knowledge of the patient's history, symptoms, and successful treatment experiences will be the foundation for future treatment planning.

Overall, facing the patient, making direct eye contact, and nodding as the patient speaks can be affirming and act as an encouragement for more conversation. During the interview, the clinician should face the patient, with the chair at the same level as the patient's chair in a room outside the treatment operatory. Patients with dental fear may find speaking about their fears or anxieties difficult in the treatment area. These initial moments are often the time when the fearful patient assesses the dentist's trustworthiness and the extent to which the patient's concerns are received. In Western culture, eye contact is the principal means of demonstrating involvement with another human being. Eye contact should be steady and frequent (without staring). Glancing elsewhere is acceptable, but the patient's face should be the focus of the clinician's attention. The clinician may take notes, but it is important to reestablish eye contact after each note is taken to reinforce the impression that the clinician cares about what the patient is saying. It is important to understand the cultural practices of your patient and adapt your practices to provide **culturally competent** patient care.

As pointed out in Chapter 1, the first step of the patient interview is obtaining accurate diagnostic information. This diagnostic information is the foundation of any evidenced based treatment plan, but to obtain that information, the dentist must first develop a relationship of mutual trust with the patient. Development of rapport and trust can begin in the first few minutes of getting acquainted. Research shows that the dentist who talks about nondental topics is more likely to be perceived by the patient as friendly and friendly dentists are more likely to produce satisfied patients. It may be helpful to start your patient visits with a conversation about the patient's topics of interest, unless the patient immediately initiates conversation about dental-related issues associated with their fear. Addressing the patient's concerns is the first priority of the conversation. Developing trust builds patient loyalty and patient loyalty is the foundation for a strong dental practice.

The second step to interviewing your patient is to practice "effective" listening. Listening is both active and reflective practice. Patients and healthcare providers listen through a filter of biases and prejudices that influence their interpretations of what is said. In this kind of interaction, it is especially important that the dentist not assume that they fully understand what the patient is saying or how the patient feels. It is a good practice for the dentist to reflect what they hear back to the patient their message by summarizing each phase of the interview. The dentist may wish to say, "Sometimes I am not as clear as I think I am or want to be. Have I said anything that is unclear or confusing to you?" Additionally, using intentional pauses or moments of silence can be a useful tool when listening to a patient. Patients may report feeling that they are not given adequate time to respond to the dentist's questions. This is especially true with older patients, who may need a bit more time to understand what is being said or asked of them. The dentist can use intentional pauses to allow the patient adequate time to collect their thoughts or to generate questions. Permitting the silence to continue may encourage the patient to provide important information that would otherwise have been missed. Overall, clinicians should encourage their patients to talk more, rather than less, during the interview. Instead, comments such as, "I understand that you are concerned about receiving dental care. Can you please tell me more about your concerns?" allows the patient to elaborate without having to justify their feelings.

The third step of building a relationship with a fearful patient is being able to understand the details of their story. One goal of the semi-structured interview is to facilitate the recollection of the patients past dental experiences. Understanding successful and unsuccessful dental experiences that they have had will help you recreate positive experiences moving forward.

Gathering this information can be accomplished by using a series of questions such as, "I am very interested in that part of your experience, which experiences have been successful for you? *[Intentional Pause]* Which experiences have been unsuccessful? *[Intentional Pause]*."

The fourth step of the interview is to practice empathy. The term **empathy** refers to the capacity and willingness to understand a situation from the other person's point of view. Using dental jargon that the patient does not understand or terms that the dentist or staff members do not clearly explain can make patients feel disrespected or not included. It is important to ensure that your patient can understand the conversation and feel empathy from the clinician. The more empathetic the clinician can be, the more likely it is that the fearful patient will accept treatment. It does not imply endorsement of another person's attitude or behavior, but it acknowledges the emotion another person, in this case the patient, is experiencing. The clinician might not have an experience similar to the patient, but empathy demonstrates that the clinician can be with the patient during theirs. Clinical empathy can be developed through a feedback loop much like hypothesis testing.[56] Successive cycles of conversation will establish what the patient believes about the nature of oral disease and treatment options available. Repeated positive conversations will allow the patient and dentist to move closer to a shared understanding about an acceptable course of treatment. If nothing else, the dentist's honest attempt to understand the patient's perspective will facilitate trust.

Treatment Plan Presentation and Informed Consent

After the interview, examination, and review of pertinent diagnoses, the dentist discusses the findings and explores possible treatment alongside the patient using a **co-diagnostic treatment planning** process. To set the stage for presenting the treatment plan to a highly stressed and fearful patient, the dentist may suggest that the patient take a few deep breaths and relax leg and back muscles. Often, it will help relieve the patient's anxiety if the treatment plan is presented and discussed during a separate appointment and in a room different from the operatory—for example, in a nearby conference room or office.

The patient's trust in the proposed treatment plan depends on the level of rapport developed, the perceived sincerity of the dentist, the level of competence that the dentist conveys, and the patient's confidence in the dentist. As the patient assumes a more active role in decision making, he or she accepts responsibility and ownership of the treatment plan. The patient's active role helps reduce anxiety and makes the patient a more willing partner in dental care. When possible, the plan should be structured to progress from least-complex treatment to more complex. This progressive increase in complexity will allow the patient to gain confidence in their ability to receive treatment. Prior to starting treatment, the patient will also sign an informed consent document and discuss the informed consent of the upcoming phases of dental care including the risks, benefits, and alternatives to treatment. Obtaining informed consent for patients with anxiety can present an ethical challenge but using the same techniques for a treatment plan presentation will help patients understand, discuss, and consent to planned treatment.

ETHICS IN DENTISTRY

Obtaining Informed Consent from an Anxious Patient

Anxiety can impact a patient's ability understand, critically evaluate, and participate in the discussion of treatment. It is the responsibility of the dentist to ensure that a fearful or anxious patient is fully informed before accepting an agreement to proceed with the next step of the treatment plan. Informed consent requires that the patient have sufficient understanding to voluntarily decide on the course of treatment. The dentist should be prepared to have multiple conversations with the patient and be prepared to revisit the treatment plan at each visit in a stepwise fashion.

The dentist's conversation with the patient is the most important component of obtaining informed consent. Discussion gives the patient the opportunity to ask questions and allows the dentist to gauge the patient's understanding of the proposed treatment. With every patient, the dentist should document the conversation and the information provided, and show that the patient's questions were addressed. The written consent form should be at an appropriate reading level and add to the conversation but not replace it. For the anxious patient, the form itself may raise further concerns because all the risks of the procedure are listed. The dentist should review the contents of the written consent form with every patient after verbal consent is obtained.

Direct Patient Care

The fearful patient is best served if the context in which care is received is based on mutual respect and concern. Many fearful patients have not previously received routine preventive care and may have extensive treatment needs, including some requiring complex, invasive treatment. If so, the patient will need reassurance that the dentist will make every effort to maintain the patient's comfort during treatment. However, no promises should be made that the treatment will be painless or free of discomfort. Pain-free dentistry is not a promise that can always be kept. It is also important to acknowledge the patient's feelings. Acknowledgment does not represent endorsement, but simply confirms that what the patient said was heard. During treatment, frequently checking on the level of comfort and keeping the patient informed of progress can help relieve anxiety.

As a part of the framework for care of a fearful patient, the dentist should work efficiently and systematically. Planning ahead and informing the patient about the next step can be reassuring. Keeping promises made to the patient will maintain the patient's trust; such promises may include the length of the appointment or the frequency of breaks. Being honest about the anticipated treatment helps both the dentist and patient. Fearful patients appreciate a frequent review of what has been accomplished, what remains to be completed, and any unanticipated deviations from the original plan.

The perception of a lack of personal control during the dental appointment can also contribute to dental fear.[57,58] Patients may perceive their inability to speak during dental treatment as a lack of control and their supine position below the level of the dentist to helplessness or vulnerability. Several studies suggest that when perceived lack of control is coupled with a heightened desire for control, patients are at risk of high levels of dental stress and pain.[59,60]

Providing fearful patients with a sense of control can facilitate compliance with the proposed care. Research has shown that fears about dental care increase when the fearful patient wants control during treatment and believes that they will not have it. Control can be provided both through information and choices about the treatment and during the treatment process. A strategy that returns some level of control to the patient involves inviting the individual to raise a hand when they would like the dentist to take a "time out." A dentist should not be surprised if a patient tests their willingness to give up control during the treatment by frequently raising their hand. Another option may include giving patients a choice of music to listen to during treatment.

Patients who manage their apprehension about dental treatment often have identified coping strategies that have worked well for them in the past. Fearful patients frequently do not have such well-defined strategies. Asking about preferred coping strategies might help the patient develop confidence in the process. Dental anxiety is often managed with conscious sedation techniques, which are described later in the chapter under "Pharmacologic Intervention." These techniques are reliable and safe, but it is important to remember that these agents do not treat anxiety; they only facilitate treatment.[61] Kvale and colleagues' meta-analysis of 38 studies using behavioral intervention to reduce either dental anxiety or anxiety-related behavior concluded that dental anxiety is treatable and that the effects of the behavioral treatment are long lasting.[62] No single intervention has emerged as significantly more effective than others. Rather, several behavioral interventions have proven effective in treating dental fear and anxiety and are reviewed in the following sections.

Refocusing

Learning to turn one's attention from anxious thoughts and engage in a more productive line of thinking is a valuable coping skill. Visually interesting artwork, décor, or tropical fish tanks can be useful when encouraging the patient to refocus on the present moment and shift away from feared stimuli. Some practitioners have used video games or a television set in the operatory as an effective and comforting distraction for anxious patients.[63,64] Additionally, two-dimensional and three-dimensional virtual-reality goggles have demonstrated reductions in blood pressure, pulse rate, and pain among patients undergoing some dental procedures,[65,66] although the effectiveness of this type of distraction may depend on patient characteristics, such as desire for control.[67]

Relaxation

The goal of relaxation is to achieve both muscular and mental relaxation. Research shows that relaxation can be an effective method of reducing patient anxiety.[68,69] Deep breathing coupled with muscle relaxation can be effective in stress reduction. Many fearful adults tend to hold their breath during basic procedures such as application of a rubber dam, injections, or impression-taking. When an individual's blood becomes poorly oxygenated because of an insufficient amount of fresh air entering the lungs, states of anxiety, depression, and fatigue arise, adding to the stressful situation. Deep breathing exercises help to reduce this unwanted stress and may consist of as little as 2 to 4 minutes of breathing deeply in, holding the breath, and then exhaling

completely. By demonstrating that deep breathing is something the patient can do independently, a new sense of control is provided to the patient, in addition to the calming effects provided by the breathing techniques. It may even be helpful to attach a heart rate monitor so that the dentist and the patient can assess this aspect of arousal and success in controlling it. Pausing during the procedure to suggest that the patient briefly repeat the deep breathing techniques can also be useful.

Muscle relaxation is also very useful in calming the patient. This method includes a series of exercises tensing and relaxing specific muscle groups (Box 15.2). Breathing and muscle techniques can be combined by tensing the muscles while breathing in and relaxing them while breathing out. Practicing this rhythmic coordination of relaxation techniques will quickly and effectively improve the patient's ability to relax.[70] Periodic reinforcement of muscle relaxation during treatment helps the patient regain composure. Pausing during the dental procedure and suggesting that the patient take several slow, deep breaths also can be useful. For some fearful patients, the mere act of

---

BOX 15.2 Muscle Relaxation Procedures

The following script can be used with patients for muscle relaxation:

"I would like to teach you a way to relax your muscles that may help you feel calm and I hope this helps you feel more comfortable during our visit today. We are going to help you feel better from your head all the way to your toes."

"We are going to start by turning on the energy in your feet, particularly your toes. If your mind wanders, that's okay. Bring your attention back to our practice. Let's start by wiggling your toes, back and forth, and notice the energy that moving your muscles creates. Now tighten your toes as if you are making a fist with your feet and notice the intensity of the energy in your feet. Hold the energy in your toes for a count of four . . . 1, 2, 3, 4. Now turn it off and relax those muscles. Notice the absence of the energy in those muscles. Make those muscles tense again as I count slowly to four . . . 1, 2, 3, 4. Notice how your muscles feel. Breathe in to turn on the energy in your toes, and as you breathe out, release your muscles, and turn off the energy.
"When you're ready, move your attention to your calves. Let's start by tightening your calf muscle, and notice the energy that moving your muscles creates. Now tighten your calves by pointing your toe, and notice the intensity of the energy in your legs. Hold the energy in your calves for a count of four . . . 1, 2, 3, 4. Now turn it off and relax those muscles. Notice the absence of the energy in those muscles. Make those muscles tense again as I count slowly to four . . . 1, 2, 3, 4. Notice how your muscles feel. Breathe in to turn on the energy in your calves, and as you breathe out, release your muscles, and turn off the energy."

After completing the procedures for the feet, calves, and thighs, move on to the next three major muscle groups: (1) hands, forearms, and biceps; (2) chest, stomach, and lower back; and (3) head, face, throat, and shoulders. The technique is often most effective when the clinician moves slowly from one muscle group to the next. It is helpful to talk slowly and softly and to provide suggestions after the relaxation phase, such as: *your muscles may feel loose, limp, or calm.* Using rhythmic breathing to coordinate the muscle tightening and relaxing is frequently a good way to help the patient fully participate in this exercise. Make suggestions such as *the sound of your breath exhaling will help remind you to relax your muscles.*

For most people, relaxing quickly and effectively requires a great deal of practice. Staying focused on the relaxation exercise may take several practice sessions; however, the benefits of the exercise can be immediately felt.

deeply inhaling and exhaling completely can help dispel negative reactions to receiving care.

Hypnosis and Guided Imagery

Hypnosis is a guided, self-controlled state of mind in which concentration and focus are directed inward. An altered level of consciousness is reached, similar to "zoning out" while daydreaming or reading a book. Guided imagery is a form of mild hypnosis that shares similarities with distraction and can be useful with fearful patients.[71] It produces a light, trancelike state from which patients can easily emerge and the procedure is less time consuming for the clinician than guiding patients into a deeper hypnotic state. Asking the patient to focus on a place where they feel very relaxed, comfortable, or safe is a good starting point for guided imagery and can be effectively combined with relaxation training.[72] Information about which type of images would be engaging can be gathered during the examination process. Current research shows that patients experience reduced pain and distress when they themselves choose the place to be imagined. The patient should be asked to choose imagery that is associated with little movement so that movements will not interfere with the provision of care. During guided imagery, the patient achieves an altered state like daydreaming or focused attention. By focusing on a calm and safe scene, positive emotions are elicited that can block or mitigate the anxiety arising from the dental treatment. An analysis of imagery topics chosen by patients showed that the topics are highly individual and further supports the efficacy of guiding patients to a "safe and comfortable place" of their own choosing.[73,74] Guided imagery is effective in managing pain during outpatient procedures and can be implemented by the dental team without disrupting the workflow in the patient care setting.[73,75]

In the past, the success of hypnosis was believed to depend on how hypnotizable the patient was and was used with a specific, "phobic" portion of the population.[76] However, more recent indications are that nearly all patients are equally able to engage in imagery during invasive outpatient procedures and that the imagery can result in reduced pain and anxiety.[76] Although nearly all patients are equally susceptible to hypnotism, attitudes, motivations, and fears relating to common misconceptions may interfere or impede the patient's willingness to be placed in a hypnotic state. The most successful conditions involving hypnotism in the clinical setting include a well-trained hypnotherapist and a patient who is highly motivated to overcome a problem.

For most mildly or moderately anxious patients, the most effective management strategy for the dentist will be taking time, actively listening to the patient's concerns and fears, and emphasizing building a trusting relationship. For more serious cases of anxiety, deep breathing techniques and hypnosis and/or guided imagery are among the most useful tools. The effectiveness of hypnosis in treating dental fear has been demonstrated. Hypnosis, however, requires specialized training and experience, and a brief "how to" belies the complexity of the strategy.[70] For dentists who are interested in receiving training in hypnosis, relevant organizations can be located via the Internet or through printed materials. Information about training opportunities may be available through local dental societies.

Altering the Treatment Approach and Sequence

If the patient begins to show high levels of stress, fear, or anxiety during treatment pausing or altering the treatment approach or sequence may be necessary. Under such circumstances, little will be gained and much could be lost in terms of the patient's trust in the dentist. If the patient expresses fear about certain, but not all, procedures, the dentist may need to alter the treatment plan. For example, if the patient fears extractions, the dentist may choose to delay that phase of the treatment until greater trust is built and the patient has experienced multiple positive experiences with the clinician. Fear and anxiety can limit the patient's ability to listen carefully so that if the treatment changes, the dentist must be sure the patient understands the change, and why the change occurred. At the end of the treatment session, reviewing the treatment completed and setting mutual goals for future appointments will improve communication.

Follow-Up Care and Referral

At any point in the care process, the dentist may refer a patient to a mental health care professional treatment. Interprofessional practice between primary care, behavioral health, and dental care is described across six levels, ranging from minimal collaboration or full collaboration in a merged and integrated practice (Table 15.1). Levels 1 and 2 are common practice among private dental offices and behavioral health professionals and include coordinated care where the key element is consistent, constant, and collaborative communication.[77] The first step in referring your patient is identifying a referral partner. If a behavioral health professional has not been identified, your team can call the county or state psychological or psychiatric association for the names of professionals who work with mental health disorders. After identifying a referral partner, safely sharing information about the patient will support collaborative care among the patients. A sample referral letter, such as the letter in Chapter 8, is included as an electronic resource (eFigure 15.3).

TABLE 15.1	Integrated Health Care: Dentists and Behavioral Health Clinicians				
COORDINATED CARE KEY ELEMENT: COMMUNICATION		CO-LOCATED CARE KEY ELEMENT: PROXIMITY		INTEGRATED CARE KEY ELEMENT: PRACTICE CHANGE	
LEVEL 1	LEVEL 2	LEVEL 3	LEVEL 4	LEVEL 5	LEVEL 6
Minimal collaboration	Basic collaboration at a distance	Basic collaboration onsite	Close collaboration onsite with some system integration	Close collaboration approaching an integrated practice	Full collaboration in a transformed/merged integrated practice

From https://www.ncbi.nlm.nih.gov/pmc/articles/PMC6797040/.

If the patient is currently in therapy, it is appropriate to ask the patient's permission to speak with the therapist. If the patient gives the dentist permission to contact the therapist, the dentist should consider maintaining an ongoing dialogue with the therapist during dental treatment. Questions that the dentist and the therapist might discuss include: How can we alter the sequence of the dental treatment plan to help our patient successfully complete comprehensive care? Which direct patient strategies could we work on together? Is sedation or pharmacotherapy recommended or contraindicated? Why? Are new anxiety treatments available that we could implement together? Based on the conversation with the therapist, the dentist can decide whether further referral is necessary or whether the patient is being treated adequately for their dental fear. If the patient's dental fear and anxiety do not subside, other measures may be necessary, including pharmacotherapy. As with all treatment, careful documentation of the anxiety treatment is important. In the United States, the dental team must adhere to the Health Insurance Portability and Accountability Act (HIPAA) privacy standards when discussing the patient's care among themselves and in sharing information with any other dentist, mental health worker, or medical care provider.

PHARMACOLOGIC INTERVENTION

Although many patients benefit from the behavioral techniques previously described, some patients will continue to experience extreme dental fear and anxiety. These patients may require *both* psychological and pharmacotherapeutic treatment to receive safe and effective dental care. The use of medications in the clinical management of apprehensive dental patients must be carefully monitored to prevent patient injury or death. The administration of any drug is never completely without risk, and therefore the use of these agents should be limited to patients who require some degree of sedation or anxiety control to undergo dental treatment.

Levels of Sedation

Pharmacologic techniques for anxiety control (**anxiolysis**) and sedation range from the use of oral antihistamines to induce drowsiness to general anesthetics, which render the patient unconscious. Depth of sedation is described as a continuum; as the level of sedation progresses, there are changes in patient responsiveness, ability to maintain an airway independently, and possible cardiovascular function impairment.[78,79]

The administration of any sedation involves an inherent unpredictability. Some patients may fall into a deeper level of sedation than intended by the practitioner. The dentist and staff must be able to recognize and manage these situations and be prepared to provide necessary airway and cardiovascular support, if needed, until the patient recovers or emergency medical assistance arrives.[79]

It is imperative that dentists who use medications for anxiety control and sedation receive comprehensive training in all aspects of patient sedation. Standards of safe sedation practice require the following:[80]

- Practitioners who are well acquainted with the dosages, adverse effects, and interaction profiles of all medications prescribed.
- Comprehensive preoperative evaluation of patients, including a thorough medical history, pretreatment evaluation, and examination.
- Physiologic and visual monitoring of the patient from the onset of sedation through the recovery period.
- The maintenance of appropriate equipment, medications, facilities, staff, and training to deal with emergency situations.
- A fully documented record of the procedure, medication(s) used, route of administration, vital signs, adverse reactions if any, recovery, and any emergency procedures used.

Routes of Administration

The **enteral** route of drug administration uses the gastrointestinal (GI) tract and includes oral, sublingual (SL), buccal, and rectal administration. The **parenteral** route encompasses all other means of drug delivery, including intravenous (IV), intramuscular (IM), subcutaneous (SC), transdermal, inhalation, and intranasal. The route of drug administration chosen for anxiolysis depends on practitioner and staff training, and patient-specific factors, such as the patient's level of cooperation, ability to swallow solid dosage forms, personal preference, and cost.

The oral route is the most common, safe, and cost-effective way to administer anxiolytic medications in the general practice setting. In the clinical practice of anxiolysis/sedation, it is important to remember that all routes of drug administration can cause any level of sedation. When medications are given via most routes, there is a "lag time" or latent period between ingestion of the drug, onset of action, and subsequent peak of clinical effect. In contrast, central nervous system (CNS) effects of drugs administered either IV or via the respiratory tract (inhalation and intranasal routes) are nearly instantaneous.

When medications are given via the oral route, both the rate and extent of absorption will vary owing to both drug and patient-specific factors. This variability is reflected in the manufacturer's package insert and drug information resources, which will indicate a range of time (1 to 2 hours or more) for the drug to reach peak plasma levels. Depending on the chemical properties of drug and the dosage form, this can mean that the sedative agent will be administered anywhere from several minutes to more than an hour before the start of the procedure.[81]

In addition, the oral route is complicated by a high degree of interpatient variability. Patient-specific factors that affect the rate and extent of drug absorption administered orally include gastric pH, vascularity, area of absorptive surfaces, GI motility, presence of other substances, and concomitant disease states. When using oral medications for anxiolysis, the dentist must take all of these factors into account when instructing the patient in the proper timing of home administration to achieve peak effects during the procedure.

When choosing a drug for anxiolysis/sedation, the practitioner must take into account the length of procedure, the patient's medical history, concomitant disease states, and current medications. In obtaining a medication history, the dentist must specifically question the patient about the use of herbal products, homeopathic agents, and dietary supplements, in addition to currently used prescription and over-the-counter medications. Many individuals do not report the use of herbal or dietary supplements to their healthcare providers. Some believe that these products are "natural" and therefore not drugs, whereas others are uncomfortable revealing self-medication practices for fear of criticism. Certain products are known to prolong bleeding times, enhance or attenuate sedation, and affect blood pressure.[82]

Impairment of cognitive and motor functioning by anxiolytics and sedative-hypnotic agents requires that all patients have a responsible escort to and from the dental office. To ensure patient safety and prevent possible litigation, it is advisable to begin the procedure only after the patient escort is in attendance. Practitioners may find it helpful to contact patients 1 or 2 days before the scheduled appointment to remind them to bring an escort and thus avoid postponement of treatment.

Therapeutic classes of drugs for the management of fearful patients include anxiolytics, sedative-hypnotics, nitrous oxide, opioids, and general anesthetics. These agents have a profound depressant effect on the CNS and may cause alteration of seizure threshold, skeletal muscle relaxation, and decreased respiratory drive.[83]

Benzodiazepines

The synthesis of benzodiazepines in the late 1950s has allowed safer and more efficacious treatment of acute anxiety over previous alternatives. Benzodiazepines are available in oral, IM, IV, and rectal dosage forms and are currently considered first-line therapy for the pharmacologic management of the fearful patient. Benzodiazepines are characterized by anxiolytic, sedative-hypnotic, anticonvulsant, amnestic, and muscle relaxant properties. These agents are used in dentistry either alone or in combination with nitrous oxide or other medications to induce sedation.

Currently, more than a dozen oral benzodiazepines are available on the US market (Table 15.2). They are often divided into either anxiolytic or sedative-hypnotic (insomnia) categories, depending on their pharmacodynamic actions. At normal therapeutic doses, anxiolytic benzodiazepines relieve anxiety and produce a mild degree of sedation without causing significant motor impairment or alteration in consciousness. At higher doses, benzodiazepines cause effects similar to alcohol intoxication in many patients, making this class of medication unsuitable for patients who are recovering alcoholics or substance abusers, because it places them at risk of recidivism.

The choice of benzodiazepine and dosage depends on the pharmacologic profile of the agent and patient-specific factors, such as age, concomitant medications, previous experience with the drug, and health status (Boxes 15.3 and 15.4).

Paradoxical (disinhibition) reactions, characterized by symptoms that can include excitement, increased talkativeness, hyperactivity, crying, or hostility, occur in fewer than 1% of patients receiving benzodiazepines and may be a dose-related phenomenon. This adverse effect occurs most frequently in patients who have underlying psychiatric conditions, a history of violent or aggressive behavior, or substance or alcohol abuse. Other risk factors for paradoxical reactions to benzodiazepines include a history of unusual reactions to sedatives, alcohol use or abuse, and age, with both the very young and the very old patient being more at risk.[81,83–85]

The dose and administration schedule of benzodiazepines is dependent on the patient's age; hepatic, renal, and pulmonary

TABLE 15.2 Select Oral Benzodiazepines for Anxiolysis

Agent	Common Oral Dosage Forms	Maximal Daily Adult Anxiolytic Dosage[a]
Alprazolam (Xanax[b])	0.25-, 0.5-, 1-, and 2-mg tablets; 1 mg/mL solution	Up to 4 mg/day in divided doses
Diazepam (Valium[b])	2-, 5-, and 10-mg tablets; 5 mg/5 mL and 5 mg/mL solutions	Up to 40 mg/day in divided doses
Lorazepam (Ativan[b])	0.5-, 1-, and 2-mg tablets; 2 mg/mL solution	Up to 10 mg/day in divided doses
Oxazepam	10-, 15-, and 30-mg capsules	Up to 120 mg/day in divided doses

[a]Maximal adult daily dosage for healthy patients younger than 50 years.
[b]Generic equivalent available.
From Facts and Comparisons eAnswers: *Benzodiazepines*. http://www.wolterskluwercdi.com/facts-comparisons-online/.

BOX 15-3 Drug Interactions with Benzodiazepines[81]

Alcohol and other central nervous system (CNS) depressants: CNS depressant effects and the risk of apnea may be increased

Clozapine: respiratory depression or arrest may occur

Itraconazole, ketoconazole, fluvoxamine, nefazodone—concurrent use may inhibit the metabolism of benzodiazepines that are metabolized by oxidation, resulting in delayed elimination and increased plasma levels

Hypotensive agents: may potentiate hypotensive effects of benzodiazepines

Opioid analgesics: additive CNS depression; must decrease the dosage of opioid by >30% and administer in small increments

BOX 15.4 Contraindications to Benzodiazepines[81,83,84]

Breast-feeding: infants cannot metabolize the agents to inactive compounds, causing sedation, feeding difficulties

Chronic obstructive pulmonary disease: ventilatory failure may be exacerbated

Geriatric patients: experience more pronounced central nervous system (CNS) effects; parenteral administration may cause apnea, hypotension, and bradycardia

Glaucoma: angle closure may be precipitated or worsened by benzodiazepines

Hepatic disease: half-life of some agents may be prolonged

Myasthenia gravis: condition may be exacerbated

Obstructive sleep apnea: exaggerates effect of apneic episodes

Pregnancy: increased risk of congenital malformations in first trimester, neonatal CNS depression

Recovering substance abusers: sensation of intoxication may promote recidivism

function; and the pharmacokinetic profile (absorption, distribution, metabolism, excretion) of the particular agent. As with paradoxical reactions, the elderly and very young are more likely to experience adverse effects with these agents. Benzodiazepines are not recommended for use in pregnant women or women who are breast-feeding.[84,85]

Nitrous Oxide

The use of nitrous oxide and oxygen (N_2O-O_2) inhalation for dental sedation and as an adjunct to dental anesthesia has been widely accepted by both patients and practitioners (Figure 15.4). The primary use in dentistry is in the management of fear and anxiety. A high degree of safety and efficacy, coupled with fast onset and termination of effect has made this form of inhalation sedation a useful option for many general dentists. The use of N_2O-O_2 requires a significant initial capital expense and proper training is required of all personnel who will be administering this form of pharmacosedation.

Nitrous oxide is the most frequently administered inhalation anesthetic by dentists. It exerts its effects on the CNS, producing cortical depression and diminishing all sensations including sight, touch, and pain. In addition to its sedative effect, N_2O possesses analgesic properties that make it a useful adjunct to local anesthetic in various clinical situations. At a concentration of 30% to 40%, N_2O produces the maximum degree of analgesia, and the patient remains able to respond to verbal commands.[86,87]

Nausea and vomiting are the most frequent complications associated with N_2O-O_2 therapy. To reduce the risk of these adverse effects, the dentist should only use concentrations of N_2O below 50%, try to limit patient exposure to less than 45 minutes, and instruct the patient to avoid food or liquid for several hours before the appointment.

The percentage of N_2O required for pharmacosedation may depend on many circumstances, including the type of procedure and the use of concomitant medications. Patient-specific factors, such as level of anxiety and pain threshold, must also be taken into consideration. The percentage of N_2O must be titrated for each patient during every procedure.

The rapid induction technique of N_2O-O_2 (also called "fixed dose") administration involves the initial use of a high percentage of N_2O (up to 50%) to sedate the patient quickly. The rapid-induction technique can result in oversedation, leading to a negative patient experience. Some of the signs and symptoms of oversedation include mouth breathing, nausea, vomiting, hallucinations, inability to move or communicate, out-of-body experiences, disassociation, combative behavior, and loss of consciousness, all of which contribute to a negative patient experience.[87] With rare exceptions, the fixed dose administration of nitrous oxide is not recommended.

The titration technique is regarded as the current standard of care when administering N_2O-O_2. After the patient is breathing 100% oxygen at an established flow rate via a nasal hood, N_2O is introduced at 10% to 20%. The gas is then titrated in 5% to 10% increments every 1 to 3 minutes until the desired level of clinical sedation is achieved. At the end of the procedure, the patient is given 100% oxygen for at least 5 minutes or until they no longer exhibit clinical signs of sedation. When completely recovered from the effects of the nitrous oxide, the patient may leave the office unescorted.[87]

To avoid hypoxia, N_2O must always be administered with at least 25% oxygen (atmospheric oxygen is 21%). The use of pure N_2O and the resultant anoxia can lead to seizures, brain damage, and death.[88,89] Nitrous oxide has low lipid solubility, which promotes rapid recovery because almost all of the gas is eliminated through the lungs within 5 minutes of halting N_2O-O_2 administration. Because N_2O is rapidly exhaled, it may cause "diffusion hypoxia" by diminishing the patient's other blood gases (oxygen and carbon dioxide). This phenomenon results in patient malaise, headache, nausea, and lethargy. To prevent this problem, it is important that the dentist provide 100% oxygen for at least 5 minutes immediately after cessation of nitrous oxide administration.[87]

Patients with many serious systemic conditions can often be managed successfully with N_2O-O_2 sedation. For patients with cardiovascular disease, the oxygen-enriched atmosphere of N_2O-O_2 therapy decreases myocardial work and reduces the risk of an ischemic event. Because N_2O does not undergo significant metabolism in the body, hepatic and/or renal dysfunction will not alter its clinical or physiologic effects. Patients otherwise unable to cooperate with dental treatment can often be managed successfully with a combination of nonpharmacologic techniques and N_2O-O_2 sedation.[87]

Anesthetic gases must be used with caution in patients with diseases or infections of the respiratory system. For patients with chronic obstructive pulmonary disease who are on hypoxic drive, elevated blood oxygen levels (from oxygen-enriched gas administration) may result in a decreased respiratory drive. Patients with upper respiratory infections, sinusitis, or other problems that compromise their ability to exchange air via the nose may have difficulty obtaining sufficient anesthetic through a nasal hood. Patients with infections, such as pneumonia and tuberculosis, can be at risk as a result of decreased lung capacity. Dental practitioners must take thorough health histories before scheduling the use of N_2O-O_2

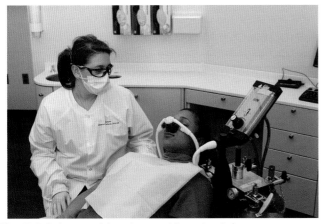

Fig. 15.4 Patient receiving nitrous oxide analgesia.

sedation and obtain physician consults when there is any concern regarding the patient's suitability for inhalation sedation and/or anesthetic.

Intravenous Sedation

The IV route is the most effective method of conscious sedation. Although IV sedation has been a mainstay for years in oral surgery practices, other dental specialists have adopted this technique for treatments involving implants and for periodontal and endodontic procedures. An advantage of IV administration is the ability to titrate the dosage rapidly to achieve the desired depth of sedation. Depending on patient need, sedation can vary from light to profound and nearly all patients can be adequately sedated with this method.

The amnestic effect of this form of sedation is particularly advantageous for the extremely fearful patient. Under conscious sedation, patients can maintain patent airways and respond to verbal commands and physical stimuli. At higher doses, the patient moves into deep sedation, in which protective reflexes (such as coughing) may be lost and the patient may no longer be able to maintain an open airway independently.

Drugs commonly used for IV sedation in dentistry include the benzodiazepines, diazepam (Valium), and midazolam (Versed). These agents may be administered alone or in conjunction with narcotics, such as fentanyl (Sublimaze) or meperidine (Demerol). In the United States, many states require a special permit to administer IV sedation. Initial investment in drugs and monitoring equipment is significant and the dentist must consider the liability issues that accompany heavier sedation. The use of IV conscious sedation requires specialized instruction in advanced cardiac life support, an extensively equipped emergency kit, appropriate monitoring equipment, and a trained support team. Iatrogenic injury, resulting from dose errors, failure to monitor vital signs, or the toxic effects of sedatives can be fatal.

Patients with respiratory, cardiovascular, or hepatic diseases and those at the extremes of age are at higher risk of developing complications while undergoing deeper sedation. Thorough patient medical histories must be obtained and informed consent given before intravenous sedation is administered.

General Anesthesia

General anesthesia offers the highest level of patient sedation. A patient under general anesthesia experiences the elimination of all sensation, accompanied by total loss of consciousness as well as loss of the ability to maintain a functional airway and, as a result, is at risk of a myriad of serious complications. This option is relatively expensive and is often reserved for young children or patients with developmental disabilities or those who have significant anxieties associated with dental treatment. Only trained dentist-anesthesiologists can perform outpatient general anesthesia in an ambulatory surgical care setting. Patients may also be admitted to a hospital for inpatient general anesthesia. In this setting, the dental procedure is carried out in an operating suite with an anesthesiologist responsible for drug delivery and patient monitoring.

Integrating Anxiolytic Therapy into the Delivery of Dental Care

For many practitioners, finding the optimal anxiety management plan for a patient often involves a trial and error approach that can be stressful for both the patient and the dentist. Although successful treatment of a fearful patient can be a time-consuming endeavor, it is often a rewarding experience for the practitioner.

The patient interview and treatment plan presentation are opportune times for the dental practitioner to assess both the need for anxiolytic measures and the patient's willingness to accept various anxiolytic management strategies. In the course of the interview, the dentist should question the patient as to their previous experiences with anxiety management. If the patient is adamant that techniques such as hypnosis and guided imagery do not work, the practitioner should avoid suggesting these modalities to preserve trust with the patient. On the other hand, a conversation that begins, "I understand that your experience with guided imagery showed that it didn't work for you. Newer techniques have been developed that may make it effective for you," may open the door for a patient to reconsider the use of guided imagery. The dentist might reassure the patient that they will not attempt to use guided imagery without telling the patient in advance. Patients who have previously had positive experiences with anxiolytic drugs are likely to request and respond positively to the same tactics.

The anxiolytic management strategy used will depend on practitioner experience and patient-specific factors. Patients with needle phobias may only require anxiolytic treatment when local anesthetic injections are necessary. Those with a history of negative dental experiences may require anxiolytic treatment for all appointments or only for those procedure(s) that resulted in discomfort in the past. Presenting the anxiolytic management plan in an empathetic, positive manner is an essential component of successful treatment because it instills confidence in the patient. Recounting examples of success with managing anxiety for other patients using the same management strategy can serve to reinforce the effectiveness of the plan and increase the patient's expectations of success.

The anxiolytic management plan may change over time because of either positive or negative patient experiences. At the conclusion of an appointment, the practitioner should inquire about the patient's perceptions of the experience. The dentist's approach should be supportive and nonjudgmental, offering positive comments that will encourage the patient to continue with treatment. If a procedure must be terminated because of anxiety or if the patient still expresses a great deal of fear, the dentist can offer alternate or additional strategies, such as adding an anxiolytic medication to guided imagery. Patients who are extremely fearful and minimally responsive to standard anxiolytic management strategies may need to be referred to practitioners qualified to perform deeper sedation.

Patients with positive dental encounters may, over time, experience a reduction in anxiety that decreases or eliminates the need for anxiolytic treatment. Although it may not be possible to eradicate dental fear, a compassionate approach to the management of these patients will enable them to obtain care with a minimum of stress.

CONCLUSION

Many factors contribute to the development of dental anxiety and fear. The dental team can select from among many tools to navigate the complex psychosocial concerns presented by the patient. If inroads are to be made in treating the high number of fearful dental patients, greater emphasis must be placed on addressing their specific concerns through effective communication and more effective pain and stress management.

The purpose of the pharmacotherapeutic management of anxiety is to provide dental care in such a manner that the patient feels relaxed and safe. Creating such an atmosphere is often best accomplished with nonpharmacologic interventions in addition to drug therapy. Ideally, positive dental experiences will lead to a reduction of fear so that the patient no longer requires anxiolytics or sedatives before dental treatment.

REVIEW QUESTIONS

- What results in dental fear, anxiety or phobias?
- What are the signs and symptoms of dental anxiety?
- How can the dental team recognize and diagnose dental anxiety?
- When should a patient be referred for professional help with dental anxiety?
- Which techniques will you use to provide comprehensive care to patients with anxiety?
- Which pharmacologic strategies (e.g., analgesia, sedation, general anesthetic) are available for managing the anxious patient and what are the advantages and disadvantages of each?

SUGGESTED PROJECTS

Develop a personalized behavioral health referral consultation letter based on the sample in eFigure 15.3 for your practice.

REFERENCES

1. White AM, Giblin L, Boyd LD. The Prevalence of Dental Anxiety in Dental Practice Settings. *J Dent Hyg.* 2017;91(1):30–34.
2. Armfield JM. The extent and nature of dental fear and phobia in Australia. *Aust Dent J.* 2010;55:368–377.
3. Nicolas E, Collado V, Faulks D, Bullier B, et al. A national cross-sectional survey of dental anxiety in the French adult population. *BMC Oral Health.* 2007;7:12.
4. Humphris G, Crawford JR, Hill K, Gilbert A, et al. UK population norms for the modified dental anxiety scale with percentile calculator: Adult dental health survey 2009 results. *BMC Oral Health.* 2013;13:29.
5. Smith TA, Heaton LJ. Fear of dental care: Are we making any progress? *J Am Dent Assoc.* 2003;134:1101–1108.
6. Ragnarsson B, Arnlaugsson S, Karlsson KO, et al. Dental anxiety in Iceland: An epidemiological postal survey. *Acta Odontol Scand.* 2003;61:283–288.
7. Moore R, Brodsgaard I, Mao TK, et al. Fear of injections and report of negative dentist behavior among caucasian American and Taiwanese adults from dental school clinics. *Community Dent Oral Epidemiol.* 1996;24:292–295.
8. Lahti S, Vehkalahti MM, Nordblad A, Hausen H. Dental fear among population aged 30 years and older in Finland. *Acta Odontol Scand.* 2007;65:97–102.
9. Folayan MO, Idehen EE, Ojo OO. The modulating effect of culture on the expression of dental anxiety in children: A literature review. *Int J Paediatr Dent.* 2004;14:241–245.
10. Ulin K, Malm D, Nygårdh A. What is known about the benefits of patient-centered care in patients with heart failure. *Curr Heart Fail Rep.* 2015;12(6):350–359.
11. Antai-Otong D. Caring for the patient with an anxiety disorder. *Nurs Clin North Am.* 2016;51(2):173–183.
12. Barlow DH. *Anxiety and Its Disorders: The Nature and Treatment of Anxiety and Panic.* 2nd ed. New York: The Guilford Press; 2002.
13. LeDoux J. Coming to terms with fear. *Proceedings of the National Academy of Sciences.* 2014;111(8):2871–2878.
14. Robin O, Alaoui-Ismaili O, Dittmar A, Vernet-Maury E. Emotional responses evoked by dental odors: An evaluation from autonomic parameters. *J Dent Res.* 1998;77:1638–1646.
15. Oosterink FM, de Jongh A, Aartman IH. What are people afraid of during dental treatment? Anxiety-provoking capacity of 67 stimuli characteristic of the dental setting. *Eur J Oral Sci.* 2008;116:44–51.
16. Freeman R. The role of memory on the dentally anxious patient's response to dental treatment. *Irish J Psych Med.* 1991;8: 110–115.
17. Lindsay S, Jackson C. Fear of routine dental treatment in adults: its nature and management. *Psychol Health.* 1993;8:135–153.
18. Lin CS. Pain catastrophizing in dental patients: implications for treatment management. *J Am Dent Assoc.* 2013;144:1244–1251.
19. Liddell A, Gosse V. Characteristics of early unpleasant dental experiences. *J Behav Ther Exp Psychiatry.* 1998;29:227–237.
20. Tickle M, Jones C, Buchannan K, Milsom KM, Blinkhorn AS, Humphris GM. A prospective study of dental anxiety in a cohort of children followed from 5 to 9 years of age. *Int J Paediatr Dent.* 2009;19(4):225–232.
21. Locker D, Liddell A, Dempster L, Shapiro D. Age of onset of dental anxiety. *J Dent Res.* 1999;78:790–796.
22. Thomson WM, Broadbent JM, Locker D, Poulton R. Trajectories of dental anxiety in a birth cohort. *Community Dent Oral Epidemiol.* 2009;37(3):209–219.
23. Locker D, Thomson WM, Poulton R. Psychological disorder, conditioning experiences, and the onset of dental anxiety in early adulthood. *J Dent Res.* 2001;80(6):1588–1592.
24. Poulton R, Waldie KE, Thomson WM, Locker D. Determinants of early- vs late-onset dental fear in a longitudinal-epidemiological study. *Behav Res Ther.* 2001;39(7):777–785.
25. Holtzman JM, Berg RG, Mann J, Berkey DB. The relationship of age and gender to fear and anxiety in response to dental care. *Spec Care Dentist.* 1997;17:82–87.

26. Davey GC. Dental phobias and anxieties: Evidence for conditioning processes in the acquisition and modulation of a learned fear. *Behav Res Ther*. 1989;27:51–58.

27. McNeil DW, Randall CL, Cohen LL, et al. Transmission of dental fear from parent to adolescent in an Appalachian sample in the USA. *Int J Paediatr Dent*. 2019;29(6):720–727.

28. Eli I, Uziel N, Baht R, Kleinhauz M. Antecedents of dental anxiety: Learned responses versus personality traits. *Community Dent Oral Epidemiol*. 1997;25:233–237.

29. Russell MW. The management of dental pain: A review of possible alternatives to drug therapy. *Tex Dent J*. 1980;98:6–8.

30. International Association for the Study of Pain *Classification of chronic pain: Descriptions of chronic pain syndromes and definitions of pain terms*. Seattle: IASP Press; 1994.

31. Sessle BJ. The neurobiology of facial and dental pain: Present knowledge, future directions. *J Dent Res*. 1987;66:962–981.

32. Litt MD. A model of pain and anxiety associated with acute stressors: distress in dental procedures. *Behav Res Ther*. 1996;34:459–476.

33. Rhudy JL, Meagher MW. Fear and anxiety: divergent effects on human pain thresholds. *Pain*. 2000;84:65–75.

34. Arntz A, van Eck M, Heijmans M. Predictions of dental pain: the fear of any expected evil, is worse than the evil itself. *Behav Res Ther*. 1990;28:29–41.

35. Caceres C, Burns JW. Cardiovascular reactivity to psychological stress may enhance subsequent pain sensitivity. *Pain*. 1997;69:237–244.

36. Klages U, Ulusoy O, Kianifard S, Wehrbein H. Dental trait anxiety and pain sensitivity as predictors of expected and experienced pain in stressful dental procedures. *Eur J Oral Sci*. 2004;112:477–483.

37. Gedney JJ, Logan H, Baron RS. Predictors of short-term and long-term memory of sensory and affective dimensions of pain. *J Pain*. 2003;4:47–55.

38. Hampton T. Pain and the brain: Researchers focus on tackling pain memories. *JAMA*. 2005;293:2845–2846.

39. Dougall A, Fiske J. Surviving child sexual abuse: the relevance to dental practice. *Dent Update*. 2009;36:294–296. 298–300, 303–304.

40. https://victimsofcrime.org/child-sexual-abuse-statistics/.

41. Willumsen T. Dental fear in sexually abused women. *Eur J Oral Sci*. 2001;109:291–296.

42. Willumsen T. The impact of childhood sexual abuse on dental fear. *Community Dent Oral Epidemiol*. 2004;32:73–79.

43. Fillingim RB, Wilkinson CS, Powell T. Self-reported abuse history and pain complaints among young adults. *Clin J Pain*. 1999;15:85–91.

44. World Health Organization. (2008). Commission on Social Determinants of Health – Final Report. https://apps.who.int/iris/bitstream/handle/10665/43943/9789241563703_eng.pdf;jsessionid=D2EB5F0D0BC71039E0E64D1450E8E5AD?sequence=1 [PDF - 7.6 MB]

45. https://hsdm.harvard.edu/files/dental/files/module_4_for_the_learner_notes.pdf.

46. Barnes-Josiah D, Myntti C, Augustin A. The "three delays" as a framework for examining maternal mortality in Haiti. *Soc Sci Med*. 1998;46(8):981–993.

47. Danna V, Bedwell C, Wakasiaka S, Lavender T. Utility of the three-delays model and its potential for supporting a solution-based approach to accessing intrapartum care in low- and middle-income countries. A qualitative evidence synthesis. *Glob Health Action*. 2020;13(1):1819052.

48. Schuller AA, Willumsen T, Holst D. Are there differences in oral health and oral health behavior between individuals with high and low dental fear? *Community Dent Oral Epidemiol*. 2003;31:116–121.

49. Wiener RC. Dental Fear and Delayed Dental Care in Appalachia-West Virginia. *J Dent Hyg*. 2015;89(4):274–281.

50. Liinavuori A, Tolvanen M, Pohjola V, Lahti S. Longitudinal interrelationships between dental fear and dental attendance among adult Finns in 2000-2011. *Community Dent Oral Epidemiol*. 2019;47(4):309–315.

51. Armfield JM, Stewart JF, Spencer AJ. The vicious cycle of dental fear: exploring the interplay between oral health, service utilization and dental fear. *BMC Oral Health*. 2007;7:1 http://creativecommons.org/licenses/by/2.0/. 14.

52. Humphris GM, Morrison T, Lindsay SJ. The modified dental anxiety scale: Validation and United Kingdom norms. *Community Dent Health*. 1995;12:143–150.

53. Armfield JM. Development and psychometric evaluation of the index of dental anxiety and fear (IDAF-4C +). *Psychol Assess*. 2010;22:279–287.

54. Yarbrough C., Nasseh K., Vujicic M. Why adults forgo dental care: Evidence from a new national survey. Health Policy Institute Research Brief. American Dental Association. November 2014. Available from: http://www.ada.org/~/media/ADA/Science%20and%20Research/HPI/Files/HPIBrief_1114_1.ashx.

55. Appukuttan DP. Strategies to manage patients with dental anxiety and dental phobia: literature review. *Clin Cosmet Investig Dent*. 2016;8:35–50.

56. Coulehan JL, Platt FW, Egener B, et al. "Let me see if I have this right...": Words that help build empathy. *Ann Int Med*. 2001;135:221–227.

57. Logan HL, Baron RS, Keeley K, et al. Desired control and felt control as mediators of stress in a dental setting. *Health Psychol*. 1991;10:352–359.

58. Law A, Logan H, Baron RS. Desire for control, felt control, and stress inoculation training during dental treatment. *J Pers Soc Psychol*. 1994;67:926–936.

59. Baron RS, Logan H. Desired control, felt control, and dental pain: recent findings and remaining issues. *Motiv Emotion*. 1993;17:181–204.

60. Logan HL, Baron RS, Kohout F. Sensory focus as therapeutic treatments for acute pain. *Psychosom Med*. 1995;57:475–484.

61. Hainsworth JM, Moss H, Fairbrother KJ. Relaxation and complementary therapies: An alternative approach to managing dental anxiety in clinical practice. *Dent Update*. 2005;32:90–92. 94–96.

62. Kvale G, Berggren U, Milgrom P. Dental fear in adults: A meta-analysis of behavioral interventions. *Community Dent Oral Epidemiol*. 2004;32:250–264.

63. Frere CL, Crout R, Yorty J, McNeil DW. Effects of audiovisual distraction during dental prophylaxis. *J Am Dent Assoc*. 2001;132:1031–1038.

64. Corah NL. Dental anxiety: Assessment, reduction and increasing patient satisfaction. *Dent Clin North Am*. 1988;32:779–790.

65. Hoffman HG, Garcia-Palacios A, Patterson DR, et al. The effectiveness of virtual reality for dental pain control: A case study. *Cyberpsychol Behav*. 2001;4:527–535.

66. Furman E, Jasinevicius TR, Bissada NF, et al. Virtual reality distraction for pain control during periodontal scaling and root planing procedures. *J Am Dent Assoc*. 2009;140:1508–1516.

67. Armfield JM, Heaton LJ. Management of fear and anxiety in the dental clinic: a review. *Aust Dent J*. 2013;58:390–407. quiz 531.

68. Corah NL, Gale EN, Illig SJ. The use of relaxation and distraction to reduce psychological stress during dental procedures. *J Am Dent Assoc*. 1979;98:390–394.

69. Corah NL, Gale EN, Pace LF, Seyrek SK. Relaxation and musical programming as means of reducing psychological stress during dental procedures. *J Am Dent Assoc*. 1981;103:232–234.

70. Milgrom P, Weinstein P, Heaton LJ. *Treating fearful dental patients: A patient management handbook*. ed 3 Seattle: Dental Behavioral Resources; 2009.

71. Bills IG. The use of hypnosis in the management of dental phobia. *Aust J Clin Exp Hypn*. 1993;21:13–18.

72. Shaw AJ, Niven N. Theoretical concepts and practical applications of hypnosis in the treatment of children and adolescents with dental fear and anxiety. *Br Dent J*. 1996;180:11–16.

73. Fick LJ, Lang EV, Logan HL, et al. Imagery content during nonpharmacologic analgesia in the procedure suite: where your patients would rather be. *Acad Radiol*. 1999;6:457–463.

74. Lang EV, Lutgendorf S, Logan H, et al. Nonpharmacologic analgesia and anxiolysis for interventional radiological procedures. *Semin Intervent Rad*. 1999;16:113–123.

75. Lang EV, Benotsch EG, Fick LJ, et al. Adjunctive non-pharmacological analgesia for invasive medical procedures: a randomised trial. *Lancet*. 2000;355:1486–1490.

76. Gerschman JA. Hypnotizability and dental phobic disorders. *Anesth Prog*. 1989;36:131–137.

77. Getch SE, Lute RM. Advancing integrated healthcare: a step by step guide for primary care physicians and behavioral health clinicians. *Mo Med*. 2019;116(5):384–388.

78. American Society of Anesthesiologists Task Force on Sedation and Analgesia by Non-Anesthesiologists: Practice guidelines for sedation and analgesia by non-anesthesiologists, Anesthesiology 96:1004–1017, 2002.

79. American Society of Dentist Anesthesiologists: Parameters of Care. Anesth Prog (2018) 65 (3):197-203.

80. American Dental Association Guidelines for the Use of Sedation and General Anesthesia by Dentists. Adopted by the ADA house of Delegates, October 2016. https://www.ada.org/~/media/ADA/Education%20and%20Careers/Files/anesthesia_use_guidelines.pdf.

81. Facts and Comparisons eAnswers: Benzodiazepines. http://www.wolterskluwercdi.com/facts-comparisons-online/. Accessed September 10, 2021.

82. Wong WW, Gabriel A, Maxwell GP, Gupta SC. Bleeding risks of herbal, homeopathic, and dietary supplements: a hidden nightmare for plastic surgeons? *Anesthet Surg J*. 2012;32(3):332–346.

83. Mihic SJ, Mayfield J, Harris RA. Chapter 19: Hypnotics and Sedatives. In: Brunton LL, Hilal-Dandan R, Knollmann BC, eds. *Goodman and Gilman's: The Pharmacological Basis of Therapeutics*. 13th ed. New York: McGraw-Hill; 2018.

84. Valium [package insert] USA. Roche Products Inc, 2008.

85. Pfizer: Xanax (alprazolam) prescribing information. New York, NY, March 2006.

86. Nitrous Oxide. In: Lexi-Drugs. Lexi-Comp, Inc. Updated: September 2, 2021. http://online.lexi.com/lco/action/doc/retrieve/docid/patch_f/7366?searchUrl=%2Flco%2Faction%2Fsearch%3Bjsessionid%3D9ED0F2138CA1CA09D2D1D3DDE1F8495E%3Forigin%3Dapi%26t%3Dglobalid%26q%3D6651%26nq%3Dtru.

87. Malamed S. *Inhalation sedation. Sedation: A Guide to Patient Management*. 6th ed. St Louis: Elsevier; 2018.

88. Facts and Comparisons eAnswers: Nitrous Oxide. http://online.factsandcomparisons.com.proxy.lib.uiowa.edu/MonoDisp.aspx?monoidfandc-hcp15266&bookDFC&fromtoptrue&search540289%7c15&isStemmedTrue&asbooks/. Accessed August 31, 2014.

89. Patel PM, Patel HH, Roth DM. General anesthetics and therapeutic gases. In: Brunton LL, Chabner BA, Knollmann BC, eds. *Goodman and Gilman's The Pharmacological Basis of Therapeutics*. 12th ed. New York: McGraw-Hill; 2011.

16

Patients With a Psychological Disorder

Sarah Getch, Erinne N. Kennedy, and Larry Segars

 Visit eBooks.Health.Elsevier.com

OUTLINE

Psychiatric disorders are common in our society and are expressed primarily as abnormalities of thought, feelings, and behaviors that cause emotional distress and result in the impairment of function. The most common classes of psychiatric disorders in the United States, in order of prevalence, are anxiety disorders, mood disorders, impulse control disorders, and substance abuse disorders.[1] Specific symptoms, as listed in the diagnostic criteria, vary in how long they must be present before a diagnosis can be made.

Epidemiologic studies indicate that 26.2% of the US adult population experience signs and symptoms of a recognized mental disorder each year. Serious mental illness is thought to

occur in nearly 6% of the population and is the leading cause of disability in the United States.[1] In 2019, the US Substance Abuse and Mental Health Services Administration (SAMHSA) reported that 43.8% or 5.8 million adults with mental illnesses who have perceived an unmet need did not received mental health services in the previous year.[2]

These statistics suggest that at any point in time a large number of patients presenting for dental care may have a treated or untreated psychological disorder and are unable to access behavioral health care services. Although the dentist will not be called on to diagnose psychological disorders, practitioners should be able to recognize patients with signs and symptoms of symptomatic psychological disorders and participate with the collaborative healthcare team for each patient. The dentist also has an important role in managing the oral effects of each disorder or the side effects of medications used to control them. A patient's behaviors and habits, for example lack of regular oral healthcare, may impact the oral cavity and result in disease. The dental team will work with the patient to manage their oral disease. Additionally, psychological needs may necessitate a marked alteration in both the nature and scope of the patient's plan of care. The adaptation of treatment plans and the provision of patient-centered care are the focus of this chapter.

PATIENT EVALUATION

The first visit for a patient with psychological disorders may be longer than for other new patients. This allows extra time for the patient to respond to questions or assimilate information provided by the dentist. It is helpful to take the perspective of a patient with an anxiety disorder. If the patient experiences a situation that includes pressure to respond quickly to questions they may feel instantly overwhelmed and have trouble concentrating, even feeling physically uncomfortable. These feelings may lead to difficulty answering questions correctly, not completing the appointment, or not returning for care because their encounter was not positive. There may be instances when the patient must be scheduled without adequate time that might otherwise be necessary for a more slowly paced interview. Developing rapport with the patient may be the best use of the time remaining after determination of the patient's chief complaint.

Obtaining A Patient History

With the social stigma that is associated with many psychological disorders, patients may be reluctant to provide information related to their social, medical, or dental history, especially information related to their psychological symptomology or disorder. The importance of establishing rapport quickly and effectively cannot be overstated. An effective way to open discussion when the dentist suspects that the patient has a psychological disorder is to mention a physical finding that may relate to the disorder. For example, because some medications for psychological disorders cause dry mouth, a nonjudgmental, nonthreatening question, such as "I notice that your mouth seems much drier than usual. Have there been any changes in your health or medications that could account for this change?" may open a discussion in which the relationship between physical findings and psychological status can be described. From the initiation of the professional relationship, honest and open communication between the dentist and the patient can ease the discomfort of discussing mental disorders. The practitioner should reassure the patient that this information is necessary to ensure provision of the best possible treatment and that the inquiry is not meant to be intrusive or embarrass the patient. The patient will be more forthcoming if questions are framed in a curious fashion with the understanding that their overall health status can affect the delivery of dental care.

Patients with psychological problems are often less defensive and more open about divulging medication history than about their psychological health history. Having an open discussion about medications can be invaluable in assisting the dentist in understanding the nature of the psychological problem, how well it is being controlled, and the severity of the disease. Such discussion can also alert the dentist to possible oral side effects of medications and potential adverse drug interactions. For these reasons, when reviewing patient medications, it is important to learn who prescribed a particular medication, its purpose and dosage, whether any recent changes in dosing have occurred, and whether the patient has suffered any adverse reactions. The clinician must ensure that the same questions are asked for all the patient's medications. Many over-the-counter remedies (antihistamines, decongestants, herbal products, and homeopathic remedies) have significant oral side effects and can increase the adverse reactions from prescription medications. It is estimated that more than 50% of patients do not voluntarily report the use of homeopathic or herbal supplements to their healthcare practitioners.[3] Many patients do not consider that herbal and homeopathic agents to be medications because they are "natural" substances, whereas others anticipate that reporting self-directed therapy will elicit a negative reaction.

Patients With a Diagnosed Psychological Disorder

Even the patient with a well-managed psychological disorder presents the clinician with the potential for related treatment planning modifications. It is essential that the dentist become knowledgeable about the diagnosis, treatment, and effectiveness of treatment of the psychological disorder before providing dental treatment. A consultation with the patient's collaborative health care team will be indicated. A sample letter drafted from the dentist to the members of the collaborative healthcare team can be found online (see eFigure 15.3). The patient may provide the dentist with information that they may have not shared with their physician. Additionally, there are several oral changes that can result from medications that warrant discussion with the physician, such as dry mouth, mouth lesions, or movement disorders. If the dentist concludes that contact with the physician is appropriate, consent must be given by the patient before the dentist communicates with another member of the collaborative healthcare team. In most instances, the patient will grant consent. Many times, simply explaining the reason for contacting the physician will be sufficient to convince the patient to provide consent. However, there will be times when the patient refuses to provide consent. The patient's refusal to allow the clinician access to information that could affect not only the dental treatment, but also their overall health, makes it inappropriate for the clinician to proceed. In such situations, the clinician should take the time to explain to the patient the importance of treating the whole person. That is, in order to provide the highest standard of care the clinician must have a thorough understanding of the patient's physical, emotional, mental, and social influences. Treatment cannot proceed without this information and the clinician should avoid giving in to the patient's wishes in this situation. The clinician should explain to the patient that the risks to both the patient and clinician far outweigh the benefits of acquiescing to the patient's wishes. If the patient remains unwilling to grant consent, the doctor-patient relationship should be terminated.

There are instances in which the patient's history and behavior suggest the presence of a psychological disorder but there is no indication of treatment in the patient's history. The explanation may be either that the patient is nonadherent to therapy or that the patient's physician and the patient are both aware of the problem, but the patient has chosen not to pursue treatment. In either case, the treating dentist must have complete health and medication histories to manage a patient with a diagnosed psychological disorder effectively. In such instances, it may be necessary for the dentist to confront the patient about their concerns and request that the patient be reevaluated by a member of their collaborative treatment team. For more information on treatment teams and interprofessional practice, see Chapter 6.

Patients With an Undiagnosed Psychological Disorder

Listening to and observing the patient helps the clinician to recognize the individual with an undiagnosed psychiatric disorder. Although a patient who displays inappropriate behaviors or responds to questions in a strange way may simply be nervous, it also may be the case that they have an undiagnosed psychological condition. Obviously, behavioral changes will be more readily recognizable in an established patient whom the dentist has seen before. When such questions are raised in the dentist's mind, it is appropriate to determine whether the patient has been recently evaluated by a member of the collaborative health care team and, if not, to suggest that such an examination be pursued. It is possible that the patient is unaware that their behavior has been changing. Codiscovering their current symptoms may be helpful in coaching the patient to access healthcare. Approaching the subject in the context of the impact of the patient's overall health on the way that oral healthcare is delivered, along with an expression of concern for the patient's health, may help the patient understand the rationale for providing the dentist with more information.

When the dentist suspects an undiagnosed psychological disorder, every effort should be made to convince the patient to see their primary care physician for a complete evaluation. Most patients will appreciate this demonstration of concern for their health. On the other hand, some patients may perceive such a referral as the dentist's refusal to treat. The patient should be reassured that the dentist will continue to provide care, but that a health status evaluation by a physician is necessary to ensure oral healthcare can be safely delivered. Although it is not ethical to withhold emergency care, a highly symptomatic patient who is a threat to themselves or others must be made aware that definitive dental treatment may be deferred until the mental health concern has been addressed. It would be dangerous to provide dental treatment when it is unclear whether the patient is reporting all current medications. The potential for an adverse drug interaction is greatly increased when treating patients taking psychotropic medications.

Patients With A Poorly Controlled Psychological Disorder

Poorly controlled psychological disorders manifest in patients in a similar manner as undiagnosed disorders, although the symptoms may be less severe. Several possible explanations may account for the behavior, including nonadherence secondary to a lack of **self-awareness** by the patient. Self-awareness refers to the patient's ability to identify the symptoms, severity, and status of their own mental illness. Patients who have self-awareness are mindful of their deteriorating mental health and will seek professional care when the condition worsens. Others, especially those with psychotic symptoms, will present with low psychological awareness and can be nonadherent in terms of taking medications and seeing a member of the collaborative healthcare team on a regular basis.

Nonadherence may also relate to financial considerations associated with healthcare costs, the misunderstanding that symptom management of a chronic disorder is permanent, or the unpleasant side effects of prescribed medications. Providing the patient with a strategy to deal with the xerostomia associated with many psychotropic medications is one way for the dental practitioner to enhance adherence. See the section on xerostomia later in this chapter.

By helping the patient recognize the deleterious oral and systemic effects of nonadherence and positively address the undesirable side effects of the therapy, the dental practitioner may be able to encourage the patient to resume medication therapy. The patient should be encouraged to discuss problems relating to the drug's effects and side effects, and the cost of treatment and medications with the psychiatric care provider. If the patient remains unwilling to adhere to the recommended therapy, it may be appropriate for the dentist to inform the medical, psychiatric, or psychological care provider about the issue. Some mental disorders are refractory to pharmacotherapy and the patient may never be completely asymptomatic despite the best available treatment. (See Video 16.1, "Interview with a Patient with Mental Disorders" on ebooks+.)

GENERAL TREATMENT PLANNING CONSIDERATIONS FOR PATIENTS WITH A PSYCHOLOGICAL DISORDER

Both long- and short-term prognoses for dental restorations and prostheses are impacted by how well the patient maintains their physical, oral, and psychological health. For oral health, the patient will be working to maintain their daily oral hygiene routine that they develop with their oral healthcare team. The dentist and dental hygienist should communicate the importance of maintaining oral health and the ways in which the disease process or its treatment can interfere with oral health (see the "Ethics in Dentistry" box). The dentist and patients will have to work together to develop a prevention plan where the protective factors will outweigh the risk factors that lead to oral disease.

Prevention and management of oral diseases should be pursued in an offensive versus a defensive manner where the patient experiences more protective factors for their oral health on a daily basis compared with risk factors for oral disease. For those patients with severe mental illness, limited definitive care (see the *Holding Phase* section in Chapter 19) may be the only option available to improve function and esthetics, especially for severely decayed and broken-down teeth. It is very important that the preventive strategy for all patients with psychological disorders is updated at every appointment. Changes in a patient's oral hygiene may result from medication changes or a change in the patient's psychological status.

The ability of a patient to cope with dental treatment should be ascertained before beginning each procedure. The patient must be compliant and cooperative and must give consent to proceed. Spending the extra time necessary to be sure that the patient is comfortable, well informed, and free of anxiety can ensure that treatment proceeds in a predictable fashion.

After receiving permission from the patient, the dentist may wish to establish a professional relationship with the clinician treating the psychological disorder. Ongoing interactions between the dentist and the mental health professional can only improve the care of the patient. The dentist needs to be aware of changes in treatment or medications so that they can adjust the treatment plan for the risk of increased oral disease. The behavioral health clinician can provide insight about patient adherence to therapy and expected patterns of patient behavior. In turn, the dentist can provide the clinician with information about the side effects of medications on oral structures and offer possible solutions to counteract xerostomia, alterations in taste, and other intraoral side effects of psychotropic medications. Contact with a physician is especially important for patients who have uncontrolled psychological symptoms or are in crisis. The patient who is contemplating suicide is an example of a patient in crisis. Signs of suicidal ideation may be overt and include verbalization of

a plan, verbalization of hopelessness, a suicide letter, or an attempt to gain access to large quantities of medications with fatal overdose implications. Other important indicators may include the experience of a recent trauma, a recent loss of a loved one, a family history of suicide, or the recent suicide of a family or loved one. If these signs or indicators are present, immediate action is necessary. The clinician should not leave the patient alone and have a team member contact the patient's friends or family members, get connected with the patient's mental health provider or primary care physician, or initiate a call for emergency services. Additionally, the clinician should have the regional or national suicide prevention phone numbers that can be shared with the patient. It is important for the clinician to remember that talking a patient out of suicide is often not successful or recommended. Instead, the clinician can let the patient know that feelings of depression and hopelessness are temporary and treatable.

Although it is not practical or appropriate for the dental clinician to diagnose psychological problems, it is helpful to have some background knowledge about the standard categorizations and treatments of common mental disorders when discussing patient histories with other healthcare professionals. In addition, it is helpful for the dentist to be aware of the approach the clinician is likely to use to evaluate the patient. Psychological problems have been categorized by the American Psychiatric Association.[4]

In the following sections, the diagnostic criteria, symptoms, and prevalence of major psychological disorders are summarized. The ramifications for dental treatment planning are also reviewed for each major category.

ANXIETY DISORDERS

Anxiety disorders are among the most common psychological illnesses encountered in clinical practice. The National Institute of Mental Health estimates that more than 40 million US adults are affected by disabling anxiety disorders each year.[1,5] In general, these illnesses are chronic, develop before the age of 30 years, and occur twice as frequently in women as in men. The etiology of anxiety disorders is thought to be based on a combination of factors, which may include genetic predisposition (family history of depression or anxiety), childhood adversity, and occupational or traumatic stress.[1,4]

The hallmark feature of anxiety disorders is excessive fear and anxiety leading to behavioral disturbances. Although the terms fear and anxiety are often used interchangeably, they are distinct entities. Anxiety results in an emotional, behavioral, cognitive, and physical response to an anticipated experience that the individual perceives as threatening. Fear[6] is a multifaceted response to an immediate and present danger and is most closely associated with a flight or fight reaction. Anxiety, however, is a response to uncertainty about the future, the unknown, or a future negative event. Research has indicated that fear and anxiety are represented by distinct neural circuitry. Fear-arousal is associated with activity in the amygdala and anxiety is associated with activity in the bed of the nucleus of the stria terminalis.

For most people, stress-induced situational fear and anxiety are usually transient, resolving when the situation or event has passed. Patients with pathologic anxiety have intense, persistent, intrusive worries and fears and develop avoidance behaviors to calm their emotions. These disorders can greatly disrupt the individual's life and result in significant disability. Worries tend to be age congruent, with younger people worried over their competence and performance, whereas older people worry about a greater range of life circumstances, making diagnosis of anxiety more likely in this population. People with anxiety disorders often also exhibit comorbidities, such as major depression or substance abuse.[4]

The differential diagnosis of anxiety disorders requires ruling out other psychiatric conditions (mood disorders, schizophrenia, dementia), physical illnesses (arrhythmias, ischemic heart disease, hyperthyroidism, seizures), and the adverse effect of drugs. Drugs whose effects may include anxiety symptoms include prednisone, bupropion, selective serotonin reuptake inhibitors (SSRIs), levodopa, cannabis, quinolone antibiotics, bronchodilators, ibuprofen, and CNS stimulants, such as caffeine, nicotine, cocaine, and amphetamines.[7]

The DSM-5 divides anxiety disorders into several categories, often with overlapping features. The categories relevant to dental practice are generalized anxiety disorder (GAD), panic disorder, social anxiety disorder, and phobias. Dental phobias and anxiety are very important to the practicing dentist and are discussed in more detail in Chapter 15.

Generalized Anxiety Disorder

The essential feature of generalized anxiety disorder (GAD) is excessive anxiety and worry (apprehensive expectation) about multiple events or activities that has occurred most days for the past 6 months. The intensity and frequency of the anxiety and worry are out of proportion to the actual likelihood or effect of the anticipated event. GAD tends to have a slow onset, with symptoms that wax and wane over the course of a lifetime. The 12-month prevalence of GAD is 0.9% of adolescents and 2.9% of adults in the United States, with women twice as likely as men to experience GAD.[4] The psychological and physical symptoms of GAD (Box 16.1) cause significant disability for patients and result in 110 million disability days per year in the United States.[4]

GAD is often comorbid with other mental disorders such as depression, panic attacks, and substance abuse. Patients report a chronic level of anxiety that is heightened during stressful events. It is important to remember that the patient's response to an external event (such as a dental visit) is very personal and should not be discounted by the clinician. Although an outsider may view the event as nonanxiety provoking and have limited understanding about why the patient has had a reaction, the patient has experienced a cognitive and emotional reaction caused by their disorder that is very real to them.

Treatment for GAD is patient specific and often consists of a combination of medications and such psychological modalities as psychotherapy, stress management, psychoeducation, and **cognitive behavioral therapy (CBT)**. CBT is a psychotherapeutic approach designed to identify and modify the dysfunctional or maladaptive behaviors and thinking patterns that cause and maintain anxiety. For patients with GAD, behavioral health clinicians and dentists can manage anxious thoughts using the technique of cognitive restructuring where patients work to replace anxiety provoking thoughts with alternative ways of thinking about the anxiety producing situation. Although highly effective, CBT is not widely available and most patients are treated with other modalities and medications.[7,8] Table 16.1 lists nonpharmacologic and pharmacologic treatment approaches for anxiety disorders.

Antidepressants belonging to the selective serotonin or serotonin and norepinephrine reuptake inhibitor classes (SSRI and SNRIs) are the first-line pharmacologic agents for many types of anxiety disorders. An alternative therapy to these classes is the medication buspirone. This medication works by being a mixed agonist and antagonist of several serotonin and the dopamine type-2 receptors in various brain regions. In contrast to benzodiazepines, these drugs do not cause dependency, have more favorable side effect profiles, manage comorbid depression (except buspirone), and reduce apprehension and worry in patients with anxiety disorders.[7]

BOX 16.1 Symptoms of Generalized Anxiety Disorder

Psychological
Excessive anxiety and worrying
Feeling "on edge" or restless
Poor concentration or mind going blank

Physical
Fatigue
Irritability
Muscle tension
Sleep disturbances

TABLE 16.1 Treatment Approaches for Anxiety Disorders

Generalized Anxiety Disorder
CBT with or without pharmacotherapy; acute efficacy is similar for both.
Psychotherapy is the preferred treatment.
Anxiolytics are indicated for patients with functional disability.

Panic Disorder
CBT; exposure and response prevention
Pharmacotherapy
Patients with agoraphobic avoidance often need CBT in addition to pharmacotherapy.
Psychological treatment with or without medications may decrease relapse when medications are discontinued.

Social Anxiety Disorder
Pharmacotherapy with or without CBT; acute outcomes are equal for both.
Drug therapy is more effective in treatment of acute symptoms, patients respond slowly, and therapy may be lifelong.

CBT, cognitive behavioral therapy

Panic Disorder

The hallmark symptom of panic disorder is recurrent, unexpected panic attacks. Full-symptom panic attacks are defined as abrupt surges of intense fear or discomfort that reach a peak within minutes and during which at least 4 of 13 defined symptoms (Box 16.2) occur. Limited-symptom attacks have fewer than four symptoms.[4] Panic attacks can arise in a calm or anxious state and can be expected or unexpected. They reach peak intensity within the first 10 minutes and resolve in 20 to 30 minutes.[7] The occurrence of panic attacks is not considered to be a mental disorder, but rather a constellation of symptoms that may occur in association with other anxiety or mental disorders (depression, substance abuse, posttraumatic stress) or medical conditions (cardiac, gastrointestinal, respiratory). The 12-month prevalence estimates for panic attacks in US adults is 11.2%, with a mean age of onset of 22 to 23 years.[4]

Panic attacks seem life-threatening to patients experiencing them. However, frightened patients often seek medical assistance only to find that their symptoms have largely resolved before they are examined. The severe nature of the symptomology can prompt healthcare providers to perform testing for a variety of serious illnesses.

Diagnostic criteria for panic disorder include recurrent, unexpected panic attacks followed by at least one of the following:

- Persistent worry about additional attacks or their consequences ("going crazy", losing control, having a heart attack)
- A significant maladaptive change in behavior related to the attacks (behaviors designed to avoid experiencing panic attacks)

Persons who suffer from panic disorder develop avoidance behaviors in an attempt to avoid/limit panic attacks or their consequences.[4] Fear of open and crowded spaces, agoraphobia, is common among patients with panic disorder and can render them homebound and completely dependent on others to perform the activities of daily living. The 12-month prevalence rate for panic disorder in the United States is 2% to 3% of adults and adolescents, with a female predominance of 2:1

over males.[4] Most patients with panic disorder have other anxiety disorders (agoraphobia), major depression, or bipolar disorder. Treatments for panic disorder include psychotherapy, CBT, SSRI antidepressants, or benzodiazepines.

Social Anxiety Disorder (Social Phobia)

Social anxiety disorder is the most common anxiety disorder, with an estimated 12-month prevalence rate of 7% in the United States.[4] The essential feature of a social phobia is the persistent distinct fear or anxiety about one or more social situations in which the individual fears being scrutinized by others (see Box 16.3). Common fears include social interactions (meeting people, conversing), being observed (eating or drinking), or performing (giving a speech, recital). Patients with social anxiety disorder fear possible embarrassment.[4] The response to the social situation must be of sufficient intensity to produce notable anxiety or fear and result in significant distress or interference with normal daily activities. Blushing is the predominant physical indicator. Social anxiety disorder is associated with increased rates of school dropout and chronic unemployment. Many patients develop concurrent mood or substance abuse disorders. Only 50% of individuals with these symptoms seek treatment, often only after 15 or more years of experiencing symptoms.[4]

Treatments for patients suffering from social anxiety disorder are specific and may involve psychotherapy, behavioral therapy, SSRI antidepressants, and anxiolytic agents.

Specific Phobias

Specific phobias are characterized by immediate and excessive fear or anxiety about a specific stimulus, object, or situation (e.g., air travel, animals, heights, seeing blood). When the fear of a particular stimulus affects an individual's life to a significant extent and the individual goes to great lengths to avoid the stimulus, it is described as a phobia. Diagnostic criteria require the fear, anxiety, or avoidance to be persistent, lasting at least 6 months and causing significant distress or impairment in daily functioning.[4] In the United States, in 2007 the 12-month prevalence estimate for specific phobia is 9.1% and is influenced by age and gender with 12.2% of females reporting a specific phobia and 5.8% of males.[9] The estimated lifetime prevalence rate in adolescents is approximately 19.3%,

---

BOX 16.2   Symptoms of Panic Attacks

Psychological
Feelings of detachment from self or surroundings
Fear of losing control or going crazy
Fear of dying

Physical
Palpitations, pounding heart, or increased heart rate
Chest pains or discomfort
Feeling dizzy, unsteady, lightheaded, or faint
Sweating
Chills or heat sensation
Trembling or shaking
Paresthesias
Feelings of choking
Nausea or abdominal distress
Sensations of shortness of breath or smothering

BOX 16.3   Symptoms of Social Anxiety Disorder

Psychological
Fears: Embarrassment, humiliation, rejection
Offending others

Physical
Blushing
Sweating
Trembling
Inadequate eye contact
Overly soft voice
"Shy" bladder

whereas the rate for adults is 12.5%.[9,10] Females are affected at a 2:1 rate over males. Certain medically related phobias are experienced equally by both genders. These include fear of receiving injections, fear of seeing blood, or fear of injury.[4] Patients with specific phobias often exhibit sympathetic nervous system arousal when faced with the phobic stimulus. Individuals with blood/injection/injury-specific phobias often experience an initial brief acceleration of heart rate and increased blood pressure, followed by a deceleration of heart rate and drop in blood pressure, which elicits a vasovagal fainting or near-fainting response.[4]

Specific phobias usually develop in childhood, although trauma-induced phobias can occur at any age. Patients are asymptomatic unless in contact with the specific stimulus to their anxiety. Although most patients simply avoid the feared objects and do not seek professional care, treatment includes desensitization therapy and anxiolytic agents for acute situations.

Medications Used to Treat Anxiety

Anxiolytic agents (Table 16.2) are used to reduce the severity, frequency, and duration of anxiety symptoms. Benzodiazepines are the most efficacious agents for the relief of acute anxiety symptoms. Although all benzodiazepines have anxiolytic effects, half of the agents marketed in the United States are used as sedative-hypnotic agents.

Serious complications of benzodiazepine therapy include physical dependence and abuse. To avoid these problems, a non-benzodiazepine agent FDA-approved for treatment of anxiety from the SSRI (citalopram, paroxetine, and sertraline) or SNRI (duloxetine) antidepressant categories or other non-benzodiazepine/non-antidepressant agent (e.g., buspirone and hydroxyzine) are prescribed for patients who require long-term pharmacotherapy for anxiety because they have been shown to decrease apprehension and worry. The lag time before onset of anxiolytic effects from the antidepressants and buspirone is 2 to 4 weeks, during which time a benzodiazepine may be needed for relief of symptoms. Ideally, benzodiazepine use for acute anxiety disorders should be limited to 2 to 4 weeks and used on a scheduled rather than as-needed basis.[1,7]

The development of physical dependence is a concern when treating patients with benzodiazepines for chronic anxiety disorders. Benzodiazepine withdrawal can manifest as worsening of preexisting anxiety, insomnia, irritability, restlessness, and muscle tension. Gradual tapering of benzodiazepines over weeks, depending on agent and length of therapy, is necessary to minimize withdrawal symptoms.

The short-term use of benzodiazepines by patients with anxiety disorders rarely results in abuse, although it is more likely to occur in patients with histories of alcohol or other substance abuse. When taking the medication history, it is important to determine the prescribed regimen, duration of drug therapy, and actual drug usage.

A number of oral side effects can accompany anxiolytic medications, including excessive salivation, or ptyalism; the perception of dry mouth, or xerostomia; difficulty swallowing, or dysphagia; and abnormalities of taste, referred to as dysgeusia. Patients experiencing the CNS adverse effects of these drugs, such as confusion or memory problems, may be unable to give adequate informed consent or understand postoperative or oral hygiene instructions. When planning to sedate a patient for dental treatment, drug dosages may need to be altered to prevent excessive sedation in patients already receiving medications that depress the CNS.

TABLE 16.2   Oral Agents to Treat Acute Anxiety

Anxiolytic Agents	Selected Adverse Effects
Benzodiazepines (BDZ) Alprazolam (Xanax, -XR) Clonazepam (Klonopin) Clorazepate (Tranxene) Diazepam (Diastat, Valium, Valtoco) Lorazepam (Ativan, Loreev XR) Oxazepam	**Significant considerations:** inability to retain new information, CNS depression, paradoxical reactions, withdrawal **Oral considerations**: xerostomia
Non-Benzodiazepines Hydroxyzine (Vistaril)	**Significant considerations:** acute generalized exanthematous pustulosis (rare), CNS depression, QT prolongation **Oral considerations:** xerostomia. Consult with physician prior to using local anesthetics.
Buspirone (Buspar)	**Significant considerations:** activation of mania, CNS stimulation, ocular effects, seizure, suicidal thinking/behavior **Oral considerations:** xerostomia, dysphagia, dysgeusia, bruxism, tongue edema, stomatitis/oral ulcers, gingivitis, glossitis

Treatment Planning for Patients With Anxiety Disorders

Treatment planning considerations for dental patients who suffer from anxiety disorders (other than dental anxiety/phobia) are summarized in Box 16.4. The decision to sedate these patients for dental treatment should be made in consultation with the patient and their behavioral health clinician. The choice of appointment length is affected by the decision regarding sedation. Short, early-morning appointments are preferred for the anxious patient who does not receive additional sedation. Long appointments are indicated when the patient will be sedated to accomplish as much treatment as possible at one visit. Allowing the patient to have control for the sequence of procedures or timing of breaks during the appointment may reduce general anxiety and help make the experience less threatening. Postoperative information should be provided both verbally and in writing to prevent any confusion about the instructions.

DEPRESSIVE DISORDERS

Mood disorders, also referred to as affective disorders, share the features of a sad, empty, or irritable mood, with physical and cognitive changes that cause significant dysfunction.[4] Depressive disorders have an unknown etiology but are understood to be the result of a complex interaction of life events, genetic predisposition, and alterations in CNS neurotransmitters.[11,12] Patients with these disorders manifest symptoms associated with changes in the neurotransmitters norepinephrine (NE), serotonin (5-HT), and dopamine. Most antidepressants exert their effects by altering the levels or effective concentrations of these neurotransmitters in various regions of the brain.[11,12]

Major Depressive Disorder

Major depressive disorder (MDD) is the most common depressive disorder. MDD is defined as experiencing feelings of sadness and/or a loss of interest in daily activities nearly all day, every day for at least two consecutive weeks. In 2018, the 12-month prevalence rate of MDD in the United States was 10.4%.[13] MDD is a disabling, often recurrent, disease with patients exhibiting significant occupational, social, and physical impairment. The onset of MDD often occurs in puberty, with incidence peaking in the twenties. Females are 1.5 to 3.0 times more likely than males to suffer from this disorder.[4] First-degree family members of individuals diagnosed with MDD have a two- to fourfold higher risk for the disorder than the general population. The course of the disorder varies widely; those with early-onset, multiple episodes, or severe or persistent symptoms are at higher risk of recurrence. The risk of recurrence of MDD decreases as the duration of remission increases.[4] Box 16.5 lists the main diagnostic criteria for MDD.

The clinician must remember that depressive illnesses are often associated with the treatment or progression of chronic physical disease. MDDs are managed with a combination of medication, behavioral therapy, and, occasionally, electroconvulsive therapy. MDD responds best to a combination of drug therapy and psychotherapy.

Persistent Depressive Disorder (Dysthymia)

Persistent depressive disorder is defined as a depressed mood for most of the day, for more days than not, for at least 2 years in adults and 1 year in children and adolescents. The disorder also includes the presence, while depressed, of at least two of the following symptoms: poor appetite or overeating, insomnia or hypersomnia, low energy or fatigue, low self-esteem, poor concentration, or difficulty making decisions, or feelings of hopelessness.[4] The disorder usually presents in childhood or adolescence with an insidious onset. The 12-month prevalence in the United States is estimated at 1.5%.[9] The effect of this disorder on functional ability varies widely and can equal or exceed the disability seen with MDD.[4] Individuals with persistent depressive disorder are at higher risk of other psychiatric comorbidity, especially substance abuse, than those with MDD.

Antidepressant Medications

Antidepressants are beneficial in up to 70% of patients and are chosen based on the patient's personal or family history of antidepressant response, any comorbid medical conditions, cost, and the potential for drug interactions.[14] A list of commonly prescribed antidepressant medications can be found in Table 16.3. The current standard of care for patients with psychiatric disorders is a combination of psychotherapy and corresponding medications.

Gaining information about who has prescribed an antidepressant and the indications for the drug's use represents an important component of the medication history, particularly because patients take antidepressants for nonpsychiatric indications. Jumping to the conclusion that a patient is depressed because of a prescribed medication can damage the mutual trust and rapport between patient and dentist. It is also important to evaluate the patient's use of herbal remedies, such as St. John's

TABLE 16.3   Antidepressant Medications

Antidepressant Medications	Selected Adverse Effects

Norepinephrine-Dopamine Reuptake Inhibitors (NDRIs)
Bupropion hydrochloride (Wellbutrin, -XL and -SR, Forfivo XL) and
    Bupropion hydrobromide ER (Aplenzin)
	Significant considerations: activation of mania, CNS stimulation, ocular effects, seizure,
	    suicidal thinking/behavior
	Oral considerations: xerostomia, dysphagia, dysgeusia, bruxism, tongue edema, stomatitis/
	    oral ulcers, gingivitis, glossitis

Monoamine Oxidase Inhibitors (MAOIs)
Isocarboxazid (Marplan)
 	
Phenelzine (Nardil)
 	
Selegiline (Eldepryl, Zelapar) and Selegiline Transdermal (EMSAM)
*Note: If the patient takes 10 mg or less, the dentist can use
    vasoconstrictors in local anesthesia.*
 	
Tranylcypromine (Parnate)
	Significant considerations: suicidal thinking/behavior, hypertensive crisis with tyramine use
	Oral considerations: avoid local anesthetics to prevent toxic reaction, orthostatic
	    hypotension, xerostomia

Serotonin-Noradrenergic Receptor Antagonists (SNRAs)
Mirtazapine (Remeron)
 	
Trazodone (Oleptro ER)
	Significant considerations: suicidal thinking/behavior, activation of mania, bleeding risk,
	    cardiac arrhythmias, orthostatic hypotension, priapism, serotonin syndrome
	Oral considerations: xerostomia, apthous stomatitis, gingival hemorrhage, oral edema,
	    glossitis, tongue discoloration, metallic taste, dysphagia, orthostatic hypotension. Consult
	    with cardiologist prior to using local anesthetic

Selective Serotonin Reuptake Inhibitors (SSRIs)
Citalopram (Celexa)
 	
Escitalopram (Lexapro)
 	
Fluoxetine (Prozac)
 	
Fluvoxamine
(only FDA-indicated for OCD)
 	
Paroxetine (Paxil, -CR, Pexeva)
 	
Sertraline (Zoloft)
	Significant considerations: activation of mania, bleeding risk, fragility fractures,
	    hyponatremia, ocular effects, QT prolongation, serotonin syndrome, sexual dysfunction,
	    suicidal thinking/behavior, withdrawal syndrome
	Oral considerations: xerostomia, abnormal taste

SSRI/Serotonin Receptor Agonist/Antagonist
Vortioxetine (Trintellix)
	Significant considerations: activation of mania, bleeding risk, fragility fractures,
	    hyponatremia, ocular effects, serotonin syndrome, sexual dysfunction, suicidal thinking/
	    behavior, withdrawal syndrome
	Oral considerations: xerostomia

SSRI/Serotonin Receptor Partial Agonist Vilazodone (Viibryd)	**Significant considerations:** suicidal thinking/behavior **Oral considerations:** xerostomia, taste perversion

Serotonin Norepinephrine Reuptake Inhibitors (SNRIs)
Desvenlafaxine ER (Pristiq, Khedezla)
 	
Duloxetine (Cymbalta, Drizalma, Irenka)
 	
Levomilnacipran ER (Fetzima)
	Significant considerations: activation of mania, bleeding risk, fragility fractures,
	    hepatotoxicity, hyponatremia, ocular effects, serotonin syndrome, sexual dysfunction,
	    suicidal thinking/behavior, withdrawal syndrome
	Oral considerations: xerostomia, bruxism

Tricyclic Antidepressants (TCAs)
 	
Tertiary Amines
 	
Amitriptyline (Elavil)
 	
Clomipramine (Anafranil)
(only FDA-indicated for OCD)
 	
Doxepin (Silenor)
 	
Imipramine
	Significant considerations: anticholinergic effects, bleeding risk, cardiac conduction
	    abnormalities, CNS depression, fragility fractures, hyponatremia, ocular effects, serotonin
	    syndrome, sexual dysfunction, suicidal thinking/behavior, withdrawal syndrome. Consult
	    with cardiologist prior to using local anesthetic
	Oral considerations: xerostomia, stomatitis, peculiar taste, orthostatic hypotension, black
	    tongue. Facial edema, tongue edema, parotid gland enlargement, and ageusia

(Continued)

TABLE 16.3 Antidepressant Medications—cont'd	
Antidepressant Medications	**Selected Adverse Effects**
Secondary Amines[a] Amoxapine Desipramine (Norpramin) Nortriptyline (Pamelor)	**Significant considerations:** anticholinergic effects cardiac conduction abnormalities, CNS depression, fragility fractures, hyponatremia, ocular effects, orthostatic hypotension, serotonin syndrome, suicidal thinking/behavior, withdrawal syndrome. Consult with cardiologist prior to using local anesthetic **Oral considerations:** xerostomia, unpleasant taste, black tongue

[a]Increased risk of bleeding (impaired platelet aggregation) especially when used with NSAIDs, anticoagulants or antiplatelets.

wort, for depression. Although the therapeutic value is questionable, there is still potential for drug interactions.

Tricyclic Antidepressants

Tricyclic antidepressants (TCAs) were considered first-line therapy for depressive disorders until the development of SSRIs, which offer an improved safety profile and equal efficacy with fewer adverse effects. TCAs interact with many neurotransmitter systems, causing a wide variety of adverse effects. In addition to inhibiting NE and serotonin (5-hydroxytryptamine; 5-HT) reuptake, they block muscarinic, histamine, and alpha-adrenergic receptors and are thus associated with strong anticholinergic effects, orthostatic hypotension, weight gain, and cardiac conduction disturbances. These agents are especially dangerous in overdose situations and must be used with caution in patients with any cardiac disease.[11] Today, TCAs are most prescribed as adjunctive agents for the management of chronic pain syndromes, including postherpetic neuralgia, peripheral neuropathy, and arthritic pain or as add-on therapy in multi-treatment resistant depression.[15]

It is important to note that TCAs exhibit a pharmacodynamic interaction with vasoconstrictors by potentiating the pressor response of direct-acting sympathomimetics (epinephrine, levonordefrin) used with local anesthetics in dentistry. Intensification of pressor activity results in raised blood pressure. This hypertensive effect is much greater with levonordefrin than with epinephrine, making epinephrine the vasoconstrictor of choice in patients who are taking TCAs.

Selective Serotonin Reuptake Inhibitors

SSRIs represent the majority of newly written prescriptions for depression and are without many of the serious side effects encountered with TCAs.[16,17] Although their cardiovascular side effects are mild, SSRI use is associated with multiple adverse effects, including nausea, fatigue, drowsiness, headache, nervousness, sexual dysfunction, insomnia, and xerostomia.[11,12] SSRIs have been linked to nocturnal bruxism (Figure 16.1).[18,19] Patients may develop bruxism and myalgia within the first few weeks of SSRI therapy.

Serotonin release by platelets is involved in hemostasis. Psychotropic drugs that decrease serotonin reuptake are known to increase the risk of upper gastrointestinal bleeding. This risk is increased by drugs that interfere with hemostasis (e.g., aspirin and other antiplatelets such as clopidogrel and prasugrel, warfarin, direct-acting anticoagulants such as rivaroxaban and

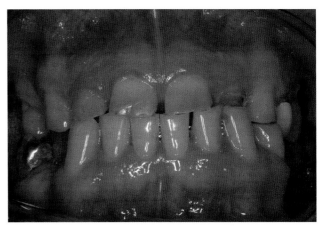

Fig. 16.1 Attrition of the mandibular teeth from nocturnal bruxism.

apixaban, and nonsteroidal antiinflammatory drugs (NSAIDs) such as ibuprofen and naproxen).[11]

Serotonin-Norepinephrine Reuptake Inhibitors

TCAs were the first SNRIs, but their effects on multiple neurotransmitter systems cause a variety of adverse effects, even at moderate doses. Newer agents have been developed that interact more specifically to inhibit the reuptake of serotonin and norepinephrine, thus avoiding many of the adverse effects associated with TCAs. These agents are prescribed for patients who have not derived an antidepressant benefit from SSRI therapy, as well as for neuropathic pain syndromes and anxiety disorders, among other indications.[11] The side effect profile of SNRIs is similar to that of SSRIs. This risk is increased by drugs that interfere with hemostasis (e.g., aspirin and other antiplatelets such as clopidogrel and prasugrel, warfarin, direct oral anticoagulants such as rivaroxaban and apixaban, and NSAIDs such as ibuprofen and naproxen).[11]

Monoamine Oxidase Inhibitors

Monoamine oxidase inhibitors (MAOIs) were the first class of antidepressants available for clinical use. Oral MAOIs are less commonly used in clinical practice because of extensive drug and food interactions. The use of these agents can result in a potentially fatal hypertensive crisis. It is crucial that patients on MAOIs avoid tyramine-containing foods (e.g., aged cheeses, fermented sausages, soy sauce, red wine). The tyramine consumption issue is less significant for the initial (low) doses of the selegiline patch indicated for depression secondary to greater selectivity for the MAO-B enzyme. Enzyme sub-type specificity is lost at increasing doses of the selegiline patch.

In addition to dietary restrictions, many common over-the-counter and prescription drugs may elicit hypertensive reactions when combined with MAOIs. Of special importance in dentistry is the interaction between these agents and indirect or mixed-acting sympathomimetics (pseudoephedrine, ephedrine, phenylephrine), which can produce a life-threatening hypertensive crisis. The direct-acting sympathomimetics (levonordefrin, epinephrine) in local anesthetics, however, react minimally when administered to patients on MAOI therapy.[20,21]

Norepinephrine-Dopamine Reuptake Inhibitors

The norepinephrine-dopamine reuptake inhibitors (NDRIs) offer an additional therapy option after, or in addition to, the SSRIs and SNRIs for the management of major depressive disorder. Based on a lack of pharmacological effect on serotonin, the NDRIs have a minimal impact on platelet activity and hemostasis. The side effect profile of the NDRIs is similar to the non-TCA SNRIs and include tachycardia and hypertension associated with sympathetic nervous system stimulation. A key concern associated with the use of bupropion is the risk of lowering the seizure threshold in patients with a history of seizure disorder. Table 16.3 lists important oral health issues of which the dentist should be aware with the use of these agents.

Serotonin-Noradrenergic Receptor Antagonists

The serotonin-noradrenergic receptor antagonists (SNRAs) are more commonly utilized as add-on therapy to SSRIs or SNRIs and work by blocking the postsynaptic serotonin and presynaptic and/or postsynaptic alpha-adrenergic (noradrenergic) receptors (alpha-1 and alpha-2). Agents in this class also block histamine receptors and have an increased likelihood of causing sedation. One agent in the class, trazodone, is most commonly utilized for its sedative properties. Patients receiving these medications should be monitored closely for increased CNS depression during dental sedation. Additionally, as a result of post-synaptic alpha-receptor blockade of some SNRAs, they can increase the risk of orthostatic hypotension.

Treatment Planning for Patients With Depressive Disorder

The dentist should address three interrelated areas of concern in the management of patients with depressive disorders: medications, mental status, and oral health needs (Box 16.6). The primary medication issue involves the determination of whether vasoconstrictors can be used safely. Cautious use of vasoconstrictors is recommended for patients taking TCAs and MAOIs. The hypertensive response to vasoconstrictors is largely dose dependent, so it is imperative that the dentist be aware of the details of the patient's current regimen. Vasoconstrictors may be used safely for patients taking SSRIs. Direct-acting sympathomimetics are the only vasoconstrictors appropriate for patients currently taking or recently withdrawn from MAOI therapy (7–14 days, depending on MAOI).

> **BOX 16.6   Treatment Planning Considerations for Patients With Depressive Disorders**
>
> - Obtain accurate health and medication histories.
> - Recommend an aggressive plaque control program.
> - Be aware of drug interactions with vasoconstrictors, NSAIDs, and others.
> - Manage diminished salivary output or xerostomia.
> - Evaluate for increased parafunctional activities and myalgia.
> - Determine whether the patient feels well enough to tolerate treatment.
> - Both written and verbal posttreatment instructions should be provided to the patient to prevent confusion.

Before beginning a procedure, the dentist should determine whether the patient feels well enough to undergo treatment. Patients with depressive disorders may have a significant challenge maintaining a regular oral hygiene routine. If the patient is experiencing a depressive episode that interferes with the ability to maintain oral health, plaque control with a pH neutral rinse or oral probiotics may be indicated. Xerostomia should be treated aggressively to prevent caries. Postoperative instructions should be given both verbally and in writing to prevent any confusion. There may be times when the depth of the patient's depression is so great that definitive treatment should be deferred until the depression is better controlled.

BIPOLAR I AND BIPOLAR II DISORDERS

Bipolar disorders are characterized by cyclical episodes of mania, or elevated mood, and, usually, depression. Epidemiologic studies show that bipolar disorders have a lifetime prevalence rate of approximately 4.4% among adults in the United States.[9] Genetic predisposition is an important determinant in the development of bipolar disorders. Environmental triggers and an unregulated relationship between the three main monoamine neurotransmitters in the brain (i.e., dopamine, norepinephrine, and serotonin) are also contributing factors to this disorder.[22]

Patients who have experienced one or more episodes of mania are classified as having bipolar I disorder. Bipolar I disorder differs from major depressive disorders in that patients experience **mania**, which is characterized by recurrent fluctuations of increased energy, expansive mood, and inappropriate behavior. During manic episodes, patients often exhibit symptoms of grandiosity, increased talking, racing thoughts, hyperactivity, and decreased need for sleep. A diagnosis of bipolar II disorder requires at least one episode of major depression and at least one hypomanic episode for diagnosis. Manic and depressive episodes are often separated by intervals in which the patient exhibits no signs or symptoms of mental illness. Multiple theories exist to explain the movement between episodes of mania and depression that occur in patients with bipolar disorders. Routine treatment should be deferred if the patient is experiencing the manic phase of bipolar disorder. Alcohol and substance abuse are frequent comorbid conditions associated with bipolar illness. Suicide attempts occur in up to 50% of patients with bipolar illness and 10% to 19% commit suicide.[22]

Lithium was the first agent used as a "mood stabilizer" for bipolar disorder. Lithium[11,22] is effective in a majority of patients with bipolar I and II disorders but has the disadvantage of having several troubling side effects and the need to monitor serum drug levels. Lithium also possesses a narrow therapeutic index, meaning there is a small range of blood levels between the likelihood of efficacy and toxicity or side effects. Currently, lithium and valproate are considered first-line medications both for the treatment of acute mania and as prophylaxis for recurrent manic and depressive episodes. Alternative or adjunctive treatments include anticonvulsants (lamotrigine, carbamazepine) and second-generation antipsychotics (quetiapine, risperidone, aripiprazole).[22] NSAIDs (e.g., ibuprofen, naproxen, aspirin), thiazide diuretics (e.g., hydrochlorothiazide, chlorthalidone), and angiotensin-converting enzyme inhibitors (e.g., lisinopril, captopril) can elevate lithium levels through decreased renal elimination. Of dental concern is the xerostomia, dysgeusia, and salivary gland swelling that may occur with lithium therapy.

SCHIZOPHRENIA SPECTRUM AND OTHER PSYCHOTIC DISORDERS

These illnesses include schizophrenia, personality (schizotypal) disorders, and other psychotic disorders. These disorders have varying effects on level of function, but often include prolonged symptoms of progressive social withdrawal, poor self-care, auditory hallucinations, delusions, disordered thinking (speech), flattened affect, and impaired concentration.[23]

Schizophrenia

The lifetime prevalence of US adult population with schizophrenia is 0.87%, with both genders equally affected.[24] The hallmark symptoms of delusions and hallucinations (psychosis) often start between 16 and 30 years of age.[4] Schizophrenia is a chronic disease that requires lifelong treatment. The long-term prognosis for this disorder is poor because patients have significant, lifelong impairment in interpersonal relationships and the ability to function in society.[25]

Symptoms of schizophrenia are usually characterized as positive, negative, and cognitive (Box 16.7). **Positive symptoms** are symptoms that occur as a result of the disease. These include hallucinations, delusions, and thought and movement disorders. Hallucinations, most commonly hearing voices when others do not, are disturbances of perception, whereas delusions are fixed, false beliefs. The most common delusions are the persecutory type, in which affected individuals may believe they are being conspired against, followed, spied on, or harassed by other individuals or organizations.[4]

Disorganized thinking (formal thought disorder) manifests as problems with speech. Difficulty in communication results from a lack of continuity of thought, in which the individual lacks concentration, focus, and logical sequence. Topics may change rapidly (derailment), and the patient may be easily distracted. Speech may suddenly stop or be garbled. Movement disorders can manifest as repetitive motions or, rarely, catatonia.[4] **Catatonia** is a movement disorder where the patient becomes

BOX 16.7   Symptoms of Schizophrenia
Positive
Delusions
Hallucinations
Disorganized thinking and speech
Movement disorders
Negative
Diminished emotional expression
Lack of drive or motivation
Diminished speech
Inability to experience pleasurable activities
Lack of desire to be social
Cognitive
Difficulty focusing
Diminished "working memory"
Difficulty understanding and using information

rigid, may stare into the distance, or have difficulty initiating movement.

Negative symptoms are disruptions in emotions and behavior. The most predominant negative symptoms of schizophrenia are diminished emotional expression, often thought of as blunted or flattened affect, a lack of drive or motivation to initiate or sustain activities. Other negative symptoms include anhedonia (an inability to experience pleasure in life), alogia (diminished speech), and being asocial (lack of desire for social interaction).[4] Cognitive symptoms include difficulty in several areas: focusing or paying attention, understanding, and using information to make decisions, and difficulty using information immediately after learning it.

Antipsychotic medications are the treatment of choice for acute psychotic episodes and to prevent relapse. Positive and negative symptoms are terms applied to aid in the categorization of symptoms associated with schizophrenia. Positive symptoms are additional experiences or behaviors, such as the addition of hallucinations, delusions, or repetitive movements that interfere with an individual's ability to function. Negative symptoms take away from an individual's ability to function and include withdrawing, an inability to display emotion, and apathy. The positive symptoms of schizophrenia respond best to pharmacotherapy, whereas the negative symptoms are more difficult to treat. The serious, debilitating nature of schizophrenia requires both comprehensive psychosocial management and continuous use of antipsychotic agents to reduce the frequency of relapse.[4,25]

Antipsychotic Medications

Antipsychotic medications are commonly divided into two groups: first-generation agents and second-generation (sometimes called "atypical") agents. Although both groups of drugs have similar efficacy, each is associated with the potential for significant adverse effects.

First-generation antipsychotics can cause extrapyramidal side effects such as pseudoparkinsonism, dystonia, akathisia, and tardive dyskinesia. These movement disorders are more likely with first-generation agents that are categorized as high-potency agents, such as haloperidol and fluphenazine, due to having a higher percentage (>78%) of dopamine receptor occupancy. Low-potency first generation antipsychotics, such as chlorpromazine and thioridazine, are known for their potential for inducing CNS effects such as sedation and their cardiovascular effects such as hypotension, tachycardia, and changes in ECG rhythm. Although second-generation agents have fewer neurologic side effects, many are associated with significant metabolic effects. These include weight gain, hyperlipidemia, hyperprolactinemia, and hyperglycemia. Choice of agent therefore depends on patient-specific factors that take into account comorbid conditions and family history of cardiovascular disease and diabetes. As with antidepressants, family and personal history of antipsychotic efficacy can aid in drug selection. Table 16.4 lists antipsychotic agents and their common side effects.

Tardive dyskinesia is characterized by persistent involuntary movement of the lips, jaws, or face and involuntary movements of the extremities, and usually occurs after prolonged use of antipsychotic medications. Risk factors include advanced age, poor drug response, the occurrence of acute extrapyramidal symptoms, diagnosis of organic mental disorder, mood disorders, and possibly female gender.[25]

Although some reports of spontaneous remission have been reported, there are two effective FDA-approved treatments for tardive dyskinesia (deutetrabenazine and valbenazine). A fine tremor of the tongue has been reported as an early indication of tardive dyskinesia and if the medication is discontinued after this finding, the full range of symptoms may not occur. The dentist may be the first healthcare provider to recognize the onset of tardive dyskinesia. Every effort should be made to identify early signs of this disorder so that the medication regimen can be altered and further symptom development or progression prevented.

The involuntary movements of the jaws that characterize tardive dyskinesia make it difficult for the patient to maintain adequate oral hygiene and may precipitate the development of temporomandibular disorders. It can also be very challenging to perform a clinical procedure on a patient with involuntary jaw movements.

Treatment Planning for Patients With a Psychotic Disorder

Treatment planning considerations for a patient with psychotic disorders are summarized in Box 16.8. The dentist has two primary responsibilities when treating a schizophrenic patient:

1. The dentist should be sure that adequate control of the disease process is being maintained by conducting a caries risk assessment at each dental visit and adjusting the preventive treatment plan to match the patient's level of risk.
2. The dentist must be alert to the development of any oral effects of the disease or the antipsychotic medications and must be prepared to either manage the oral side effects or communicate with the health care professionals if the side effects are severe (e.g., extrapyramidal effects).

All but emergency treatment must be deferred for the patient with uncontrolled or poorly controlled psychoses. Using oral probiotics to maintain the oral microbiome should be considered with the understanding that the patient may not be able to cope with a task such as swishing and expectorating.[26,27]

TABLE 16.4 Common Antipsychotic Medications

Antipsychotic Medications	Selected Adverse Events
Examples of First-Generation Antipsychotics	
Chlorpromazine	**Significant considerations:**
Haloperidol (Haldol)	hypotension, anticholinergic effects
Loxapine (Adasuve)	(confusion, memory loss, psychotic
Thioridazine	behavior, and agitation), sedation.
Thiothixene	Consult with cardiologist prior to
	using local anesthetic
	Oral considerations: xerostomia,
	tardive dyskinesia
Second-Generation Antipsychotics	
Aripiprazole (Abilify, Aristada)	**Significant considerations:**
Asenapine (Saphris, Secuado)	anticholinergic effects, dyslipidemia,
Cariprazine (Vraylar)	extrapyramidal symptoms, fever,
	gastrointestinal hypomobility,
Clozapine (Clozaril, Versacloz)	hepatic effects, hyperglycemia,
Iloperidone (Fanapt)	mortality in older adults,
Lumateperone (Caplyta)	myocarditis, neuroleptic malignant
	syndrome, orthostatic hypotension,
Lurasidone (Latuda)	QT wave prolongation, sedation,
Olanzapine (Zyprexa)	agranulocytosis, sialorrhea,
Olanzapine/Fluoxetine (Symbyax)	temperature dysregulation, venous
Olanzapine/Samidorphan (Lybalvi)	thromboembolism, weight gain.
Paliperidone (Invega, -Sustenna (1 month); -Trinza (3 month); -Hafyera (6 month)	Consult with cardiologist prior to using local anesthetic
	Oral considerations: xerostomia
Quetiapine (Seroquel, -XR)	
Risperidone (Risperdal, -Consta, Perseris)	
Ziprasidone (Geodon)	

BOX 16.8 Treatment Planning Considerations for Patients With Psychotic Disorders

- Obtain an accurate health and medication history.
- Implement an aggressive plaque control program.
- Manage diminished salivary output or xerostomia; encourage the patient to maintain adequate hydration.
- Determine whether the patient feels well enough to tolerate treatment.
- Both written and verbal posttreatment instructions should be provided to the patient to prevent confusion.
- Defer treatment if necessary because of poor mental status. Be alert for adverse effects of psychotropic medications, especially (1) orthostatic hypotension and (2) extrapyramidal effects, such as pseudoparkinsonism, acute dystonia, akathisia, or tardive dyskinesia.

Xerostomia, orthostatic hypotension, anticholinergic effects, and extrapyramidal effects are the primary treatment planning considerations for a medicated patient with a psychotic illness. Because most antipsychotic medications are associated with salivary gland hypofunction, adequate plaque removal and caries control is of critical importance. Cholinergic agonist medications, such as cevimeline and pilocarpine, will stimulate saliva production in patients with diminished salivary flow rates. Because of the potential for serious drug and disease state interactions, consultation with the prescribing healthcare provider should be made before use of a cholinergic agent. Orthostatic hypotension is possible in patients treated with antipsychotic agents and its manifestation—syncope—can be prevented by minimizing rapid changes in patient positioning and by keeping the patient in a seated position until any sensation of dizziness has dissipated.

The extrapyramidal effects of psychotic medications may necessitate modification of the dental treatment plan. These effects include tardive dyskinesia; pseudoparkinsonism, similar to the tremor disorder seen with Parkinson's disease; dystonia, an irregular and sometimes sustained contraction of muscles; and akathisia, a constant perception to move and the inability to sit still. Patient sedation or the use of general anesthesia may be considered as strategies for diminishing the effects of tardive dyskinesia, but the interaction between sedative, anesthetic, and antipsychotic medications must be carefully evaluated. Definitive dental care should be deferred if the patient is experiencing a psychotic episode.

OTHER PATHOLOGIC DISORDERS

Obsessive-Compulsive and Related Disorders

Obsessive-compulsive disorder (OCD), body dysmorphic disorder, hoarding, excoriation (skin picking), and substance/medication-induced OCD have a close relationship to anxiety disorders. OCD is a psychiatric condition in the United States with a 12-month prevalence rate of 1.2% of the population.[9] **Obsessions** are defined as recurrent persistent thoughts, urges, or images that the patient recognizes as inappropriate. Attempts to suppress these unwanted thoughts produce significant anxiety. **Compulsions** (or rituals) are repeated behaviors or mental acts that the patient feels compelled to perform in response to an obsession (e.g., ritualistic washing because of fears of contamination). Box 16.9 lists some common symptoms of OCD.[4,28]

The onset of OCD usually occurs in late adolescence or early adulthood, with most patients exhibiting both obsessive and compulsive symptoms. Patients with OCD usually have some level of insight, recognizing that their thoughts and behaviors are irrational, but are unable to control them (Figure 16.2). Common themes are cleaners and checkers. Checkers spend much of their day making sure that lights or the stove are turned off or that all of the doors and windows are locked, owing to an underlying fear of catastrophe. Cleaners may continually clean themselves in an attempt to avoid illness.[4] This ritualistic cleansing may involve every waking hour.

BOX 16.9   Symptoms of Obsessive-Compulsive Disorder

Obsessions

Repetitive thoughts:
Contamination (germs/disease, bodily fluids, dirt)
Unwanted sexual thoughts
Repetitive images:
Violent or horrific scenes
Inappropriate sexual conduct
Repetitive urges:
Fear of acting on impulse to harm self/others
Perfectionism (fear of losing important information, need to put objects in specific order)

Compulsions

Cleaning: constantly washing self or objects, excessive toothbrushing
Checking: that nothing terrible happened, that a mistake has not been done or harm to self/others
Repeating: rewriting, repeating bodily movements, repeating activities in exact/safe numbers
Collecting: hoarding items
Mental: counting while performing a task

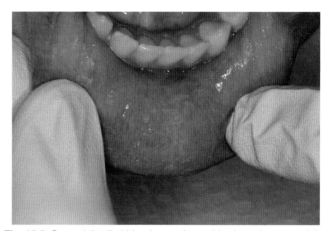

Fig. 16.2 Compulsive lip biting in a patient with obsessive-compulsive disorder.

OCD usually presents with other mental disorders.[29] Cognitive behavioral therapy is the treatment of choice for mild OCD. Many patients also require pharmacologic intervention in the form of high doses of SSRIs. Even with pharmacologic treatment, many OCD patients still suffer from lifelong disabling symptoms.[4]

Treatment planning considerations for patients with OCD are similar to those for patients with anxiety disorders. The length of appointment and the use of sedation are important considerations when treating these patients. When providing instructions to the patient, the clinician must be very specific about how long or how many times a particular activity should be performed. A technique for helping patients with OCD during the appointment is to ask the patient to rate their current anxiety level and check in on their anxiety level periodically throughout the visit. By acknowledging, labeling, and attributing their symptoms to OCD the patient can then identify ways to refocus during the visit. It can be helpful for the patient and clinician to acknowledge that the symptoms are linked to OCD: "It's not me, it's my OCD." With consistent and collaborative hard work, anxiety levels should drop within 30 minutes. If the patient cannot participate in at least 15 minutes of the appointment, the clinician can stop and reschedule.

Posttraumatic Stress Disorder

Posttraumatic stress disorder (PTSD) was once thought to be primarily a disorder of war veterans because approximately 30% of individuals who have spent time in a war zone manifest signs or symptoms of PTSD.[30,31] Although direct exposure to actual or near death, serious injury, or sexual violence are all precipitants of PTSD, individuals can also develop PTSD after witnessing these events happening to others, or learning that the traumatic event(s) have happened to someone close to them, or after repeated exposure to traumatic situations (emergency medical personnel, police).[4] PTSD is now recognized in many different population groups, such as survivors of natural disasters and victims of mugging, rape, or automobile accidents.

An estimated 7.7 million US adults are affected by PTSD every year.[30] The disorder may occur at any age. The symptom clusters identified in the DSM-V include reexperiencing, avoidance, persistent negative alterations in cognition and mood, and arousal and reactivity. These can manifest as nightmares, flashbacks, avoidance of pleasurable activities, difficulty with social interactions, lack of trust, irritability, and aggression. This disorder is often associated with anxiety, depression, or substance abuse. Symptom onset most frequently occurs within the first 3 months after the trauma but may be delayed. Fifty percent of adults will completely recover within 3 months, whereas others continue to experience chronic symptoms that fluctuate in response to life stressors, new trauma, or reminders of the event.[4]

Treatment for PTSD is dependent on presenting symptoms and often consists of psychoeducation or psychosocial/therapy, including CBT. Antidepressants, usually SSRIs, are first-line pharmacotherapeutic agents in the management of this disorder, because they also treat the associated anxiety and depression that often accompany PTSD.

Patients with PTSD require many of the basic treatment planning considerations used for patients with anxiety or depression. It is important to determine whether the patient can identify their "good" or "bad" days so that appointments on "bad" days can be avoided. Additionally, there is a high level of substance abuse associated with PTSD, therefore the clinician should be cognizant of the potential for drug interactions as well as illicit drug use. Patients with PTSD have a high prevalence of bruxism and other parafunctional activities. Bruxism in the presence of a dry mouth may result in more rapid loss of tooth structure than would be the case in a patient with normal salivary output. Additionally, bruxism places a greater occlusal load on existing and planned restorations.[32,33]

Attention-Deficit/Hyperactivity Disorder

Central to the diagnosis of attention-deficit/hyperactivity disorder (ADHD) is a continuous pattern of inattention and/or hyperactivity-impulsivity that affects functioning or development.[4] This disorder occurs in approximately 5% of US children and persists into adulthood for 50% of affected individuals. Inattention can present as difficulty staying focused or on task, a lack of persistence, inability to follow through on instructions, or being disorganized. Hyperactivity manifests as excessive motor activity, fidgeting, or talkativeness. Impulsivity can be seen in an inability to delay gratification, interrupting conversations, or intrusive behavior. Intrusive behavior could be repeatedly raising their hand, speaking to loudly, or not respecting personal boundaries.

This disorder has a strong genetic component and occurs more frequently in males, at a 2:1 ratio in childhood and a 1.6:1.0 ratio in adulthood.[4] Children with ADHD often experience lower academic achievement and problems with peer relationships. Adults exhibit fewer symptoms of ADHD than children; impairment is seen in decreased employment, occupational performance and attendance, and higher levels of interpersonal conflict.[4]

Stimulant medications are considered first-line pharmacologic therapy for ADHD, as they modulate neurotransmitter activity and target the core symptoms of the disorder. These agents are short-acting, immediate-release dosage forms and commonly must be taken two or three times daily to sustain efficacy throughout the day. Extended-/sustained-release formulations (-XL, -XR, -ER, -SR) are preferred because once-daily dosing improves adherence and can diminish breakthrough symptoms during the day. Nonstimulant agents are also used in the management of ADHD and may be effective for a patient intolerant to or unwilling to be treated with a stimulant medication. A list of the oral agents used to treat ADHD is given in Table 16.5. A combination of ADHD-specific cognitive and behavioral interventions and pharmacotherapy produces better outcomes than pharmacotherapy alone.[34] Common adverse effects of stimulants include reduced appetite, weight loss, stomachache, insomnia, an increase in blood pressure and heart rate, headache, irritability, and xerostomia.[11,34] Appetite suppression has potentially disastrous dental consequences when combined with dry mouth. Parents frequently allow the child to eat anything as long as they eat something, with dietary choices often including foods high in fat and refined carbohydrates. A refined carbohydrate diet and dry mouth constitute strong risk factors for dental caries. Clenching and bruxism seem to be more prevalent in children with this disorder, but it is unclear whether these behaviors are the result of the disorder or the treatment.

Patients with ADHD may exhibit widely disparate behaviors. Untreated persons may exhibit hyperactivity, impulsivity, and distractibility. They may have difficulty staying in one place for any length of time, making it difficult to complete a complex dental procedure. Persons who are under treatment for the disorder tend to be more sedate but may suffer from the adverse effects of their medications—dry mouth, bruxism, and anorexia (Box 16.10).

Children and adolescents are the age groups most likely to be affected with this disorder and the age groups also more likely to have a higher incidence of dental caries. Most medications[35] used in the management of the disorder affect the patient's behavior but do not address any underlying learning disabilities. Patient instructions must be given with this fact in mind. Instructions should be provided in both verbal and written form and may need to be shared with a family member or caregiver as well. Some dental schools and offices have oral self-care websites with videos that patients can visit (see Chapter 4). Bruxism

and dental attrition are more common in these patients. If the use of a night guard is considered, the age of the patient and potential for growth of the dental arches must be evaluated and taken into account.

SOMATIC SYMPTOM AND RELATED DISORDERS

This diagnostic class includes individuals with a diagnosis of somatic symptom disorder, factitious disorder, illness anxiety disorder, or conversion disorder. These disorders share the feature of predominant somatic (body) symptoms that are associated with a disproportionate degree of patient distress and impairment.[4] Somatic symptom disorder diagnostic criteria include at least one somatic complaint (most patients have more than one) that is distressing or causes a disruption in daily life. According to the DSM-V, at least one of the following symptoms must also be present:[4]

1. Disproportionate and persistent thought about the seriousness of one's symptoms.
2. Persistently high level of anxiety about health or symptoms.
3. Excessive time and energy devoted to these symptoms or health concerns.

The prevalence of this disorder in the United States is estimated at 5% to 7% and it is more common in females.

Somatic Symptom Disorder

For these individuals, an underlying excessive fear of illness and preoccupation with the state of their health leads to overuse of medical care as the individual seeks confirmation of their fears and symptoms. Health concerns assume a dominant role in the lives of patients with severe disease, adversely affecting their interpersonal relationships and quality of life.[4] Patients with somatic symptom disorder do not fabricate the symptomatology. An underlying medical disorder may or may not be present. When physical illness is present, the level of impairment is markedly higher than expected.[4]

For the dentist, these patients may be demanding with regard to diagnostic testing and may attempt to dictate treatment. It is important for the dentist to identify the problem and provide reassurance that appropriate tests will be performed to help diagnose complaints. Many patients may also have been diagnosed with other psychological problems, such as depression or an anxiety disorder. Patients with somatization disorder sometimes have several physicians and may be receiving different treatments from each. Identification of all prescription medications and prescribers minimizes the possibility of creating an adverse response to a medication prescribed in the course of dental treatment.

When the patient presents with symptoms that do not match the physical signs, it is important for the dentist to confer with the patient's primary care physician. The patient may have omitted pertinent information regarding their general health status that will explain the complaint, or the dentist may be able to provide the physician with a new piece of information that facilitates a formal diagnosis. In either instance, clear lines

TABLE 16.5 Oral Agents to Treat Attention Deficit-Hyperactivity Disorder

ADHD Agents	Selected Adverse Effects
Stimulants	
Mixed Amphetamine Salts (Adderall, -XR, Mydayis)	**Significant considerations:** use vasoconstrictors with caution, tachycardia, hypertension, and heart palpitations
Amphetamine (Adzenys XR, Dyanavel XR, Evekeo)	
Dextroamphetamine (Dexedrine, ProCentra, Zenzedi)	**Oral considerations:** bruxism, speech disturbances, and xerostomia
Dexmethylphenidate (Focalin, -XR)	
Lisdexamfetamine (Vyvanse)	
Methamphetamine (Desoxyn)	
Methylphenidate (Adhansia XR, Aptensio XR, Concerta, Cotempla XR, Daytrana, Jornay PM, Metadate ER, Methylin, QuilliChew ER, Quillivant XR, Relexxii, Ritalin, -LA)	
Serdexmethylphenidate/ Dexmethylphenidate (Azstarys)	
Non-Stimulants	
Atomoxetine (Strattera)	**Significant considerations:** QTc prolongation, consult with physician prior to using local anesthetic
Clonidine (Kapvay)	
Guanfacine (Intuniv)	
Viloxazine (Qelbree)	**Oral considerations:** xerostomia, abnormal taste, orthostatic hypotension

BOX 16.10 Treatment Planning Considerations for Patients With Attention Deficit/Hyperactivity Disorder

- Obtain an accurate health and medication history.
- Recommend an aggressive plaque control program.
- Manage xerostomia and encourage adequate hydration. Recommend maintaining an adequate diet (reduce high carbohydrate content foods).
- Provide written and verbal patient instructions.
- Recommend judicious use of a night guard to avoid any effect on facial development in children.

of communication must remain open between the dentist and primary care physician. The patient may insist that the dentist make a diagnosis and recommend a specific treatment for the complaint at the time of presentation. In such instances, it is prudent to defer both diagnosis and/or treatment until adequate data are collected to ensure that an accurate diagnosis is made.

The identification of patients with any of the somatoform disorders often takes months or years and is easier to see in retrospect. Complaints that do not coincide with the physical signs or symptoms that transcend normal anatomic and physiologic boundaries (e.g., neurogenic pain in the mandible that crosses the midline, pain that jumps from maxillary to mandibular teeth) should raise the index of suspicion that a somatoform disorder exists. However, appropriate diagnostic procedures should be performed to rule out a true oral pathologic entity or emergent condition.

Factitious Disorder

Factitial injuries are oral lesions created by the patient that are not attributable to oral disease or accidental trauma. The patient may or may not be aware of having caused the injury. In a patient suffering from OCD, the injury may be a part of a ritual; in a psychotic patient, a form of self-mutilation; or the lesion may simply be the result of an innocent habit in a mouth rendered susceptible because of inadequate saliva. The common types of dental factitial injuries include gingival abrasion with a fingernail (Figure 16.3), obsessive tooth brushing, use of inappropriate aids to clean the teeth, and burns caused by aspirin placement over sore tissue. Although factitial injuries are usually minor, there have been reports of self-extraction of teeth and even autoglossectomy in schizophrenic patients.[36,37] Dental treatment for the more minor forms of factitial injury will involve patient education and symptomatic care.

OTHER PSYCHOLOGICAL PHENOMENA

Denial

A patient's refusal to accept a particular diagnosis is characterized as denial. Although more commonly manifested in association with the diagnosis of a life-threatening disease, denial can also occur in the dental setting. Many patients will deny

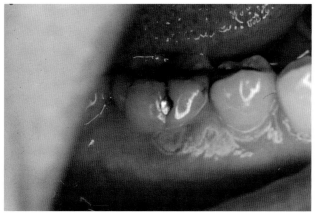

Fig. 16.3 Gingival irritation as a result of repeated abrasion with a fingernail.

that their teeth need to be removed when faced with a hopeless prognosis resulting from severe periodontitis and bone loss. The dentist can help the patient deal with difficult diagnoses by recognizing denial and providing the patient with a mechanism by which they can either confirm or disprove the initial diagnosis such as obtaining a second opinion.

The very fact that the dentist offers the option of securing a second opinion helps diminish anxiety and may allow the person to process the available information in a logical manner. Avoidance of a power struggle or a "my way or the highway" confrontation helps the patient deal with difficult diagnoses and may diminish the effect of denial on dental treatment.

Collusion

Sometimes the patient attempts to manipulate the dentist into performing a task "as a favor" and at the same time withholds specific information that would in all likelihood have a negative effect on the dentist's willingness to provide the favor. The request may seem trivial, such as if a patient says, "Let's not tell my doctor what happened today," when discussing a syncopal episode, vomiting, or a behavior outburst. It could very well be that the physician has told the patient that if such an episode recurs, changes will be made in the treatment regimen. Becoming involved in this type of patient conspiracy, regardless of how trivial it may seem, can have disastrous consequences for both the dentist and patient. It is best to explain to the patient that you will need to speak to the involved persons (e.g., caregiver, physician) to ensure that the patient's health is not compromised. It is difficult for a patient to be upset with a dentist who is truly concerned about their overall health.

Delusions

Sometimes a patient reports a complaint for which no physical signs are apparent. The complaint may be a prodrome for an emergent condition—for example, tingling of the lip before the onset of recurrent herpes labialis, trigeminal neuralgia, or ongoing pulpal necrosis. Adequate diagnostic procedures help identify these conditions. Some oral complaints may be delusional, however. Patients may report that insects are in their gums or that their teeth are disintegrating. Delusional oral complaints may signal the onset of a psychotic episode or the failure of treatment for an existing psychotic disorder. In either instance, referral to or consultation with the primary care physician or therapist is essential. Oral health complaints, no matter how unlikely, must be adequately explored because a series of bizarre symptoms may in fact reflect a genuine physical pathologic condition. Diabetic neuropathies, for example, can often produce uncommon symptoms that could be mistakenly interpreted as delusional.

Secondary Gain

Secondary gain occurs when a patient seeks the reward of attention or avoidance of unpleasant tasks as an outcome of their illness. Gains include securing time off work, avoiding unpleasant responsibilities, obtaining sympathy, and procuring medications. This behavior is fairly common in persons with multiple chronic illnesses, but can also manifest in dental patients, especially those with a chronic pain complaint. The index of suspicion should be raised when the patient continues to report pain despite multiple, apparently adequate treatments. These patients may be unable to drive and must be transported to the office. They may report that they can no longer carry out the activities of daily living. It becomes apparent that if these patients ever recover from their perceived illness, they may lose their captive audience and need to take care of themselves. This cycle can have untoward effects on the patient, family, and dentist. Consultation with the primary care physician may provide insight into the management of such patients.

MEDICATION EFFECTS THAT AFFECT DENTAL TREATMENT

Interactions of Psychotherapeutic Drugs With Medications Used in Dentistry

Many psychotherapeutic agents interact with medications commonly used in dentistry. Although a thorough discussion of dental drug interactions with psychotherapeutic agents is beyond the scope of this text, practitioners must be aware of the drug–drug and drug–disease state interactions that can occur with the medications they prescribe or use in clinical practice. Many interactions relate to the potentiation of the sedative or anticholinergic actions of the psychotherapeutic medication (e.g., dry mouth, orthostatic hypotension, additive sedation). Consultation with the physician prescribing the psychotherapeutic medications should be made when any sort of sedation is planned so that dosage can be adjusted to prevent adverse events.

Confusion

Many psychotropic medications can cause confusion. More prevalent in older patients, confusion can occur in any age group. Patient confusion is an important factor to consider when providing dental treatment. The onset of confusion may be a sign that the patient is overmedicated. It is not unusual for the patient with these problems to report that they had forgotten whether the medication had been taken at the appropriate time and took a second dose just in case.

Oral hygiene and postoperative instructions should be given both verbally and in writing. Make sure that the patient understands the instructions and if in doubt, also give the instructions to a family member or care provider. If possible, avoid prescribing medications that cause CNS depression and may exacerbate patient confusion. When confusion is a concern, nonopioid analgesics are a more prudent choice than a centrally acting analgesic medication.

Orthostatic Hypotension

Many medications used to manage psychological disorders diminish sympathetic tone and cause lowered blood pressure. As a result, sudden changes in position can produce dizziness and a feeling of light-headedness. Syncope is a common occurrence after dismissal of a patient who has spent an hour reclined in a dental chair. Orthostatic hypotension cannot be completely avoided but can be minimized by allowing the patient to acclimate slowly to the seated and standing position after a dental procedure. Orthostatic hypotension may be exacerbated with the use of intravenous sedation or with nitrous oxide conscious sedation. Monitoring preprocedural and postprocedural blood pressure readings or continuously measuring blood pressure is considered the standard of care in management of a sedated patient.

Intraoral Effects of Psychotherapeutic Agents

Many prescription, over-the-counter, and herbal medications have intraoral effects. Adverse effects include, but are not limited to, problems such as dysgeusia, stomatitis, lichenoid reactions, halitosis, and xerostomia. Most psychotherapeutic agents can cause xerostomia, which is the most common adverse intraoral effect of all drugs. (See the section on xerostomia, later in this chapter.)

Dysgeusia, or altered taste sensation, can be an adverse effect of many drugs, including psychotherapeutic agents. Patients may report a persistent unpleasant taste, altered taste of foods, or generalized loss of taste sensation, referred to as ageusia. Patients suffering from dysgeusia should be questioned extensively regarding the nature, severity, and persistence of the altered taste sensation. For some patients, an alteration in taste sensation may be a nuisance; for others, it may interfere with nutritional intake and hydration. Some patients eat constantly in an attempt to eliminate an unpleasant taste in the mouth. Others eat nothing because food "doesn't taste the same." Because large carious lesions, severe periodontal disease, or oral ulcerations can also produce a persistent bad taste in the mouth, the practitioner must rule out intraoral disease as a causative factor in dysgeusia before considering patient medications as the primary cause. Every effort should be made to diminish the effects of dysgeusia so that it does not interfere with the patient's well-being.

The clinical presentation of reactions to lichenoid drugs may be very similar to erosive lichen planus and can be intensely painful (Figure 16.4). The discomfort is exacerbated when the patient also suffers from a dry mouth. Such reactions may occur with both phenothiazine first-generation antipsychotic agents (e.g., chlorpromazine, fluphenazine), lithium, and TCAs, but are not specific to psychotropic medications. Lichenoid drug reactions have also been reported with a variety of antihypertensive medications (e.g., beta-blockers, angiotensin-converting enzyme inhibitors, methyldopa, and thiazides), antitumor necrosis factor agents used for inflammatory bowel disease, rheumatoid and psoriatic arthritis (e.g., infliximab), and NSAIDs. The dentist may want to refer the patient to an oral surgeon or periodontist to obtain an incisional biopsy for an oral pathologist to evaluate the sample to confirm the clinical diagnosis.

Treatment for lichenoid drug reactions should be directed toward switching to a medication that does not produce the reaction. If a medication change is not possible, symptomatic areas should be treated with topical corticosteroid agents.

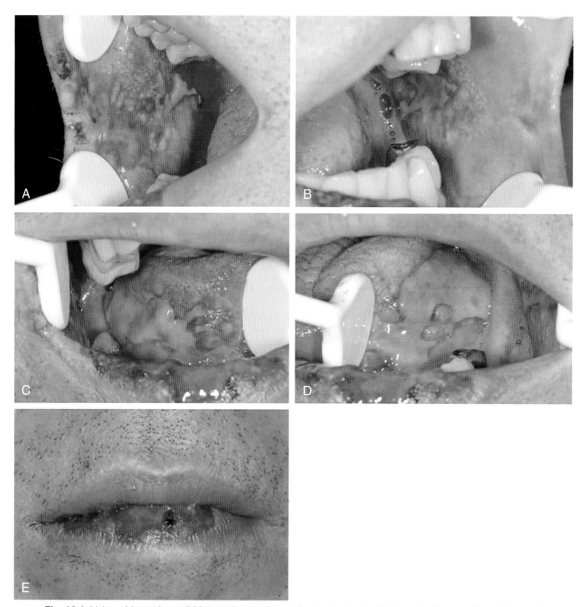

Fig. 16.4 Lichenoid reaction to lithium carbonate in a patient being treated for bipolar disorder. (From Kumagai A, Matsuo S, Hoshi H, Sato H, Takeda Y, Sugiyama Y. Oral lichenoid drug reaction with autoantibodies in peripheral blood: Case report. 2011;8(1):29–33.)

However, the use of topical corticosteroids in a dry mouth may predispose the patient to candidiasis. For some patients, it may also be necessary to prescribe topical or systemic antifungal medications.

EFFECT OF PSYCHOLOGICAL DISORDERS ON THE ORAL CAVITY

Many changes in the environment of the oral cavity can be directly related to certain psychological disorders. Common examples include the patient with a psychotic disorder who develops oral ulcers because of self-inflicted trauma, or the patient with an OCD who has severely abraded teeth caused by excessive brushing. In many other cases, although the relationship between the mental health condition and oral pathology is indirect, the results can be devastating and pervasive—as with

dental caries or progressive periodontal disease. Recognition of and differentiation between direct and indirect disease-related and medication-related oral conditions will be important elements in developing such a patient's treatment plan.

Xerostomia and Dental Caries

Saliva serves many purposes in the oral cavity, including acting as a lubricant, buffer, digestive aid, and other roles seen in Figure 16.5. As salivary flow diminishes, the beneficial effects of saliva also diminish resulting in oral disease. After a few days of a patient experiencing inadequate salivary flow they may report a sore, erythematous oral cavity. Patients may also report that they bite themselves, their dentures do not fit, and food does not taste the same. Additional symptoms include having a feeling of slime or a gritty sensation in their mouth, and/or halitosis or bad breath. Not only is saliva needed for patient comfort and function, but it is also needed to maintain a healthy oral microbiome.[38]

Although psychological disorders do not cause dental caries formation, the consequences of and treatments for many of these disorders impact the salivary composition and flow, diet, and oral health behaviors of the patient. Without adequate preventive care, these changes can result in an increased number and rate of progression of carious lesions.[39] The effect of xerostomia on other oral tissue is shown in Figure 16.6. A frequent side effect of most psychotropic medications, xerostomia can also result from numerous psychological disorders.[40]

Stress not only diminishes salivary flow, but also influences the components of saliva. Because salivary immunoglobulin A (IgA) levels and buffering capacity are diminished in patients experiencing high levels of stress or depressive events, an oral environment favorable to caries development may result (Figure 16.7). For patients with removable prostheses, inadequate saliva can affect denture retention and predispose the patient to denture injuries through inadequate lubrication of the oral tissue. Patients should be informed of the adverse effects of inadequate salivary flow before any extensive dental treatment.

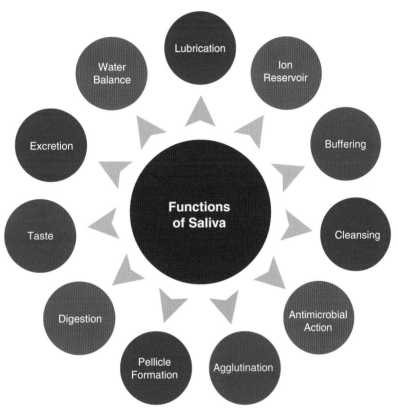

Fig. 16.5 Functions of saliva.

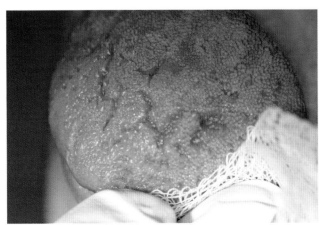

Fig. 16.6 Furrowed tongue in patient complaining of dry mouth.

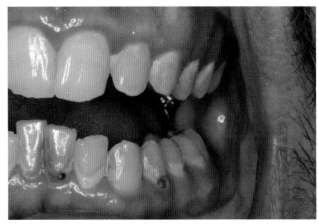

Fig. 16.7 Caries and hypomineralized smooth surface lesions in a patient with xerostomia, poor plaque control, and a diet high in refined carbohydrates.

BOX 16.11 Saliva Stimulants and Substitutes

Saliva Stimulants

Over-the-Counter
SalivaSure tablets (Scandinavian formulas)

Prescription
Pilocarpine Hydrochloride (HCl) tablets, ophthalmic drops
Cevimeline HCl capsules
Bethanechol tablets

Saliva Substitutes

Over-the-Counter
SalivaMAX (Forward Science)
Salivart (Gebauer)
Dentiva or Salese (Nuvora)
Mouth Kote (Parnell)
XyliMelts (OraCoat)

Diminished salivary flow can be the result of many diseases and medications. Without objective measurement of salivary flow, it is difficult to equate patient reported symptoms with the availability of needed quality and quantity of saliva. Chairside salivary testing can help dentists evaluate the quantity and quality of the patient's saliva before recommending treatment.[41]

Management of dry mouth can be complex. Chapter 18 outlines the treatment of hyposalivation and symptom management. It is best to begin with strategies that lend themselves to patient adherence. Adequate hydration is essential. Decreasing caffeine intake is helpful in alleviating the symptoms, although adherence can be a problem. Avoidance of alcohol-containing mouthwashes and mouthwashes with a low pH is essential. If these preliminary interventions do not provide adequate relief, the next step is the use of artificial saliva. Patients need to use the saliva substitutes frequently (one to two times per waking hour) for the substitute to be effective. The dentist should provide the patient with several saliva substitute options (Box 16.11). Patients with xerostomia sometimes have an altered sense of taste and may not be adherent because of the flavoring in the substitutes. The next stage of therapy involves requesting that the patient's physician either alter the medication regimen or add a cholinergic agent, such as pilocarpine, bethanechol, or cevimeline. In recalcitrant cases of xerostomia secondary to antipsychotic or antidepressant medications, it may be desirable to confer with the prescribing mental health therapist to determine whether a less-xerogenic medication can be used to control the disorder.

CONCLUSION

Providing successful oral healthcare for patients with psychological disorders requires trust building, collaborative care, and the practice of person centered care. Learning to successfully manage these patients' often complex oral problems can be of inestimable value to the patients and their caregivers and can be both satisfying and rewarding to the dentist and the entire dental team.

REFERENCES

1. Kessler R, Chiu W, Demler O, et al. Prevalence, severity, and comorbidity of twelve-month DSM-IV disorders on the National Comorbidity Survey Replication (NCS-R). *Arch Gen Psychiatry.* 2005;62:617–627.
2. Substance Abuse and Mental Health Services Administration *Key substance use and mental health indicators in the United States: Results from the 2019 National Survey on Drug Use and Health (HHS Publication No. PEP20-07-01-001, NSDUH Series H-55).* Rockville, MD: Center for Behavioral Health Statistics and Quality, Substance Abuse and Mental Health Services Administration; 2020. https://www.samhsa.gov/data/.
3. Mishra S, Stierman B, Gahche JJ, Potischman N. *Dietary supplement use among adults: United States, 2017–2018. NCHS Data Brief, no 399.* Hyattsville, MD: National Center for Health Statistics; 2021.
4. American Psychiatric Association *Diagnostic and Statistical Manual of Mental Disorders.* ed 5 Arlington, VA: American Psychiatric Publishing; 2013.
5. National Institute of Mental Health: Anxiety disorders, NIH publication 09-3879, 2009.
6. Barlow DH. *Anxiety and Its Disorders: The Nature and Treatment of Anxiety and Panic.* 2nd ed. New York: The Guilford Press; 2002.
7. Melton ST, Kirkwood CK. Anxiety disorders: generalized anxiety, panic, and social anxiety disorders. In: DiPiro JT, ed. *Pharmacotherapy: A Pathophysiologic Approach.* ed 11 New York: McGraw-Hill Education; 2020.
8. Katzman MA. Current considerations in the treatment of generalized anxiety disorder. *CNS Drugs.* 2009;23(2):103–120.
9. Harvard Medical School, 2007. National Comorbidity Survey (NCS). (2017, August 21). Retrieved from https://www.hcp.med.harvard.edu/ncs/index.php. Data Table 2: 12-month prevalence DSM-IV/WMH-CIDI disorders by sex and cohort.
10. Merikangas KR, He JP, Burstein M, et al. Lifetime prevalence of mental disorders in U.S. adolescents: results from the National Comorbidity Survey Replication--Adolescent Supplement (NCS-A). *J Am Acad Child Adolesc Psychiatry.* 2010 Oct;49(10):980–989.
11. Elsevier/Gold Standard: *Clinical pharmacology* [database online]. https://www.clinicalpharmacology.com/.
12. Wolters Kluwer Health: *Lexicomp online* [database online]. https://online.lexi.com/.
13. Hasin DS, Sarvet AL, Meyers JL, et al. Epidemiology of Adult DSM-5 Major Depressive Disorder and Its Specifiers in the United States. *JAMA Psychiatry.* 2018;75(4):336–346.
14. VandenBerg AM. Major depressive disorder. In: DiPiro JT, ed. *Pharmacotherapy: A Pathophysiologic Approach.* ed 11 New York: McGraw-Hill Education; 2020.
15. Offson M, Marcus S. National patterns in antidepressant medication treatment. *Arch Gen Psychiatry.* 2009;66:848–856.
16. Trivedi M, Maurizio F, Wisniewski S, et al. Medication augmentation after the failure of SSRIs for depression. *N Engl J Med.* 2006;354:1243–1252.
17. Muskens E, Eveleigh R, Lucassen P, et al. Prescribing antidepressants appropriately (PANDA): a cluster randomized controlled trial in primary care. *BMC Family Practice.* 2013;14:6.
18. Tanda G, Carboni E, Frau R, et al. Increase of extracellular dopamine in the prefrontal cortex: a trait of drug with antidepressant potential? *Psychopharmacology (Berl).* 1994;115: 285–288.
19. Bostwick JM, Jaffee MS. Buspirone as an antidote to SSRI-induced bruxism in 4 cases. *J Clin Psychiatry.* 1999;60:857–860.

20. Yagiela JA, Duffin SR, Hunt LM. Drug interactions and vasoconstrictors used in local anesthetic solutions. *Oral Surg Oral Med Oral Pathol Oral Radiol Endod*. 1985;59:565–571.

21. Malamed SF. *Handbook of Local Anesthesia, ed 6. St. Louis.* : Mosby; 2012.

22. Drayton SJ, Fields CS. Bipolar disorder. In: DiPiro JT, ed. *Pharmacotherapy: A Pathophysiologic Approach*. ed 11 New York: McGraw-Hill Education; 2020.

23. National Institute of Mental Health: Schizophrenia, NIH publication 09-3517, 2009.

24. Perälä J, Suvisaari J, Saarni SI, et al. Lifetime Prevalence of Psychotic and Bipolar I Disorders in a General Population. *Arch Gen Psychiatry*. 2007;64(1):19–28.

25. Crismon ML, Smith T, Buckley PF. Schizophrenia. In: DiPiro JT, ed. *Pharmacotherapy: A Pathophysiologic Approach*. ed 11 New York: McGraw-Hill Education; 2020.

26. Suganya K, Koo BS. Gut-brain axis: role of gut microbiota on neurological disorders and how probiotics/prebiotics beneficially modulate microbial and immune pathways to improve brain functions. *Int. J. Mol Sci*. 2020;21:7551.

27. McCann K.: Assessment and management of dental patients with mental health issues. http://www.oralhealthgroup.com/news/.

28. March JS, Foa E, Gammon P, et al. *Cognitive Therapy for Obsessive-Compulsive Disorder: A Guide for Professionals*. Oakland CA: New Harbinger Publications; 2006.

29. March JS, et al. Cognitive-behavior therapy, sertraline, and their combination for children and adolescents with obsessive-compulsive disorder. *JAMA*. 2004;292:1969–1976.

30. National Institute of Mental Health: Post-traumatic stress disorder (PTSD), NIH publication 08-6388, 2008.

31. Friedlander A, Friedlander I, Marder S. Posttraumatic stress disorder: Psychopathology, medical management and dental implications. *Oral Surg Oral Med Oral Pathol Oral Radiol Endod*. 2004;97:5–11.

32. Wright E, Thompson R, Paunovich E. Post-traumatic stress disorder: Considerations for dentistry. *Quintessence Int*. 2004;35: 206–210.

33. Botko G. Post-traumatic stress disorder. Understanding and treating patients with PTSD. *AGD Impact*. December 2013:24–27.

34. Dopheide JA, Stutzmann DL, Pliszka SR. Attention deficit/ hyperactivity disorder. In: DiPiro JT, ed. *Pharmacotherapy: A Pathophysiologic Approach*. ed 11 New York: McGraw-Hill Education; 2020.

35. Broadbent JM, Ayers KM, Thomson WM. Is attention-deficit hyperactivity disorder a risk factor for dental caries? A case-control study. *Caries Res*. 2004 Jan-Feb;38(1):29–33.

36. Tenzer JA, Orozco H. Traumatic glossectomy: report of two cases. *Oral Surg Oral Med Oral Pathol*. 1970;30:182–184.

37. Altom RL, DiAngelis AJ. Multiple autoextractions: oral self-mutilation reviewed. *Oral Surg Oral Med Oral Pathol*. 1989;67: 271–274.

38. Kaidonis J, Townsend G. The 'sialo–microbial– dental complex' in oral health and disease. *Ann Anat - Anat Anz*. 2016;203:85–89.

39. Kisely S. No Mental Health without Oral Health. *Can J Psychiatry*. 2016;61(5):277–282.

40. Heaton LJ, Swigart K, McNelis G, Milgrom P, Downing DF. Oral health in patients taking psychotropic medications: Results from a pharmacy-based pilot study. *J Am Pharm Assoc (2003)*. 2016;56(4):412–417. e1.

41. Novy B, Kennedy E, Donahoe J, Fournier S. Minimizing aerosols with non-surgical approaches to caries management. *Journal of the Michigan Dental Association*. July 2020:48–56.

17

Adolescent Patients

Lorne D. Koroluk, and Tate H. Jackson

 Visit eBooks.Health.Elsevier.com

OUTLINE

Before reaching adulthood, every individual passes through the stages of infancy, childhood, and adolescence. **Adolescence** is the developmental period between childhood and adulthood and is characterized by major physical, psychological, and social changes. Adolescence begins at the onset of puberty, a well-defined physiologic milestone that occurs as a result of increased levels of various hormones and results in significant physical growth and the development of secondary sexual characteristics. The timing of the initiation and completion of adolescence is highly variable among individuals. Humans have a prolonged adolescent development in which the conclusion is not defined by physiologic milestones, but rather by less clear-cut sociologic parameters that may vary widely among different cultures and societies.

THE ADOLESCENT IN THE WORLD

An adolescent must achieve several emotional or developmental milestones before becoming a psychologically normal functioning adult (Box 17.1). Erikson's psychosocial theory of development describes the identity crisis as the major event of adolescence. During this phase, adolescents must discover who they are and develop a unique identity, separate from family and other adults. According to this theory, the attainment of a realistic self-identity is a milestone for the passage into adulthood.

Stages of Adolescence

The psychosocial development of the adolescent can be divided into three distinct phases: early, middle, and late adolescence. During early adolescence, childhood roles are cast aside and dependent emotional ties with the family severed. In Western culture, the first signs of independence may occur when an adolescent becomes less involved and less interested in long-standing family activities and routines. It is common at this stage for an adolescent to bristle and become resistant when criticized or given unsolicited advice by adults or other authority figures. Within a short period, the once-obedient child may become rebellious and belligerent, heightening tensions and anxiety within the family. At times, an adolescent may be fearful of relinquishing the security of childhood and, when stressed, may revert to childlike behavior. To ease the transition into the early phase of adolescence, parents and other adults must recognize this assertion of independence as a part of normal development and, when possible, allow the teenager some degree of freedom of choice.

During the middle phase of adolescence, the teenager begins to seek a new identity through peer group involvement. New emotional ties with the peer group fill the psychological void left by the abandonment of childhood dependence on parents. Participation in peer group activities reinforces the sense of separation from parents and facilitates emotional separation

BOX 17.1   Adolescent Milestones

- A realistic, stable, positive adult self-identity must be established.
- The adolescent must become emancipated from parents and other adults (often leading to the classic dependence-independence struggles that occur between adolescents and their parents).
- Skills for future economic independence must be acquired. During adolescence, much time is spent developing the skills and talents that will guide individual career and vocational plans.
- Psychosexual differentiation must occur, enabling function in adult sexual roles. Once the adolescent develops a stable self-identity with which they are confident, mature intimate relationships with other adults can be entered into without the fear of losing self-identity.

TABLE 17.1   US Population Trends

Year	Age Group (Years)	Total Population (%)
2020	14–17	5.03
	65 and older	18.84
2040	14–17	4.67
	65 and older	25.55
2060	14–17	4.43
	65 and older	28.26

Adapted from US Bureau of the Census: 2012 National Population Projections: Summary Tables. https://www.census.gov/data/tables/2017/demo/popproj/2017-summary-tables.html.

from them. Adolescent groups may adopt outlandish clothes, hairstyles, piercings, tattoos, speech patterns, or other behaviors to differentiate themselves clearly from their parents and other adults. Paradoxically, peer groups discourage individuality and the development of self-identity. Adolescents must either conform to the ways of the peer group or cease to be a member. At this stage, however, adolescents are not seeking a distinct identity but rather a *stable* one. Interpersonal relationships in the peer group are often superficial and individual identity is highly compromised by pressures to conform to group standards. At the conclusion of middle adolescence, peer groups dissolve as individuality and self-identity increase. An adolescent with no friends, or poor peer group ties, may experience problems in facilitating the development of self-identity and independence.

In late adolescence, physical ties with the family are severed as the adolescent moves out of the home, becomes financially more self-sufficient, and accepts adult roles and responsibilities. With the eventual attainment of a stable self-identity and independence, the young adult accepts mature relationships with other adults without experiencing fear of losing control of their self-identity. Problems in these relationships may occur when an individual seeks to maintain peer group ties and/or family dependence.

Although these stages describe adolescent development in most North American and European families, considerable variation in the sequence may exist in other areas of the world. In many cultures, extended multigenerational families living together are the cultural norm. In some cultures, the passage into adulthood is clearly defined by a ritual passage or event. Once the adolescent has demonstrated completion of the rite of passage, acceptance as an adult member of the society occurs.

Adolescent Population

Adolescents are a significant proportion of the US population. According to US Census Bureau estimates, in 2019 there were 41,852,838 young people aged 10–19 years in the United States, 13% of the total US population.[1] Between 2016 and 2050, the total number of 10- to 19-year-olds is projected to increase by 5.2% and the number of 60- to 79-year-olds will increase by 35.5%.[2] These projections are based on the expectation of a relatively stable birth rate and an increased life expectancy,

resulting in an increased number of persons older than 65 years of age (Table 17.1). As a result, the size of the adolescent population will remain relatively stable, but as more people live longer, the proportion of the total population who are adolescents will become smaller.

The United Nations Population Division estimates that the percentage of 10- to 19-year-olds in the world population based on a medium fertility rate will decline from 16.1% in 2020 to 11.9% in 2100.[3] In developing nations, because of higher birth rates and shorter life expectancy, a larger proportion of the population is composed of children and adolescents. The United Nations estimates that 21.9% of the population of the least-developed countries in the world will be comprised of 10- to 19-year-olds in 2025 and will decline to 14.2% by 2100. These estimates are based primarily on the increased life expectancy in these countries because of global health initiatives and medical innovations.

LIFESTYLE ISSUES THAT MAY AFFECT ADOLESCENT HEALTH

Diet and Nutrition

Significant physical growth occurs during the pubertal growth spurt. The age at which this spurt occurs varies among individuals. As a general rule, females tend to begin puberty and the growth spurt at a younger age than males. Proper nutrition is essential to ensure adequate development during this period and to maximize genetically determined growth potential. In response to rapid growth, total caloric intake may be increased significantly. Although a nutritionally balanced diet is important, teenagers may develop poor nutritional habits by filling the increased demand for calories with a diet high in refined carbohydrates, fats, and salt. Peer group pressures may influence the type of diet an adolescent maintains. Increased social, academic, and leisure demands also may limit the amount of time a teenager has available to eat well-balanced meals in a home environment.

At-Risk Behaviors

Rejection of adult authority may cause some adolescents to show reduced interest in or abandon both oral and general preventive health practices. Pressures from peer groups may encourage teenagers to take risks, such as experimenting with tobacco, alcohol, or drugs. Peer pressures to engage in dangerous risk-taking activities with automobiles, motorcycles, off-road vehicles, bicycles, or skateboards may lead to physical injury. Traumatic brain injury is the leading cause of death and disability among adolescents in the United States.[4] Motor vehicle accidents, firearm injury, and opioid overdoses account for the majority of fatalities in adolescents and young adults in spite of recent injury prevention initiatives.[5]

Traumatic dental injuries are common in adolescents and risk factors include behavioral, environmental, and oral factors. Oral factors include increased overjet, incisor protrusion, and lip incompetence and environmental factors include socioeconomic status and unsafe environments.[6] Behavioral factors include risk taking, attention deficit/hyperactivity disorder and executive function disorder which entails poor self-control and impulsivity.[7]

Tattoos and body piercing have gained popularity among adolescents as a way of demonstrating independence and separation from the adult population. The jewelry associated with a pierced tongue or lip may cause damage to teeth or create a source of intraoral infection. Some individuals may also go to extremes to modify the shape or appearance of the maxillary incisors. Radical changes in the shape of the incisors or the insertion of oversized poorly contoured metal crowns may increase the risk of periodontal disease and caries.

Mental Health Issues

During adolescence most individuals struggle to find their own identity and their place in the world. The extensive exposure to social media has shifted standards of physical development and behavior away from traditional family- and community-based norms to much broader expectations and aspirations that may be unrealistic and in some cases destructive. For many teens this leads to a sense of isolation, deep feelings of inadequacy, and lack of self-worth. Mental health issues commonly seen in adolescents include anxiety, body (and/or dentofacial) dysmorphia, depression, and suicide.[8]

In 2020, the National Institute for Mental Health [https://www.nimh.nih.gov/Statistics/MajorDepression/Prevalenceof MajorDepressiveEpisodeAmongAdolescents] reported that an estimated 4.1 million adolescents aged 12 to 17 years had at least one major depressive episode; this represented 17.0% of that population. The prevalence was higher in females and highest in adolescents reporting two or more races. The 2019 Youth Risk Behaviors Survey [CDC-2019-ncvc.dspacedirect.org] revealed that 8.9% of US youths in grades 9–12 reported that they had made at least one suicide attempt in the last 12 months and female students attempted suicide almost twice as often as male students. In 2020, the World Health Organization [https://www.who.int] reported that, globally, depression is one of the leading causes of illness and disability among adolescents and, worldwide, suicide is the fourth leading cause of death in 15- to 19-year-olds.

During treatment, dentists may identify adolescents who are exhibiting signs of nonsuicidal self-injury (NSSI), which is

defined as the self-inflicted damage to the surface of the body without suicidal intention. Commonly, NSSI presents as cutting, scratching, carving, or scaping. The prevalence rate is 15%–20% in mid-adolescence and tends to decline toward late adolescence. Psychiatric disorders and suicide attempts are common comorbidities in a subset of adolescents with NSSI behaviors.[9]

Sexually Transmitted Disease and HPV

With the onset of puberty, many adolescents will become sexually active. When engaging in unprotected sex, teenagers will be vulnerable to developing sexually transmitted diseases (STDs). Although manifestations of syphilis or gonorrhea in the oral cavity are relatively rare, HPV infection has become more prevalent.[10] Because oral HPV infection, whether contracted via sexual activity or other means, can lead to the development of oral cancer, we have a professional responsibility to counsel our adolescent patients and their parents to have the adolescent vaccinated against HPV by the age of 11 or 12 years [https://www.cdc.gov>HPV].

Physical Abuse

Teens may find themselves living in an abusive home environment or while escaping an untenable home life, they may be in a vulnerable or unsafe living situation "on the street." In the presence of signs of abuse the dental team will need to manage and treat the effects of trauma to the head, face, or mouth, and to report the signs of abuse to appropriate authorities (see Chapter 7).

PATIENT ASSESSMENT

Confidentiality Issues

Practitioners must be aware that the relationship between a dentist and adolescent patients is confidential, although, as with adults, situations may arise in which a breach of that confidentiality is ethically justified, such as when the patient poses an obvious threat to others or to him or herself. The discovery of information through history taking or physical examination may place the practitioner in an ethical dilemma with respect to the issue of disclosure to parents or legal guardians. In addition, during treatment, the practitioner may gain information concerning sexually transmitted diseases, illicit drug use, pregnancy, or emotional disorders. In such situations, the dentist is not legally obligated to inform the parents or guardian of such findings. In some US states, the law allows adolescents to receive treatment without parental consent for conditions such as sexually transmitted diseases and drug addictions.

To avoid the development of difficult situations, at the initial appointment the practitioner can discuss these confidentiality issues with the adolescent and parents or guardian. The adolescent can be informed that findings will not be disclosed without their knowledge, but that it may be in their best interest to disclose certain kinds of information to their parents so that they can be supportive. The parents or guardian can then be advised that the practitioner is bound to respect the confidentiality of the dentist–patient relationship, unless an immediate direct threat to the well-being of the adolescent or others is present. If, in the judgment of the practitioner, the adolescent patient does become a threat to self or others and refuses to inform the parents or guardian, the practitioner must discuss the findings with the parents or guardian so that appropriate treatment or referral can be pursued.

If, at some point, disclosure of other confidential information would seem to be in the patient's best interest, the first step should be to discuss frankly with the patient the benefits of including the parents in planning for future treatment or referral. After this discussion, the adolescent should be encouraged to provide the information to their parents or guardian. The dentist can offer to be present when the patient discusses these issues with their parent.

Patient History

Although with pediatric dental patients, parents or guardians provide most if not all the information gathered during the health history, obtaining an accurate patient history for an adolescent requires the tactful involvement of both the parents or guardian and the adolescent. The parents or guardian can be asked to supply the majority of the historical recall of past medical history for an adolescent. Surprisingly, however, some pediatric and adolescent patients may have a more accurate recall of events than their parents, and therefore it is wise to have all parties present during the history taking.

With this age group, it is important that the chief concern be clearly stated by both the adolescent and the parents or guardian. Ideally, the adolescent can be asked to articulate the chief concern and treatment expectations in their own words at a time or location away from parents or guardian. A major discrepancy between the two versions may indicate differing expectations for treatment and treatment outcomes and, unless resolved, may lead to future conflicts between the parents or guardian, adolescent, and dentist.

The components of the patient history and process for obtaining the history in the adolescent patient are like those of the adult patient, and are described in detail in Chapter 1.

Clinical Examination

As the patient evaluation process transitions from history taking to the physical examination, the dentist will typically gather information about recent growth changes and physical signs of puberty. The adolescent is asked to describe recent physical growth changes and current height and weight can be plotted against normal growth curves or used to calculate an age and gender-adjusted body mass index (BMI) percentile to assess weight status.[11] The US Centers for Disease Control and Prevention defines an "overweight" child as having a BMI percentile between the 85th and 95th percentile, with a BMI percentile greater than the 95th percentile defined as "obese." Physical signs, such as voice changes, presence of facial hair, initiation of menstrual cycles, and breast development, can be used to evaluate whether puberty has begun or how advanced it is.

The physical examination process in the adolescent is similar to that for adult patients (see Chapter 1). Extraoral and intraoral examination of soft tissue is completed, along with an assessment of temporomandibular joint function and range of motion. The periodontal and dental examinations are identical to those used for adults except that, in the adolescent, examination may reveal the presence of newly erupted teeth. To screen for the presence of aggressive periodontitis, periodontal probing is important, especially on first molars and incisors, the most commonly involved sites.

A radiographic survey for an adolescent patient with age-appropriate dentition and no clinical signs of periodontal disease or need for extensive restorative treatment includes a panoramic radiograph plus bite-wings. The panoramic image can be used to assess third molar development as well as the presence of any unerupted teeth. Bite-wings should be taken at appropriate intervals in adolescents to assess the occurrence of proximal caries after posterior contacts have been established. During the transition period between the loss of primary teeth and the eruption of the permanent teeth in the posterior segments, bite-wing radiographs are unnecessary if no proximal contact exists.

Because most definitive orthodontics are completed in adolescence, general dentists should be well versed in assessing the need for such treatment in these patients. Visually evaluate the patient's anteroposterior and vertical skeletal relationships from the frontal and lateral positions. With the patient standing and looking forward, position the patient's head so that the Frankfort horizontal (line joining the external ear canal and infraorbital rim) is parallel to the floor. A vertical line dropped down from the nasal bridge (soft tissue nasion) can be used to assess maxillary and mandibular anteroposterior relationships (Figure 17.1). Discrepancies may indicate underlying skeletal disharmonies, which may require orthognathic

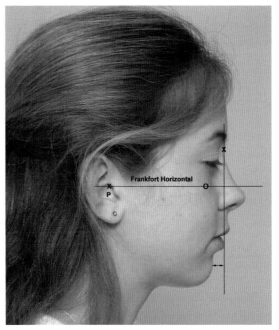

Fig. 17.1 Profile analysis using Frankfort horizontal and the anteroposterior relationship of the mandible and maxilla in relation to a vertical reference line through the bridge of the nose. *P,* porion; *O,* orbitale.

surgery plus orthodontics to improve facial esthetics. Vertical skeletal relationships may also be evaluated at the same time. The mandibular plane angle (normal: 30 degrees) can be estimated by the angle formed by the lower border of the bony mandible and Frankfort horizontal. Assess the symmetry of structures from the frontal view. The position of the chin button relative to the midsagittal plane can identify significant mandibular skeletal asymmetry, whereas observing the dental midlines relative to the midsagittal plane can indicate any dental arch asymmetry. If lip incompetence at rest is more than 4 mm, a significant vertical skeletal discrepancy may be present or the incisors may be excessively proclined to accommodate the teeth in the dental arch. In such cases, extractions or orthognathic surgery may be necessary to reduce lip incompetence and incisor or gingival display.

Evaluate the dental arches for any overretained primary teeth, which may signify impacted or congenitally missing permanent teeth. The most commonly impacted teeth are the maxillary canines and the mandibular second premolars.

Overjet and overbite should be assessed. Excessive overjet usually indicates an underlying Class II skeletal relationship, whereas a negative overjet indicates a Class III skeletal relationship. A deep bite may result in stripping of palatal attached gingiva around the maxillary incisors, compromising their periodontal status. An anterior open bite usually indicates a skeletal vertical discrepancy and may require orthognathic surgery to affect a permanent correction.

Dental occlusion is then assessed as part of the orthodontic examination. Class II or Class III canine and molar relationships may indicate a skeletal discrepancy. In adolescents, dental malocclusions with an underlying mild skeletal discrepancy can be treated with growth modification or **camouflage**. Growth modification uses various appliances, such as headgear, to differentially control mandibular and maxillary growth. Camouflage relies on the extraction of permanent teeth to correct the dental malocclusion while masking the underlying minor skeletal discrepancy. To be effective, growth modification treatment for Class II patients requires a period of active growth. In late adolescence, if minimal further growth can be anticipated, treatment options may be limited to orthognathic surgery or extractions to camouflage the underlying Class II skeletal relationships. Treatment of patients with Class III malocclusion caused by mandibular prognathism is usually delayed until skeletal growth is nearly complete. Because mandibular growth does not cease until late adolescence or early adulthood, patients may outgrow early treatment in the mixed or early permanent dentition. However, patients with Class III malocclusion caused by a retrognathic maxilla and well-positioned mandible may be treated in the mixed dentition or early permanent dentition with reverse pull headgear or bone anchor maxillary protraction with class III elastics.

A posterior cross-bite with a functional shift of the mandible is indicative of a skeletal or dental transverse discrepancy. The correction of transverse problems is more easily accomplished with maxillary expansion appliances in early adolescence, as the midpalatal suture is less organized and less interdigitated than it will become in late adolescence or adulthood. After the suture has fused in adulthood, surgery is usually required to correct significant transverse problems.

If skeletal or dental disharmonies exist, early adolescence or the late mixed dentition is usually an appropriate time to consider orthodontic referral and intervention. Whereas many general dentists may consider undertaking adjunctive or limited tooth movement orthodontic treatment, most will elect to refer patients with Class II or III dental and skeletal malocclusions or Class I malocclusions with severe tooth/arch discrepancies to an orthodontist. The orthodontic screening referral form (Figure 17.2) can be a helpful aid to the general dentist both in assessing the patient's orthodontic needs and in facilitating the referral to an orthodontist.

ORAL HEALTH PROBLEMS IN THE ADOLESCENT

Dental Erosion

Dental erosion is widespread in adolescents in the developed world, owing to the ubiquitous exposure to acidic foods, beverages, and condiments.[12] Common acidic substances for adolescents to ingest include sodas (carbonated soft drinks), both sugared and diet; energy drinks; sports drinks; citrus fruits and juices; ketchup; hot sauce; and other vinegar-based products. Wine can also be a contributing factor, as can (to a lesser extent) coffee.

Erosion causes loss of tooth enamel and tooth structure and it can contribute to both occlusal attrition and cervical notching. Some of the significant problems associated with dental erosion include discoloration of the teeth (as the enamel thins and dentin is exposed), tooth sensitivity, pulpal pathology, and, in severe cases, the need for extensive restorative work.

The role of the dental team in managing this condition is threefold: prevention, mitigation of the symptoms, and restoration of the tooth defects. Prevention entails a detailed dietary analysis (see *In Clinical Practice: Diet and Nutritional Counseling for Adolescents* box), discerning which frequent acid exposures the patient is exposed to and counseling the patient about how to minimize those exposures, especially between meals. Three simple recommendations are usually helpful in this regard:

- Minimize the frequency and duration of any between-meal acid exposures.
- Rinse with water immediately after any between-meal acid exposures.
- Refrain from brushing teeth for 30 minutes after a known acid exposure.

If the teeth become symptomatic, most commonly becoming sensitive to cold, the dentist can usually provide relief with the application of fluoride varnish, Gluma, or other desensitizing product while the patient is in the dental office. Often, the use of a desensitizing dentifrice on a daily basis as part of the oral self-care regimen is beneficial.

A restoration may be needed if cervical notching becomes unsightly to the patient, persistent sensitivity cannot be resolved with conservative means, or pulpal pathology or tooth fracture are thought to be imminent.

Orthodontic Screening Referral Form

Patient Name: _____

Parent/Guardian Name: _____

Address: _____

_____

Phone: Daytime: _____ **Evenings:** _____

Date of Birth: _____

To be lled out by the referring dentist:

This patient has been in my (our) practice since: _____

Date of last examination: _____

Decay currently present: Yes: _____ **No:** _____

If yes, is restorative treatment scheduled: Yes: _____ No: _____

Oral hygiene status: Excellent: _____ Good: _____ Fair: _____ Poor: _____

Periodontal status: _____

	Right	Left

Molar Relationship (I, II, III) _____ _____

Canine Relationship (I, II, III) _____ _____

Overjet _____ mm

Overbite _____ mm

Estimated Crowding: Upper Arch _____ mm, Lower Arch _____ mm

Missing Permanent Teeth: Yes _____ No _____

If yes, which teeth are missing: _____

What are your main concerns for treatment: _____

_____

_____

Name of Referring Dentist: _____

Address of Referring Dentist: _____

Office Phone Number: _____

Dentist Signature: _____ Date: _____

Fig. 17.2 Orthodontic screening referral form.

Diet and Nutritional Counseling for Adolescents

The prevalence of overweight and obese teenagers in the United States has dramatically increased over the past few decades. A recent study of adolescents seen for orthodontic treatment found that 12% were judged to be obese, whereas 18% were categorized as at least overweight.[13] This trend appears to become established early, as a study in a similar population of 6- to 9-year-old children seen for a new patient dental examination found 13% to be obese and 15% to be at least overweight.[14] Overweight and obese children and adolescents are more likely to become overweight or obese adults who will be at risk for the development of such serious health conditions as cardiovascular disease, type 2 diabetes, hypertension, orthopedic problems, and sleep apnea.[15] Owing to demanding academic, sports, and social schedules, teenagers may develop poor dietary habits and be unaware of the potential hazards. Teenagers with weight, caries, or periodontal issues will benefit from dietary analysis and nutritional counseling.

Dietary Analysis

Ask the adolescent to keep a record of all food consumed during a 3- to 7-day period, including when and how much. Compare the number of food group servings consumed per day with the recommendations shown in this box. In particular, observe the extent of exposure to fermentable carbohydrates (sugars and sweets) and acids (citrus fruits and carbonated or other low pH beverages) with respect to the form (solution versus solid), time of ingestion (during meal, end of meal, or between meals), and length of exposure. Adolescents and their parents should be advised that minimizing exposure to fermentable carbohydrates, especially between meals, reduces acid production by cariogenic bacteria. Compliance and accuracy of diet records may be a problem, however, in adolescents who are not interested in the process.

Nutritional Goals

The recommended daily servings of each food group are as follows:
Milk group: 2 to 4 servings
Meat group: 2 to 3 servings
Vegetable group: 3 to 5 servings
Fruit group: 2 to 4 servings
Grain group: 6 to 11 servings

The total recommended caloric intake for adolescent boys and girls is 2200 to 2800 calories per day. Because of increased calcium demand, adolescents should receive three or four servings of milk per day, depending on the total caloric intake.

Affecting Change

Helping a patient to make behavioral changes, such as altering their diet, can be a challenging undertaking. But when effective strategies are purposefully engaged, the chances of success are good. Modifying the diet for an adolescent is more complex, because the dental team must take into account that meals are often prepared by a parent or other family member, many meals may be consumed away from the home setting, and there may be minimal time allowed for meal preparation. Many adolescents have virtually unlimited access to snack foods and beverages throughout the day. Any recommended change must be made in the context of what is appropriate for the patient's culture, religion, and family setting. Often, an effective beginning point is a straightforward conversation with the patient (and family member or other person who is the primary meal preparer) about perceptions of the benefit to be derived by the proposed change. This conversation must be open, candid, and tailored to the patient's and/or food preparer's education level and life experience. An important companion question is to ask, "What is the likelihood (on a scale of 0 to 10) that you will be able to carry out the desired diet changes?" Again, if the response suggests a low likelihood, further candid discussion about the barriers to change should take place. Often,

it is helpful to set small, realistic goals for change, followed by sequential reinforcement of the progress and ratcheting upward to higher and more difficult-to-achieve goals. The patient needs to be a partner in this process of goal setting and their efforts should be reaffirmed at each stage. Through this process, the adolescent can and should accept ownership of their own dietary choices and the consequences of those choices. As the adolescent experiences and comes to value the benefits of the change, it is more likely that the new pattern will become internalized and continue in the months and years to come.

Dental Caries

Although dental caries have declined significantly in the adolescent population in the United States during the past two decades, some individuals continue to be susceptible. It is expected that the incidence of dental caries will increase in many developing countries as a result of an increase in the consumption of sugars and inadequate exposure to fluorides.[16] Although many adolescents present with no caries or with only isolated pit and fissure caries, some individuals will have rampant caries and will be at high risk of new lesions. This latter group can be a major treatment challenge.

Several explanations for adolescent caries risk can be identified. With the eruption of the permanent premolars and the permanent second molars, the number of susceptible occlusal and proximal tooth surfaces exposed to the oral environment increases. The crystalline structure and surface characteristics of these newly erupted teeth make them more susceptible both to the initiation of caries and to the rapid advancement of the lesions once formed. The fact that adolescents often consume cariogenic diets and may maintain less-than-adequate oral hygiene increases the risk of caries.[17]

Adequate plaque control is essential to the maintenance of good oral health. Effective oral self-care has the dual benefit of creating an environment that is less conducive to the formation of carious lesions and more favorable to the maintenance of optimum periodontal health. Oral health instruction must be provided in a tactful manner that the adolescent patient will readily accept and implement. Just as important, the patient must perceive the information to be relevant. The importance of good oral self-care can be emphasized through discussion of the microbiologic basis of dental caries and periodontal disease. Informing the patient about the possible sequelae of poor oral home care—including halitosis, painful teeth or gums, and unattractive or missing teeth—will reinforce the perception of the value of good oral self-care.

Traditionally oral hygiene instruction occurs through one-on-one communication in the dental office. Now patients can easily access healthcare information through the Internet via Facebook, Twitter and You Tube. In 2016, 85% of surveyed individuals in the United Kingdom accessed You Tube. Another UK study found that a substantial number of You Tube sites related to oral hygiene were produced by lay people without professional qualifications and lacked evidence-based material. Dentists should be cautious when recommending on-line resources for oral hygiene instruction and carefully assess all content before making recommendations to patients.[18]

For a patient with a high caries rate history who is at risk of developing new lesions, the dentist may recommend a diet analysis. The cooperation of the parents and adolescent may be needed to obtain an accurate representation of dietary intake (see the box *In Clinical Practice: Diet and Nutritional Counseling for Adolescents*). If, after obtaining the diet history, it is determined that changes are needed, it is often necessary to counsel the parents and the adolescent to effect those changes.

Interim protective direct-fill restorations can be a valuable tool in the overall management of an active caries problem. By excavating gross caries and placing interim restorations, the dentist can help arrest the caries process, creating an environment in which a preventive program can be effective. Before placing any definitive indirect restorations, adequate oral self-care, diet control, and fluoride use must be established. If such an approach is not followed, in the near future the dentist will see an older adolescent or young adult returning with multiple recurrent and new lesions (see the *In Clinical Practice: Management of Adolescents With High Caries Rates* box).

IN CLINICAL PRACTICE

Management of Adolescents With High Caries Rates

Multiple existing restorations and/or new or recurrent carious lesions are markers of adolescents who are at risk for the development of future caries. Caries development on the proximal surfaces of lower incisors or the cervical areas of the facial and lingual surfaces indicates elevated risk. Individuals who continue to develop multiple new carious lesions between periodic visits should also be classified as high risk. The chronically ill or immune-compromised patient may develop increased significant caries risk as a result of the underlying systemic condition or therapy. An in-depth preventive program to control the caries process is an essential element in the treatment of the high-risk individual. The program must include all the elements described in the following paragraphs.

Diet analysis and counseling: Initially, the patient needs to be queried about sugar and acid exposures. If there is suspicion by the dental team that the patient is at elevated risk for dental caries or erosion, and that the diet is a contributing cause, it is appropriate to do a formal diet analysis. The findings from that analysis will become the basis for counseling the patient about their diet and making recommendations for change.

Oral self-care improvement: Adequate plaque control measures must be instituted and maintained to reduce caries susceptibility. Proper, timely brushing and flossing are essential elements of any oral self-care regimen.

Fluoride use: Both professionally applied and self-applied topical fluoride can be helpful in preventing the development of new lesions and encouraging remineralization of decalcified surfaces. Daily rinses or self-applied gels in custom trays may be warranted.

Restoration of all active lesions: Active lesions should be excavated and provisional or definitive direct-fill restorations placed to stop the progression of caries. Reinforced zinc oxide eugenol (IRM) or glass-ionomer cements can be used effectively in these cases to stop the site-specific caries process. Restoration of lesions without an intensive preventive program will almost certainly result in new and recurrent carious lesions and treatment failure. (For additional management considerations, see Chapter 10.)

Periodontal Diseases

Adolescents are at risk of developing gingival and periodontal diseases. Identifiable risk indicators or risk factors for loss of periodontal support include gingival bleeding, calculus, abundance of certain microbiota, decreased immune response or immune deficiencies, diabetes, and tobacco use.[19] Many periodontal problems, such as puberty-associated gingivitis, aggressive periodontitis (currently known as periodontitis Stage III or IV, Grade C), necrotizing ulcerative gingivitis (NUG), and pericoronitis, are more prevalent during adolescence. Most 14- to 17-year-olds in the United States have gingivitis, usually affecting the soft tissue supporting the maxillary molars and the mandibular incisors. The prevalence of gingivitis during adolescence is slightly higher in females than in males[20] and tends to decline with increasing age. Supragingival calculus is found on the maxillary molars and the mandibular canines in approximately one-fourth to one-third of adolescents. Gingival bleeding and periodontal pocketing are also prevalent in teenagers. When periodontal attachment loss occurs in the adolescent, it most often affects the maxillary molars and premolars, with the mandibular molars and canines the next-most-likely teeth to be involved.[21]

Proper sequencing of periodontal treatment is essential to ensure optimal periodontal health in adolescents. Initial periodontal therapy (see Chapter 10) should emphasize conservative measures, including the institution and maintenance of good oral self-care and reduction of the detrimental microbiota. Hopelessly involved teeth that can compromise adjacent healthy teeth should be extracted in the disease control phase. It is essential that periodontal disease be managed effectively before the initiation of comprehensive orthodontic treatment or definitive indirect restorative procedures.

After initial therapy, patients should be reevaluated to determine whether additional periodontal therapy would be beneficial or necessary (see *Periodontal Reevaluation* section in Chapter 10). Patients with more severe periodontitis may require surgical intervention to eliminate unresolved active disease and/or establish a state of periodontal health. Patients with minimal attached gingiva may be at risk for further loss of attachment resulting from the combined effects of orthodontic treatment and poor oral hygiene practices. Gingival grafting may be necessary in areas of insufficiently attached gingiva.

Puberty-Associated Gingivitis

The increase in gingival inflammation that occurs during puberty has been called **puberty-associated gingivitis** and is a generalized form of gingivitis characterized by inflamed, enlarged gingival papillae that are susceptible to bleeding (Figure 17.3). Clinical findings are typically more profound than would normally be expected based on the magnitude of existing local factors, such as plaque, calculus, or caries. The **bleeding index**, a measure of sites with gingival bleeding during periodontal probing, has been shown to increase significantly at the onset of puberty and to decrease after the age of 14 years in both males and females. Both the papillary bleeding index and the percentage of interdental sites with bleeding have been found to correlate with the development of secondary sexual characteristics.[22] Increased levels of sex hormones may lead to the development of an aggravated form of gingivitis, with increased inflammatory response and altered microbiology.[23,24]

Treatment of puberty-associated gingivitis involves the removal of any local irritants, such as plaque or calculus. The level of gingival inflammation can be reduced with normal oral hygiene procedures, such as tooth brushing and flossing. In some patients, however, inflammation may persist even with meticulous oral hygiene. The presence of orthodontic appliances may complicate the maintenance of adequate oral self-care and increase the risk of puberty-associated gingivitis. Fortunately, the process is usually self-limiting and does not cause permanent damage to the periodontium. The use of topical or systemic antibiotics usually is not indicated.

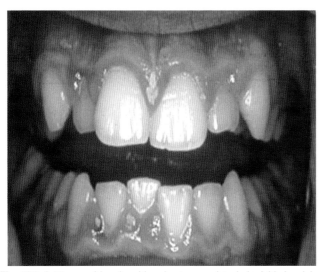

Fig. 17.3 A 14-year-old male with puberty-associated gingivitis involving the maxillary and mandibular incisors. (Courtesy Dr. M. Roberts, Chapel Hill, NC)

Eruption Gingivitis

Gingival inflammation and enlargement are common with the emergence of the early permanent dentition around 6 to 7 years of age and young adolescents may develop **eruption gingivitis** during emergence of the premolars and permanent second molars. Because the gingival margins receive no protection from the coronal contours of partially erupted teeth, food impingement on the gingiva can cause a localized inflammation of the tissue. Animal studies have confirmed that plaque accumulation at the newly formed gingival margins is responsible for leukocyte infiltration and the changes in vascular morphology associated with gingivitis.[25] Once the permanent tooth has fully erupted and plaque control measures are instituted, eruption gingivitis usually resolves without intervention.

Periodontitis

The terms periodontosis, juvenile periodontitis, early-onset periodontitis, and, more recently, **aggressive periodontitis**[26] have been used to characterize rapid attachment loss and bone destruction in otherwise clinically healthy adolescents and young adults (Figure 17.4). This condition is commonly associated with an abnormal host response and/or a highly virulent periodontal microbiota and can occur even in the presence of good oral hygiene. Bone/attachment loss commonly occurs in one of two patterns: (1) a localized form, involving the permanent first molars and incisors, or (2) a generalized form, in which the entire dentition may be affected.

Based on contemporary knowledge, a recent consensus workgroup consolidated the various forms of periodontitis (eliminating aggressive periodontitis) and developed a periodontitis classification system utilizing *stages* and *grades* for all forms of the disease. The *stages* define severity using

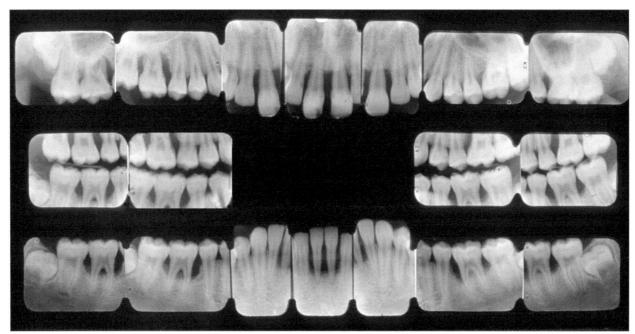

Fig. 17.4 Intraoral radiographs of an adolescent patient with **aggressive** with ***Stage III Grade C*** periodontitis showing vertical bone loss in the molar and incisor regions. (Courtesy Dr. John Moriarty, Cary, NC)

interproximal attachment loss, radiographic bone loss, and tooth loss while *grading* reflects the rate of disease progression (risk assessment) and anticipated responsiveness to therapy (prognosis). The majority of these patients will likely have stages of III or IV, but this assignment will largely depend on the timing of disease detection. Most patients will be given a grade of C to reflect their rapid rate of disease progression.[27] All forms of periodontitis require the challenge of a pathogenic microbiota and an immune response from a susceptible host leading to tissue destruction. The same is true in periodontal diseases that affect adolescents and young adults, but these patients tend to have the following:

- a more virulent microbiota (such as *Aggregatibacter actinomycetemcomitans*),[28]
- a stronger genetic predisposition influencing the host immune response at the level of connective tissue/bone metabolism,[29] and
- the presence of various syndromes (e.g. congenital or cyclic neutropenia, Down syndrome, etc.) that negatively influence the host immune response or the susceptibility of periodontal tissues to breakdown.[30,31]

The strong influence of genetic factors on the host immune response result in familial clustering being common in these forms of the disease.[32]

In the past, this disorder was thought to affect females more than males, but more recent epidemiologic studies across the globe have challenged this theory. Older adolescent and young adults are more commonly affected compared with younger adolescents. Although forms of this disease are quite rare (typically less than 1% of the global population), certain forms of the disease disproportionately affect different racial/ethnic groups, with patients of African or Middle Eastern descent having a 10-fold higher rate of disease prevalence.[33,34]

Treatment is aimed at stopping disease progression by eliminating the pathogenic bacteria and reducing periodontal inflammation. As with other standard periodontitis treatment protocols, initial therapy begins with the establishment of good oral self-care. A regimen of scaling and root planing with concomitant administration of systemic antibiotics (most commonly amoxicillin and metronidazole) has been most successful in treating these patients.[35] Surgical treatment is frequently required and is aimed at reducing probing depths and, when possible, regenerating lost periodontal tissues through the use of various biomaterials. The prompt referral of a patient with this form of disease to a periodontist is strongly encouraged to ensure proper evaluation and management of these complex cases.

Necrotizing Periodontal Disease

Necrotizing Ulcerative Gingivitis (NUG)/Necrotizing Ulcerative Periodontitis (NUP), previously termed acute necrotizing ulcerative gingivitis, can be found in adolescents and young adults. Along with this age predilection, several classic risk factors can be cited, including low socioeconomic status, poor nutrition, poor oral hygiene, preexisting marginal gingivitis, cigarette smoking, and increased psychosocial stress. Temporarily immunocompromised patients with viral infections such as herpes, measles, chickenpox, and febrile illness

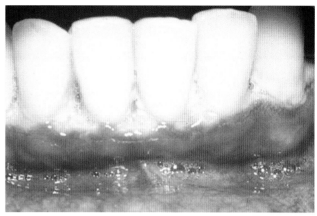

Fig. 17.5 Adolescent with necrotizing ulcerative gingivitis showing gingival enlargement with pseudomembrane. (Courtesy Dr. J. Moriarty, Chapel Hill, NC)

may be affected. Commonly, college students at examination time and new military recruits are sometimes afflicted. Signs and symptoms may include fever and malaise, accompanied by a loss of appetite. Gingival tissues are inflamed, enlarged, and painful, and bleed easily. The interproximal gingiva tends to be more involved than other soft tissue areas and may show signs of necrosis and ulceration. The tips of the papillae are often missing or blunted and may be covered with a gray pseudomembrane (Figure 17.5). The necrotic tissue results in a fetid odor from the oral cavity. Plaque from these patients often contains large numbers of spirochetes and fusiform bacteria. An association between the disorder and a generalized viral infection, specifically cytomegalovirus, has also been proposed.[36]

Treatment includes removal of plaque and calculus and local debridement of the diseased tissues using hand or ultrasonic instrumentation. Significant resolution is usually seen after the initial local therapy. Penicillin, metronidazole, and/or chlorhexidine rinses are effective in severe cases when the patient is debilitated.

Eliminating predisposing factors, such as poor nutrition, smoking, or stress and establishing good oral self-care practices shortens the clinical course of NUG. When gingival health has been restored, corrective periodontal procedures, such as a gingivectomy, may be required to reestablish normal gingival contours.[37,38]

Pericoronitis

Pericoronitis is a localized inflammation of the tissue surrounding an erupting tooth (Figure 17.6). As the tooth erupts, an operculum of tissue overlaying the distal portion of the occlusal surface may form. The operculum becomes inflamed, enlarged, and painful because of the accumulation of debris and microorganisms under the tissue. Trauma caused by mastication can lead to further irritation of the sensitive tissues. During adolescence, the most commonly involved teeth tend to be the mandibular third molars, but occasionally mandibular second molars are involved. Typically, patients present with localized tenderness of the surrounding tissue and some degree of trismus. More severely affected patients are febrile and show signs

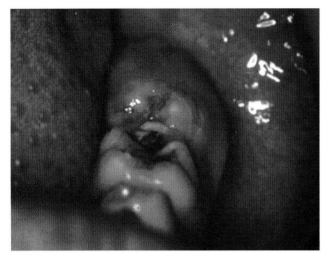

Fig. 17.6 Pericoronitis associated with an erupting mandibular molar. (Courtesy Dr. M. Roberts, Chapel Hill, NC)

of facial cellulitis. Treatment depends on the degree of involvement and clinical signs and symptoms. Local measures, such as analgesics and irrigation of the involved tissue, are usually effective in reducing symptoms. In some cases, an operculectomy on the involved tooth, or extraction of an opposing tooth, may provide moderate to long-term relief. In more involved cases with signs of overt infection of the soft tissues, antibiotics may be recommended. When symptoms subside, extraction of partially erupted or impacted third molars may be indicated to prevent recurrence.

Malocclusion

Malocclusion is seen in many adolescents. A large-scale survey in the United States found that approximately 15% of subjects had severe malocclusion that could affect social acceptability or function.[39] Most comprehensive orthodontic treatment is carried out during adolescence. With the eruption of the permanent canines and premolars, dental crowding becomes more evident. Significant maxillary crowding may lead to labial eruption of the canines into highly visible and unesthetic positions. During this period, adolescents and parents become more aware of esthetics and self-image. Skeletal discrepancies may become more obvious as a result of accelerated growth. Excessive mandibular or vertical growth may accentuate existing relationships, such as mandibular prognathism or excessive facial height. Comprehensive orthodontic treatment that relies on growth modification procedures must be carried out during a phase of active growth.

The desire on the part of the patient (and the family unit) to treat a malocclusion can vary greatly and is dependent on cultural and societal norms. Malocclusions rarely result in functional issues that interfere with speech or mastication, whereas esthetics and self-image usually influence the decision to pursue treatment. The cost of treatment may preclude treatment for some adolescents with significant malocclusions, whereas more economically advantaged teens with minor treatment needs obtain treatment owing to peer pressure and the perception in some cultures that orthodontic treatment in adolescence is a necessity.

Without proper patient cooperation, comprehensive orthodontics is destined to fail. Meticulous oral self-care and plaque control are essential to prevent the decalcification of tooth surfaces and development of periodontal problems. Lack of compliance with the use of extraoral and intraoral appliances may compromise the final treatment result. The necessary degree of cooperation may be difficult to achieve, particularly in early adolescence, when parent-teen confrontations are common. Practitioners must persuade the teenager to appreciate the benefits of treatment and accept responsibility for daily oral self-care and the maintenance of appliances. Offering some degree of participation in the treatment planning and some control in the direction of treatment can encourage this. An autocratic approach by the practitioner is often met with resistance by the patient and is more likely to fail.

Dentofacial Trauma

Adolescents typically engage in an active lifestyle and are prone to facial trauma from team sports, independent activities such as skateboarding or 4-wheeling; motor vehicle accidents while driving (or riding with a driver who is) impaired; or aggravated physical confrontations. As a result they may suffer facial lacerations or contusions; fractured jaws or condyles; avulsed, displaced or fractured teeth. It is incumbent on the dental team to assess, diagnose, and manage all such injuries. Treatment may range from a composite repair of a simple tooth fracture to referral to an oral and maxillofacial surgeon to reposition and stabilize a fractured and displaced jawbone. Other services the dental team may be called upon to provide include debridement of wounds, suturing lacerations, stabilizing and splinting mobile teeth, root canal therapy, tooth reconstruction, and tooth replacement.

Tobacco-Related Problems

Tobacco use among adolescents is a major public health concern. Intense peer pressures are placed on teenagers to use tobacco. Curiosity and a desire to be different from one's parents also may drive teenagers to experiment with tobacco use. In addition to these pressures, adolescents are bombarded with well-funded multimedia advertising glamorizing tobacco use. The use of smokeless tobacco by high-profile professional athletes sends the message to adolescents that tobacco use is acceptable and that success in sports is associated with its use. Federally mandated warning labels on cigarette packages have been shown to be ineffective in curtailing tobacco use among teenagers and paradoxically may be associated with an increase in smoking rather than the expected reduction.[40]

In recent years the use of traditional tobacco cigarettes by adolescents decreased but at the same time the use of e-cigarettes for the delivery of nicotine is increasing. A large study in the United States found that 14.2% of 16- to 19-year-olds had used e-cigarettes in the past month.[41]

The oral sequelae of smoking and smokeless tobacco use are well documented. Tobacco products can lead to gingival recession and staining of dental enamel. Soft tissue changes, such as hyperkeratosis and oral leukoplakia, can result and have the potential to undergo malignant transformation into squamous

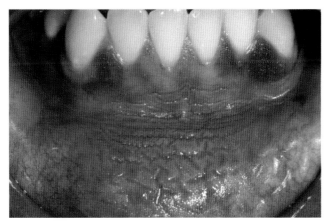

Fig. 17.7 Tobacco pouch keratosis; also known as snuff pouch. (Neville BW, Damm DD, Allen CM, et al. *Oral and Maxillofacial Pathology*. 4th ed. St. Louis: Elsevier; 2016.)

cell carcinoma (Figure 17.7). Patients with suspected malignant or premalignant changes require a biopsy by the general dentist or an appropriate specialist.

Parents and dentists should counsel teenagers to avoid the use of tobacco products. Once regular use has been established, the addiction can be very difficult to break. The tactics used to approach the issue are crucial if success is to be achieved. A nonauthoritarian, informative approach that allows the teenager to actively participate in the process offers the best chance of success. Discussion should address the negative implications of tobacco use: significant health risks, including lung cancer, emphysema, chronic bronchitis, and heart disease; addiction; financial cost; reduced esthetics; and poor physical performance. The parent or dentist should convey a degree of empathy and concern for the teenager at this crucial decision point. Teenagers are under enormous pressure to fit into a routine, behavior, and appearance prescribed by peer groups. The prospect of exclusion from a peer group and the potential loss of friends may inhibit the adolescent from giving up smoking or tobacco use. Counseling may be more effective if the deeper meaning of friendship is stressed, including reminders of the minor role that appearance and behavior play in true friendship. "If they are your real friends, they will still like you if you do not smoke."

Major public health initiatives are required to reduce the number of teenagers who use tobacco and discourage the development of new users in this age group. If progress is not made, the healthcare system will be further strained by future generations of adults who suffer from serious tobacco-related conditions arising from long-standing habits acquired in adolescence. Dentists, as part of the healthcare system, must accept the responsibility of becoming active in counseling adolescent patients against the use of tobacco (see Chapter 10 for discussion of tobacco use cessation).

Alcohol and Substance Use and Abuse

Along with tobacco use, abuse of alcohol and a widening array of illegal street drugs are major problems in some segments of the adolescent population. Glamorous advertising campaigns associate alcohol consumption with feelings of power, control, attractiveness, freedom, comfort, and "being cool." Peer pressure, natural curiosity, and presentations in written, visual, and audio media act as strong inducements for adolescent experimentation with alcohol and drugs. A large US national study in 2019 showed that 24.5% of surveyed adolescents (12–17 years of age) reported having used illicit drugs previously and 13% had used marijuana in the past year.[42]

Binge drinking (five or more alcoholic drinks on the same occasion) was reported by 5.8% of adolescents aged 12 to 17 years old in the past month.[43]

During the initial examination and at subsequent visits, the dentist should be alert to potential physical and behavioral signs of substance abuse. Patients may exhibit a wide range of behaviors, from excitation to central nervous system depression, depending on the type of agent used. Intravenous drug use may be confirmed by the presence of multiple venipuncture sites. Solvent abuse and inhalation of cocaine or other drugs can lead to chronic rhinitis and inflammatory changes of the nasal mucosa. Pupillary constriction, hypertension, and tachycardia may indicate current use of narcotic drugs such as cocaine. Changes in behavior, such as depression, impulsiveness, lack of motivation, unresponsiveness, or concealment, may accompany drug abuse. Altered sleeping patterns and eating habits or weight loss may be indicative of substance abuse. Many of these changes may be mistakenly identified as part of the normal psychological development of teenagers.

If the practitioner suspects that the patient abuses substances and may be a threat to themselves or others, they have a professional responsibility to intervene. When interacting with patients who are minors, the dentist may be faced with the dilemma of breaching patient–dentist confidentiality to inform the parents of possible substance abuse. If the abuse is significant and if referral for treatment or counseling is appropriate, the latter will be difficult to accomplish if the parents are not informed. One approach can be for the dentist to describe the suspicions and concerns to the teenager. After this, the dentist can ask permission to inform the teenager's parents of the suspicions. Informing the parents without the teenager's input will certainly have a negative effect on the patient–dentist relationship and may produce a long-term distrust of dentists by the patient. Therefore, this step should be taken only after careful weighing of the benefits and potential problems. In general, this is a last resort that should be pursued only when the patient's substance use/abuse is thought to be potentially life threatening. If the adolescent patient is diagnosed with substance use disorder the dentist needs to consult with their physician before prescribing pain medications. (See Chapter 14 for extended discussion of how to manage patients who are alcohol or substance dependent.)

Anorexia Nervosa and Bulimia

Anorexia nervosa and **bulimia** are unfortunately common in the adolescent age group, especially among females. Anorexia nervosa is defined as a pathologic psychosocial disorder characterized by extreme aversion to food and the intense fear of gaining weight. Inordinate attention is given to efforts to lose weight, even when the individual is already below a normal body weight. Bulimia is defined as episodic binge-eating followed by purging in an attempt to prevent weight gain. The process of purging most often takes the form of self-induced vomiting but can also involve the use of laxatives and diuretics. A significant number of anorexic patients may also practice bulimic behavior. A systematic review found weighted lifetime eating disorders to be 8.4% for females and 2.2 % for males. Eating disorders were also found to be prevalent in Western countries but also in Asia and developing Middle Eastern countries.[44]

Psychological profiles of anorexic patients reveal some common features. These individuals tend to have a distorted self-image, perceiving themselves as overweight even when they are emaciated. Compulsive physical activity may be pursued to further reduce body weight. Affected individuals tend to be overachievers who set high performance standards for themselves—for example, in academic pursuits. The individual may be guilt ridden and irritable while at the same time maintaining a steadfast denial of any physical or emotional problems (Box 17.2).

The dentist should be alert to potential physical changes that may be apparent on examination. Several clinical findings can result from significant weight loss:

- Amenorrhea (the cessation of menstruation in females)
- No detectable body fat
- **Bradycardia** and **hypotension** resulting from electrolyte imbalances
- **Hypothermia** as a result of the lack of insulating body fat Orofacial manifestations can include the following:
- Decreased salivary flow and lowered salivary pH
- Increased dental caries, primarily because of salivary changes
- Increased incidence and severity of gingivitis, resulting from vitamin deficiencies and xerostomia

Bulimia, like anorexia, tends to occur in young adult females who have a history of dieting and a fear of obesity. In their compulsion to maintain a normal or near-normal body weight, purging follows binge-eating episodes (Box 17.3). During episodes of binge-eating, bulimics may have extremely high caloric intakes, approaching 20,000 to 50,000 calories per day, depending on the food ingested. Favored binge foods tend to be those that require little chewing and are high in carbohydrates, starches, fats, and calories. Significant electrolyte disturbances can result from the loss of gastric hydrochloric acid during vomiting. This disruption can lead to serious sequelae, such as metabolic acidosis,

muscle weakness, and cardiac abnormalities. As with anorexia, bulimia often has significant orofacial manifestations. The palatal and pharyngeal oral mucosa may exhibit signs of trauma, erosion, ulceration, and inflammation as a result of self-induced gagging and exposure to stomach acid. The lingual surfaces of the maxillary incisors and the occlusal surfaces of the posterior teeth may exhibit **perimolysis**, a characteristic type of enamel erosion caused by a decreased oral pH resulting from the reflux of acidic stomach contents (Figures 17.8 and 17.9). In this form of erosion, dental restorations appear to stand out from the tooth surface because of the notable discrepancy between the eroded enamel surface and the restoration surface. **Cheilitis** of the lips may result from acid irritation and vitamin B deficiencies. Salivary gland enlargement and xerostomia can occur. Enlargement of the parotid gland can make the patient appear to have cherub-like cheeks, which may trigger additional, more-intense episodes of bulimic behavior, thereby exacerbating an already-serious condition.

An interdisciplinary team is usually needed to effectively manage a patient with anorexia or bulimia. Since the dentist may be the first health care professional to recognize the physical signs, the dental team should cultivate referral sources and

---

BOX 17.3 Common Signs of Bulimia Nervosa[a]

- Recurrent episodes of binge-eating.
- Self-induced vomiting.
- Misuse of laxatives, diuretics, or other medications in an attempt to lose weight.
- Fasting.
- Excessive exercise.
- The behaviors listed above occur, on average, at least once a week for 3 months.
- Distorted self-image based on body shape and weight.

[a]Comprehensive diagnostic criteria are located in the American Psychiatric Association: Diagnostic and Statistical Manual of Mental Disorders, 5th ed. Arlington, VA: American Psychiatric Association; 2013. Reprinted with permission from the American Psychiatric Association.

BOX 17.2 Common Signs of Anorexia Nervosa[a]

- Conscious restriction of food intake leading to a significant low body weight relative to developmental norms.
- Intense fear of gaining weight or becoming fat.
- Distorted self-image based on body shape and weight.
- Inability to recognize a significant low body weight relative to developmental norms.

[a]Comprehensive diagnostic criteria are located in the American Psychiatric Association: Diagnostic and Statistical Manual of Mental Disorders, 5th ed. Arlington, VA: American Psychiatric Association; 2013. Reprinted with permission from the American Psychiatric Association.

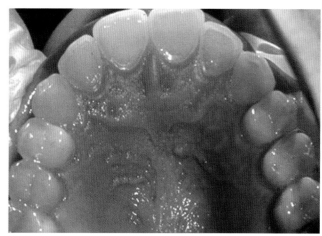

Fig. 17.8 Early perimolysis involving the lingual surfaces of the maxillary incisors of a patient with bulimia. (Roberts MW, Tylenda CA. Dental aspects of anorexia and bulimia nervosa, *Pediatrician.* 1989;16(3-4):178-184. Reprinted with permission of S. Karger AG, Basel.)

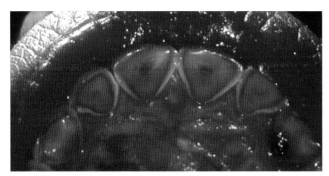

Fig. 17.9 Advanced perimolysis of the maxillary incisors in which the pulp chambers of the teeth are visible. (From Johnson GH, Powell LV, Gordon GE. Dentin bonding systems: a review of current products and techniques. *J Am Dent Assoc.* 1991;122(7):37-41.)

establish working relationships with a psychologist, psychiatrist, social worker or other mental health professional who can confirm the diagnosis and provide counseling, support and mental health therapy for the afflicted individual.

The dental treatment of anorexic and bulimic patients can be challenging and complex. Initial dental treatment should include oral self-care instruction and diet counseling. The use of sodium bicarbonate mouth rinses can be prescribed to reduce oral acidity after episodes of vomiting. Patient-applied neutral (not acidulated) fluoride gels in custom trays can also be used to reduce enamel solubility and enamel erosion. Prescribing increased fluid intake, artificial saliva, or sugarless gums or mints can reduce xerostomia. In cases of rampant caries, initial restorative care should be aimed at caries control through the use of protective (or definitive) direct-fill restorations. Only after the condition has stabilized should indirect definitive restorations be placed. (See Chapter 10 for more specifics on management of the caries active patient.)

TREATMENT PLANNING

Informed Consent

When performing any treatment on a patient who is under the legal age of consent, practitioners must first obtain permission from the parent or legal guardian to complete diagnostic procedures, including radiographs, and any treatment procedures. Although it is not unusual for another relative, such as a grandparent, to accompany a younger adolescent to a dental appointment, the dentist must remember that grandparents are usually not the legal guardians and cannot provide valid consent to proceed. When an individual telephones to make a new patient examination appointment for an adolescent, staff must remind the caller that a parent or guardian must accompany the patient to the initial examination appointment to provide valid consent. In some jurisdictions, an exception to this rule is allowed for **emancipated minors**—persons under the legal age of consent who function as independent adults, living apart from their parents and supporting themselves. In such instances, the emancipated teenager may give valid consent to proceed with the chosen treatment. Once a formal plan of care

has been established and consented to by the parent, guardian, or emancipated minor, subsequent treatment that is on the plan of care can be rendered without the parent or guardian being present.

Although parents or legal guardians must give consent for treatment of adolescents, the adolescent should also be involved in the treatment planning process (see the *Ethics in Dentistry* box). All treatment options and the associated risks and benefits for each option should be explained to both the parents and patient. To ensure successful outcomes, adolescents should actively participate in the selection of the appropriate treatment plan and assent to the agreed-on treatment.

Special Considerations for the Adolescent Patient

Esthetics are particularly important to adolescent patients, caught between the conformist world in which they are expected to maintain the behavior and appearances of childhood and the rebellious world in which alternative appearances are essential to seeking new identities. In the majority of cases, adolescents remain acutely aware of their own physical appearance and wish to achieve and maintain good oral and dental health. Heightened awareness of their own sexual identity and exploring interpersonal relationships in a more adult way during puberty may motivate teenagers to pay more attention to physical appearance, including the appearance of their teeth.

Techniques such as resin bonding, veneers, and orthodontics offer adolescents the opportunity to improve oral health and appearance and encourage development of a healthy and positive self-image. Resin bonding and veneers can provide an esthetic and functional reconstruction for teeth marred by developmental or traumatic defects. Orthodontic treatment has also become a widely accepted part of dental treatment during adolescence.

Esthetic restorations may be required on anterior teeth that have been traumatically fractured or that have enamel hypoplasia. Restoring these teeth with composite resin materials can provide good esthetic results, require minimal chair time, and can be done at modest cost to the patient. These materials can also provide an acceptable interim alternative to full-coverage restorations. When a full-coverage restoration is required, it is often preferable to delay the process for a period of months or years to reduce the likelihood of encroachment on the pulp and to allow the age-related migration of the gingival attachment to occur.

For patients with congenitally missing permanent teeth, a definitive treatment plan should be developed during adolescence. In these situations, two basic treatment choices exist. One option is to maintain the space for a prosthetic replacement, such as a removable or fixed partial denture or an implant. The second option is to consider using orthodontic appliances to close the space, thus eliminating the need for a future prosthesis. If comprehensive orthodontics with extractions are already indicated, the latter treatment plan may be more cost effective.

With the eruption of the premolars and second permanent molars, the number of caries susceptible occlusal surfaces increases. Recently erupted premolars and molars with deep pits and fissures should receive pit and fissure sealants when it has been determined that the individual is at risk of occlusal caries. Second molars tend to have less well-defined occlusal fissures than the first permanent molars, but they should also receive sealants when the patient is at risk of caries. Appropriate placement of pit and fissure sealants during adolescence can help these individuals transition into and through adulthood caries free or with fewer restorations than would otherwise have been needed.

In adolescents, the design of cavity preparations may need to be modified to accommodate certain oral conditions that are common in this age group. Because pulp chambers in newly erupted teeth are comparatively larger than those of more mature adult teeth, in which secondary dentin has been deposited, cavity preparations should be configured to prevent noncarious exposures of the pulp. Gingival tissue height on the teeth of adolescents is more coronally placed than in adults. Also, because clinical crowns in adolescents may be shorter as a result of partial eruption of the teeth, establishing adequate apical extension of extracoronal restorations can be difficult. The design of restorations may also need to be modified because of inadequate oral self-care. In Class II and III preparations, cavosurface margins may need to be extended into self-cleansing areas to reduce the chance of recurrent caries. The use of fluoride-releasing restorative materials may aid in the prevention of recurrent caries in high-risk adolescents (see discussion of this topic in Chapter 10).

In adolescents, posterior teeth needing full-coverage restoration may also present restorative challenges. Short clinical crowns and high gingival attachment may compromise the retention of onlays or crowns. Interim restorations, such as stainless steel crowns, may need to be used until gingival tissue height has stabilized and an adequate level of plaque control has been established. Care must be taken, however, because the use of improperly adapted stainless steel crowns for long periods of time may compromise the long-term gingival or periodontal health of these teeth.

TREATING THE ADOLESCENT PATIENT

Adolescent patients should be treated as individuals, unique and separate from their parents. During appointments, the dentist should try to focus on the patient and their desires rather than on the parents. If the parents are present during the dental visits, the dentist should avoid spending an inordinate amount of time relating to them. Successful dialogue and interactions are easier to establish if the dental team shows interest in topics that the adolescent regards as important. Such simple gestures as providing Internet access in the office and video selection in the waiting room, or offering the adolescent the opportunity to select the type of music to listen to during the appointment, can be an effective means of improving rapport. If the office has a website or social media interface, posting invitations specifically to adolescent patients and links to educational materials geared to their needs can be helpful in making the adolescent patient feel accepted and valued for who they are.

Wide-ranging behaviors may be encountered among adolescents, depending on their developmental phase. Unlike young children, adolescents are capable of understanding the scientific basis of disease. Knowledge of biology and science gained from the school curriculum allows the adolescent to comprehend the microbiologic basis of caries and periodontal disease. As a result, most adolescents are aware of the importance of good oral hygiene and the sequelae of failing to comply with such practices. To encourage good oral self-care in younger adolescents, parents can offer a choice of a regular toothbrush versus an electric toothbrush with the premise that the decision to brush or not to brush is not debatable, but that other options are under the young person's control.

At the same time, as a normal part of development, adolescents tend to question or reject adult authority. In the dental setting, the adolescent may relate poorly to the dental team because of this conflict. The acceptance or rejection of dental counseling and treatment may depend on the manner in which the information is conveyed. An authoritarian approach is more apt to be a "turnoff" and to impede the development of a trusting and positive dentist-patient relationship. A nonthreatening, understanding approach that conveys respect for the individual's approaching maturity and allows some freedom of choice increases the chances for successful communication. Oral hygiene and diet instruction should be discussed in a straightforward and factual manner, rather than with a threatening or demanding tone. Instead of making appointments for adolescents, parents can give the teenager a choice of dates and allow them to choose the one that works best for them.

With advances in technology, teenagers are more accustomed to communicating digitally using text messaging and online chat rooms. An explosion of social networking sites allows teenagers to communicate and share common interests on a global level. Smartphones and computers allow instant access to the content of the World Wide Web and all its resources, whether good or bad. Modern dentists must be digital savvy and willing to use these electronic resources to their advantage to educate and motivate technologically connected teenagers. Text messages or office social media sites can be used to stress healthy lifestyles and the importance of good oral hygiene.

FOLLOW-UP AND MAINTENANCE

As with adult patients, adequate follow-up and maintenance are crucial to the success of the adolescent's treatment plan. Periodic visits are essential to ensure that previous treatment has been effective, assess the patient's current condition, and develop strategies to address new and continuing oral health needs.

Issues relating to planning for and executing the recall visits, discussed in Chapter 12, are equally applicable to the adolescent patient. Because of the changing physiology, metabolism, self-image, and lifestyle that characterize this group, the need for regular periodic dental visits takes on an added dimension. Dental disease—most notably dental caries—can initiate and progress extremely rapidly. Significant occlusal changes occur as a result of growth and development. Periodic visits provide an opportunity to manage these and other emerging oral health problems proactively and effectively. The patient's interest in oral health and receptivity to oral healthcare instructions may rise or fall throughout adolescence. At periodic visits, the dental team can provide positive reinforcement in good times, and provide encouragement when the patient's enthusiasm has flagged. The team can also use these periodic visits as opportunities to explore new strategies—recognizing that previous methods and techniques may no longer be effective, and that other, more-adult strategies may now be relevant and useful. As the adolescent patient's interests, motivation, and perspectives change, so too will desires and expectations concerning oral function and appearance. Periodic visits provide the ideal opportunity to revisit or raise new treatment options to improve on oral esthetics, correct malocclusion, and permanently restore or replace individual teeth.

CONCLUSION

This chapter has outlined some of the problems the dentist is likely to encounter in planning treatment for adolescents. Although many of the disease processes encountered in adolescents are not unique to this age group, and procedures that are followed during diagnosis and treatment planning parallel those used in adults, the psychosocial and physical changes that occur during this period of development may require modification of routine clinical techniques. Lack of motivation and compliance are frequently encountered as adolescents seek to establish an autonomous, stable self-identity. Open communication and understanding of these issues are essential requirements for successful interaction with and treatment of the adolescent patient.

REVIEW QUESTIONS

- What are the three phases of psychosocial development in the adolescent? How might each phase influence the adolescent's view of dentistry and expectations regarding dental treatment?
- List some lifestyle issues that may have an effect on an adolescent's oral condition and dental treatment.
- How does patient–dentist confidentiality affect the dentist–adolescent–parent relationship?
- Why are many adolescents attracted to using tobacco, alcohol, and other substances? What oral problems can these behaviors create? How might alcohol or substance abuse affect the delivery of dental care?
- Why are some adolescents highly caries prone?
- What forms of periodontal disease are found in the adolescent? How are these diseases treated?

- Delineate common occlusal problems in adolescents. How are they identified? How are they treated?
- What are the signs of anorexia and bulimia? Why are adolescents more at risk of developing these disorders? How are they treated?
- Are the processes of developing a plan of care and achieving consent different in adolescent and adult patients? If so, how?

Practice Enhancements

- Develop a management strategy for adolescents at high caries risk.
- Develop an office protocol for identifying and managing adolescent patients in your practice who are at risk for obesity.

REFERENCES

1. Google Search: *Percent of US population between 10 and 19 years old*. https://actforyouth.net/YouthStatistics/U.S. Teen Demographics. Accessed October 2, 2021.
2. 2017 National Population Projections Tables: Main Series. http://www.census.gov/data/tables2017/demo/popproj/2017-summary-tables.html. Table 3.
3. United Nations Population Division. http://population.un.org/wpp/Download/Probabilistic/Population/TotalPopulation. Accessed May 7, 2021
4. Asemota AO, George BP, Bowman SM, et al. Causes and trends in traumatic brain injury for United States adolescents. *J Neurotrauma*. 2013;30(2):67–75.
5. Dodington J, Violano P, Baum CR, Bechtel K. Drugs, guns and cars: how far we have come to improve safety in the United States; yet we still far to go. *Pediatric Research*. 2017;81(1):227–232.
6. Glendor U. Epidemiology of traumatic dental injuries – a 12 year review of the literature. *Dental Traumatology*. 2008;24:603–611.
7. Nyquist JM, Phillips C, Stein M, Koroluk LD. Executive function as a risk factor for incisor trauma. *Dent Traumatol*. 2018;34(4):229–236.
8. Pelkonen M, Marttunen M. Child and adolescent suicide. *Pediatric Drugs*. 2003;5:243–265.
9. Brown RC, Plener PL. Non-suicidal self-injury in adolescence. *Curr Pyschiatry Rep*. 2017;19:20.

10. Bacopoulou F, Karakitsos P, Kottaridi C, et al. Genital HPV in children and adolescents: Does sexual activity make a difference? *J Pediatr Adolesc Gynecol.* 2016;29:228–233.

11. Centers for Disease Control and Prevention: *Adult BMI calculator.* http://www.cdc.gov/healthyweight/assessing/bmi/adult_bmi/english_bmicalculator/bmi_calculator.html. Accessed September 26, 2021.

12. Okunseri C, Okunseri E, Gonzalez C, et al. Erosive tooth wear and consumption of beverages among children in the United States. *Caries Res.* 2011;45(2):130–135.

13. Mack KB, Phillips C, Jain N, Koroluk LD. Relationship between body mass index percentile and skeletal maturation and dental development in orthodontic patients. *Am J Orthod Dentofacial Orthop.* 2013;143:228–234.

14. Werner SL, Phillips C, Koroluk LD. Association between childhood obesity and dental caries. *Pediatr Dent.* 2012;34:546–550.

15. Wardle J. Understanding the aetiology of childhood obesity: Implications for treatment. *Proc Nutr Soc.* 2005;64:73–79.

16. World Health Organization: *What is the burden of oral disease?* http://www.who.int/news-room/fact-sheets/detail/oral-health. Accessed October 2, 2021.

17. Kallestal C. The effect of five years' implementation of caries-preventive methods in Swedish high risk adolescents. *Caries Res.* 2005;39:20–26.

18. Smyth RS, Amlani M, Fulton A, Sharif MO. The availability and characteristics of patient focused YouTube videos related to oral hygiene instruction. *Br Dental J.* 2020;228:773–781.

19. Caplan DJ, Weintraub JA. The oral health burden in the United States: a summary of recent epidemiological studies. *J Dent Educ.* 1993;57:853–862.

20. Bhat M. Periodontal health of 14-17-year-old United States schoolchildren. *J Public Health Dent.* 1991;51:5–11.

21. Brown L, Brunelle J, Kingman A. Periodontal status in the United States, 1988-91: Prevalence, extent and demographic variations. *J Dent Res.* 1996;75:672–683.

22. Mombelli A, Gusberti FA, van Oosten MA, Lang NP. Gingival health and gingivitis development during puberty. *J Clin Periodontol.* 1989;16:451–456.

23. Nakagawa S, Fujii H, Machida Y, Okuda K. A longitudinal study from prepuberty to puberty of gingivitis. *J Clin Periodontol.* 1994;21:658–665.

24. Mombelli A, Lang NP, Burgin WB, Gusberti FA. Microbiological changes associated with the development of puberty gingivitis. *J Periodontal Res.* 1990;25:331–338.

25. Hock J. Gingival vasculature around erupting deciduous teeth of dogs and cats. *J Clin Periodontol.* 1975;2:44–50.

26. Albandar JM. Aggressive periodontitis: case definition and diagnostic criteria. *Periodontology 2000.* 2014;65:13–26.

27. Papapanou PN, Sanz M, et al. Periodontitis: Consensus report of Workgroup 2 of the 2017 World Workshop on the Classification of Periodontal and Peri-Implant Diseases and Conditions. *J Clin Periodontol.* 2018;45(Suppl 20):S162–S170.

28. Faveri M, Figueiredo LC, Duarte PM, Mestnik MJ, Mayer MP, Feres M. Microbiological profile of untreated subjects with localized aggressive periodontitis. *J Clin Periodontol.* 2009;36(9):739–749.

29. Shaddox LM, Morford LA, Nibali L. Periodontal health and disease: The contribution of genetics. *Periodontol 2000.* 2021;85(1):161–181.

30. Albandar JM, Susin C, Hughes FJ. Manifestations of systemic diseases and conditions that affect the periodontal attachment apparatus: case definitions and diagnostic considerations. *J Clin Periodontol.* 2018;45(Suppl 20):S171–S189.

31. Khocht A, Albandar JM. Aggressive forms of periodontitis secondary to systemic disorders. *Periodontol 2000.* 2014 Jun;65(1):134–148.

32. Meng H, Ren X, Tian Y, Feng X, Xu L, Zhang L, Lu R, Shi D, Chen Z. Genetic study of families affected with aggressive periodontitis. *Periodontol 2000.* 2011 Jun;56(1):87–101.

33. Fine DH, Armitage GC, Genco RJ, Griffen AL, Diehl SR. Unique etiologic, demographic, and pathologic characteristics of localized aggressive periodontitis support classification as a distinct subcategory of periodontitis. *J Am Dent Assoc.* 2019;150(11):922–931.

34. Susin C, Haas AN, Albandar JM. Epidemiology and demographics of aggressive periodontitis. *Periodontol 2000.* 2014;65(1):27–45.

35. Teughels W, Feres M, Oud V, Martín C, Matesanz P, Herrera D. Adjunctive effect of systemic antimicrobials in periodontitis therapy: A systematic review and meta-analysis. *J Clin Periodontol.* 2020;47(Suppl 22):257–281.

36. Sabiston CB. A review and proposal for the etiology of acute necrotizing gingivitis. *J Clin Periodontol.* 1986;13(8):727–734.

37. Wade DN. Acute necrotizing ulcerative gingivitis-periodontitis: a literature review. *Military Med.* 1988;163:337–342.

38. Hodgdon A. Dental and related infections. *Emerg Med Clin North Am.* 2013;31:465–480.

39. Proffit WR, Fields Jr HW, Moray LJ. Prevalence of malocclusion and orthodontic treatment need in the United States: estimates from the NHANES III survey. *Int J Adult Orthodon Orthognath Surg.* 1998;13(2):97–106.

40. Robinson TN, Killen JD. Do cigarette warning labels reduce smoking? Paradoxical effects among adolescents. *Arch Pediatr Adolesc Med.* 1997;151:267–272.

41. Hammond DH, Wackowski OA, Reid JL, O'Connor RJ. Use of JUUL E-cigarettes among youth in the United States. *Nicotine & Tobacco Res.* 2020;22(5):827–832.

42. US Department of Health and Human Services. 2019 National Survey of drug use and health. Substance Abuse and Mental Health Administration. 2019

43. Chung T, Creswell KG, Bachrach R, Clark DB, Martin CS. Adolescent binge drinking: Developmental context and opportunities for prevention. *Alcohol Res.* 2018;39(1):5–15.

44. Galmiche M, Dechelotte P, Lambert G, Tavolacci MP. Prevalence of eating disorders over the 2000-2-18 period: a systematic literature review. *Am J Clin Nutr.* 2019;109:1402–1413.

45. Katz AL, Webb SA. Informed consent in decision-making in pediatric practice. *Pediatrics.* 2016;138(2). e 20161484.

SUGGESTED READINGS AND WEBSITES

McDonald RE, Avery DR. *Dentistry for the child and adolescent.* 11th ed. St Louis: Mosby; 2021.

Nowak A, Christensen J, Mabry T, Townsend J, Wells M. *Pediatric dentistry: infancy through adolescence.* 6th ed. St. Louis: Elsevier; 2019.

Orthodontics: https://www.aaoinfo.org/EducationalMaterial

Dental Care per American Academy of Pediatric Dentistry: https://www.mychildrensteeth.org

American Dental Association Information for Patients: https://www.mouthhealthy.org>teens

18

Geriatric Patients

Jennifer E. Hartshorn, Gretchen Gibson, and Linda C. Niessen

 Visit eBooks.Health.Elsevier.com

OUTLINE

Globally the number of elderly people continues to increase as a result of increasing life expectancy and decreasing levels of fertility. The United Nations estimates that there were 727 million persons aged 65 years or older in the world in 2020.[1] This number is projected to double to 1.5 billion by 2050. Globally the share of the population aged 65 years or older is expected to increase from 9.3% in 2020 to ~16% in 2050.[1] Figure. 18.1 demonstrates the change in demography of the world population from 1950 to 2018 including population projections through the year 2100. The number of older adults over the age of 65 years projected in 2050 is significantly greater than in 2018 and vastly greater than 1950.

Table 18.1 shows the percentage of the population who are older than 65 years in selected countries throughout the world in 2013 and in 2019. The table shows the continued increase in the global population older than 65 years during these years. Japan leads the world with 28% of its population over the age of 65 years.[2] Many countries on the European continent have populations at or over 20% aged 65 years or older. Australia,

Canada, Russia, and the United States have seen their populations over the age of 65 years increase to 15%–18%.

Mexico and India have much younger populations than Europe and the United States, and have seen their populations over the age of 65 years increase to 7% and 6% respectively.[2] It must be noted, however, that 6% of India's population represents more than 60 million adults who are older than 65 years, which is more than the entire population of Canada. China's "one child" policy and a rapidly increasing older population has resulted in China's population over the age of 65 years increasing to 11% in 2019, which is up from 9% in 2013. It is of interest to note that China is changing its "one child" policy perhaps as a result of the increasing aging of its population. These global data suggest that oral healthcare for an increasingly large number of older adults will be a fact of life for dentists everywhere.

In 1900 life expectancy at birth in the United States was approximately 47 years. By the beginning of the 21st century, life expectancy had increased to almost 80 years. Life expectancy at the age of 65 years refers to how many years you can expect

The Demography of the World Population from 1950 to 2100

Shown is the age distribution of the world population – by sex – from 1950 to 2018 and the *UN Population Division*'s projection until 2100.

Our World in Data

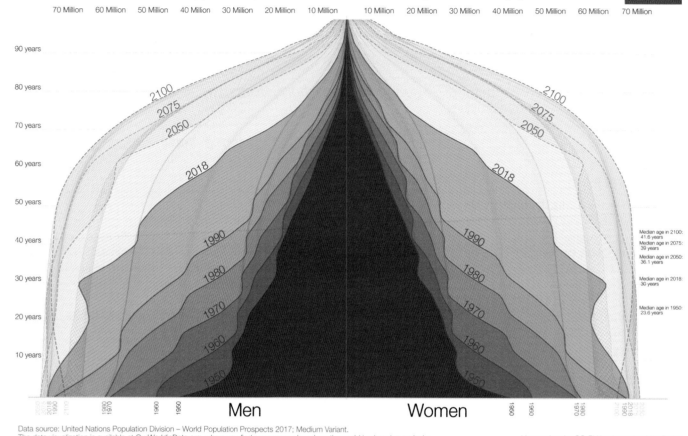

Data source: United Nations Population Division – World Population Prospects 2017; Medium Variant.
The data visualization is available at OurWorldinData.org, where you find more research on how the world is changing and why.
Licensed under CC-BY by the author Max Roser.

Fig. 18.1 Demography of the World Population from 1950 to 2100. (From Ritchie H, Roser M. Our world in data: Age structure (2019). https://ourworldindata.org/age-structure.)

to live, once you reach the age of 65 years. For the past several decades, life expectancy at birth and at the age of 65 years have increased each year. In 2020, the rapid spread of the COVID-19 virus resulted in over 600,000 deaths in the United States. The virus disproportionately killed older adults, Black and Latino populations and was the third leading cause of death in the United States in 2020. Demographers are now reporting reductions in life expectancy at birth of 1.13 years because of COVID-19.[3]

Older adults are the fastest growing segment of the US population. Currently, 16% (52.8 million) of the US population is older than 65 years and this number will increase throughout the 21st century.[4] The segment of the population older than 85 years is projected to triple from 6.7 million in 2020 to over 19 million in 2060. The number of centenarians in the United States is expected to reach 600,000 by 2060.[5] Dentists in the mid-21st century will be providing dental care for many more people over 65 years than ever before.

In the United States and throughout the world, most older adults (85%) are healthy and live in community settings. In the United States, approximately 10% are described as homebound (i.e., able to leave their homes only with great difficulty), and 5% of US seniors (1.5 million) reside in nursing homes. In the United States, people older than 65 years have a one in four chance of spending some time in a nursing home during their lifetime. The proportion of older adults living in nursing homes varies by age, only 1% of the 65- to 74-year-old group reside in nursing facilities, compared with 15% of those older than 85 years. Of the 1.5 million US seniors living in nursing homes, approximately 50% are over the age of 85 years, ~72% are women, and many have never married or no longer have a spouse.[6] As will be discussed later in this chapter, access to oral healthcare can be difficult for nursing home residents, as well as for health-compromised homebound persons and the provision of treatment may become more complex as a result of chronic systemic illnesses.

Because of the differential in life expectancies between men and women, aging is sometimes described as a women's issue. As the population ages, the ratio (number of men to women) decreases. In 2020 in the United States, there was parity between men and women in the 18- to 64-year-old age group (100 men for 100 women).[5] In this group, there are 84 men per 100 women and, at age 85 years and older, there are only 56 men for every 100 women.[5] Globally, older men are more likely to be married (81%) compared with older women (50%).[1] Older women are more likely to be single, divorced, or widowed and are more likely to live in poverty.

TABLE 18.1	Changes in Global Aging 2009–2013; 2019	
Country	Estimated % of the Population ≥ 65 years 2019	2013
Australia	16	14
Canada	18	15
China	11	9
Greece	22	19
India	6	5
Ireland	14	12
Israel	12	11
Italy	23	21
Japan	28	24
Korea	15	9
Mexico	7	6
Peru	8	6
Russian Federation	15	13
Singapore	12	10
Sweden	20	19
United States	16	14

World Bank: *UN Population Division's World Population.* http://data.worldbank.org/indicator/SP.POP.65UP.TO.ZS/.

Poverty rates in 2019 overall were lower for older adults (8.9%) than for children under 18 years (14.4%) and adults 18–64 years old (9.4%).[7] Although 8.9% of adults aged 65 years and over had incomes below poverty, the number of aged poor has increased to 4.9 million as a result of the increase in the number of older adults.[7] Poverty rates in older adults vary by gender, race, and ethnic background. The rate also increases with age, with retirees over the age of 88 years, women over the age of 80 years, and older people who have never married having the greatest financial needs.

This chapter will discuss treatment-planning issues that have particular relevance to this age group. The terms "senior," "geriatric," "elderly," and "older adult" are used interchangeably, all referring to persons over the age of 65 years. Although the authors recognize the arbitrariness of this designation, the age of 65 years has become a common marker for retirement and therefore serves as a standard and convenient reference.

ORAL HEALTH IN THE AGING POPULATION

Oral health can be both a benchmark for, and a determinant of, the quality of life. Currently, for example, people in the United States who are 85 years old can expect to have at least another 6.7 years of life, but more important than the length of life span will be the quality of life that can be afforded to individuals in those later years. In the United States over the past 20 years, the oral health of older adults has improved considerably, from that of a generation that was predominantly edentulous to one in which each individual in that age group has an average of 20 teeth.

Perhaps as a result, older adults in the United States have greater dental needs, use dental services at higher rates, and incur higher average costs per visit than do younger people. A recent report by the American Dental Association's (ADA) Health Policy and Research Division noted that although adjusted per patient dental expenditures were flat among children; they had increased among adults, especially older adults and higher-income adults. The authors concluded that "due to the aging of the baby boomers, the percent of the population over age 65 will grow and dental expenditures among this segment of the population could buoy up the dental economy for years to come."[8]

On the less-optimistic side, it must be noted that most US dental insurance benefits cease when retirement begins because they are work-related benefits. With the exception of some Medicare Advantage plans, Medicare includes no dental benefits. Dental offices may need to alert baby boomers planning for their retirement to this upcoming change in their dental benefit status.

For the affluent elderly, dental expenditures will continue to be made from discretionary or expendable income, but for the low-income elderly in the United States, financial options to pay for dental care are limited. Medicaid, available to some, varies from state to state both in the types of dental care reimbursed and in the age groups covered. Even when the patient does qualify, few services are covered beyond basic preventive therapy, direct-fill restorations, extractions, and dentures. A mechanism does exist for using Supplemental Social Security Income to pay for needed dental services if the patient resides in a long-term care facility, termed Incurred Medical Expenses. However, this benefit is often difficult to access. (See *Suggested Readings and Resources* at the end of this chapter.)

Two-thirds of those seniors who are considered poor are not eligible for any type of Medicaid dental coverage. For those persons, the prospects for receiving definitive dental care are limited.

The trend worldwide is for individuals to live longer and retain more of their natural teeth; as a result, there are more older adults with more complex medical needs who also have dental needs. Access to dental care for homebound elderly and nursing home residents is even more difficult, even in countries with national healthcare systems. Developed countries with national health systems that include dental care have seen increased costs as their population ages. As oral health costs have increased for aging populations, some governments have examined new ways of preventing oral diseases, particularly root caries.

Changing Needs and Values

In their book *Successful Aging*, Rowe and Kahn suggest that lifestyle choices may be more important to the aging process than genes.[9] Globally, attitudes about oral health in older adulthood vary considerably. In some regions, edentulism may be viewed as an inevitable fact of aging. In other areas, good oral health is considered essential to successful aging. Japan, for example, has undertaken a health promotion program called "20 by 80."[10] The goal of this program is for Japanese adults to retain 20 teeth by the time they reach the age of 80 years. In the United States, the baby boomers' approach to aging differs dramatically from that of their parents and grandparents. They are the best-educated age group in the US population (almost 25% have attended college) and with more leisure time, discretionary income, knowledge of wellness issues, and opportunity to engage in healthful activities, this group is expected to live longer and have greater expectations for their health than did their parents. They are demonstrating an increasing demand for discretionary healthcare services, particularly plastic surgery. Similarly, the cosmetic services that dentistry can provide have increased popularity with this group. As the first generation to benefit from the widespread fluoridation of water supplies and availability of fluoride toothpaste, boomers generally have a strong appreciation for the benefits of preventive oral healthcare. Already using dental services at a relatively high rate, they are predicted to seek out and benefit from high-quality oral healthcare. As the baby boom generation ages further, many in that segment will reach older adulthood with a relatively complete dentition.

Although the expectations for what older individuals want and can afford in dental care can and do vary widely, there are also commonalties. Many health problems—both oral and systemic—are more likely to occur in this population. How are these problems recognized and diagnosed? How are they managed? What are the specific dental treatment needs of the elderly, and how is dental treatment planning shaped by the characteristics of aging? These questions are the focus of this chapter.

A movement within healthcare, termed Whole Health includes broad principles that are key to geriatric treatment planning. This movement incorporates a paradigm shift from "find it and fix it" to consideration of a full range of physical, emotional, mental, social, spiritual, and environmental issues that could affect a patient's life.[11] A key to this form of treatment planning is understanding what a patient's values, needs, and goals are for their life and health. As this chapter will point out, Systemic disease, the effects of aging on the body, and social determinants of health will all have a significant impact on patients' health and treatment outcomes.

Physiology of Aging

As the body ages, changes in organ function occur as seen in Table 18.2. Some of these changes occur with the aging process but sometimes these changes occur as a result of disease. These changes make it more difficult for the organs to compensate when variations to normal occur. They also make it more difficult for older adults to maintain homeostasis.

The inability to maintain homeostasis lowers the physiologic threshold for systemic disease to occur.[12] For example: as kidneys age, their ability to filter and excrete waste begins to slow. If an older adult then experiences high levels of salt in the diet, it takes longer for the kidney to filter and excrete the dietary salt causing high blood pressure. Whereas, that same dietary salt in a younger individual with a normal functioning kidney would not cause high blood pressure and the kidney would be able to

maintain homeostasis. Aging's effect on normal organ function becomes very important in dentistry when considering a patient's risk of aspiration of oral bacteria, the risk and effects of increase in systemic inflammatory markers as a result of periodontal disease, and risks associated with repeated trauma to the oral mucosa.

Changes associated with aging can be seen in both hard and soft oral tissues of the oral cavity. Physiologic changes in the teeth include a decrease in pulpal size, decreased pulpal cellularity, and loss of enamel from functional, chemical, and mechanical forces. As the pulp recedes, teeth typically darken in color, may become more brittle, and are at increased risk of fracture.[12] Attrition, a natural function of aging, leaves the affected teeth more vulnerable to dentinal sensitivity, erosion, caries, and fractures. Gingival recession is common in the elderly, which can lead to root sensitivity, periodontal disease, root caries, and pulpal necrosis.

The oral mucosa continues to play a critical role as a barrier organ for the body throughout life. Although there is little change in the thickness of stratified squamous epithelium on the surface (except under dentures), the connective tissue layer below becomes thinner and loses elasticity, decreasing the effectiveness of the barrier function. In addition, a reduced immune response may increase the vulnerability of oral tissues to infection and trauma. The incidence of oral mucosal disorders increases with advancing age. Such diseases include vesiculobullous disorders, ulcerative lesions secondary to medication use, and lichenoid, infectious, or malignant lesions.

TABLE 18.2	Physiology of Aging
Organ System	**Physiology Changes**
Cardiovascular system	Decrease cardiac output Decrease baroreceptor activity Increase total peripheral resistance
Central nervous system	Decrease neuronal density Decrease reflexes Decrease sympathetic response
Gastrointestinal system	Decrease gastric emptying Decrease gastrointestinal motility Increase gastric pH Decrease intestinal blood flow
Immune system	Decrease neurohumoral response Decrease white blood cells Decrease cell-mediated immunity
Renal System	Decrease renal blood flow Decrease glomerular filtration Decrease tubular secretion
Respiratory System	Decrease tidal volume Decrease vital capacity Increase residual volume Decrease lung capacity

Modified from: Ouanounou A, Haas DA. Pharmacotherapy for the elderly dental patient. *J Can Dent Assoc*. 2015;80:f18.

EVALUATION OF OLDER PATIENTS

Geriatric patients, in general, and the frail elderly in particular, will need very individualized plans for care. Simply looking in a patient's mouth and at radiographs will not be sufficient for determining a treatment plan. Many factors must be considered in the decision-making process and these factors hold much more significance in older adults than with other age groups.

The best time to determine whether these factors apply, and how significant they may be, is during the patient evaluation. Important factors that may affect treatment plans for the elderly include the living situation (e.g., independent community living, assisted living, nursing home), the patient's hand skills and coordination, the cognitive ability of the patient, the need for and availability of a caregiver to assist with oral hygiene, distance traveled to the office, type of transportation required, social schedule, consistency of the diet (e.g., regular, soft, mechanical soft, pureed), the constituents of the diet (amount of carbohydrates and sugars), health history and medications, the patient's vision and auditory status, and volume and quality of saliva present. A comprehensive understanding of the patient will be needed to formulate the best treatment plan.

Patient Interview

To develop a good relationship with the patient and an appropriate treatment plan, it is important to recognize social issues associated with the elderly. If these issues are discussed during the original patient interview, both treatment planning and scheduling of future appointments can be facilitated more effectively. For instance, although retired, many seniors, especially the younger members of this age group, find themselves with as complex a schedule as they had while working; with involvement in organizations, volunteer work, travel, and hobbies filling busy days and weeks. Many older adults have become full-time caregivers for an aging spouse, grandchildren, or other family members. Such caregiving can be time consuming and exhausting and lead to difficulty finding time to devote to their own personal health needs. This, in turn, can result in infrequent and/or shorter dental appointments for these patients. Many older adults still place a high priority on punctuality and expect the dentist to respect their time. Some older adults spend winter or summer in different places, which may affect the continuity of medical and dental care.

Age-related memory loss is a part of the lives of many seniors. Appointment reminders become more important and some elderly persons may wish to involve another family member, such as a spouse or adult child, in treatment-planning decisions. It is appropriate to ask the patient whether they would like to discuss treatment options with another family member before making a decision, simultaneously acknowledging the patient's autonomy.

With increasing frailty may come special transportation requirements. The clinician should not hesitate to raise these issues during the patient interview. If an individual depends on a family member to provide transportation to appointments, the frequency or length of visits may become a treatment-planning modifier. Some patients may require an Uber or taxi, adding to the expense of the treatment, or require appointments to be scheduled at particular times to accommodate public transportation schedules. Treatment sequencing may need to be altered to accommodate such special situations.

Because the older-than-65 segment of the population spans several generations, individual perceptions of dental needs and treatment choices will differ, based in part on past experiences. It is imperative to ask about past dental care and what the patient's expectations are for their teeth and their oral health overall. Based on their previous experiences, some may have low expectations. Providing information about the more recent alternatives in dentistry may help enlighten patients about available options. As a group, baby boomers may be more likely to have higher expectations than individuals in previous generations.

Visual and auditory disabilities are among the most common chronic conditions reported by seniors. Although the office staff should never assume that a patient is unable to see or hear well, it is wise to be aware that these conditions may be present. If the patient has removed their glasses for the examination, they should be returned before any written materials are reviewed. Black print on a white background is the most easily read. Developing health history forms and written take-home instruction materials in slightly larger print will be helpful.

Close contact with a hearing aid can occur during the initial examination or dental treatment and may cause unpleasant ringing in the patient's ear. The patient may turn off the hearing aid during treatment and a reminder to turn the aid back on may be needed before beginning any discussion. Lip reading can be an important tool for healing impaired seniors and removing a mask (or using a mask that has a clear face) when talking to a patient is helpful. Written treatment plans or postoperative instructions can assist in the presentation of the information and can be shared with family or friends later.

Alterations in mastication, swallowing, and sensory function occur with age. Mastication and swallowing difficulties can also occur as sequelae of systemic diseases seen more frequently in older adults, such as stroke or Parkinson's disease, or as the result of prolonged use of antipsychotic medications causing involuntary and uncontrollable muscle spasms. The sense of taste (salt, sweet, bitter, sour) appears to undergo few age-related alterations but is commonly affected by chemotherapy, opioids, and antibiotics. The sense of smell, however, appears to decrease with age and that change is thought to account for loss of flavor perception in older adults. In the case of COVID-19, loss of taste and smell occurred early in the infection. Fortunately, most patients recovered both when they recovered from the viral infection.

Patient's Health History

Because older adults are more likely to have chronic health problems, more time is generally required to obtain a thorough and accurate health history. Questioning is necessary to gather additional information about each positive response on the health history form. If a comprehensive health history form is used (see Chapter 1), an ideal format includes space for patient responses and for the dentist to record notes pertaining to each affirmative answer. It is advisable to assume that the patient can provide a reliable health history until otherwise demonstrated. If the patient seems unable to supply the necessary information, a tactful request for assistance should be made to family or caregivers. It may also be advisable to obtain a verbal or written consultation from the patient's physician, regarding specific issues that require further clarification.

The following guidelines should be observed when obtaining health-related information about the patient from caregivers or healthcare providers:

- Be attentive to federal Health Insurance Portability and Accountability Act or any applicable confidentiality regulations that may apply (see Chapter 7). Obtain permission from the patient (or guardian or Health Care Power of Attorney) to seek information from a caregiver or healthcare provider and document that consent.
- Use *specific* open-ended questions when seeking further information from a guardian or healthcare provider in response to positive answers on the health history. For example, "Mr. Smith reports having a heart problem, can you tell me more about that?" A general, "Is there anything I need to know?" query is less likely to elicit all the important or relevant information needed to carry out dental treatment safely.
- If a patient has a diagnosed illness, but the presentation is unusual, or if a patient develops new manifestations or conditions, a consultation with the physician should be requested.
- Contact the correct physician or specialist. Many older patients see more than one healthcare provider. When in doubt, it is often best to begin with the internist, family physician, or geriatric specialist, because the individuals in these disciplines often serve as the medical care coordinators.
- Access to laboratory, radiology, pharmacy and medical data is often required during the data collection phase and before the initiation of treatment. Although this was traditionally done through the request of paper copies of records, the advancement of electronic health records (EHR) with patient portals provide patients a way to access readily their personal health information, physician notes, and even send messages to their physician directly. This has now made it possible for more patients to share their health data electronically with providers outside their physician network. Assessing how to access necessary health data should now become a part of the initial interview process. If the patient is undergoing anticoagulation (Coumadin) therapy, a recent prothrombin level or international normalized ratio (INR) measurement is needed. Therefore, a flag will be required in this patient's chart to assure the test is always ordered and reviewed within 48 hours prior to any invasive dental treatment. Diabetic patients should obtain copies of their most recent hemoglobin A1c values. Patients with chronic kidney disease will need a recent estimated glomerular filtration rate (eGFR) before prescribing medications. For patients receiving radiation therapy or chemotherapy, it should be determined whether the patient has been given an antiresorptive agent, such as an intravenous bisphosphonate, or for patients receiving radiation, the total amount and location of radiation should be documented. Reported laboratory values need to be evaluated carefully, because "normal" may vary more in seniors and an addendum or additional normal range for older patients may be listed on the report.

Medication History

Medications play an important role in maintaining the health and quality of life for many older patients. More than 88% of older patients take at least one prescription medication and approximately 37% of older adults take five or more.[13] The patient should be instructed to bring the medications to the appointment or the physician or pharmacy may have supplied a printed list the patient can bring. "Over-the-counter" remedies can affect the patient's mood, coagulation rate, or oral condition and the dentist should therefore also ask for a list of those.

A thorough review of the patient's medication list is an essential component of the health history review and a requisite for the formulation of a comprehensive diagnosis and plan of care. A complete understanding of the types and dosages of an older dental patient's medications can aid in the differential diagnosis of oral conditions or lesions and can be a useful indicator of the level of severity of a specific disease. Such information may alert the dentist to potential medical emergencies that may arise during treatment. Because the patient's medical status and the types and dosages of medications can change frequently, it is often helpful to have the patient or care provider bring a list (or the medication containers themselves) at least once a year to update the medication history.

It is important to ask whether the medications are being used according to the physician's directions. For various reasons, including cost, side effects, and difficulty with the timing of multiple medications, patients may not be compliant with the prescribed regimen. If a patient is taking multiple medications, they may become confused and simply forget to take one or more. In any of these situations, the dentist should advise the patient and/or the caregiver to share this information with the patient's physician. In addition, the dental team should be watchful for signs of under- or overmedication. For example, if the patient has chosen to lower the dose of a hypertension medication because of side effects, the dentist should closely monitor the patient's blood pressure, particularly during a stressful dental procedure. As dentists, some of the issues that we should be aware of include hypotension associated with nifedipine, as well as falls and delirium that can be induced by benzodiazepines or narcotics.

For older patients, overmedication can be an issue and the law of multiples applies when reviewing or adding medications for these patients. In other words, multiple medications from multiple providers and even multiple pharmacies can lead to poor compliance and adverse drug interactions. The Beers Criteria, developed by the American Geriatric Society, is a published list of medications that can be dangerous for older adults.[14] (See *Suggested Readings and Resources* at the end of this chapter.)

This panel of geriatricians and pharmacists made a point of urging caution when prescribing any of the more than 50 medications that have strong anticholinergic effects. These include many antihistamines, antidepressants, antipsychotics, and muscle relaxants. Such medications can have a significant effect on oral health, owing to their high xerostomic potential.

Opioid use disorder is not confined to younger generations. Although dentists make up 9% of providers of opioids, some US research has shown they account for up to 45% of opioid prescriptions,[15] and therefore should be a contributing partner in opioid stewardship efforts. Older adults are at higher risk of harm from opioid use, compared with younger adults. This includes psychological and physiological changes, falls, adverse drug events, and uncoordinated care issues, such as coprescribing with a benzodiazepine.[16] Approximately one-third of adults over 65 years of age used prescription opioid pain relievers in 2017–18 and opioid deaths in seniors rose 217% between 2008 and 2018.[17] There are appropriate and effective options for pain control besides, or in addition to, short-term opioids. The first step of opioid stewardship is including pain assessment as part of your health history, identifying issues such as those noted in Table 18.3[18] with a discussion of the increased risks of opioid use with your geriatric patient.

Examination

A careful initial interview ensures that the dentist becomes familiar with the patient's health history and is primed to look for signs of any reported diseases or conditions during the examination. Box 18.1 provides a list of oral problems more common among older patients. Procedures for the oral examination and radiographic selection criteria are the same for older patients as for any adult patient, but certain aspects of the examination are more important for this group.

BOX 18.1 Common Oral Problems in Older Adults by Disease Category

Medication-Related Problems
Xerostomia (medication or radiation induced)
Gingival hyperplasia (mediation induced)

Infectious Conditions
Caries
Periodontal disease
Oral Candidiasis

Inflammatory Conditions
Sjögren's syndrome
Pemphigoid
Lichen planus

Neoplastic Disease
Oral cancer
Oral complications of cancer therapy

TABLE 18.3 Pre-Procedural Pain Assessment Checklist

Evaluate medical diagnoses that would affect patient's postprocedural acute pain	☐ Medical DX, which might increasepostprocedural acute pain:
Evaluate current medications for potential adverse drug interactions	☐ Potential druginteractions noted:
Evaluate psychiatric diagnoses that would affect patient's postprocedural acute pain	☐ Mental health DX whichmight increase acute pain:
Current or past abuse of drugs or alcohol	Drug abuse (other than opioids): ☐ Current ☐ Past Opioid Abuse: ☐ Current ☐ Past Alcohol abuse: ☐ Current ☐ Past
Use of opioids for chronic pain management	☐ Current If current, list type and dosage: ☐ Past
Provider responsible for pain contract or chronic pain management	☐ Provider and contact info: OR ☐ n/a
Does the patient have any other pain management strategies they are currently using (e.g., nonmedication strategies or daily over-the-counter medications)?	☐ Nonmedication strategies patient uses for chronic pain control: ☐ Current over-the-counter medication strategies patient uses for chronic pain control:

Preoperative Dental Pain Score (use Pain Numeric Rating Scale)	Score: 0 1 2 3 4 5 6 7
	         8 9 10
	         No pain **Worst pain imaginable**

Preoperative General Pain Score (use Pain Numeric Rating Scale)	Score: 0 1 2 3 4 5 6 7
	         8 9 10
	         No pain **Worst pain imaginable**

Preoperative pain management education completed with patient	☐ Yes ☐ No

Document positive findings in column 2.

Reprinted from Wehler CJ, Panchal NH, Cotchery DL, 3rd, et al. Alternatives to opioids for acute pain management after dental procedures: A Department of Veterans Affairs consensus paper. *J Am Dent Assoc* 2021;152(8):641–652.

A complete oral examination requires a thorough evaluation of both extraoral and intraoral structures. Because skin cancer is more prevalent in the older population, the examination must always include evaluation of the face, neck, and all exposed skin surfaces. Important findings include basal cell carcinomas or melanomas of the skin; or solar cheilosis, carcinoma in situ, or squamous cell carcinoma of the lower lip.

Oral cancer is predominantly a disorder of the elderly, with the median age of diagnosis at 64 years.[19] Currently, oral cancer accounts for 2.8% of all new cases and 1.8% of all cancer deaths. Unfortunately, the incidence of oral and pharyngeal cancer is on the rise for both men and women over the past few years.[20] Because other smoking-related cancers are decreasing, this increase might be attributable to cases related to the HPV virus. Therefore it is important to monitor older adults carefully and frequently for signs of such disease.

Radiographic examinations can show evidence of osteoporosis and panoramic images can reveal carotid calcifications—both abnormalities more common in the elderly.

Part of the oral examination should include a thorough evaluation of salivary function. Salivary gland dysfunction is more common in seniors than in younger patients. Signs of chronic xerostomia include a desiccated mucosa; a red, fissured, denuded, or shiny tongue; caries around the gingival margins and cusps of teeth; demineralization around the gingival margins, even without obvious caries; bubbly saliva; frequency of soft tissue trauma; and adherence of a gloved finger or mouth mirror to the buccal mucosa. Salivary glands should always be palpated extraorally while viewing the duct to make sure an adequate flow of saliva occurs when the glands are massaged.[21] Patients should also be questioned about any history of pain or swelling in the glandular areas that could indicate infection, blockage, or neoplasm.

Risk Assessment

As James Beck has noted, the relative importance of risk factors changes as people age.[22] For older adults, systemic disease and medications play a far greater role in oral health than is true of younger adults. A key to geriatric treatment planning is understanding the concept of multimorbidity, the progression of chronic diseases. **Frailty** is defined as increased vulnerability as a result of a decline in the individual's reserve capacity. In the dental setting, frailty means that the patient's ability to access dental care, tolerate dental procedures, and manage the home care required after treatment may all be compromised. One surrogate for frailty is the patient's level of dependency. Using previous systemic definitions of dependency, a large group of geriatric dentists from around the world developed and published a list of five levels of dependency to help the dentist determine the appropriate clinical pathway or necessary care modifications for geriatric patients.[23] These ranged from no dependency, which requires really no change in care decisions, through pre, low, medium, or high dependency. As the level of dependency rises, the modifications that must be considered in assessment, prevention, and even communication will also rise.

Frail elderly patients, in particular, are much more susceptible to a full range of oral health disorders. In the presence of diminished mental capacity, a weakened physical condition, poor nutritional intake, dehydration, need for a soft diet, and inability to engage in effective oral self-care and other activities of daily living (ADL), these patients are much more vulnerable to the ravages of caries, periodontal disease, and other forms of oral pathology.

When assessing the risk of oral disease associated with frailty and dependency, there are several assessments that clinicians may find beneficial. The traditional caries risk assessment (see Chapter 3) can be beneficial when assessing caries in older adults and uses risk groups of high, moderate, and low to describe a patient's specific risk. The Rapid Oral Health Deterioration (ROHD) risk assessment is another assessment tool that builds on the traditional caries risk assessment by relating future risk of oral disease based on the patient's general and physical health with particular focus conditions that cause progressive cognitive or functional decline and the current level of oral disease present in the mouth. The ROHD assessment was developed to identify quickly those individuals who are at risk of frailty with the goal of establishing adequate preventive recommendations early before the progression of oral disease can take hold.[24] In Japan, researchers introduced the term oral frailty to describe poor oral health in older adults who are experiencing adverse health outcomes, including overall frailty, long-term care needs, and individuals at risk of premature mortality among community-dwelling older adults. This includes an oral frailty screening questionnaire that assesses older adults' tooth loss, poor oral function, oral health-related behaviors, and declining social participation in order to identify individuals at risk of poor oral health and in need of oral care with a dental professional.[25]

For periodontal disease, clinicians often use the 2018 guidelines for the classification of periodontal and peri-implant diseases and conditions to assess a patient's periodontal disease. However, establishing risk and prognosis often becomes increasingly challenging in older adult patients because dentists often have to consider the additional risks associated with oral systemic link, quality of life, and maintenance of functional status especially when patients systemic diseases make adaptation to complete dentures challenging.

When evaluating older adults, it is important to look beyond the traditional risk assessments for oral diseases and also predict a patient's risk of oral health decline based on a patient's predicted end of life trajectory. When categorizing patients at the end of life, patients can be grouped into three categories based on functional decline in the last several years prior to death and the associated common oral conditions prior to death. These categories include: (1) older adults who die suddenly. This group experiences little to no functional or oral health decline toward the end of life. (2) Older adults diagnosed with a terminal illness. These patients can experience some functional decline, which can be minimal to severe depending on the time remaining to death, and can experience oral conditions such as xerostomia, mucositis, stomatitis, oral soft tissue pathology, and again pending the time until death possibly increased dental caries, oral pain, and tooth loss. (3) Older adults with progressive functional disability. This group includes patients experiencing organ failure and/or frailty, which results in a functional decline that can last several years before death. Often in this group patients can experience changes in oral hygiene, increased dental caries, dental pain and infection, decreased chewing function, xerostomia, and oral soft tissue pathology.[26] For patients with terminal illness and progressive functional loss, it is important to provide stage appropriate treatment strategies as shown in Table 18.4. By understanding these categories and the associated oral conditions, dentists can begin to provide recommendations and treatment options that will address the patient's present needs, institute prevention recommendations early, and assist in treatment planning for the future.

Identifying Health Problems That May Affect Dental Treatment

As described earlier, there is an intimate relationship between oral and systemic health. Treatment planning must therefore include an assessment of any chronic conditions and the likelihood that such conditions will increase the patient's risk of oral disease. For example, a systemic disease that compromises the immune system may result in a *Candida* infection in the oral cavity. Patients with chronic gastrointestinal problems may have a lower oral pH because of constant acid reflux, leading to increased risk of oral disease or an unusual pattern of oral disease (Figure. 18.2). Each time an older patient's health history is reviewed, the dentist must consider what effect any new illness may have on the patient's oral cavity.

Box 18.2 lists the most likely chronic conditions with which an older patient will present to an examining dentist, many of which can have a direct effect on oral health and dental care. Arthritis may affect an individual's ability to perform daily brushing or flossing. Patients with uncontrolled diabetes are more prone to severe periodontal disease.

Because senior patients are more likely to be taking medications, they are also more likely to develop medication-related oral changes. Patients taking medications for high blood pressure, depression, or antipsychotic disorders may suffer from dry

mouth. An online medication database (examples: *Mosby's Dental Drug Reference* and *Lexicomp Online for Dentistry*) can be used by the dental team to identify the oral side effects of medications and a printout of that information can be given to the patient.

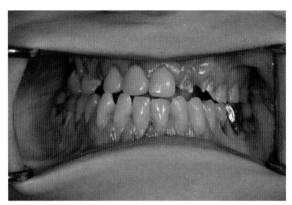

Fig. 18.2 Patient with oral problems caused by severe acid reflux. The effect of systemic disease can be devastating to the oral cavity. This patient, who was diagnosed with severe gastroesophageal reflux, exhibits a high caries rate around the gum line and on the cusps because of the low pH in the oral cavity.

BOX 18.2 Top 10 Chronic Conditions in Older Adults

High blood pressure
High cholesterol
Ischemic heart disease
Arthritis
Diabetes
Heart failure
Chronic kidney disease
Depression
Chronic obstructive pulmonary disease
Alzheimer's disease and dementia

From Center for Medicare and Medicaid Services: Chronic conditions among Medicare beneficiaries chartbook: 2018 Edition.

TABLE 18.4 Stage Appropriate Dental Care for Patients with Terminal Illness or Progressive Functional Disability

Stage	Decline Stage	Preactive Dying Stage	Actively Dying Stage	
Duration	------------>Years — Months	------------>Months — Weeks	------------>Weeks — Days	Death
Major Oral Health Problems	• Xerostomia • Loss of oral function • Oral infection • Oral pain	• Xerostomia • Oral infection • Oral pain	• Xerostomia • Oral infection • Oral pain	
Treatment Goals	• Improve quality of life • Maintain function and nutrition • Prevent pain and infection • Prevent systemic complications of oral disease • Meet personal needs	• Improve comfort • Manage oral pain • Control infection	• Improve comfort • Manage oral pain	
Approach	• May consider in-office treatment if tolerant • Cautious with invasive procedures • Avoid aggressive, intensive treatment	• Bedside management • Avoid in-office treatment • Avoid invasive procedures	• Bedside comfort care	

Reprinted from Chen X, Kistler CE. Oral health care for older adults with serious illness: when and how? *J Am Geriatr Soc* 2015;63(2):375–378.

TABLE 18.5	Possible Adverse Drug Reactions and Drug–Drug Interactions	
Drug or Drug Class	**Possible Adverse Drug Reaction or Interaction**
Aspirin	May reduce platelet aggregation or increase warfarin levels, resulting in possible excessive bleeding
Antibiotics (long-term 7 days or more)	May reduce intrinsic intestinal bacteria levels with resultant reduced absorption of vitamin K; may increase warfarin levels, resulting in a deficiency of certain clotting factors
Anticoagulants	Excessive bleeding, especially with periodontal disease
Bisphosphonates	Risk of osteonecrosis of the jaw
Benzodiazepines	Taken with other CNS depressants (codeine, alcohol, antihistamines), can cause excessive CNS depression, sedation, respiratory depression, and loss of consciousness
Narcotics	Nausea, constipation, risk of falls
Nonsteroidal anti-inflammatory drugs	May increase warfarin levels, resulting in excessive bleeding; may reduce effects of hypertension medications
Warfarin	Reduction of production of vitamin K clotting factors; risk of excessive bleeding

Adapted from Hersh EV, Moore PA. Adverse drug reactions in dentistry. *Periodontol.* 2000;46:109–142.

As more medications are taken, the potential for drug–drug interactions increases. It is estimated that 50% of patients taking at least four medications will have some type of drug–drug interaction. Qato and colleagues[27] concluded that approximately one in every 25 older adults was taking concurrent drugs with the potential for harm from serious drug–drug interactions. A significant portion of these interactions occurs with antibiotics, analgesics, and sedatives—medications that are all commonly prescribed by dentists. Most side effects and interactions are mild and many go unnoticed. Nevertheless, it is important for the clinician to be alert to the possibility of this type of problem. Table 18.5 lists some of the common adverse drug reactions and drug–drug interactions that may impact on the patient's oral health or treatment in the dental setting.

Need for Antibiotic Premedication

Treatment planning and pretreatment evaluation of any patient requires the dentist to assess the need for antibiotic premedication. Antibiotic premedication is utilized in dentistry to reduce the likelihood of either systemic or local post-surgical infections. Guidelines for reducing the risk of systemic infections, such as viridans group streptococcal (VGS) infective endocarditis (IE), or infections around prosthetic joints are fairly succinct. More than one-half of all cases of infective endocarditis in the United States occur in persons older than 60 years and 42% of institutionalized elderly may have at least one cardiac risk factor for infective endocarditis.[28,29] The American Heart Association's

(AHA) 2021 update to the 2007 statement regarding prevention of VGS IE kept the same categories of highest risk patients who required antibiotic premedication prior to invasive dental procedures, but also added conditions that do not require premedication (See Box 8.4).[30]

For those highest risk patients, the AHA Guidelines recommend the use of antibiotic premedication 30–60 minutes before any dental procedures that include tissue manipulation. One of the changes in 2021 is the removal of clindamycin as a prescription choice for penicillin allergic patients. Because of the higher risk of adverse drug effects including *Clostridioides difficile* infection, which can lead to hospitalization and death, the newer guidelines no longer recommend prescribing clindamycin prior to dental appointments. The updated drug regimen can be found in Table 8.5.[30]

Both the American Dental Association (ADA) and the American Academy of Orthopedic Surgeons (AAOS) provide documents stating there are very limited circumstances where a patient with a prosthetic joint will require antibiotic premedication. The ADA recommendations state, "in general, for patients with prosthetic joint implants, prophylactic antibiotics are not recommended prior to dental procedures to prevent prosthetic joint infection. The evidence showing the benefits of this prophylactic treatment is not strong and these benefits may not exceed the potential harms, such as antibiotic resistance and opportunistic infections, such as *Clostridioides difficile*."[31] In general, older patients will carry a higher burden of poor systemic health. For patients who have issues that put them at higher risk of prosthetic joint failure, the AAOS has developed an online Appropriate Use Criteria tool that allows you to answer several questions related to your patient's health history and see whether antibiotic premedication is recommended prior to a patient's invasive dental care. This tool can be accessed at OrthoGuidelines. (See *Suggested Readings and Resources* at the end of this chapter.) In general, the questions will focus on the patient's immunocompromised status, diabetic condition and control, history of a previous prosthetic joint infection and timing since the joint was replaced. There are few situations where either group would recommend premedication for prosthetic joint patients. If either the patient or the orthopedic surgeon request antibiotic premedication when a patient does not meet the Appropriate Use Criteria, it is suggested that you request the orthopedic surgeon to provide the prescription for the premedication.

Bacteremias occur on a daily basis as a result of normal activities, such as tooth brushing or chewing when a patient has poor oral health. For this reason, the latest AHA guidelines for VGS IE have a powerful statement that the best way to prevent systemic infections caused by oral issues is to help assure good oral health and access to oral healthcare for patients who are at highest risk of systemic infections.[30]

As stated at the beginning of this section, antibiotic prophylaxis is also used prior to, or on the day of invasive surgeries such as surgical extractions, implant placement, or periodontal surgery to prevent a localized postoperative infection. The use of antibiotics for these purposes carries the same risks as noted earlier when used to prevent systemic infections, but the literature supporting their use is not nearly as clear. A 2021 Cochrane Review found low certainty evidence that prophylactic antibiotics prior to surgical extractions may reduce the risk of postoperative infection. Unfortunately, there was no evidence to judge the effects of preventive antibiotics for extractions due to severe decay or periodontal disease or in patients who are medically compromised.[32] There is also a 2013 Cochrane Review that looked at the benefit of antibiotic prophylaxis prior to implant placement. This review found antibiotics were beneficial in reducing implant failures and suggested a single dose much like the IE recommendations 1 hour prior to the surgery. However, they note that antibiotics would need to be given to 25 patients undergoing surgery to avoid 1 person experiencing the loss of an implant, suggesting that this also raises the risk of adverse events from antibiotics.[33] More definitive guidelines regarding antibiotic prophylaxis to prevent postoperative localized infections are desperately needed for practitioners. Until that time, consider issues such as immunosuppression, diabetic control, and ability to care for the wound postsurgery when deciding whether premedication is necessary and have an open discussion with the patient regarding the risks and benefits of antibiotics in these situations.

SYSTEMIC PHASE DENTAL TREATMENT PLANNING

Links Between Oral Infection, Chronic Inflammation, and Systemic Diseases

Research has shown that oral diseases, particularly periodontal (gum) disease, can affect systemic health through the mechanisms of chronic inflammation.[19] CDC estimates that more than 45% of all US adults over the age of 30 years (64.7 million) have periodontal disease. Of these, 30% have moderate periodontitis and 8.5% have severe periodontitis.[34] Smoking, genetics, malnutrition, systemic disease, and local factors can contribute to patients developing gum disease. With more than 45% of US adults having periodontal disease, it is estimated that periodontal disease is the number one cause of inflammation in the body.[34]

Studies from mice to humans implicate inflammation and oxidative stress in the mechanism linking obesity and cardiovascular risk.[35] Obesity affects roughly 42% of US adults[36] and contributes to metabolic disorders such as diabetes mellitus (DM) type II. Research has shown a two-way relationship between DM and periodontal disease. Diabetic patients who had their periodontal disease treated showed improved blood glucose control and patients with well-controlled DM showed improved periodontal health.[37] With obesity affecting 42% of the US population, it is now the second most common cause of inflammation in the United States.

Regardless of the cause of chronic inflammation whether periodontal disease, obesity, diabetes mellitus, or a combination, it contributes to cardiovascular disease, which remains the leading cause of death in older adults in the United States.[38] Research by Bale, Doneen and Vigerust reports that high-risk periodontal pathogens are a contributory cause of the pathogenesis of atherosclerosis.[39]

Periodontal pathogens also contribute to chronic inflammation through oral infections. A study by Konig et al. reported on the role that *Aa*, a periodontal pathogen, plays in linking periodontal infection to autoimmunity in rheumatoid arthritis.[40] A follow-up editorial suggested that to "prevent rheumatoid arthritis, look past the joints to the gums."[41]

A study by Dominy et al. demonstrated that *Porphyromonas gingivalis* (PG), a key periodontal pathogen, was recently identified in the brain of Alzheimer's patients.[42] The article identified that the toxic proteases from PG, called gingipains, were also identified in the brain. The levels of the proteases correlated with brain pathology. The study further demonstrated that gingipain inhibitors reduced the PG brain infection and neuroinflammation, suggesting that effective management of periodontal disease may be helpful in preventing neurodegeneration in Alzheimer's disease.

By understanding the role of oral infections and chronic inflammation, clinicians can develop preventive strategies for patients, which include smoking cessation, blood pressure control, oral self-care, and treatment for periodontal disease to decrease pathogenic bacteria and reduce inflammation.

The leading causes of death in US adults older than age 65 include heart disease, cancer, stroke, and Alzheimer's disease. In 2020, COVID-19 was among the top three causes of death in the US population overall. Approximately four of five patients older than age 65 who present for oral healthcare suffer from at least one chronic systemic condition. The following sections include brief discussions of the more common chronic systemic diseases and their potential impact on the dental treatment plan and the way oral health care is delivered to the patient.

Cardiac Disease

Cardiac conditions are not only the most common type of chronic disease among seniors but also the most likely to be the cause of death. The standard of care requires an initial assessment of the patient's blood pressure in the dental office to evaluate for **hypertension**. Stage 1 hypertension is defined as a blood pressure reading greater than 130/80. With the most recent hypertension guidelines, a systolic blood pressure of 120 to 129 or diastolic blood pressure more than 80 is classified as elevated blood pressure.[43] A discussion of blood pressure measurement and implications for referral is presented in Chapter 1. Often, individuals are unaware of the gradual onset of hypertension and several studies have shown that with a large number of people, this condition may not be well controlled. Every older patient's blood pressure should be checked at each visit. A preoperative blood pressure reading is mandatory if a scheduled procedure can be anticipated as stressful, or if the patient has a known history of hypertension, or if drugs such as a local anesthetic will be administered.

Congestive heart failure (CHF), in simplest terms, is failure of the heart to pump blood adequately. This condition has various causes and varying degrees of severity. An affirmative answer to any of the following questions signals that the patient's condition warrants special consideration.

- Do you become out of breath easily while walking or performing light household chores?
- Do you need to rest if you are climbing even one flight of stairs?
- Do you have trouble breathing at night or need to prop yourself up in the bed to sleep?

For patients with CHF, adaptations in treatment planning and the provision of dental care will commonly include strategies to maintain comfort during treatment and reduce stress. The patient may be unable to tolerate a reclining position in the dental chair. Appointments should be kept relatively short and a particular effort should be made to control anxiety. Supplemental oxygen must be available in preparation for a possible medical emergency.

Coronary artery disease results from the development of atherosclerotic lesions affecting the blood supply to cardiac muscle. The onset is usually slow and may go unnoticed until it becomes severe enough to cause an episode of pain or discomfort. Coronary artery disease can lead to **angina, myocardial infarction (MI)**, or sudden death. Patients who present with a diagnosis of angina should be assessed during treatment planning to determine the severity of their disease. Does the patient experience angina during times of rest or only in times of activity? The frequency of use of nitroglycerin tablets and the size of doses used will provide clues about the stability of the condition. The patient should be reminded to bring this medication to each appointment. Anginal pain sometimes radiates to the jaw and on occasion will produce the sensation of a toothache. When the patient reports pain radiating from the neck to the lower angle of the jaw or lower jaw pain for which the dentist cannot discern a dental or oral source, the possibility of a cardiac problem should be included in the differential diagnosis.

More worrisome in the aging population is the frequent absence of pain during an MI. Studies of nursing home residents found that, unlike younger adults, more than 50% did not experience pain during an MI (referred to as a "silent" MI). In some instances, minimal symptoms such as hiccups were the only sign of an MI. Current research has shown that although heart disease is the number-one killer of older women, symptoms of cardiac disease often go unrecognized in women and the disease tends to be treated less aggressively than it is in men.

When considering when to have patients resume dental treatment after an MI, it is important to note dental procedures are considered minor surgical procedures and have a low cardiac risk. However, most authorities suggest that patients should not undergo elective outpatient dental care until at least 4–6 weeks after an MI to allow time for a post infarction scar to form, to create collateral circulation, and to restore contractility of damaged myocardium.[44,45] After any severe systemic episode, consultation with the patient's physician can provide the most appropriate way to determine when the patient is ready to undergo dental treatment. The physician's response should be documented in the patient's record.

Neurologic Disorders

Neurologic disorders encompass abnormalities of the brain or nervous system. Neurologic diseases can cause sensory or motor neuron impairment. Diseases with motor impairments, such as multiple sclerosis, amyotrophic lateral sclerosis, or stroke with hemiparesis, will make getting in and out of the dental office and operatory more difficult. Neurologic diseases can also affect speech and/or memory loss or cause other cognitive decline. Patients with dementia, stroke, or Parkinson's disease may have difficulty understanding the dental treatment plan and communicating their acceptance of the treatment plan. Patients with these diseases may require assistance from a family member to help them understand the required treatment and making the decision to accept treatment.

In older patients, acute situations such as infections or medication side effects can also cause a state of confusion, which is typically temporary and can be managed without complication. In the dental setting, it is important to keep this in mind if an older patient presents with an acute oral infection *and* an obvious change in cognitive function.

Alzheimer's Disease

Alzheimer's disease (AD) is marked by a loss of cognitive function in the affected person. One in nine individuals older than 65 years currently has AD in the United States and with the increased number of aging individuals in the population, this number can be expected to rise rapidly. Women with AD outnumber men 2:1, and older African-Americans and Hispanics are disproportionately more likely to have the disease.[46] The two main risk factors are age over 65 years and a genetic predisposition.

Dental treatment planning for patients with AD must take into account the following issues[47]:

- *Stage and trajectory of AD*. When dental treatment planning and treatment are undertaken in the earliest stage of the disease, the dentist is afforded the opportunity for long-range planning. The dentist, patient, and caregiver all need to recognize that invasive treatment will be easiest at this stage. It must be anticipated that the patient will, over time, have a diminished capacity to undergo treatment and perform effective oral home care. It should be assumed that eventually the teeth, periodontium, and any restorations or prostheses would have to be cleaned and maintained by a caregiver. Therefore, if needed, consider recommendations for treatment that involves simple, prostheses that are easy to insert and remove, easy to clean, require minimal maintenance, are relatively caries and periodontal disease resistant, and have a good long-term prognosis. This often means recommending a removable rather than a fixed prosthesis, if the latter would include crowns or bridges that require meticulous home care.

The patient's ability to cooperate during dental care in the midstages of AD is unpredictable. Appointments should be short and midmorning versus later afternoon is better to avoid "sun downing" or increased agitation as the day wears on. Treatment options should focus on maintaining or improving the patient's quality of life, which often means ensuring that the individual is free from pain and infection and can chew as well as possible.

In the final stages of AD, patients may no longer be able to voice their oral health concerns. This will necessitate a scheduled dental evaluation with a caregiver or family member at regular intervals to make sure any potential problems are identified and addressed early. Treatment planning at this stage of AD will focus primarily on relief of pain.

- *Caries risk.* For patients with AD, oral care becomes more difficult to perform and/or provide as the disease progresses. At the same time, AD patients often have an increased appetite for foods and beverages containing high amounts of refined sugar. Because eating is a function that many AD patients still enjoy, caregivers often make these foods available for consumption throughout the day. Although few of us would have the heart to remove this pleasure, one option may be to suggest that the caregiver/long-term care staff dispense this type of food only two to three times per day and that the patient be encouraged to drink water afterward to help reduce the length of the acidic assault on any remaining dentition.

Parkinson's Disease

Parkinson's disease (PD) is a chronic disorder that progresses slowly. Approximately 1% of persons between the ages of 50 and 65 years develop Parkinson's. The disease affects the nerve cells in the midbrain that control body movement. Movements become jerky and the individual develops a shuffling gait, along with a resting tremor. In the later stages, the voice is often reduced to a whisper, swallowing problems occur, and the face takes on a masklike appearance as the body becomes increasingly rigid. When treatment planning dental care for patients with PD, it is helpful to keep the following issues in mind:

- *Stage and trajectory of the disease.* Like AD, PD is a condition that will worsen with time. Although there are treatments to limit the effects of the disease, there is no cure for it. It will be imperative that, for all treatment options weighed, post-delivery care be taken into consideration. Patients with PD will have periods in which they have difficulty using their hands to manipulate a toothbrush and, as with AD, there will probably come a time when the dental team will need to train a caregiver in daily oral care for the PD patient. An electric toothbrush, two-times daily use of a prescription fluoride toothpaste, and interproximal cleaning aids are frequently recommended for such patients.
- *Swallowing disorders and compliance during dental visits.* Patients in the later stages of PD may exhibit reduced swallowing ability or dysphagia. No treatment should begin until the dentist has established whether this is an issue for the patient. Treatment planning can accommodate the condition if required. Strategies for treatment decisions involving dysphagia are shown in Box 18.3. Use of a rubber dam may be helpful during dental treatment if the patient has a swallowing disorder. Timing treatment to occur approximately 1 hour after the patient has taken an antiparkinson medication may be helpful. Midmorning appointments and shorter appointments can be more accommodating for PD patients. Bite blocks can help reduce tremors with the mandible allowing for better patient comfort and compliance during dental treatment. In addition, if treatment is planned on both arches at the same visit, it is recommended to start on the lower arch since muscles of mastication may fatigue and tremors with the mandible worsen later in the appointment.
- *Understanding the effect medications may have on both PD and the oral cavity.* Medications prescribed for the disease, such as L-dopa, may become ineffective over time, allowing the physical symptoms to worsen. In addition, medications for this disease are often associated with dry mouth, which, if not managed effectively, can have devastating oral consequences.

Respiratory Illness

Chronic obstructive pulmonary disease (COPD) is a chronic respiratory disease that makes emptying the lungs progressively more difficult and can be associated with mucus production, cough, wheezing, and breathlessness. COPD is estimated to affect between 12% and 32% of elderly adults worldwide, which is higher than any other age group.[48] As dentists work within the respiratory system, it is important to facilitate an open airway and ease of breathing while completing dental work. With severe cases of COPD, dentists may have to avoid the supine position, avoid or limit use of rubber dams, and avoid use of nitrous oxide.[49]

Aspiration pneumonia is another respiratory illness occurring primarily in older adults. It is associated with significant morbidity and mortality especially in frail and dependent older adults. Aspiration pneumonia occurs when foreign material (food debris, saliva, and oral biofilm) descend into the lungs causing pneumonia. With age and functional decline, the body's protective mechanisms including ciliary movement, coughing reflex, and immune response become impaired. Additionally, certain conditions can increase the risk of developing aspiration pneumonia. These include lung diseases, dysphagia, diabetes mellitus, severe dementia, malnutrition, and Parkinson's disease. Poor oral health has also been linked to aspiration pneumonia, and studies have also shown that good oral hygiene can reduce the risk of occurrence. No specific oral health interventions have proved more efficacious than others, but it is currently recommended that oral care include tooth brushing after each meal, cleaning dentures daily, and frequent professional oral health care.[50]

BOX 18.3 Treatment Recommendations for Patients With Dysphagia

Use a minimum volume of oral irrigation. A dental assistant should always be available to provide diligent suction if water is required during treatment.

Keep the patient in an upright position during treatment to reduce the risk of aspiration.

Use a pretreatment antimicrobial rinse, such as chlorhexidine gluconate, to reduce the oral flora as much as possible in the event a small amount of aspirated fluid reaches the patient's respiratory system.

Allow frequent breaks during treatment and encourage the patient to cough or clear the throat.

Avoid use of an ultrasonic scaler to prevent generating an oral aerosol.

Use a slow-speed handpiece to the extent possible rather than high speed with aerosol.

If possible, use a rubber dam during restorative procedures.

In 2020, the world experienced a new deadly virus previously unseen, **COVID-19**. This respiratory disease was transmitted fairly easily by respiratory droplets. It has affected over 192 million people resulting in over 4.1 million deaths (as of July 2021). This respiratory illness, like the flu, disproportionately affected adults over the age of 65 years and members of racial and ethnic minority groups including Hispanic or Latino and non-Hispanic Black populations. The risk of requiring hospitalization, intensive care, or a ventilator to assist with breathing increases for older adults in their 60 s, 70 s, and 80 s with people aged 85 years and older being the most likely to require these services. More than 80% of the deaths associated with COVID-19 occur in older adults over the age of 65 years. Additionally, older adults with certain medical conditions are at an increased risk of morbidity and mortality associated with COVID-19. These conditions include diabetes, cancer, chronic kidney disease, chronic respiratory diseases (COPD), dementia, heart conditions (heart failure, coronary artery disease, and cardiomyopathy), liver disease, history of cerebrovascular disease, and autoimmune diseases.[51]

Older adults living in long-term care facilities were particularly affected during the pandemic. Given the congregate nature of the facilities and a resident population that includes older adults with underlying chronic medical conditions, long-term care facility residents are at high risk of the morbidity and mortality associated with COVID-19.[51] During the pandemic, facilities instituted visitor and travel restrictions for residents, which isolated these individuals from their families and the general public and prevented many from obtaining dental services during this time. The extent to which the pandemic has impacted the oral health of both older adults and long-term care residents is still not fully known. However, with the introduction of COVID vaccines, older adults who are fully vaccinated have shown a 94% reduction in risk of COVID-19 hospitalizations.[51] This has allowed many of these previously isolated individuals to reenter society and resume dental services.

Cerebrovascular Accident

Cerebrovascular accident (CVA), or stroke, is a leading cause of death and a major cause of disability among persons older than 65 years. A stroke is defined as the sudden onset of a neurologic deficit. In approximately 80% of cases, the deficit results from an ischemic event—that is, a blockage of blood flow to the brain. Risk factors include hypertension and a previous history of a stroke, or ministrokes, known as **transient ischemic attacks (TIAs)**. Stroke is the leading cause of long-term disability in the United States. Fourteen percent of those who survive a first stroke or TIA will have another within 1 year.[49]

For those who survive a stroke, the effects can be both devastating and long-lasting. The residual functional effects in the extremities can result in an increase in oral disease and any previous levels of oral dysfunction may be intensified. Oral hygiene is often impaired following a stroke as a result of residual functional impairment and dental treatment and maintenance becomes increasingly important to maintain oral hygiene and prevent oral diseases. There is no definitive guidance on a time frame for beginning elective dental treatment following a stroke. The American Heart Association's perioperative care guidelines consider minor surgical procedures including those performed with local anesthesia to be associated with a low risk of complications for vascular events.[52] A consult with the patient's physician is the optimal way to assess when the individual is ready to undergo dental care. Such consultation can provide the dentist with information about the patient's rehabilitation and help frame a timetable for resumption of urgent and definitive dental treatment.

Muscle weakness often follows a stroke and may affect the muscles in and around the oral cavity. If the facial nerve is involved, the muscles of facial expression may be impaired. An affected trigeminal nerve results in weakness in the muscles of mastication, causing pouching or food packing in the oral cavity. In addition, a stroke patient may lose the ability to clear food with the tongue on the affected side. As a result, heavy debris may build up on the affected side, resulting in an oral environment susceptible to bacterial overgrowth (Figure. 18.3). When considering replacement of a removable prosthesis, delaying until maximum muscle strength has returned will help ensure a better fit.

Patients may come in for dental treatment before the completion of rehabilitation. For these patients, the primary goals of an interim treatment plan are to help maintain the ability to consume a healthy diet and to ensure prevention of oral infection and pain. The following are common strategies:

- If an existing removable prosthesis no longer fits well, tissue conditioning or a temporary reline may provide a better fit and improve comfort. Often, the patient complains that a denture fit well before the stroke but is now unusable. The most likely explanation is loss of control of oral muscles that before the illness had helped retain marginally fitting dentures.
- If the patient has lost some or all use of the dominant hand, provide both patient and caregiver with instruction in modified oral home care techniques.

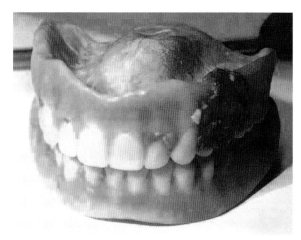

Fig. 18.3 Food packing on the denture of a stroke patient. Post-stroke patients may exhibit areas of food packing around the buccal surfaces of the affected side. (Courtesy Dr. Gretchen Gibson.)

- Prescribe an antimicrobial rinse for use during the first few months to mitigate periodontal disease, prevent oral infection, and promote a healthy oral environment.
- Instruct the patient to rinse after each meal to clear any food and debris that may result from pouching.

Two other important after-effects of stroke, **aphasia** and **dysphagia**, must be considered when providing a dental treatment plan for the post-CVA patient. Aphasia is defined as a deficiency in the ability to understand or communicate the spoken or written word. Dysphagia involves difficulty in swallowing and may be indicative of damage to the 9th, 10th, and/or 12th cranial nerve. Strategies for planning treatment for patients with either of these disabilities are discussed in Boxes 18.3 and 18.4.

Post stroke patients benefit from an interdisciplinary approach to treatment planning (see Chapter 6). The dentist should not hesitate to confer with the physician and any rehabilitation therapists to determine when the patient has achieved the maximum level of rehabilitation possible. The speech pathologist may be able to provide information about a swallowing or speech disorder after a stroke and may provide suggestions on how best to communicate with the patient.

Late-Life Depression

The elderly experience many types of loss, which naturally may elicit sadness. When this sadness persists beyond a normal time period for grieving, the condition may be defined as late-life depression. Common among seniors, depression, unfortunately, is underdiagnosed in many primary care settings. Although the rate of depression among all age groups is approximately 18%, at least 20% of those older than 65 years suffer from this affective disorder. Because dental professionals often schedule longer clinical visits with patients than do physicians, they may be the first to recognize depression. As a result, taking note of changes in the patient's attitudes and demeanor that could represent symptoms of depression and making appropriate referrals become critical responsibilities. In general terms, seniors suffering from depression may resist comforting, display irritability, and express feelings of hopelessness, low self-esteem, and guilt. Suicide is one of the most devastating results of depression. The rate of lethal suicide attempts among the elderly is higher than in any other age group.[53] In the United States, elderly white men are at the greatest risk of suicide and the elderly in general are the most likely population group to follow through with a suicide attempt.[54,55] Fortunately, depression is treatable and appropriate referrals may be lifesaving.

During the diagnosis and treatment planning process and in the course of delivering dental care, the dental team must be able to recognize clinical depression and be prepared to use strategies to mitigate its effect. Because dental treatment can result in positive changes that are visible to the patient, the prospect of improved oral health and appearance can sometimes act as an incentive for the patient to comply with treatment recommendations. In some cases, it can also become an antidote to the depression. In instances of severe depression, however, it may be appropriate simply to strive to maintain the patient's current level of oral health, postponing more aggressive treatment until the depression has lifted.

Oral Cancer and Other Malignant Neoplasms

Oral cancer causes high morbidity and mortality in older adults. The treatment and resulting oral disabilities are devastating and 60% of patients with diagnosed oral cancer survive for 5 years. This 5-year survival rate has steadily improved since 1975.[56] Like most cancers, survival rates are linked to stage of disease at the time of diagnosis. Lip cancers have the best survival rates because they are more readily seen and diagnosed. Most oral cancers (90%) are squamous cell carcinoma (SCC), and the average age at diagnosis is approximately 60 years, making this an important issue in the geriatric population.

Twenty-five percent of oral cancer lesions are not associated with the typical risk factors of tobacco and alcohol. Research on risk factors is demonstrating important new information about the link between SCC and human papillomavirus (HPV). Cleveland et al. note that HPV-associated oropharyngeal cancers are increasing, whereas other head and neck cancers are decreasing.[57] HPV-positive lesions appear to have a better prognosis than those that are negative.

Because the prognosis depends on the stage of the malignancy at the time of diagnosis, early detection represents the most significant contribution the dentist can make in the treatment of oral cancer. Although, like skin, the oral cavity provides an easily accessible site for identification of a cancerous lesion, oral cancers are often not diagnosed until the lesion is quite large and has metastasized to the lymph nodes or other regions.

Oral cancer lesions are believed to occur most often in areas of frequent trauma and where saliva pools. Common sites include the lateral border of the tongue, the floor of the mouth, the retromolar area, and the soft palate. Having the patient fully extend the tongue, grasping it with gauze, and viewing the posterior lateral borders is an essential component of an oral soft tissue

BOX 18.4 Communication Recommendations for Patients With Aphasia

Keep questions and instructions simple, addressing only one task or topic at a time.

Begin the session with two or three yes-or-no questions to which you know the answer. This will allow you to assess whether the patient is able to respond appropriately. If they can answer with an appropriate head nod, phrase questions in the yes-or-no format.

Give the aphasic patient extra time to respond, but do not persist if they cannot respond. A different form of communication, such as writing, may be an option. If the patient tries to speak but cannot, ask whether written responses can be made.

Do not overreact if the patient swears or cries. These responses are common after a stroke and are usually not directed toward the healthcare provider, but simply reflect the frustration the patient feels because of the inability to communicate.

Remember that communication is also visual. If the patient does not seem to understand a request, such as "Stick out your tongue," use a visual cue. Lower your mask and ask the patient again; then demonstrate the movement yourself. This may trigger the correct response.

examination in the geriatric patient. Good lighting, gauze, and a mouth mirror or tongue depressor are the only instruments required for this potentially lifesaving screening examination.

Patients should be encouraged to conduct a self-examination at regular intervals in conjunction with daily oral care. Oral lesions are common in older patients, mostly related to trauma. However, all patients should be taught how and what to look for in their mouths. They can be advised that anything that does not appear normal, is not seen on both sides of the mouth, and does not go away within 7 to 10 days warrants a check by the individual's dental professional.

DISEASE CONTROL PHASE AND PREVENTION STRATEGIES

The objectives of the disease control phase in this age group are the same as with any adult population: to eradicate active disease and to reduce or eliminate the risk of new or recurrent disease (see Chapter 10). However, because older adults have more systemic illnesses, use more medications, and are at higher risk of new and recurring oral disease, the management of disease control issues is more complex. Definitive treatment, if it is to be provided, often proceeds in the presence of ongoing medical problems and, in some cases, in the presence of oral disease. Understanding the stage and trajectory of the patient's systemic conditions is critical and will aid the dentist in formulating the disease control phase. Furthermore, the dentist must be vigilant in monitoring the effects of these changes and be willing to alter the original treatment plan accordingly. For some patients, the goals, objectives, and nature of the treatment must be changed significantly on more than one occasion.

Future generations of older adults can be expected to retain more of their teeth and thus to have more tooth-related treatment needs. Because they do not have the physical capacity or stamina that they had when they were 20, 30, or 40 years of age, older people understand the concept of functional decline. Many of these individuals will have a strong desire to resist that trend and will work hard to maintain their teeth and a healthy oral condition. Furthermore, virtually all older adults with normal cognitive function will strive to remain pain and infection free and most will seek regular preventive care as long as it is within their means to pay for it.

Management of Xerostomia

Xerostomia has long been thought to be a natural part of aging. We now know that although changes associated with aging occur in the salivary glands in healthy older adults, normally, adequate salivary flow is maintained throughout life.[58] Salivary hypofunction is the diagnosed loss of salivary flow. Generally, flow will be decreased by at least 50% before the person becomes symptomatic or complains of oral dryness. Treatment planning for older adults must address the complaint of xerostomia by identifying the underlying causes of the condition and include strategies to mitigate or cope with the problem.

More than 400 medications can cause xerostomia or dry mouth. Sedatives, antipsychotics, antidepressants, antihistamines,

diuretics, and some hypertension medications are among the most frequently cited offenders. The actual mechanisms for xerostomia associated with medication use vary and are not always well understood. Medications with anticholinergic activity neurologically reduce saliva flow. Other drugs may dehydrate the oral tissues, causing the sensation of oral dryness.

Box 18.5 lists some of the most common conditions associated with xerostomia. Medication side effect is the most frequently cited cause, but in the differential diagnosis, many systemic diseases may also contribute to the problem. As with many other geriatric issues, the underlying cause may prove to be a combination of multiple issues. Some systemic diseases, such as Sjögren's syndrome, actually damage the glands and preclude any stimulated flow. This chronic inflammatory autoimmune disorder affects primarily the salivary and lacrimal glands. Glandular tissue is permanently destroyed by lymphocytic infiltration. The disease is often associated with other autoimmune disorders and is accompanied by systemic symptoms, such as dryness of pulmonary, genital, and dermal tissue; dry eyes; and/or dry mouth.

Many insulin-dependent diabetic patients are xerostomic, but the literature to date has been inconclusive as to whether salivary gland function is reduced in all diabetics. For many diabetic patients, poor glycemic control and subsequent dehydration may be the underlying cause of the hyposalivation.

Generalized dehydration is also more common in the senior population and probably contributes more to xerostomia than previously understood. With aging comes a decrease in the sense of thirst, increasing the chance of dehydration and subsequently decreasing fluid output of all types.

Radiation treatment for head and neck malignancies destroys salivary gland tissue within the radiation field. Oral dryness can begin as early as 2 weeks into the radiation treatment. The remaining salivary flow is often described as being "thick" and it is frequently associated with an alteration in the sense of taste. Serous acini are more susceptible to radiation than the mucinous acini and therefore the affected glands produce more viscous and mucinous saliva. Reduced saliva production has devastating consequences in the oral cavity. Without the protection of adequate saliva flow, the mouth lacks minerals and fluoride to remineralize hard tissues, a reduced ability to buffer

---

BOX 18.5   Conditions Frequently Associated With Xerostomia

Alcoholism
Medication side effects
Autoimmune disorders
Parkinson's disease
Cognitive impairment
Psychological disorders
Dehydration
Radiation of salivary glands
Diabetes
Sjögren's syndrome
Habitual oral breathing
Surgery affecting salivary glands

acidic conditions, and the ability to clear debris. As a result, bacterial overgrowth occurs and can lead to rampant post radiation caries as early as 3 months after radiation therapy.[59]

Without proper lubrication, patients may complain frequently about biting their cheek. Inadequate saliva can also lead to a chief complaint of heightened sensitivity of the oral tissues. Rough or broken restorations are more likely to cause trauma or discomfort. Oral prostheses are more likely to be uncomfortable without salivary lubrication to the underlying soft tissue, and because of the reduction in surface tension, retention of a maxillary denture may be greatly reduced.

Treatment for xerostomia can be divided into two categories: (1) treatment of hyposalivation, aimed at increasing the flow of saliva from the gland, and (2) palliative treatment, aimed at relieving the symptoms caused by xerostomia. Treatment for hyposalivation includes use of medications such as pilocarpine, as well as direct stimulation resulting from chewing sugarless gum or sucking on sugarless candies or lozenges, such as SalivaSure tablets. Proper hydration of the whole body is also important. Saliva is mostly composed of water and if the patient is dehydrated, as may be the case with many elderly persons, salivary output will be diminished.

Palliative treatment provides comfort for the patient during oral dryness. Salivary substitutes are manufactured in a wide variety of formulations and are available in liquid, spray, and gel forms. All are designed to enhance lubrication and relieve the sensation of dryness in the mouth. Dentifrices have been formulated for use by xerostomic patients that will clean the teeth without drying the mucosa. It is important for patients to avoid toothpastes containing sodium lauryl sulfate, which will remove the mucous layer from the mucosal surface. Topical gels, in addition to temporarily lubricating the mucosa, may temporarily help with retention of complete dentures.

Patients should also limit ingesting foods and beverages that contain caffeine and products containing alcohol, which are dehydrating to the body. It is important to avoid sipping acidic beverages, and instead to sip water throughout the day. Salivary stimulants, alcohol-free chlorhexidine rinses, prescription concentration fluoride toothpastes or gels (1.1% sodium fluoride = 5000 ppm fluoride), and fluoride varnishes on root surfaces used separately, sequentially, or in combination can negate the cariogenic potential of xerostomia.

Treatment planning for patients with long-term xerostomia should include frequent evaluation for candidiasis, a common comorbidity with hyposalivation. This infection can exacerbate the symptoms of oral dryness. In addition, if the xerostomia continues, the *Candida* infection may recur, even after it has been successfully treated. Table 18.6 lists various prescription regimens that may be used to manage an oral candidiasis infection. Most often, topical treatment, such as nystatin, will be the best choice. If this treatment is insufficient or if the infection has spread down into the esophageal passage, a systemic antifungal, such as fluconazole, may be necessary. Although nystatin oral suspension is frequently prescribed, it contains nearly 50% sugar and is not recommended for patients who have a natural dentition and would need to use this medication repeatedly.

TABLE 18.6 Therapeutic Agents for Management of Oral Candidiasis

Description	Comments
TOPICAL SUSPENSIONS	
RX: Nystatin oral suspension 100,000 U/mL *Disp:* 14-day supply (300 mL) *Sig:* Rinse with 5 mL for 1 min and expectorate 4 times daily PC (after meals) and HS (before retiring). NPO 30 min after use	Products usually contain 30%–50% sucrose Sulfur-like aftertaste may not be palatable to some patients Not a first-line choice Ineffective as a denture soak
OINTMENTS AND CREAMS	
RX: Nystatin ointment 100,000 U/g *Disp:* 15 g *Sig:* Apply thin film to inner surfaces of dentures and angles of mouth 3 or 4 times daily, PC and HS; NPO 30 min after use	• Inexpensive • Can be applied to tissue surface of dentures for localized effect • Bright yellow color may be objectionable for some patients for treatment of angular cheilitis
RX: Clotrimazole 1% cream (Lotrimin, g Rx, Lotrimin AF, g OTC) *Disp:* 15 g Rx or 12 g OTC *Sig:* Apply thin film to inner surface of denture and angles of mouth 2–4 times daily; NPO 30 min after using	• Less expensive than ketoconazole cream • Has some activity against *Staphylococcus aureus* and *Streptococcus pyogenes* • Good choice for angular cheilitis • Available OTC, but labeled for athletes foot and jock itch, which may cause some patients to hesitate
LOZENGES	
RX: Clotrimazole 10 mg oral troches *Disp:* 70 tabs *Sig:* Dissolve 1 tab in mouth every 3 hours while awake (5 tablets per day) for 14 days; NPO 30 min after using	• Compliance problems • Patients must be instructed to dissolve tablets slowly in mouth and not to chew • Does not work well in patients with severe xerostomia
SYSTEMIC	
RX: Fluconazole 100-mg tablets (Diflucan, g) *Disp:* 8 tablets *Sig:* Take 2 tablets on day 1, then take 1 tablet daily for 5–7 days	• Inhibitor of CYP2C9 and CYP3A4 isoenzymes; ALWAYS check for drug interaction before prescribing • Clinical symptoms resolve in 3–4 days; longer therapy decreases relapse rate
RX: Itraconazole 10 mg/mL oral solution (Sporanox) *Disp:* 150 mL *Sig:* Rinse with 10 mL for 20 seconds two times daily. Swish solution vigorously in mouth and swallow.	• Capsules should not be used for oral candidosis • If possible, administer in fasting condition to improve bioavailability • Multiple drug interactions • May require 14 days of therapy • Expensive

g, Generic.
Courtesy Cindy L. Marek, PharmD.

Oral Physiotherapy

Oral physiotherapy is defined as the use of aids such as toothbrush, floss, or other adjunctive armamentaria to maintain the oral health. Older adults should be given advice and assistance in support of their continued efforts to maintain good oral home care. This can be accomplished by providing each patient with the tools, knowledge, and skills required to maintain a healthy oral environment. To be successful, it is crucial to offer oral health education (more than simply brushing and flossing instruction) in a manner that respects the patient's autonomy and is not embarrassing because of any disease-related impairment. For patients who are unable to engage in effective oral self-care, it is essential to inform the caregiver about the importance of effective plaque control and provide specific instruction and demonstration on how to assist with or perform oral physiotherapy on the patient.

Toothbrushes and Interdental Cleaning Aids

Because many older adults have difficulty achieving effective daily plaque control, manufacturers have developed, produced, and marketed several different toothbrushes designed to facilitate tooth cleaning. Various bristle and handle designs are available in either manual or powered (electric or sonic) brushes. Powered brushes have heads that clean groups of teeth (traditional brush head) or one tooth surface at a time and may be very effective for some patients. The use of a powered toothbrush may help to reduce plaque in older adults with compromised oral hygiene. A systematic review of 29 trials found that powered toothbrushes with a rotation oscillation action (brush head rotates in one direction and then the other), used more than 3 months, reduced plaque by 7% and gingivitis by 17%.[60] In a study of individuals aged 68 to 85 years, the powered toothbrush was more effective than a regular manual toothbrush in removing plaque and controlling gingivitis.[61] In a study of 40- to 90-year-old long-term-care facility residents, a powered toothbrush was superior to a manual toothbrush in removing plaque when oral hygiene was performed on a regular basis by a caregiver.[62] Not all elderly individuals can tolerate the stimulation of an electric toothbrush and the cost and availability must also be taken into account when recommending powered toothbrushes to the elderly.

For patients with difficulty holding a toothbrush because of arthritis or stroke, devices are available to facilitate brushing. An occupational therapist can assist the dentist in identifying grips that will make oral care easier for patients. Wider floss, Teflon-coated floss, floss holders, proximal brushes, and even an electric flosser are now available. When prescribing any of these aids, it is important that someone on the dental team take the time to demonstrate the product and to be sure that the patient can use it safely and effectively. Adaptive aids are available for patients who lack manual dexterity and need to be able to clean a removable prosthesis

Chemotherapeutic Agents

Older adults are more susceptible to dental caries for multiple reasons. Gingival recession often occurs in the elderly, leaving root surfaces exposed. Many elderly people take medications for hypertension or psychological disorders with side effects

of decreased saliva flow, altered saliva composition, and dry mouth, leading to a higher caries rate.[63,64] The 1980s provided strong scientific evidence that fluoride benefits older adults. Those with lifelong residence in a community with water fluoridation have experienced reduced incidence of root caries and tooth loss compared with those who have lived in communities with nonfluoridated water supplies.[65]

Topically applied fluoride in many forms is important, not only to prevent new carious lesions from developing but also to arrest developing carious lesions. Both professionally applied fluoride varnish and 5000 ppm fluoride toothpaste applied daily have been shown to prevent the development of carious lesions and arrest existing carious lesions when compared with over-the-counter toothpastes. Some older adults prefer fluoride toothpastes without sodium laurel sulfate, which can cause a burning sensation in individuals suffering from dry mouth. In addition, professionally applied chlorhexidine varnish compared with placebo varnish has been shown to reduce the initiation of root caries lesions. Chlorhexidine is an antimicrobial agent that chemically controls plaque formation and thus has been shown to decrease the initiation of carious root lesions.[66]

While many of these modalities have been used throughout the years, **silver diamine fluoride** (SDF) is becoming more common and studies in older adults have shown that SDF can both successfully prevent and arrest carious root lesions. Silver diamine fluoride 38% is an alkaline colorless solution containing 24%–27% silver, 8.5%–10.5% ammonia, and 5%–6% fluoride. It can be applied in minutes before being rinsed away. Patients should be made aware that any carious lesion will become black in color because of the silver component. Both the protective and arresting capabilities of SDF diminish over time. Therefore follow-up applications are recommended to prevent arrested carious lesions from becoming active again.[67] SDF can be particularly useful for treatment of caries in older adults with transportation barriers, dependent older adults such as nursing home residents, patients experiencing a rapid decline in oral health, and palliative care or end-of-life patients.

For patients with gingivitis or gingival overgrowth secondary to medication use, chlorhexidine may be indicated. Chlorhexidine has been shown to have bacteriocidal, fungicidal, and some virus-killing properties. Many dentists prescribe chlorhexidine for elderly patients who are at risk of aspiration pneumonia. Although research in this area is limited, some studies have shown it to be beneficial in preventing aspiration pneumonia in patients who are on ventilators in hospital settings, as well as for improving the cough reflex.[68] Many practitioners prescribe chlorhexidine for patients after tooth extractions or for patients undergoing immunosuppressive treatment. Use of chlorhexidine can range from simply swabbing the buccal mucosa, using it in place of a dentifrice when brushing, or using it as a mouth rinse. However, chronic use of chlorhexidine may cause unpleasant staining of the teeth.

Dietary Modification

Dietary assessment must be included as a part of the caries risk analysis. Older adults often increase their intake of refined carbohydrates, thereby increasing the risk of caries. Assessment of refined carbohydrate consumption should include a review of any possible hidden sugars, including those found in over-the-counter medications or sugared lozenges to manage xerostomia. Patients are often unaware that many of these compounds, such as antacid tablets, contain a high sugar content. Esophageal reflux can increase on lying down and patients may therefore place an antacid in their mouth at night and allow it to dissolve through the night, when saliva is at its lowest. This and other sugar-based substances should be reduced as much as possible. When it is not possible or practical to eliminate these sources, less cariogenic alternatives can be suggested. (see Chapter 10)

As noted earlier in this chapter, as an individual ages, thirst may decrease, resulting in dehydration. Therefore, older adults should be encouraged to drink water and stay away from acidic and sugary beverages. Increased hydration has multiple health benefits, including decreased caries risk.

Research, mostly in children, has also shown a reduction in caries rates with the use of xylitol as a sugar substitute. Patients at high risk of caries who also suffer from salivary dysfunction are known to benefit from chewing a xylitol-containing chewing gum or xylitol candies or lozenges. For effective caries prevention, it is recommended that a patient be exposed to 6 g of xylitol daily divided into three or more consumption periods. Products on the market such as Spry gum contain 0.72 g of xylitol per piece so that the patient would need to chew nine pieces daily to have the optimal exposure. It should also be noted that chewing gum stimulates saliva, thus adding another layer of prevention. Caution should be used because higher amounts of xylitol may cause gastrointestinal disturbance in some patients. Owing to the risk of choking, caution should be used when recommending xylitol gum or lozenges in patients with neurologic or swallowing disorders.

Oral Health Care Provided by Caregivers

Oral home care for a frail elderly person is an important and frequently neglected service. Providing daily oral physiotherapy to long-term care residents is often considered an unpleasant task and is delegated to nursing auxiliaries, who have even less oral health training than the registered nursing staff. The dentist delivering care in a long-term care setting must take a leadership role in educating the staff about the importance of good daily oral care for their patients. Annual oral health in-service training and continuous communication with nursing staff, once positive rapport has been established, help ensure compliance with recommended therapy. Often, providing the staff with oral disease prevention information for themselves and their families may help increase interest in oral care for their patients.

In the United States, the Omnibus Budget and Reconciliation Act of 1987 (OBRA) contained legislative language intended to ensure that long-term care patients receive adequate care to live to their full potential. Included in the act is the requirement that all such patients, if covered at least in part by either Medicare or Medicaid programs, undergo a comprehensive needs evaluation. The result of the evaluation determines the services the patient will receive. Box 18.6 illustrates Section L of the Minimum Data Set, the oral assessment instrument, which is included in that evaluation. The nurse answers the dental

---

BOX 18.6 Section L of the Minimum Data Set for Long-Term Care Patients (Version 3.0)

Intent: This item is intended to record any dental problems present in the 7-day look-back period.

L0200: Dental

↓ Check all that apply:

- 1. A. Broken or loosely fitting full or partial denture (chipped, cracked, uncleanable or loose).
- 2. B. No natural teeth or tooth fragments (edentulous).
- 3. C. Abnormal mouth soft tissue (ulcers, masses, oral lesions, including under denture or partial denture).
- 4. D. Obvious or likely cavity or broken natural teeth.
- 5. E. Inflamed or bleeding gums or loose natural teeth.
- 6. F. Mouth or facial pain, discomfort or difficulty with chewing.
- 7. G. Unable to examine.
- 8. Z. None of the above was present.

---

questions in Section L, which are rudimentary at best; completes the form; and determines whether follow-up oral care is required. However research demonstrates when nurses were educated to identify oral disease, they completed an oral assessment more thoroughly and identified more oral problems in patients.[69] Efforts have been made to educate those who monitor nursing home care to help identify obvious neglect of oral health needs. Recognition of the patient's oral health needs by the nursing home staff is the first step in developing solutions for the widespread unmet dental needs of long-term residents.

For homebound patients, daily oral self-care may require the assistance of a family member or other caregiver and/or the use of aids designed for patients with disabilities. For a patient who only has use of one hand or for whom a conventional flossing technique is not feasible, large-handled toothbrushes, large Y flossers, and/or denture brushes with suction on the bottom may be useful.

DEFINITIVE TREATMENT PLANNING FOR OLDER ADULTS

Treatment Planning for Active and Independent Elderly Patients

As mentioned early in this chapter, the concepts of whole health and person-centered care provide the context and the foundation for the treatment planning process. A treatment plan must include the patient's goals and attempt to address anticipated medical, social or psychological impediments to a successful outcome. One way to do this is always to make sure the treatment plan has answered the following five questions:

1. Does the treatment we have planned fit the patient's goals and expectations for their oral health?
2. Did I make sure I appropriately addressed the issue of informed consent for the treatment we have planned?

3. Can the patient physically and mentally go through all the treatment steps to reach our final goal?
4. What are any potential adverse outcomes to the planned treatment and have I addressed them to the extent possible?
5. Can the patient or caregiver realistically take care of the outcome or prosthesis we have planned?

General Principles for Devising Plan of Care

Although dental treatment planning for the elderly, as with other age groups, is patient-specific, the following general guidelines may be helpful:

- Chronologic age is not indicative of biologic health. The dentist should not make assumptions about the patient's dental treatment needs based on age alone. The average 85-year-old who has another 5 years of life expectancy may be quite interested in, and benefit from, elective dental treatment.
- The dentist should not make judgments about what treatment the patient wants to have or can afford without discussion. Treatment should be planned with the goal of achieving optimal oral health and the patient should be given the opportunity to select the best of all feasible treatment options.
- In planning treatment, the dentist should make every effort to "do no harm." The benefits of the oral healthcare provided should always outweigh the risks. An internal question for the oral healthcare provider should be whether the proposed treatment will improve or maintain the patient's quality of life. When dental treatment becomes more of a problem than a solution, it is time to reevaluate the treatment. In some cases, it is acceptable to do less rather than more. Palliative care for patients who are terminally ill may be more humane than dental treatment that causes the patient more inconvenience and suffering.
- The treatment plan should be devised to ensure success. If extensive restorative treatment will be provided, a predetermination must be made that the patient can maintain it. If the patient needs additional help with oral home care, maintenance visits should be scheduled at more frequent intervals to assess compliance and the help of family and caregivers should be enlisted, if necessary.

Treatment options for senior patients with periodontal disease do not differ from those for a younger patient, but the optimal choices and the manner in which treatment is provided may differ. For example, periodontal surgery may be contraindicated because of poor systemic health and the possibility that poor healing will compromise the outcome. Locally, topically, or systemically administered antimicrobials offer a less-invasive option for the patient who needs, but is not a candidate for surgery. Other typical strategies include more frequent appointments for scaling (e.g., every 3 to 4 months) and helping the patient find better ways to improve daily oral care. As with any patient, the dentist must work with the individual to eliminate or modify risk factors such as tobacco use.

In theory, all treatment options should be available to the patient regardless of age, but in reality, the social conditions, systemic health, and oral health of the patient may require the dentist to alter the usual treatment protocol. Person-centered treatment planning becomes even more important when treating older adults as there are often more issues that need to be considered that will have a significant impact on the delineation of the reasonable treatment options. This means the dentist may need to assess the patient's frailty status and life expectancy, physical or cognitive conditions that limit the patient's ability to sit in a dental chair for extended periods of time, neuromuscular skills required to use and maintain the proposed treatment options, the patient's availability to attend dental appointments in addition to other medical appointments, and any travel considerations especially if the patient no longer drives themselves and must rely on others for travel. For frail or dependent older adults, this treatment planning philosophy is called *rational dental care* as alternative methods of dental treatment become more appropriate than technically idealized dental care.[70]

Presentation of Treatment Options

Engaging the patient in an open comprehensive discussion of all the reasonable treatment options is essential to achieving informed consent (see Chapter 7) and is necessary in order to arrive at a mutually agreed upon plan of care that is best for the patient. In the treatment planning discussion the dentist must respect the patient's autonomy as the decision maker, even in the presence of an adult child, spouse, or other caregiver. It should not be assumed that the patient has hearing or visual problems, but neither should the dentist hesitate to ask questions to be sure that the patient can read all materials, including the consent form, and understands what is being said. If the patient fails to fully comprehend the treatment options, informed consent cannot be achieved.

In addition to possible hearing or vision deficits, it is important to assess whether the patient is capable of making an informed decision about the treatment plan. Such cues as a spouse or adult child's always accompanying the patient to appointments, someone else's taking care of the financial matters relating to dental treatment, or the patient's inability to discuss the treatment options may suggest that another responsible person should be included in the discussion to help make the decisions (see the *Ethics in Dentistry* box). If the patient's mental disabilities are severe, special informed consent may be required. Especially in practices in which the elderly constitute a substantial portion of the patient population, the dentist may consider including an additional line to the treatment plan so that, along with the patient's signature, a legal guardian can also provide consent.

ETHICS IN DENTISTRY

Surrogate Decision Making for the Elderly

If an adult patient lacks the capacity to make decisions, the dentist must determine who the appropriate surrogate decision maker should be. Although it is often easiest to turn to the person accompanying the patient, this may not be the person the patient trusts to make important health decisions. Many countries provide a formal mechanism that allows people to name a proxy (or surrogate) decision maker. For example, in the United States, an adult can complete a Durable Power of Attorney for Health Care form naming another person to serve as decision maker for all health-related decisions. The surrogate decision maker assumes that role *only* if the patient becomes unable to participate in decision making.

Written advance directives are typically kept on file in care facilities by the primary care physician and by family members. Dental health professionals may not routinely receive copies of these documents but should make it a common practice to inquire whether an adult patient has written directives. If the patient has not named a decision maker, the dentist should ask the individual to identify a primary contact for the dentist to consult with if they are ever unable to participate in the clinical decision-making process. This step is particularly helpful when patients have a condition, such as dementia, in which capacity may fluctuate or be expected to diminish over time. However, any adult can sustain an acute neurologic injury, such as stroke, that can temporarily or permanently reduce their decision-making skills. If the dentist has already documented the patient's preference for a surrogate decision maker to authorize treatment decisions and consult with the dentist, this can reduce uncertainty about who should make decisions on behalf of the patient.

If a patient lacks decision-making ability and no clear surrogate has been identified, then decisions usually default to "next of kin." Some jurisdictions have formalized a hierarchy for identifying decision makers as follows: legal guardian, spouse, adult child, parent, adult sibling, adult grandchild, close friend, and last, the guardian of the patient's estate.[71]

Delivery of Care

Dental care for the active and independent elderly is very similar to dental care for younger adults and treatment can be delivered in much the same way. The dentist will still need to take into consideration the patient's current health status and its impact on the delivery of dental treatment, and assess whether any systemic conditions are likely to affect the nature of treatment or the manner that oral health is delivered to the patient in the future.

Matching the properties of restorative materials to patient needs is one key to successful dental treatment in senior patients. In recent years, the range of available materials has expanded to permit more specific and appropriate matching of patient and restoration. For example, in restoring root caries, which is primarily a disease of the elderly, several options are available. The adhesive properties and potential for fluoride release with glass ionomer make this material an effective alternative for restoring root surface lesions. Although the true glass ionomer materials offer the potential for the greatest amount of fluoride release, glass ionomer–resin hybrid materials provide better esthetics and may be a more appealing to the patient in visible areas of the mouth. Full-coverage restorations may be appropriate especially if extensive tooth structure is missing. Amalgam can be used in areas where moisture control is poor or when patient cooperation does not allow the provider to maintain the isolation needed for materials such as composite.

For older adults, the goal is for the patient to maintain their current functional status for as long as possible. However, as you provide treatment, it is also important to plan for failure. Dental professionals should understand that the patient's current oral hygiene and caries risk may change for the worse. This recognition allows the dentist to make some adjustments in the

delivery of care. For instance, if a removable partial denture is being fabricated, it can be designed in a way that will allow the addition of teeth at a later time if other extractions are required.

It is important to be aware that the transition from being an active and independent elderly person to becoming a frail and dependent elderly person can happen rather quickly. In an aging population, a patient can have good oral hygiene and keep regular dental visits and then suddenly stop coming to the dentist. This may be because the patient has experienced a significant medical event affecting mobility and/or dependency, such as a heart attack, stroke, or fall resulting in a fractured bone. The patient's spouse may fall ill and the patient may become a full-time caregiver. Such events may prevent the patient from attending dental appointments as scheduled. The difficulties that arise from this change can create an added burden on daily life and can start the patient on the downward slope to poor oral self care and infrequent professional dental care visits. It is not possible to predict that such an event will occur, but it is important to recognize that when a regularly scheduled patient misses their recall appointments, a follow-up with the patient is in order. This conversation may reveal new barriers to care, and can facilitate a discussion with the patient, and other interested parties, regarding emerging oral disease risk and appropriate preventive measures to be considered.

Treatment for Frail and Dependent Elderly Patients

Long-term care patients and those who are homebound may be defined as functionally independent or dependent. One of the primary ways function is assessed is in terms of the capability to perform the activities of daily living (ADLs) (see Chapter 13), the tasks that must be performed to maintain daily life. The ADLs include eating, bathing, dressing, transferring, and toileting. A person's ability to perform these tasks will be established by a healthcare provider, usually a physical or occupational therapist. The results of this evaluation will help establish how much intervention will be required on a daily basis and whether the person can continue to reside at home or must have more constant care in a nursing home.

Options for Delivering Care

Although the science of dentistry has seen considerable advances, the old-fashioned concept of the house call is returning. The use of mobile and portable dental care is slowly increasing across the United States, although not always quickly enough to meet the growing needs of patients. Two distinct categories of elderly patients require dental care outside the usual confines of the traditional practice setting: (1) residents of long-term care facilities and (2) homebound seniors, those who still live in their own homes but are unable to leave without great difficulty. Residents of long-term care facilities often cannot travel to a dental office except in an ambulance or specially designed wheelchair-accessible van and the transporting may upset both the mental and systemic health of the frail elderly patient.

Varying levels of dental treatment can be provided in alternative settings. The dentist must decide before undertaking

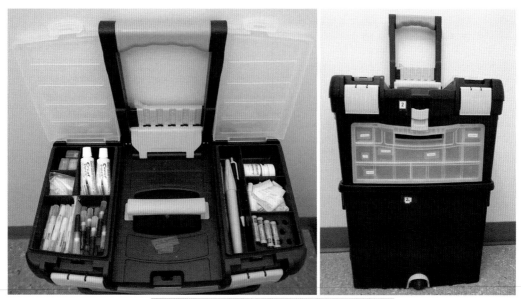

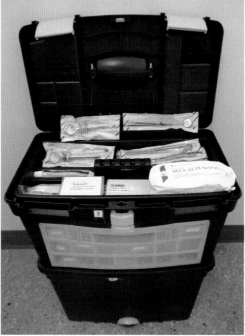

Fig. 18.4 "Black bag" dental supplies and equipment to treat a patient of record in a residential setting.

such a practice what services he or she wishes to provide. Some dentists make portable dental care a full-time endeavor, purchasing a complete portable dental unit that includes handpieces, air, suction, water, and a separate portable radiographic unit. The scope of service that can be provided with this type of equipment includes preventive care, restorative care, extractions, removable prostheses, and, in warranted cases, limited fixed prostheses.

The "black bag" approach is a minimalist method of providing this type of care on an as-needed basis and usually only for patients of record. Here the dentist transports the dental supplies and equipment necessary for immediate care to a residential or other nonresidential institutional setting (Figure. 18.4).

For more complex procedures, the patient is brought to the dental office. Even this type of approach offers an opportunity to provide a moderate range of services. Dentures can be fabricated without a traditional dental unit. Portable lights, such as loupe lights, fiberoptic headlamps or portable fiberoptic lighted mirrors, are available. Radiographic capabilities have portable options when using a laptop, digital sensor, and handheld battery operated x-ray systems. Portable ultrasonic units with their own irrigation source can be acquired, in addition to battery operation prophy polishing handpieces. All long-term care facilities have portable suction units that can be pushed into the patient's room or into a makeshift operatory, often the beauty parlor or space provided for the podiatrist. Some restorative

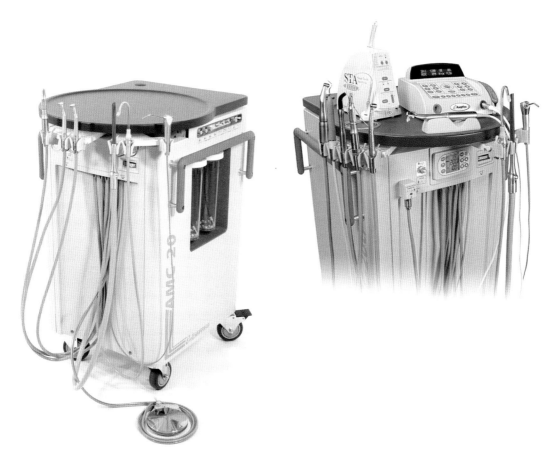

Fig. 18.5 Dental operatory equipment designed for easy transport to nursing homes or assisted living facilities. (AMC-20 mobile dental cart shown.) (Courtesy Aseptico, Inc., Woodinville, WA.)

dentistry can be performed using hand instruments and self-curing or light cured glass ionomer material. Many extractions can be performed with minimal instruments, as long as the root anatomy is confirmed radiographically in advance.

Another form of mobile care uses a portable operatory that can be quickly broken down and carried from house to house or room to room, to be set up in small spaces within a nursing home facility (Figure. 18.5). Provision of this type of practice removes the barriers to accessing dental care for frail elderly patients. Implementation requires additional time to drive from place to place and set up the portable equipment. Additional expenditures of time are also necessary to transfer the patient from bed to chair and to gather and assess a more comprehensive health history. These expenditures must be reflected in the cost of dental care to this special population.

The highest level of care can be provided in a fully equipped self-contained dental operatory housed in a bus or truck built for that purpose. This format has the advantage of providing all of the necessary infrastructure required to support a complete range of dental services and allows moving the operatory from one distant site to another at will. In this venue, the patient need only be transported to the dental van or bus, which is typically driven to the parking lot at the care facility.

Disadvantages of this approach include the high initial cost, necessity of transporting patients through various weather conditions (rain, snow, and ice) into the vehicle, patient's access up into the vehicle via steps, ramps, or wheelchair lifts, and limited space inside to accommodate wheelchairs and walkers. As a result of these limitations, the dental van approach has been used predominantly by institutions whose mission is to serve patients in multiple locations using multiple care providers (including dental students). Some individual practitioners have also used this venue, particularly in urban areas where there is higher demand and less travel time is required. As a full-time endeavor, the dental entrepreneur can make this an effective cost center.

Teledentistry is an alternative option that can be used to improve access and care to some older adult patients. Teledentistry is the use of technology to deliver virtual oral health services via synchronous (live video) interactions with patients or asynchronous (e.g., taking a photo to forward to your dental provider) communications. It is very important to be aware of any local, regional, or national regulations involving teledentistry in order to conduct communications properly and in a way that protects patient's protected health information. Older adults are becoming more technologically savvy every day and are becoming more open to teledentistry to be able to access a dental clinician quickly. This includes using teledentistry services to gather diagnostic information, triage, to improve planning and preparation for an in-person appointment, conduct postoperative evaluations, and to provide patient specific instructions or recommendations. In addition, teledentistry can be used to improve access to care for patients with transportation barriers including those living in a nursing home or care facility. Pending local regulations, teledentistry could be used in the following three scenarios. (1) Dentists could educate nursing facility staff to assist in conducting a telehealth synchronous or asynchronous visit. (2) Dental offices could send dental team members to nursing homes to assist in the teledentistry visit either synchronously or asynchronously. (3) Dental offices could use mobile or portable equipment to send hygienists to nursing facilities to gather diagnostic information and to provide preventive treatment while on site. Unlike our medical colleagues, it is not possible to conduct all dental treatment using teledentistry, but with a little effort, teledentistry can be used to eliminate transportation barriers to a dental office, treatment plan prior to the dental visit, to gain consent for treatment prior to the dental office visit especially if the patient is unable to make their own decisions, to minimize disruptions to residents with dementia, and to expedite treatment while a patient is in the dental office.[72]

No matter the location, the provision of dental care for frail elderly patients necessitates thought and planning about emergencies that may arise during treatment. A thorough knowledge of the patient's systemic health history and medication use will assist in preventing such situations. This highlights the need for all staff to be familiar with the office protocol for emergencies. The dentist should become familiar with the emergency protocol at each long-term care facility and the location of the "crash" or emergency cart. During home visits, the dentist should always carry an emergency kit and a small portable oxygen unit. The risk of adverse events exists with all patients. Frail patients and their families must be made aware of such risks before initiating treatment. Treatment planning for this group requires recognition that the benefits of dental treatment must be weighed against the risks to the health of the patient.

Providing care in alternative practice settings can be complex but offers significant rewards, including the opportunity to function as a vital part of an interdisciplinary healthcare team and the satisfaction gained in improving the quality of life for a challenging group of patients.

Interdisciplinary Geriatric Healthcare Team

Even a general dentist in a private practice has the opportunity to participate in the delivery of dental treatment to elderly patients as part of an interdisciplinary healthcare team. Many non-dental disciplines have a vested interest in the oral health of their patients. As an increasing number of physicians and other professionals understand the links between oral health,

systemic health and the quality of life, they will be prepared to refer their patients and to work with dental professionals during treatment planning to identify to the dental team to manage oral health problems and provide clearance prior to medical and surgical procedures. Similarly, they will be receptive to our referral of dental patients to them to diagnose and manage general health problems, consult with us as how we can provide oral health services to our patients within the context of their medical and psychosocial problems, and work with us in a collaborative effort to help our patients achieve an optimal state of health and wellness (see Chapter 6).

Occupational therapists, trained to help patients learn alternative approaches to daily activities, can assist the patient with tasks such as tooth brushing, denture cleaning, and denture insertion and removal. This assistance can significantly augment the limited teaching opportunities the dental team may have with the patient. Speech pathologists can assess the patient's swallowing ability and may be the first to consult the dentist if the patient has speech problems during therapy because of a poor-fitting prosthesis. Others on the team, including the nursing staff, psychologists, physical therapists, and social workers, can offer valuable information on the patient's condition, progress, long-term prognosis, and inform us regarding the individual's abilities to perform tasks of daily living. (See Chapter 6 for more information.)

Palliative care teams are interdisciplinary teams where dentists can greatly impact a patient's quality of life during end of life care. A dentist's main goal in a palliative care team is to assist in providing oral comfort for patients. This can be achieved by addressing painful oral conditions such as mucositis, stomatitis, xerostomia, and candidiasis. Teeth can be restored and periodontal therapy provided to improve patient's comfort or intake of food. Replacement of missing teeth can be accomplished to improve the patient's masticatory efficiency and nutritional intake.[73]

Documentation Requirements

Documentation of findings in a traditional private setting for healthy older patients will not differ from those concepts described in previous chapters. Frail elderly patients seen in a nursing home, home, or hospital setting, however, will require more data evaluation and documentation. Provision of care to patients in any of these settings requires a thorough evaluation of the individual's systemic and mental health and an assessment of other social issues. Although the health history for a patient in a long-term care facility may be lengthy, it is also easily accessible. Each patient has a chart that can be found at the facility's nursing station. The chart can be expected to include the following information:

- A written health history, including documentation of any predisposing conditions for endocarditis
- A current list of all medications and documentation of any known drug allergies
- A problem list (list of all current medical and psychological diagnoses)

- A personal contact if the patient requires follow-up for consent to treatment
- Progress notes documenting recent changes in the patient's health
- A description of the type of diet the patient receives (e.g., pureed versus soft mechanical versus regular consistency)

Regulations that apply to documentation of patient assessment and care in the traditional acute care hospital setting also apply in long-term care facilities. The patient's chart should be reviewed at each visit to learn whether any changes have occurred since the previous visit. After each dental visit, the dentist must provide a written record of any findings and the treatment provided in the care facility's patient chart. This can be accomplished by putting the original oral health evaluation sheet in the chart and retaining a copy for the dentist's own records. A progress note is required for all subsequent dental treatment and is most appropriately written in the form of a SOAP note (Subjective findings, Objective findings, an Assessment, and a Plan), the common format used by the medical profession. (For a more complete discussion of the SOAP note format, see Chapter 9.) Because patients in long-term care have serious systemic health problems and receive healthcare from various health professionals, the oral health history, dental treatment plan, and progress notes inform and educate all of the patient's health professionals about the role of oral health and dental care in the patient's overall care.

Homebound patients will not have such easily accessible health information. Discussions with caregivers, the patient's physicians, or the family social worker are advisable before any invasive dental treatment. If the verbal health history provided by the homebound patient raises questions in the clinician's mind, periodic calls to the geriatrician or primary care physician may be necessary before invasive care is provided to rule out any significant limitations or contraindications to the proposed dental treatment. The mode of documentation for treatment rendered to the patient is comparable to that carried out in a conventional dental setting.

MAINTENANCE PHASE TREATMENT PLANNING

Assessment of daily oral care for senior patients should be an ongoing process for the dental treatment team. It is important to assess the patient's oral hygiene and to ask the patient which movements or tasks are becoming difficult and why. Such disabilities may be episodic, for example, as a result of a recent hospital stay or because of intermittent pain from osteoarthritis in the upper extremities that limits oral care. Based on this assessment, the dental team can tailor recommendations to the particular situation. Examples include proximal brushes and automated flossing devices that require less dexterity than traditional dental floss. Automated toothbrushes, even the least expensive, will help reduce the amount of arm movement required and circumvent dexterity problems that

may preclude effective use of a manual brush. In seeking solutions to daily oral care problems, autonomy is always a goal. Recommendations by the dental team should be focused on helping the patient to maintain their own oral care whenever possible.

As patients become more debilitated or dependent on caregivers, the dental team may be required to train the caregiver in providing good daily oral hygiene for the patient. Because a caregiver's day is long and can be difficult, the simpler the regimen, the better. Again, automated toothbrushes are desirable because they require less effort or movement on the caregiver's part. Use of a prescription high-fluoride toothpaste may be recommended, especially when the oral care is provided by a busy caregiver and performed no more than once per day. Unfortunately, the additional cost of a prescription toothpaste may be prohibitive for some patients. Oral rinses, such as chlorhexidine, can be recommended after brushing if gingivitis or high caries risk has been diagnosed. It should be stressed to caregivers, however, that rinses are an adjunct and rarely a replacement for brushing.

CONCLUSION

Because seniors span such a wide age range (65 years to older than 100 years), it is difficult to make social or health generalizations. Many older adults view themselves as youthful, energetic, and forward looking. They prefer to be referred to as adults or seniors. Older adults visit their dentists more frequently than in the past and expect higher levels of oral health throughout their lives. A general guideline for treatment planning that is especially appropriate for the older individual is to "give the patient the opportunity to say yes" to a full range of treatment options. However, no matter how simple or extensive the treatment plan, it should be designed to establish and maintain optimum oral health.

To plan treatment appropriately, you must know your patient and their goals. Then you will need to consider the medical/dental indications, patient preferences, quality of life issues, and factors within the contextual scope of their current life situation. As stated earlier in this chapter, it is important to end each treatment planning session by making sure you have answered the following questions:

- Does the treatment we have planned fit the patient's goals and expectations for their oral health?
- Did I make sure I appropriately addressed the issue of informed consent for the treatment we have planned?
- Can the patient physically and mentally go through all the treatment steps to reach our final goal?
- What are any potential adverse outcomes to the planned treatment, and have I addressed them to the extent possible?
- Can the patient or caregiver realistically take care of the outcome or prosthesis we have planned?

Affirmative answers to each of these questions helps ensure that you have addressed both the immediate needs and the long-term best interests of your patient.

REVIEW QUESTIONS

- Describe demographic oral health characteristics of the elderly patient population.
- Describe the aspirations of healthy older adults regarding their oral health.
- Describe the oral health needs and desires of the frail elderly.
- Do interview and examination procedures differ for the elderly patient? If so, how?
- List three common systemic conditions that occur in older adults and the implications these health issues may have on the person's dental care.

- Which medications contribute to xerostomia in older adults?
- Which medications are used to treat oral candidiasis?
- How do strategies for oral disease control and prevention differ for the aging population compared with younger cohorts?
- Does restorative treatment planning in the elderly differ from that for younger patients? If so, how?
- How will the treatment plan presentation differ for older patients?
- Which dental services might you provide to elderly persons who are homebound or in a nursing home?

SUGGESTED READINGS AND RESOURCES

American Dental Association: Incurred Medical Expenses. https://www.ada.org/en/member-center/member-benefits/practice-resources/paying-for-dental-care-a-how-to-guide-incurred-med. Accessed August 9, 2021.

American Geriatric Society: American Geriatric Society 2019 Updated AGS Beers Criteria for potentially inappropriate medication used in older adults. https://sbgg.org.br/informativos/13-02-19/1_Updated_AGS_Beer.pdf. Accessed August 9, 2021

Chen X, Chen H, Douglas C, Preisser JS, Shuman SK. Dental treatment intensity in frail older adults in the last year of life. *J Am Dent Assoc.* 2013;144(11):1234–1242.

Little JW FD, Miller CS, et al. *Little and Falace's Dental Management of the Medically Compromised Patient.* 9th ed. St. Louis: Mosby; 2017.

Napenas JJ, Kujan O, Arduino PG, et al. World Workshop on Oral Medicine VI: Controversies regarding dental management of medically complex patients: assessment of current recommendations. *Oral Surg Oral Med Oral Pathol Oral Radiol.* 2015;120(2):207–226.

Pretty IA, Ellwood RP, Lo EC, et al. The Seattle Care Pathway for securing oral health in older patients. *Gerodontology.* 2014;31(Suppl 1):77–87.

REFERENCES

1. United Nations Department of Economic and Social Affairs PD. World Population Ageing 2020 Highlights: Living arrangements of older persons; 2020.
2. The World Bank. Population ages 65 and above (% of total population). 2019. https://data.worldbank.org/indicator/SP.POP.65UP.TO.ZS/.
3. Andrasfay T, Goldman N. Reductions in 2020 US life expectancy due to COVID-19 and the disproportionate impact on the Black and Latino populations. *PNAS.* 2021;118(5). e2014746118.
4. United States Census Bureau. Quick Facts: Population Estimates April 1, 2020; 2020. https://www.census.gov/quickfacts/fact/table/US/RHI225220
5. PRB. The U.S. population is growing older and the gender gap in life expectancy is narrowing. 2020. https://www.prb.org/resources/u-s-population-is-growing-older/#:~:text=The%20Sex%20Ratio%20at%20Older%20Ages%20Is%20Narrowing&text=In%20the%20United%20States%2C%20as,patterns%20vary%20across%20age%20groups.
6. Aging Hi Nursing Homes. 2020. https://www.healthinaging.org/age-friendly-healthcare-you/care-settings/nursing-homes. August 4, 2021.
7. Li Z. DJ. Poverty among the population aged 65 & older. In: Service CR, editor; 2021.
8. Wall T.N.K., Vujicic M. The per-patient dental expenditure rising, driven by baby boomers. In: Institute ADAHP, editor; 2014.
9. Rowe JW, Kahn RL. Successful aging. *Gerontologist.* 1997;37(4):433–440.
10. Shinsho F. New strategy for better geriatric oral health in Japan: 80/20 movement and Healthy Japan 21. *Int Dent J.* 2001;51(3 Suppl):200–206.
11. Taylor SL, Bolton R, Huynh A, et al. What Should Health Care Systems Consider When Implementing Complementary and Integrative Health: Lessons from Veterans Health Administration. *J Altern Complement Med.* 2019;25(S1):S52–S60.
12. Abrams AP, Thompson LA. Physiology of aging of older adults: systemic and oral health considerations. *Dent Clin North Am.* 2014;58(4):729–738.
13. Gu Q, Dillon CF, Burt VL. Prescription drug use continues to increase: U.S. prescription drug data for 2007-2008. *NCHS Data Brief.* 2010(42):1–8.
14. American Geriatrics Society Beers Criteria Update Expert Panel American Geriatrics Society 2019 Updated AGS Beers Criteria(R) for potentially inappropriate medication use in older adults. *J Am Geriatr Soc.* 2019;67(4):674–694.
15. McCauley JL, Hyer JM, Ramakrishnan VR, et al. Dental opioid prescribing and multiple opioid prescriptions among dental patients: Administrative data from the South Carolina prescription drug monitoring program. *J Am Dent Assoc.* 2016;147(7):537–544.
16. US Department of Health and Human Services, SAaMHSA. State data tables and reports from 2018-2019 NSDUH. Detailed Tables. 2019. https://www.samhsa.gov/data/nsduh/state-reports-NSDUH-2019
17. Statistics NCfH. 2018 Current Multiple Causes of Death Data. 2019.
18. Wehler CJ, Panchal NH, Cotchery 3rd DL, et al. Alternatives to opioids for acute pain management after dental procedures: A Department of Veterans Affairs consensus paper. *J Am Dent Assoc.* 2021;152(8):641–652.

19. Oral health in America A report of the Surgeon General. *J Calif Dent Assoc*. 2000;28(9):685–695.

20. National Cancer Institute Surveillance, Epidemiology and End Results Program. Cancer Stat Facts: Oral Cavity and Pharynx Cancer; 2021.

21. Gibson G. Identifying and treating xerostomia in restorative patients. *J Esthet Dent*. 1998;10(5):253–264.

22. Beck JD. Periodontal implications: older adults. *Ann Periodontol*. 1996;1(1):322–357.

23. Pretty IA, Ellwood RP, Lo EC, et al. The Seattle Care Pathway for securing oral health in older patients. *Gerodontology*. 2014;31 (Suppl 1):77–87.

24. Marchini L, Hartshorn JE, Cowen H, Dawson DV, Johnsen DC. A teaching tool for establishing risk of oral health deterioration in elderly patients: development, implementation, and evaluation at a U.S. dental school. *J Dent Educ*. 2017;81(11):1283–1290.

25. Tanaka T, Takahashi K, Hirano H, et al. Oral frailty as a risk factor for physical frailty and mortality in community-dwelling elderly. *J Gerontol A Biol Sci Med Sci*. 2018;73(12):1661–1667.

26. Chen X, Kistler CE. Oral health care for older adults with serious illness: when and how? *J Am Geriatr Soc*. 2015;63(2):375–378.

27. Qato DM, Alexander GC, Conti RM, et al. Use of prescription and over-the-counter medications and dietary supplements among older adults in the United States. *JAMA*. 2008;300(24):2867–2878.

28. SI H. Definitions and Demographics Characteristics . In: Kaye D, ed. *Infective Endocarditis*. New York: Raven Press; 1992.

29. Felder RS, Nardone D, Palac R. Prevalence of predisposing factors for endocarditis among an elderly institutionalized population. *Oral Surg Oral Med Oral Pathol*. 1992;73(1):30–34.

30. Wilson WR, Gewitz M, Lockhart PB, et al. Prevention of viridans group streptococcal infective endocarditis: A Scientific Statement From the American Heart Association. *Circulation*. 2021;143:e963–e978.

31. Sollecito TP, Abt E, Lockhart PB, et al. The use of prophylactic antibiotics prior to dental procedures in patients with prosthetic joints: Evidence-based clinical practice guideline for dental practitioners—a report of the American Dental Association Council on Scientific Affairs. *J Am Dent Assoc*. 2015;146(1): 11–16. e8.

32. Lodi G, Azzi L, Varoni EM, et al. Antibiotics to prevent complications following tooth extractions. *Cochrane Database Syst Rev*. 2021;2:CD003811.

33. Esposito M, Grusovin MG, Worthington HV. Interventions for replacing missing teeth: antibiotics at dental implant placement to prevent complications. *Cochrane Database Syst Rev*. 2013(7):CD004152.

34. Eke PI, Dye BA, Wei L, et al. Update on Prevalence of periodontitis in adults in the United States: NHANES 2009 to 2012. *J Periodontol*. 2015;86(5):611–622.

35. Schmidt AM. The growing problem of obesity: mechanisms, consequences, and therapeutic approaches. *Arterioscler Thromb Vasc Biol*. 2015;35(6):e19–e23.

36. Hales CM, Carroll MD, Fryar CD, Ogden CL. Prevalence of obesity and severe obesity among adults: United States, 2017-2018. *NCHS Data Brief*. 2020(360):1–8.

37. Winning LLG. A Review of the Relationship between chronic periodontitis and diabetes. *US Endocrinol*. 2018;14(2):80.

38. Kochanek K.D., Xu J., Arias E. Mortality in the United States, 2019. NCHS Data Brief 2020(395):1-8.

39. Bale BF, Doneen AL, Vigerust DJ. High-risk periodontal pathogens contribute to the pathogenesis of atherosclerosis. *Postgrad Med J*. 2017;93(1098):215–220.

40. Konig MF, Abusleme L, Reinholdt J, et al. Aggregatibacter actinomycetemcomitans-induced hypercitrullination links periodontal infection to autoimmunity in rheumatoid arthritis. *Sci Transl Med*. 2016;8(369). 369ra176.

41. Abbasi J. To prevent rheumatoid arthritis, look past the joints to the gums. *JAMA*. 2017;317(12):1201–1202.

42. Dominy SS, Lynch C, Ermini F, et al. Porphyromonas gingivalis in Alzheimer's disease brains: Evidence for disease causation and treatment with small-molecule inhibitors. *Sci Adv*. 2019;5(1). eaau3333.

43. Whelton PK, Carey RM, Aronow WS, et al. 2017 ACC/AHA/ AAPA/ABC/ACPM/AGS/APhA/ASH/ASPC/NMA/PCNA Guideline for the Prevention, Detection, Evaluation, and Management of High Blood Pressure in Adults: A Report of the American College of Cardiology/American Heart Association Task Force on Clinical Practice Guidelines. *Hypertension*. 2018;71(6):e13–e115.

44. Silvestre FJ, Miralles-Jorda L, Tamarit C, Gascon R. Dental management of the patient with ischemic heart disease: an update. *Med Oral*. 2002;7(3):222–230.

45. Samulak-Zielinska R, Dembowska E, Lizakowski P. Dental treatment of post-myocardial infarction patients: A review of the literature. *Dent Med Probl*. 2019;56(3):291–298.

46. Alzheimer's Association. 2021 Alzheimer's Disease facts and figures: Special report race, ethnicity, and Alzheimer's in America; 2021.

47. Niessen LC, Jones JA. Alzheimer's disease: a guide for dental professionals. *Spec Care Dentist*. 1986;6(1):6–12.

48. Ntritsos G, Franek J, Belbasis L, et al. Gender-specific estimates of COPD prevalence: a systematic review and meta-analysis. *Int J Chron Obstruct Pulmon Dis*. 2018;13:1507–1514.

49. Little JWFD, Miller CS, et al. *Dental Management of the Medically Compromised Patient*. 8th ed. St. Louis: Mosby; 2012.

50. van der Maarel-Wierink CD, Vanobbergen JN, Bronkhorst EM, Schols JM, de Baat C. Oral health care and aspiration pneumonia in frail older people: a systematic literature review. *Gerodontology*. 2013;30(1):3–9.

51. Prevention CfDCa COVID-19: Older Adults. 2021. https://www. cdc.gov/coronavirus/2019-ncov/need-extra-precautions/older-adults.html.

52. Elad S, Zadik Y, Kaufman E, et al. A new management approach for dental treatment after a cerebrovascular event: a comparative retrospective study. *Oral Surg Oral Med Oral Pathol Oral Radiol Endod*. 2010;110(2):145–150.

53. Spicer RS, Miller TR. Suicide acts in 8 states: incidence and case fatality rates by demographics and method. *Am J Public Health*. 2000;90(12):1885–1891.

54. Control CfDCaPNCflPa Web-based inquiry statistics query and reporting system (WISQARS). http://www.cdc.gov/injury/wisqars

55. Murphy S.L.X.J., Kochanek K.D. Deaths: Final data for 2010, National Vital Statistics Report 2012.

56. Surveillance EaERSP, National Center Institute Surveilance Research Program, based on previous submissions of SEER data (1977-2003). Oral Cancer 5-Year Survival Rates by Race, Gender, and Stage of Diagnosis. In: Research NIoDaC, editor; 2018.

57. Cleveland JL, Junger ML, Saraiya M, et al. The connection between human papillomavirus and oropharyngeal squamous cell carcinomas in the United States: implications for dentistry. *J Am Dent Assoc*. 2011;142(8):915–924.

58. Dawes C. Physiological factors affecting salivary flow rate, oral sugar clearance, and the sensation of dry mouth in man. *J Dent Res*. 1987;66. Spec No:648–653.

59. Dreizen S, Brown LR, Daly TE, Drane JB. Prevention of xerostomia-related dental caries in irradiated cancer patients. *J Dent Res*. 1977;56(2):99–104.

60. Heanue M, Deacon SA, Deery C, et al. Manual versus powered toothbrushing for oral health. *Cochrane Database Syst Rev*. 2003(1):CD002281.

61. Verma S, Bhat KM. Acceptability of powered toothbrushes for elderly individuals. *J Public Health Dent*. 2004;64(2):115–117.

62. Day J, Martin MD, Chin M. Efficacy of a sonic toothbrush for plaque removal by caregivers in a special needs population. *Spec Care Dentist*. 1998;18(5):202–206.

63. Sreebny L.M., Schwartz S.S. A reference guide to drugs and dry mouth—2nd edition. Gerodontology 1997;14(1):33–47.

64. Papas AS, Joshi A, MacDonald SL, et al. Caries prevalence in xerostomic individuals. *J Can Dent Assoc*. 1993;59(2):171–174. 77-9.

65. From the Centers for Disease Control and Prevention Achievements in public health, 1900-1999: fluoridation of drinking water to prevent dental caries. *JAMA*. 2000;283(10): 1283–1286.

66. Slot DE, Vaandrager NC, Van Loveren C, Van Palenstein Helderman WH, Van der Weijden GA. The effect of chlorhexidine varnish on root caries: a systematic review. *Caries Res*. 2011;45(2):162–173.

67. Hendre AD, Taylor GW, Chavez EM, Hyde S. A systematic review of silver diamine fluoride: Effectiveness and application in older adults. *Gerodontology*. 2017;34(4):411–419.

68. Watando A, Ebihara S, Ebihara T, et al. Daily oral care and cough reflex sensitivity in elderly nursing home patients. *Chest*. 2004;126(4):1066–1070.

69. Lin CY, Jones DB, Godwin K, et al. Oral health assessment by nursing staff of Alzheimer's patients in a long-term-care facility. *Spec Care Dentist*. 1999;19(2):64–71.

70. Ettinger RL. Rational dental care: part 1. Has the concept changed in 20 years? *J Can Dent Assoc*. 2006;72(5):441–445.

71. State of Illinois Health Care Surrogate Act, 755 ILCS 40/1

72. Aquilanti L, Santarelli A, Mascitti M, Procaccini M, Rappelli G. Dental care access and the elderly: what is the role of teledentistry? A systematic review. *Int J Environ Res Public Health*. 2020;17(23).

73. Mulk BS, Chintamaneni RL, Mpv P, Gummadapu S, Salvadhi SS. Palliative dental care- a boon for debilitating. *J Clin Diagn Res*. 2014;8(6). ZE01-6.

19

Patients Who Are Motivationally or Financially Challenged

Lewis Lampiris, Zachary Brian, and Samuel Nesbit

 Visit eBooks.Health.Elsevier.com

OUTLINE

The focus of this chapter is on patients who are motivationally challenged and those who are financially challenged. Although there are frequent commonalities between the two groups the reader should be aware that the motivationally challenged patient is not always financially limited and the financially challenged patient is not necessarily motivationally challenged. The body of the chapter focuses on the psychological, emotional, and social factors that are common threads in both groups and management strategies that are applicable to both. The chapter then offers additional information regarding motivational interviewing and options relating specifically to the financially limited patient.

Also woven into this chapter is a focus on **social determinants of health**, **health disparities**, and **health equity**. Such determinants as socioeconomic status, level of education attained, and **health beliefs** can be important for any patient but are more likely to have a significant effect on the oral health status of these patients. Social inequality in oral health status and the use of services is in many ways universal across the globe.[1]

As identified by the World Health Organization, approximately 3.5 billion people are affected by oral diseases.[2] Accessing preventive, diagnostic, and treatment services is unattainable for millions.[3]

Structural and interpersonal racism and lack of health equity often result in poor health outcomes for these populations. The entire dental team must be cognizant of ways in which the patient may be affected by these issues, keeping them in mind as efforts are made to relate to, communicate with, educate, and deliver care to this vulnerable and important segment of the population.

Both motivationally and financially challenged patients may be fatalistic about their teeth. They may have serious doubts as to whether their teeth can or should be saved. They commonly see the challenge of attempting to rehabilitate their dentition as insurmountable, believing that they do not have the time, energy, ability, or financial resources to accomplish the task. These are all perceptions; sometimes they are realistic and sometimes they are not. In some cases, historic mistrust of the health care system, displays of microaggressions and discrimination by healthcare providers can play a role in patients' acceptance of treatment recommendations.[4,5]

In many cases, significant improvements in oral health can be accomplished that are within the patient's financial means and capacity to handle (Figure 19.1). For treatment to be successful, however, patients must be willing to participate actively in the management of their own oral health and have trust in the dental team providing care. Unfortunately, some patients are unwilling or unable to do so—at least initially. Herein lies one of the greatest challenges to the practicing dentist—learning how to motivate a patient to engage actively in their own oral health care and to demonstrate to the patient that the practice has their oral health and well-being as their top priority. Indeed, although some patients will become enthusiastically engaged, others will do so only after much education and encouragement, and some never will.

The challenges in treating these patients are significant, but the rewards can be extraordinary. With a caring, committed, and sometimes adventuresome approach to treatment planning and treatment, the practitioner can achieve notable success in this arena. Furthermore, if the rewards and sense of accomplishment for the dental team are great, they can be even greater for the patient. The value to the patient who regains a functional, esthetic dentition is inestimable. The associated benefits to the person's self-esteem and overall quality of life may last a lifetime.

ORAL HEALTH MYTHS AND BELIEFS

Several commonly encountered situations illustrate the kinds of health beliefs and myths that a motivationally or financially challenged patient may hold. Many of these are related to cultural beliefs about oral health.[6] Listening carefully, the dentist can attempt to glean the health beliefs contributing to the patient's oral disease, while avoiding the temptation to immediately dispel myths and misunderstandings on the spot. The patient may resent the insensitivity of a healthcare professional who quickly dismisses their beliefs and values.[7] The careful listener allows the patient sufficient latitude to characterize their perceptions concerning oral disease. As rapport and trust build in the relationship, the dentist will find opportunities to add to the patient's knowledge base. Providing patients with information to modify their own beliefs is a more effective strategy than trying to substitute entirely new ones. The latter approach often does not work at all or if it does, apparent acceptance is more often incomplete or short-lived, failing for two critical reasons. First, the patient may perceive such a wholesale substitution as a dismissal of their total belief system. Second, this approach ignores the essential psychological and emotional investment that the beliefs represent for the patient. Several beliefs commonly held by such patients are discussed in the following section. Moving forward, we will also explore how a unique approach to listening and guided modification (called "motivational interviewing") can be applied to improve the relationship between patient and dentist and affect positive outcomes.

Soft Teeth

Patients who believe their teeth are "soft" often report numerous visits to the dentist beginning in their early teens and a long succession of teeth restored and restored again because of new and recurrent caries. By the time this patient reaches middle adulthood, some teeth may be missing, and others have large restorations (Figure 19.2). Recurrent caries continues to be a problem. Although a dentist may have even told the patient as a child, "You have soft teeth," the most frequent explanation is a cariogenic diet and poor oral hygiene. The patient may now believe that the teeth can no longer hold fillings and doubts that they are worth saving.

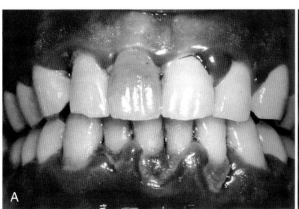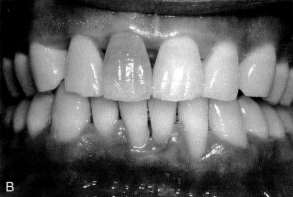

Fig. 19.1 Motivationally compromised and financially limited patient before **(A)** and after **(B)** treatment. (From Newman MG, Takei HH, Klokkevold PR, et al. *Carranza's Clinical Periodontology*, 12th ed. St. Louis: Saunders; 2015.)

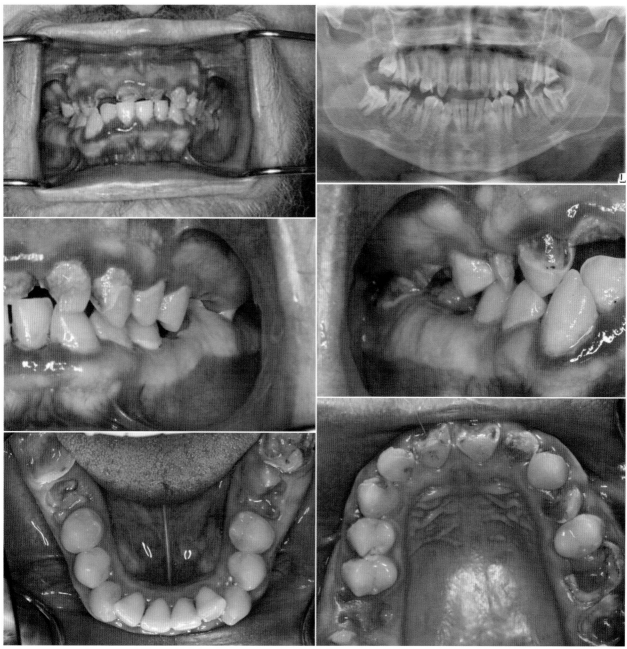

Fig. 19.2 Patient with "soft teeth." (Courtesy Dr. Scott Eidson, Chapel Hill, NC.)

Pregnancy and Breast-Feeding

Female patients who have carried and delivered babies and later breast-fed them may relate a history of rampant caries developing during that time. It is imperative that the dentist engage in active listening, as well as provide scientific evidence in explaining potential causes for an increase in caries burden, including nausea and vomiting etiology, which occurs in 70% of pregnancies. In addition to the belief that pregnancy directly leads to an increase in tooth decay, many patients will also present with concern that pregnancy resulted in bone loss and ultimately the loss of dentition. There is currently no scientific basis, however, to support the myth that calcium needed for fetal growth is obtained from the oral dentition and/or surrounding structures.[8]

In some cases, the caries may have become less active, but the patient continues to suffer from the ill effects of the earlier decay (Figure 19.3). Large restorations are often present, some teeth may now be fractured, and multiple full-coverage restorations may be necessary. Some may continue to suffer from the rampant caries that they attribute to the earlier period of pregnancy and lactation. The patient may have been reluctant to replace missing teeth out of concern for the perceived poor prognosis or because of a maternal desire to take care of the needs of her children first.

Family Dentures

Some patients, often those with extensive restorative needs or those suffering from severe periodontal disease, are certain that

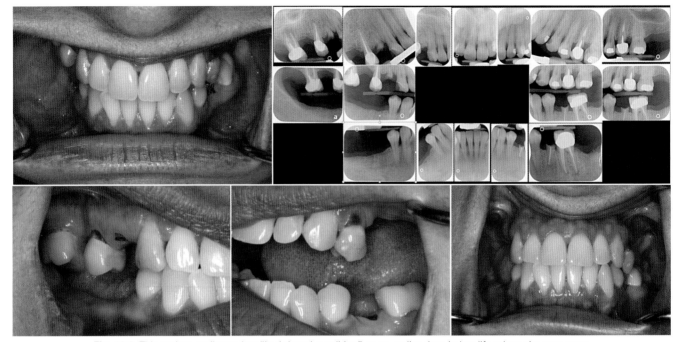

Fig. 19.3 This patient attributes her "bad dental condition" to an earlier time in her life when she was pregnant and a single parent with limited time and financial resources for dental treatment. She is now motivated and very interested in improving her oral condition. (Courtesy Dr. Christina Shaw, Chapel Hill, NC.)

dentures are inevitable. Because numerous family members have experienced this fate, they see becoming edentulous as unavoidable. Those who are most fatalistic often observe that they have inherited the condition. The dentist may be hard pressed to convince such patients that they have alternative options.

A variant of this explanation comes from a patient who refuses the option of replacing missing teeth with a removable partial denture, arguing that the retentive clasps will harm the abutment teeth. The patient often relates stories of friends or family members who wore partial dentures and eventually lost all remaining teeth. It is not surprising that partial dentures may sometimes fail when one considers the often questionable prognosis of some abutment teeth, the added burden of removing plaque around the clasps and other partial denture components, and the continuing risk of caries or periodontal disease. When a patient witnesses such a failure, it only confirms the belief that the family wisdom is correct and the patient also will end up in dentures (Figure 19.4).

Fear of the Dentist

The management of anxious or fearful patients is discussed in Chapter 15. Patients who have been unable to come to terms with this problem often avoid dental treatment altogether. Those with untreated active caries suffer from gross tooth destruction, fractures, abscesses, and toothaches. They typically have a history of episodic visits for pain relief. Similarly, patients with untreated, rapidly progressive, or severe periodontal disease become afflicted with pain, infection, and tooth loss. Despite the physical discomfort and loss of self-esteem, the patient comes to believe that overcoming fear is a greater obstacle than they can surmount, resulting in grave consequences to teeth, health, and self-image.

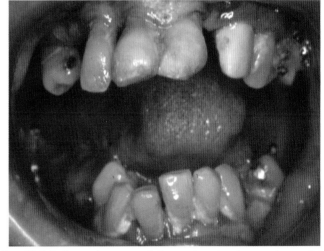

Fig. 19.4 Patient who wants full mouth extractions and complete dentures. (From Zarb G, Hobkirk JA, Eckert SE, et al. Prosthodontic Treatment for Edentulous Patients: Completed Dentures and Implant-Supported Prostheses. 13th ed. St. Louis: Mosby; 2013.)

IDENTIFYING UNDERLYING PROBLEMS

The patient's history and the clinical examination will be indispensable, not only in determining the clinical condition, but also in helping to reveal how the condition evolved. At the initial visit, a motivationally challenged patient is often apologetic about the condition of their mouth. It is not unusual for such a patient to express embarrassment and self-consciousness about gross caries, fractured or missing teeth, periodontally involved teeth, and halitosis. It is imperative that the dentist project a nonjudgmental demeanor, assuring the patient that their oral condition is not unique, that improvement can be achieved, and that the dentist and staff will do their best to correct the problems and eliminate disease. In many cases, it will have taken great courage for the patient to come to the appointment. Any comments, stringent office policies regarding payment, or body language by the dentist or staff that the patient interprets as patronizing, unsympathetic, or demeaning can be devastating to an individual's self-esteem. Many motivationally challenged patients are extremely vulnerable at this point and may overreact to the smallest slight. On the positive side, if such patients are treated with respect and dignity and if their concerns are dealt with professionally and sensitively, they can become appreciative, cooperative, and loyal to the practice. As the history is taken and the examination conducted, the patient usually begins to open up and share concerns and perspectives. Box 19.1 includes useful questions to ask that may help to facilitate discussion with the patient.

As this process unfolds, specific causes for the compromised oral health will become apparent. The following includes many of the common underlying causes for the patient's condition. It is noteworthy that there is rarely a single cause for the patient's lack of motivation to address oral problems. Rather, it is not unusual for the motivationally challenged patient's history to include several of the following causes, and many of these patients may be affected by two or more of these factors at any moment in time.

Genetic and Developmental Factors

Genetic and developmental factors affecting the dentition may include conditions such as hypocalcification, hypoplasia, amelogenesis imperfecta, and severe fluorosis (Figure 19.5). Recent research illustrates the complex interaction between an individual's genetic profile and the environment in the development of caries.[9] Periodontal disease affects approximately 90% of the population in its mildest form (gingivitis) and, like caries, stems from both genetic and environmental causes.[9] Identifying such factors can be useful in two important respects: helping the dentist develop treatment strategies that target the root causes of the patient's oral disease and providing positive psychological benefit to the patient who now sees a logical reason for the condition of his or her teeth and may come to find hope that there is a solution.

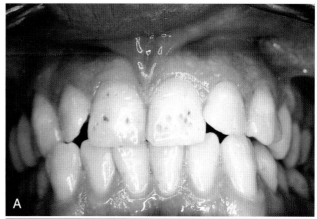
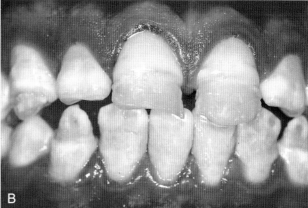

Fig. 19.5 Enamel hypoplasia. **(A)** Maxillary central incisors with a mild form of pitted enamel. **(B)** Multiple teeth with horizontal band of severe form of enamel hypoplasia. (From Sapp JP, Eversole LR, Wysocki GP. *Contemporary Oral and Maxillofacial Pathology.* 2nd ed. St. Louis: Mosby; 2004.)

Metabolic, Endocrine, and Immune Deficiency Factors

Hormonal changes are known factors in the development of pubertal and pregnancy gingivitis (Figure 19.6). Both endocrine disorders and altered immune function can contribute to periodontal disease and other intraoral abnormalities and infections. Identifying these issues and sharing that insight with the patient will have the same potential benefits as noted previously, relating to genetic and developmental factors.

Oral Health Literacy

Some patients are fully capable of understanding the relationship between their behavior and the oral disease but suffer from a lack of information or, perhaps worse, from misinformation. Sometimes they have correct information but are reluctant to act on it. There is an emerging body of literature regarding the effect of oral health literacy on an individual's ability to maintain good oral health.[10,11] **Oral health literacy** has been defined as "the degree to which individuals have the capacity to obtain, process and understand basic oral and craniofacial health information and services needed to make appropriate health decisions."[12] Careful listening to what the patient has to say, use of

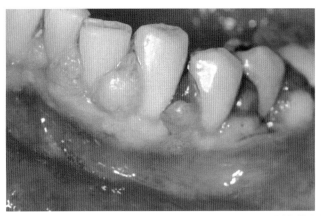

Fig. 19.6 Pregnancy-associated gingivitis. (From Newman MG, Takei HH, Klokkevold PR, et al. *Carranza's Clinical Periodontology.* 12th ed. St. Louis: Saunders; 2015.)

plain language rather than dental or technical terms, asking the patient to confirm that what they understand aligns with what the dentist has communicated, and using visual aids with verbal explanations are strategies that have been shown to be effective techniques in addressing health literacy issues.

As the examination continues, the dentist will have an opportunity to gain a sense of the patient's level of knowledge about oral health and disease. This may not be the best time to try to educate or reeducate the individual, however. Only after a full understanding of all problems has been reached and a conscious decision made as to the most effective intervention should the dentist attempt to modify the patient's knowledge base.

In some instances, the intellectually challenged patient may be unable to grasp the connection between oral disease and deleterious habits, including poor oral self-care. Intellectually, psychologically, or physically challenged patients also may have care providers who are unaware that they are contributing to oral disease by supplying highly cariogenic snacks as rewards or pacifiers in the management of their clients. In such a situation, the caregiver must be counseled with appropriate information that will help improve the patient's oral health. Dentists should take care to remember that oral health literacy is equally important for both the patient and caregiver.[13,14]

Interrelationship of Oral Health and Self-Image

A poor self-image often diminishes an individual's interest in good oral health and reduces willingness to absorb the cost and discomfort of dental treatment. If the patient is not happy with themselves or with life in general, it is unlikely that enthusiasm for dental care will be generated. Unfortunately, such patients are more likely than most to need extensive and complex treatment, reinforcing this negative perception. Some may barely cope with the issues of daily life and it may be too much for them to deal with the fear and expense of dental treatment, much of which they may consider elective. It is also important to consider the social stigma the patient may be experiencing or has experienced in the past. Poor oral health is sometimes viewed by society as a reflection of diminished self-worth, potentially impacting the patient's self-esteem and image. This may directly influence the patient's motivation.[15] A rarely vocalized but often

perceived sentiment is, "My bad teeth are just one more bad thing in my life." This negative perspective might have redeeming value if some tangible benefit to avoiding dental treatment could be described. Unfortunately, this is almost never the case. Left unattended and untreated, oral disease worsens, the likelihood of pain and infection increases, and, apart from full denture construction, the costs and complexity of treatment continue to grow. Furthermore, as the oral condition deteriorates, the patient's appearance becomes less attractive and the self-image suffers even more.

Behavioral and Nutritional Factors

The motivationally challenged patient is also likely to have poor dietary habits, engage in self-destructive behaviors, and be less likely to engage in health-promoting practices, such as effective oral self-care or regular physical exercise. These behaviors are most often a consequence of the underlying social determinants that affect the individual's health.[16] In the case of a patient with limited financial resources, dire economic conditions may hinder the ability to participate adequately in healthy behaviors. Regardless of the cause, the end result will be a significant negative effect on the patient's sense of wellness and the actual state of oral, mental, and physical health. Poor nutrition contributes to dental caries and, to a lesser extent, periodontal disease. Self-destructive habits, such as smoking and excessive alcohol consumption, also contribute to oral disease (see Chapter 14). Behavioral causes can be the most complex and difficult to solve, because the environmental and social factors underlying these behaviors are often beyond the control of the patient. Such patients can be a challenge for the dentist to manage (see *In Clinical Practice: Enhancing Relationships With Patients Who Have Oral Health Challenges* box). In extreme cases, such persons may be clinically depressed and have the expectation that they will not live a normal life span. In this situation, antidepressant therapy may be necessary and integral to any attempts to modify behavior relating to oral health. For more on managing patients with clinical depression, see Chapter 16.

IN CLINICAL PRACTICE

Enhancing Relationships With Patients Who Have Oral Health Challenges

Although many patients with oral health challenges are prompt, polite, and engaged, others are not. When patients are inconsistent in their own oral healthcare, erratic in keeping appointments, and/or appear to be disinterested or resistive to oral hygiene instructions, they may be labeled as "difficult," "noncompliant," or "problematic." Although these behaviors by patients pose real problems in clinical settings, it is also important to recognize the importance of the response to these behaviors. As professionals, we must always remember that our own experiences, standards, and values influence what we perceive as acceptable or unacceptable behavior and that we must not allow our own prejudices and stereotypes to affect the way we treat patients. It is also noteworthy that when members of the dental team first encounter a patient who is anticipated to be a "problem," the overt and subconscious body language, expressions, tone of voice, and manner in which information is delivered to the patient may actually promote and foster the predicted negative behaviors.

Continues

Healthy professional relationships require mutual effort on the part of both the clinician and the patient. Rather than blaming the "difficult patient," it can be valuable to explore why the behaviors occur. Missing appointments or frequently arriving late may be because of dependence on a family member or friend for transportation or because of an unexpected event that took precedence over the dental visit. Some patients will cancel or fail to appear for an appointment because of a lack of financial resources. Patient rudeness may represent frustration with any number of issues encountered before arriving for the dental appointment or could simply be a part of the patient's acquired response to a lifetime of unfulfilled expectations, hopes, and dreams. Acknowledging that the professional's response to patient behavior may contribute to a dysfunctional clinical relationship balances the responsibility for finding reasonable solutions.

Exploring the reasons for the patient's behavior can help the clinician understand the patient's perspective. Setting clear boundaries or reaching agreements (e.g., contracts) with patients can also improve clinical relationships. When a dentist–patient relationship is perceived as difficult, the clinician and staff should attempt to identify the underlying reason or source of the difficulty. Once the clinician is able to pinpoint the problem, the issue can be addressed directly with the patient. For example, the clinician could say, "Forgive me if I am interpreting incorrectly, but you seem skeptical (or doubtful) about all of this; please help me to understand what you are thinking." and "Can you think of ways you can help me help you?"[17] Building strong clinical relationships requires time and commitment from both dentist and patient. Clear documentation of discussions with the patient regarding the expectations of the office that are designed to improve and maintain good oral health, such as keeping appointments and following postoperative instructions, may help the dentist support a decision to discontinue a clinical relationship in the event that efforts to build a workable relationship fail.

Psychological Gain

Some individuals find a psychological benefit in being impaired. They may garner sympathy for their poor oral health from family members, friends, and coworkers, using it to avoid work or other responsibilities. For such patients, a health-related disability may have become part of a defense mechanism, used as a shield to deflect blame or limit expectations. Sometimes, it may actually be safer or more comfortable for the patient to believe that the situation is hopeless. In situations where it seems possible that the patient has a significant psychological investment in poor health, the dentist has the challenging but essential task of determining whether the patient genuinely seeks improved oral health. If so, do they want a temporary fix or a genuine solution? How much emotional energy is the patient capable of investing in dental treatment? Motivational interviewing, as we will explore further, provides a lens through which the dentist may seek an informed answer.

EVALUATING POTENTIAL FOR CHANGE

Maslow's hierarchy is a model frequently used to explain an individual's value system and priorities at a particular point in life (Figure 19.7). This hierarchy is also an excellent tool to help determine how a patient might be encouraged to improve their oral health condition. If, in fact, satisfaction of the person's needs is restricted to Level 1, physiologic (most basic human needs), it is unlikely that efforts to convince the patient of the value of long term improved dental health will be persuasive. By the same

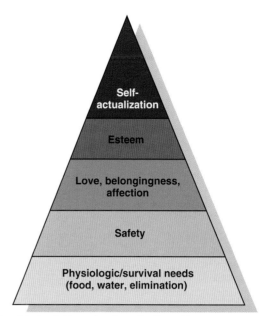

Fig. 19.7 Maslow's hierarchy of needs. (From Maslow, AH.; Frager, RD.; Fadiman, James, *Motivation and Personality*, 3rd ed. ©1987. Reprinted by permission of Pearson Education, Inc.)

token, a patient who has all their basic needs met and is now motivated by Level 5, self-actualization, is more likely to be amenable to a sophisticated intellectual rationale supporting the benefits of optimal oral health for a lifetime. But even if the discussion is appropriately directed at the patient's level on the hierarchy, there is no guarantee that those efforts will be successful because the patient retains the autonomy to accept or reject the rationale that is being put forth for their (unrelated) personal reasons. The patient may also choose to reject the logic because other self-actualizing concepts are more appealing or take precedence. Therefore, while not applicable in all situations, Maslow's hierarchy can often be a useful instrument to determine whether a patient is likely to be amenable to change, and if so, how to frame that discussion.

Some factors contributing to the patient's motivational challenges cannot be altered, most notably those relating to heredity or physical and mental development. Some environmental factors, such as job stress, have the potential to be improved, whereas others realistically cannot, such as chronic unemployment and poor housing. Behavioral factors are strongly influenced by the patient's psychological perspective and sense of self-worth. When psychological barriers to change are not overwhelming and when the patient has a positive sense of self-worth, the potential for eliminating mutable deleterious behaviors and promoting positive ones is good. The potential for eliminating or minimizing psychological barriers to change is highly variable and may not be completely under the patient's control. When circumstances that contribute to deleterious behaviors cannot be eliminated, the best the dentist may hope to accomplish is to raise the patient's consciousness to the recognition that the barriers exist and help motivate the individual to work around or through them. With time and a professional and supportive approach, such patients may be able to change and to improve both their oral and general health.

Attempting to improve the patient's sense of self-worth is a similarly difficult undertaking with no guarantee of success.

However, if early in the treatment the dentist can bring about a positive change in the patient's appearance, the person may be buoyed by an improved sense of self and begin to develop the belief that the effort is worthwhile. When these issues are dealt with effectively, educating the patient about the benefits of dental treatment is much easier.

It is also important to evaluate the patient's potential for improving oral self-care. The motivationally challenged patient often has poor oral home care, creating an unfavorable environment for the long-term success of any treatment. Most patients are receptive to some level of oral health instruction. How much they absorb and how effectively they implement that instruction varies, however. It is particularly important for the office staff to be attuned to the patient's dental history, cultural beliefs, knowledge base, and other factors that affect the individual's oral health status, including any specific barriers to care. When crafting an instructional plan, the dental staff and the hygienist, in particular, must have an understanding of the patient's individual needs and take those needs into account. The routine impersonal approach to oral physiotherapy instruction is unlikely to succeed with the motivationally challenged patient. A compassionate, thoughtful, and individualized approach to educating the patient regarding effective oral self-care is much more likely to produce the desired result and may also give the patient a greater appreciation for the benefits of comprehensive oral health care.

MAKING A TREATMENT DECISION

Once the dentist has determined that a motivationally challenged patient genuinely wishes to improve their oral health status, a plan of care must be developed and informed consent obtained. If the patient remains unmotivated or is unwilling or unable to modify the circumstances and attitudes that led to the oral problems, there may be no alternative but to recommend the extraction of questionable teeth and transition the patient to complete dentures. If the individual is receptive and motivated to change, however, then more comprehensive treatment can be proposed. Some of these treatment options are discussed later in this chapter.

The presentation of treatment options is critical with the motivationally challenged patient. At the outset, such a patient is more likely to have an unusually pessimistic view of the treatment and its chances of success. The same patient may also have unrealistic expectations about how long or how demanding the dental treatment will be. Although candid, the discussion must not be coercive, threatening, or intimidating. The patient must feel comfortable enough with the dentist to be able to share what are often deep-seated concerns and reservations.

For this patient, informed consent also carries greater-than-normal significance. In addition to the usual presentation of treatment options, their risks and benefits and advantages and disadvantages, and the costs in time and money required for each additional subjective component must be carefully and clearly presented. These include a patient-specific estimation of (1) the likelihood of successful treatment and (2) the consequences of failure. For these patients, the rewards of success are generally greater and the risks of failure often far more devastating than for other patients. After such a discussion, the patient is more likely to be engaged in the treatment plan decision making in a meaningful way.

Likelihood of Successful Treatment

Having presented to the practice in what is often a self-described "deep dark hole," the motivationally challenged patient is in a position to have an extraordinary appreciation for the value of specific restorations and the importance of improved overall oral health. Successful treatment may significantly increase the individual's comfort level, enjoyment of life, and self-esteem. For the dentist, an accurate estimation of prognosis guides the selection of treatment options for presentation to the patient and may also shape the manner that the options are presented. For the patient, such information helps determine which option to pursue and whether to accept a plan. Unfortunately, with these patients, it can often be difficult to determine the likelihood of success with any or all dental treatments, making it more difficult for patient and dentist to evaluate and compare the various options.

Often, dentist and patient must make a treatment decision without a clear idea of the disease or treatment prognosis. In these situations, the dentist must be sure the patient receives all the available information and that the information and discussion of prognosis, although limited, are documented thoroughly.

In the process, some patients will become able to recognize and correct preconceived notions about dental disease and dental treatment. On completion of the plan of care and having achieved a good state of oral health, as well as a value of and a wish to preserve it, this patient is likely to be an appreciative and committed participant in the practice for the long term.

Having an honest, realistic discussion is also helpful in another important way. Even if the treatment outcome is not what the patient and dentist hoped it would be, at least the patient will have been fully informed of that possibility and can, in most cases, appreciate that although one approach has not worked, there are other treatment options to be tried and success may still be achieved.

Consequences of Failure

For the motivationally challenged patient, the consequences of treatment failure may go far beyond such concerns as infection or loss of a tooth. The dentist may need to assess what effect treatment failure could have on the patient's self-worth and sense of well-being. If the patient is already fragile psychologically or emotionally, a dental treatment failure could result in an emotional breakdown or a severe depressive episode.

While developing the plan of care, it is useful to be mindful of the patient's future or anticipated concerns about treatment failure. The motivationally challenged patient is more apt to attach greater-than-normal (sometimes inappropriately or excessively) significance to each step or to any unexpected event in the treatment process. This patient is likely to regard even minor setbacks as abject failures and be tempted to give up entirely on the process. Appropriately detailed explanations and gentle positive persuasion by the dental team can be effective tools in reassuring the patient, encouraging continued participation, enhancing self-esteem, and moving the process forward. If the dentist believes that the patient's anxiety about treatment failure cannot be overcome, it is preferable to suggest a more aggressive or robust treatment plan involving extraction of any questionable teeth. This stratagem has dual benefits: increasing the probability of treatment success and simultaneously reducing both the number and intensity of the patient's concerns about treatment failure.

Patient Participation

It is not unusual at this juncture for some patients to attempt to distance themselves from the discussion and seek to pass the decision making to the dentist, with expressions such as, "You're the doc. Whatever you recommend is fine with me." Because the dental problems seem overwhelming, the options complex, and the prognosis guarded, it is not surprising that the patient has difficulty making decisions. The older practitioner with a paternalistic approach to treatment plan presentation may be inclined to drive the decision making, whereas a less-experienced practitioner may find it flattering that the patient has that level of confidence in their skills and may fill the apparent vacuum with their personal treatment recommendation. However, an astute provider will try to avoid both of these pathways. By abdicating the decision-making role, the patient, consciously or unconsciously, also abdicates responsibility for their own oral health. If the treatment fails, no matter how many disclaimers have been made and no matter how complete the informed consent, the patient is likely to attribute the failure to the dentist. Even when the treatment is ultimately successful, if the patient has cast the burden of success fully on the dentist, unanticipated costs in time, money, stress, and energy may be resented and blamed on the dentist. For these reasons, and particularly with this type of patient, the dentist must *not* make final treatment decisions *for* the patient. The dentist may guide, assist, or provide recommendations, but at the same time must encourage the patient to take responsibility for making the ultimate decision. In some circumstances, a family member, trusted friend, or caregiver may be willing to participate in the discussion and provide support for the patient's decision.

MOTIVATING THE PATIENT

After the dental problems have been identified, the root causes and contributing factors brought to light, and the patient and practitioner have agreed together to embark on a serious attempt to deal with the oral disease, a strategy for motivating the patient must still be developed. The patient and practitioner may design and carry out this strategy jointly or more often the dentist undertakes it alone. Often, this aspect of planning, although a part of the dentist's thought process, is not formalized in conversation or in the patient record. The fact that it is not externalized, however, does not mean that it is not important. When this part of the process is carried out with forethought and purpose, the chances of successful treatment are greatly enhanced. Without it, the likelihood of success is poor. The development of an effective strategy is generally a two-part process: (1) identifying an approach to motivating the patient and (2) discerning how to apply those motivators to greatest effect.

Several issues may motivate a patient to improve his or her oral condition and overcome deep-seated barriers to care. Although these can be categorized separately as external or internal factors, to a great degree, they overlap.

Internal Motivators
Immediate Pain Relief

Pain relief is a powerful motivator in the short term but unfortunately, when the pain is gone, the patient may resume old habits and patterns that will delay treatment until the next painful episode arises. Occasionally, suggestions by the dentist or other members of the dental team at the episodic visit will induce the patient to commit to comprehensive care.

Long-Term Pain Relief

The prospect of long-term pain relief is a less powerful but still potentially effective motivator, especially if the patient has had a notably traumatic episode that they wish never to repeat.

Prospect of a More-Positive Self-Image

The desire for or expectation of a more positive self-image can be an effective long-term motivator and works best with the patient who functions at or near the top of Maslow's hierarchy.

Improved Appearance and Elimination of Halitosis

The prospect of improved appearance and elimination of halitosis are powerful motivators; however, in the absence of other longer-term motivators, the patient may lose interest and discontinue treatment once the esthetic goal is achieved or the halitosis eliminated.

Improved Function

For persons at any level of Maslow's hierarchy who "want to chew better," the prospect of improved function can be an extremely effective short-term and long-term motivator.

Eliminating Disease

For a few patients, the prospect of eliminating disease can be a strong and all-sufficient motivator. Care must be taken to temper enthusiasm and avoid self-destructive or obsessive cleaning behaviors. For patients who function at the upper levels of Maslow's hierarchy, eliminating oral disease can sometimes be an effective short- and long-term motivator.

Improved Wellness

Although an abstract concept to most patients, improved wellness is a powerful priority for some persons, especially those functioning at the upper level of Maslow's hierarchy.

External Motivators
Family Pressure

Expressed through the wishes of parents, children, or significant others, family pressure can be a powerful short- and long-term motivator. In the absence of concurrent internal motivation, however, this influence may wane over time.

Career Advancement/Positive Employment Outcomes

Associating improved oral health and appearance with career advancement may generate enthusiasm for treatment and willingness to undergo considerable sacrifice and cost. Additional benefits may include fewer lost days at work because of dental pain.[18] Studies have shown a favorable employment outcome in welfare recipients after completion of dental treatment.[19]

Impending Changes in Life Companion

Dating, marriage or remarriage, and the social pressures associated with impending changes in personal relationships can be among the most powerful of motivators, but the manner in which patients react to those forces and the duration of their effects are highly variable. Affairs of the heart can be fickle and so can this patient's compliance with and enthusiasm for dental treatment.

Implementation

To be effective, the issues mentioned must be matched specifically to the patient's needs and circumstances. The dentist must articulate clearly how the dental treatment will benefit the patient's particular circumstances. The dental team also needs to share these views with the patient in a manner that will both engage and motivate the individual. The patient may require frequent reminders of the critical issues and relationships. Key issues in motivating and managing the motivationally challenged patient are summarized in Box 19.2.

Some patients will fail to maintain a new oral health program despite the dentist's best efforts. Some will lose interest; others will suffer personal or financial difficulties that preclude continuation of treatment. Still others will delay or discontinue care with the expectation of resuming later. The dentist must be prepared for the possibility that a comprehensive plan of care must be terminated. This unfortunate outcome is more common with the motivationally or financially challenged patient than with others. Should the situation arise, the dentist must handle it with tact and professionalism and should not take the failure personally.

MOTIVATIONAL INTERVIEWING

Many of the approaches discussed in this chapter encompass a methodology known as motivational interviewing (see Chapter 12 for additional discussion). Motivational interviewing has been described as "a collaborative, patient-centered approach evoking the patient's own motivation to change, thereby enhancing the relationship between the clinician and patient and improving patient outcomes."[20] The practice of motivational interviewing is the subject of many dedicated studies and articles (see Suggested Readings at the end of this chapter) and it is worth briefly exploring the four processes critical to the technique's success: engaging, focusing, evoking, and planning.

Engaging

No treatment plan, no matter how well prescribed, may reasonably be expected to succeed without patient–dentist rapport. In the Engaging phase of motivational interviewing, the dentist should invite open dialogue with the patient, with an emphasis on open-ended questions and listening: "I'm glad you're here. What brings you in today?" or "Thanks for coming in. Was there

---

> **BOX 19.2 Some "Dos and Don'ts" When Motivating a Compromised Patient**
>
> **Do**
> - Present information in clear segments that the patient can understand and retain.
> - Set realistic and incremental goals.
> - Reward the patient for positive behavior and achievement of goals.
> - Add new goals sequentially. Giving the patient too many goals too quickly can be counterproductive.
> - Strive to build the patient's confidence.
> - Work to dispel the perception that the problems are insurmountable.
>
> **Do not**
> - Overwhelm the patient with information.
> - Rush the process to completion if the patient is not responding.
> - Let yourself get discouraged or give up. The patient is looking to you to keep the process going. A resetting of goals or a change of course may be necessary, but as long as the patient is trying, the dentist must stay engaged.
> - Make a half-hearted effort. A half-hearted effort is an invitation to failure and simply confirms the patient's earlier suspicions.

a specific concern that brought you to our office?" The motivationally or financially challenged patient will often arrive at the clinic in a state of ambivalence or resistance and the dentist should take this opportunity to build trust and present themself as empathetic and actively engaged in the patient's success.

Focusing

Having fostered a comfortable and nonjudgmental environment for the patient in the Engaging phase, the dentist can now help guide the patient toward the target behavior or condition to change. In the Focusing phase of motivational interviewing, the dentist again uses open-ended questions to steer, but not force, the conversation. Nonthreatening questions such as "Would you like to talk about that tooth pain now?" or "Should we see what we can do about your bleeding gums?" help reinforce a collaborative relationship and focus the conversation on the problem or behavior to be modified.

Evoking

This critical phase of motivational interviewing is designed to leverage "change talk" (a patient's own statements about their desire or need to change) to highlight the need for modifying behavior and explore potential solutions.[20] In the Evoking phase, the dentist draws upon the patient's own words to underscore the problem and possibility for change. For example, the dentist might ask, "It sounds like you're concerned about the possibility of losing that tooth. Is that right?" or "If you continue smoking, how do you think that might affect the health of your gums?" Clarification is important. Some practitioners may find it useful to ask the patient to rate their commitment or confidence. For instance, "On a scale of 1 to 10, how confident are you that you could floss more regularly?" By reflectively listening to the patient's own thoughts, the dentist can help guide the patient toward an agreeable solution.

Planning

The Planning phase of motivational interviewing offers the chance to increase the odds of success dramatically by giving the patient the opportunity to modify their own behavior, with the dentist simply serving as a guide. As has been said, "It is important that the patient commits to change rather than the clinician telling them how to change." Open-ended questions such as "How can I help you with that?" or "What do you think is a reasonable first step?" reinforce respect for the patient's autonomy and help motivate change.

Motivational interviewing is both an art and a science and when properly applied can dramatically enhance the patient–dentist relationship, reduce ambivalence or resistance to behavior change or treatment, and improve oral health outcomes among motivationally and financially challenged patients.

MANAGEMENT OPTIONS

The motivationally or financially challenged patient may still have multiple treatment options. Any limitations or barriers to treatment should not necessarily limit the breadth or scope of treatment. In some cases, the barriers to care may stimulate innovative solutions to the patient's unique difficulties. Occasionally, during discussion, the patient may be inspired to suggest their own treatment solution, which can be exciting and productive for both the patient and dentist.

Selecting the right plan for such a patient is often more difficult and has a greater chance of failure than with the average person. Given that reality, it is important for the dentist to modify his or her own standards and expectations as discussed in the accompanying *In Clinical Practice: The Need to Redefine "Success"* box. As with most patients, the possibilities range from ideal treatment to no treatment. Additional approaches to be considered for the motivationally or financially challenged patient include the limited treatment plan and the extraordinary efforts plan to maintain a dentition with a questionable prognosis.

Ideal Treatment

The dentist may assume that the motivationally challenged patient is not really interested or committed to ideal treatment, but it may be the case that the patient has never been *offered* ideal care and is unaware of its potential advantages. All patients deserve to at least hear about an optimal treatment option. In some clear instances, information about available alternatives may provide the motivation and incentive necessary to encourage the patient to participate in such treatment.

On the other hand, it is unwise to tantalize the patient with the prospects of ideal comprehensive care when the disease control phase has not been successfully completed. For example, a patient with rampant caries and severe periodontal disease may inquire about replacing a missing tooth with an implant. Although it is desirable to offer replacement options, an implant would not be a viable immediate option in the presence of an overall deteriorating oral condition.

IN CLINICAL PRACTICE

The Need to Redefine "Success"

When dealing with a motivationally or financially challenged patient, the dentist's barometer of success must be reset. With this type of patient, it is almost guaranteed that achieving goals will come less often and goals will be harder to reach. The reason for this is self-evident. By definition, these patients have significant barriers to care. Most have sporadic dental histories and are anxious or phobic about receiving dental treatment. It can be extremely difficult to reverse this cycle of behavior and its effects. When dealing with such patients, the specific goals must be clear, realistic, and attainable. The goals should be neither too high, increasing the failure rate and discouraging the patient, nor too low, appearing simplistic and therefore meaningless.

The process of redefining treatment success for the motivationally challenged patient must often include a shift in the perspective of both the patient and the dentist.

Patient's Perspective

The dentist and patient must engage in honest discussion. If the patient has an overly pessimistic view of their condition and the possibility of overcoming problems, the dentist must help to raise those expectations. Conversely, if the patient has an overly optimistic or fanciful view of the situation, the dentist must encourage lower expectations and lead the patient to view the situation more realistically.

Practitioner's Perspective

The dentist should recognize that the more complicated or heroic the proposed plan, the less likely the chance of success. The obvious response to this predicament is to simplify the plan, but this approach can become counterproductive if the patient is asked to give up personally important elements. If too much is sacrificed for the sake of simplicity, the patient may forego the attempt altogether or enter into it with so little enthusiasm that there is little chance of success. The dentist must avoid the temptation to simplify all such treatment plans to improve their own personal success rate.

The dentist must accept the fact that not all cases will yield *immediate* success. For some patients, it may take months or years and active treatment may be in on-again, off-again cycles before the patient and dental team are satisfied with the achieved level of oral health.

The following suggestions can improve the odds of attaining success with this patient:

- At the outset, offer ideal treatment to those patients who are motivated to change destructive behaviors and determined to undergo the treatment. Patients who initially are not motivated or committed to receive ideal treatment should be offered acute care or limited care. After acute needs are addressed, active disease stabilized or resolved, and trust and rapport established, ideal treatment options should then be thoroughly investigated.
- Give your best effort and encourage the patient to do the same. If treatment fails, it should be for reasons other than lack of trying. The patient will usually appreciate your effort and may then choose to work with you on a revised plan.
- Do not take shortcuts or compromise the standard of care. Not only can this jeopardize the success of the plan, but it also may be hard to justify to other care providers or licensing boards.
- Document thoroughly, because with good documentation the provider can substantiate whatever was done, even if the treatment does not succeed.
- Do not take the failure of treatment personally. Other opportunities will present themselves and other patients will need you to go to the same lengths for them.
- Be realistic about your chances of helping the patient to achieve an optimal state of oral health. You can expect that approximately one-third of the motivationally and financially challenged patients will discontinue care. Despite your best efforts, multiple issues and confounding circumstances will prohibit their continuance with dental treatment. You can expect another one-third of this group to have an uneven, largely episodic experience. With perseverance, patience, compassion, and understanding on your part, you can expect that approximately one-third of these patients who come to your practice will become motivated and conscientious comprehensive care patients. Recognizing that turning one-third of these patients around is a significant success should serve as a realistic goal for the dentist and keep the dental team motivated to continue this important endeavor.

No Comprehensive Treatment (Provision of Acute Care Only)

Dentists are conditioned to intervene when a problem is encountered. When a patient displays the ravages of oral disease, the dentist is not inclined to wait and see what happens. As uncomfortable as that alternative may be, however, sometimes it is best for all concerned not to intervene, except for acute care to eliminate current active infection. At least three situations can be described where comprehensive care would not be the best alternative.

1. *The patient has been brought in for treatment for the sole purpose of making someone else happy.* If the patient has no personal interest whatsoever in undergoing treatment, the treatment is almost certain to fail. A good case in point is the patient confined in a nursing home who has no desire for dental treatment, but whose family members seek to improve their appearance. In such a situation, a simple cosmetic compromise that the patient can tolerate may satisfy the family. To attempt comprehensive care for this patient would be ill advised.

2. *The patient suffers from extensive oral disease and believes they want comprehensive care but are unrealistic about the demands of the task.* This patient may have unrealistic expectations about the amount of time and effort necessary to complete the treatment, as well as about the outcome. The patient's financial resources may not be adequate to pay for such a complex treatment plan. If the dentist initiates comprehensive treatment under these circumstances, the likelihood of patient discontent, treatment failure, and a host of negative outcomes for the dentist is great. Again, the most prudent course of action is to provide acute care for pain or swelling and then educate the patient about the demands and commitment required to complete the comprehensive treatment plan. If the patient is still unrealistic about what is entailed in the treatment or the expected outcomes of the treatment, the dentist may have no alternative but to decline treating the patient.

3. *The patient desires extensive restorative work but has several missing teeth, severe attrition, and decreased vertical dimension of occlusion.* The patient does not want dentures and does not have the financial resources to pay for a full mouth reconstruction. This is often an onerous situation for both patient and practitioner. Difficult though it may be, if the patient is asymptomatic and has no active disease, the best approach may be to defer treatment until more teeth have been lost and the patient accepts the idea of a complete denture or dentures. An occlusal guard or cast partial overdenture may represent a compromise approach, but such treatment has significant risk for the dentist. It may raise the patient's expectations unrealistically and obligate the dentist professionally and legally to maintain the patient in a "holding phase" for an indefinite period. If the patient's finances truly preclude comprehensive treatment and the patient continues to decline complete or partial denture options, the only recourse may be to dismiss the patient from the practice.

Unfortunately, the *no treatment* option is sometimes used improperly by the dentist. Following are descriptions of two situations to be avoided.

First, when confronted by a patient with limited finances or who is motivationally challenged and who suffers from overwhelming oral disease, the dentist may be drawn to the *no treatment* option simply because it is the easiest solution for *the dentist.* The shortsighted perspective is "Why waste time explaining options and considering treatment for a patient who doesn't really want or can't afford comprehensive care anyway?" But all patients deserve to be given an honest and complete perspective on all the reasonable options available and to be offered the opportunity to make an informed choice. The patient should not be discouraged from reasonable treatment options simply because of the *dentist's* reluctance to get involved. Refusal to treat a patient because it is inconvenient for the dentist would be a violation of several ethical principles (see Chapter 7).

However, there are legitimate reasons for a dentist to refer a patient to another provider for comprehensive treatment. If the patient desires comprehensive care, but the dentist does not believe that he or she has the knowledge, skill, or expertise to complete the treatment successfully, then the patient can, in good conscience, be referred to another practitioner for treatment. If the encounter and referral are handled well by the dental team, the patient will leave better informed and appreciative of the time and respectful manner with which they were dealt.

The second difficulty to avoid is the temptation to use the *no treatment* option as a method of scaring the patient into treatment. It is appropriate and wise to caution the patient about the ill effects and hazards of declining treatment, but that presentation must be honest and realistic and should never be used to coerce.

If the patient, dentist, or both choose the *no treatment* option, the dentist still has several obligations to the patient. Any acute needs must be addressed and all reasonable efforts should be made to eliminate current active infection. The patient must be informed about the risks and hazards associated with deferring treatment. The dentist must thoroughly document this discussion in the patient's record, including options presented, risks and benefits, the choice of no treatment, and the rationale for the decision.

Limited (Disease Control Phase) Treatment

A reasonable option for many motivationally and financially challenged patients is limited treatment, which may eventually lead to complete care when the limitations or barriers to treatment have been reduced or eliminated. A limited treatment plan provides the practitioner and patient with maximum flexibility. A disease control phase plan represents one form of limited treatment, the details of which are described in Chapter 10. The goals of limited care are similar to those of a disease control phase but may include more than disease and infection control. A limited treatment plan typically includes temporary or definitive management of the chief concern, resolution of any acute problems, and disease control phase treatment for teeth that are certain to be retained (including behavioral, chemotherapeutic, and restorative treatment). Any specific barriers to treatment must be addressed. As with a standard disease control phase plan, it is imperative to have clear goals and an established endpoint to the treatment. In most cases, it is necessary to follow with a posttreatment assessment or equivalent mechanism to reassess the extent to which established goals have been achieved. At that assessment appointment, patient and dentist can come to a decision about whether to discontinue treatment altogether, go into a holding phase, or proceed with some form of definitive phase care. In any case, it is essential that full and informed consent is achieved and that the patient does not have any illusions about the prospect or promise of treatment beyond the limited plan that has been agreed to.

Extraordinary Efforts to Maintain Dentition With Questionable Prognosis

Virtually all patients who are motivationally challenged come to the dentist seeking some form of treatment and sometimes have very specific treatment requests. They may not have the interest or the financial resources to embark on an ideal treatment plan. They may be overwhelmed with oral problems and oral disease to such an extent that they are unwilling to engage in a classic disease control phase plan of care. In such situations, are there other alternatives that can be offered? Here the dentist is challenged to come up with a creative, sometimes adventuresome, sometimes unconventional approach to treatment planning. For some patients, limited financial resources will be the driver in this exploration, but that is not always necessarily the case. Rarely will this involve untried experimental techniques. Most frequently, established techniques will be selected for treatment, but in this setting, there is uncertainty with the prognosis and lack of predictability in the outcome.

This approach has sometimes been described as **compromise treatment**. Unfortunately, this term is often misinterpreted and the concept often abused. In this context, *compromise* does not mean that the work fails to meet professional standards. Indeed, there should be no diminution in the quality of the individual restorations or in the way in which care is delivered or documented. Examples of this type of treatment include the following:

The dentist and patient agree:
- To save a key tooth (see Chapter 5), even though there is significant bone loss and mobility.
- To attempt to salvage the existing dentition despite advanced generalized periodontitis.
- To provide a large protective cusp direct fill restoration (rather than a full coverage indirect restoration) in an effort to save a badly broken-down tooth.
- To enlist heroic measures to maintain an existing fixed partial denture.

Before engaging in such treatment, several essential elements must be in place:
- Informed consent: The patient must have complete understanding of the limitations of treatment and the significant possibility of failure resulting in loss of the tooth or teeth.
- Agreement of both parties: The dentist and patient must both agree to the plan and be firmly committed to it.

- Documentation of the nature of the compromise, the rationale behind it, and contingency plans in case of a negative or adverse outcome.

It is important to recognize that compromise treatment plans involve an element of risk—and in some cases, a high degree of risk—for both parties. A compromise plan is not for the faint of heart—dentist or patient. From the dentist's perspective, the plan will often push the limits of the "comfort zone" and may encourage trying techniques and/or materials that are innovative or new to the practitioner. Similarly, the patient must be, at least to some degree, a risk taker, preferably an adventuresome spirit, who is willing to face the possibility of a fractured tooth, lost restoration, broken appliance, or even toothache at an inopportune time.

Proper patient selection is critical. Compromise treatment should only be attempted when there is complete trust and entirely open communication between the parties. An anxious patient who has had previous unsatisfactory dental experiences, who has mistrusted dentists in the past, or who is rattled by the prospect of unscheduled emergency dental visits is not a candidate for a compromise plan.

It is important to keep in mind that a compromise plan does not supplant the need for disease control therapy. In reality, most compromise plans will be an amalgam of specific heroic treatments within the framework of a disease control plan of care. As with all dental patients, a definitive phase treatment plan should never be undertaken without confirming that the patient's active oral disease is being controlled.

With careful patient selection, open communication, complete informed consent, and ideal documentation, a compromise plan can be successfully accomplished with minimal legal risk. Consideration of a compromise plan can drastically expand the range of possible therapies. The process can be exciting, dynamic, and creative for both patient and provider. But in the absence of the required elements (patient flexibility and understanding, informed consent, and thorough documentation), a compromise plan can be a recipe for disaster, inviting patient anxiety and disappointment, peer criticism for the dentist, and the potential for malpractice litigation.

As with the limited care plan, the compromise plan may be followed by a complete array of definitive therapies as the clinical situation evolves, the patient's finances improve, and the patient's attitude, interests, and expectations mature and come into clearer focus.

CARING FOR PATIENTS WITH LIMITED FINANCIAL MEANS

Financially limited patients have many of the characteristics described for motivationally challenged patients. They often suffer from the ill effects of poor oral hygiene and inadequate professional care. They may be afflicted with extensive oral disease. In addition, their financial limitations color their perceptions of the treatment they can obtain. Such patients may feel intimidated by the cost of dental care. Financial limitations, whether real or perceived, can be a significant barrier to a patient's ability to seek and obtain dental treatment and may severely limit the nature and scope of treatment that the patient may be able to afford.

Having spent many hours and much energy learning how to improve the oral health of their patients, most dentists find the discussion of costs and finances intrusive and potentially damaging to the doctor–patient relationship. At no time is this more necessary, however, than with patients who have limited financial means. Such patients may have very real financial limitations or they may simply perceive financial limitations because dental treatment falls below other priorities for use of their discretionary income. To complicate matters further, the patient may use the perceived financial limitation to mask other barriers to care. In any case, the issue of finances must be dealt with forthrightly before treatment can begin.

In general, patients who describe themselves as having financial limitations fall into one of four groups:

1. Patients on a fixed or bare subsistence income with no discretionary resources available to spend on dental care.
2. Patients who can afford a minimal level of care.
3. Patients who can afford comprehensive dental care but prefer to use their discretionary income for other things.
4. Patients who previously had financial means (whether through employer-sponsored insurance or out-of-pocket payments) but are now unemployed or underemployed.

For most patients, the easiest and most effective approach is to separate the discussion of finances into two parts and deal with each part individually and at different times. During the first part of the discussion, focus simply on the question of how much the patient can reasonably afford to spend on dental care in the foreseeable future (usually in the next 6 to 12 months). The question must be raised with discretion and only after ample opportunity has been provided to develop rapport and trust between the dentist and patient. This should be a value-based discussion with the dentist placing emphasis on the perceived benefit to the patient in terms of their health, function and appearance, and couched in terms identified in the patient's previously reported concerns and desires. Usually, this stage is reached toward the end of the initial examination visit, but in some cases, it may need to be deferred to a later time. It does need to occur before or during the informed consent treatment planning discussion with the patient. But if financial issues are raised too early, or insensitively, the patient may perceive the queries as an intrusion into their private life and conclude that the dentist is "after my money." Such a breach in the dentist–patient relationship may be irreparable.

Some questions from the dentist's perspective that will commonly come up in this discussion include: Does the patient have the financial resources to engage in some level of minimalist (i.e., disease control phase) treatment? Should outside financial assistance for the patient be sought? Is the reported financial limitation an expression of some other underlying barrier to treatment?

Without such information, the dentist cannot determine which type of treatment plan (acute, disease control, limited care, extraordinary efforts to maintain a dentition with a questionable prognosis, or comprehensive care) is most appropriate, much less its details and sequence. With financial information, the dentist can, in a professional and sympathetic manner, begin to establish a range of feasible options for the patient to consider.

The second part of the discussion addresses the issue of how payment for the services will be resourced and sequenced. This part of the discussion occurs most appropriately after the treatment plan has been developed and agreed to by patient and dentist. The office manager often handles the specific arrangements. Like all other aspects of the patient's records, the financial information must remain confidential between dentist, administrative staff, and patient. Conversation about financial affairs must reaffirm the patient's dignity regardless of their financial means. It is always important that the treatment be provided in a compassionate manner, with an appreciation for the patient's individual needs and circumstances.

Many patients are unable to afford the optimum treatment plan. Some will be unwilling to accept even the limited treatment alternatives proposed by the dentist. What then? Options that can be considered are discussed in the following sections.

Staged Treatment

Staged treatment may be a workable alternative and is particularly appropriate for a patient whose treatment needs are not acute or urgent. A patient with a stable oral condition who needs multiple indirect restorations can be offered a plan where the restorations are placed sequentially over a period of years.

Payment Plans

Payment plans are certainly an option if the patient has good credit and the needs are urgent, or if the patient, for whatever reason, does not want staged treatment. Through various different sources, including local or national financial institutions or credit cards, the patient or the practice can establish payment plans or loans, or in-office individualized arrangements.

Outside Resources

Family members may be a source of financial aid, particularly if the family has a vested interest in the patient's improved oral health. Outside funding sources, including religious organizations, philanthropic organizations, and social services, can sometimes augment the patient's limited resources.

Other Practice Settings

All of the aforementioned options represent possible alternatives if the patient wants to stay in the practice and the practitioner wishes to keep the patient in the practice. Many financially limited patients take a long time to build a trusting relationship with a particular care provider and, once that relationship is established, are extremely loyal and do not wish to leave the practice under any circumstances. If it becomes desirable or necessary for the patient to seek care elsewhere, however, the following options remain:

- Colleges of dentistry in academic health centers and their associated satellite clinics
- Community, county or state sponsored public health clinics
- Federally Qualified Health Centers (FQHCs)
- Clinics for low-income patients that have been established in some localities by local or state dental societies and are staffed by volunteer practitioners.

The principal limitations to these programs may be lack of universal availability, relative inaccessibility, and limitations to the scope of services they may provide. A dental college, for example, represents a source for good-quality care but requires some remuneration and substantially more time to complete the treatment and may not be accessible to some patients. Local, regional, state, or private, not-for-profit public health clinics or volunteer clinics may have restricted hours, long waiting lists and may provide only a limited range of services. (For more information regarding FQHCs, see *Suggested Readings* at the end of this chapter.)

Reducing or Waiving Fees

Reducing or waiving fees should be an option of last resort and considered only for the most worthy and reliable of patients. For more details, see the accompanying *In Clinical Practice: Should I Do Pro Bono Work in My Office?* box.

IN CLINICAL PRACTICE

Should I Do Pro Bono Work in My Practice?

Many reasons can be cited for choosing to provide free or reduced-fee dental treatment for selected patients. Many dentists are motivated by the altruistic desire to give something back to the community because their lives have been enriched by their experience in the profession. Some, who would like to do charitable or mission work but are unable to go outside their community, see this as an alternative. Others report doing it simply because they feel an obligation to society, a sort of social contract. The personal rewards from philanthropic work come in many forms. They include positive responses from appreciative patients and the self-satisfaction that comes from knowing that a disadvantaged patient is healthier because of one's own efforts. In addition, there may be spiritual rewards and the satisfaction of building a positive image in the community and among one's peers.

There are also many reasons why a practitioner might choose not to provide dental care at waived or reduced fees. It may be viewed that providing this care to a few patients has no real effect on the overall societal need. Furthermore, it may provide false hope to other patients or perhaps cause bitterness among those not able to benefit from such philanthropy. An argument can be made against such work on financial grounds. Fee reductions may not be possible for patients who have dental insurance. Waiving the patient's copayment or accepting the insurance contribution as full payment is usually forbidden by insurance companies and is illegal in many jurisdictions.

Ideally, the decision about whether to offer treatment at a reduced rate or *gratis* is made with thoughtful consideration after the establishment of a formal office policy. Written guidelines in office policies, clearly delineating the circumstances in which waivers of fees (and fee reductions) will be granted, can help the practitioner avoid ambiguity. This can also make clear to staff that a consistent policy exists that is fair and equitable.

The following list of suggestions summarizes a rational approach to free or reduced-fee dental work:

- Establish a clear office policy and maintain consistency.
- Select patients who have compelling oral health needs and legitimate financial constraints.
- Consider a patient's reliability and motivation to improve his or her oral health.
- Confirm with the office manager or other staff that the patient meets the established criteria for this kind of assistance.
- Carefully plan the case with a clear timetable for both the dental treatment and payment schedule. Include appropriate stipulations concerning expected appointment and home care compliance. Put this information in writing and have both the patient and provider sign it.
- Carefully document the treatment, outcomes, and the patient's compliance with recommendations.
- In all cases, provide treatment that meets the professional standard of care.

Government-Sponsored Programs/Public Assistance Programs

In the United States, Medicaid is the primary government-sponsored public assistance program that supports the dental treatment of children who fall below the poverty line, the disabled, and the impaired. Medicaid also supports a limited range of dental services for adults who qualify based on limited financial means. The intent of the Medicaid dental program is to provide low-income individuals with dental insurance, because individuals with such insurance, including children, are more likely to receive dental care than those without dental insurance.[21-32]

Medicaid, a joint federal and state healthcare program, began in 1965 and, with its inception, became the largest public dental insurance program in the United States.[33] To qualify for Medicaid, a family must demonstrate that their income is a certain percentage of the Federal Poverty Level (FPL). For example, in 2021, 100% of the FPL for a family of four is $26,500.[34] Many states have expanded coverage, particularly for children, above the federal minimums. The Affordable Care Act of 2010, signed by President Barack Obama on March 23, 2010, created a national Medicaid minimum eligibility level of 133% of the federal poverty level ($29,711 for a family of four in 2011) for nearly all Americans younger than 65 years. States have the option to expand Medicaid coverage with federal support for a limited time period.[33]

Although the program covers both medical and dental care, considerably fewer federal and state dollars are allocated to Medicaid dental care compared with medical care.[35] Although the federal government requires that state Medicaid programs include dental services for children, the type and extent of dental services for adults are left to the discretion of each state.[33] States vary in the services they cover, eligibility criteria, and reimbursement levels.[36] Most states have the goal of providing a full range of dental services to all individuals who are eligible for Medicaid.[37] The cost of such provisions is expensive and often not recognized when funding allocations are made. Instead of reducing the number of services provided by Medicaid or the number of individuals who are eligible, states often decide to reduce the level of reimbursement for services.[35,37] As a result, in many states, dental services for adults under the program are limited or nonexistent. The dental practitioner in the United States makes the decision whether to participate or abstain from providing care to patients with dental Medicaid insurance (see *In Clinical Practice: Should I Accept Medicaid in My Practice?* box).

In most high-income countries, treatment for oral health care services is expensive and usually not part of universal health coverage.[38]

IN CLINICAL PRACTICE

Should I Accept Medicaid in My Practice?

Many dentists report that they do not accept Medicaid patients because of low reimbursement levels, the limited number of reimbursed procedures, cumbersome claims administration, delays in reimbursement, and problematic patient behavior, such as missed appointments and lack of compliance with professional recommendations.[35,37-47]

Continues

Those who accept Medicaid reimbursement for services rendered do so for multiple reasons. Some feel a desire to "give back," others feel a responsibility as a practitioner to provide care for a certain number of low-income individuals, some have been in less-than-ideal economic situations themselves, and others accept it when the practice is young and regular patients are few.

Although the administrative burden of filing Medicaid claims has decreased dramatically in most states, some dentists opt out of Medicaid and instead provide pro bono care in their offices (see the *In Clinical Practice: Should I Do Pro Bono Work in My Office?* box). Nevertheless, when children living below the poverty level do receive dental care, it is most likely to be through the Medicaid program.[48]

Given the option of participating in the Medicaid program, dentists usually choose one of the three following courses of action:

1. *Declining the option*, perhaps waiting for a time when the reimbursement will be more reasonable.
2. *Accepting a limited number of Medicaid patients* and making such patients an adjunctive part but not the focus of the practice. This approach serves some patients that otherwise would not receive treatment and the practice minimizes some of the expenses incurred.
3. *Establishing a practice that focuses on Medicaid.* With this option, the goals and mode of operation are modified somewhat from the typical private practice. Patients are typically overbooked owing to anticipation of higher no-show rates and every effort is made to complete as many procedures as possible at one visit. Other models of care receive a per-visit Medicaid rate reimbursement, giving the dentist more choice in determining the number of procedures to be completed at each visit. By increasing production volume and decreasing expenses and overhead costs, some dentists have been successful in a practice that generates its revenues from Medicaid insurance.

DISPARITIES IN ORAL HEALTH AND ACCESS TO CARE

Oral Health Disparities and Social Determinants of Health

The landmark report "Oral Health in America: A Report of the Surgeon General" makes it clear that there are "profound and consequential disparities in the oral health of our citizens."[49] The report describes a "silent epidemic" of oral disease affecting our most vulnerable populations, many of whom are motivationally and financially disadvantaged. The disparities are found within specific population groups, including those with lower levels of income and education, racial and ethnic minorities, indigenous populations and First Peoples, the older adult population, those living with disabilities and other health conditions, and those living in rural areas.[50]

Good health, including oral health, begins at home and is directly related to the physical and social environment in which one lives, works, and plays.[51] Living in a community in which the water is fluoridated, nutritious foods are readily available, and dental offices are conveniently located facilitates good oral health for the general population. Access to reliable transportation, good schools, and safe environments in which to participate actively in physical activities affects person's ability to maintain their health.

Multiple barriers exist to accessing oral health services. These include but are not limited to socioeconomic status, oral health literacy, geography, availability of dental insurance, and location of dental offices.[52] The issues surrounding the lack of access to dental care are complex and require collaborative and coordinated action by the private and public sector. Dentists must consider the social determinants of health (sometimes called "non-medical drivers of health") when evaluating patient motivation, modifying patient beliefs that may reduce the chances of success, and treatment planning.

Role of the Profession

As a profession, dentistry has done a remarkably effective job of treating the ravages of oral disease in those patients who seek treatment and have the financial resources to pay for it. The record in the United States for managing care for those who are both motivationally and financially challenged has been far less impressive. The reasons for this failure are myriad and are found on multiple levels. In the United States, dental treatment is generally perceived as a privilege rather than a right. Oral health, or lack thereof, has traditionally been viewed as something within the purview and responsibility of the individual. Most dental treatment in the United States is still delivered through a private practice, fee-for-service system, and overtures to move to a single payer (government based) delivery system continue to be met with vigorous political opposition.

On the positive side, the American Dental Association's and other dental professional codes of ethics (see Chapter 7), clearly espouse the need for dental professionals to help alleviate this problem. To their credit, many dental organizations and societies and individual practitioners have tried to make a contribution to this cause. But much need remains.

Role of Government

Historically, in the United States, the dental sections of state departments of public health have focused their efforts on prevention of oral disease and provision of preventive dental services. Many county and municipal governments have established community-based dental clinics to provide services for the underserved in their area. When direct therapeutic care has been made available, the focus almost always has been on the needs of children and those with acute dental problems. Few of these programs provide definitive care for adults beyond direct-fill restorations, extractions, and uncomplicated removable prostheses. The admissions criteria, availability, and level of services, and fees charged may vary greatly from locality to locality, even within the same jurisdiction.

The federal government has partnered with local communities to establish permanent medical and dental public health clinics in some designated areas of need, and has recently expanded funds to provide dental services in some established FQHCs.

In many instances, community-based clinics and FQHCs also operate school-based dental programs. These programs, where screening and preventive oral health care services are provided by dental hygienists, efficiently increase access to care. In certain situations, comprehensive, restorative dental services may also be provided by dentists. Oral healthcare in school-based programs may be delivered via portable equipment, mobile vans parked on school property, and sometimes through fixed clinics located within the schools themselves. Research has shown that "incorporating dental care into a school-based health center resulted in improved oral health in underserved children while overcoming barriers that typically restrict access."[53]

Medicaid funds administered through state government are available to the practitioner who chooses to provide dental services to low-income patients. The range of covered services is limited and the provider must agree to accept Medicaid fees as payment in full. Typically, adult patients are required to make a minimal copayment to cover the administrative costs for each visit; there is often no copayment for child patients. Although much of the administrative process (such as submitting claims and prior authorizations) has been streamlined in some jurisdictions in recent years, the enrollment process for the practitioner can be slow and cumbersome. For these and other reasons, many private practitioners have chosen to opt out from participating in Medicaid.

Some state governments, sometimes in cooperation with the federal government, have made available scholarships and low-interest loans and used partial forgiveness of health profession loans to encourage dental providers to settle in underserved areas. The future of many of these programs is uncertain because they may need periodic legislative approval for continuation and funding.

The Canadian healthcare system is similar to that of the United States in that oral healthcare delivery is separate from the medical delivery system. Limited governmental oral health benefits, at the federal level, are available to veterans, refugees, and First Nations People.[54] The majority of public oral health programs fall under the jurisdiction of provincial governments.[55]

Across the European Union, out-of-pocket costs are much greater for oral health services than those for other healthcare services. As in the United States, this leads to limited access to care for low-income individuals. Most of the countries provide minimum scope of services (emergency care, children), but there is large variation in terms of restriction as to who qualifies for services and the range of services, from very limited, to partial, to comprehensive coverage.[56]

In Nordic Countries (Sweden, Finland, Norway, Iceland, Denmark) universal availability and high-quality oral health programs are funded through taxation and public provision. Access and utilization rates are generally high.[57]

In the UK, dental services are provided through the National Health Service (NHS).[58] Unlike the other components of the NHS, patients are expected to contribute toward the cost of care. Patients receiving care through the NHS face long waiting lists and increased costs. The portion of household spending on dental services has doubled over a recent 10-year period. Along with fear, the most common reason for not accessing dental care in the UK is cost.[58]

In Australia, as seen in the United States and in Canada, socially disadvantaged individuals across all ages have poor oral health and have difficulty finding timely dental treatment.[59] Care is provided both in the public and private sectors. Public services are primarily provided by states and territories. As in Canada, the scope of services varies by state. A common denominator across all of the public programs in Australia are

the significant waiting times to get care, which can range from 2–5 years in some areas.[60]

Role of Third-Party Payers

In the United States, private dental insurance carriers are profit driven. Patients in vulnerable populations, with a need for extensive services, do not offer an attractive revenue stream. Because cost containment is achieved via high premiums and high co-pays or limiting services and reducing reimbursement rates, dental insurance is often not very beneficial to these patients.

With dental managed care plans, patients are enrolled in a private health plan that receives a fixed monthly premium from the state or employer. The health plan is then responsible for providing all or most of the recipient's healthcare needs. The managed care model embraces a concept often referred to as value-based care. This approach to payment is intended to base reimbursement on clinical outcomes, as well as incentivize lowered health care costs and increased efficiency in clinical care delivery.[61] Although the potential for benefit from such plans to the motivationally or financially limited patient is great, uncertainties remain concerning the extent of benefits, level of care to be provided, and accessibility of care. Many states are embracing managed care plans. At this time, it is difficult to predict the effect these plans will have on this group of patients.

A LOOK TO THE FUTURE

What does the future hold for financially or motivationally challenged patients? As the general population continues to increase, the number of these patients can also be expected to increase. Our society places a high value on a healthy mouth and an esthetically pleasing dentition. Government intervention may be required if the dental profession, individual dentists, insurance carriers, and managed care plans fail to serve this population's oral health needs. It is difficult to predict how the autonomy of the treatment planning experience or the dentist–patient relationship will be affected. However, a change seems certain.

What is not expected to change is the existence of a group of patients with both complex treatment needs and significant barriers to care influenced by the social determinants of health. These patients will continue to require significant demands on the dental team in terms of time, expertise, and financial considerations. Fundamentally, it will be important for the dentist and dental team to acknowledge and deepen their understanding of the social and economic barriers that exist among these populations such as lack of reliable transportation, housing insecurity, or food insecurity. These nonmedical drivers of health may impact the patient's ability to address their non-acute oral health needs adequately and/or to make their ability to seek services that much more difficult. To serve the patient and community better, it is advisable for the dental team to take an integrated approach, helping connect the patient with social support services and resources that can help mitigate or eliminate barriers to care (see Chapter 6).

The challenges that the motivationally challenged or financially limited patient present to the individual dentist and to the dental profession as a whole are significant. These challenges deserve to be met in a responsible and meaningful way. Altered societal values will be necessary to create a climate where the needs of these patients are recognized and public resources applied to the task. The dental profession, allied health workers, third-party payers, and public health agencies at all levels of government will need to engage in a cooperative effort if this complex problem is to be addressed. In the meantime, it is the individual dentist who, with an open, caring, and

compassionate approach, can often make the difference in the lives of these patients. Guided by ethics discussed in Chapter 7, it is a moral imperative that dentists consider the disadvantaged patient's individual circumstances and motivations in treatment planning. Although the patient's care requires a significant investment of energy on the part of the dentist, the professional satisfaction that comes with a successful outcome is immeasurable. For the patient, the positive effect on their well-being and self-esteem can have lifelong benefits.

REVIEW QUESTIONS

- What common perceptions (or misperceptions) about their own oral health and oral healthcare limit or preclude patients from seeking dental treatment?
- Describe some of the frequently encountered causes for an individual to develop a severely compromised oral condition.
- How can the dentist assess a patient's potential for developing a realistic and positive attitude toward oral healthcare?
- What techniques and strategies can the dentist use to motivate a patient to improve their oral condition?
- What dental treatment options are available in your community for the patient with limited financial resources?
- Does the profession of dentistry have an ethical obligation to address the needs of the underserved? If so, how far does that obligation extend (what populations need to be served? What treatment should be provided? Under what circumstances should that treatment be provided?).

- Do you have an ethical responsibility as an individual practitioner to serve patients who have limited financial resources? If so, how will you fulfill that responsibility?

Practice Assessment

Do a self-assessment of your current practice setting. When patients present who have extensive oral health needs and limited financial resources, how are those patients managed in your practice? Are those patients welcomed into the practice? What are the provider and staff attitudes and behaviors toward these patients? Does the dental team effectively discern, appreciate, and address the individual patients' social determinants of health? What efforts are being made to help patients overcome their past and present barriers to care? After such an assessment, analyze how office policies, culture, and behaviors might become more responsive to the needs of your patients.

REFERENCES

1. Pitts N, Amaechi B, Niederman R, et al. Global Oral Health Inequalities Dental Caries Task Group research Agenda. *Adv Dent Res.* 2011:211–220.
2. Global, regional, and national incidence, prevalence, and years lived with disability for 354 diseases and injuries for 195 countries and territories, 1990–2017: a systematic analysis for the Global Burden of Disease Study 2017. Lancet 2018;392:1789–8583
3. World Health Organization Consolidate report by the Director-General 2021. https://apps.who.int/gb/ebwha/pdf_files/WHA74/A74_10Rev1-en.pdf
4. Flores G, Lin H. Trends in racial/ethnic disparities in medical and oral health, access to care, and use of services in US children: has anything changed over the years? *Int J Equity Health.* 2013; 12(10).
5. Almond AL. Measuring racial microaggression in medical practice. *Ethn Health.* 2019;24(6):589–606.
6. Butani Y, Weintraub JA, Barker JC. Oral health-related cultural beliefs for four racial/ethnic groups: assessment of the literature. *BMC Oral Health.* 2008;8:26.
7. Mofidi M, Rozier RG, King RS. Problems with access to dental care for Medicaid-insured children: what caregivers think. *Am J Public Health.* 2002;92(1):53–58.
8. Yenen Z, Atacag T. Oral care in pregnancy. *J Turk Ger Gynecol Assoc.* 2019;20(4):264–268.
9. D'Souza RN, Dunnvald M, Frazier-Bowers S, et al. Translational genetics advancing fronts for craniofacial health. *J Dent Res.* 2013;92(12):1058–1064.

10. Lee JY, Divaris K, Baker AD, et al. The relationship of oral health literacy and self-efficacy with oral health status and dental neglect. *Am J Public Health.* 2012;102(5):923–929.
11. Baskaradoss JK. Relationship between oral health literacy and oral health status. *BMC Oral Health.* 2018;18:172.
12. Institute of Medicine *Oral Health Literacy.* Washington, DC: The National Academies Press; 2013.
13. Miller E, Lee JY, DeWalt DA. Impact of caregiver literacy on children's oral health outcomes. *Pediatrics.* 2010;126(1):107–114.
14. Baskaradoss JK, AlThunayan MF, Alessa JA, et al. Relationship between caregivers' oral health literacy and their child's caries experience. *Community Dent Health.* 2019;36(2):111–117.
15. Otto M. *Teeth: The Story of Beauty, Inequality, and the Struggle for Oral Health in America.* New York: The New Press; 2017.
16. Watt RG. From victim blaming to upstream action: tackling the social determinants of oral health inequalities. *Community Dent Oral Epidemiol.* 2007;35(1):1–11.
17. Niselle P. Difficult doctor-patient relationships. *Aust Fam Phys.* 2000;29(1):47–49.
18. Hall JP, Chapan SL, Kurth NK. Poor oral health as an obstacle to employment for Medicaid beneficiaries with disabilities. *J Public Health Dent.* 2013;73:79–82.
19. Hyde S, Satariano WA, Weintraub JA. Welfare dental intervention improves employment and quality of life. *J Dent Res.* 2006;85(1):79–84.
20. Gillam DG, Yusuf H. Brief motivational interviewing in dental practice. *Dent J.* 2019;7(2):51.
21. Ahlberg J, Tuominen R, Murtomaa H. Dental knowledge, attitudes towards oral health care and utilization of dental services

among male industrial workers with or without an employer-provided dental benefit scheme. *Community Dent Oral Epidemiol.* 1996;24(6):380–384.

22. Bloom B, Jones LI, Freeman G. Summary health statistics for US children: National Health Interview Survey, 2012. *Vital Health Stat.* Dec 2013;10(258):1–81.

23. Eklund SA, Pittman JL, Smith RC. Trends in dental care among insured Americans: 1980 to 1995. *J Am Dent Assoc.* 1997;128(2):171–178.

24. Grembowski D, Conrad D, Milgrom P. Utilization of a prepaid plan of commercial dental insurance. *J Public Health.* 1985;75(1):87–89.

25. Macek MD, Wagner ML, Goodman HS, et al. Dental visits and access to dental care among Maryland schoolchildren. *J Am Dent Assoc.* 2005;136(4):524–533.

26. Manski RJ, Edelstein BL, Moeller JF. The impact of insurance coverage on children's dental visits and expenditures, 1996. *J Am Dent Assoc.* 2001;132(8):1137–1145.

27. Manski RJ, Magder LS. Demographic and socioeconomic predictors of dental care utilization. *J Am Dent Assoc.* 1998;129(2):195–200.

28. Manski RJ, Macek MD, Moeller JF. Private dental coverage: who has it and how does it influence dental visits and expenditures? *J Am Dent Assoc.* 2002;133(11):1551–1559.

29. Manski RJ, Moeller JF, Mass WR. Dental services, use, expenditures and sources of payment, 1987. *J Am Dent Assoc.* 1999;130(4):500–508.

30. Manning WG, Bailit HL, Benjamin B, et al. The demand for dental care: evidence from a randomized trial in health insurance. *J Am Dent Assoc.* 1985;110(6):895–902.

31. Eklund SA. The impact of insurance on oral health. *J Am Coll Dent.* 2001;68(2):8–11.

32. Sweet M, Damiano P, Rivera E, et al. A comparison of dental services received by Medicaid and privately insured adult populations. *J Am Dent Assoc.* 2005;136(1):93–100.

33. Medicaid: http://www.Medicaid.gov/.

34. Office of the Assistant Secretary for Planning and Evaluation: 2021 poverty guidelines: https://aspe.hhs.gov/2021-poverty-guidelines.

35. Manski RJ, Moeller JF, Maas WR. Dental services. An analysis of utilization over 20 years. *J Am Dent Assoc.* 2001;133:655–664.

36. White BA. Toward improving the oral health of Americans: an overview of oral health status, resources, and care delivery, Oral Health Coordinating Committee, Public Health Service editor. *Public Health Rep.* 1993;108(6):657–672.

37. Manski RJ. Access to dental care: a call for innovation. *J Am Coll Dent.* 2001;68(2):12–15.

38. World Health Organization Oral Health https://www.who.int/news-room/fact-sheets/detail/oral-health Accessed June 7, 2021.

39. Lang WP, Weintraub JA. Comparison of Medicaid and non-Medicaid dental providers. *J Public Health Dent.* 1986;46(4):207–211.

40. Nainar SM. Dentists' ranking of Medicaid reimbursement rates as a measure of their pediatric Medicaid participation. *ASDC J Dent Child, Nov-Dec.* 2000;67(6):422–424. 375, 407.

41. Venezie RD, Vann Jr WF, Cashion SW, et al. Pediatric and general dentists' participation in the North Carolina Medicaid program: trends from 1986 to 1992. *Pediatr Dent.* 1997;19(2):114–117.

42. Iben P, Kanellis MJ, Warren J. Appointment-keeping behavior of Medicaid-enrolled pediatric dental patients in eastern Iowa. *Pediat Dent.* 2000;22(4):325–329.

43. Damiano PC, Brown ER, Johnson JD, et al. Factors affecting dentist participation in a state Medicaid program. *J Dent Educ.* 1990;54(11):638–643.

44. Blackwelder A, Shulman JD. Texas dentists' attitudes toward the dental Medicaid program. *Pediatr Dent Jan-Feb.* 2007;29(1):40–46.

45. Im JL, Phillips C, Lee J, Beane R. The North Carolina Medicaid program: participation and perceptions among practicing orthodontists. *Am J Orthod Dentofacial Orthop Aug.* 2007;132(2):144e15–144e21.

46. Morris PJ, Freed JR, Nguyen A, et al. Pediatric dentists; participation in the California Medicaid program. *Pediatr Dent Jan-Feb.* 2004;26(1):79–86.

47. Shulman JD, Ezemobi EO, Sutherland JN, Barsley R. Louisiana dentists' attitudes toward the dental Medicaid program. *Pediatr Dent.* Sep-Oct 2001;23(5):395–400.

48. U.S. Congress *Office of Technology Assessment. Children's dental services under the Medicaid program: background paper.* Washington, DC: Congress Report OTA-BP-H-78; 1990.

49. U.S. Department of Health and Human Services. *Oral health in America: a report of the Surgeon General.* Rockville, MD: U.S. Department of Health and Human Services, National Institute of Dental and Craniofacial Research, National Institutes of Health; 2000.

50. Shaw J, Farmer J. (2016). An environmental scan of publicly financed dental care in Canada: 2015 Update. 2016. doi: 10.13140/RG.2.2.16001.86888.

51. U.S. Department of Health and Human Services: Secretary's Advisory Committee on health promotion and disease prevention objectives for 2020. Healthy people 2020: an opportunity to address the societal determinants of health in the United States. http://www.healthypeople.gov/2010/hp2020/advisory/SocietalDeterminantsHealth.htm/.

52. Institute of Medicine and National Research Council. *Improving Access to Oral Health Care for Vulnerable and Underserved Populations.* Washington, DC: The National Academies Press; 2011.

53. Carpino R, Walker MP, Liu Y, et al. Assessing the effectiveness of a school-based dental clinic on the oral health of children who lack access to dental care. *J Sch Nurs.* 2017;33(3):181–188.

54. The State of Oral Health in Canada. https://www.cda-adc.ca/stateoforalhealth/

55. Canadian Association of Public Health Dentistry Government Dental Programs. https://www.caphd.ca/programs-and-resources/government-dental-programs.

56. Winkelmann J., Henschke C., Scarpetti S., Panteli D. Dental care in Europe: financing, coverage and provision. September 2020 The European Journal of Public Health 30(Supplement_5)

57. Widström E., Ekman A., Liljan S. Aandahl L.S., Malling Pedersen M. Developments in Oral Health Policy in the Nordic Countries February 2005 Oral Health & Preventive Dentistry 3(4):225–35

58. Dental care in the United Kingdom - Statistics & Facts https://www.statista.com/topics/3350/dental-care-in-the-united-kingdom/

59. Oral Health and Dental Care in Australia (Australian Institute for Health and Welfare) https://www.aihw.gov.au/reports/den/231/oral-health-and-dental-care-in-australia/contents/dental-care

60. Australian Government Department of Health Report Of The National Advisory Council On Dental Health. https://www1.health.gov.au/internet/publications/publishing.nsf/Content/report_nacdh~report_nacdh_ack

61. Boynes S, Nelson J, Diep V, et al. Understanding value in oral health: the oral health value-based care symposium. *J Public Health Dent.* 2020;80(S2):27–34.

SUGGESTED READINGS/WEBSITES

Association of Clinicians for the Underserved
www.clinicians.org
Health Resources and Services Administration
http://www.nidcr.nih.gov/DataStatistics/SurgeonGeneral/
National Association of Community Health Centers
www.nachc.com

National Network for Oral Health Access
www.nnoha.org
US Department of Health and Human Services: Oral health in
America: a report of the Surgeon General. Rockville: National
Institute of Dental and Craniofacial Research, National Institutes
of Health; 2000.
www.surgeongeneral.gov/library/oralhealth/

A

Abfraction A wedge-shaped lesion occurring in the cervical third of the tooth attributed to occlusal loading and tooth flexure in this area.

Abrasion The wearing away or notching of teeth by mechanical means; for example, because of excessive toothbrushing.

Abscess A consolidated collection of polymorphonuclear leukocytes (pus) characterized by pain and swelling.

Access to care The timely use of personal health services to achieve the best health outcomes.

Acquired immunodeficiency syndrome (AIDS) The most severe manifestation of disease due to infection with human immunodeficiency virus (HIV). The criteria established by the Centers for Disease Control and Prevention for the diagnosis of AIDS include (1) presence of certain opportunistic infections indicating an underlying defect in cell-mediated immunity in the absence of known causes of underlying immunodeficiency or other host defense defects; or (2) CD4+ cell count of less than 200/mL; or (3) CD4+ cell percentage of less than 14%.

Actinic keratosis A precancerous lesion on the skin caused by excessive exposure to the sun. The lesion may be red or skin colored, flat or elevated, and verrucous or keratotic.

Active caries lesion A caries lesion that continues to progress; not arrested.

Active treatment plan A document that lists the disease control and definitive procedures sequenced in the order in which they will be provided. The active treatment plan has an endpoint, in contrast to the perpetual treatment plan.

Activities of daily living (ADL) Activities that require basic skills and focus on self-care tasks such as bathing/showering, bowel and bladder management, dressing/undressing, eating/swallowing, feeding, functional mobility, sexual activity, toilet hygiene, and the care of personal devices.

Acute apical abscess Pulpal infection and necrosis that lead to tooth sensitivity, abscess formation, and eventual swelling of associated tissues.

Acute phase of care Diagnostic and treatment procedures aimed at solving urgent problems.

Acute pulmonary edema Fluid accumulation in the lungs causing difficulty in breathing; often seen in patients with congestive heart failure.

Acute sinusitis A severe infection in one or both maxillary sinuses characterized by a constant, "heavy," debilitating pain that changes intensity with changes in head position and may be accompanied by heavy discharge of mucus or pus from the affected sinus.

Addiction Physical or emotional dependence, or both, on a substance such as alcohol or drugs.

Adenocarcinoma A carcinoma derived from glandular tissue.

Administrative law Type of law governing state and federal regulatory areas that define the qualifications required for a specified profession.

Adolescence The period of life beginning with the appearance of secondary sex characters and terminating with the cessation of somatic growth, roughly from 11 to 19 years of age.

Adrenocortical crisis An emergency situation caused by inability of the adrenal cortex to produce sufficient corticosteroids in the presence of stress, such as during a dental appointment. Symptoms include weakness, headache, nausea, and confusion.

Advance directives Instruction about a person's wishes, goals, and values regarding what will be done in case the person becomes incapable of making decisions about medical care. Also called *living will, durable power of attorney for healthcare*, and sometimes *advance healthcare directive* or *healthcare advance directive*.

Affective disorders Mood disorders.

Ageusia A generalized loss of taste sensation.

Aggressive periodontitis A type of periodontal disease that leads to rapid attachment loss and periodontal bone destruction. Most commonly seen in younger individuals.

Agoraphobia A fear of open and crowded spaces that often renders patients homebound.

Akathisia The inability to sit still.

Alcohol use disorder (AUD) A medical condition characterized by an impaired ability to stop or control alcohol use despite adverse social, occupational, or health consequences.

Algorithm A series of definable processes or instructions that can be implemented by a computer to solve a problem or accomplish an action.

Alogia Diminished speech.

Alzheimer's disease (AD) A presenile dementia characterized by confusion, memory failure, disorientation, restlessness, agnosia, hallucinosis, speech disturbances, and the inability to carry out purposeful movement. The disease usually begins in later middle life with slight defects in memory and behavior that become progressively more severe.

Amalgam An alloy, composed chiefly of silver, tin, and copper, that is mixed with mercury to form dental amalgam.

Amalgam bluing A flat, bluish-gray lesion of the oral mucosa that results from introducing amalgam into the oral tissues. Also referred to as an amalgam tattoo.

Amelogenesis imperfecta A hereditary abnormality characterized by defects in the formation of enamel.

Amotivational syndrome A loss of interest and desire to study or work, decreased energy or productivity, and generalized apathy, sullenness, moodiness, and inability to concentrate. Frequently seen in chronic marijuana users.

Anesthesia A temporary but complete loss of sensation.

Angina A spasmodic, often severe pain in the chest caused by reduced blood flow to the heart. Symptoms of stable angina are predictable and usually occur after stress or physical exertion. Unstable angina is chest pain that is unpredictable and often occurs without exertion and at night.

Angle classification II relationship Advancement of the maxillary teeth relative to the mandibular teeth; often identified by the intercuspal relationship between the maxillary first molars and the mandibular first molars on the same side of the patient's mouth; frequently accompanied by a large anterior overjet.

Angle classification III relationship Advancement of the mandibular teeth relative to the maxillary teeth; often identified by the intercuspal relationship between the maxillary first molars and the mandibular first molars on the same side of the patient's mouth; frequently accompanied by a minimal or nonexistent anterior overjet or an anterior crossbite.

Angular cheilitis Inflammation with fissuring at the labial commissure; *Candida albicans* infection and loss of vertical dimension of occlusion are commonly recognized are contributing causes.

Anhedonia The inability to experience pleasure in life.

Ankyloglossia A short lingual frenum that limits tongue mobility; may contribute to difficulty with speech, mastication, swallowing. Also referred to as *tongue tied*.

Ankylosed teeth Teeth that are fused to the alveolar bone.

Anorexia nervosa A pathologic, psychosocial disorder manifested by extreme aversion to food and an intense fear of gaining weight.

Anterograde amnesia A form of amnesia in which new events are not transferred to long-term memory.

Antibiotics Medications used to treat or prevent infection.

Anxiety A response to an anticipated experience that the person perceives as threatening in some way.

Anxiolytics Anxiety-relieving medications used in the management of fearful patients.

Aphasia A deficiency in the ability to understand or communicate the spoken or written word.

Aphthous ulcer An ulcerative lesion on the oral mucosa generally believed to be autoimmune in origin and recognized in some patients to be initiated by stress, nutritional deficiency, or food allergy. Also referred to as canker sores.

Apical microsurgery   The excision of the apical portion of a tooth through an opening made in the overlying labial, buccal, or palatal alveolar bone to provide access for placement of a retrograde endodontic filling.

Apical periodontitis   An inflammatory reaction of the tissues near or at the tooth root apex; evident on a radiograph as a widening of the periodontal ligament space.

Apical rarefying osteitis   A radiographic term that is applied to a radiolucent area at the apex of a tooth. Also referred to as periapical radiolucency (PARL).

Apical sclerosing osteitis   A radiographic term that is applied to a radiopaque area at the apex of a tooth; similarly, a chronic confined inflammatory response of bone is referred to as a *focal sclerosing osteomyelitis* or *condensing osteitis*.

Apical rarefying and sclerosing osteitis   A radiographic term that is applied to a radiolucent and radiopaque area at the apex of a tooth.

Appointment plan   A document that lists the activities and procedures that will occur at each patient visit and is useful for providing an estimate of the number of appointments that will be necessary to complete the treatment plan.

Arrested caries   A carious lesion that is no longer active or progressive. It often appears as a dark, stained pit or fissure on the teeth or as a cavitation with hard, dark dentin at its base.

Artificial intelligence (AI)   The use of computer algorithms to simulate human thought and other activities.

Asociality   A lack of desire for social interaction.

Aspiration pneumonia   Pneumonia due to the entrance of foreign matter, such as food particles or oral secretions, into the respiratory passages or lungs.

Asymptomatic apical periodontitis   The inflammation and destruction of the apical periodontium that is of pulpal origin but the patient does not have any symptoms and does not have sensitivity to percussion or palpation or other signs of infection.

Asynchronous communication   Any type of communication where there is a time lag between the sender of information and the person receiving the information. Examples include email and most text message systems.

Assent   An agreement to a plan of treatment based on a freedom of choice and a reasonable knowledge of the options and expected outcomes.

At risk/at increased risk   A phrase used to describe individuals who have an innate predisposition for a particular disease or condition or who engage in behaviors that are known to promote that disease or condition.

Attrition   The wearing of occlusal or incisal surfaces of the teeth because of functional or parafunctional occlusal contact.

Atypical odontalgia   Chronic pain in a tooth or teeth, or in a site where teeth have been extracted or following endodontic treatment, without an identifiable cause. Also referred to as idiopathic continuous neuropathic pain.

Autotransplantation   The transplantation of a tooth from one location in the mouth to another location in the same mouth.

B

Baby boomers   The cohort of persons born in the United States between 1946 and 1964.

Beneficence   One of the five core principles of the *Principles of Ethics and Code of Professional Responsibility* published by the American Dental Association; requires dentists to maximize the patient's welfare at all times.

Biofilm   A thin layer of microorganisms adhering to the surface of a structure, which may be organic or inorganic, together with the polymers that they secrete. Also referred to as *plaque*.

Biopsy   The removal and examination of bodily tissue performed to establish a diagnosis.

Bipolar disorder   Also known as manic-depressive illness, this disorder is characterized by cyclical episodes of mania, or elevated mood, often alternating with depression. During episodes of mania, patients experience recurrent fluctuations of increased energy, expansive mood, and often inappropriate behavior.

Bite guard/occlusal guard   A custom-fabricated hard or soft acrylic device that fits over the occlusal and incisal surfaces of the maxillary or mandibular teeth for the purpose of protecting the teeth from fracture or excessive wear.

Black triangles   Gingival esthetic issue caused by gingival recession and the exposure of interproximal spaces at the cervical portion of the teeth.

Bleeding index   The percentage of examined sites that bleed upon periodontal probing.

Bounded edentulous spaces   An edentulous space with at least one tooth on either side of it.

Brachytherapy   A form of radiation therapy in which radioactive material is inserted directly into the tumor.

Bradycardia   A slow heart rate as evidenced by a pulse rate of less than 60 beats per minute.

Breach of duty   Failing to do something that the ordinary, prudent, or "reasonable" dentist would do in the same or similar circumstances; also, failure to not do something that the ordinary, prudent, or "reasonable" dentist would not do in the same or similar circumstances.

Bruxism/bruxing   A condition in which a patient grinds their teeth.

Bulimia   Episodic binge eating followed by purging in an attempt to prevent weight gain. The process of purging most often takes the form of self-induced vomiting, but can also involve the use of laxatives.

Burning mouth syndrome   A disorder characterized by persistent burning pain perceived in the oral mucosa, tongue, and/or lips.

Burnout   A state of emotional, mental, and often physical exhaustion brought on by prolonged or repeated stress or frustration.

C

Calcified canals   The presence of calcified material in the root canal space, often making such teeth more difficult to treat endodontically.

Calculus   A concretion of mineral salts that adheres to teeth or restorations.

Camouflage/camouflaging   Orthodontically displacing teeth relative to the supporting bone to compensate for an underlying jaw discrepancy. This technique is used primarily to improve facial esthetics and as an alternative to orthognathic surgery.

Candidiasis   An infection of the mucosa caused by *Candida albicans*.

Cannabis use disorder   The continued use of cannabis despite clinically significant impairment.

Carcinoma   A malignant growth of epithelial tissue.

Caries control/caries management   Any and all efforts to prevent, arrest, remineralize, or restore carious lesions.

Caries control restoration   A direct-fill provisional or definitive restoration placed during the disease control phase of treatment for the purpose of eliminating an active caries lesion and halting the caries progression in that site.

Caries control protocol   A comprehensive plan designed to arrest or remineralize early carious lesions, to eradicate overt carious lesions, and to prevent the formation of new lesions in a person who has a moderate or high rate of caries formation or who is at significant risk for developing future caries.

Caries risk assessment   Evaluation of the likelihood or probability that a patient will develop caries.

Caries susceptibility tests   Salivary tests designed to assist in determining a patient's risk for caries; may include salivary flow rate, buffering capacity, *Streptococcus mutans* count, and lactobacillus count.

Cellulitis   A diffuse soft tissue infection with swelling and poorly defined borders. Often accompanied by pain, fever, and malaise.

Cerebrovascular accident (CVA)   A neurologic deficit caused by a sudden interruption of oxygenated blood to the brain; also known as a stroke.

Cervical notching   A common noncarious abnormality of the teeth often seen in middle-aged and older individuals that may be caused by abfraction, erosion, or abrasion.

Cheilitis   An inflammatory condition of the lips and angles of the mouth characterized by chapping and fissuring.

Chemotherapeutic agent   Chemical agents used to treat pathologic conditions.

Chemotherapy   Treatment of cancer with chemical agents.

Chief complaint/chief concern (CC)   A symptom or request that becomes the motivating factor for seeking dental treatment.

Chronic apical periodontitis   An inflammatory process at the apex of a tooth, characterized by radiographic change in the form of a widened periodontal ligament space, usually in the absence of pain.

Chronic apical abscess   An asymptomatic and persistent inflammation and destruction of the apical periodontium that is of pulpal origin; signs of systemic involvement (fever, malaise, lymphadenitis) are absent; commonly there is an apical radiolucency, and a parulis or sinus tract (also referred to as *fistula*) will be present.

Chronic obstructive pulmonary disease (COPD)   Any disorder characterized by persistent or recurring obstruction of bronchial air flow, such as chronic bronchitis, asthma, or pulmonary emphysema.

Civil law   Type of law that governs the private legal relationships between two or more parties.

Clenching   Holding the teeth together and tightening the muscles of mastication; a parafunctional habit that can be a cause of attrition and myositis.

Clinical decision support (CDS)   A group of informatic tools that provide clinicians, staff, patients, or other individuals with knowledge and person-specific information, intelligently filtered, or presented at appropriate times to enhance healthcare.

Closed questions   Questions that usually can be answered with one or two words. In the dental interview they permit specific facts to be obtained or clarified, but do not give insight into patient beliefs, attitudes, or feelings.

Coagulopathies   Any disorders of blood coagulation. Also called *bleeding disorders.*

Cognitive disorders (CD)   A category of mental health disorders that primarily affect cognitive abilities including learning, memory, perception, and problem solving. Alzheimer's disease accounts for the majority of cases of CD in the US.

Combination factors   Factors about which the dentist and patient have legitimate, though sometimes differing, interests and perspectives that are critical to making the correct treatment decision.

Combination syndrome   A condition sometimes seen in patients with a mandibular distal extension partial denture opposing a complete maxillary denture; if occlusal force is not evenly distributed throughout the mouth during chewing, excessive load may be placed on the anterior part of the maxillary denture, causing loss of the anterior maxillary alveolus.

Complete denture   A dental prosthesis replacing all natural teeth and associated mandibular and maxillary structures; it is completely supported by the tissues. Also called *full denture.*

Complete (displaced) fracture   A fracture that involves the entire cross section of the bone so that the bone snaps into two or more parts.

Composite resin   A tooth-colored restorative material usually composed of glass or porcelain filler particles in a resin matrix.

Compromise plan   A treatment plan that intentionally does not meet all of the patient's or practitioner's goals but that provides some level of care at a lower overall cost to the patient.

Computed tomography (CT)   An x-ray technique used to create cross-sectional images of the body or area of the body. This technique provides more detailed images than can be obtained with conventional x-rays. May be used to help pinpoint the exact location of a tumor or to help guide procedures such as biopsies, surgery, and/or radiation therapy. Also called CT, CT scan, or CAT scan.

Computer-aided design (CAD)   The use of computers and computer software to create and analyze a design of an object.

Computer-aided manufacturing (CAM)   The use of computer software to control machinery in the manufacturing of a designed object.

Condensing osteitis   *See apical sclerosing osteitis.*

Cone-beam CT   An imaging technique in which a cone-shaped beam of x-rays makes a single revolution around the head during exposure. The resultant transmission data collected by the x-ray detector are manipulated with a computer to produce images of the head in multiple planes to provide three-dimensional information.

Confidentiality   The expectation that the disclosure of patient information made to healthcare professionals will not be made public.

Congestive heart failure   A failure of the heart to pump blood adequately; has various causes and degrees of severity.

Consultation   The referral of a patient to another clinician for an opinion or treatment. A dentist may also seek specified information from another clinician regarding a patient's case.

Contingency management   A treatment program that provides immediate rewards for desired changes in behavior. Often used in the treatment of drug and alcohol abuse.

Contract   A legally enforceable agreement that creates, defines, and governs mutual rights and obligations among its parties.

Conversion hysteria   A mental disorder characterized by symptoms of a physical illness for which there is no demonstrable physiologic cause.

Convolutional neural network (CNN)   A class of artificial neural network that is most commonly applied to analyze visual imagery.

Continuous positive airway pressure device (CPAP)   A method of positive pressure ventilation used with patients who are breathing spontaneously, in which pressure in the airway is maintained above the level of atmospheric pressure throughout the respiratory cycle. The purpose is to keep the alveoli open at the end of exhalation and thus increase oxygenation and reduce the work of breathing.

Core buildup/foundation   Restoration of a severely fractured or carious, or heavily restored, tooth for the purpose of (1) replacing missing tooth structure and (2) providing retention and resistance form for a definitive indirect restoration.

Corrosion   Surface destruction of a metal restoration, most commonly amalgam, in the oral environment by a chemical or electrochemical reaction.

COVID-19   A respiratory disease caused by SARS-CoV-2, a coronavirus discovered in 2019. The virus spreads mainly from person to person through respiratory droplets produced when an infected person coughs, sneezes, or talks. Some people who are infected may not have symptoms.

Cracked tooth   A tooth with a visible nondisplaced fracture; the presence of a large intracoronal restoration may be a precipitating factor; transient acute pain experienced while biting on the affected tooth or cusp.

Craze line   A small, vertical hairline crack that only affects the outer enamel on a tooth.

Credentialing   The process of assessing and confirming the qualifications of a healthcare practitioner.

Criminal law   Type of law that governs wrongful acts against society or the public.

Cross-bite   An occlusal relationship in which the maxillary facial surface of one or several teeth is positioned lingual to the facial surface of the opposing mandibular tooth.

Cross-tolerance   A phenomenon in which tolerance to one drug induces tolerance to another drug.

Crown   An indirect restoration that covers the coronal portion of a tooth; can be fabricated ingold, resin, porcelain-fused-to-metal (PFM), or ceramic material.

Cytology   The microscopic study of cells obtained by aspiration, smearing, or scraping.

D

Damage/damages   In a lawsuit, an undesired result that must be shown to be directly related to a breach of duty and must be quantifiable.

Database   An organized collection of data stored and accessed electronically.

Decision-making capacity   An ability to make informed decisions about proposed treatment, risks and benefits, alternatives, and consequences of nontreatment. The patient must exhibit rationality in weighing the options and be able to communicate a choice.

Decision pathways   Protocols that provide direction in identifying the range of treatment options, indicating some of the key decision points leading to an appropriate treatment decision.

Decision trees   Protocols that specify key decision points and treatment options; may also include research-based success rates for each of these options.

Decreased vertical dimension of occlusion (see VDO)   A diminished interarch space when jaws are closed in maximum intercuspation position. Also referred to as *overclosure.*

Deep learning (DL)   A type of machine learning that applies algorithms in a layered fashion to extract higher level data from the original raw data.

Definitive diagnosis   A pattern of findings from the patient history, examination, and clinical tests that leads to the identification of a specific disease entity.

Definitive phase of care Treatment aimed at comprehensive, long-term rehabilitation of a patient's oral condition. Depending on the patient, procedures in the various disciplines of dentistry, such as prosthodontics, periodontics, and endodontics may be required.

Degenerative joint disease (DJD) A disorder resulting from destruction of the articular surfaces of the condyle and fossa caused by inflammation of the joint, also known as osteoarthritis. It may result from traumatic injury or a prior surgical procedure involving the joint.

Dental evaluation and clearance Routine practice in some areas of medicine to ensure that any necessary dental treatment is rendered before certain surgeries, chemotherapy, or organ transplant to minimize the risk of infection and oral complications after the medical procedures.

Dental practice guidelines Specific suggestions (parameters of care) for how patients should be managed or their treatment planned. These suggestions may be the work of governing bodies, agencies, councils, or any professional organizations or societies within or outside of dentistry.

Dentist-patient relationship The relationship between dentist and patient that is initiated when the dentist moves beyond the examination stage and implements treatment.

Dental surveyor A paralleling instrument used in construction of a prosthesis to locate and delineate the contours and relative positions of abutment teeth and associated structures.

Dental caries Localized destruction of calcified tissue initiated on the tooth surface by decalcification of the enamel of the teeth, followed by enzymatic lysis of organic structures, leading to cavity formation that, if left unchecked, penetrates the enamel and dentin and may reach the pulp.

Designated record set Information that is used to make decisions about an individual patient and that they have a legal right to see.

Developmental delay An individual who has not gained the developmental skills expected of them, compared to others of the same age. Delays may occur in the areas of motor function, speech and language, cognitive, and social skills.

Diagnoses Precise, scientific terms used to describe variations from normal.

Diagnostic and Statistical Manual of Mental Disorders A classification system for mental disorders, published by the American Psychiatric Association, that delineates objective criteria to be used in diagnosis.

Diastema A noticeable space between two teeth.

Dietary counseling/nutritional counseling Counseling on food and beverage selection, and dietary habits, as a part of treatment and control of oral health problems.

Differential diagnosis The determination of which one of two or more diseases or conditions a patient is suffering from, by systematically comparing and contrasting their clinical characteristics.

Dilaceration Sharply bent or angular-shaped roots.

Direct-fill restoration Usually a composite, amalgam, or glass ionomer filling that is placed, shaped, set, and finished directly in the cavity preparation.

Direct pulp cap A medicated dressing placed over an exposed vital pulp for the purpose of promoting dentinal bridge formation and maintaining pulp vitality.

Disc displacement (DD) Abnormal position of the articular disc. A condition in which the articular disc is displaced and remains fully displaced in open and closed jaw positions.

Disc displacement with reduction (DDR) A displacement of the articular disc against the mandibular condyle and the articular eminence during jaw movements, accompanied by clicking sounds and, in some cases, pain and/or limitation of mandibular movement.

Disease control phase of care That portion of a treatment plan that focuses on the elimination of active disease and its causes.

Disease risk The probability that an individual or population will develop a certain disease or condition. It is usually expressed as a general category, such as high/low or high/moderate/negligible.

Distraction osteogenesis A surgical process for the reconstruction of skeletal deformities and the lengthening of bones. A bone fracture is surgically created and the two ends of the bone are moved apart, slowly enough so that new bone can grow in the gap. Distraction osteogenesis is useful in simultaneously expanding both bone volume and the surrounding soft tissues.

Do not intubate (DNI) Physician's orders written in conjunction with the wishes of a patient (and their care provider and family if the patient is incapacitated) instructing that if the patient goes into respiratory arrest, they will not be intubated and placed on a respirator. DNI orders are usually written only for terminally ill patients or those with severely diminished quality of life and no expectation of recovery.

Do not resuscitate (DNR) Physician's orders written in conjunction with the wishes of a patient (and their care provider and family if the patient is incapacitated) instructing that if the patient goes into cardiac arrest, they will not be given cardiopulmonary resuscitation (CPR) or placed on artificial life support. DNR orders are usually written only for terminally ill patients or those with severely diminished quality of life and no expectation of recovery.

Drug tolerance A condition in which an individual's reaction to a drug, such as alcohol or narcotics, decreases over time so that larger doses are required to achieve an equivalent effect.

Duty to treat An understanding that arises from the doctor-patient relationship for all dentists to properly diagnose and appropriately treat disease.

Dysgeusia Abnormalities of the sense of taste.

Dysphagia Difficulty in swallowing that may be indicative of 9th, 10th, and/or 12th cranial nerve damage.

Dysplasia Abnormal tissue development. Pathologic alteration in size, shape, and organization of cells.

Dysthymic disorder A depressed mood that persists for at least 2 years, but that is not severe enough to meet the criteria for major depression.

Dystonia An irregular contraction of the muscles.

E

Ectopic eruption The abnormal direction of tooth eruption; teeth most commonly afflicted include first and third molars, mandibular lateral incisors, and maxillary canines; may lead to abnormal resorption of the adjacent tooth.

Edentulous/edentate Without teeth.

Electronic health record (EHR) Health information relating to the patient's past, present, or future physical and mental health condition maintained in electronic format, usually involving computer systems, for the primary purpose of providing and documenting healthcare and health-related services. Also referred to as electronic patient record (EPR).

Emancipated minors Persons who are under the legal age of consent, but who function as independent adults, living apart from their parents and supporting themselves.

Emergency problem A situation that incapacitates the patient and has the potential to become life threatening.

Empathy The capacity and willingness to understand a situation from another person's point of view.

Encrypted Converted information, such as with a web page or an email message, that allows only authorized access.

Erosion Chemical dissolution of the tooth enamel often seen in patients with a high-acid diet, gastric acid reflux disease, or bulimia.

Eruption gingivitis Plaque-induced gingivitis associated with tooth eruption.

Erythroplakia A rare, slow-growing, homogenous red plaque or patch on the oral mucosa with well-defined margins. It has predilection for middle-aged to older adults. The most common location is the floor of the mouth, followed by the retromolar area, tongue, and palate. Histologically, this lesion is either invasive carcinoma, carcinoma in situ, or dysplasia at the time of biopsy.

Erythroleukoplakia A leukoplakia with a red component in it. The malignant potential is considered higher than pure leukoplakia. A biopsy is always warranted.

Esthetic A term that refers to the extent to which a specific treatment restores or enhances physical appearance.

Esthetic zone Any dentoalveolar segment that is visible upon full smile.

Evidence-based dentistry   Assessing clinical findings, making diagnoses, and recommending treatment based on a combination of the clinician's expertise, the patient's particular needs, and the best and most relevant published research.

Excess buccal corridor display   A patient with a narrow maxillary arch and upon smiling reveals the facial surfaces of most or all of the posterior teeth on the affected side or sides.

Excessive gingival display   Showing too much of the gingiva to be esthetically pleasing when the lip raises above the gingival margins of the maxillary anterior teeth as the patient is speaking or smiling.

Exostoses   Developmental, nonmalignant bony overgrowths.

Explicit bias   Conscious thoughts or actions that demonstrate bias against an individual or group.

Express contract   An exchange of promise in which the terms by which the parties agree to be bound are declared either orally or in writing, or a combination of both, at the time it is made.

External resorption   Resorption of a tooth initiated in the periodontium and affecting the external root surfaces.

Extracoronal restorations   A restoration, such as a gold crown or a ceramic onlay, that covers most, or all, of the visible external surface of a tooth.

Extrapyramidal effects   Movement disorders that may include tardive dyskinesia, pseudoparkinsonism, dystonia, and akathisia; can result from long-term use of certain antipsychotic medications.

Extravasation phenomenon   A fluid-filled lesion most commonly found on the mucosal surface of the lower lip caused by blockage of the duct from one or more minor salivary glands. Also referred to as mucocele or mucous extravasation phenomenon.

Extrinsic staining   Stains on the surface of tooth enamel caused by exposure to substances such as coffee, tea, or tobacco products.

F

Factitial injuries   Self-inflicted lesions not attributable to accidental trauma or other oral disease.

Failing restoration   A dental restoration that is not serviceable because of cracks and fractures; open margins with known, suspected, or anticipated recurrent caries; voids in material; loose restorations; or restorations with poor contours.

Fear   An emotional response to a perceived threat or danger.

Fever lines   A developmental anomaly that can occur to the developing teeth of a fetus if the mother suffers a serious virus or infection during pregnancy. The lines appear when the teeth later erupt into the mouth.

Fiduciary relationship   Any relationship grounded in assumed trust.

Findings   Pieces of information about the patient that have been gathered by asking questions and reviewing forms, observing and examining structures, performing diagnostic tests, and, if appropriate, consulting with physicians and other dentists.

Fistula   See sinus tract.

Fixed partial denture (FPD)   A prosthetic dental appliance that replaces lost teeth and is held in position by attachments to adjacent prepared natural teeth, roots, or implants. Also called bridge and fixed bridge.

Florid osseous dysplasia   Multiple radiopaque and radiolucent lesions in the periapical regions throughout one jaw or in several quadrants; a more extensive form of periapical cemental dysplasia.

Fluorosis   Chronic overexposure to fluoride.

Focal sclerosing osteitis   The radiographic diagnosis of a zone of increased radiopacity in the maxilla or mandible. The condition is also known as condensing osteitis.

Full code   Physician's order that stipulates that in the case of a cardiac arrest, the patient is to be resuscitated and placed on artificial life support if necessary to sustain life.

Functional history   Patient history that includes activities of daily living (ADL) and instrumental activities of daily living.

Furcation involvement   Bone loss in the area where the roots divide on a multirooted tooth.

Fractured cusp   A cusp on a posterior tooth that has broken and is displaced.

Frailty   The condition of being weak and delicate.

G

General anesthesia   A reversible state of unconsciousness, produced by anesthetic agents, with absence of pain sensation over the entire body and a greater or lesser degree of muscular relaxation; the drugs producing this state can be administered by inhalation, intravenously, intramuscularly, or rectally.

Generalized anxiety disorder (GAD)   A disorder characterized by excessive anxiety and worry about multiple events or activities that is out of proportion to the actual likelihood or effect of the anticipated event. This condition is often comorbid with other mental disorders such as depression, panic attacks, and substance abuse.

GERD   Gastroesophageal reflux disease.

Gingival zenith   The most apical aspect of the free gingival margin.

Gingivitis   Inflammation of the gingival tissue.

Goals   In the context of treatment planning, patient or practitioner expectations that can be either short- or long-term in nature, or both.

Guided bone regeneration (GBR)   Surgical procedure associated with implant placement performed in edentulous sites with insufficient bone volume or in cases where the ridge volume is deficient. GBR increases the ridge dimension using a variety of materials including bone grafts, barrier membranes, biologic agents, and/or space maintaining devices.

H

Halitosis   Breath that has an unpleasant odor; "bad breath."

Headache   A pain in the head; also called cephalalgia, cephalgia, and cephalodynia; many different causes have been identified including headache attributed to TMD (TMDH).

Health beliefs   What people believe about their health, what they think constitutes their health, what they consider the cause of their illness, and ways to overcome their illness.

Health disparities   Preventable differences in the burden of disease, injury, violence, or opportunities to achieve optimal health, which are experienced by socially disadvantaged populations.

Health equity   A belief that everyone has an equal opportunity to be healthy; it is achieved when patients have access to the social determinants of health, specifically those that derive from wealth, power, and prestige.

Health Insurance Portability and Accountability Act of 1996 (HIPAA)   A US law that requires practitioners and healthcare organizations to prevent unnecessary use and release of protected health information.

Heritable condition   A disease or condition transmitted from parent to offspring.

Herpes zoster   An acute viral disease involving the dorsal spinal root or cranial nerve and producing vesicular eruptions in areas of the skin corresponding to the involved sensory nerve. Pain is a prominent feature and may persist, although skin lesions subside in 1 to 2 weeks.

Herpetic ulcer   A recurring vesicular lesion caused by herpes simplex virus (HSV) that progresses to an ulceration; usually on keratinized tissue, such as the lips or gingiva.

History of present illness   The history of the chief concern or complaint.

Holding period   Not a formally recognized phase of treatment; an interval during which the patient is in a stable oral health condition but is unwilling or unable (for financial or other reasons) to proceed with additional elective or recommended dental treatment. During this hiatus the patient continues to have a professional relationship with the practice and be appointed for ongoing preventive therapy and oral health maintenance.

Hospice care   Palliative and supportive care for terminally ill patients and their families, in a facility or at home, either directly or on a consulting basis.

Host modulation   A treatment concept that reduces tissue destruction and stabilizes or even regenerates inflammatory tissue by modifying host response factors.

Hybrid prosthesis   Nonremovable fixed complete denture prosthesis composed of cast alloy framework with denture teeth and resin for completely edentulous patients, which compensates for moderate bone loss and missing soft tissue contours.

Hyperactive lip   Excess lip mobility evident when the lip raises above the gingival margins of the maxillary anterior teeth as the patient is speaking or smiling.

Hypercementosis   An excessive formation of cementum on the roots of one or more teeth.

Hypererupted   A tooth that protrudes out of the occlusal plane, usually because there is no antagonist. Also referred to as *supraeruption*.

Hyperesthesia   Increased sensation.

Hyperkeratosis   Hypertrophy of the stratum corneum of the skin, oral mucosa, or gingiva.

Hypertension   An abnormal elevation of systolic and/or diastolic arterial pressure.

Hyperventilation   Rapid or excessive breathing.

Hypocalcification   A developmental anomaly that results in the incomplete calcification or hardening of the enamel of a tooth.

Hypoglycemic   Being in a state of low blood glucose level. Early signs and symptoms include hunger, weakness, trembling, pallor, and a rapid heartbeat. Condition is sometimes seen in diabetic patients when glycemic control is altered.

Hypoplasia   A developmental anomaly that results in the incomplete development of the teeth.

Hyposalivation   A diminished secretion of saliva.

Hypotension   Abnormally low blood pressure.

Hypothermia   Body temperature significantly below 98.6°F (37°C).

I

Iatrogenic problem   An adverse condition in a patient that occurs as a result of treatment by a dentist or physician. An amalgam, composite, or a crown with an overhang is an example of an *iatrogenic restoration*.

Iatrosedation   A mode of anxiety control that can be simply and routinely applied by the dentist in the course of treating the patient; it is independent of pharmacologic forms of anxiety control or traditional forms of psychosedation (as administered by a psychologist or psychotherapist). Common elements include a calm, soothing, and compassionate demeanor on the part of the dentist; voice control; and suggestions that evoke a positive and relaxing environment and that minimize aversive stimuli. Giving the patient control over breaks and the power to interrupt or terminate the procedure can also be an effective form of iatrosedation.

Ideal treatment plan   The treatment plan that provides the best, or most preferred, treatment for each of the patient's problems regardless of time or financial concerns.

Immediate loading   Placing an abutment and the prosthesis attached to the abutment at the time of the implant fixture placement. Placing a provisional restoration at the time of implant fixture placement is also known as *immediate provisionalization*.

Immediate placement   Placing an implant fixture in the tooth socket at the time of the tooth extraction.

Immunosuppression   The diminution or prevention of the immune response.

Immutable risk factor   Those risk factors that are not within the patient's ability to alter. Examples include heritable or genetic conditions. Also referred to as a *nonmodifiable risk factor*.

Impacted tooth   A tooth that is prevented from erupting by a physical barrier.

Implicit bias   Unconscious thoughts or actions that demonstrate bias against an individual or group.

Implied contract   A legally binding obligation that derives from actions, conduct, or circumstances of one or more parties in an agreement. It has the same legal force as an *express* contract.

Incidence   The number of new cases of a specific disease occurring during a specified period.

Incipient   Beginning, initial, commencing.

Incomplete (nondisplaced) fracture   Fracture that does not go across the entire width of the bone; the bone cracks but does not break all the way through.

Indirect restoration   A dental restoration such as a crown, inlay, or porcelain veneer that is fabricated outside of the patient's mouth for later placement.

Infective endocarditis   An infection by microorganisms of the valves and/or lining of the heart.

Informed consent   A verbal or written agreement by a patient to have a procedure performed after being informed in sufficient detail of possible risks, benefits, and options.

Initial therapy   In dentistry, this usually refers to the management of active periodontal disease during the disease control phase of treatment. Common procedures include oral hygiene instructions and either localized or complete mouth scaling and root planing.

Inlay   An indirect, intracoronal restoration made of gold, composite resin, or ceramic material.

Inspection   The visual examination of the body or portions thereof. It is an integral part of the physical or dental examination.

Intensity modulated radiation therapy (IMRT)   A treatment method using a computer-directed radiation source to deliver precisely targeted high doses of radiation directly to cancer cells.

Interarch space requirement   The minimum required vertical space between the dental arches to place a dental prosthesis.

Internal resorption   A pathologic process of tooth structure loss from within the pulp space that may perforate the external root surface.

International normalized ratio (INR)   A standardized laboratory value used to assess a patient's coagulation time.

Interprofessional care   The collaborative care provided by dentists, other healthcare professionals, the patient, family members, and patient caregivers all working together for the patient.

Interproximal or bite-wing radiographs   Intraoral radiographs that show the coronal portion of the teeth and the alveolar crestal bone in both arches.

Intracoronal restoration   A direct or indirect restoration placed within the outer confines of a tooth; the restoration does not cover any of the tooth cusps.

Intraprofessional care   The collaborative care provided by multidisciplinary healthcare providers within the same profession.

Intravenous (IV) sedation   Analgesic or anesthetic medication delivered through the blood stream to allow a patient to better tolerate a procedure.

Intrinsic staining   Staining within the enamel, dentin, or pulp space of a tooth.

Irreversible pulpitis   A clinical diagnosis, based on subjective and objective findings, that the pulp is incapable of healing. The condition is characterized by prolonged dental pain that appears to arise spontaneously. The tooth may have marked sensitivity to cold, air, or heat.

J

Justice   One of the five core principles of the *Principles of Ethics and Code of Professional Responsibility* published by the American Dental Association; prohibits dentists from discrimination against individual patients or groups of people, and obligates dentists to assure access to oral health services for all members of society.

K

Key teeth   Important teeth that often serve as abutments for fixed or removable partial dentures or to add stability to a dental prosthesis. Such teeth are favorably positioned in the dental arch, are restorable, and often improve the prognosis for other teeth or the case as a whole. Loss of a key tooth or teeth may adversely affect the treatment options and prognosis.

L

Lateral window sinus elevation (lift)   A commonly used technique for sinus floor elevation. The bone is removed from the lateral aspect of the alveolus overlying the planned implant site, permitting access to the underlying Schneiderian membrane lining the sinus cavity.

Legal competence   A legally defined age of majority at which the right to make certain binding commitments is granted. The mental capacity and condition a person must have to be responsible for their own decisions or acts.

Legal risk   The risk of financial or reputational loss that can result from lack of awareness or misunderstanding of, ambiguity in, or reckless indifference to, the way law and regulation apply to the practice of dentistry.

Lesions   Tissue abnormalities.

Leukoplakia   A white patch on a mucous membrane that will not rub off.

Lichen planus (LP) An autoimmune disorder of skin and/or mucous membranes; may present in multiple forms and either with or without erosion. In the oral cavity it commonly appears with white lines in a reticular pattern known as *Wickham's Striae*.

Lichenoid reaction Lesions on the oral mucosa that are clinically reminiscent of lichen planus but do not have a confirmed histologic diagnosis of LP.

Linea alba A white line; linear hyperkeratosis frequently found on the buccal mucosa, or lateral border of the tongue, adjacent to the plane of occlusion.

Linear gingival erythema (LGE) A distinctive red band of free gingiva that is the result of a fungal infection; often seen in immunocompromised patients.

Lip incompetence A short upper lip.

Longitudinal study The process of evaluating a group of subjects over time. This process may be used to determine whether persons with a particular risk factor develop a disease or other problem. Contrasts with cross-sectional studies that evaluate patients or other subjects at one point in time.

Lymphadenitis The inflammation of one or more lymph nodes, usually caused by infection; usually manifests as a discrete swelling that is tender to patient on palpation.

Lymphadenopathy An abnormality of a lymph node or nodes in size, shape, texture, or mobility; most commonly this is a form of benign lymphoid hyperplasia (scarring) residual from a previous infection in the orofacial region. A lymph node that is fixed, hard, and irregular in shape is often associated with oral cancer.

Lymphoma Any neoplastic disorder of the lymphoid tissue.

M

Machine learning (ML) A subcategory of artificial intelligence that is based on the idea that systems can learn from data, identify patterns, and make decisions with minimal human intervention.

Macroabrasion The removal of minute amounts of enamel with a high-speed carbide bur in order to correct tooth discoloration.

Magnetic resonance imaging (MRI) An imaging technique that uses a magnetic field and radio waves to create cross-sectional images. These images can be combined to create a three-dimensional image. The detailed, clear images assist in the diagnosis and treatment of many conditions including oral cancer.

Maintenance phase of care That portion of a comprehensive dental treatment plan that is intended to promote the long-term oral health of the patient and manage any persistent or chronic oral problems.

Maintenance therapy Preventive and therapeutic measures instituted to sustain and ensure long-term oral health.

Major depressive disorder A disabling, often recurrent disorder defined as a depressed mood, loss of interest, and other symptoms occurring almost daily for at least 2 weeks.

Malignancy A cancerous growth.

Mandibular advancement device (MAD) A removable prosthesis that is retained on both dental arches and designed to position the mandible more anteriorly. The purpose is to improve airflow, reduce or eliminate sleep apnea, and improve sleep.

Masticatory myalgia A regional manifestation of musculoskeletal disorders. Common symptoms include tenderness with the muscles of mastication, limited opening, decreased masticatory function, The etiology is multifactorial.

Maximum intercuspation A patient's unguided natural position of mouth closure when the maxillary and mandibular teeth are in full contact.

Medicaid A US social healthcare program, defined by the federal government, but administered by the states, to provide health insurance for low-income individuals and families. Among the groups of people served by Medicaid are eligible low-income parents, children, seniors, and people with disabilities.

Medicare A US health insurance program that helps pay medical costs for individuals aged 65 and older, some disabled individuals under age 65, and individuals with end-stage renal disease (permanent kidney failure treated with dialysis or a transplant).

Melanoma A malignant tumor composed of melanin-pigmented cells.

Metastasis The transfer of disease cells from one organ or area to another not directly connected to it; characteristic of malignant tumors.

Meta-analysis Any systematic method that uses statistical analysis to integrate the data from a number of independent studies.

Metal ceramic restoration A restoration composed of a ceramic layer fused to a metal substructure (coping). Also referred to as *a porcelain-fused-to-metal (PFM) crown*.

Microabrasion The removal of minute amounts of dental enamel using an abrasive compound in order to correct enamel defects.

Microdonts Abnormally small teeth.

Microleakage Microscopic space located at the interface of the tooth structure and the sealant or restoration.

Microstomia A congenital or acquired reduction in the size of the oral opening that is severe enough to compromise physical appearance, nutrition, and quality of life.

Migraine headache Type of headache characterized by recurrent, severe, and disabling attacks of head pain, often unilateral and pulsating, along with symptoms of sensory disturbance, such as photophobia, phonophobia, and hyperosmia. *Orofacial migraine* is specific to the orofacial complex.

Modified treatment plan A variation from an ideal treatment plan that balances the patient's treatment objectives with those of the dentist.

Morsicatio A shaggy white lesion caused by chronically biting or chewing the cheek, tongue, or lips. The term for chewing one's cheek is *morsicatio buccarum*.

Motivational interviewing It is directive, patient-centered, counseling style for eliciting behavioral change by helping to explore and resolve ambivalence.

Mucocele A nonneoplastic lesion most commonly found on the mucosal surface of the lower lip. It is caused by trauma to, and blockage of, minor salivary glands.

Mucogingival condition or defect The location where there is minimal or no attached gingiva adjacent to a tooth; often accompanied by marked gingival recession and/or frenal pull.

Mucositis An inflammation of a mucous membrane.

Mutable risk factor Those risk factors that are within the patient's purview to change. Examples include tobacco smoking, lack of exercise, and an unhealthy diet. Also referred to as a *modifiable risk factor*.

Myalgia Muscular pain.

Myelosuppression A reduction in the ability of the bone marrow to produce blood cells.

Myocardial infarction (MI) Blockage of one or more coronary arteries leading to necrosis of a localized area of the myocardium, commonly referred to as a heart attack.

N

Natural history The typical course of events; the sequence and progression over time of a disease process in the absence of treatment or medical intervention.

Necrotizing periodontal disease (*formerly necrotizing ulcerative gingivitis [NUG] or acute necrotizing ulcerative gingivitis [ANUG]*) Historically referred to by the public as "trench mouth." Distinctive clinical features include marked gingival inflammation, foul breath, and "punched-out" papillae with a pseudomembrane. Contributing factors include stress, poor diet, sleep deprivation, tobacco use, and poor oral self-care.

Neoplasm Any new and abnormal growth; may be benign or malignant.

Neuritis A deep, constant, burning pain that runs the course of a nerve trunk.

Nicotine A poisonous colorless soluble fluid alkaloid. It is the psychoactive and addictive chemical agent found in all forms of tobacco.

Nicotine replacement (NRT) A product used to reduce or eliminate withdrawal symptoms in individuals with nicotine addiction. These products may be over the counter or prescription agents.

Nitrous oxide and oxygen analgesia The administration of nitrous oxide and oxygen to reduce patient pain and anxiety.

Nonmaleficence   One of the five core principles of the *Principles of Ethics and Code of Professional Responsibility* published by the American Dental Association; requires dentists to act to avoid harm or risk to patients and recognize their own limitations.

Nondiscoverable   Records kept by a dentist that are not admissible in court because they are not a part of the patient record and therefore subject to the confidentiality between attorney and client (dentist).

Nonreducing anterior disc displacement (NADD)   A condition where the articular disc of the temporomandibular joint has been abnormally displaced in a forward, medial, or lateral position. The condition often limits the opening of the mouth.

Nonvital bleach   A noninvasive technique to treat the intrinsic discoloration of nonvital, root canal treated teeth.

NSAIDs   The acronym for nonsteroidal antiinflammatory drugs/agents used in the control of pain and inflammation.

O

Obsessive-compulsive disorder   Abnormal behavior involving performance of repetitive acts or rituals, usually as a means of releasing tension or relieving anxiety.

Obstructive sleep apnea (OSA)   An intermittent airflow obstruction during sleep; more common in older individuals and those with obesity.

Obturator   A prosthetic appliance used to close a congenital or acquired opening in the palate.

Occlusal equilibration   Occlusal adjustment through selective grinding of tooth surfaces with the goal of improving tooth contact patterns.

Occlusal guard/bite guard/night guard   A custom-fitted device commonly used to prevent additional occlusal wear in patients who have marked bruxism or attrition.

Occlusal radiograph   A radiographic exposure during which the film is placed over the teeth in the occlusal plane.

Occlusal/functional risk assessment   The evaluation of the likelihood or probability that a patient will develop occlusal or functional problems such as bruxism, occlusal trauma, tooth fracture, or impaired ability to chew.

Occlusal splint/bite splint   A custom-fitted device that fits over the occlusal and incisal surfaces of the maxillary or mandibular teeth typically used for patients with temporomandibular disorders.

Occlusal trauma   An injury to any part of the masticatory system as a result of occlusal dysfunction.

Odontoma   An odontogenic tumor composed of mature enamel, dentin, cementum, and pulp tissue.

One-stage technique   A surgical technique in which the implant fixture is placed in the bone and a healing cap is screwed into place leaving the coronal portion exposed to the oral environment. After an appropriate healing time, the healing cap is removed and an impression of the fixture and surrounding tissue is taken.

Onlay   An indirect restoration that covers most, but not all, of the coronal surface of the tooth.

Open questions   Questions that cannot be answered with a simple response, such as "yes" or "no," but instead generate reflection by asking for opinions, past experiences, feelings, or desires.

Operculum   A soft tissue flap covering the crown of an erupting tooth.

Oral cancer   Cancer that occurs in any part of the oral cavity, including lips and oropharynx.

Oral cancer risk assessment   Evaluation of the likelihood or probability that a patient will develop oral cancer.

Oral health literacy   The ability to obtain, read, understand, and use oral healthcare information in order to make appropriate health decisions and follow instructions for treatment.

Oral hygiene instruction (OHI)   Patient education regarding plaque/biofilm removal. Examples include teaching of how to brush the teeth and tongue, floss, and use special oral hygiene aids. (Also referred to as *oral home care instructions*, *oral self-care instructions*.)

Oral physiotherapy   The use of aids such as toothbrush, floss, or other adjunctive armamentaria to maintain the oral health.

Oral sedation   Use of a medication taken orally (i.e., a tablet or liquid) to reduce anxiety and relax the patient.

Oropharynx   The part of the pharynx that lies between the soft palate and the upper edge of the epiglottis.

Orthognathic surgery   Surgical realignment of the jaws or repositioning of dentoalveolar segments.

Orthostatic hypotension   Low blood pressure and a feeling of light-headedness that occurs when an individual arises quickly from a supine position.

Osseointegration   The process of introducing certain metals, such as titanium, into living bone and forming a biocompatible bond with living bone.

Osteoarthritis (OA) of the temporomandibular joint   A degenerative disease of the jaw joint. It is characterized by breakdown of the articular cartilage, architectural changes in bone, and degeneration of the synovial tissues causing pain and/or dysfunction in functional movements of the jaw.

Osteomyelitis   An infection of the bone.

Osteoradionecrosis   Bone destruction and sloughing as a result of therapeutic radiation to the area.

Otorhinolaryngologist   A surgeon specializing in treatment of ears, noses, and throats; commonly called an ENT doctor.

Outcomes   Specific, tangible results of treatment.

Outcomes assessment   The analysis of data leading to an understanding of the effects of a treatment and the determination of whether the treatment is having the desired result.

Outcomes expectations   The results that a patient and practitioner anticipate will occur as a consequence of a course of treatment.

Overhang   An overcontoured portion of a restoration on a proximal surface.

P

Pack year   The number of years someone has smoked multiplied by the number of packs smoked per day. This may have different significance in various countries. For example, a pack of cigarettes in the United States contains 20 cigarettes, whereas in Canada a pack can contain 25 cigarettes.

Painful posttraumatic trigeminal neuropathy (PPTTN)   A uni- or bilateral oral and/or facial pain secondary to peripheral injury of the trigeminal nerve (e.g., following orthognathic surgery, facial trauma, tooth avulsion, endodontic treatment).

Parafunction   A situation of disordered or abnormal function. Habits that exercise a body part in a way that is other than its most common use. Biting fingernails, chewing ice cubes, using teeth to open packaging are common parafunctional habits for teeth. *See also parafunctional habits.*

Patient portal   A secure online website that gives patients access to their personal health information and allows them to interact and communicate with healthcare providers, such as physicians, nurses, and hospitals.

Palliative care   Treatment to relieve, rather than cure, a patient's symptoms.

Palpation   An examination procedure in which the sense of touch is used to gather data for diagnosis.

Palpitation   The sensation by a patient of a rapid or irregular heartbeat.

Panoramic radiograph   An extraoral radiographic film image that displays a wide area of the jaws and enables evaluation of some structures not visualized by intraoral projections. Also referred to as a pantomograph.

Papillary-bleeding index   Measure of sites with gingival bleeding during periodontal probing.

Parafunctional habits   Jaw movements and their accompanying tooth contacts, such as bruxism, that are considered outside or beyond masticatory function and that can result in damage to the oral soft or hard tissues.

Paresthesia   Altered sensation.

Parkinson's disease (PD)   A degenerative neurologic disease characterized by tremor, rigidity, slow movement, and postural instability.

PARQ note   An acronym representing the components of informed consent: procedure, alternatives, risks, questions; can be documented in a patient's health record before treatment.

Partial caries excavation (PCE)   A conservative procedure to manage caries encroaching on the pulp of a tooth that is done during the disease control phase and ideally results in the formation of secondary dentin and also maintaining the vitality of the tooth.

Partial luxation   Slight loosening of a single tooth.

Partially erupted teeth Teeth that have not fully erupted.

Parulis A localized abscess of the gingiva. Also referred to as a gum boil.

Patient autonomy One of the five core principles of the *Principles of Ethics and Code of Professional Responsibility* published by the American Dental Association; asserts that dentists "have a duty to treat the patient according to the patient's desires, within the bounds of accepted treatment, and to protect the patient's confidentiality."

Patient considerations Modifiers to treatment planning that are derived exclusively from information about the patient.

Patient database Information gathered about the patient from which treatment planning decisions are made.

Patient factors (or modifiers) Patient concerns, issues, or attributes that have a bearing on treatment plan formulation.

Percussion A diagnostic procedure that involves tapping a tooth or other body part.

Peri-implant mucositis An infection of the gingiva or mucosa adjacent to an implant.

Peri-implantitis Infection of the peri-implant soft tissues and bone.

Periapical cemental dysplasia A localized, usually benign change in the periapical bone that results in a characteristic radiolucent and/or radiopaque appearance.

Periapical radiograph An intraoral radiographic film or image that includes the tooth and surrounding bone.

Pericoronitis An infection of the soft tissue covering a partially erupted tooth.

Perimolysis A characteristic type of enamel erosion caused by a decreased oral pH resulting from the reflux of acidic stomach contents.

Periodic visit/recare visit/recall visit The visits prescribed after completion of all active treatment during which the patient returns to the dental office for maintenance therapy. The visit commonly includes an examination and periodontal maintenance procedures.

Periodontal abscess A localized collection of pus that originates in the periodontal pocket.

Periodontal/endodontic lesion An inflammatory process that simultaneously involves a necrotic pulp, the periapical area, and the marginal periodontium.

Periodontal probing A diagnostic technique that measures the depth of the periodontal sulcus.

Periodontal reevaluation The reassessment of the patient's periodontal condition 4 to 8 weeks after initial periodontal therapy has been completed.

Periodontal regenerative therapy A surgical procedure to place bone or bone substitute material into a bone defect with the objective of producing new bone and possibly the regeneration of periodontal ligament and cementum.

Periodontal risk assessment Evaluation of the likelihood or probability that a patient will develop periodontal disease.

Periodontitis Inflammatory disease of the supporting tissues of the teeth.

Perpetual oral healthcare Treatment and care delivered, and education imparted, by the oral healthcare team; and procedures and activities carried out by the patient, that cumulatively help the patient sustain optimal oral health for their lifetime.

Perpetual treatment plan A document that addresses patient concerns, issues, and needs beyond the completion of the active treatment plan, and may continue for the life of the doctor-patient relationship. Perpetual treatment plans commonly include specific systemic and maintenance procedures and actions, and have no endpoint.

Persistent depressive disorder (dysthymia) Being in a depressed mood most of the day, for more days than not, for at least 2 years in adults and 1 year in children and adolescents.

Phases Segments of a treatment plan.

Phobia A fear of a specific stimulus. The response to such a fear may dominate a person's life.

Physical addiction A physiologic adaption to the use of a substance in which the absence of the substance produces symptoms and signs of withdrawal.

Pixel Area elements (squares) that comprise a two-dimensional digital image.

Pleomorphic adenoma The most common type of salivary gland neoplasia, which presents as a dome-shaped mass without ulceration or symptoms.

Pontic The suspended member of a fixed partial denture.

Porcelain-fused-to-metal crown (PFM) *See metal ceramic restoration.*

Porcelain jacket crown A full-coverage indirect restoration made of lithium disilicate.

Porcelain veneer A thin porcelain restoration designed to cover the facial and incisal surfaces of anterior teeth and premolars for esthetic purposes.

Positron emission tomography (PET) A type of diagnostic imaging that detects a small amount of radioactive material injected into the bloodstream that has concentrated in areas of cancer.

Post and core A directly or indirectly fabricated foundation restoration that is anchored in the root canal space of an endodontically treated tooth and provides a resistance and retention form for a final restoration, usually a crown.

Postherpetic neuralgia Pain that develops during the acute phase of herpes zoster and recurs or persists for more than 3 months after the onset of herpetic eruption.

Postinitial therapy evaluation An evaluation of the disease control phase of periodontal therapy. It serves to assess the effectiveness of periodontal therapy to date and to provide guidance for future treatment.

Posttreatment assessment examination A comprehensive evaluation of the patient's oral condition and the treatment performed to date. The assessment is typically made at the conclusion of the disease control and definitive phases of treatment.

Posttreatment assessment protocol A formalized process for accomplishing the posttreatment assessment.

Pregnancy gingivitis Inflammatory gingival changes during pregnancy.

Prescription drug monitoring programs An electronic database that tracks controlled substance prescriptions for patients in each US state.

Prevalence The total number of cases of a disease in existence in a population at a certain time.

Preventive trajectory The dynamic (changing) course of health and illness as impacted by the patient's ability and/or willingness to effectively carry out behavioral and therapeutic preventive measures.

Primary caries An initial caries lesion on an unrestored tooth surface.

Primary occlusal trauma Injury to a previously healthy periodontium, in the absence of inflammation, caused by excessive occlusal forces. This may be caused by a "high" restoration or prosthetic device.

Privacy In healthcare, a patient's rights and expectations that personal health information is shared only between individuals who need it to manage the patient.

Privileging The process that healthcare organizations employ in authorizing practitioners to provide specific services to patients.

Problem A significant finding that may have an important effect on the treatment plan, but that does not fit the classic definition of a diagnosis.

Professional factors Medical, physiological, and technical parameters identified by the dentist that have a bearing on the formulation of the treatment plan.

Prognosis An estimation of the probable outcome for a disease, condition, or treatment.

Protected health information (PHI) Health-related findings, diagnoses, treatment notes, or demographic data that could identify the patient, and needs to be protected.

Protective cusp restoration A direct-fill (amalgam or composite) or indirect restoration that covers or "shoes" the cusps of a posterior tooth. This design is usually undertaken when there has been significant undermining of the cusp(s) due to caries, fracture, root canal treatment, or previous restorative work.

Provisional/provisional restoration A prosthesis or individual tooth restoration intended to serve only for a limited period of time.

Proximate cause A legal term for the initial act or event that produces an injury.

Pseudoparkinsonism A side effect of some antipsychotic drugs that resembles symptoms of Parkinson's disease.

Psychological addiction A person's need to use a drug out of desire for the effects it produces, rather than to relieve withdrawal symptoms.

Ptyalism Excessive salivation.

Puberty associated gingivitis/puberty gingivitis An increase in gingival inflammation that sometimes occurs during puberty. It is a generalized form of gingivitis characterized by inflamed, enlarged gingival papillae that are susceptible to bleeding.

Pulp vitality testing Techniques for evaluating the condition of pulp tissue in a tooth.

Pulpal necrosis A clinical diagnosis that indicates the death of dental pulp tissue.

R

Radiation caries Decalcification, decay, and disintegration of tooth structure after radiation therapy, typically affecting the cervical and coronal root surfaces of a tooth. The condition is attributed to decreased salivary function and an alteration of the saliva's buffering capacity.

Radiation ports The areas of radiation exposure during radiation therapy.

Radiation therapy The use of ionizing radiation to treat cancer.

Randomized controlled trials (RCT) A test in which subjects are assigned to groups in a random manner. In a clinical trial, an appropriate control group is used, such as to receive placebo or sham treatment or the standard well-established therapy, and this is compared with a group receiving experimental therapy; patients are assigned in a random manner to one of the groups, usually with blinding. This method is generally considered to yield the strongest scientific evidence of any well-designed trial.

Ranula A mucous-filled lesion associated with the submandibular or sublingual glands and located on the floor of the mouth.

Reasons for treatment The foundation of a treatment plan, justified by one or more diagnoses.

Recall/recare interval The appropriate length of time before the patient's next periodic visit and examination.

Reciprocal click A pronounced snap or pop in the temporomandibular joint both on opening and closing.

Recurrent caries Caries occurring at the restoration-tooth interface or under an existing restoration. Also referred to as secondary caries.

Reduced periodontium Clinical appearance of the breakdown of the structures that surround, support, and are attached to the teeth, resulting in loss of tissue attachment and destruction of alveolar bone.

Reducing anterior disc displacement (RADD) Anterior displacement of the intraarticular disc when the posterior teeth are fully occluded.

Remineralization The reintroduction of complex mineral salts into bone, enamel, dentin, or cementum.

Removable partial denture A denture replacing one or several of the natural teeth, made so that it can be readily removed from the mouth; it may be entirely supported by the residual teeth, or supported by both the teeth and the tissue of the residual area.

Repose A neutral facial expression.

Res ipsa loquitur Latin for "the thing speaks for itself." This legal term refers to situations in which it is assumed that a person's injury was caused by the negligent action of another party because the accident was otherwise unlikely to have occurred.

Residency Where the patient lives; their domiciliary arrangements.

Resin infiltration A minimally invasive restorative technique to treat white-spot lesions; the procedure entails etching and drying the lesion and applying a resin infiltrant.

Respondeat superior Latin for "let the master answer," a legal term that provides that an employer is responsible for those actions of their employees performed within the scope of their employment.

Retainer An orthodontic appliance placed at the completion of active orthodontic therapy to maintain the position of the teeth. Also, the *fixed partial denture component (crown) that attaches to an FPD abutment.*

Retreatment Providing further treatment; often applied to endodontics when there is apparent recontamination of the root canal system, and the original root canal filling is removed and replaced with another root canal filling via conventional (nonsurgical) means.

Reversible pulpitis A clinical diagnosis that describes an inflamed dental pulp judged capable of recovery.

Review of systems That portion of the patient history in which the clinician evaluates the major organ systems.

Ridge augmentation The placement of bone graft materials to enhance the height and/or width of the alveolar ridge in preparation to receive dental implants, or to better retain a dental prosthesis.

Risk assessment Evaluation of the likelihood or probability that a patient will develop a particular condition or disease.

Risk factors Identifiable conditions known to predispose individuals to an undesirable condition; for example, oral disease. Ideally, this causal biologic link is confirmed from longitudinal studies.

Risk indicators Identifiable conditions that are known to be associated with a higher probability of the occurrence of a disease. They are typically identified from cross-sectional studies.

Robust treatment planning An aggressive approach to treatment planning that involves removal of all teeth with a questionable prognosis and simplification of the treatment plan.

Root caries A caries lesion apical to the cemento-enamel junction on a tooth.

Root dilacerations A condition characterized by a crease or band at the junction of the crown and root, or by tortuous roots with abnormal curvatures.

S

Sarcoma Cancerous tumors that develop from mesenchymal tissues, such as fat, bone, muscle, nerve, joint, blood vessel, or deep skin tissue.

SBIRT A three-step process used when confronting a patient with a substance abuse problem that consists of (1) *s*creening, (2) *b*rief *i*ntervention, and (3) *r*eferral to *t*reatment.

Search engine A software system that is designed to carry out web queries for information.

Secondary caries Caries that occurs adjacent to an existing restoration.

Secondary occlusal trauma Injury to the periodontium in the presence of inflammation and attachment loss; caused by excessive occlusal forces.

Secondhand smoke The environmental smoke produced by tobacco smokers. Secondhand smoke exposes nonsmokers to the adverse effects of tobacco smoking.

Security In healthcare, protecting the integrity of patient information and preventing unauthorized access.

Sedative-hypnotics Medications that reduce the excitability of patients and induce an altered state of consciousness.

Sedative restoration An interim, direct-fill restoration placed with the dual purpose of decreasing pulpal sensitivity and arresting the progression of caries in the tooth.

Selective caries removal The excavation technique in which peripheral dentin is removed until only hard dentin is left, while the pulp wall is excavated until reaching firm or soft dentin.

Shared decision making The process of making informed treatment choices between dentist and patient based on the dentist providing the proper information to the patient.

Sialagogue A medication used to promote the flow of saliva.

Signs Findings discovered by the clinician during an examination.

Silver diamine fluoride (SDF) A topical medication used to treat and prevent dental caries and relieve dentin sensitivity.

Sinus tract A chronic or persistent abscess that drains purulent exudate. Also referred to as a fistula or fistulous tract.

Site preservation Placement of bone fill materials in a new extraction site for the purpose of preserving ridge height and contour and preventing bone loss. Also referred to as socket preservation.

Sjögren's syndrome An autoimmune condition usually occurring in middle-aged or older women, marked by the triad of keratoconjunctivitis sicca with or without lacrimal gland enlargement, xerostomia with or without salivary gland enlargement, and the presence of a connective tissue disease, usually rheumatoid arthritis but sometimes systemic lupus erythematosus, scleroderma, or polymyositis.

Sliding board A smooth wooden board used to help a disabled patient transfer from a wheelchair to the dental chair.

Smokeless tobacco A form of tobacco designed to be used without smoking. Also referred to as spit, topical, snuff, or chewing tobacco.

SOAP note A method of organizing information to document a patient visit. The component parts are *s*ubjective findings, *o*bjective findings, *a*ssessment, and the *p*lan for treatment. The SOAP note is frequently used to document treatment for acute conditions.

Social determinants of health Conditions in the environments in which people are born, live, learn, work, play, worship, and age, which affect a wide range of health, functioning, and quality-of-life outcomes and risks.

Social phobias A persistent distinct fear of social or performance situations in which embarrassment may occur.

Solar cheilitis/solar cheilosis A premalignant lesion of the lip caused by excessive ultraviolet exposure; often appears as a mottled white and red lesion with chapping and a loss of definition of the vermillion border of the lower lip.

Somatoform disorders A set of conditions in which, although the patient does not fabricate the symptomatology, the symptoms described by the patient appear to greatly exceed the physical signs of a particular disease process.

Specific phobias Excessive fear of a specific object or situation, such as heights, flying, snakes, or insects. Patients are asymptomatic unless in contact with the specific "trigger" to their anxiety.

Split tooth The end result of a vertically cracked tooth. The root surface, or the roots of a multirooted tooth, is/are completely separated.

Squamous cell carcinoma A malignant tumor developed from squamous epithelium.

Staging The classification of cancers according to the extent of the tumor. Staging is based on three basic components: primary tumor (T), regional nodes (N), and metastasis (M).

Standard of care An established measure or model for treatment to which a health practitioner should conform. In legal proceedings, it would be defined as treatment that the reasonable or average dentist might have provided under the circumstances.

Stomatitis Generalized oral lesions, such as vesicles, bullae, erosions, or ulcers commonly found in patients in debilitated health or suffering from an autoimmune disorder.

Stress A disturbance in a person's normal homeostasis resulting from events that may be physical, mental, or emotional in nature.

Substance use disorders A group of disorders in which psychoactive substance use or abuse repeatedly results in significantly adverse consequences.

Sun protection factor (SPF) A measure of the effectiveness of a sunscreen product. The higher the SPF the more protection an individual will receive.

Supernumerary tooth Any tooth in excess of the 32 normal permanent teeth. The tooth may be normal in size but is frequently small and poorly developed.

Surgical stent A device usually made of acrylic or thermo-formed material that may be used to hold a graft in place. May also be used during imaging or surgery to assist in the planning and placement of implants or other prosthodontic devices.

Surrogate decision maker/proxy A patient's representative who speaks for the patient in situations when a patient if unable to make an informed choice.

Symptoms Findings that are apparent to a patient, usually because the findings are causing a problem.

Symptomatic apical periodontitis (SAP) Periapical inflammatory process associated with necrosis of the tooth pulp; manifests with sensitivity to biting, and on clinical examination a positive response to percussion; radiograph may or may not exhibit periapical radiolucency.

Symptomatic irreversible pulpitis A clinical diagnosis based on subjective and objective findings indicating that the vital inflamed pulp is incapable of healing.

Synchronous communication Any type of communication where there is no time lag between the sender of information and the person receiving the information. Examples include telephone calls and meeting in person.

Systematic review A detailed and comprehensive plan and search strategy with the goal of reducing bias by identifying, appraising, and synthesizing all relevant studies on a particular topic. A systematic review is the highest level of evidence in the hierarchy of evidence.

Systemic phase of care The aspects of a treatment plan aimed at establishing and maintaining the best possible state of physical health for a patient before, during, and after dental treatment. This aspect of the plan takes into account the effect that any systemic illness or condition will have on dental treatment.

T

Tachycardia A heart rate that is greater than 100 beats a minute.

Tachyphylaxis The decrease in the effectiveness of a given dose of a drug in response to long term use.

Tardive dyskinesia An adverse reaction to certain antipsychotic drugs, characterized by persistent involuntary movement of the lips, jaws, or face, and the extremities.

Teledentistry The use of information and communication technologies for providing dental care.

Telemedicine The use of information and communication technologies for providing healthcare.

Temporization The process of fabricating and placing a provisional restoration.

Temporomandibular disorder (TMD) An abnormality of the temporomandibular joint complex characterized by pain and altered function.

Tentative diagnosis A presumed diagnosis when there is insufficient information to determine a definitive diagnosis.

Tetracycline stain Staining of teeth that occurs when tetracycline is absorbed during tooth development.

Therapeutic index A measure of the safety of a medication.

Thin gingival biotype When the gingiva is delicate, friable, highly scalloped, and translucent in appearance; there is often a minimal amount of attached gingiva.

Third parties Other persons or organizations that may modify the dentist-patient relationship. Examples include dental insurance companies and a patient's parent or guardian.

Tooth mobility Visible movement of a tooth or teeth when external pressure is applied.

Tooth fracture A crack or break in a tooth that may occur when heavy occlusal forces are applied to a vulnerable tooth.

Tort law/torts The body of the law that allows an injured person to obtain compensation from the person who caused the injury.

Torus mandibularis A benign bony exostosis located on the lingual side of the mandibular premolars.

Torus palatinus A benign bony exostosis located on the median of the hard palate.

Transalveolar sinus elevation (lift) A commonly used technique for sinus floor elevation in which the Schneiderian membrane is gently elevated through the socket immediately following tooth extraction. Also referred to as osteotome sinus lift.

Transient ischemic attack (TIA) A temporary disturbance in blood supply to a localized area of the brain.

Transillumination The passage of light between the teeth to help identify dark areas of proximal caries, especially in the anterior region.

Traumatic brain injury Brain dysfunction caused by an outside force, usually a violent blow to the head.

Traumatic ulcer A localized area on the skin or mucosa in which the surface epithelium has been disrupted as a result of trauma.

Treatment objectives Certain goals that represent the intent or rationale for a treatment plan.

Treatment notes Documentation of each appointment recorded in the patient record. This documentation can include appointment-specific diagnoses, evidence of a health history review, details of treatment provided, patient behavior, and plans for the next appointment. Also referred to as progress notes.

Treatment outcomes The actual results of treatment.

Trigeminal autonomic cephalalgias (TAC) Idiopathic headaches involving activation of trigeminovascular nociceptive pathways along with reflex cranial autonomic activation.

Trigeminal nerve injury/deafferentation The pain that follows the loss of normal afferent input to the central nervous system.

Trigeminal neuralgia An exquisitely severe, electric-like, lancinating pain whose location is related to the distribution of the trigeminal nerve.

Trismus Spasms of the muscles of mastication that result in the inability to open the mouth.

Tumor board A multidisciplinary group of healthcare providers who convene to discuss and coordinate cancer therapy for individual patients.

Two-stage technique Surgical technique in which the implant fixture is placed and covered with oral tissue at the first surgical appointment. The patient returns for another visit, usually 3 to 6 weeks later, to uncover the fixture. At that time a fixture or abutment level impression is taken using an impression post.

U

Unbounded edentulous spaces An edentulous space that does not have a tooth on at least one side of it.

Uneven gingival zeniths The gingival crest on the maxillary anterior teeth is not in harmony with the horizontal plane.

Unintentional torts An unintended accident that leads to injury, property damage, or financial loss.

Urgent problem A situation that does not require immediate attention for health reasons but is a problem that the dentist, or more commonly the patient, thinks should be attended to "now" or "soon."

V

Varicosity/varix A varicose vein visible in the oral cavity; commonly found on the floor of the mouth or ventral surface of the tongue.

Vasodepressor syncope A loss of consciousness that may be caused by the stress and fear associated with receiving dental treatment or by rapid positional changes such as sitting or standing up quickly.

Veneer A layer of tooth-colored material, usually ceramic or acrylic resin, placed on the facial surface of a tooth for esthetic reasons.

Veracity One of the five core principles of the *Principles of Ethics and Code of Professional Responsibility* published by the American Dental Association; stipulates that dentists maintain truthfulness in all professional relationships.

Vertical dimension of occlusion (VDO) The superior-inferior relationship of the maxilla and the mandible when the teeth are situated in maximum intercuspation.

Vertical root fracture A complete or incomplete fracture line, initiated from the root, running parallel or slightly oblique to the long axis of the tooth.

Vestibuloplasty The surgical modification of the gingival–mucous membrane relationships in the vestibule of the mouth, including deepening of the vestibular trough, repositioning of the frenum or muscle attachments, and broadening of the zone of attached gingiva.

Vision An image or idea of what the patient's mouth will look like when treatment is complete.

Voxel Volumetric elements (cubes) that comprise a three-dimensional digital image (the 3D equivalent of a pixel).

W

Withdrawal syndromes A predictable group of signs and symptoms resulting from abrupt removal of, or a rapid decrease in, the regular dosage of a psychoactive substance.

Working diagnosis A preliminary diagnosis made before beginning treatment, when the actual diagnosis is questionable.

X

Xerostomia Dry mouth.

Z

Zirconia indirect restoration Ceramic restoration made of zirconium dioxide; because of its relative strength and fracture resistance, less tooth reduction is required for the preparation compared with other ceramic materials.

Note: Page numbers followed by "*b*" indicate boxes; "*f*" figures; and "*t*" tables.

Pulp vitality
    loss of, 228, 228b
    testing, 198–199
Pulse
    irregular, 27–28
    maintenance phase of treatment and, 297
Pulse rate, 10
Punitive damages, 170
Pyogenic granuloma, 31–32, 72.e4

Q

Quadrant/sextant, sequencing by, in disease
        control phase, 213
Questionnaire(s)
    on examination process, 4
    health, 170, 170b
    history, updating, 296
    minimal questions necessary for, 197b

R

Radiation treatment, oral cancer, 80
Radiographically evident abnormalities and
        pathologies management, 303
Radiographic images
    maintenance phase and, 295–296, 295f
    procuring and interpreting, 297–298
    selection for common acute dental problems, 200t
Radiographs
    bite-wing, 17
    interproximal, 17
    occlusal, 17
    panoramic radiograph, 17–18
    periapical radiographs, 16
    pregnancy and, 189
    refusal to update, by patient, 297b–298b
Ranula, 32, 34–35, 72.e7
Rapid induction technique, nitrous oxide and
        oxygen (N_2O-O_2) therapy, 369
Rapid Oral Health Deterioration (ROHD), 420
Rapport
    building, 292
    development of, in patients, 363
RAU. See Recurrent aphthous ulcers (RAU)
"Reasonable" dentist, 168–169
Recall interval, 296
Recare interval, maintenance phase and, 296
Recare visit, maintenance phase, 296–306
    evaluation, 296–302
Recession
    defects, 249f
    gingival, 416
Reciprocal click, 234
Recording information, in dental records, 167
Recreational drugs, patients using, 339
Recurrent aphthous stomatitis (RAS). See
        Aphthous ulcers
Recurrent aphthous ulcers (RAU), 33. See also
        Aphthous ulcers
Recurrent caries, 50–51
Recurrent herpes, 32
Reduced periodontium, 44, 44f
    concept, 44
Reducing fees, for financially limited patient, 455
Referral, of fearful patient, 366–367
Refined carbohydrates, limiting exposure to, 217
Registered nurses (RNs), 142, 333
Reinforced zinc oxide eugenol (IRM), caries and, 403
Relaxation, for fearful patients, 365–366
Remote patient monitoring, teledentistry, 111
Removable partial dentures (RPD), 100.e3, 134,
        276–278
Removable prostheses, 300–301

Replacement of silver filling, 259b
Residency, special care patients and, 313
Resin-based composite restorations, 100.e1–100.e2
Resin-bonded bridges, 300
Resin-bonded fixed partial denture, 100.e3, 277f
Resin infiltration, 262, 262f
Resin modified glass ionomer cement (RMGI),
        217–218
Res ipsa loquitur doctrine, 169
Respiratory illness, geriatric patients and, 425–426
Respondeat superior, 160–161
Restoration
    adjusting, 304
    amalgam, 100.e2, 258–259
    caries control, 217–218
    cast gold, 100.e2, 259, 260f
    composite resin, 255f, 257–258
    defective, 225
        replacement, 90
    direct fill, 231, 258
    extracoronal, 256
    glass ionomer (GI), 217–218, 218b, 258
    iatrogenic, elimination of, active periodontal
            disease and, 226
    inlay, 259
    intracoronal, 256
    longevity, 257
    maintenance phase and, 295
    metallic, 229f
    onlay, 259
    provisional, 133
    resin-based composite, 100.e1–100.e2
    single tooth, 231, 257–261
Restraints, special care patients and, 331
Retained root(s), 56t–57t
Retainers, 276
Retention, factors favoring, 92b–93b
Retreatment, 268–269
Reversible pulpitis, 45, 200, 228–229
Review of systems (ROS), 8, 8t
    of special care patients, 316, 316b
Rewards, patient with acute problems and, 194
Rheumatoid arthritis, 27, 72.e8f
Ridge augmentation procedures, 274
Ridge preservation, 274
Risk. See also Risk assessment; Risk factor
    for caries, 218–220
    vs. causality, 76–77
Risk assessment, 74–75
    caries, 81–82, 82f
    in dentistry, 76–80
    geriatric patients and, 420–421
    maintenance phase and, 294
    occlusal/ functional, 84–85
    oral cancer risk assessment, 80–81
    periodontal disease, 82–84
Risk factor, 75–77
Risk indicators, 76–77
    behavioral, 77–79
    environmental, 79
    related to stress and anxiety, 79
Risk management, 172–173
RMGI. See Resin modified glass ionomer cement
        (RMGI)
RNs. See Registered nurses (RNs)
ROHD. See Rapid Oral Health Deterioration
        (ROHD)
Root canal, failed, 92–93
Root canal therapy, 269, 269f
    retreatment, 269f
Root caries
    lesions, 51
    radiographic findings, 52t–53t
Root dilacerations, 270
Root planing, active periodontal disease and, 226

Root proximity problem, 232, 232f, 247
Root surface caries lesions, 51
Routes of administration, 367–368
RPD. See Removable partial dentures (RPD)

S

Saliva, functions, 393f
Salivary gland abnormalities, 34–36
    neoplastic lesions, 35–36
    nonneoplastic lesions, 34–35
Salivary gland swelling, alcoholic patient, 341f
Salivary stone, 35
SBIRT. See Screening, Brief Intervention, and
        Referral to Treatment (SBIRT)
Scaling, 200t, 226
SCCA. See Squamous cell carcinoma (SCCA)
Scheduling appointments, 329
Schizophrenia, 385–387
    symptoms, 385, 385b
SCR. See Selective caries removal (SCR)
Screening, Brief Intervention, and Referral to
        Treatment (SBIRT), 351
Screening, for oral cancer, 198b
SDF. See Silver diamine fluoride (SDF)
SDH. Social Determinants of Health (SDH);. See
        Social determinants of health (SDH)
Sealants, 217, 257
Search engines, digital information, 102, 102b
Seborrheic keratosis, 28, 72.e1
Secondary caries, 50–51
Secondary gain, 390–391
Secondary occlusal trauma, 58t–59t, 232–233, 247
Security, patient health information, 110
Sedation
    anxiety control, 367
    intravenous, 370
    levels of, 367
    need for, 323–324
    oral, 323
    for uncooperative patient, 320
Sedative-hypnotics, 331
Sedatives, 338
Selective caries removal (SCR), 217–218, 228
Selective serotonin reuptake inhibitors (SSRIs),
        382t–383t, 383
Self-awareness, 376
Self-image, interrelationship of oral health and, 446
Self-neglect, 332b
Sequencing
    dental treatment, guidelines for, 131–136, 132b
    of periodontal treatment, 403
    the plan for special care patients, 325–326
Serotonin-noradrenergic receptor antagonists
        (SNRAs), 382t–383t
Serotonin norepinephrine reuptake inhibitors
        (SNRIs), 382t–383t, 383
Sertraline, 382t–383t
Settings, alternative, geriatric patients treatment
        planning in, 436
Severe coagulopathies, 314–315
Sextant, sequencing by, in disease control phase of
        treatment, 213
Sexual abuse, 332b
Sexually transmitted diseases (STDs), 341–342
    adolescents, 398
Sexual/physical abuse history, dental anxiety, 360
Shade matching equipment, 117
Shade selection function, intraoral scanners, 117f
Shared decision making, 141, 163
Shingles, 29
Sialolithiasis, 35
Signs, 2
"Silent" myocardial infarction, 424